45 00

January 1980

- Oakwood -

Ampicillin x 3days

Len

THE MANAGEMENT OF TRAUMA

Third Edition

Edited by

GEORGE D. ZUIDEMA, M.D.

Warfield M. Firor Professor of and Director, Section of Surgical Sciences, The Johns Hopkins University School of Medicine; Surgeon-in-Chief, The Johns Hopkins Hospital, Baltimore

ROBERT B. RUTHERFORD, M.D.

Professor of Surgery, University of Colorado School of Medicine, Denver

WALTER F. BALLINGER, II, M.D.

Professor of Surgery, Washington University School of Medicine, St. Louis; Surgeon, Barnes and Allied Hospitals, St. Louis

1979

W. B. SAUNDERS COMPANY

Philadelphia
London
Toronto

W. B. Saunders Company: West Washington Square
                           Philadelphia, PA 19105

                           1 St. Anne's Road
                           Eastbourne, East Sussex BN21 3UN, England

                           1 Goldthorne Avenue
                           Toronto, Ontario M8Z 5T9, Canada

Listed here is the latest translated edition of this book together with
the language of the translation and the publisher:

Spanish — *Third Edition*   Nueva Editorial Interamericana S.A. de C.V.
                           Mexico 4 D.F., Mexico

The Management of Trauma   ISBN   0-7216-9722-4

Last digit is the print number: 9   8   7   6   5   4   3   2   1

CONTRIBUTORS

CHARLES B. ANDERSON, M.D. Professor of Surgery, Washington University School of Medicine; Surgeon, Barnes Hospital, St. Louis, Missouri
Abdominal Injuries

SUSAN P. BAKER, M.P.H. Associate Professor of Health Services Administration and of Environmental Health Services, The Johns Hopkins University School of Hygiene and Public Health; Research Associate, Office of Chief Medical Examiner of Maryland, Baltimore, Maryland
The Epidemiology and Prevention of Injuries

THOMAS J. BALKANY, M.D. Assistant Professor, University of Colorado Medical Center; Chairman, Department of Otolaryngology, Denver Children's Hospital; Attending Physician, Colorado General, Denver General, Mercy, Saint Joseph, and General Rose Memorial Hospitals, Denver, Colorado
The Management of Neck Injuries

WALTER F. BALLINGER, II, M.D. Professor of Surgery, Washington University School of Medicine; Surgeon, Barnes and Affiliated Hospitals, St. Louis, Missouri
Abdominal Injuries

PERRY BLACK, M.D., C.M. Professor and Chairman, Department of Neurosurgery, Hahnemann Medical College and Hospital, Philadelphia, Pennsylvania
Injuries of the Head and Spinal Cord

CONRADO C. BONDOC, M.D. Lecturer in Surgery, Harvard Medical School; Assistant Surgeon, Massachusetts General Hospital; Associate Surgeon, Shriners Hospitals for Crippled Children–Burns Institute, Boston Unit, Boston, Massachusetts
Wound Sepsis: Prevention and Control

CHARLES A. BUERK, M.D. Associate Professor, Department of Surgery, University of Colorado Medical School, Denver, Colorado
The Pathophysiology of Trauma and Shock

JOHN F. BURKE, M.D. Helen Andrus Benedict Professor of Surgery, Harvard Medical School; Visiting Surgeon, Massachusetts General Hospital; Chief of Staff, Shriners Hospitals for Crippled Children–Burns Institute, Boston Unit, Boston, Massachusetts
Wound Sepsis: Prevention and Control

JOHN LEMUEL CAMERON, M.D. Professor of Surgery, The Johns Hopkins University School of Medicine; Professor of Surgery, The Johns Hopkins Hospital, Baltimore, Maryland
Initial Evaluation and Resuscitation of the Injured Patient

MILTON L. COBB, M.D. Assistant Professor of Anesthesiology, Washington University School of Medicine; Assistant Anesthesiologist, Barnes Hospital and St. Louis Children's Hospital, St. Louis, Missouri
Anesthetic Management of the Trauma Victim

JOHN A. COLLINS, M.D. Chidester Professor and Chairman, Department of Surgery, Stanford University School of Medicine, Stanford, California
The Treatment of Shock

RAYMOND M. CURTIS, M.D. Chief of the Division of Hand Surgery, The Union Memorial Hospital; Associate Professor of Plastic and Orthopaedic Surgery, The Johns Hopkins University School of Medicine; The Consultant in Hand Surgery to the Surgeon General of the Army, Baltimore, Maryland
Injuries of the Hand

JAMES J. DELANEY, M.D. Associate Clinical Professor of Obstetrics and Gynecology, University of Colorado Medical Center; Attending Physician, Colorado General Hospital, General Rose Hospital and Saint Joseph Hospital, Denver, Colorado
Obstetrical and Gynecological Injuries

PARK ELLIOT DIETZ, M.D., M.P.H. Assistant Professor of Psychiatry, Harvard Medical School; Director of Medical Criminology Research Center, McLean Hospital, Belmont, Massachusetts
The Epidemiology and Prevention of Injuries

MILTON T. EDGERTON, JR., M.D. Professor and Chairman, Department of Plastic Surgery, University of Virginia School of Medicine; University of Virginia Medical Center; National Clinical Center, NIH; Veterans Administration Hospital, Salem, Virginia
Emergency Care of Maxillofacial Injuries

JARED M. EMERY, M.D. Associate Professor, Baylor College of Medicine; Attending Physician, Veterans Administration Hospital; Associate Attending Physician, Ben Taub Hospital and The Methodist Hospital; Attending Physician, St. Luke's–Texas Children's Hospital, Houston, Texas
Injuries of the Eye, the Lids and the Orbit

RAINER M. ENGEL, M.D. Associate Professor of Urology, The Johns Hopkins University School of Medicine; Active Staff Urologist, Union Memorial Hospital, Greater Baltimore Medical Center, and Children's Hospital; Consultant Urologist, U.S. Public Health Hospital, Baltimore, Maryland
Trauma of the Genitourinary System

EDWARD E. ETHEREDGE, M.D., Ph.D. Associate Professor of Surgery, Washington University School of Medicine; Staff Surgeon, Barnes Hospital and St. Louis Children's Hospital; Consultant Surgeon, St. Louis City, St. Louis County, and Cochran Veterans Administration Hospitals, St. Louis, Missouri
Acute Renal Failure in the Surgical Patient

MARGARET M. FLETCHER, M.D. Clinical Assistant Professor, The Johns Hopkins University School of Medicine; Clinical Associate Professor, University of Maryland School of Medicine, Baltimore, Maryland
Tracheostomy

DONALD S. GANN, M.D. Professor and Chairman, Section of Surgery, Brown University, Division of Biology and Medicine; Surgeon-in-chief, Department of Surgery, Rhode Island Hospital, Providence, Rhode Island
Emergency Department Organization; Mass Casualty Management

JORDAN H. GINSBURG, M.D. Assistant Professor of Orthopedic Surgery, Washington University School of Medicine; Attending Surgeon, Barnes and Affiliated Hospitals and St. Louis Children's Hospital; Chief of Orthopedic Service, St. Louis County Hospital; Assistant Surgeon, Shriners Hospital for Crippled Children, St. Louis, Missouri
Injuries of the Lower Extremities

MORTON F. GOLDBERG, M.D. Chairman, Department of Ophthalmology, University of Illinois College of Medicine; University of Illinois Eye and Ear Infirmary, Chicago, Illinois
Injuries of the Eye, the Lids and the Orbit

HUBERT T. GURLEY, M.D. Acting Director, Emergency Medicine Department, Assistant Professor of Medicine, Director of Permanent Pacemaker Laboratory, The Johns Hopkins University School of Medicine, Baltimore, Maryland
Cardiopulmonary Resuscitation

J. ALEX HALLER, JR., M.D. Robert Garrett Professor of Pediatric Surgery, The Johns Hopkins University School of Medicine; Children's Surgeon-in-charge, The Johns Hopkins Hospital, Baltimore, Maryland
Trauma and the Child

JOHN E. HOOPES, M.D. Professor and Chairman, Division of Plastic Surgery, The Johns Hopkins University School of Medicine, Baltimore, Maryland
Soft Tissue Injuries of the Extremities

KEITH A. HRUSKA, M.D. Assistant Professor of Medicine, Washington University School of Medicine; Associate Physician, Barnes Hospital and Jewish Hospital of St. Louis, St. Louis, Missouri
Acute Renal Failure in the Surgical Patient

JAMES LANGSTON HUGHES, M.D. Chairman, Division of Orthopaedic Surgery, University of Mississippi Medical Center, Jackson, Mississippi
Initial Management of Fractures and Joint Injuries: Thoracic and Lumbar Spine, Pelvis and Hip

MICHAEL E. JABALEY, M.D. Professor of Surgery and Chairman, Division of Plastic Surgery, University of Mississippi School of Medicine, Jackson, Mississippi
Injuries of the Hand

BRUCE W. JAFEK, M.D. Professor and Chairman, Department of Otolaryngology, University of Colorado Medical Center; Attending Physician, Colorado General, Denver Children's, Denver General, and General Rose Hospital, Denver, Colorado
The Management of Neck Injuries

GLENN L. KELLY, M.D. Associate Clinical Professor of Surgery, University of Colorado Medical Center; Head, Division of Vascular Surgery, Denver General Hospital, Denver, Colorado
Peripheral Vascular Injuries

THOMAS J. KRIZEK, M.D. Professor of Surgery, College of Physicians & Surgeons of Columbia University; Chief, Plastic Surgery Division, Columbia–Presbyterian Medical Center, New York, New York
Care of the Thermally Injured Patient

EDWARD R. LAWS, JR., M.D. Associate Professor in Neurologic Surgery, Mayo Medical School; Consultant in Neurologic Surgery at Mayo Clinic, St. Marys Hospital of Rochester, and Rochester Methodist Hospital, Rochester, Minnesota
Injuries of the Head and Spinal Cord

PAUL R. MANSKE, M.D. Research Assistant Professor of Surgery, Washington University School of Medicine; Director, Hand Clinic, Shriners Hospital; Orthopedic Surgeon, St. Louis County Orthopedic Group, St. Louis, Missouri
Fractures and Joint Injuries of the Upper Extremities

G. PATRICK MAXWELL, M.D. Instructor, Division of Plastic Surgery, The Johns Hopkins Hospital, Baltimore, Maryland
Soft Tissue Injuries of the Extremities

T. CRAWFORD McASLAN, M.D.   Associate Professor of Anesthesiology, The Johns
  Hopkins University School of Medicine; Professor of Anesthesiology, University
  of Maryland Hospital; Anesthesiologist-in-chief, Baltimore City Hospitals,
  Baltimore, Maryland
  Cardiopulmonary Resuscitation

J. DONALD McQUEEN, M.D.   Professor of Clinical Neurological Sciences, Neuro-
  surgeon-in-chief, University of Saskatchewan, University Hospital, Saskatoon,
  Saskatchewan
  Injuries of the Head and Spinal Cord

EUGENE L. NAGEL, M.D.   Professor of Anesthesiology, The Johns Hopkins Uni-
  versity School of Medicine; Director, Anesthesiology, Anesthesiologist-in-chief,
  Department of Anesthesiology, The Johns Hopkins Hospital, Baltimore, Maryland
  Cardiopulmonary Resuscitation; Mass Casualty Management

WILLIAM D. OWENS, M.D.   Associate Professor of Anesthesiology, Washington
  University School of Medicine; Associate Anesthesiologist, Barnes Hospital and
  St. Louis Children's Hospital; Medical Director, Respiratory Therapy Depart-
  ment, Barnes Hospital, St. Louis, Missouri
  Anesthetic Management of the Trauma Victim

DAVID PATON, M.D.   Professor and Chairman, Baylor College of Medicine;
  Chief of Ophthalmology Service, The Methodist Hospital, Houston, Texas
  Injuries of the Eye, the Lids and the Orbit

CHARLES D. RAY, M.D.   Clinical Associate Professor of Neurosurgery, University
  of Minnesota; Consulting Neurosurgeon, Department of Neuroaugmentive
  Surgery, Sister Kenny Institute, Minneapolis, Minnesota
  Injuries of the Head and Spinal Cord

MARTIN C. ROBSON, M.D.   Professor of Surgery, Pritzker School of Medicine,
  University of Chicago; Chief, Section of Plastic and Reconstructive Surgery and
  Director of Burn Center, University of Chicago Hospitals and Clinics, Chicago,
  Illinois
  Care of the Thermally Injured Patient

ROBERT B. RUTHERFORD, M.D.   Professor of Surgery, University of Colorado
  Medical Center, Denver, Colorado
  *The Pathophysiology of Trauma and Shock; The Management of Neck Injuries;
  Thoracic Injuries; Peripheral Vascular Injuries*

JAMES J. RYAN, M.D.   Assistant Professor of Plastic Surgery, The Johns Hopkins
  University School of Medicine, Baltimore, Maryland
  Injuries of the Hand

HENRY STEWART SABATIER, M.D.   Assistant Professor of Surgery and Emer-
  gency Medicine, The Johns Hopkins University School of Medicine; Emergency
  Physician, Fallston General Hospital, Baltimore, Maryland
  Initial Evaluation and Resuscitation of the Injured Patient

MARLA ELIZABETH SALMON WHITE, Sc.D.   Assistant Professor, Projects in
  Nursing Administration, Associate Project Director, School of Public Health,
  University of Minnesota, Minneapolis, Minnesota
  Emergency Department Organization

CHESTER W. SCHMIDT, JR., M.D.   Associate Professor of Psychiatry, The Johns
  Hopkins University School of Medicine; Chief, Department of Psychiatry, Balti-
  more City Hospitals, Baltimore, Maryland
  Psychiatric Management of Acute Trauma

PERRY L. SCHOENECKER, M.D. Assistant Professor of Orthopedic Surgery, Washington University School of Medicine; Attending Surgeon, Barnes and Affiliated Hospitals, St. Louis Children's Hospital and St. Louis County Hospital; Chief Surgeon, Shriners Hospital for Crippled Children, St. Louis, Missouri
Injuries of the Lower Extremities

GEORGE FRANK SHELDON, M.D. Associate Professor of Surgery, University of California, San Francisco; Chief of Trauma and Hyperalimentation Service, San Francisco General Hospital, San Francisco, California
The Treatment of Shock

DENNIS W. SHERMETA, M.D. Associate Professor of Pediatric Surgery, The Johns Hopkins University School of Medicine; Pediatric Surgeon, The Johns Hopkins Hospital, Baltimore, Maryland
Trauma and the Child

JOHN D. STAFFORD, M.D. Lecturer, Epidemiology, Emergency Medicine; The Johns Hopkins Hospital, Baltimore, Maryland
Mass Casualty Management

JAMES L. TALBERT, M.D. Professor of Surgery and Pediatrics, University of Florida School of Medicine; Chief, Division of Pediatric Surgery, J. Hillis Miller Health Center, University of Florida, Gainesville, Florida
Trauma and the Child

DONALD D. TRUNKEY, M.D. Professor of Surgery, University of California, San Francisco; Chief of Surgery, San Francisco General Hospital; Director of Burn Center, San Francisco General Hospital, San Francisco, California
The Treatment of Shock

GEORGE B. UDVARHELYI, M.D. Professor of Neurosurgery, Associate Professor of Radiology, The Johns Hopkins University School of Medicine; Staff Neurosurgeon, The Johns Hopkins Hospital; Chief, Neurosurgery, Veterans Administration Hospital; Consultant, Baltimore City Hospitals, Baltimore, Maryland
Injuries of the Head and Spinal Cord

A. EARL WALKER, M.D. Professor Emeritus of Neurological Surgery, The Johns Hopkins University School of Medicine; Professor (visiting) of Neurology and Neurosurgery, University of New Mexico School of Medicine, Albuquerque, New Mexico
Injuries of the Head and Spinal Cord

FREDERICK W. WALKER, M.D. Assistant Professor of Emergency Medicine, The Johns Hopkins University School of Medicine; Active Staff, Emergency Medicine and Surgery, Department of Emergency Medicine, The Johns Hopkins Hospital, Baltimore, Maryland
Mass Casualty Management

MYRON L. WEISFELDT, M.D. Professor of Medicine, The Johns Hopkins University Medical School; Director of Cardiology Division, The Johns Hopkins Hospital; Visiting Physician, Baltimore City Hospitals, Baltimore, Maryland
Cardiopulmonary Resuscitation

ROBERT CHRISTIE WRAY, JR., M.D. Associate Professor of Plastic and Reconstructive Surgery, Washington University School of Medicine; St. Louis, Missouri
Care of the Thermally Injured Patient

GEORGE D. ZUIDEMA, M.D. Professor and Chairman, Department of Surgery, The Johns Hopkins University School of Medicine; Surgeon-in-chief, The Johns Hopkins Hospital, Baltimore, Maryland
Initial Evaluation and Resuscitation of the Injured Patient

PREFACE

The battleground, with its insistent pressure for immediate yet thoughtful and considered management of injury, has traditionally been a rich medium for development of surgical principles and procedures. The progressive decrease in the mortality rate of the wounded from World War I, World War II, the Korean War and the Vietnam conflict offers striking evidence of advantages, not only in the surgical management of trauma but also in general supportive care and rapid means of transportation to centers where definitive management is possible.

But just as disease patterns and epidemiology change with the passage of time, so has the spectrum of trauma altered in recent years. We can now speak of the epidemiology of trauma with at least as much assurance as of the epidemiology of hepatitis, and we can state with precision that since the turn of the century the contribution of motor vehicles to the annual accidental death rate has steadily risen to the point where it now exceeds 45 per cent. As a result, blunt trauma, frequently producing multiple injuries, has taken a dominant position in our accident wards, and therefore in the surgeon's training and experience.

While our methods of treatment have improved and continue to improve, our means of producing injury are also being perfected. Ever increasing horsepower, coupled with an unchanging degree of human error, has exceeded the rate of our willingness or ability to incorporate safety features into our automobiles. Furthermore, new weapons and changing methods of waging war continue to demand much of our resources. In our opinion, these factors provide clear evidence of the large and continuing need for investigation of the mechanism of injuries and for a methodology for their prevention and management.

Although impressive progress has been made recently in a number of areas, such as organ transplantation, mechanical cardiopulmonary assistance and prosthetic valves and vessels, we have not paid sufficient attention to another area—one that involves the death or disability of large numbers of our population every year. The following statistics bear sobering insight into the serious impact of trauma in this country. Accidents injure more than 50 million people and kill more than 100,000 in the United States each year. Trauma is exceeded only by cardiovascular disease and cancer as a cause of death in this country, and it is the leading cause of death among persons between the ages of 1 and 37. Thus, in terms of productive man-years lost, trauma can be considered our leading "killer." Moreover, for every person killed accidentally, approximately 100 suffer a temporarily disabling injury, and 10 to 15 require hospitalization. Accident patients occupy 12 per cent of the total general hospital space, requiring more hospital bed days than all heart patients and four times more than all cancer patients.

The challenge continues to be great.

All the material in the previous two editions of *The Management of Trauma* has been reviewed, updated and, in many cases, completely rewritten, incorporating newer concepts of diagnosis and management. Particular attention has been paid to increasing coverage of cardiopulmonary resuscitation, anesthesia, acute renal failure and injuries of the neck. Furthermore, entirely new chapters have been added, emphasizing the importance of post-traumatic pulmonary insufficiency, organization of the emergency department, epidemiology and prevention of injuries, and the psychiatric management of the injured patient.

In order to confine the almost limitless scope of trauma from injury through rehabilitation, we have urged our associates to stress the principles and techniques of early management as opposed to those of late reconstructive care. We have asked them to pay special attention to interpretation of the constellation of physiologic disturbances that inevitably accompany serious injury, and to describe the ways they have found effective for restoring body functions quickly and gently to a normal pattern.

To each of the contributors the editors express their sincere appreciation.

Walter F. Ballinger
Robert B. Rutherford
George D. Zuidema

CONTENTS

CHAPTER 1

INITIAL EVALUATION AND RESUSCITATION OF THE INJURED PATIENT

George D. Zuidema, M.D.
John L. Cameron, M.D.
Henry S. Sabatier, Jr., M.D.

GENERAL PRINCIPLES

There is no task in surgery more difficult or more important than the initial evaluation of a trauma victim. When dealing with acute trauma it is often impossible to separate diagnostic and therapeutic measures; in fact, it is improper to attempt to dissociate them. The care of the acutely injured patient imposes certain important time restrictions upon the physician. He must not only carry out his usual diagnostic evaluation but must also attend to the urgent therapeutic needs of his patient. It is frequently impossible and impractical to obtain a detailed history. He is forced to rely heavily on physical findings for diagnosis, and the initial examination may well be performed with an agitated, uncooperative patient making the task even more difficult.

The initial priority in the evaluation of an injured patient is an immediate search for rapidly fatal but reversible conditions (Table 1–1). When these have been excluded or treated, a complete inventory of injuries that will require further diagnostic studies will help the physician to form an orderly plan of management. Then, based on the known pattern of injury, the physician conducts an aggressive search for occult injuries. Finally, consideration is given to likely future complications and the available preventive measures to be instituted.

Following severe trauma there are only a few situations that are reversible but produce death within minutes if left unattended. The first of these is inadequate ventilation; the second is hypoxia resulting from circulatory insufficiency; and the third, which often accompanies the second, is rapid, continuing bleeding. Other types of reversible injury lead to slower deterioration of the patient's condition and therefore are not given the same priority for emergency management.

Inadequate Ventilation

Inadequate ventilation leads immediately to hypoxemia and insufficient oxygen delivery to tissues. This state is tolerated poorly, and if complete asphyxia follows, the brain suffers irreversible anoxic damage within 5 minutes. If ventilation is to be re-established, it must be done quickly.

Inadequate ventilation can result from

TABLE 1–1.   Priorities in Evaluation and Resuscitation of the Injured Patient

Rapidly fatal conditions	Inadequate ventilation Inadequate circulation Rapid bleeding
Injuries requiring prompt therapy or diagnostic studies	Closed head trauma Long bone fractures Arterial injury Urinary tract injury
Occult injuries	Blunt abdominal trauma Facial bone fractures Cervical spine injuries Aortic tears Myocardial contusion
Complications	Progressive pulmonary insufficiency Sepsis Withdrawal from drugs

several sources, but in acute trauma upper airway obstruction is the most common. If obstruction is complete, all methods of resuscitation fail until the obstruction is removed. Frequently, such obstruction can be relieved simply. In an unconscious, apneic patient obstruction is frequently caused by the relaxation of the soft tissue of the pharynx, the falling back of the tongue, or blockage of the upper airways by mucus, blood or vomitus. If foreign material is discovered in the mouth or oropharynx, suctioning should be performed immediately. The head should be tilted backward so that the jaw is pointing upward, and the jaw should be pushed or pulled into a jutting position (Fig. 1–1). This maneuver relieves obstruction in the airway by moving the base of the tongue away from the back of the throat. If these measures fail to restore adequate ventilation — if the patient remains apneic or cyanotic, displays retractions of the chest with ventilatory effort, or has only shallow and inadequate respiratory movements — the cause is probably not simple upper airway obstruction. Such a situation occurs in severe neurological damage, in obstruction of the trachea below the glottis, in flail chest injury, in bilateral pneumothorax and in laryngeal fracture. Precise diagnosis is often impossible in the short time allowed to restore adequate ventilation and therefore should not delay treatment. An oral or nasal endotracheal tube should be inserted immediately, preferably with direct laryngoscopy, and positive pressure

ventilation should be instituted with a compressible bag. If an endotracheal tube and laryngoscope are not available, an esophageal airway (Fig. 1–2) is a satisfactory alternative, and its prompt use may be lifesaving.

Only in the case of direct laryngeal trauma will an endotracheal tube be inadequate. A direct tracheal airway should then be established. This can be done most quickly by creating a temporary opening in the subcutaneously located cricothyroid ligament in the midline of the neck. The classic tracheostomy performed below the cricothyroid ligament is too time-consuming in real emergency situations. The introduction of large bore needles into the cricothyroid membrane has been recommended, but these needles are frequently not available. Resuscitation by this technique can be continued until an artificial ventilatory apparatus becomes available. At this point, with an endotracheal or tracheostomy tube in place, chest tubes can be inserted if part of the ventilatory inadequacy is secondary to intrapleural air or blood.

Circulatory Insufficiency

Two varieties of circulatory insufficiency are seen with acute trauma. The first is associated with marked hypovolemia secondary to blood loss, resulting in inadequate delivery of oxygen to tissues, and the second is cardiac arrest.

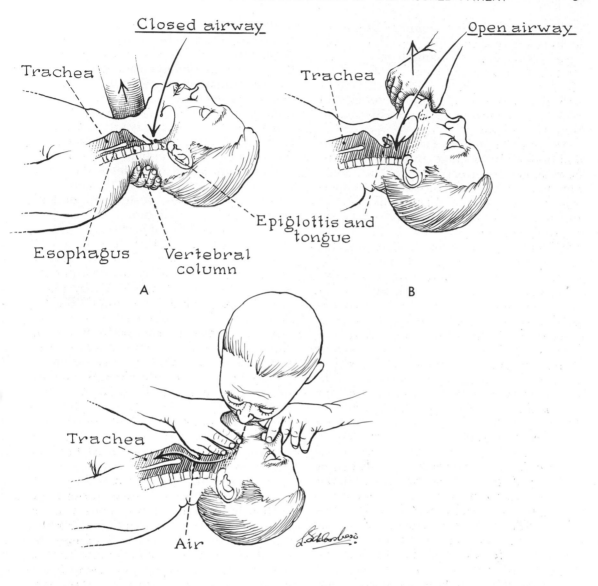

Figure 1–1. A, *Illustrates the wrong way of supporting the head during resuscitation. Note that the tongue and epiglottis fall back to obstruct the airway.* B, *Shows the correct way of handling the patient's airway. Supporting the jaw and tongue provides for an unobstructed airway during resuscitation.* C, *Demonstrates how support of the patient's jaw is properly combined with mouth-to-mouth resuscitation.*

Figure 1–2. *Illustration of an esophageal airway in place. Note the cuff occluding the esophagus, so that air enters the trachea.*

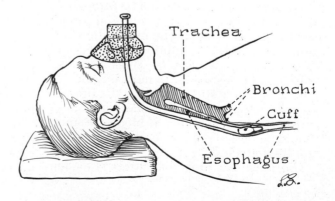

If shock is present or imminent, traumatic hypovolemia requires aggressive volume replacement immediately. This should follow establishment of air exchange and effective cardiac rhythm if only one physician is present, and should proceed concurrently if a resuscitation team is available.

Multiple large-bore (at least 16 gauge and preferably 14 gauge) intravenous catheters should be placed rapidly. The choice of veins may be left to the individual operator, depending on the pattern of injury of the individual patient and the operator's skill, speed and experience in venous catheterization techniques. Percutaneous introduction of short (2 to 6 inches) catheters into large peripheral veins (antecubital, external jugular, femoral, saphenous) or central veins (subclavian or internal jugular) is usually most practical. Cutdowns are frequently time-consuming and should be reserved for situations in which circumstances in either the patient or the physician contraindicate percutaneous methods. Intravenous solutions in plastic bags can be delivered under pressure quite rapidly with the help of a blood pump inflated to moderate pressures. Use of the above equipment (large-bore catheters and pressurized intravenous solutions) will permit delivery of several liters of fluid within the first 5 or 10 minutes of resuscitation.

The use of central venous lines for delivery of fluid and measurement of venous pressure has achieved almost universal acceptance. However, if the resuscitation team is composed of few or inexperienced members, they should take care to ensure that inordinate time is not wasted trying to establish these lines before adequate volume replacement through easily accessible peripheral routes is well under way.

If chest trauma is present, at least one of the intravenous routes should be through a lower extremity in case a superior vena caval injury is present. The rapid administration of electrolyte solutions and plasma substitutes is adequate for short periods until blood is available. In most instances, if heart action is still present by the time a trauma victim reaches an emergency department, the restoration of blood volume should be possible if care is efficiently and rapidly delivered.

The diagnosis of cardiac arrest is made initially by the detection of pulselessness. It can be confirmed by cardiac auscultation or an electrocardiogram. Usually, however, resuscitative efforts are begun without EKG confirmation. Since ventilatory insufficiency is always an accompanying condition, its treatment is an integral part of the management of circulatory arrest. External cardiac massage is the best way to restore the circulation immediately. Circulation without ventilation is useless. The treatment of circulatory arrest, therefore, involves two features: restoration of both ventilation and circulation.

Basic cardiac life support (cardiopulmonary resuscitation [CPR]) has been well described in the medical literature and is being taught to ancillary medical personnel and the general public. Every physician should be able to perform CPR alone or as part of a two-man team.

A single rescuer can perform manual closed chest compressions at a rate of 80 per minute. Respiration can be maintained by two mouth-to-mouth positive pressure breaths after each 15 chest compressions. This technique results in about 60 compressions and eight breaths per minute. Of course, this technique is rapidly tiring and cannot be continued for a long period of time. It may, however, be necessary in order to permit a second operator to perform other essential procedures, such as intubation or intravenous cannulation. Two operators can perform CPR in a more effective fashion if one compresses the sternum 60 times per minute and the partner provides ventilation every 5 seconds. The rhythm of cardiac compression should not be interrupted for ventilation. A tidal volume of approximately 800 to 1000 ml. must be insufflated within an interval of less than 1 second. The use of face masks, compressible bags or manually triggered high-flow valves may be helpful. The use of pressure cycled ventilators during CPR is condemned because they will deliver inadequate tidal volumes and cannot be synchronized with external cardiac compression. The effectiveness of compression can be monitored by the palpation of pulses in the groin or in the neck.

In the absence of intrinsic cardiac disease or injury there are a few situations in which such a resuscitative effort will be unsuccessful. These include bilateral tension pneumothorax and severe injury to the thoracic wall that renders it incapable of rebound when compressed. In these situations circulation can be restored by emergency thoracotomy and direct manual massage of the heart.

In the most experienced hands, CPR will achieve a cardiac output of 25 to 30 per cent of normal. As soon as possible, the full array of advanced cardiac life-support measures — countershock, drug therapy, and volume replacement — should be used with the goal of re-establishing normal cardiac contractions. In the trauma patient, recurrent or refractory cardiac arrest is most frequently due to hypovolemia or hypoxia or both. As long as positive pressure ventilation, external cardiac massage, and blood volume support are continued, life can be supported for long periods of time. It is possible to transport patients during these resuscitative efforts to an area where definitive therapeutic measures are available. The most important aspects of emergency treatment of respiratory and circulatory failure are immediate recognition of the problem and the instantaneous application of simple therapeutic measures. This condition must be assessed and treated where it occurs, whether on the highway, in a casualty clearing station or in the emergency ward of a hospital.

Bleeding

The last condition that has to be controlled within a very short time is continuing rapid bleeding. In the past a great deal was taught about the application of tourniquets and the use of pressure points to control arterial bleeding. Both of these techniques are more cumbersome than necessary, and much misunderstanding has resulted from their use. External bleeding can almost always be adequately controlled by direct pressure over the bleeding site. Any clean cloth will do in providing this pressure. Unfortunately, patients are still brought into the hospital with proximal tourniquets in place and continued bleeding that can easily be stopped by removal of the tourniquet, which has impeded venous return and produced excessive venous bleeding. Occult bleeding will be discussed completely in the later section on hypovolemia.

There is increasing use of inflatable pressurized trousers (MAST trousers) in pre-hospital care of trauma victims. It is imperative that the physician recognize that these trousers, when inflated, give the patient an autotransfusion of up to 2 liters of his own blood. Therefore, fluid resuscitation must be complete before consideration is given to deflation. If deflation is premature or too hasty, hypotension will develop. Needless to say, these expensive trousers should not be cut away in a hasty effort to examine the lower extremities! (Use of this device is discussed in Chapter 4.)

Rapid Estimation of the Extent of Injury

When ventilatory and circulatory competence are assured and external bleeding sources have been controlled, rapid evaluation of the patient's injuries is necessary to determine what precautions are necessary in the subsequent handling and moving of the patient. Movement of the patient should be accomplished with great care. Simple splinting of limb fractures is advisable to prevent more serious compounding of these injuries. Medications to relieve pain should not be given before a more detailed examination is performed.

When adequate ventilation and circulation have been assured and rapid bleeding has been controlled, a complete and rapid history and physical examination, supplemented by laboratory and radiologic studies, should follow. The objectives of these evaluations are: elucidation of the full extent of other apparent injuries, discovery of additional injuries not immediately observed, definition of pre-injury conditions that may affect later management, and anticipation of complications, to permit institution of preventive measures in a timely manner. This is also the time to begin longitudinal monitoring of various cardiovascular, respiratory, metabolic, and neurologic parameters, so that early detection of deteriorating status can lead to prompt intervention. To omit a rapid survey for additional injuries in eagerness to treat an obvious one is an error that often leads to catastrophe. Most medical institutions have insisted that major trauma cases be supervised by general surgeons, hoping that they would be less prejudiced toward a specific organ system. Only rapid overall evaluation of the patient will avoid such disasters as a patient overwhelmed by an incipient cardiac tamponade during evaluation of a minor cerebral injury or irreversible shock produced by intra-abdominal hemorrhage during operative repair of a long bone fracture. Brief but accurate and thorough records of the initial evaluating examination should be kept for later comparison. Changes in vital signs or late appearance of abdominal tenderness when the initial examination showed none is evidence of progressive injury. The following brief outline is a reliable guide for such a rapid survey of injuries:

1. Examination of the head will determine the state of consciousness. The skull should be palpated for evidence of laceration and fractures. The nose and ears should be inspected for evidence of oozing blood or fluid. The size and symmetry of the pupils should be ascertained and noted. The neck should be palpated to determine the position of the trachea and to ascertain the presence of air in the soft tissues. The patient should be questioned to establish level of consciousness, orientation, and recall of circumstances.

2. Examination of the chest will disclose any thoracic wounds. Wounds of the thorax should be covered immediately with petrolatum gauze. Auscultation will determine whether breath sounds can be heard on both sides of the chest. The thoracic cage should be compressed to determine whether rib fractures have occurred. The quality of heart sounds and the pulse rate should be noted.

3. The abdomen should be examined for evidence of muscle spasm and abdominal tenderness. A thorough search should be made for subtle signs of blunt abdominal trauma. Wounds that have permitted herniation of abdominal contents should be covered with moist packs.

4. The patient should be asked to move all parts of his extremities. If he is unable to cooperate, the extremities should be gently moved and palpated for evidence of fracture.

5. The wings of the ilium should be compressed to discover whether the pelvis has been fractured.

6. The legs should be separated. The perineum should be inspected for evidence of extravasated blood and urine.

7. The patient should be moved sufficiently to inspect the back and buttock areas for previously undisclosed wounds.

8. The extremities should be examined for temperature and color. The quality and rate of the peripheral pulse should be determined bilaterally and in all extremities.

9. A record of serially determined blood pressure, pulse, respiration and level of consciousness should be started immediately and maintained until it has become clear that the patient's condition is stable.

From this point the initial evaluation of the injured patient is determined by the results of the rapid survey of injuries and by the condition of the patient. The more detailed evaluation of specific injuries is now begun and carried on simultaneously with specific therapy for already discovered injuries.

SPECIAL PROBLEMS IN DIAGNOSIS AND MANAGEMENT

Hypovolemia

Injury is almost always associated with the loss of some fluid from the fluid-containing compartments of the body. Hemorrhage at a wound site is a simple and classic example of rapid fluid loss. Even in the absence of hemorrhage, however, and without disruption of the integrity of the vascular system, tissue injury produces a sequestration of fluid into the area of the wound. Such sequestered fluid is, of course, derived from the fluid-containing compartments of the body, which are in dynamic equilibrium. The amount of fluid that is lost into a wound depends upon the size of the wound, the extent of tissue damage produced and the type of tissue injured. Whenever the fluid lost into the wound is of sufficient magnitude, depletion of all the fluid compartments of the body results. The distribution of the loss between intracellular, extracellular and intravascular compartments probably also depends upon the magnitude and severity of the wound, the type of wounded tissue, and the interval between time of injury and commencement of replacement therapy. The complex syndrome of physiologic derangement resulting from the sudden loss of fluid from the fluid-containing compartments of the body has been called hypovolemic shock. Before discussion of the signs, symptoms and function tests that are useful in the evaluation of the hypovolemic state, it is necessary to consider the pathologic physiology that results from the acute loss of body fluids. Although a complete discussion of the shock state follows in a later chapter, basic information is pertinent here.

Compensatory Mechanisms. Following an acute injury fluid is lost first from the vascular space. This is true whether the fluid is whole blood, as in the severance of a major artery, or interstitial fluid flowing into an extensive burn area and producing edema. The initial response to such a loss is a fall in the pressure within the cardiovascular system. Such a response is immediately monitored by a complex baroreceptor system in the aortic arch and carotid sinus and relayed to the medullary vasomotor center. Reflexes then effect changes that restore the pressure to its normal level. In general, this effect is mediated through the sympathetic nervous system and is achieved by arterial constriction that raises the peripheral resistance in the vascular system and by an increase in the cardiac output resulting from an increase in the force of cardiac contraction and an increase in the heart rate. An additional effect is constriction within the venous portion of the vascular system, mobilizing blood from reservoirs to the central portion of the vascular system. During these sympathetically induced restorative efforts, blood is mobilized from the extremities, the intestine and the kidney to provide sufficient volume for the heart and brain. This set of reactions reduces the size and changes the shape of the vascular compartment.

Other responses act to restore the plasma volume to the vascular compartment. Small increases in the osmolarity of the blood plasma are detected in the hypothalamic region; this stimulates the release of antidiuretic hormone and this, in turn, influences the kidney to conserve both water and sodium. It has been postulated that the juxtaglomerular apparatus in the kidney is also stimulated, possibly by a narrowing of the pulse pressure, to release renin, which in turn releases an octapeptide, angiotensin, from plasma protein precursors to stimulate the adrenal cortex to release aldosterone. This also has the effect of producing water and sodium conservation by the kidney. Further shifts of fluid between the vascular compartments are dictated by tension at the capillary level.

A fall in pressure in an arteriole produces a reduction of transmural capillary pressure so that extracellular fluid is moved into the capillary to restore blood volume. However, following the sympathetic response when venoconstriction has been established, the pressure relationships at the capillary level are such that in areas where constriction is prominent, plasma is lost from the capillary into the extracellular space. The inadequate perfusion following hypovolemia produces an elevation of carbon dioxide tension in the blood, a fall of the oxygen tension and a rise in hydrogen ion concentration. These chemical changes are immediately sensed by chemoreceptors located in the carotid and aortic bodies that signal the respiratory center. The response is hyperpnea, which is effective in reducing the carbon dioxide tension and returning pH values toward normal. The respiratory compensation for metabolic acidosis is illustrated in Figure 1–3.

All of these compensatory mechanisms function as an emergency reaction to preserve life. When hypovolemia is not corrected and these compensatory changes are allowed to persist, they themselves produce irreversible damage. The heart will eventually fail under these circumstances. Studies in experimental shock indicate that left atrial pressure rises after severe hypotension even when the blood volume has been restored. In the shock-dog preparation following the reinfusion of blood, cardiac output can be sustained only by progressive increase in the left atrial pressure. It has been a clinical finding with patients in advanced shock that intravenous infusion sometimes results in a rapid rise of central venous pressure without a concomitant increase in the cardiac output. The pulmonary edema characteristic of advanced shock has been attributed to progressive left heart failure and also to the redistribution of blood volume in which the pulmonary circulation is regarded as preferential circulation. It has also been attributed to the destructive ac-

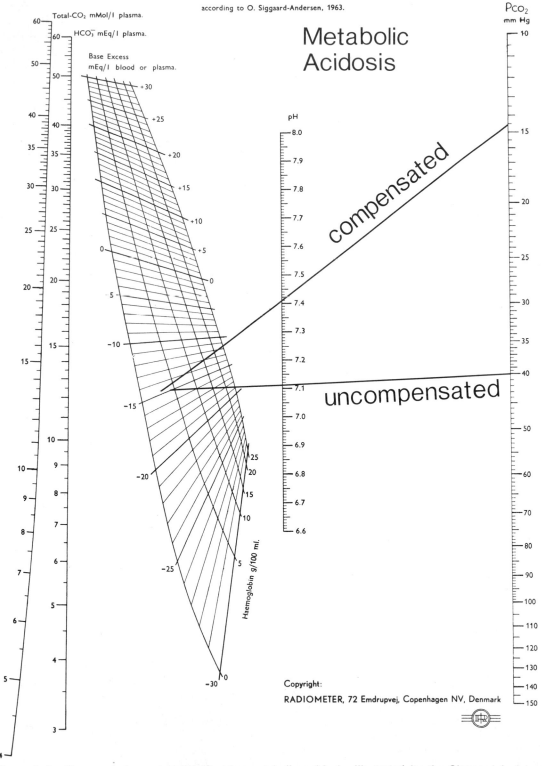

Figure 1–3. *The respiratory compensation for metabolic acidosis, illustrated by the Siggaard-Andersen nomogram. (Reprinted by permission. From Siggaard-Andersen, O.: Blood acid-base alignment nomogram. Scand. J. Clin. Lab. Invest. 15:211, 1963.)*

tion of certain humoral agents released into the blood stream that alter the permeability of lung capillaries.

Recently it has been suggested that certain phospholipid substances having surface-active properties are diminished in prolonged hypovolemia. These phospholipid substances are known to be important in maintaining the patency of pulmonary alveoli. Evidence of the impairment of renal function during prolonged hypovolemia has been obtained from experimental shock preparations. This information indicates that the renal vascular constrictive response that results in a high renal vascular resistance may continue inappropriately after the restoration of depleted blood volume. The renal cortical circulation, which under normal circumstances is rapid and requires a high oxygen concentration, may be especially impaired by the constrictive response. Thus, renal function may remain impaired long after the successful restoration of hemodynamic variables.

The profound gastrointestinal alterations that have been noted frequently in shock-dog preparations have never been an important feature of profound hypovolemic shock in patients. It is probable, however, that the function of almost all organ systems is affected by the changes resulting from inadequate tissue perfusion in hypovolemia and from the compensatory mechanisms called into play to preserve life.

The Diagnosis of Hypovolemia

SYSTEMIC BLOOD PRESSURE. Systemic hypotension is still frequently regarded as essential for the diagnosis of shock. In order to evaluate a single pressure recording as hypotensive it is necessary to know previous levels. Patients who normally function with a severe hypertension may be profoundly hypotensive with a blood pressure that would generally be regarded as normal. Because a fall in blood pressure is rapidly compensated by sympathetic responses, it is a poor indication of the severity of shock. Indeed, a patient's blood volume may be decreased by as much as 25 per cent with no change in blood pressure. Under these circumstances, a small additional hemorrhage, hypotensive agents (morphine, meperidine, general anesthetics) or positive end expiratory pressure may precipitate rapid and profound cardiovascular collapse.

Serial determinations of the systemic blood pressure, however, do reflect the course of developing hypovolemic shock in relation to compensatory mechanisms. It is for this reason that the blood pressure should be monitored during the evaluation of a patient with suspected hypovolemia at intervals of not longer than 15 minutes. The data should be evaluated in relation to other data such as pulse rate, central venous pressure and urine production. The instrument most commonly used to determine blood pressure is the sphygmomanometer. In patients with unstable cardiovascular systems and intense vasoconstriction secondary to endogenous catecholamines, there may be errors of 30 mm. Hg in either direction. Therefore, there is a tendency to earlier use of indwelling arterial catheters for monitoring purposes.

SIGNS OF INCREASED SYMPATHETIC ACTIVITY. As noted, the earliest compensatory mechanism following the loss of a significant amount of fluid from the vascular space is a profound sympathetic response. For this reason detection of sympathetic activity forms the most reliable basis for the early diagnosis of hypovolemic shock. Evidence includes pallor of the skin and mucous membranes, coolness of extremities, increased sweating, anxiety, collapse of veins on the dorsum of the hand and in the neck, tachycardia and a reduction in the pulse pressure. The combination of tachycardia and reduced pulse pressure produces what has become known as the rapid, weak and thready pulse. These signs should be observed at periodic intervals and an appropriate record kept. Following the institution of therapy, color and warmth return to the skin, anxiety disappears, the pulse rate reduces and the pulse pressure widens.

CENTRAL VENOUS PRESSURE. In hypovolemic shock the central venous pressure is low but can be raised by an infusion of saline. The heart will respond to such an infusion with an increased cardiac output. At the beginning of this century, Yandall Henderson insisted that observation of the central venous pressure was a reliable guide to the treatment of shock. At the present time there is considerable enthusiasm for the use of venous pressure measurements. The technique can be easily performed and is an effective guide for the measurement of fluid replacement in the therapy of shock. An improvement in systemic blood pressure with no rise in the central venous pressure strongly suggests that a hypovolemic state still exists. In general, it is safe to continue therapy under close observation until a rapid rise in the venous pressure indicates that the heart is loaded to its capacity. Failure to detect this rise may result in dangerous overloading. It must also be pointed out that venous pressure is determined not only by the volume on the venous side but also by the contractile force of the heart; at the stage at which myocardial failure complicates hypovolemia, the measurement fails as an indicator of volume deficits.

HYPERPNEA. The hyperventilation seen in hypovolemia is an important compensatory mechanism and is a good indication of hypoxia as well as metabolic acidosis. It has been suggested that the hypocapnea resulting from hyperventilation may have injurious effects by producing increased fatigue and decreased myocardial function. This suggestion is of minor theoretical importance in the acutely traumatized patient. Because hyperpnea may indicate hypoxia or metabolic acidosis, it is important that this compensatory response not be abolished by inappropriate sedation. Under such circumstances, respiratory depression may be fatal.

OLIGURIA. Because of the renal vasoconstriction which is part of the compensatory mechanism in shock, a diminution of urinary output is noted. Periodic measurements of urinary output are a helpful guide to the course of hypovolemic shock and the efficacy of therapy. An indwelling urinary catheter provides for hourly determinations of volume and specific gravity. A urinary output of less than 30 milliliters per hour is generally accepted as indicating an inadequate renal blood flow.

The advisability and timing of insertion of an indwelling catheter continues to be a source of anxiety to those who are less experienced in trauma resuscitation. Inspection of the external genitalia for evidence of urethral injury should be done first, along with a search for physical and radiographic evidence of pelvic fractures.

In the male, the urethra should be "milked"; if blood is obtained, a urethral injury is likely. The prostate should be palpated per rectum. If disruption of the membranous urethra has occurred, the gland will be floating in a hematoma, and its outlines will be indistinct. If there is any suspicion of a urethral injury, an emergency urethrogram should be performed. A normal urethrogram should then be followed by insertion of a catheter. With proper technique, a urethral catheter can be inserted without trauma. Therefore, any hematuria can be interpreted as evidence of urinary tract injury. Waiting for an injured patient to void spontaneously because of fear of possible false-positive hematuria is unacceptable: it may delay the diagnosis of significant urinary tract injury and will deprive the physician of a valuable monitoring system.

CHEMICAL MEASUREMENTS. As noted, chemical determinations are static, whereas responses to hypovolemia, both untreated and during therapy, are dynamic. For that reason, chemical determinations have little value unless they are repeated frequently. Techniques are now available for measuring blood volume with the aid of albumin labeled with radioactive iodine or red blood cells tagged with radioactive chromium. The chief objection to these techniques is that they are time consuming, and there is some difficulty in obtaining consistent and reproducible determinations. The hematocrit is not a reliable test of volume but indicates only the concentration of red blood cells. Its value in acutely developing hypovolemia is sharply restricted, but it has considerable value in slowly developing hypovolemia in which shifts of fluid between compartments gradually compensate for the loss of whole blood. The hematocrit is a good indicator of *which* intravenous fluid to give, but it is a poor guide to *when* it should be given.

Arterial blood gas determinations are useful in the traumatized patient and should be obtained early and often until resuscitation is complete. Hypoxemia may be an immediate problem or a progressive complication in a patient with multiple injuries. Color and other physical signs are notoriously late in warning the physician of the presence of a hypoxic state. Serial measurement of pH and pCO_2 and calculation of base deficit will indicate the severity of metabolic acidosis and the efficacy of therapeutic measures. Experience has shown that a metabolic acidosis may persist for several hours after apparent correction of blood volume deficit.

The patient presenting in a state of advanced hypovolemic shock usually presents no diagnostic challenge. However, if the diagnosis of hypovolemia is delayed until most of the classic manifestations of shock are present — systolic pressure of less than 80 mm. Hg severe oliguria, cold and clammy skin, cloudy sensorium — there will be extensive deterioration of vital organs, and the chances of successful therapy will be greatly reduced. There is a danger that the patient in a state of compensated hypovolemia — i.e., near normal blood pressure, tachycardia, tachypnea and decreased urine volume of high specific gravity — may be inadequately evaluated and therefore may go on to develop severe shock while in the emergency department. It is tragic for such a deterioration to occur in a hospital, particularly if it follows a superficial evaluation or slow-paced therapeutic program. The effect of shock on mortality from injury is significant: going into shock may double mortality, and staying in shock for more than 15 minutes may double it again. A realistic goal for the physician dealing with traumatized patients is the prevention of shock in patients under his care.

SUMMARY.   The proper diagnosis of hypovolemia in an injured patient depends upon the continuous monitoring of a variety of signs related to volume deficit and a series of compensatory mechanisms that attempt to protect the patient. Because of the dynamic nature of these mechanisms, estimates of loss and simple replacement are not adequate. A graphic record of the variables provides continuous evaluation and permits adequate therapy. In advanced shock many organ systems are damaged and demonstrate extreme malfunction. The primary aim of therapy in patients with hypovolemic shock is to restore tissue perfusion and thereby restore function. However, such therapy becomes extremely complicated since it depends on the time and course of development of the hypovolemia, the type of fluid loss, the

degree of organ damage and the advancement of compensatory mechanisms. The therapy of acute hypovolemia will be discussed in a later chapter.

The Evaluation of Thoracic Injuries

Careful evaluation of patients with thoracic injuries is important because apparently insignificant injuries are potentially lethal. Injuries of the chest may be obvious because of the position of the wound or the complaints of the patient. Alternatively, especially in a severely injured patient, they may be obscure. A history of the nature of the injury is extremely important; the approach to a penetrating injury of the thoracic cage differs from that to a blunt injury without penetration. The proper evaluation and successful management of various thoracic injuries depend upon an understanding of physiological aberrations that result from the different types of wounds.

Diagnosis is made largely by observation of the patient and a satisfactory x-ray examination of the chest. In evaluating thoracic trauma an upright radiograph, if the patient is able to sit or stand, is preferable to one obtained flat. The established techniques of physical diagnosis for detection of thoracic abnormalities (percussion and auscultation) are probably less valuable than a satisfactory x-ray examination. The physician must be careful not to order "routine" x-rays before he examines the patient. The trip to the radiology department may take quite a while, and x-ray technicians are not trained to monitor severely injured patients. In urgent circumstances, it may be advisable to proceed with treatment in the absence of confirmatory radiologic studies, as in the case of tension pneumothorax and pericardial tamponade. The most important part of a good evaluation for thoracic injury is the physician's awareness of the potential of all thoracic wounds and systematic elimination of such potential damage.

Injury of the Thoracic Wall Without Penetration.   Injury to the thoracic wall without penetration usually results from a blow, a contusion or a crush injury. Such injuries are commonly associated with deceleration injuries. The automobile steering wheel is a special offender.

Rib Fractures. Rib fractures may be single or multiple. They may occur spontaneously in the presence of osteal disease but usually are the result of a fall or a blow on the chest. Patients complain of pain in the region of the fracture. This pain is aggravated by deep inspiration, and there is usually an associated voluntary restriction of respiratory activity on the side of the rib fracture. The patient should be stripped to the waist, examined and the painful site carefully palpated. A crunchy sensation of air in the subcutaneous space is sometimes detected, and movement of the fractured rib fragments produces exquisite pain. Identification of the injured rib is made by counting ribs. The recommended techniques are identification of the second rib at the angle of Louis with downward counting or identification of the twelfth rib where it is palpable with upward counting. On occasion, fractures of the ribs are occult and, in such cases, the diagnosis usually can be made by gently compressing the chest in the anteroposterior direction, which usually elicits pain at the site of the rib fracture. A fracture of the rib may be associated with significant intrathoracic damage as the result of lacerations of the lung or tears of intercostal vessels. A remarkable degree of hemothorax may be produced by a single rib fracture; therefore, percussion and auscultation of the chest should be carried out to detect the signs of pneumothorax and pleural effusion. Every patient with suspected rib fracture should have an x-ray of the chest to rule out the presence of air or fluid within the pleural space.

Multiple rib fractures that result from severe compression injuries of the chest frequently show two fracture sites for each rib and result in a complete separation of a portion of the chest wall, producing loss of stability. This condition is known as traumatic flail chest. The mobile portion of the chest wall moves paradoxically, being sucked in with inspiration and expanding outward with expiration. Thus, expired air from the lung within the undamaged hemithorax passes into the lung on the injured side, increasing the amount of dead space and decreasing the effectiveness of ventilation. Patients with flail chest injuries usually complain of great pain. Ventilation is difficult, and cyanosis frequently develops. On close inspection the paradoxical movement of the chest cage is obvious. However, patients with this injury who appear to be quite well may develop an insidious hypercapnia, resulting in sudden cardiac arrhythmias and death. Because of the severe injury necessary to produce such a flail chest, underlying pulmonary damage is a frequent complication, and the development of bronchial spasm, excessive bronchorrhea, interstitial hemorrhage and edema results in a situation known as traumatic wet lung and further interferes with adequate ventilation. Traumatic flail chest therefore is a surgical emergency requiring immediate treatment.

Adequate stabilization of the chest can sometimes be accomplished with sandbags. Techniques of external fixation of separated portions of the chest wall have been largely abandoned in favor of tracheostomy and artificial ventilation. The former reduces dead space and permits an adequate clearing of accumulated secretions; the latter encourages adequate ventilation. Separation of the costochondral junction is frequently an occult injury that cannot be detected by x-ray or definite physical signs and is usually detected by careful palpation and gentle compression of the costochondral areas.

Still another injury that can result from a blow of great violence is fracture of the sternum. This injury produces extreme pain in the region of the sternum. The patient breathes shallowly and assumes a characteristic posture in which the head and neck are held forward rigidly. Inspection of the sternal area may reveal evidence of depression and ecchymosis over the fracture site. The diagnosis of sternal fracture is established by palpation in the region of the injury and detection of movements of the ends of the bone. X-ray examination of the sternum with special views makes possible a definite diagnosis. It has frequently been noted that patients with sternal fractures are subject to severe cardiac contusion, with the development of sudden cardiac arrhythmias. Therefore, all patients suffering blunt anterior chest trauma should have a twelve-lead electrocardiogram and rhythm strip, regardless of age. Enzyme studies (CPK isoenzymes) may also be helpful.

Injuries to the Chest Wall with Penetration. In civilian practice penetrating injuries of the chest are usually produced by stab wounds or gunshot wounds. The evaluation of such wounds depends upon information concerning the damage most frequently produced by various weapons. Stab wounds are usually made with knives, daggers or ice picks. Most of the weapons are short and narrow and cause minimal destruction. However, the external appearance of a wound may be misleading because it does not reflect the degree of damage within the chest. In general, the wider the blade, the greater the possibility of severe injury. Ice pick wounds have a tendency to seal off quickly and, even when they penetrate the lung, they usually do not produce a severe air leak. The angle of entry should be determined and a search made for a site of exit. In general, women tend to stab downward, whereas men tend to stab in an upward direction. When the line of entry points toward the diaphragm the possibility of intra-abdominal damage should be considered; when an abdominal site of entry points upward, there is the possibility of intrathoracic damage. It is well recognized that high thoracic wounds can penetrate the diaphragm if the injury was produced during deep expiration.

Civilian gunshot wounds are usually caused by revolvers, high velocity rifles or shotgun pellets. A variety of high velocity everyday accidents simulate shotgun injuries, notably the propulsion of fragments by the blades of a rotary mower. The path of a missile injury is usually a straight line, although deflection by various tissues, particularly bone, is not uncommon. Bullet wounds penetrate more deeply than stab wounds and produce an area of damage around the tract of the bullet resulting from compression injury within the tissue. A jacketed slug produces less damage than a soft-nosed slug, which has a tendency to produce ragged tears within the tissue. A complication of missile injuries occurs when fragments of wadding and clothing are carried inward with the missile. Shotgun injuries received at close range produce injury by blast as well as by the penetrating missile.

The Pathophysiology of Penetrating Wounds of the Thorax. A wound that permits an open communication between the pleural space and the exterior atmosphere causes collapse of the lung as air under atmospheric pressure enters the chest. With inspiration, additional air is drawn into the chest, producing further collapse of the lung and a shift of the mediastinum toward the uninjured side. With expiration, the mediastinum is pushed toward the injured side, and air passes from the lung on the uninjured side to the lung on the injured side. Some air is then forced by partial inflation of the collapsed lung out through the open wound. Such to-and-fro movement of the mediastinum is known as mediastinal flutter.

The movement of air from one lung to the other has been referred to as "pendelluft," and the situation is known to be extremely deleterious and often lethal. Such an inefficient movement of air reduces tidal exchange by a volume equal to that entering and escaping through the wound in the chest wall. There is then an inefficient exchange of oxygen and carbon dioxide. Open wounds that produce mediastinal flutter and "pendelluft" have been referred to as sucking wounds. It is important to recognize that all wounds of the chest have the potential to produce this abnormality. No effort should be made to determine whether a significant collapse of the lung has occurred or whether there is significant mediastinal flutter; instead, all wounds of the chest should be immediately closed with a sterile dressing. The closure of a large sucking wound must be regarded as an emergency procedure; in desperate cases the wound should be closed with any available material without regard for sterility.

In the most extreme situations a sucking wound of the chest produces the following picture: The patient is in considerable distress with signs of asphyxiation. His respirations are labored and his expiratory efforts seem forced. He may be cyanotic and hypotensive. Tachycardia is usually present. Frothy material may appear with expiration, and the sound of air rushing in and out of the wound can usually be detected. If there has not been significant injury to the lung, the patient's condition should stabilize when a sucking wound of the chest has been closed. His respiration will improve, and diagnosis and evaluation may proceed at a more leisurely pace. If a sucking wound of the chest has been complicated by the penetration of the underlying lung with a leak of air from pulmonary tissue, closure of the sucking wound will permit more rapid development of two other severe complications. The most important of these is tension pneumothorax. The other is the development of subcutaneous and mediastinal emphysema.

Tension Pneumothorax. In the presence of a significant parenchymal leak of air and maintained integrity of the chest wall, air is drawn from the lung into the pleural space with each inspiration and trapped there. As more air is drawn into the pleural space, collapse of the injured lung occurs and the mediastinum begins to shift toward the uninjured side. This reduces the function of the uninjured lung as well. As pneumothorax becomes increasingly severe, it produces collapse of the major veins in the thorax. Many wounds of the lung stabilize without the development of these lethal abnormalities, but it is important to recognize that every patient with a penetrating wound of the chest that has been closed may develop tension pneumothorax. In the most severe form of tension pneumothorax, the patient is markedly dyspneic and appears to be suffocating. Cyanosis may be produced, and there is vascular collapse resulting from the cardiac embarrassment that occurs when there is prevention of an adequate venous return to the heart. This results in systemic hypotension, tachycardia and a reduction in the pulse pressure, which is easily confused with hypovolemic shock.

The diagnosis of tension pneumothorax is made by detecting the physical signs of pneumothorax as well as by tracheal shift and displacement of the apical heart beat. Tracheal shift is discovered by simple palpation of the trachea in the neck just above the thoracic inlet. The diagnosis can be made with certainty by radiographic examination of the chest, which will demonstrate pulmonary collapse and mediastinal shift. However, it is important that patients be positioned properly for this examination, since rotation of the patient will produce confusing x-rays that obscure the

diagnosis. Recognition of developing tension pneumothorax requires immediate aspiration of trapped air from the pleural space. If the patient is cyanotic or unconscious, it is advisable to proceed with life-saving therapy in the absence of confirmatory radiographs. A quick bedside test of increased intrapleural pressure can be made using a moistened glass syringe with attached needle. As the needle enters the pleural cavity, the plunger is moved by the air trapped under pressure in the pleural space. A plastic syringe, half filled with saline and without a plunger, can be substituted. Vigorous bubbling of air is a positive sign.

PHYSICAL SIGNS OF PNEUMOTHORAX. Physical signs of pneumothorax depend upon its extent and are minimal when only a small amount of air is trapped in the pleural space. Consequently, radiographic examination of the chest is a more reliable diagnostic tool than physical examination. The physical signs described here are those seen with extensive pneumothorax. Inspection of the patient reveals diminished respiratory excursion of the chest wall on the affected side. There is usually an increase in ventilatory rate. The patient complains of pain in the chest and, frequently, of shortness of breath. Percussion reveals hyperresonance and tympany and, if done with care, a mediastinal shift. Tactile fremitus is absent. Various signs of air and fluid in the pleural space have been described, including the "coin" test in which a coin is laid against the chest wall and tapped with another. This produces a particular metallic sound. In addition, one can frequently hear a succussion splash in which fluid in the pleural space moves about when the patient is moved. In addition to these signs, tension pneumothorax will produce mediastinal shifts and tracheal deviations.

Subcutaneous Emphysema and Mediastinal Emphysema. The combination of a chest wall wound and an underlying lung wound permits air under pressure in the pleural space to dissect into the tissue planes about the wound, especially when there is no open external communication. The presence of air in the subcutaneous tissues is called subcutaneous emphysema. The classic situation in which this condition develops is a compression injury of the chest that produces fractures of the ribs. These may result in stab wounds of the lung at moments of extreme thoracic pressure. Air is then injected into the tissues about the fractured ends of the ribs. Mediastinal emphysema occurs most commonly when there is a rupture of the pulmonary parenchyma without significant damage to the visceral pleura. Air can leak along the peribronchial planes during inspiration, enter the mediastinum and travel toward the superior outlet of the thorax, continuing as subcutaneous emphysema that spreads over the neck, face, chest and anterior abdominal wall. When fully developed the condition produces a frightening appearance but is usually not serious. On occasion, mediastinal emphysema has produced compression of mediastinal structures and has required cervical mediastinotomy for its relief. The physical signs of subcutaneous and mediastinal emphysema are swelling and crepitation in the subcutaneous tissues; frequently, it can be diagnosed before it progresses to cervical subcutaneous emphysema by the detection of a so-called crunching sound on auscultation over the sternum.

Hemothorax. In addition to pneumothorax and subcutaneous emphysema, penetrating wounds of the chest frequently produce hemothorax because of associated injuries to blood vessels in the lung or chest wall. Hemothorax, of course, occurs as a complication of injuries that do not destroy the integrity of the chest wall, such as severe crush injuries in which fractured ribs damage the underlying pleura and the lung parenchyma. When hemothorax occurs as a complication of a penetrating wound, pneumothorax is usually associated — a combination known as hemopneumothorax. The extent of bleeding within the pleural space depends upon the type of injury. When major vessels have been damaged, bleeding may be massive and death may occur quickly; lacerations of the lung, however, do not usually produce excessive bleeding. Blood pressure in the pulmonary circulation is low, and the elastic qualities of pulmonary tissue allow for collapse and vessel retraction in areas of injury. Rapidly developing hemothorax usually indicates damage to a small systemic vessel or an intercostal artery. Blood in the pleural space, like air,

produces collapse of the lung and eventual shifting of the mediastinum, so that signs of respiratory embarrassment are combined with the signs of developing hypovolemia and also include percussion dullness and diminished or absent breath sounds. In cases of hemopneumothorax the signs of the pneumothorax tend to dominate, and rather extensive collections of blood within the pleural space produce minimal physical signs. Consequently, the most reliable tool in the diagnosis of hemothorax as well as pneumothorax and hemopneumothorax is x-ray examination.

Penetrating Wounds of the Mediastinum. All penetrating wounds of the chest must be regarded as possible penetrating wounds of the mediastinum. Damage to the major airways, major vessels, esophagus and heart can occur, and such injury can be surprisingly occult. Mediastinal hemorrhage can be contained temporarily in a hematoma, but rupture may later produce fatal exsanguination. Undetected esophageal injuries can produce fatal mediastinitis, and major airway injuries produce rapidly developing and fatal mediastinal emphysema if not relieved by proper venting. Penetrating injuries of the heart with contained bleeding in the pericardium produce cardiac tamponade, which results in progressive compression of the heart and obstruction of the great veins with diminished cardiac output and ultimate death. The most reliable sign of developing cardiac tamponade is a rise in the central venous pressure. In the evaluation of a patient with a penetrating wound of the chest, therefore, serial monitoring of venous pressure is essential.

A variety of other signs produced by cardiac tamponade either are unreliable or are also produced by other injuries. Examination for mediastinal widening is not reliable, for example, because rapid effusions may occur that do not appreciably enlarge the area of cardiac dullness or significantly change the size of the cardiac shadow on x-ray examination. Dyspnea and pallid cyanosis, which occur in cardiac tamponade, are also complications of hemopneumothorax and tachycardia; systemic hypotension and diminution of the pulse pressure also appear in hypovolemia. Pulsus paradoxus, in which the systolic blood pressure falls with each inspiration, is a difficult physical sign to detect and so is considerably less reliable than serial monitoring of the venous pressure. The diagnosis of pericardial tamponade may be confirmed by aspiration of nonclotting blood from the pericardial sac. The pericardium may be reached by precordial or subcostal routes. Unfortunately, a negative result is not trustworthy: patients have expired from pericardial tamponade after negative pericardiocentesis. In such cases, autopsy has revealed that the heart was "floating" on 200 to 300 ml. of clotted blood in a posterior, and therefore inaccessible, location. If strong suspicion of pericardial tamponade exists, a limited pericardiotomy through a subcostal extrapleural approach may be diagnostic and life-saving.

Whenever mediastinal injury is suspected, a gastrograffin swallow should be obtained to rule out injury to the esophagus. Serial x-rays should be obtained to follow any changes in the contour of the mediastinal shadows. Foreign bodies lodged within the mediastinum should be observed fluoroscopically for evidence of movement; if it is noted, the relationship between such foreign bodies and the great vessels within the mediastinum should be determined through angiocardiography.

The management of cardiac tamponade and other mediastinal injuries is discussed in a later chapter.

Intrathoracic Injury with No Visible Evidence of Chest Wall Damage. Frequently, decelerating and crushing injuries produce intrathoracic damage without any visible evidence of chest wall damage. Such injury should always be suspected in high velocity accidents and fall and crush injuries.

Lacerations of the Aorta. A syndrome of aortic laceration following deceleration is now well recognized. This laceration usually occurs at points of fixation of the aorta, most notably at the level of the left subclavian artery. The injury can be occult, at first producing only a small hematoma, but if unrecognized it will lead to fatal exsanguination or formation of a traumatic aortic aneurysm. The diagnosis is suspected from observation of abnormal contours of the mediastinal shadows on roentgenographic examination and is confirmed by aortography. It is important to

remember that full and symmetrical pulses may be present in a patient with total transection of the aorta.

Contusion of the Lung. Contusion injuries of the lung without evidence of chest wall damage produce intrapulmonary hemorrhage with dyspnea and hemoptysis. Physical signs are those of localized consolidation with diminished breath sounds and crepitant rales. Marked hypoxemia will usually precede physical and radiographic changes by several hours. There is good reason to believe that early detection of shunting secondary to pulmonary contusion accompanied by prompt initiation of positive pressure ventilation or positive end expiratory pressure may decrease morbidity and mortality.

Contusion of the Heart. Contusion injury of the myocardium with intramyocardial hemorrhage occurs following blunt trauma to the chest. Such injury may be followed by cardiac arrhythmias and sudden death. When this condition is suspected, the patient should be followed with serial electrocardiograms to determine the presence of injury currents.

The Diagnosis of Intra-abdominal Injury

Intra-abdominal injury may be produced by blunt trauma or by a penetrating wound of the abdomen. When external wounds are evident, the examiner should immediately consider the possibility of intra-abdominal injury. A nasogastric tube should be passed in all patients with suspected abdominal trauma. Gastric contents should be analyzed for blood and toxic substances. If there is a disturbance of consciousness, the tube should be kept in the stomach to prevent aspiration of gastric contents. Experience has shown that apparently trivial abrasions and contusions of the abdominal wall may be associated with major blunt injury to the intra-abdominal organs.

Closed Abdominal Injuries. The spleen, liver, stomach, intestines and pancreas are vulnerable to blunt injury. This may occur when the viscus is crushed against the vertebral column or is violently displaced on its mesenteric attachments. It is not unusual to see little or no evidence of intra-abdominal injury at the time of primary examination. Frequent examination of the abdomen may reveal early signs of injury. Solid organs — such as the liver, spleen and kidneys — and major vessels are most frequently injured in blunt abdominal trauma, resulting in accumulation of blood within the peritoneal cavity. In many circumstances, blood is not very irritating to the peritoneum, especially if there is no contamination by bile or bowel contents. Consequently, early physical signs of peritoneal irritation — muscle spasm, rebound tenderness, absent bowel sounds — may be absent, or they may be too late to be of use. The first indication of significant organ injury may be hypovolemic shock.

Routine laparotomy was recommended in the past in cases of suspected blunt abdominal trauma. This resulted in excessive morbidity from negative laparotomies in addition to injuries that were missed owing to hesitation in performing this drastic diagnostic maneuver. Four-quadrant and flank taps had a very high false-negative rate. These methods have been largely replaced by early use of diagnostic peritoneal lavage. Briefly, this involves the atraumatic insertion of a peritoneal dialysis catheter into the peritoneal cavity, followed by instillation of normal saline. When the fluid is returned by siphon action, it is analyzed for blood by any of several methods. The accuracy of this technique in the detection of significant intra-abdominal hemorrhage approaches 98 per cent; a negative result carries a 99 per cent probability that there is no significant intra-abdominal injury. The technique is especially useful in unconscious patients and those who require prolonged operative intervention for other injuries. Of course, patients who have an indication for laparotomy should not undergo this test. Lavage may be performed with minimal discomfort on conscious patients. Patients may be discharged after a negative lavage if their other injuries do not require hospitalization.

Injuries to the intra-abdominal viscera are usually classified in certain general groups. One of these is laceration of the liver, resulting in intraperitoneal hemorrhage. The extent of hemorrhage varies widely, but if it is extensive — involving the major hepatic or portal veins — exsan-

guination and death may ensue. Minor degrees of laceration may produce bile peritonitis with serious consequences. In either instance, the physical signs shown by the patient may be those of peritoneal irritation, possibly with shifting dullness, rebound tenderness and generalized peritonitis. An examination of the abdomen may also be normal, particularly in the early hours after injury.

Splenic rupture is a very common injury and should be suspected when patients report blows on the left flank or left lower chest. The ribs overlying the area may or may not be fractured. Early physical signs may be unimpressive and may consist only of tachycardia and minimal abdominal tenderness. Later, abdominal pain may be severe and may be associated with shock and referred pain in the left shoulder. Physical examination usually reveals some indication of peritoneal irritation, which is most marked in the left upper quadrant. Diaphragmatic irritation may contribute to dyspnea. When there are minor lacerations of the spleen and continued slow bleeding, diagnosis may be difficult. Peritoneal lavage will detect such injuries before hypovolemia makes them obvious.

Mild degrees of trauma may produce subcapsular hematoma of the spleen, which may rupture several days or weeks later. Lateral abdominal x-rays may aid in differentiating this from retroperitoneal tumor masses, and an upright film of the abdomen after injection of a small amount of air through a nasogastric tube may reveal irregular margins of the hematoma in the gastrosplenic ligament. Recently, splenic scans and celiac axis arteriography have been of great help in making this difficult diagnosis. It is often helpful to know whether the patient had some preexisting disease such as malaria, leukemia, infectious mononucleosis or other hematological disorder in which splenomegaly may be a prominent feature. In such patients splenic rupture may occur spontaneously or may accompany minor degrees of trauma. There is increasing suspicion that "delayed rupture" of the spleen may in fact be missed rupture. The incidence of this condition should decrease with wider acceptance of early diagnostic lavage.

Compression of the intestine, particularly when filled with fluid, may lead to its rupture. The small intestine is more frequently involved than the large; and the commonest locations for perforation are at the ligament of Treitz, the terminal ileum, or at a point where an adhesion is present from previous surgery. These points are related to areas of fixation, which presumably limit the mobility of the bowel and contribute to the rupture. The duodenum and pancreas lie anterior to the spine and may be involved in a crush injury against this bony structure. Pancreatic and duodenal injuries commonly occur together and carry a very high mortality. Laceration of the duodenum permits bowel contents to leak posteriorly into the retroperitoneum. Associated physical signs, such as spasm and abdominal rigidity, may be delayed.

Rupture of the large intestine is infrequently encountered. Lacerations of the large bowel mesentery may occur, however, resulting in hemorrhage, necrosis and gangrene. Patients with this type of injury may have considerable abdominal pain without early signs of peritonitis, and this diagnosis may be particularly difficult to make preoperatively.

Penetrating Wounds of the Abdomen. All patients with penetrating wounds of the abdominal wall caused by missiles that could have entered or traversed the peritoneal cavity require surgical exploration. This is not true, however, for stab wounds. With a high degree of accuracy it is possible to demonstrate penetration of the peritoneal cavity by the injection of radiopaque contrast material into the wound tract under local anesthesia, or by direct exploration of the wound with minor extension of the laceration, also under local anesthesia. This technique permits one to rule out superficial, non-penetrating stab wounds and possibly avoid unnecessary operation. If penetration is demonstrated, however, early operation is recommended. An alternative approach, called selective conservatism, requires admission to the hospital of all patients with abdominal stab wounds. Vital signs, the abdominal examination and the leukocyte count are monitored closely. If changes occur that suggest intraperitoneal injury, the patient is explored. Otherwise, the patient is discharged in 24 to 48 hours.

In performing the abdominal examination on a patient with a penetrating injury, several points are worth noting. When there are multiple wounds it is easy to overlook small wounds of entrance. It should be routine to inspect carefully the buttocks, perineum and anal canal as well as the obvious areas of the back, abdomen and flanks. Under certain circumstances, the appearance of the wound and discharge from it may provide information regarding the nature of the injury; the presence of intestinal contents or bile denotes specific visceral injury and indicates the need for prompt exploration. Small entrance wounds necessitate a search for minor degrees of peritoneal irritation, including careful examination of the rectum and, when necessary, sigmoidoscopy without the use of air insufflation. The examiner must coordinate abdominal findings with those of the neurological examination, since spinal cord injuries may either obscure or produce abdominal pain, rigidity and hypotension.

The development of pallor, sweating, restlessness and thirst following injury is significant, for it may indicate intra-abdominal hemorrhage resulting from laceration of the liver, spleen, mesenteric vessels or retroperitoneum. Other physical signs include the development of hypotension, rapid pulse rate with thready quality, dyspnea or "air hunger," shifting dullness and rebound tenderness. When there is massive hemorrhage the abdomen becomes progressively dull and distended. When the rate of hemorrhage is slower, normal blood pressure may be maintained for several hours. It is obviously important to follow pulse pressure and pulse rate with great care and not to be completely dependent upon the absolute systolic and diastolic arterial pressures. The course of the indices and physical signs is more significant in most instances than the actual initial value. With slow, continued bleeding, for instance, progressive abdominal tenderness and spasm may be evident.

Perforation of a hollow viscus is associated with abdominal rigidity, tenderness and absence of bowel sounds; it may be accompanied by abdominal pain and vomiting. These features tend to become more prominent as time elapses following injury. It is possible to overlook early signs of visceral perforation in the presence of multiple injuries and when analgesics or sedatives have been administered. When shock develops 8 to 12 hours after injury, generalized peritonitis must be considered as a cause. In this instance tachypnea and the characteristic anxious facies may be present.

Continuing blood loss with or without peritonitis may lead to "irreversible shock." The examiner should not be too quick to pronounce the hypotension irreversible, for he may simply be underestimating fluid losses. It is true, however, that failure of vital signs to return to normal after what appears to be adequate replacement transfusion carries with it a poor prognosis. One must be certain that a remediable lesion is not contributing to the patient's deteriorating clinical condition. Tension pneumothorax or cardiac tamponade may easily occur in association with intra-abdominal injury. Continual re-evaluation of the patient is required to be certain that the working diagnosis is accurate.

The Evaluation of Arterial Injury

The diagnosis of injury to a major artery is not usually a problem since such injury frequently produces a pulsatile hemorrhage or obvious acute ischemia in the part supplied by the damaged vessel. However, this is not always the case; the injury to a major vessel may sometimes be occult, with no signs or only slowly developing signs of ischemia and without much evidence of severe external hemorrhage. It is no longer a tenable view that the primary concern in major arterial injury is the adequate control of hemorrhage. With the development of adequate techniques for arterial reconstruction, it has become increasingly important to make an early and accurate diagnosis of arterial injury so that circulation can be completely restored. Pulsatile and excessive wound hemorrhage should be controlled with pressure until an appropriate exploration of the wound can be performed under operating room conditions. Major vessels that can be reconstructed should never be blindly clamped and sutured.

In the absence of pulsatile hemorrhage, the most accurate sign of major vessel damage is distal pulselessness. For this reason an important part of the physical examination of the acutely injured patient is an examination of the pulses bilaterally in the neck and in the upper and lower extremities. Although it is true that in the absence of pre-existing arterial disease pulselessness is a definite sign of acute arterial injury, such injury may occur without the development of this sign. It is even possible to have a completely severed artery in conjunction with maintenance of distal pulses, and thus it is important that pulses be compared with their opposite member. The small portable Doppler instrument has facilitated quantitative measurements of extremity pulses. Ischemia of a part produces pallor or pallid cyanosis and changes in temperature, with the ischemic part being cooler than the perfused part. In the conscious patient pain is a prominent symptom of ischemia; in time, associated neurological ischemia will produce sensory changes of paresthesia and anesthesia as well as motor changes of weakness and paralysis.

Major arterial damage occurs in a variety of ways, including laceration without loss of substance, laceration with loss of substance, external compression when an artery is impinged upon by a bony fragment or occlusion without loss of continuity due to subintimal hemorrhage or fracture of the vascular intima with arterial dissection. These latter two types of injury were formerly frequently attributed to arterial spasm and treated inappropriately.

Because of the occult nature of major vascular injuries, the suggestion has been made that all wounds in the vicinity of major vessels deserve a surgical exploration. Such a policy is at times impractical, and, with the availability of arteriography, usually unnecessary. It is certainly true, however, that all wounds with pulsatile hemorrhage, rapidly expanding hematomas or pulsatile hematomas deserve surgical exploration. It is also true that the finding of pulselessness with signs of distal ischemia is an indication for surgical exploration. When the diagnosis of major vessel damage is in doubt, serially recorded observations related to the quality of pulse, temperature, color and sensory and motor activity of the affected part should be made. Serial pressures using the

Doppler method are particularly useful in detecting the early stages of ischemia from arterial injury. Arteriography has a definite and important part to play in the evaluation of arterial injury. It provides a certain diagnosis without long observation, precise localization of the wound and an estimate of collateral circulation. False negative results in arteriographic evaluation of vascular injury have been noted, but they are extremely rare. The technique has the disadvantage of being somewhat time-consuming, but when properly performed, it carries little hazard.

Initial Evaluation of the Burned Patient

A later chapter in this text deals with the complex subject of the management of the burned patient. The successful management of such a patient can be carried out only with the aid of repeated evaluation of the patient's wound and the burn shock that it has produced. The initial evaluation of such a patient, which is only the first of many evaluations, has two main functions. It must first be established whether or not the burn has produced respiratory injury. This is done by examining the nasal and oral airways for evidence of burn and by detecting evidence of hoarseness, crowing, coughing or ventilatory abnormality. Initial and subsequent arterial blood gas determinations will provide early evidence of progressive hypoxemia. When a severe burn has been sustained in a closed space and when there are significant burns of the face, head or neck, such respiratory damage must be anticipated. The diagnosis of respiratory burn alerts one to the possible need for ventilatory assistance.

The other objective of the initial examination is estimation of the severity of the burn. It must be remembered that all burns of the hands, feet or face, all burns of the aged and the very young, and all burns that involve more than 10 per cent of the body area must be considered serious and therefore require hospitalization. A record of the seriously burned patient's vital signs should be established early in the period of evaluation. This should include the pulse rate, rate of respiration, blood pressure and weight when these measurements can be obtained. In planning and

initiating treatment of burn shock, an estimate of the percentage area of the body burned and of the depth of burn are valuable. The "rule of nines," by which portions of the body are assigned 9 or 18 per cent, is a helpful and adequate technique for quickly estimating the area of the burn.

The depth of the burn is considerably more difficult to gauge and is likely to be underestimated. Flame burns may be assumed to be full thickness. Full thickness burns may assume a variety of appearances, including a brown color with a leathery charred appearance, white and cadaveric, or oily and transparent with the obvious thrombosed vessel or with large broken blisters. Blister formation, which was formerly considered characteristic of second degree burns, is frequently seen with deeper burns. The fluid shifts accompanying burns may be rapid and extensive. The dynamics involved in their estimation and correction are those associated with hypovolemia. The situation is further complicated by infection and by heat, water and energy losses through the damaged skin. Detailed consideration of these special problems is included in Chapter 23.

Diagnosis of Neurological Injury

A thorough history of the circumstances surrounding craniocerebral trauma and the postinjury behavior of the patient often provide information that is significant in diagnosis and treatment. Witnesses of the accident or people who have observed the patient immediately after injury should be carefully questioned regarding his state of consciousness, duration of unconsciousness, ability to move his extremities, ability to speak, confusion or disorientation and the presence of convulsions.

It is obvious that complete evaluation of the patient's physical condition is necessary and that initial treatment must be instituted as indicated. Patients with craniocerebral trauma frequently have associated airway obstruction or difficulties with ventilation that require primary attention. Once the pressing demands for evaluation of the patient's overall condition and emergency treatment of life-threatening injury are cared for, neurological examination may be performed. This type of emergency neurological examination has three objectives: to obtain base line neurological information for later comparison, to establish the diagnosis of the existence of a head injury and to determine the need for emergency surgical intervention.

A few carefully selected neurological studies will often offer sufficient information to permit adequate initial treatment. A time-consuming and detailed neurological examination is not appropriate for the early care of head injury patients. The state of consciousness should be carefully evaluated, as well as the patient's response to painful stimulation. This may be obtained by noting response to supraorbital pressure, pinprick or pressure on the sternum. The relative size, equality and response to light of the pupils of the patient's eyes should be observed early and carefully recorded. Small contracted pupils that do not respond to light may be associated with midbrain damage. The administration of medication or the patient's recent consumption of alcohol may render this sign misleading. The presence of dilated fixed pupils usually indicates a poor prognosis. Inequality of the pupils may reflect local brain damage. Unilateral dilatation of the pupils, particularly when it occurs under observation, is strongly suggestive of intracranial hemorrhage.

The character of ventilation may assist in diagnosis, since irregular or depressed ventilations frequently accompany severe intracranial injury. If ventilatory alterations persist with an adequate airway, the prognosis is grave.

The degree of the patient's motor activity should be evaluated. If the patient is conscious, motor activity can be easily appraised by having the patient squeeze the examiner's hands or by testing his ability to resist passive motion of the extremities. In the comatose patient motor activity should be tested by determining the degree of flaccidity by lifting the extremity slightly and letting it drop. It should be emphasized that both sides of the patient should be tested. This permits comparison and provides base line information that is helpful as observation of his condition continues. Extensor rigidity of the extremities also carries a poor prognosis. Alcoholism or drug intoxication may confuse

this issue, but complete flaccidity and areflexia are usually indications of severe central nervous system damage.

Body temperature should be recorded early and followed with care. When associated with evidence of intracranial injury, the development of hyperthermia is significant. Fever in excess of 103° Fahrenheit indicates a bad prognosis. Profound hypothermia, with temperatures less than 92° F., may be the sole explanation for severe generalized neurological deficit. Such patients may have no detectable signs of life. Cardiopulmonary resuscitation and other life-support measures should be continued until the temperature exceeds 95° F. *per rectum* before a diagnosis of death or severe neurological injury can be certain.

Simple evaluation of the deep tendon reflexes is adequate for the initial examination. The triceps, biceps, radial-periosteal, plantar, knee and ankle reflexes, with a test for the presence of ankle clonus, should be sufficient for initial evaluation and later comparison.

One should be particularly cautious in handling a patient who is able to move his arms but whose legs are immobile. He should be regarded as having a fractured spine and spinal cord injury until it is proved otherwise. Evaluation of the level of injury should include determination of a sensory level and response to painful stimuli. X-rays of the spine should be included among the diagnostic procedures, and care should be taken to apply manual traction to the neck and feet to avoid flexion of the spine during movement. The portable lateral cervical spine film, with visualization of all seven vertebral bodies, should be obtained before movement of any kind is allowed.

The patient's head should be carefully inspected and palpated for lacerations and depressions in the skull. Bleeding from the ear without an obvious source of laceration strongly suggests basilar skull fracture, involving the temporal bone. The eardrums should be inspected routinely for the presence of blood in the middle ear. Bleeding from the nose, which is often due to local trauma, may also indicate involvement of the paranasal sinuses by a fracture. Many of these fractures are difficult to visualize on skull films, and one should be acutely aware that a blood or cerebrospinal fluid leak into the middle ear or the sinuses provides ready access for invasion of the subarachnoid spaces, leading to meningitis or brain abscess. Consequently, antibiotic coverage is indicated in patients with these findings.

The significance of a simple linear skull fracture as seen on x-rays of the skull depends on possible injury to the central nervous system, signs and symptoms of which would be present in the individual patient. This finding should not in itself alter the overall program of management. A depressed skull fracture is a result of direct trauma with an instrument or missile of some kind. The resulting brain damage may be extremely variable and, again, the importance of the finding depends on the neurological signs and symptoms present in the individual patient. One should, however, suspect a depressed skull fracture in all patients with lacerated or contused wounds of the scalp. The diagnosis of a depressed skull fracture is usually an indication for prompt surgical intervention. Failure to perform surgery may result in progressive neurological deterioration or infection.

Penetrating wounds of the skull may be particularly misleading. Extensive intracranial injury may be associated with a very small entrance wound that is obscured by hair. Early surgical exploration and debridement are indicated.

Cerebral concussion is associated with loss of consciousness and, often, with memory loss regarding the time of the accident. Although the patient may appear to be well when first seen, careful repeated observation is of vital importance because the possibility of delayed intracranial hemorrhage is always present.

Intracranial hemorrhage may be either extradural or subdural in location. Characteristically, a brief period of unconsciousness may be noted, followed by a "lucid interval" and then by confusion, drowsiness and progressive coma. When the hemorrhage is extradural in location, the sequence of events tends to be fairly rapid — often developing over a period of minutes or hours. With the development of a subdural hemorrhage the course may be extended over several weeks or even months. In either event, the presence of lateralizing neurological signs, asymmetrical dilatation of the pupils and alteration in the deep tendon reflexes and motor responses should be sufficient evidence to prompt neurosurgical and operative steps.

Attention is often so focused on a head injury that associated injuries such as those of the cervical, dorsal or lumbar spine may be overlooked. A thorough evaluation is essential to the patient's overall well-being. Fractures or fracture dislocations of the spine usually result from violent trauma and may occur independently or in association with head injury. Evaluation of suspected spine injury must be completed without disturbing the patient. This applies to his initial evaluation and transportation from the scene of the injury as well as to his diagnosis and therapy upon entrance into the hospital. Failure to observe this rule may result in irreversible injury to the spinal cord. The cervical spine, because of its mobility, is particularly susceptible to injury, and it is essential that gentle traction be exerted on the head and the long axis of the spine whenever a patient with a suspected spinal injury is moved. Flexion of the neck or any portion of the spine must be avoided. In general, the patient should be permitted as little motion as possible and transported in the prone or supine position without rotation, flexion or extension of the spine.

Patients with suspected cervical spine injuries who also have a compromised airway or laryngeal trauma require special care. Laryngoscopy for endotracheal intubation may be impossible without a dangerous degree of cervical spine extension. Therefore, the physician may wish to employ an esophageal obturator airway (EOA), which can be inserted rapidly in a blind fashion without cervical motion. Cricothyroidotomy is an alternative method of rapid tracheal intubation that requires no cervical motion.

Injury of the spinal cord may be evaluated by asking the patient to move his legs and toes. If he can do this, he has escaped major cord damage. If the legs are paralyzed but the patient is able to move his hands, the spinal cord injury is located below the cervical region. If arm function is faulty, cervical spine involvement is likely. More precise localization of cord injury may be obtained by testing for loss of sensation to pinprick.

Diagnosis of Peripheral Nerve Injuries

Extensive wounds of the soft tissues and long bones of the extremities occur in both military and civilian life. Peripheral nerve injuries frequently accompany these injuries; the radial nerve, for example, may be injured if there are fractures about the elbow. Common peroneal nerve involvement may occur with fractures, soft tissue wounds or tight casts that produce pressure about the knee; and the sciatic nerve may be damaged by dislocations or fractures of the hip. Lacerations about the wrist may produce damage to median or ulnar nerves, and traction on the upper extremity may result in damage to the brachial plexus.

Peripheral nerve damage involves lower motor neuron axons as well as sensory nerves. The result is a flaccid type of paralysis. Early diagnosis may depend on loss of voluntary muscle power or absence of perception of pinprick. Inadequate treatment produces such late results as muscular atrophy, sensory loss and autonomic changes. Distally, the skin becomes thinned and smooth, often pale or mottled. Sweating is absent, and fingernails and toenails become brittle.

Partial damage to a peripheral nerve may result in causalgia, which develops soon after injury or requires several days to make its appearance. This condition is characterized by constant intense burning pain and is worsened by touching or moving, minor trauma, excitement or temperature change. The sciatic and median nerves are those commonly involved. Characteristically, in this lesion peripheral nerve injury is incomplete, although the skin often tends to be shiny and glossy. Blocking the related sympathetic pathways may produce prompt relief of the pain of causalgia, and this observation may assist in making the diagnosis.

Diagnosis of Musculoskeletal Injury

Injuries to the musculoskeletal system are among the most common injuries encountered in emergency services. Fractures, often including joint involvement, make up the bulk of these injuries. Certain general physical signs, including local tenderness, deformity, loss of function, abnormal range of motion and crepitus, are common to all fractures. There may be additional physical findings associated with injury to soft tissue, peripheral nerves and blood vessels. In many instances, the diagnosis will be apparent on the basis of simple physical examination. If this is the case, it is unnecessary and indeed contraindicated to demonstrate such physical signs as abnormal range of motion or crepitus. To do so may simply cause the patient extreme discomfort and increase local soft tissue damage. Prompt x-ray examination is of much greater value in determining the extent of the injury.

Fractures should be splinted before the patient is moved from the scene of the accident. If standard external splints are not readily available, improvised splints may be prepared from pillows, boards or doors. Early splinting minimizes discomfort, limits local extravasation and loss of blood and prevents the secondary damage that may occur from displacing fracture fragments, with associated laceration of blood vessels, nerves or other soft tissues. Careful evaluation of the patient for fractures should be included as a part of the general evaluation of the patient upon his arrival in the emergency service. Because of the often dramatic deformities associated with long bone fractures, early fracture care may distract the traumatologist from investigating signs or symptoms of other, possibly more serious injuries, such as progressive deterioration of consciousness, blunt trauma to abdominal organs or bladder rupture. Compound fractures and those resulting in neurological or vascular compromise require immediate therapy. Others can be splinted while the complete evaluation of the patient is carried out. Detailed description of diagnosis and treatment of fractures is included in Chapter 20.

Injury of the Urinary Tract

Upper urinary tract injuries primarily involving the kidney are usually encountered with either blunt or penetrating abdominal trauma. Renal injuries may vary from simple contusion to severe laceration of the renal parenchyma. The latter may also involve extensive damage to the vascular pedicle of the kidney. In adults the kidney is protected to some degree from direct trauma. The bony chest cage, the lumbar spine and the vertebral muscles as well as the perinephric fat and Gerota's fascia offer protection. In infants and children the kidney occupies a lower position and is less well protected by perirenal fat and a poorly developed Gerota's fascia. As a result, children are more susceptible to renal injury. Renal trauma in adults is more often seen in men because of their greater exposure to automobile injury, athletic activities and industrial accidents.

Renal trauma can usually be detected by the presence of flank pain and hematuria. The amount of blood loss varies but is rarely exsanguinating. This obviously depends on the extent of the renal injury, whether parenchymal damage is accompanied by laceration of the renal capsule and the extent of involvement of the vascular pedicle. When parenchymal damage is associated with damage to the collecting system, hematuria and sometimes extravasation of urine into the renal fossa and flank result. The combination of hemorrhage and urinary extravasation may produce muscle spasm, tenderness and flank dullness A mass may be palpable and, in some instances, detectable on inspection. Additional physical signs include ecchymoses in the flank, nonshifting flank dullness, and a positive psoas sign produced by extravasation of blood and urine over the psoas muscle.

Renal trauma is often associated with injury of the spleen or liver. If it can be accomplished with safety, an intravenous pyelogram is of great assistance in evaluating the patient's condition. This furnishes information about the extent of injury to the involved kidney as well as the functional state of the kidney on the uninvolved side. If the contrast medium is injected intravenously into a femoral vein at the same time, a flat abdominal x-ray is obtained, and additional information about the state of the inferior vena cava can be obtained. The need for direct surgical intervention depends on the extent of the injury involved. The presence of an enlarging renal mass associated with signs of blood loss may make operation necessary, but this requires careful evaluation and depends somewhat upon the patient's condition. Recently, arteriography has proved vitally important in evaluating the extent of renal injury and is essential if an attempt is to be made to preserve renal mass by a partial nephrectomy. The presence of extravasated urine makes surgery mandatory to provide adequate drainage and conserve renal tissue.

Injuries to the lower urinary tract are usually associated with fractures of the pelvis. Rupture of the bladder is the most common injury of the lower tract and is present in about 10 per cent of cases of pelvic fracture. In most instances, rupture of the bladder is extraperitoneal, although in about 20 per cent of cases the rupture is intraperitoneal. Extraperitoneal rupture is usually produced by chips of bone perforating the bladder wall and is associated with extravasation of urine into the extraperitoneal tissues, causing infection. Intraperitoneal rupture of the bladder is associated with a laceration of the dome of the bladder due to sudden compression of the full viscus; this, too, is associated with serious infection. The diagnosis is usually not difficult; the patient is unable to void or perhaps voids only a few drops of bloody urine. If the patient successfully voids clear urine after the accident, it is reasonably safe to assume that no serious injury to the lower urinary tract has resulted. Physical findings include deep tenderness, spasms of the lower abdominal muscles and peritoneal irritation, usually with rebound tenderness. Rectal examination demonstrates diffused tenderness with a normal prostate and membranous urethra. Catheterization should be performed early, and if bloody urine is obtained, urinary tract damage should be suspected. A cystogram should be performed in the anteroposterior and, in some instances, lateral positions. Intravenous pyelography should be performed if the initial evaluation and treatment indicate absence of other critical injury.

Injury of the bladder neck or membranous urethra is also common. The membranous portion of the urethra is particularly prone to injury at the level at which the urethra perforates the triangular ligament. Fractures of the pubic bone frequently disrupt this ligament and result in displacement of the proximal and distal segments of the lacerated urethra. This injury results in extravasation of urine into the tissues surrounding the bladder and lower abdominal wall. The extravasation extends laterally and the area is markedly tender; rectal examination is helpful in localizing the area of injury. When the prostatic urethra is damaged, the prostate gland is surrounded by a boggy tender mass. With laceration of the urogenital diaphragm, urine and blood are extravasated into the perineum. These physical findings are indications for early surgical intervention involving suprapubic exploration to permit re-establishment of urethral continuity.

Rupture of the vesical neck and prostatic urethra combine the physical findings of both rupture of the bladder and rupture of the urethra. Since injuries of the lower urinary tract occur in conjunction with pelvic fractures, simple testing for lateral compression of the pelvis is useful in diagnosis. Once fracture of the pelvis is suspected, diagnostic measures to determine the extent of urinary tract injury should be undertaken.

THE SEARCH FOR OCCULT INJURY

Certain regions of the body do not readily permit the usual techniques of physical examination. These may include the cranium, the vertebral column and the bony thorax. Under certain circumstances these protective bony envelopes or their contents may be injured without demonstrating classic clinical signs. For example, linear skull fractures or compression fractures of the spine may not be accompanied by neurological changes; in other instances, x-ray examination is much more accurate and effective in detecting subtle pulmonary mediastinal or cardiac changes than are the usual techniques of percussion and auscultation. Reference has been made to selected x-ray studies in relation to a variety of injuries. Certain general examinations are of considerable value and, as a general rule, should be obtained. Common sense should dictate when radiological studies will contribute to successful management. Under certain urgent circumstances, operative intervention is more important than

obtaining a complete set of films. In situations of this kind only films that vitally affect important decisions are indicated.

With this understanding it is clear that the standard-sized chest film is of great value in providing accurate information about the condition of the heart and lungs. If the clinical situation permits, the film should be obtained in the upright position. A flat film of the abdomen is important if abdominal trauma has occurred. Free air from a perforated viscus may be detected by an upright or a lateral decubitus film. Intraperitoneal or retroperitoneal fluid may be detected by local loss of psoas shadow. Pleural effusion may indicate subdiaphragmatic irritation, and so on.

X-ray examination of the skull is an important part of the evaluation of patients with head injury. It should be emphasized, however, that proper timing is important. To obtain satisfactory films of good quality, the cooperation of the patient is essential, and this is frequently impossible early after injury when manipulation of the patient may be hazardous. Skull films should be obtained when the patient's condition is stable, but since the principal value of these films lies in the recognition of skull fractures that require specific treatment, these studies should be completed as soon as the general condition permits. It should also be recognized that the types of intracranial hemorrhage requiring prompt surgical intervention will be detected by observation of vital signs and neurological examination rather than on the basis of an x-ray study alone.

It should be noted that radiologists are frequently helpful consultants in the diagnosis and management of injured patients. On many occasions the radiologist can recommend the films and techniques that will be of greatest value with least risk to the patient. Whenever possible, the case should be discussed with him for suggestions for obtaining the most meaningful data. Failure to enlist the cooperation of the radiologist may result in much wasted time and effectiveness at the expense of the patient's welfare.

ANALGESIA AND SEDATION

Patients with major injuries have variable degrees of pain. Many factors influence the subjective pain experience, including age, sex, extent of injury, time elapsed since injury, ethnic background, movement, diagnostic maneuvers performed, previous painful experiences, presence of hysterical bystanders, sedation due to alcohol or drugs, secondary pain, and fears of loss of body image or function. The judicious use of sedatives and analgesics should be integrated with the overall diagnostic and therapeutic plan for the injured patient. It has been stressed that restlessness and anxiety may be signs of air hunger, metabolic acidosis or cerebral hypoperfusion. All sedative and analgesic agents in common use are synergistic with general anesthetics and with hypovolemia. Therefore, these agents should be used cautiously, with definite indications, and only after ruling out the complicating conditions already listed. The intravenous route is definitely preferred: a rapid effect is achieved with a smaller dose, and the possibility of erratic absorption from intramuscular or gastric sites is eliminated.

The Toxic Patient

The delirious, intoxicated or violent patient may be a danger to himself and others. If the physician feels that the patient's behavior may aggravate or cause injuries or preclude needed diagnostic and therapeutic procedures, aggressive measures must be instituted. Often the best course is to paralyze the patient with a short-acting reversible agent, providing ventilatory support by means of endotracheal intubation and positive pressure ventilation. One must be careful to exclude treatable causes of delirium. In addition, it may be necessary to maintain a very abnormal ventilatory pattern if this is required as compensation for metabolic acidosis or treatment of thoracic injuries. The intoxicated or poisoned trauma patient requires the usual toxicologic studies, antidotes and other measures to hasten the metabolism or elimination of toxic substances.

The common association of trauma and

TABLE 1–2. Tubes for the Trauma Patient: Have You Used Enough?

TUBE	INDICATIONS FOR USE
1. Large-bore IV cannulas	Most patients need one; more may be needed with more extensive and severe injuries
2. Supplemental oxygen cannula	Probably useful in most patients
3. Endotracheal tube or oral airway	Patients with compromised airway or in need of ventilatory assistance
4. Urethral catheter	Suspected urinary tract injury; monitoring hypovolemia; inability to void (unconsciousness)
5. Nasogastric tube	Disturbances of consciousness; toxic substance ingestion; possible aspiration of gastric contents; possible gastroesophageal injury
6. Arterial catheter	Accurate monitoring of blood pressure; frequent blood gas samples
7. Chest tube	Evacuation of blood, fluid or air in the pericardial cavity
8. Pericardiocentesis or pericardiostomy	Suspected pericardial tamponade
9. Peritoneal lavage catheter	Suspected blunt abdominal trauma
10. Tubes of blood to laboratory	Baseline studies; crossmatching blood; arterial blood gases
11. X-ray tube	Confirm findings on physical examination search for occult injury

ethanol abuse may present the traumatologist with a postoperative patient, attached to numerous therapeutic and monitoring machines and with tubes in many places, who develops delirium tremens and threatens to undo much of the progress he has made. The major alcohol withdrawal reactions (seizures, hallucinosis, delirium) usually occur about 24 to 60 hours after cessation of drinking, whereas injury is usually associated with the intoxicated state. However, the physician in the emergency department should be familiar with the manifestations of the acute intoxicated state as well as with the complications of withdrawal.

SUMMARY

The initial evaluation and resuscitation of an injured patient should be done according to a logical plan. If each member of the trauma team is familiar with the priorities of effort and is experienced in the performance of the various technical procedures that may be required, as well as with the indications, contraindications and complications of each, there will be a minimum of panic, and the optimum plan for definitive care of the patient will result. In stressful and ambiguous situations, it is helpful to employ mental checklists to be sure that important steps are not omitted. Step-by-step protocols for the management of trauma patients are appearing in the literature. A simplistic but sometimes helpful concept of trauma management is related to the number and timing of a variety of tubes. The tubes listed in Table 1–2 need not all be employed in any given patient, and the list is certainly not exhaustive. A quick mental run-down may help the traumatologist avoid serious errors of omission.

CHAPTER 2

CARDIOPULMONARY RESUSCITATION

Hubert T. Gurley, M.D.
T. Crawford McAslan, M.D.
Eugene L. Nagel, M.D.
Myron L. Weisfeldt, M.D.

CARDIAC RESUSCITATION

Diagnosis of Cardiac Arrest

Recognition of cardiac arrest or of a totally inadequate cardiac output is more difficult in injured patients than in those in the operating room or the hospital ward. The presence of severe shock frequently complicates the picture. Nevertheless, the rescuer must make some immediate evaluations concerning the adequacy of circulation. The first and most frequently utilized measure is the pulse. In the severe shock of hypovolemia, pulses may be undetectable in the more peripheral vessels such as the radial artery, but they may be felt in central arteries such as the femoral or carotid arteries. However, even these pulses may be absent in some instances, and heart sounds may be very difficult to hear.

Another reliable sign of circulatory inadequacy is the degree of dilatation of the pupil of the eye. This is a fairly sensitive sign, since the pupil usually dilates rapidly when cardiac arrest occurs. Patients with severe head trauma may have dilata-tion of one or both pupils in the presence of adequate cardiac and circulatory activity; however, in patients with absent peripheral arterial pulses or other similar indications of shock, the presence of a dilated pupil strongly suggests an inadequate circulation that must be supported promptly. A third sensitive measure of the adequacy of circulation is respiration. If cardiac arrest is present or if cardiac output is so low that the brain is moderately deprived of oxygenated blood, respiration will usually cease. Thus, if a patient is breathing on his own and pulses cannot be felt, there must then be some circulatory activity that is at least partially adequate. Again, it must be remembered that trauma complicates the picture, since many forms of trauma may in themselves cause cessation of respiration.

The absence of electrical activity of the heart on the electrocardiogram certainly is indicative of cardiac arrest, but one should not delay cardiopulmonary resuscitation to obtain an electrocardiogram. A seemingly normal electrocardiogram can exist in the presence of an extremely low cardiac output that is inadequate for cerebral or coronary perfusion. Often CPR is necessary in a patient with an apparently normal electrocardiogram.

Chest Compression

The goal of chest compression is to provide sufficient circulation of the blood to maintain organ viability in a patient with ineffective or absent intrinsic cardiac function. Optimally performed CPR will maintain viability of the brain, heart and other organs until definitive correction of a compromised circulation state occurs. Since brain viability is lost within 6 minutes of the complete cessation of circulation, this is the organ of most direct concern. Other organs can survive more prolonged periods of ischemia without permanent loss of function. In general, if total cessation of circulation has lasted for longer than 6 minutes, resuscitation measures should not be undertaken. Survival after more prolonged periods of cardiac arrest has been reported when the patient is initially hypothermic, when barbiturate intoxication is present, and following electrocution.

Clearly, even when optimally performed, cardiopulmonary resuscitation is only a temporary measure that will ultimately be unsuccessful unless the primary etiology of the patient's compromised circulatory state is identified and corrected. The most dramatically successful resuscitative efforts are often those in which hypoxia, blood loss or pericardial tamponade is the primary etiology. In the setting of trauma, hypoxia may result from pneumothorax or hypoventilation, as discussed previously. Loss of blood from a large vascular structure will also quickly result in apparent cardiac arrest. In addition, loss of blood into the pericardium will result in tamponade and cardiac arrest. If the blood is accumulating rapidly within the pericardium the loss of only 100 to 200 ml. of blood is required to produce severely compromised output.

One clue to the presence of these causes of trauma-associated cardiac arrest (hypoxia, blood loss and tamponade) is sinus bradycardia rather than ventricular fibrillation. Skin color, the type of injury and the status of the neck veins also suggest the presence of these complications. Absent neck vein distention suggests hypovolemia and blood loss, and unusually severe distention suggests tamponade. Brief periods of CPR with correction of hypoxia will often be followed by spontaneous restoration of effective cardiac activity and effective circulation.

Cardiac arrest due to pneumothorax or hypoxia due to other causes will require chest tube placement or correction of the hypoxic state prior to effective reestablishment of cardiac function. Evidence of ineffective chest compression (e.g., inability to palpate a femoral or carotid pulse during chest compression) should again serve as a clue to the possible presence of tamponade, inadequate vascular blood volume or pneumothorax. Tamponade must be relieved by needle aspiration or a more definitive approach with thoracotomy should blood be accumulating rapidly. Indwelling percutaneous pericardial catheters have also been used in this setting. If severe hypovolemia or blood loss is suspected, rapid administration of available intravenous fluids may be life-saving. The definitive management of cardiac arrest due to ventricular tachycardia or ventricular fibrillation is clearly the treatment of the arrhythmia by countershock. Viability should be maintained by cardiopulmonary resuscitation until defibrillation equipment is available.

Internal cardiac massage has no established advantage over external chest compression except when the patient's condition dictates the usefulness of a thoracotomy. These conditions include (1) the presence of pneumothorax that cannot be corrected sufficiently by routine measures, (2) indications of rapid blood loss within the chest cavity, particularly with evidence of pericardial tamponade and a high likelihood of direct heart or aortic injury or rupture, and (3) gross chest wall injury where external chest compression might be highly likely to result in further internal organ injury. Internal cardiac massage obviously requires a thoracotomy that is time consuming and delays the essential restoration of effective cerebral perfusion, which can be achieved in almost all subjects by external compression.

Performance of External Chest Compression During CPR. Using the heel of the hand with the patient in the supine position on a firm surface, the sternum is compressed rhythmically by extending the elbow and leaning on the extended arms. The sternum should be compressed 2 to 2.5 inches with each compression. Classic recommendations and instruction of cardiopulmonary resuscitation have emphasized achievement of a precise chest compression rate. The recommended rate is 60 compressions per minute.[19] Recent studies have suggested that rates of between 40 and 80 compressions per minute are equally effective if each compression is sufficiently prolonged.

Although written standards for cardiopulmonary resuscitation include the statement that chest compression should be prolonged to 50 per cent of cycle time, this fact is rarely mentioned by instructors and is rarely carried out in practice.[23] This is unfortunate because recent evidence clearly identifies prolonged compression time as the most important simple determinant of effectiveness of CPR in man and in animal models.[21] Compression duration of slightly more than 50 per cent of cycle time appears to maximize carotid blood flow. During manual chest compression, prolongation of compression time to 50 per cent of cycle time requires a distinct pause at the maximum point of chest deflection, but this is easily performed if practiced. In learning this technique it is most helpful to record the compression force or the arterial blood pressure in the patient so that the approximate compression duration from the period of increase in force or pressure can be measured retrospectively. Standard recommendations for chest compression include the concept that compression should not be interrupted for ventilation. It is our experience that patients with pulmonary edema or congestion, chronic obstructive pulmonary disease or other factors increasing resistance to lung inflation require a pause in compression for ventilation. This pause need be only a half-second delay in compression.

It is most important to monitor either the carotid or the femoral artery pulse to be certain that blood flow is occurring during chest compression. Should the pulse not be palpable the possibilities of hypovolemia, pericardial tamponade or pneumothorax should be considered. The fact that the pulse is palpable is not assurance of adequate compression duration since it is the sharp rise in pressure rather than the duration of pressure rise that is sensed during pulse palpation. Further, the presence of a palpable pulse does not insure adequacy of cardiac output or regional organ perfusion.

Mechanical chest compression devices have been available for nearly 10 years. These devices have not had broad clinical use until recently as more extensive out-of-hospital resuscitative efforts have been undertaken. Also, until recently there was no distinct clinical evidence that such mechanical resuscitation devices were in fact effective; however, a recent prospective randomized trial[20] comparing long-term mechanical with long-term manual chest compression showed that the two methods were essentially equally effective. Thus, in the setting of the traumatized patient, when transportation is essential or when available physicians are either untrained or need to attend to other aspects of the patient's injury, a mechanical resuscitation device would seem to be a reasonable choice.

Major complications of chest compression during CPR include traumatic injury to bony and visceral structures. The chance of laceration or contusion of the liver, heart, spleen or other organs can be minimized by compression well above the xyphoid process and by avoiding excessive compression force. Chest compression can lead to severe traumatic injury to the sternum and ribs that may result in a flail sternum, multiple bony injuries, and pneumothorax and/or lung contusion.

Newer Concepts of Movement of Blood During CPR

Kouwenhoven, Jude, and Knickerbocker[10] originally proposed that blood moved during chest compression because of the compression of the heart between the sternum and the vertebral column. This compression was thought to squeeze blood out of the heart. Because of anecdotal clinical observations that did not appear to be consistent with this theory, the question of the mechanism of the movement of blood during CPR was recently re-examined. These efforts were stimulated by the observations of Criley and his associates, who showed that patients who were able to cough continuously would maintain consciousness despite absent cardiac activity.[5] Cyclic increases in intrathoracic pressure induced by coughing were sufficient to maintain cerebral blood flow at a level compatible with a conscious state. From such studies, it appears that the heart is compressed between the sternum and vertebral colum during CPR in only 30 per cent of patients with cardiac arrest on a medical service in an in-hospital setting. In the remainder of patients, the major mechanism for movement of blood is the increase in intrathoracic pressure that results from chest compression.

In the dog[16] it has been shown that all intrathoracic intravascular and intracardiac pressures during chest compression are similar to general intrathoracic pressure and that interventions that increase intrathoracic pressure usually increase blood flow also. Detailed studies in the animal model demonstrated that intrathoracic pressure is transmitted to arteries outside the chest. Because of this transmission and the simultaneous collapse of venous structures at the exit of the thorax, an arterial-venous pressure gradient is established outside the chest. Measurements of venous flow show that after a brief period of retrograde jugular venous flow, venous flow during chest compression falls to zero. The pressure gradient between the arteries and veins outside the chest results in antegrade flow through the capillaries of the brain.

In the animal model interventions such as abdominal binding or increases in airway pressure tend to increase blood flow, since a higher pressure is transmitted to the carotid arteries. Under sufficiently high intrathoracic pressure the carotid arteries may also collapse. Once carotid collapse occurs, there is no further forward flow. It is unclear at this point how frequently carotid collapse is a problem in a human under conditions of increased intrathoracic pressure. This new understanding of the mechanism of movement of blood during CPR holds considerable promise for identifying more effective methods of moving blood to the brain during CPR in the majority of patients. Application of these principles must await assessment of the problem of arterial collapse in man and careful examination of other potential complications of any new technique.

Drug Therapy

The appropriate use of drugs in CPR for the traumatically injured patient is vital to the success of the resuscitative effort. A basic understanding of the physiologic derangements and the mechanisms of drug action is essential for the proper use of these agents (see Table 2–1). This overview represents a simplified and basic approach that will help to facilitate rapid assessment and proper therapy of cardiopulmonary arrest. No one standard regimen is appropriate to all cases, and drugs must be chosen to produce specific effects in a given situation.

Tissue perfusion is the ultimate concern in treating the clinical shock syndrome, and all pharmacologic manipulations must be directed toward achieving this end with minimal drug-related toxicity. The support of the blood pressure will be a major goal in the initial resuscitative effort. The physician must understand that blood pressure alone is not a reliable indicator of tissue perfusion. However, once a blood pressure has been obtained and maintained, attention can be given to the validity and reliability of the numerical reading, and to the adequacy of vital organ perfusion as evidenced by the clinical correlates of level of consciousness, skin color and temperature, and urine flow. When some level of blood pressure has been restored, the physician's work has just begun — the patient's survival depends as much on subsequent therapy as on the initial resuscitative effort.

Parameters amenable to manipulation during the early resuscitative effort include stroke volume, heart rate and peripheral resistance. These parameters are closely inter-related as follows:

Cardiac output = stroke volume × heart rate

Systemic blood pressure = cardiac output × peripheral resistance

Combining these two relationships yields the following equation:

Systemic blood pressure = (stroke volume × heart rate) × total peripheral resistance

TABLE 2–1. Drugs in Cardiopulmonary Resuscitation

DRUG	OBJECTIVE	DILUTION	DOSE (INTRAVENOUS)	TOXICITY	COMMENTS
Atropine	Increase HR	none	0.5 mg. every 5 min.; 2.0 mg. maximum	Tachycardia Ventricular fibrillation	Use only when bradycardia is accompanied by hypotension or heart rates below 40 per min.
Isoproterenol	Increase HR Increase HF	1.0 mg. in ½ liter D5W = 2 μg./ml.	2–20 μg./min.	Tachycardia Tachyarrhythmias Ventricular fibrillation	Markedly increases myocardial oxygen consumption; contraindicated in acute myocardial infarction except to increase rate while placing pacer.
Calcium chloride or gluconate	Increase HF	10%	5.0 ml. chloride 10 ml. gluconate	Bradycardia Sinus arrest	May aggravate digitalis toxicity; precipitates in IV tubing with sodium bicarbonate.
Epinephrine	Increase BP Increase HR Increase HF Increase TPR	1:10,000	5 ml. = 5 mg. every 5 min. p.r.n.	Tachycardia	Inactivated in tubing by sodium bicarbonate; may be given directly into the heart but risks tamponade, laceration of coronary artery, pneumothorax, and interruption of CPR; intramyocardial injection may produce intractable ventricular fibrillation; may be injected into endotracheal tube if no IV is available
Norepinephrine	Increase BP Increase TPR	8.0 mg. base in ½ liter D5W	8–32 μg./min. to achieve 90 mm. Hg systolic	Constricts skin and renal and splanchnic vessels	Always use large bore catheter in central vein; infiltration results in sloughing, which should be treated by local injection of phentolamine; renal failure and mesenteric or hepatic infarction may follow prolonged administration.

Drug	Action	Preparation	Dose	Toxicity	Remarks
Dopamine	Increase BP Increase TPR Increase HR Increase HF Increase RBF	$10 \times$ weight in kg. = mg to be added to 1 liter to achieve 10 μg. per kg. per ml.	2.5–10 μg/kg./min. to increase RBF; 20–50 μg./kg./min. to support BP	Vasoconstriction	Renal effects are dose related; less potent for BP support than norepinephrine.
Sodium bicarbonate	Correct acidosis	—	1 mEq./kg. initially, then ½ dose every 10 min.	Alkalosis, hypernatremia, hyperosmolality, myocardial depression	May inactivate other drugs if mixed in same IV tubing. Adequate ventilation and frequent ABG's are essential to avoid elevated pCO_2 with myocardial depression and increased serum osmolality.
Lidocaine	Suppress ventricular arrhythmias	1 gm. in 250 ml. D5W = 4 mg./ml.	50–100 mg. (or 1 mg./kg.) IV bolus followed immediately by infusion of 1–4 mg./min.	CNS depression, seizures, paresthesias, disorientation, agitation, heart block	Chronic heart failure predisposes the patient to high plasma levels and early toxicity. Total bolus injection in excess of 300 mg. predisposes to toxicity. Repeat administration can produce complete heart block or abolish an adequate nodal rhythm.
Propranolol	Control recurrent ventricular tachycardia or ventricular fibrillation	—	1.0 mg. per minute over 5 min., not to exceed 3–5 mg. total	Acute congestive heart failure, bronchospasm	Use only after lidocaine failure. May worsen bradyarrhythmias or heart block. Use with extreme caution in patients known to have bronchospasm.
Morphine	Produce analgesia, decrease pulmonary congestion after initial successful resuscitation	As required to produce 1 mg./ml.	Up to 4 mg. initially, then 2 mg. every 5 min.	Respiratory depression, hypotension, vomiting	Titrate small doses at frequent intervals. Toxic effects antagonized by naloxone (0.4–0.8 mg. IV).

HR = Heart rate
HF = Heart-force of contraction
BP = Blood pressure
TPR = Total peripheral resistance
RBF = Renal blood flow

Pharmacologic intervention almost always affects more than one of these parameters. Each drug affects them in its own particular fashion, and it is for this reason that the basic pharmacology of the commonly employed agents must be understood by the treating physician.

The stroke volume of each cardiac contraction, whether in the normal state or during cardiac massage, depends upon the filling pressure of the heart and the contractile force generated by the myocardium. To develop optimal squeeze, the heart must have adequate filling. This phenomenon is described by the well-known Frank-Starling relationship. In the traumatically injured patient, attention must be given to the adequacy of the circulating blood volume. Blood replacement or other means of volume expansion (discussed elsewhere in this volume) is therefore of critical importance if the heart is to generate adequate pressure through the vital coronary, cerebral, renal and splanchnic circulations. The central venous pressure is invaluable in assessing the degree of volume expansion. Catheterization of the pulmonary artery with a balloon-tipped flow-directed catheter may be expected to give more reliable information in the patient with primary cardiac disease or injury. This technique is most appropriately utilized after the success of the initial resuscitative effort. Drugs that increase the contractile state of the myocardium and hence increase the stroke volume include ionized calcium, isoproterenol and epinephrine.

The optimal heart rate for healthy adults is between 70 and 120 beats per minute. Rates of below 60 may be associated with signs of inadequate tissue perfusion. Rates in excess of 140 result in decreased diastolic filling due to the shortened duration of diastole and to an unacceptable ratio of oxygen supply to demand, which may lead to myocardial ischemia, failure or infarction. Agents that may be employed to increase the heart rate include atropine, isoproterenol, and placement of a temporary pacing wire. Propranolol may be used to slow the heart rate, although the administration of this agent to the patient with cardiovascular instability has the potential to further decrease myocardial performance by direct suppression of myocardial contractility. It should be employed to slow the heart rate only when the rapid rate is believed to be the primary cause of diminished myocardial performance. This drug is also useful in terminating repeated episodes of ventricular tachycardia accompanied by signs of decreased myocardial function and inadequate tissue perfusion.

Peripheral resistance can be dramatically increased by the administration of norepinephrine or dopamine, both of which are primarily alpha-adrenergic agents, in doses employed for the treatment of cardiac arrest. Norepinephrine is the more potent of these agents and is the drug of choice in the patient who has no blood pressure but an adequate cardiac rhythm. Norepinephrine is also the more toxic agent, and its use must be limited to the briefest period possible to avoid the sequelae of renal failure or ischemia of the splanchnic circulation. Dopamine is the preferred agent when the necessity of prolonged blood pressure support is anticipated. It has the additional theoretical benefit of protecting the renal, splanchnic and coronary circulations by selectively increasing the circulation to these areas through stimulation of specific dopaminergic receptors. Dopamine increases urine flow and induces a natruresis; it may be of particular value in the patient with fluid overload, congestive heart failure or myocardial infarction. Both norepinephrine and dopamine modestly increase heart rate and the force of myocardial contractions.

Isoproterenol is the most potent agent for increasing the force of myocardial contraction. It is also the agent most likely to cause ventricular arrhythmias and to be inactivated by acidosis. Isoproterenol, a pure beta-adrenergic agent, increases blood flow through the peripheral muscles and may thereby significantly decrease the circulating blood volume. The resulting effect on blood pressure is dependent on the balance achieved between increased contractility, increased heart rate and increased muscle blood flow. The blood pressure in a given patient receiving an infusion of isoproterenol may increase, remain unchanged or decrease, depending upon the overall effect of this agent. The physician must not be misled by the warm, pink appearance of the patient receiving isoproterenol. The vital perfusion pressures may be unacceptably low in spite of the patient's appearance.

Epinephrine has both alpha- and beta-adrenergic action. The drug has proven utility in the setting of cardiac arrest, although it may be less useful for long-term support of the circulation. Clinically, epinephrine elevates perfusion pressure generated during cardiac compression, improves myocardial contractility, stimulates spontaneous contractions, and facilitates conversion of a fine fibrillation to a coarse one more amenable to termination by countershock.

The so-called pressor agents —norepinephrine, epinephrine, isoproterenol and dopamine — are valuable for temporary support of the circulation. It must be remembered that no patient presents to the physician suffering from an acute deficiency of a pressor agent. That is to say, these agents are not curative in any sense. Each of them has its own significant toxicities, and it is encumbent upon the physician to initiate a plan for withdrawal of these drugs almost as soon as the patient has achieved some degree of cardiovascular stability. At best, these agents can be regarded as a means of buying a small amount of additional time while the basic underlying physiologic derangements are restored to normal. The optimal dose of each of these agents is the lowest possible dose that will achieve the desired effect, administered over the briefest possible period. Mechanisms of action differ for each agent, and they are sometimes used in combination. Their therapeutic effects are cumulative, but so are their toxicities.

Each of the pressor agents functions within a fairly narrow pH range. Hence, they cannot be expected to be of use in the patient who is severely acidotic and hypoxemic. Proper ventilatory support and the intermittent administration of sodium bicarbonate may facilitate the actions of these agents and decrease the occurrence of pressor-induced cardiac arrhythmias.

The patient undergoing cardiopulmonary arrest rapidly manifests metabolic and respiratory acidosis. Hypoperfusion and subsequent hypoxemia result in the generation of lactic acid, while ventilatory failure results in carbon dioxide retention and respiratory acidosis. Effective ventilation of the lungs is essential for the excretion of carbon dioxide as well as for oxygenation, and is absolutely necessary for the management of the acidosis of cardiac arrest. The importance of prompt and adequate ventilation cannot be overemphasized.

The administration of intravenous sodium bicarbonate can be a useful adjunct to managing the metabolic component of acidosis during cardiac arrest. Bicarbonate combines with excess hydrogen ion to produce water and carbon dioxide by the following reaction:

$$HCO_3^- + H^+ \rightleftarrows H_2CO_3 \rightleftarrows CO_2 + H_2O$$

However, bicarbonate administration raises the pH of the blood only if the carbon dioxide produced is excreted through the lungs.[1] Administration of sodium bicarbonate in the absence of adequate ventilation does not result in a rise in the arterial pH but only in substantial increases in the arterial pCO_2 and serum osmolality. Elevation of the pCO_2 may aggravate intracellular acidosis and result in further depression of myocardial performance. Therefore, administration of small amounts of sodium bicarbonate should be followed by sustained CPR to overcome an initial period of depressed myocardial function resulting from increased pCO_2 consequent to bicarbonate administration. Blood gas measurements should be made frequently during the resuscitative effort. The adequacy of ventilation must be reassessed prior to the repeated administration of sodium bicarbonate.

Electrical Defibrillation

Ventricular fibrillation is a random, disorganized firing of individual myocardial fibers that produces no heart beat and no forward blood flow. The rhythm is rapidly fatal unless the circulation is adequately supported by ventilation and cardiac massage or unless the rhythm is terminated by the application of electrical countershock.

The electrical defibrillator is a life-saving device that also has the potential to produce severe injury and even death to the patient and to medical personnel. Capacitor-induced direct current (DC) defibrillators are in common use in medical facilities. The older alternating current defibrillators should be replaced by DC defibrillators, which are more reliable and safer, and pose less of a threat to patients and personnel alike.

The DC defibrillator consists of an adjustable, high-voltage DC power supply used to charge an energy storage capacitor that is connected to paddles through a current-limiting inductor. The monophasic current delivered is of the order of several thousand volts but lasts for only a few milliseconds. All units have some method for measuring energy. Newer units indicate the actual energy delivered, while others indicate the maximum energy stored. Stored energy may differ markedly from delivered energy. All units should be checked to determine actual energy delivered across a 50 ohm load at each energy setting. The amount of energy delivered may be a critical factor in determining the success of the defibrillation attempt. Energy is delivered through two paddles following activation of one or more switches. Saline soaked 4×4 gauze pads or, preferably, electrode paste applied to the surface of the electrodes may be used to reduce skin resistance and allow adequate energy to reach the heart. If one allows electrode paste or saline to cover the skin area between the two electrodes, the current will travel the path of least resistance and flow across the chest surface, "bridging" the area between the electrodes, and adequate current will not reach the heart. Care must be taken to wipe off excess electrode paste or saline from the skin surface between the two electrodes.

Placement of the defibrillator paddles is important for proper energy delivery. The standard positions are one paddle just to the right of the upper sternum and below the clavicle and the other just to the left of the apex, or just lateral to the left nipple in the anterior axillary line. Electrodes should never be placed directly over the nipple or over ECG-monitoring electrodes or wires because burns may result.

Once the paddles are in place, firm pressure of 20 to 25 pounds is exerted on each paddle in order to make good contact with the skin, reduce the chance of skin burns, and increase the efficiency of passage of electrical current through the skin. Failure of the instrument to discharge is most often due to inadequate time for the capacitor to recharge following activation of the capacitor circuit or inadvertent use of the synchronizer circuit. The synchronizer must be turned off or else the instrument will await the detection of a QRS complex before delivering its energy. The synchronizer is useful in cardioversion but must be turned off for defibrillation.

Immediately after the delivery of the defibrillation current, the pulse and electrocardiogram should be checked. If there is no pulse or if an electrocardiographic pattern does reappear, basic life support with closed chest cardiac compression should be reinstituted without delay.

Myocardial damage may follow the application of defibrillatory current and is related to three factors: energy level, frequency of shocks and recovery time between shocks, and electrode paddle size. The higher the energy level, the greater the likelihood of myocardial damage. The lowest effective energy level should be used. For patients weighing less than 50 kilograms, 3.5 to 6.0 watt/seconds per kilogram of delivered energy is suggested. For patients weighing 50 kilograms or more, the maximum output of the defibrillator should be used. The suggested output for open chest defibrillation is 20 to 60 watt seconds. Each defibrillator should be tested to determine the amount of actual energy delivered through a 50 ohm test load at given dial settings. Larger paddles produce less myocardial damage. Paddles intended for external use are generally satisfactory. Paddles designed for application to the surface of the heart in open chest defibrillation should never be used as external paddles. The anoxic or acidotic myocardium may be refractory to electrical defibrillation. Closed chest cardiac massage and optimal ventilation are often effective in improving the likelihood of successful defibrillation and are to be preferred to repeated application of defibrillatory current at close intervals.

SUMMARY

There are many definitive aspects of basic and advanced life support that are not described in this chapter. The reader is referred to the many excellent articles, texts and course manuals that are listed in the references. The early management and resuscitation of the victim of traumatic injury depend on preparedness, a trained team, and a well-identified and rehearsed protocol. Hesitation, diffusion of authority, confusion and conflict will negatively affect the outcome.

REFERENCES

1. Bishop, R.L., and Weisfeldt, M.L.: Sodium bicarbonate administration during cardiac arrest—effect on arterial pH, pCO_2 and osmolality. J.A.M.A. 235:506–509, 1976.
2. Civetta, J.M., et al.: Prehospital use of the military anti-shock trouser (MAST). J. Am. Col. Emergency Physicians 5:581–587, 1976.
3. Cole, W.H.: The need for improved first aid care in motor vehicle accidents. (editorial). J. Trauma 10:184, 1970.
4. Cowley, R.A., Hudson, F., Scanlan, E., Gill, W., Lally, R.J., Long W., and Cuhn, A.O: An economical and proved helicopter program for transporting the emergency critically ill and injured patient in Maryland. J. Trauma 13:1029, 1973.
5. Criley, J.M., Blaufuss, A.H., and Kissel, G.L.: Cough-induced cardiac compression. J.A.M.A. 236:1246, 1976.
6. Frey, C.F., Heulke, D.F., and Gikas, P.W.: Resuscitation and survival in motor vehicle accidents. J. Trauma 9:292, 1969.
7. Gertner, H.R., Baker, S.P., Rutherford, R.B., and Spitz, W.U.: Evaluation of the management of vehicular fatalities secondary to abdominal injury. J. Trauma 12:425, 1972.
8. Gill, W., Champion, H.R., Long, W.B., Jamaris, J., and Cowley, R.A.: Abdominal lavage in blunt trauma. Br. J. Surg. 62:121, 1975.
9. Kaplan, B.C., Civetta, J.M., Nagel, E.L., et al.: The military anti-shock trouser in civilian prehospital emergency care. J. Trauma 13:843–848, 1973.
10. Kouwenhoven, W.B., Jude, J.R., and Knickerbocker, G.C.: Closed chest cardiac massage. J.A.M.A. 173:1064–1067, 1960.
11. McAslan, T.C., and Cowley, R.A.: The preventive use of PEEP in major trauma. (In press, 1979.)
12. McSwain, N.E., Jr.: Pneumatic trousers and the management of shock. J. Trauma 17:719–723.
13. Manual for Instructor-Trainers and Instructors of Advanced Cardiac Life Support (ACLS). Dallas, American Heart Association, 1975.
14. Manual for Instructor-Trainers and Instructors of Basic Life Support (BLS). Dallas, American Heart Association, 1974.
15. Nagel, E.L., and Schofferman, J.: Preliminary observations during mechanical external heart compressions. In Safar, P., and Elam, J. O. (eds.): Advances in Cardiopulmonary Resuscitation. New York, Springer-Verlag, 1977, p 99–101.
16. Rudikoff, M.T., Freund, P., and Weisfeldt, M.L. Mechanisms of blood flow during cardiopulmonary resuscitation. Circulation 56:111, 1977.
17. Shapiro, H.M.: Intracranial hypertension: Therapeutic and anesthetic considerations. Anesthesiology 43:445–471, 1975.
18. Shin, B., Isenhower, N.N., McAslan, T.C., and Mackenzie, C.F.: Early recognition of renal insufficiency in post-anesthetic trauma victims. (In press, 1979.)
19. Standards for Cardiopulmonary Resuscitation (CPR) and Emergency Cardiac Care (ECC). J.A.M.A. (Suppl.) 227:833–868, 1974.
20. Taylor, G.J., Rubin, R., Tucker, M., Greene, H.L., Rudikoff, M., and Weisfeldt, M.L.: External cardiac compression: A randomized comparison of mechanical and manual techniques. (In press, 1979.)
21. Taylor, G., Tucker, W.M., Greene, H.L., Rudikoff, M.T., and Weisfeldt, M.L.: Importance of prolonged compression duration during cardiopulmonary resuscitation in man. N. Engl. J. Med. 296:1515, 1977.
22. Van Wagoner, F.H.: Died in hospital — three year study of deaths following trauma. J. Trauma 1:401, 1961.
23. Waller, J.A.: Control of accidents in rural areas. J.A.M.A. 201:94, 1967.

CHAPTER 3

THE PATHOPHYSIOLOGY OF TRAUMA AND SHOCK

Robert B. Rutherford, M.D.
Charles A. Buerk, M.D.

TRAUMA

The term "trauma" encompasses a wide range of insults to the body. Even individual wounds take a wide variety of forms — a crushing blow, a jagged laceration, a missile penetration, a burn, a bite. It is natural to consider trauma primarily as the result of the body's striking, or being struck by, some object; but one must also consider injuries inflicted by chemical, electrical or thermal insult and those caused by changes in environmental pressure or gravitational force. Some injuries have diffuse systemic effects; others mainly involve one or two organ systems. Considerable variation is possible even among wounds of the same type. For example, the local damage from a gunshot wound depends on the mass and particularly the velocity of the missile; the degree of burn varies with the temperature and duration of contact with the burning agent; and deceleration injuries are largely determined by the victim's mass, the rate of deceleration and the surface area of the body over which the energy is dissipated. Finally, the effects of an injury may be modified significantly by personal and environmental factors such as age, sex, nutritional status, intercurrent disease, local contamination, ambient temperature, and so forth.

It is not possible to incorporate such an array of variables into a simple, uniform description of the effects of trauma on the body. In this chapter, emphasis is placed only on the general, local and systemic effects and responses to trauma. The specific effects of other contributing factors will be discussed in the presentation of the injuries to which they pertain.

LOCAL RESPONSE — THE WOUND

As Rhoads and Howard have emphasized, "It is incorrect to assume (after the initial wounding) that the injury has now been inflicted."[136] The injury will continue to be inflicted until its components have been corrected or arrested. The major components of injury are tissue destruction, blood loss, mechanical defects and superimposed infections. Their local effects can be better appreciated if one first considers the events that normally occur in healing a simple, clean incision — a wound in which the contributions of these components are minimal.

Phases of Healing. The initial phase of wound healing is the period before tensile strength develops in the wound — the "lag" phase. However, it is by no means a quiescent period. There is increased vascularity with an outpouring of plasma and a diapedesis of leukocytes and macrophages into the wound area. Trauma always invokes a true inflammatory reaction that is at least initially indistinguishable from that caused by bacterial infection or physical or chemical agents. Damaged tissue is broken down and removed. Hexosamines derived from plasma glycoproteins accumulate locally and, in turn, are converted into mucopolysaccharide ground substance by a process that appears to involve mast cells and requires methionine.[75] Because of these activities, this period has been called the "inflammatory," "catabolic" or "substrate" phase.

The second phase, called the "collagen," "productive" or "fibroblastic" phase, is characterized by the deposition of collagen and a progressive increase in the tensile strength of the wound. Fibrin deposition in the injured area provides the lattice-work for the invasion of fibroblasts derived from neighboring, undifferentiated mesenchymal cells. It is thought that the mucopolysaccharide ground substance provides the medium in which procollagen, a protein component of the fibroblast, is converted into collagen fibrils.[49] This process can be quantitated by the hydroxyproline content of the wound.

Hydroxyproline is found, ostensibly, only in collagen and its precursors. It is not incorporated into the collagen molecule as such. Rather, proline is first incorporated and later hydroxylated as the molecule is being built up into triple helical coils held together by hydrogen bonds.[7, 171] Hydroxyproline and hydroxylysine are important factors in the stability of this helical structure. This ability to hydroxylate proline and lysine appears to be limited to fibroblasts, and this process appears to be the site of the essential action of ascorbic acid (vitamin C) in wound healing. The reaction also requires ferrous ion and alpha-ketoglutarate as well as molecular oxygen. The collagen content begins to level off at 10 to 12 days, and tensile strength reaches a temporary plateau by 10 days to 2 weeks.

In the final phase, there is a maturation of the collagen into a strong weave by a process of remolding and inter- and intramolecular cross-linkages. This is more important than the amount of collagen itself in determining the final tensile strength of the wound, for, as Douglas has shown, the wound's tensile strength at the end of 2 weeks is only one fifth its eventual maximum.[46] This maturation process may take 6 weeks or more.

Adverse Influences of Trauma on Wound Healing. The major components of injury — tissue destruction, blood loss, mechanical defects and superimposed infection — all influence wound healing adversely. Destroyed tissue delays wound healing because of the additional time required for its catabolism and clearance. Along with extravasated blood plasma, it is an ideal medium in which bacteria can multiply beyond the body's first line of defense. The pressure effects of hematomas and seromas are greater than generally appreciated and, along with the mechanical effects of tissue disruption, interfere significantly with wound healing. Avoiding tension is, of course, one of the cardinal rules in promoting wound healing. Extravasated blood has been shown to have a synergistic effect on the activity of certain bacteria, particularly *Escherichia coli.* Furthermore, if enough blood is lost so that shock ensues, the body's defense mechanisms against bacterial invasion may be greatly impaired.[123] Simple bacterial contamination of the wound is not, in itself, a significant deterrent to normal wound healing. It occurs to some degree in nearly all "clean" surgical wounds.[24] However, in the presence of a dead space, foreign body, extravasated blood or devitalized tissue, bacterial multiplication will occur. This not only perpetuates the inflammatory phase of wound healing but delays the accumulation of factors essential to wound healing, since these factors also serve as bacterial substrates.

Local vascularity normally influences the rate of wound healing, as contrasted in the healing rates of facial and extremity wounds. Similarly, any factor that interferes with circulation to the wound, from arterial occlusion to anti-inflammatory drugs, will retard healing. The vascular bed in the area of the wound may be damaged directly by a sharp blow, a crushing injury or a burn, or it may be compromised later by the pressure of extravasated blood and edema. Similarly, a laceration may interrupt a significant portion of the circulation to the wound area. This is particularly true of oblique lacerations and partial avulsions. Interruption of the major arterial supply to the wound area, even if it does not produce actual ischemia, may impede the vascular response that assembles the elements necessary for wound healing at the wound site. Experience with pedicle flaps has shown that impaired venous outflow with secondary edema is equally harmful.

Because of difficulties in controlling the various components of injury independently and because the underlying mechanisms of wound healing have not yet been fully elucidated even in the simplest of wounds, very little actual investigation into the healing of wounds of violence has been made. Although it is clear that the cumulative effects of these components of injury are a significant deterrent to wound healing and, in turn, magnify and prolong the systemic effects of injury, we do not yet have any quantitative estimates of these effects on which to base our care of such wounds (e.g., the proper time for suture removal, for resumption of normal use of the injured part, and so on).

Certain drugs and a few disease states may have an adverse influence on wound healing.[75] Among the most important of these are cortisone therapy, some cancer chemotherapy and immunosuppressive drugs, diabetes, congestive heart failure, uremia,[119] scurvy and severe hypoproteinemia. More remarkable, however, is how little systemic conditions interfere with wound healing. "The primacy of the wound," the ability to heal a wound even while the body is in a continued state of catabolism, is still one of the great wonders and mysteries of the body.

THE SYSTEMIC EFFECTS OF INJURY

Just as there are gradations in the severity of the wound itself, so there are corresponding variations in its systemic effects. Following Churchill's concept that the severity of a wound is the sum of all factors acting in the direction of deterioration, Moore and Ball used a scale of ten in grading various forms of trauma (mainly operative procedures) according to se-

verity.[114] Howard and Ladd devised a point system in evaluating battle casualties of the Korean War based on the injury itself, treatment delay and response to therapy.[82] Recently, the AMA's Committee on the Medical Aspects of Automotive Safety has developed a more comprehensive rating system, an abbreviated outline of which is presented in Table 3–1. Such systems are valuable in correlating studies on systemic responses to trauma but are of only relative value in quantitating the response of an individual patient to trauma.

Metabolic Response to Injury. Systemic or metabolic effects of trauma are commonly described in terms of fluid and electrolyte shifts, endocrine activity, nitrogen balance and weight change. Most investigators in this field, with certain justification, equate operative and nonoperative trauma and, for the sake of simplicity, concentrate on responses to common surgical procedures to obtain reasonably comparable data.

Most traumatic states are not suitable for this type of study, not only because of problems in quantitating the severity of the injury but also because of the lack of baseline values and the variable nature of measures required in resuscitation and definitive treatment. The other important distinction is that operative trauma, particularly abdominal procedures, causes a greater degree of interference with alimentation than nonoperative trauma. Nevertheless, the basic patterns that have been observed after operation are felt to be reasonably representative of post-traumatic states as well. Moore's original description of the endocrine response to trauma provided the basic framework and the stimulus for definitive investigation into the metabolic response to trauma.[112]

The Metabolic Response to Trauma

The most basic requirement for sustaining life is energy. Metabolism is the sum of the physical and chemical processes by which living substance is produced and maintained. This includes the transformations by which energy is made available for these procedures. In the normal adult the constructive processes (anabolism) and the destructive processes (catabolism) are

TABLE 3–1. Injury Description

INJURY CATEGORY SEVERITY CODE	GENERAL	HEAD AND NECK	CHEST	ABDOMINAL	EXTREMITIES
No Injury	None	None	None	None	None
Minor 1	Minor lacerations, contusions and abrasions. All 1-degree, small 2- and 3-degree burns.	Cerebral injury without loss of consciousness. "Whiplash" without vertebral damage. Ocular abrasions and contusions.	Minor chest wall contusions, abrasions.	Muscle contusions; seat belt abrasion.	Minor sprains and fractures, and/or dislocation of digits.
Moderate 2	Extensive contusions, abrasions; large lacerations; avulsions (<3" diameter) 10-20% 2- or 3-degree burns.	Cerebral injury with <15 minutes' unconsciousness; no amnesia. Undisplaced skull or facial bone fractures. Eye lacerations, retinal detachment. "Whiplash" with vertebral injury.	Simple rib or sternal fractures. Major contusions of chest wall without hemo- or pneumothorax, or respiratory embarrassment.	Major contusion of abdominal wall without intraabdominal injury.	Compound fractures of digits or nose. Undisplaced long bone or pelvic fractures. Major joint sprains.
Severe 3 (not life-threatening)	Extensive contusions or abrasions; large lacerations or avulsions (> 3" diameter). 20-30% 2- or 3-degree burns.	Cerebral injury with unconsciousness >15 minutes without severe neurologic signs; <3 hours' post-traumatic amnesia. Displaced closed skull fractures without signs of intracranial injury. Loss of eye, or avulsion of optic nerve. Facial bone fractures, displaced or without antral or orbital involvement. Cervical spine fractures without cord damage.	Multiple rib fracture without respiratory embarrassment. Simple hemo- or pneumothorax. Rupture of diaphragm. Moderate pulmonary contusion.	Contusion of abdominal organs. Extraperitoneal bladder rupture. Retroperitoneal hemorrhage. Avulsion of ureter. Laceration of urethra. Thoracic or lumbar spine fractures without neurologic involvement.	Displaced simple long bone fractures, and/or multiple hand and foot fractures. Single open long bone fractures. Pelvic fractures with displacement. Dislocation of major joints. Lacerations of major nerves or vessels of extremities.
Severe 4 (life-threatening, survival probable)	Severe lacerations and/or avulsions with dangerous hemorrhage. 30–50% 2- or 3-degree burns.	Cerebral injury with or without skull fracture, with unconsciousness of >15 minutes with definite abnormal neurologic signs; post-traumatic amnesia 3-12 hours. Compound skull fracture.	Open chest wounds; flail chest; pneumomediastinum; myocardial contusion and pericardial injuries without circulatory embarrassment.	Minor lacerations of intra-abdominal viscera including kidney, spleen and tail of pancreas. Intraperitoneal bladder rupture. Avulsion of genitals. Dorsal and/or lumbar spine fractures with paraplegia.	Multiple closed long bone fractures. Amputation of limbs.
Critical 5 (survival uncertain)	Over 50% 2- or 3-degree burns.	Cerebral injury with unconsciousness of >24 hours; post-traumatic amnesia >12 hours; intracranial hemorrhage; signs of increased intracranial pressure. Cervical spine injury with quadriplegia. Major airway obstruction.	Chest injuries with major respiratory embarrassment (laceration of trachea, hemomediastinum, etc.). Aortic laceration. Myocardial rupture or contusion with circulatory embarrassment.	Rupture, avulsion, or severe laceration of abdominal vessels or organs, except kidney, spleen or ureter.	Multiple open limb fractures.

in essential equilibrium. The organism is in a dynamic state in which there is a constant interplay of cell and substrate destruction and rebuilding. Trauma and shock upset this finely balanced equilibrium and produce alterations in the important biochemical pathways that affect the metabolic responses of the organism.

The hallmark of the metabolic response to trauma is increased energy expenditure. The amount and duration of this increased energy utilization is proportionate to the severity and duration of the insult. Minor injury results in minor or even undetectable changes in metabolism, whereas severe injury results in a proportionately severe energy drain (Fig. 3–1). The apogee of severe injury is an extensive burn, which can require an energy expenditure approaching two times the resting metabolic rate and requiring up to 5000 kilocalories per day and a nitrogen loss of some 20 to 30 grains per day.[91] The advent of intercurrent sepsis imposes further energy demands. In fact, each degree of centigrade elevation over normal increases energy expenditure an average of 13 per cent.[48]

The significance of this severe energy drain is the eventual depletion of energy stores, leading to the exhaustion of certain important physiologic processes. The human organism has a limited potential for energy storage, and unless constantly replenished energy is rapidly depleted.

Carbohydrate Metabolism. The prime

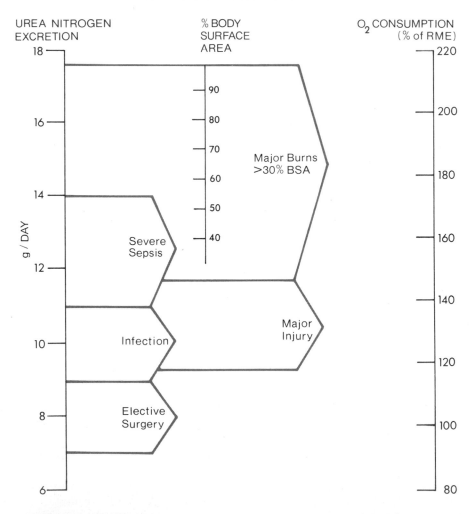

Figure 3–1. *Rates of hypermetabolism associated with trauma and infection as estimated from urinary urea nitrogen excretion. (From Blackburn, G. L., Bistrian, B. R., Maini, B. S., Schlamm, H. T., and Smith, M. F.: Nutritional and metabolic assessment of the hospitalized patient. J. Parent. Ent. Nutr. 1:11–22, 1977.)*

energy source in humans is glucose, which is stored mostly as liver glycogen. The amount of this stored liver glycogen totals only about 300 grams or 1200 kilocalories. Without other exogenous or endogenous sources of glucose, this supply could be totally depleted in less than 24 hours.

Following trauma, there is almost invariably an abrupt rise in blood glucose levels. The initial phase of this hyperglycemia seems to consist of the outpouring of hepatic glucose secondary to increased adrenergic activity and increased circulating catecholamines, including epinephrine.[131] In addition to this effect of epinephrine on hepatic glycogen, Porte has reported inhibition of insulin secretion during epinephrine infusion.[132] This corresponds to the finding that this early phase of hyperglycemia is characterized by a lack of increased insulin secretion[88] and by antagonism of the peripheral action of insulin, thus further decreasing utilization of insulin and increasing the hyperglycemia.[87] The antagonism leads to a state of pseudodiabetes with an abnormal glucose tolerance curve.[2]

This decrease in insulin secretion and activity is orchestrated primarily by the sympathetic hormones and means that at least initially in trauma, the metabolic importance of glucose is diminished. Despite this decreased role of glucose, certain tissues (brain, white cells and reparative tissue) must still rely on it as their main energy source. In response to this need an increase in gluconeogenesis is associated with trauma.[68]

Fat Metabolism. A major supply of energy is contained in the adipose tissue. An average 70-kilogram man contains approximately 15 kilograms of body fat, which amounts to approximately 140,000 calories of stored energy. Because fat is stored in the extra-aqueous phase, 1 gram of fat yields approximately 9 calories, compared to carbohydrates and protein which yield only 2 calories per gram of tissue catabolized. Fat as energy obviously affords the organism a much more efficient weight to energy ratio.

The major metabolic pathway by which fats are catabolized for energy is through free fatty acids. These fatty acids are controlled by the same hormonal interplay activated by the stress response as described above, and increased serum levels of free fatty acids are typically observed following injury.[178] These fatty acids are metabolized by the successive cleaving of two carbon fragments, which produce acetyl coenzyme A (CoA) and thus ultimately carbon dioxide and water.

During severe trauma and sepsis this catabolism of fatty acids can account for some 80 per cent of the total energy balance; however, fatty acid cannot be converted to glucose and therefore cannot be utilized for energy by the brain, white cells and reparative tissue. Under certain circumstances the brain can adapt to the utilization of another metabolite of fatty acids, the ketones. These are partially oxidized metabolites of fatty acids and, unlike the fatty acids themselves, can cross the blood-brain barrier. This adaptation to the utilization of ketones is particularly important in starvation, for it results in the sparing of glucose and ultimately protein. Insulin appears to play an important role in this adaptation because, in addition to its other important metabolic roles, it also has an *antilipolytic* action. As blood sugar levels fall in starvation, insulin levels also fall, allowing release of fatty acids from adipose tissue.

Protein Metabolism. Another major characteristic of the metabolic response to trauma is the increased utilization of protein as an energy source. This phenomenon of increased protein catabolism following injury was well known in the later part of the nineteenth century but received little attention until the 1930's, when Cuthbertson began detailed studies of nitrogen metabolism following peripheral trauma.[41]

An average 70-kilogram male has approximately 13 kilograms of body protein. This could conceivably be translated into 52,000 kilocalories but for the fact that proteins cannot be considered to be an energy resource. Every protein molecule appears to have a specific physiologic role as a structural, enzymatic or transport protein. Increased protein expenditure then, if prolonged, could create serious metabolic consequences. Skeletal muscle is the major site of the protein catabolism that occurs following trauma.

A possible reason for the increased catabolism of protein is to supply glucose to meet metabolic demands; this process is called gluconeogenesis. A major source of these new glucose molecules is protein and ultimately amino acids such as alanine from skeletal muscle. Thus alanine appears in much greater concentration than could be calculated from the other protein constituents of actin and myosin.[64]

The characteristic hormonal environment of trauma plays an important although not fully elucidated role in protein catabolism. Insulin has long been known to increase incorporation of amino acids into skeletal protein.[57] Insulin, used in an isolated forearm preparation in man, has been clearly shown to inhibit amino acid release from skeletal muscle.[133] The relatively depressed insulin levels and the peripheral antagonism of insulin following trauma allow peripheral protein to be mobilized for energy expenditure.

Glucagon, which is increased in response to trauma, also plays an important role in post-traumatic metabolism. Normally, the fine tuning of metabolism is controlled by the interplay of insulin and glucagon. Unger[173] noted that the hypermetabolism that occurs following severe trauma may be related to a decreased molar ratio of insulin to glucagon. Although glucagon per se is not a catabolic hormone and does not have any direct action on muscle,[3] its importance in the catabolic response lies in its relationship to insulin.

Cortisol, although necessary for the normal catabolic response to trauma, does *not* in itself stimulate gluconeogenesis[51] or protein catabolism.[124] Cortisol seems to play a permissive rather than a direct role in post-traumatic catabolism.

Nutritional Management of the Post-Traumatic State. Given the above metabolic consequences of trauma, one of the obvious goals of management is to meet the increased energy requirements of the patient and not allow exhaustion of mechanical and immunological processes. It is particularly important to counteract the hormonal initiators of the hypermetabolism of trauma. After surgery and injury, metabolism is best served by reducing the catecholamine response and returning the insulin-glucagon ratio to normal. The first consideration, therefore, is not the provision of calories but aggressive support of the circulating volume and maintenance of cardiovascular function. These efforts can be augmented by the debridement of necrotic tissue, the drainage of abscesses, the correction of electrolytes and acid-base imbalance, and the alleviation of pain. It is of little value to supply the patient with a well-balanced menu of nutrients while the continuing stress response inhibits the utilization of external substrates.

Once the stress is under control, one can concentrate on supplying the necessary nutrients to meet the metabolic needs of the patient. Although sophisticated tests are available to determine this energy expenditure, a more practical clinical focus is to supply enough calories (and nitrogen) to retard weight loss and develop a positive nitrogen balance.

The manner in which these nutrients are supplied is important clinically. If the patient's intestinal tract is functioning and the patient can take food orally, it is best to use enteral nutrition. This can be augmented by supplemental feedings by mouth or nasogastric tube. Premature feeding, however, usually leads to vomiting and possibly aspiration and therefore should be avoided. If gastrointestinal function is not adequate but is expected to return within 7 days and the anticipated metabolic drain will not be too great, a peripheral intravenous line will usually suffice. The usual regimen is to supply needed fluids as a 5 or 10 per cent glucose solution. The administration of 400 to 700 grams of glucose by this means will markedly reduce nitrogen loss.[60, 122] A new approach is to provide the patient with isotonic amino acids as a method of decreasing endogenous protein catabolism. Blackburn and co-workers have shown that when given amino acids without concomitant glucose the body will convert to a starvation pattern of metabolism utilizing fat and conserving protein.[16]

If the patient is suffering a severe metabolic drain or will not be able to tolerate enteral feedings within 7 days, plans should be made to institute parenteral alimentation as soon as the stress response is under control.

SHOCK

The largest portion of this chapter is devoted to shock in keeping with the intense investigative and clinical interest in this condition. Despite great advances made in this century in understanding the pathophysiology of shock, the refractory hemodynamic state that develops during protracted shock and the multiple organ failure that follows adequate resuscitation still constitute the greatest remaining barriers to the successful management of the severely traumatized patient.

Definition. The term "shock" embraces a group of conditions with grossly similar physiologic derangements but a wide variety of inciting causes. Originally, it was represented in the English language by the word "collapse" from the Latin *conlapsus*. This connotation persists in the descriptive German word *Zusammenseukung*. The word "shock" itself first appeared in English medical literature in a 1743 translation of LeDran's "Reflections Drawn from Experiences with Gunshot Wounds," in which it implied a sudden violent impact. Its present connotation did not develop until the mid-nineteenth century.[40]

The earliest definitions of shock were descriptive expressions, such as Gross's "a rude unhinging of the machinery of life," and Warren's "a momentary pause in the act of death."[67] There followed many attempts to define it in precise terms. These usually failed to encompass its many facets or were too complex to be generally adopted. For this reason, it is expedient to define shock simply as *a generalized state of severe circulatory inadequacy.* It should be noted that this definition avoids reference to blood pressure or volume deficits, since *inadequate tissue perfusion,* which is the essence of shock, may occur when either of these parameters is within generally accepted normal limits.

Historical Background

Until the advent of the era of experimental physiology at the end of the nineteenth century, our concept of shock was based almost entirely on clinical description. Under the influence of the then popular spheres of physiologic interest, there followed periods of emphasis on the nervous, toxic, hemodynamic and metabolic aspects of shock. Many of the impressions of the pioneers in this field are interesting today

because their significance was not fully appreciated at the time and have only recently been popularized by new and independent observations.

Early in this century, physiological studies on the neural control of circulation spawned the concept that shock represented an inhibition of the vasomotor center, producing weakened heart action and peripheral pooling of blood. In 1914, George W. Crile, one of the first to carry out extensive experiments on shock, stated: "There is a group of organs whose function is the conversion of potential to kinetic energy. This kinetic system includes the brain, thyroid, suprarenals, muscle and liver. If the stimuli are overwhelmingly intense, the kinetic system, particularly the brain, is exhausted, even permanently injured. This condition is acute shock."[36]

The concept of exhaustion of the central nervous system and its vasomotor control was one of the earliest physiological explanations of the mechanisms of shock. However, its popularity waned after evidence indicated that, if anything, vasomotor activity was heightened in response to hypovolemia. Nevertheless, vasomotor tone *is lost* late in shock. However, the mechanisms involved appear to be intrinsic or humoral rather than of central nervous origin. As for Crile's "kinetic systems," a modern parallel can be found in current work on the effects of shock on the energy-producing intracellular enzyme systems.

Crile did much work in support of the use of saline as a temporary replacement for blood. Even earlier, in 1901, Roswell Park had suggested the infusion of a liter of saline in patients with significant blood loss. This, too, has regained popularity from the work of Shires et al.[148] and of Moyer and his associates,[118] which suggests that the loss of extracellular fluid in shock and burn states is much greater than previously appreciated.

In 1909, Henderson presented an "acapnia" theory of shock.[76] In spite of the misconception of his central theme, he was one of the first to recognize the importance of venous return in shock. He stated: "Venous pressure is, so to speak, the fulcrum of the circulation. Shock, as surgeons use the word, is due to the failure of the fulcrum. Because of diminished venous supply, the heart is not adequately distended in diastole." Judging by their frequent reliance on the central venous pressure as a diagnostic and therapeutic guide to the management of shock, this statement would be soundly endorsed today by most surgeons.

Physiologists and surgeons combined their efforts in the study of shock during World War I. Measurements of the volume of fluid lost into a crushed limb in the experiments of Cannon and Bayliss suggested that this alone could not account for the degree of shock observed.[26, 27] It was implied that a toxic agent liberated from the crushed tissue might be responsible. The prestige of these investigators did much to advance the "toxic" theory of traumatic shock. Since it had been shown by Dale and Richards only a few years earlier that histamine resulted in profound hypotension when injected into cats, this substance was the principal suspect.[42]

However, the popularity of the toxic theory waned in 1930 when Blalock, and Parsons and Phemister, independently repeating Cannon and Bayliss's experiments, showed that if one included in the estimates the volume of fluid lost into tissues just proximal to the level of the crush injury, this volume did correspond to that required to produce an equivalent degree of shock by slow withdrawal from the venous system.[17, 127] Their observations restored the position of inadequate circulating volume as the leading factor in most forms of traumatic shock, a position supported by the extensive clinical experiences of World War II and one that has not been seriously challenged since.

However, interest in toxic humoral substances in shock was soon restored, not only in regard to bacterial endotoxins as the etiologic agents in septic shock, and, as championed by Fine, the final cause of irreversibility in shock of any etiology, but in relation to the contributor roles played by endogenously released vasoactive humoral substances such as histamine, serotonin, bradykinin, prostaglandins and other vasoactive substances such as the myocardial-depressant factor, and lysosomal enzymes.

Since World War II, experimental studies have continued the development of standard shock preparations, with particular emphasis on a common denominator in irreversible shock. In recent years, the practice of characterizing the events in shock solely in terms of *macrocirculatory* hemodynamics has decreased; the focus is being shifted more and more toward changes in regional blood flow, the microcirculation, and the metabolic effects of shock as reflected by changes in organ function, cellular metabolism, intracellular enzyme systems and ultrastructure. The literature on shock has reached staggering proportions since World War II, and although many questions have been answered, at least an equal number have been raised.

Classification of Shock

The nomenclature encountered in shock literature can be very confusing. This is exemplified by Table 3–2, which lists some of the forms of clinical and experimental shock commonly mentioned. However, a simpler classification is desirable from both physiological and therapeutic points of view. The following is a simplified classification of shock similar to that conceived by Blalock in 1934.[18]

Hypovolemic Shock. Hemorrhagic shock is the classic example of this type of shock, but in addition to blood loss, any uncompensated loss of extracellular fluid — like that from intestinal obstruction, major burns, crushing injuries, peritonitis or fistulas — can produce it.

Cardiogenic Shock. This category implies shock primarily due to ineffective cardiac pumping action. It occurs in instances of myocardial insufficiency (e.g., massive myocardial infarction), with certain cardiac arrhythmias, or when there is mechanical obstruction of the flow of blood into or out of the heart (e.g., cardiac tamponade, massive pulmonary embolism).

TABLE 3–2. Forms of Shock Commonly Referred to in the Literature

Allergic shock	Peptone shock
Anaphylactic shock	Septic shock
Burn shock	Spinal shock
Cardiogenic shock	Surgical shock
Endotoxin shock	Tourniquet shock
Hematogenic shock	Toxin shock
Hemorrhagic shock	Traumatic shock
Histamine shock	Tumbling shock
Neurogenic shock	Vasogenic shock
Oligemic shock	Vasovagal shock

Vasogenic Shock. The most common clinical example of this type of shock is septic shock, although a number of toxic agents or the sudden release of allergic mediators may produce a similar state (e.g., hymenopterous insect bites, reactions to local anesthetics).

Actually, Blalock included, as a fourth category, "neurogenic shock," but many if not most current treatises on shock disregard this as a separate category and consider it as a "central" form of vasogenic shock. This de-emphasis probably stems in large part from the classic description by Grant and Reeves, in their World War II study of traumatic forms of shock, of a condition called "warm hypotension" in which, despite abnormally low blood pressure, adequate tissue perfusion was maintained, as evidenced by skin of normal color and temperature and adequate urinary excretion.[65] This apparent state of reflex vasodilatation with decreased peripheral vascular resistance is not uncommonly seen briefly immediately after significant trauma and cannot truly be considered a form of shock. Otherwise, neurogenic shock is rarely encountered clinically outside of the iatrogenic examples provided by "spinal" anesthesia. Of course, if it were of sudden onset and serious magnitude, neurogenic shock might not be so innocuous, particularly if an arteriosclerotic or otherwise diseased heart was the victim of the sudden loss of venous return it would cause.

Although this classification implies that the cause of the circulatory inadequacy that is called shock can be traced to the function of the pump (heart), the volumes of fluid it circulates (blood and extracellular fluid), or the tone of the conducting vessels (vasomotor activity), it should be emphasized that shock, as it is encountered clinically, frequently represents a *combination* of two or more of these forms.

Thus, when a patient develops shock following a myocardial infarction, a massive gastrointestinal hemorrhage, or the rigors of ascending cholangitis, there is little question that one is dealing, initially at least, with a simple form of shock — in these instances, cardiogenic, hypovolemic and septic shock respectively — and one can initiate appropriate therapy with some degree of confidence in the diagnosis if not the outcome. However, it is just as common

for the etiology to be uncertain, particularly in the postoperative or late post-traumatic periods. Even more perplexing are the frequent instances in which a mixture of contributing elements exists. Next to inadequate volume restoration, failure to recognize later contributions by factors other than the primary etiology factor is probably the most common cause of "refractory shock." One common example is hypovolemia associated with septic shock, resulting from a failure to recognize the magnitude of "third space" and "insensible fluid losses" associated with sepsis. In fact, most cases initially diagnosed as septic shock will turn out to be a combination of hypovolemia and sepsis, the hypovolemia having been made relatively more significant by the increased circulatory demands imposed by the sepsis. A final common example of misdiagnosis occurs in the patient being treated for cardiogenic shock secondary to myocardial infarction, who develops unrecognized hypovolemia, either from rigid fluid restriction or the shift of extracellular fluid from the intravascular to the extravascular compartment caused by vasopressor therapy. However, as long as one recognizes the limitations of this oversimplified approach to etiologic classification of shock, the attempt to make this categorical distinction clinically is justified by the therapeutic implications, as indicated by the experience of MacLean et al.[103]

Experimental Versus Clinical Shock Research. Even a casual perusal of shock literature reveals that much disagreement exists in this field. One can find differences of opinion among reputable investigators studying the same problem. One of the most important factors contributing to this disagreement is the necessity of studying most aspects of the pathophysiology of shock in animals. It is extremely difficult, if not impossible, to conduct truly controlled shock studies on humans. Patients accepted for study in special units have varying medical backgrounds complicated by a variety of intercurrent diseases. Not only do they enter their state of shock by diverse routes, but almost invariably they have undergone a variety of treatments before entering the study unit.

However, in carrying out more detailed controlled studies of experimental animals, equally formidable barriers are encountered. As Zweifach has indicated, differences in the comparative physiology of laboratory animals present very complex problems in the interpretation of experimental shock studies.[185] Even among animals obtained from a common source, factors such as age, sex, season, nutritional state and intercurrent infection are difficult to control. More important, however, are species differences that limit the extrapolation of findings to human shock.

The animals commonly used in shock experiments differ in the organ system that constitutes their "weak link" in response to shock. For example, the hepatic vein sphincters of the dog are extremely sensitive to changes in pH, adrenergic stimuli and vasoactive substances. The effects of their constriction in shock led many to the impression that severe hepatosplanchnic congestion was a critical factor in determining the lethality of shock. However, these sphincters are not as well developed in most other species and appear to have little significance in primates.[120, 176]

Studies of the hemodynamic response to hypovolemia have often been performed in dogs and cats. However, it has been shown that contraction of the liver and spleen of these animals can add as much as 30 per cent to the active circulating volume. These organs do not have nearly that propensity in man and subhuman primates, in whom the cutaneous circulation appears to act as such a depot.

The intense peripheral vasoconstriction seen in most forms of shock is not uniformly distributed throughout the circulation, and the pattern of distribution varies from species to species. For example, in the shocked rabbit renal cortical ischemia is marked, whereas in the rat or monkey it is mild or absent.

There are also marked species differences in sensitivity to bacterial products, and the relative contents of the vasoactive substances released by certain key organs in response to bacterial toxins are quite variable. The rabbit and cat are extremely sensitive to the lipopolysaccharide extracts of certain bacteria, but the rat and mouse are usually quite resistant to these same endotoxins.

The histological picture of acute endotoxemia varies considerably among species. In the rat, a massive accumulation of leukocytes is seen in the lung; in the rabbit, focal necrosis of the liver and splenitis are encountered; and in the dog, submucosal hemorrhage throughout the intestinal tract appears to be a major pathological event. In the dog an injection of *Escherichia coli* endotoxin will cause shock characterized by severe vasoconstriction; in the monkey it causes shock with vasodilatation.[184]

Another major problem in experimental shock investigations occurs in experiments that isolate a particular factor for study. The difficulty lies in interpreting the significance of changes in the factor studied in relation to the overall pathogenesis of shock. In focusing on one aspect, overall perspective can be lost as the trail of investigation is followed further and further in that direction. For this phenomenon, Simeone has coined the word "ideolepsis," meaning to be captured by an idea.[154] This has been particularly common in experiments studying the nature of irreversible shock.

The Effects of Shock on Organ Systems

Shock affects every tissue in the body, but because of selective compensatory mechanisms, the tissues of some organs are affected more than others. One of the most controversial issues in medical research has been the relative importance of the functional deterioration of certain vital organ systems in the final capitulation of the body's compensatory and recuperative mechanisms to severe prolonged shock. The hope that this "irreversibility" is merely a function of our limited state of knowledge has encouraged an intense research interest in this state of shock, which in turn has greatly extended our knowledge of the effects of shock on the various organ systems. Another effect of improved shock therapy has been to open the door to the entire spectrum of sequential organ failure. That is, patients who used to die from hemodynamic causes or recover with renal shutdown are now surviving to the point where pulmonary insufficiency, gastrointestinal hemorrhage and sepsis are playing major roles in the eventual outcome.

The following discussion summarizes what is known of these effects as well as the conflicting opinions about their significance. The effects of shock on the more important organ systems described below are those resulting from *hypovolemia,* unless otherwise noted. This emphasis is deliberate, since hypovolemic shock is the type initially encountered in the injured patient. However, in discussing the cardiac effects of hypovolemic shock, some comments will also be made regarding the characteristics of cardiogenic shock. The problem of endotoxin or septic shock, as an example of vasogenic shock, will be given separate consideration.

In shock, the endocrine organs are more important for the responses they mediate than for the effects they suffer. Consequently, they will not be treated separately but dealt with in discussing the organ systems they affect, mainly their circulatory and renal effects.

The Effects of Shock on the Circulatory System. Isolation of the responses of the heart from those of the vessels conducting the blood and lymph and consideration of changes in regional distribution of blood flow separately from changes in the distribution of body fluids are justified only in an attempt to bring some order to the complexities of the circulatory responses to shock. In addition, the coagulation changes attending shock are considered here because of their potential effects on microcirculation.

THE INITIAL CARDIOVASCULAR RESPONSE TO HYPOVOLEMIA. In general, the rate and volume of fluid lost from the effective circulation determine the cardiovascular responses to hypovolemia. At one extreme is a rapid exsanguinating hemorrhage from a large artery, and at the other, the insidious venous ooze or the seeping sequestration of extracellular fluid. In the "open artery" type of bleeding, a profound loss of peripheral vascular resistance occurs in spite of compensating mechanisms. Hypotension is out of proportion to volume loss. Coronary flow, robbed of the driving force of diastole, is greatly impaired, and the rate of deterioration of cardiac function is rapid. The importance of recognizing this form of shock is evident, for prolonging efforts to "catch up" with volume-expanding fluids before surgical intervention in behalf of hemostasis is futile. At the other extreme, the gradual loss

of volume, unless quite prolonged, may be entirely compensated for by fluid retention by the kidney and the repartition of body fluids without grossly discernible hemodynamic disturbances.

Between these two extremes lies the more common situation, typified by a combined loss from small arteries, veins and capillaries. Unless the blood loss is arrested, this condition will progress successively through recognizable stages of compensated hypovolemia, impending shock, hypotensive shock and, finally, refractory shock. The volume losses necessary to reach these stages depend on many factors other than the rate of blood loss, among them body position, the stress of other trauma, age and cardiovascular reserve. It has been stated that a 10 to 15 per cent gradual volume loss usually produces minimal changes, that a 20 to 30 per cent loss may be compensated for without hypotension, and that a 30 to 50 per cent loss is required to produce progressive hypotension to a level of 50 mm. Hg.[112] However, these volume estimates were based largely on studies of the physiologic responses to venesection conducted on healthy young volunteers and were not meant to be applied too literally to patients encountered in the emergency department. Nevertheless, the progression of events demonstrated in these studies can be applied to equivalent stages of circulatory impairment seen clinically.

COMPENSATION. Initial increments of volume loss are compensated by adjustments in venous tone. To some extent this response is an intrinsic one that is not well maintained later in shock.[1] Its mechanism is poorly understood. As hypovolemia progresses, sympathetic neurohumoral activity also contributes to the increased venomotor tone. The capacity of the venous system to adjust for volume loss can be appreciated from the fact that fourteen times as much blood normally resides in the systemic veins and venules as in the capillary bed. For this reason venomotor mechanisms are called the "capacitance" system and the "volume effectors," in contrast to arteriolar sphincters that are "pressure effectors" and constitute the "resistance" system.

Even with modest degrees of hypovolemia that can be compensated by adjustments in venous capacity without grossly discernible hemodynamic changes, volume receptors within this system will initiate plasma refilling mechanisms (to be described later).

When reduction in the capacity of the venous system can no longer compensate for the volume loss, sequential decreases in venous pressure, diastolic filling, stroke volume and arterial pressure result. These effects are short-lived and quickly counterbalanced. They stimulate baroreceptors that respond through the sympathetic neurohumoral axis. These baroreceptors probably exist throughout the circulatory system, but those in the atrium and in the carotid and aortic sinuses are best known. However, their relative sensitivity and their contribution to vasomotor adjustment are not fully understood. Impulses are relayed first to hypothalamic regulator centers and then to the vasomotor center in the medulla. The efferent arm of this response, the sympathetic nervous system, increases the release of catecholamines at its nerve endings and in the adrenal medulla. The result is an inotropic and chronotropic effect on the heart and a widespread but selective vasoconstriction by which flow is decreased through certain regions of the circulation (e.g., skin, muscle and adipose tissue) but not to the heart or brain. Splanchnic, and therefore portal venous, flow is also reduced, but overall hepatic blood flow is supported by an increased distribution of cardiac output to the hepatic artery.[89] It has also been shown that the heart is capable of some degree of intrinsic response, that is, independent of nervous and humoral stimuli.

Initially, the combined effect of these compensatory mechanisms is the restoration of arterial pressure, but not without a quickening of the pulse and a narrowing of the pulse pressure. The skin becomes cool and urinary output decreases. Other expressions of sympathetic overactivity are evident — dry mouth, sweating, pupillary dilation and restlessness. At this stage hypotension may be precipitated by postural elevation or other manipulation of the patient, such as a Valsalva maneuver.

This adrenergic response can counterbalance a considerable degree of acute blood loss (up to 30 per cent) and maintain the integrity of the organism while volume replenishment goes on. If this compensatory capacity is exceeded, generalized circulatory inadequacy (shock) will result. When the blood pressure is used as a reference, the transition into the actual state of shock may seem abrupt; however, most physiologic parameters change gradually throughout the preceding period. Finally, in addition to a redistribution of regional blood flow, there is an increased uptake of oxygen from the blood flowing at a reduced rate through the tissues. Thus, the available circulating volume of blood is speeded along by the heart, strategically redistributed by the vascular tree and more efficiently utilized by the tissues.

DECOMPENSATION. Once a certain stage of inadequate tissue perfusion is reached, a series of vicious cycles is initiated; these progressively interfere with the organism's ability to restore its own integrity. There is a shift to anaerobic metabolism, a depletion of existing energy stores and the development of metabolic acidosis. Acidosis reduces myocardial contractility, depresses the vascular response to catecholamines and promotes intravascular clotting. Reduced flow to the kidney results in a functional shutdown which, in time, will become permanent. This compounds the acidosis and may lead to significant electrolyte disturbances, such as hyperkalemia. Similarly, poor perfusion of the hepatosplanchnic bed may weaken the intestinal mucosa's barrier against bacterial invasion and reduce the reticuloendothelial system's ability to inactivate toxins. These toxins and tissue ischemia itself cause the release of lysosomal enzymes and other vasoactive humoral substances (histamine, serotonin, bradykinin, prostaglandins and possibly myocardial-depressant factor), which in turn profoundly affect vascular tone and integrity, with further volume losses resulting from sequestration and capillary permeability. Initially in shock, there is little arterial hypoxemia unless there is associated trauma. Eventually, however, hypoxemia develops despite a degree of compensatory hyperventilation sufficient to produce hypocarbia, probably because of an elevation of the ventilation-perfusion ratio with shunting around the pulmonary vascular bed and also because of an increased arteriovenous difference in the systemic circulation. There is no evidence that this reversal in the arteriovenous oxygen difference seen late in shock is due to the shunting of blood through true arteriovenous communications. In fact, microsphere studies by the author[141] indicate that this does *not* occur in uncomplicated hemorrhagic shock. Rather, there is a failure of exchange at the microcirculatory level that cannot be explained on the basis of such things as depletion in 2,3-diphosphoglycerate (as discussed later) and that may well simply reflect the inability of the defective mechanisms of "sick" or dying cells to utilize oxygen and other substrates.

The continuation of this trend (to hypoxia and hypocarbia) eventually weakens the respiratory drive and may interfere with the autoregulatory capacity of the pulmonary microcirculation. Hypotension decreases coronary flow, which in turn further depresses myocardial contractility. The eventual consequences of a weakened heart trying to pump a progressively reduced effective circulating volume to disabled tissues requires no further explanation.

THE ROLE OF THE HEART. It is natural and correct to consider the heart an organ of prime importance in shock. However, whether or not the heart constitutes the weak link in the body's struggle against shock is disputed. Those who contend that cardiac deterioration is *the* factor that determines irreversibility point out that myocardial flow, contractility and oxygen consumption deteriorate progressively as hemorrhagic shock deepens. Cardiac output falls steadily, and terminally there are arrhythmias and a rise in the right atrial pressure. Using serial pressure-output curves. Crowell has demonstrated a progressive weakening of the heart's action.[37] In addition, myocardial structural disintegration has been demonstrated in irreversibly shocked animals.

Nevertheless, the impression has been equally strong that the heart possesses remarkable recuperative powers and responds strongly to an expansion of circulating volume long after a recognizable point of irreversibility has been passed. It has also been shown that cardiac function can be maintained as long as venous return is supported.[179] Indeed, the most impressive evidence of cardiac dysfunction appears only terminally. Even the late elevation of right atrial pressure may be related to pulmonary vasoconstriction.

Thus, experimental evidence to date suggests that although cardiac function deterioration is a striking event late in hemorrhagic shock, it occurs when other organs are also showing evidence of terminal decompensation. However, this impression must be tempered by the realization that what may be true for young laboratory animals may not be valid in older human subjects whose cardiac reserve has been lowered by age or disease.

Finally, in resuscitated hemorrhagic shock victims, both experimental and clinical investigations have shown supranormal cardiac outputs despite evidence of inadequate tissue perfusion (e.g., rising blood lactate levels and increasing lactate-pyruvate ratios). Just as an effective circulating blood volume after prolonged hypovolemia may significantly exceed normal limits, so may the circulatory requirements of this post-shock state be excessive. The question that still remains unanswered is whether this hyperdynamic circulatory failure represents a failure of the heart, in spite of supranormal effort, to meet the excessive demands placed on it, or whether the cardiac response is appropriate but peripheral factors, such as indiscriminant vasodilation, abnormal oxygen transport, or widespread cellular dysfunction, are to be blamed.

CARDIOGENIC SHOCK. Shock may, of course, result from primary cardiac lesions, such as myocardial infarction, severe arrhythmias, and acute myocardiopathies, as well as conditions that mechanically interfere with the heart's action, such as cardiac tamponade and pulmonary embolism. Cardiogenic shock can lead to a refractory state by the same series of vicious cycles described for hypovolemic shock. In cardiogenic shock, the pumping action of the heart is not able to maintain a sufficient pressure head for adequate tissue perfusion. There are conflicting opinions regarding the direction in which peripheral vascular resistance changes in response to this so-called forward heart failure. In laboratory preparations of cardiogenic shock, particularly in the dog, peripheral resistance appears to rise, and some clinical success has been claimed with vasodilators, particularly in the "low-output" failure encountered after open-heart surgery. Clinical studies, however, report variable changes in peripheral resistance; many patients stay in the normal range and the high peripheral resistances characteristic of hemorrhagic shock rarely occur. The answer may lie in the acuteness with which this failure develops: with slower development some compensation may be afforded by volume expansion and increased tissue extraction of substrates, but in the acutely developing situation, a certain degree of selective vasoconstriction would seem necessary to protect the more vital regional circulations. However, one would not expect the extreme degrees of vasoconstriction and elevated peripheral resistance invoked to compensate for major volume losses.

In earlier years, the direction in which peripheral vascular resistance changed in cardiogenic shock attracted much attention because of its therapeutic significance in regard to the choice of drugs. At that time, a stalemate existed concerning the choice of vasopressor vs. vasodilator drugs. Vasopressors were recommended because they were thought to increase coronary flow and perfusion pressure, but this benefit was offset by the increased work of the heart secondary to increased peripheral resistance. Vasodilators on the other hand were felt to decrease cardiac work and increase perfusion through deprived regions of the circulation by decreased resistance to flow; yet a disproportionate reduction in diastolic pressure and therefore coronary flow was feared to further weaken the diseased heart. This conflict has waned with the loss in popularity of both pure vasodilators and vasopressors in favor of drugs that singly or in combination have a positive inotropic effect on the heart with either little effect on the peripheral resistance (glucagon, dopamine) or vasodilation (isoproterenol), or selective vasoconstriction (mephentermine, epinephrine in small doses). Finally, the earlier reported successes of "vasodilators" in cardiogenic shock preparations may be quite valid but are related to the relief of "afterload" on the heart provided by some of these agents rather than to the relief of pathologic degrees of vasoconstriction.

THE MICROCIRCULATION. Capillary flow is impaired in shock by a combination of factors. As significant hypovolemia occurs, the perfusion pressure is decreased. Sympathetic neurohumoral activity causes a constriction of arteriolar sphincters in most vascular beds. Theoretically, flow into these capillary beds may be further diminished by the passive opening of arteriovenous shunts proximal to the constricted arterioles, but labeled microsphere studies indicate that there is no significant degree of anatomic arteriovenous shunting in pure hypovolemic shock.[141] Normally, flow through the capillary circulation is intermittently phased so that only about one third of the channels are open at any one time. This "winking circulation" appears to result from each capillary opening intermittently on demand, probably mediated by locally released vasoactive substances such as the kinins or prostaglandins. However, when the perfusion is inadequate, all the capillaries "demand" blood so that the capacitance of the capillary circulation is roughly trebled. The combination of low perfusion pressure and increased precapillary arteriolar resistance allows very little blood into this wide-open capillary bed. The result is a marked degree of stagnation in the microcirculation. This is compounded later in shock by further loss of volume by sequestration and by changes in permeability secondary to ischemia so that fluid shifts into the cell. This offsets the forces contributing to capillary refill, and the end result is partial restoration of intravascular volume, an increase in intracellular volume and a contraction in the extracellular, extravascular fluid compartment,[148] as will be discussed more fully later (p. 55).

Lillehei et al. explain the microcirculation events somewhat differently at this point.[100] They contend that constriction of both the precapillary arteriolar sphincters and the postcapillary venular sphincters is present early in shock. Then the loss of precapillary arteriolar tone occurs while the postcapillary venous sphincters remain constricted so that a "stagnant anoxia" replaces an "ischemic anoxia." The sequestration losses in protracted shock are thus explained by an imbalance between vascular tone on the "resistance" and "capacitance" sides of the capillary bed. This mechanism may apply in the dog and other animals in which the venous sphincters are well developed, but its occurrence in man is highly questionable. Indeed, such an explanation is not necessary. This effect can be just as easily explained by a *relaxation* of tone on the venous side of the circulation. Normally, 25 per cent of the blood volume is present in the heart and pulmonary circulation, 15 per cent in the arterial system and only 4 per cent in the capillary bed. Over 26 per cent of the blood volume resides in the postcapillary venules and 30 per cent in the larger veins. Thus, the venous circulation has the greatest capacity for sequestering blood. The latter contention is supported by the observation that a progressive loss of venous tone occurs in advancing stages of shock. An explanation for this late loss of tone in vascular smooth muscle may be found in the electron microscopic studies of Ashford.[4] He has demonstrated remarkable increases in the intracellular fluid of vascular smooth muscle in advanced stages of shock. It is not hard to understand the inability of the myofibrils to contract when they are separated and disoriented by this abnormal accumulation of cell sap.

Other factors that may be important in these microcirculatory events are the critical closing pressures of arterioles and precapillary sphincters and the increasingly significant effects of changes in viscosity under low-flow situations. Thus, evidence is accumulating that obviates the need to explain the microcirculatory changes in shock entirely on the basis of "sphincters," an explanation that has been very popular in the past decade.

COAGULATION CHANGES. The clotting changes associated with shock are considered here because of their implications on the microcirculation. There is little doubt that changes in coagulability occur in response to stress, trauma and shock. The state of coagulation represents a dynamic system of checks and balances that acts to prevent the development of extremes of hyper- and hypocoagulability. As early as the 1830's Hewson noted that the "blood which was drawn last clotted first in men and animals being venesected."[79] The hypercoagulable state that follows blood loss has a valuable homeostatic function and, in combination with vasoconstriction, helps to stem the loss of blood.

The cause of this increased coagulability has not been fully elucidated, but several factors play a role. Locally, damaged tissues and platelets release thromboplastic substances. Platelets also release serotonin, which is thought to contribute to the local vasoconstriction. This probably explains the common observation that a cleanly incised wound bleeds longer than a jagged laceration. However, the clotting response is more than a local one, since venesection alone leads to hypercoagulability, particularly if shock supervenes. There is information to suggest that the release of catecholamines and even lysosomal enzymes may contribute to this. The acidosis that accompanies shock appears to be important also. Experimental lowering of the pH by intravenous lactate has been shown to shorten the clotting time.[38] Even heparinized blood can be made *hypercoagulable* if the pH is sufficiently lowered.[72] Finally, if the acidosis of hemorrhagic shock is prevented by buffering with trishydroxymethanolamine, the severity of the associated clotting changes is greatly ameliorated.[142]

The rate of mobilization of clotting factors is greatly accelerated in response to trauma, although the mechanisms involved are not known.[74] Changes in electric potential, the release of activators and the factors involved in platelet agglutination and red cell cohesiveness are all under study. An increase in platelet aggregation occurs after stress, trauma or shock, and platelet microthrombi have been demonstrated in movies of the microcirculation by Robb.[137] Similarly, Bjork et al. have shown clumping of red cells,[15] and Knisely and his associates have shown sludging of the blood in postoperative and shock states.[92]

Although the initial response is that of hypercoagulability, this tendency is reversed later if shock is severe and prolonged, and an extreme degree of *hypocoagulability* may result. To some extent this may reflect a loss of clotting factors through hemorrhage and a decrease in production and mobilization of clotting factors secondary to inadequate tissue perfusion. However, the most important factor appears to be the consumption of clotting factors. This is not only a local process at the site of injury, but a disseminated intravascular coagulation as well. Hardaway feels that this results from a combination of capillary stasis and hypercoagulability and that it may contribute greatly to the development of irreversibility as microthrombi block the circulation through vital organs.[72]

In the dog, fibrinolytic activity and circulating anticoagulants do not appear to contribute significantly to this hypocoagulability, which may develop to extreme degrees after 2 to 4 hours of hemorrhagic shock.[142] However, clinical observations suggest that these processes may be initiated later when shock is prolonged. One source may be the by-products of coagulation themselves. In the proteolytic reaction that produces fibrin from fibrinogen, a fibrin monomer is first released along with two polypeptide fragments. Fibrin is then formed by polymerization of this monomer. These polypeptide byproducts have fibrinolytic activity, and one may have vasoconstrictive properties.[94, 114]

Whether these changes in the state of coagulation can lead to significant deleterious effects in clinical shock by a process of disseminated intravascular coagulation is debatable. In histologic studies of human cases of refractory shock, Hardaway et al. have shown that microthrombi and peculiar "globular clots" can be found frequently if looked for.[73] In addition, they presented circumstantial evidence for occlusion of the microcirculation in the form of microinfarcts and petechial hemorrhages. These findings were absent in control patients who died suddenly without passing through a period of protracted shock.

The work of Attar and his associates suggests that there are natural oscillations in coagulability, which, by a system of negative feedbacks, strive to maintain a normal level.[6] In cases of refractory shock they found oscillations that exceeded normal limits in both directions. The magnitude of these oscillations correlated very well with mortality; in nonsurviving patients, they increased progressively to a point of extreme hypocoagulability instead of gradually returning to a normal range.

Simmons et al. recently reported a thorough study of coagulation disorders in Vietnam combat casualties.[156] They studied the acute changes after wounding, after massive transfusion and later in the postresuscitative period. In the acute phase following wounding and before intravenous therapy, changes in the state of coagulability correlated closely with the degree of hypotension, acidosis and lactacidemia. Those with wounds of mild to moderate severity had normal or shortened prothrombin and partial thromboplastin times. The more severely wounded patients, including those in shock, had normal or prolonged prothrombin and partial thromboplastin times. In general, the severity of the coagulation defects were milder than those seen in experimental canine studies but showed the same initial phase of hypercoagulability followed by a return to normal or progression into a phase of hypocoagulability. Following the administration of intravenous fluids and blood, a dilutional coagulation picture was produced with the pattern of depression of coagulation factors similar to that of stored bank blood. Platelet levels fell during transfusion to about 100,000 per cubic millimeter. Prothrombin times, partial thromboplastin times and fibrinogen levels were less severely affected. Severe operative bleeding was not associated with these relatively mild dilutional changes and the use of fresh blood was rarely warranted. Finally, during early convalescence, coagulation abnormalities were found in approximately one half of the casualties. These could be correlated with the presence of shock on admission to the hospital, transfusion of *large* quantities of blood and the presence of abnormalities in clotting parameters prior to operation. The prolongation of prothrombin and partial thromboplastin times was much greater than that seen earlier. In 20 per cent of the patients, the pattern of recurring cycles of hypocoagulability occurred, and the presence of four or more of these peaks could be correlated with the appearance of life-threatening complications. All the patients who died had clotting abnormalities at some time prior to death. Bleeding episodes requiring reoperation, however, could not be blamed on coagulation abnormalities. Fibrinogen levels were greater than normal in all patients in this third phase. Platelet counts returned to normal over the first week in almost all patients, and fibrinolysin values returned toward normal but remained elevated in most patients during the first convalescent week. It was concluded that the coincidence of abnormalities of prothrombin and partial thromboplastin times with thrombocytopenia and fibrinolysis and a relative deficiency of fibrinogen in most seriously wounded patients was consistent with the contention that nonlethal episodes of disseminated intravascular coagulation occurred during recovery from severe trauma and shock.

In summary, there is a hypercoagulable response to hemorrhage that may serve an important homeostatic function. However, when shock is extreme and prolonged, a state of hypocoagulability may ensue as a result of extravasation of clotting factors, decrease in their production and mobilization and, particularly, disseminated intravascular coagulation. This may be aggravated by an increase in fibrinolytic activity and the release of circulating anticoagulants and by the transfusion of blood deficient in clotting factors. If extreme, this hypocoagulability poses a threat to the bleeding patient and compromises any surgical efforts that may be made on his behalf.

CHANGES IN BODY FLUID DISTRIBUTION. Repartition of body fluids is one of the most important responses to hypovolemia. The translocation of extravascular fluid into the vascular compartment results in a hemodilution that has long been recognized by clinicians in the hematocrit changes that follow hemorrhage.

Volume replenishment can be detected within minutes after a moderate but nonshocking venous hemorrhage (10 to 20 per cent). After reaching a peak 6 to 10 hours after such a hemorrhage, the rate of refill gradually decreases and is usually completed in 20 to 40 hours. Electrolyte adjustments take a few days longer, and restoration of the red cell mass goes on over approximately a 6-week period at rates of 15 to 50 ml. a day.[113]

Only recently have the mechanisms involved in this response finally begun to be uncovered. For years plasma refilling has been explained solely on the basis of Starling's principle — that is, the lowering of intravascular pressure promotes the ingress of fluid from the extravascular space. Starling suggested that the balance between intravascular and extravascular pressure controlled extracellular fluid movements so that an egress of intravascular fluid occurred with the higher pressure at the arteriolar end of the capillary bed and an ingress of extravascular fluid occurred

with the lower pressures at the venular end. Although attractive, there is evidence to suggest that the process is not this simple. Guyton[70] has pointed out that the interstitial fluid, which constitutes one sixth of the total tissue mass, is almost entirely (99 per cent) in a sol-gel state with very little free fluid. This gel tends to imbibe fluid and has an average imbibition pressure of −7 mm. Hg. This is offset by an interlacing interstitial reticulum whose fibers tend to push cells apart and exert a *positive* pressure. These two forces work in concert to maintain a normal interstitial fluid volume and are assisted in this by the action of the lymphatics, which rhythmically pump out tissue lymph. The endothelial cells of the lymphatics are constructed in overlapping fashion to serve as one-way valves. Their outer surfaces are attached to anchoring filaments of the interstitial reticulum, so that they are only pulled open when the interstitium swells with excess fluid. While lymph flow normally accounts for only 10 to 15 per cent of the egress of interstitial fluid, it significantly controls the remainder, which is drawn back into the capillaries by osmosis, to the extent that it controls the protein content of this fluid. Capillary walls are impervious to protein, which must therefore leave via the lymphatics. In doing so the protein concentration of the interstitial fluid is lowered along with tissue oncotic pressure, allowing more fluid to be drawn back into the capillaries.

The above mechanisms act in the primary phase of restitution of blood volume, but they quickly reach an equilibrium (in one half hour to 6 hours), when secondary changes in interstitial hydrostatic and capillary oncotic pressures offset the initial fall in capillary hydrostatic pressure. There follows an important second phase of blood volume restitution that depends on the simultaneous restitution of plasma protein, primarily from preformed albumen. As mentioned previously, since capillaries are impervious to protein, protein can be mobilized into the circulation only via the lymphatics. Cope and Litwin[33] have shown that the volume and rate of fluid replacement correlated well with the increases in flow of thoracic duct lymph. The lymphatics, which are closed during the initial phase by decreased interstitial fluid volume, can be opened only in the absence of exogenous input in the form of intravenous fluids, by a shift in fluid from the cells to the interstitium. This in turn implies an osmotic gradient between the intracellular and the extracellular compartments. Boyd and Mansberger[21] first called attention to the increase in plasma osmolality that occurred in severely injured or shocked patients and experimental animals. Gann et al.[130] have confirmed this and have shown that it is hormonally induced, as it can be prevented by prior adrenalectomy. Also, the infusion of sufficient colloid-free fluid can induce complete restitution of plasma protein and volume in the absence of this shift, but without this exogenous input the described processes are essential for volume restitution.

The adrenal participation consists primarily of the effects of cortisol and the renin-angiotensin-aldosterone axis. These hormonal effects are in turn controlled by hypothalamic-pituitary activity, at least partly expressed in the output of ACTH. These responses are initiated by the same mechanisms described earlier for the vasoconstrictive responses mediated by the sympathetic nervous system — namely, signals from atrial receptors in response to decreased venous return and atrial filling are relayed via the vagus nerve to the hypothalamus and special medullary nuclei. An overall view of this neurohu-

moral control of blood volume restitution, as reconstructed by Gann,[61] can be seen in Figure 3–2. Once initiated, these mechanisms can be interrupted only by exogenous volume restoration in the form of intravenous fluids, and this has the important additional advantage of also interrupting or greatly ameliorating the adverse metabolic responses to shock and trauma described elsewhere in this chapter.

The final aspect of fluid compartment shifts associated with shock that deserves detailed discussion and that has received intense interest in the last two decades is the question of so-called "hidden" extracellular fluid losses. In the 1950's, a number of clinical experiences indicated that intravenous saline infusions could be used to replace lost blood. Experimental investigations indicated that saline infusions were as effective as blood in hemorrhagic shock preparations if three to four times the volume of lost blood was given. Indeed, the survival of shock and burn preparations was often better when crystalloid infusions were given instead of blood. This challenged two time-honored concepts of surgical care: (1) that electrolytes or saline solutions could only incompletely and transiently restore blood volume and (2) that saline solutions were undesirable during or immediately after operation or trauma because of the associat-

THE NEUROHUMORAL CONTROL OF VOLUME RESTITUTION

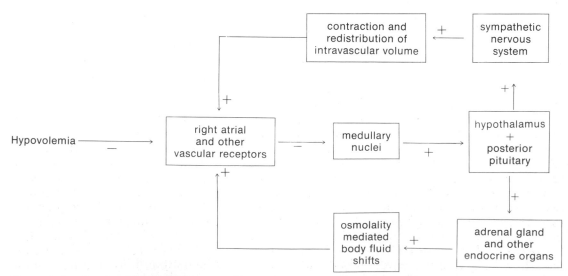

Figure 3–2. *An algorithm depicting the neurohumoral control of blood volume restitution, as viewed by Gann.*[61]

ed tendency toward salt and water retention. Since, up until the early 1960's, support for this approach was based on equal or better survival rates in animal studies and physiologic tolerance in clinical experiences, it was felt by most that this approach represented something one could get away with but was not necessarily best for the patient. However, in the early sixties, triple isotope studies by Shires indicated that in severe *shocking* degrees of hemorrhage (25 per cent volume loss), there was a much greater reduction in the extracellular fluid space than one would expect from the actual volume lost, a phenomenon that was not observed with lesser, nonshocking degrees of hemorrhage (10 per cent volume loss).[147] There followed a series of reports by other investigators using just about every known isotope technique for measuring extracellular fluid volume, the majority of which refuted Shires' claim. The most common explanation offered for this disagreement was that there was a shift to the right between the control and the posthemorrhagic radiosulfate equilibration curves so that estimation of the extracellular fluid space from a single 20-minute equilibration sample, as Shires had done, would indicate a reduction, whereas extrapolation from the total curve indicated little change in extracellular fluid volume. However, in fairness, most isotope studies that disputed Shires' conclusions were performed on milder or less prolonged shock preparations.

At the time of this impasse, Borden et al. investigated this problem using an entirely different approach, monitoring interstitial fluid pressure using Guyton's technique.[81] They showed that after prolonged shock, the interstitial fluid pressure was considerably more negative than it was normally, and that restoration of shed blood and even additional colloid solutions did not restore the interstitial fluid pressure to prehemorrhage levels, whereas an additional infusion of a crystalloid solution, in an amount equal to 5 per cent of the body weight, did accomplish this end. They contended that whether one could demonstrate it by isotope techniques or not, there was at least a functional ECF deficit following profound hemorrhage shock as demonstrated by the interstitial fluid pressures. Mathews, using an improved radiosulfate technique and multiple serial samples, was then able to

demonstrate two components to the radiosulfate equilibrium curve: an initial fast-equilibrating component representing the "functional" extracellular fluid volume, and a later, more slowly equilibrating component representing the total extracellular fluid volume.[110] He demonstrated that in moderate shock there was a decrease in the fast-equilibrating or functional compartment, and in severe shock there was a decrease in both the functional and total ECF volume. Restoration of shed blood after severe shock restored total ECF volume. However, only treatment with additional crystalloid solutions restored both slopes to normal. This work appeared to resolve much of the conflict between previous isotope studies.

From the beginning, Shires had claimed that these changes in ECF volume represented a shift of sodium and water into the cells during profound shock, whereas others had claimed that this shift was more apparent than real and actually reflected changes taking place in the interstitium.

It now begins to look as if there is justification for both points of view. Cunningham and Shires finally succeeded in showing both a drop in the transmembrane potential of skeletal muscle and an increase in the potassium content of microaspirates of interstitial fluid in severely shocked rats, with the change in membrane potential preceding the rise in potassium in interstitial fluid.[67] This was felt to represent primarily a depression in the activity of the cell membrane sodium pump, with the potassium shift occurring secondarily as a result of a diffusion potential. Hageberg and Haljamäe in Sweden had reached the same conclusion in a series of earlier experiments.[71] They had shown consistent decreases in the transmembrane potential in hemorrhagic shock but had been unable to show significant changes in the sodium and potassium content of skeletal muscle samples. Finally, it became apparent that if diffusion between the interstitium and the vascular compartment was extremely restricted, shifts between the intracellular and extracellular compartments could take place without being reflected in peripheral plasma samples and without being uncovered by analysis of macrotissue samples, which reflect a combination of cellular and interstitial electrolyte composition. They confirmed this suspicion by analysis of washed single cells and showed an average decrease of 26 per cent of intracellular potassium after hemorrhagic shock. Later, directly sampling nanoliter volumes of interstitial fluid, they confirmed the suspected cation shifts. They also showed that skeletal muscle cells taken from severely shocked animals were not able to reaccumulate potassium during prolonged incubation as could cells subjected to milder degrees of shock. Their studies indicated that there was something going on in the interstitial fluid or ground substance that was interfering with the movement of water or at least the diffusion of cations and anions. It is this, it appears, that is responsible for the "functional changes" in extracellular fluid volume.

Some years earlier, Moyer and Butcher, in trying to explain an apparent major expansion in the distribution space of sodium in burns, suggested that connective tissue might trap water in shock and other traumatic states.[17] They pointed out that collagen swelled whenever the pH was altered away from either of its two isoelectric points. Fulton subsequently studied subcutaneously implanted collagen strips and showed that their salt and water content increased after shock, a situation that persisted even after volume restoration.[58] Slonim and Stahl compared the sodium and water contents of cellular tissue (muscle) and connective tissue (tail) in a group of control rats, a group that was severely shocked, and a group that was moderately shocked.[158] In the severely shocked group there was an increase in sodium and water content of both cellular and noncellular tissue, but in the milder shock group these changes occurred only in the noncellular or connective tissue. As we have previously pointed out, the interstitium consists of both a ground substance and a free fluid phase. The ground substance consists of a macromolecular mesh of mucopolysaccharides in which there is "bound" water, and the free fluid phase exists between these aggregates. It has been suggested that, in addition to the homeostatic balance between the negative pressure of the sol gel and the positive pressure of the interstitial reticulum fibers, this sol-gel state can increase its "osmotic activity" in response to a number of circulating substances such

as acid metabolites, lysosomal hydrolysates and certain hormones like catecholamines, which are known to be increased in shock. Thus, one currently popular theory is that the "functional" changes in ECF volume can be blamed on changes in the sol-gel state of the interstitial tissues. Drucker's group have made some interesting empiric observations that further support this impression of a functional impairment of extracellular fluid in shock.[59] In their experiments, minute amounts of patent blue dye were injected intradermally through a 25-gauge needle, using a constant infusion pump, and the size of the dye spots was measured microscopically over extended periods of time. Migration of this dye was resolved in multi-exponential curves with two major phases. The earliest phase of dye spread was solely dependent on available free water in the tissue, that is, interstitial diffusion as opposed to capillary uptake, the latter affecting mainly the later rate of spread and disappearance. They found that both rates were reduced in severe untreated shock subjects, that the administration of blood had little benefit on interstitial diffusion but improved capillary uptake, whereas administration of salt solutions improved interstitial diffusion but, even when given in three times the volume of shed blood, did not effectively restore capillary uptake and (presumably) flow.

In summary, current thinking favors the existence of deficits in extracellular fluid volume in shock and suggests that there may be a breakdown of the cell membrane ion pump in profound or prolonged shock with a shift to sodium and water to the cells and a diffusion of potassium out of them, but that in milder degrees of hemorrhage where this shift does not occur, there are "functional" changes in extracellular fluid volume that may be related to changes in the sol-get state of the ground substance.

The Effect of Shock on the Kidney. Since 1941, when Bywaters first drew attention to the syndrome of posttraumatic renal shutdown, the effects of shock on the kidney have come under careful scrutiny.[25] The kidney's response to hypovolemia is more complex than originally thought.

One of the most striking effects of a moderate, nonshocking venous hemorrhage is the decrease in urinary excretion of both water and sodium. Farrell has demonstrated volume receptors in the right atrium that take part in this response.[53] Aldosterone appears to play an important role here, and Barter et al. have shown that phlebotomy is a potent stimulus to aldosterone release.[8] Ganong and Mulrow pointed out the importance of the intact kidney in this aldosterone response.[62] The response appears to involve the juxtaglomerular apparatus and macula densa. Renin is released at this site, and this proteolytic enzyme acts on a plasma substrate to produce angiotensin, which in turn increases the adrenocortical release of aldosterone.

Aldosterone causes active tubular reabsorption of sodium with obligatory retention of water. It is also thought to be necessary for the recruitment of intracellular water in the repartition process. In addition to this aldosterone effect, antidiuretic hormone, released by the hypothalamic-posterior-pituitary axis, effects a net retention of sodium-free water, a response that lasts as long as hypovolemia. As the hypovolemia progresses into shock, decreased glomerular filtration further reduces urinary excretion until finally, in deep shock, renal excretion comes to a standstill. However, while these renal mechanisms conserve water and reduce excretory losses, they cannot participate in the restoration of lost blood volume in the absence of increased fluid intake.[61]

In addition to these aldosterone and antidiuretic effects, Stahl observed a considerable degree of autoregulation.[160] Many of the early investigations measured total renal blood flow. However, it has become apparent that the partitioning of blood flow between the cortex and medulla plays an important role in regulating renal function. The renal responses to hypovolemia are activated before there is significant hypotension or even generalized vasoconstriction. Initially, the kidney receives an *increased* distribution of cardiac output and, in addition, maintains cortical flow by constriction of efferent arterioles. This is important not only for the maintenance of glomerular filtration but of sodium and water reabsorption. Most renal oxygen consumption takes place in the cortex, where it is utilized largely for the process of sodium resorption in the proximal convoluted tubules. This preferential support of renal cortical flow helps to maintain the osmotic gradients necessary for the countercurrent mechanism of sodium and water reabsorption, a process that has a high energy requirement and is important in combating hypovolemia.

However, in the face of greater degrees of hypotension, the kidney's share in the distribution of cardiac output abruptly drops and there is a disproportionate reduction in renal blood flow. It is reduced from almost 25 per cent of the cardiac output to 7 per cent when the blood pressure is reduced to the 40 to 60 mm. Hg range, and renal vascular resistance increases as much as sevenfold.[63] Once initiated, this renal vasoconstriction may be maintained by intrinsic mechanisms, independent of neutral and humoral control, long after hypovolemia is corrected. In studies of regional blood flow in hemorrhagic shock, Rutherford has shown that renal blood flow is the slowest organ flow to return to normal after restoration of blood volume.[141] This supports the earlier observation of Cournand et al. that renal blood flow sometimes did not return to normal in shocked patients for 12 hours after volume restoration.[35]

Thus, although renal cortical flow can be relatively well maintained in the face of moderate degrees of hypovolemia, these compensatory mechanisms do not suffice in profound or prolonged shock. Selkurt's measurements of cortical flow at this stage show that it is severely impaired.[145] Boyland and Ashauer have shown that a washout of the medullary hyperosmotic zone occurs.[22] This event is marked by sodium in the renal venous blood that exceeds that of the arterial blood and signals a breakdown of the countercurrent concentrating mechanism. Restoration of blood flow at this stage may result in inability to concentrate urine, which would explain the polyuria that sometimes follows lesser periods of shock. However, as time progresses, ischemic damage to the nephron produces renal shutdown. At one time, the more striking histological changes in the lower part of the nephron led to the impression that the damage was quite selective, hence the long-popular term "lower nephron nephrosis." Further study, aided by electron microscopic techniques, has established that the entire nephron shares the damaging effect of renal ischemia. Although this damage may be aggravated by the deposition of hemoglobin pigments in transfusion reactions, myoglobin in severe crush injuries, and a proteinaceous material under other circumstances, there is little agreement concerning the extent to which such tubular deposits are cause or effect in the renal shutdown that follows hypovolemic shock.

The Effect of Shock on the Lungs. Although a great deal of attention has been given to respiratory impairment at the cellular level, the effects of shock on the organs of respiration received little attention until the late 1960's. Since World War I, descriptions of heavy, wet, congested or hemorrhagic lungs have been given in postmortem examinations of shock victims. Since, to a certain degree, similar findings are present in 80 per cent of all autopsies, particularly in dependent areas, these observations were usually passed off as being due to a combination of prolonged recumbency and terminal congestive failure. After World War II, the term "congestive atelectasis" was used to describe the histological counterpart of this condition. More recently, many casualties of the Vietnam conflict, resuscitated by rapid transportation and aggressive intravenous therapy from what would previously have been a lethal degree of injury, were observed to develop a progressive and often lethal form of pulmonary insufficiency that did not reach full bloom until 24 to 48 hours after resuscitation. The apparent narrow margin between early death and survival without pulmonary complications may be one of the reasons this pulmonary shock lesion was not fully appreciated before. It is suspected by some that newer approaches to intravenous fluid therapy employing voluminous amounts of crystalloid solutions, particularly in association with loss of pulmonary autoregulatory mechanisms during general anesthesia or hyperventilation, may have converted a relatively innocuous lesion into a serious clinical problem. Nevertheless, there does appear to be a genuine pulmonary shock lesion. Furthermore, since similar findings associated with progressive pulmonary insufficiency have also been noted following cardiopulmonary bypass, inhalation burns, fat embolism, and other lesions, the lung appears to show a commonality of response to a wide variety of insults.

These forms of pulmonary insufficiency associated with shock, as well as trauma that is not directly inflicted on the thorax, have achieved an extremely important position in terms of incidence, morbidity and mortality in trauma victims now that improved resuscitation methods have achieved hemodynamic recovery in patients who previously would have "died in shock." This subject is dealt with in Chapter 6.

The Effects of Shock on the Liver. The liver ranks high in the chain of vital organs that maintain the organism's integrity. It is the metabolic factory and warehouse of the body. In addition, it is the clearing station for many of the body's endogenous toxins. The importance of its many functions is underscored by the early lethality of hepatectomy. It lies at the estuary of portal flow, the origins of which are that bacterial jungle, the gut. Its well-developed reticuloendothelial system reflects its function in guarding against bacterial assault from within. Finally, it has a unique mixed inflow system. Normally, the arterial inflow supplies only 40 to 50 per cent of the oxygen consumed by the liver. The portal venous blood, contributing between two thirds and four fifths of hepatic blood flow, supplies the remainder. Because the larger portion of the liver's blood and oxygen supply is subject to the physiological demands of viscera lying upstream from it, the liver is unusually susceptible to shock and hypoxia. McMichael's observation in cats is pertinent in this regard.[105] When the arterial pressure was dropped from 140 to 80 mm. Hg, the oxygen saturation in the portal vein decreased from 68 to 29 volume percentage. It is not surprising, then, that the liver has been called the body's "Achilles heel" in shock. The pathological changes observed in the livers of dogs dying after a period of hemorrhagic hypotension tend to re-enforce this suspicion. The livers are heavy and congested, and, microscopically, the sinusoids are packed with red cells. There is central necrosis in the hepatic lobules. Blood drawn from such animals prior to death shows evidence of hepatocellular damage, and levels of blood ammonia are elevated.

As previously noted, many of these changes can be explained by constriction of hepatic vein sphincters, which in the dog are well developed and very sensitive to acidosis and to certain vasoactive substances released in shock. Anatomic and hemodynamic studies of subhuman primates suggest that these sphincters are not a significant factor in humans.[120, 176] Another species difference that may play a role is the degree of bacterial contamination of the hepatic blood and bile found in the dog. These same factors may be involved in the dog's greater degree of susceptibility to acute occlusion of the hepatic artery or portal vein as well as to shock. However, regional blood flow studies show that the distribution of cardiac output to the hepatic artery increases as it does to the cerebral and coronary vessels in hemorrhagic shock, and that this greatly offsets the reduction in flow and oxygen to the liver caused by splanchnic vasoconstriction.[89] Furthermore, in the primate, splanchnic vasoconstriction is not as marked as it is in the dog, and after resuscitation there appears to be a reactive hyperemia in the liver.

Thus, there is reason to believe that the liver may play a more prominent role in the lethality of shock in dogs than it does in humans. This does not mean that hepatic damage does not contribute significantly to the late deterioration that follows protracted shock. It probably does, but convincing evidence of the significance of hepatic dysfunction in clinical shock has not been developed.

The Effect of Shock on the Gastrointestinal Tract. Striking changes in the gastrointestinal tract occur in dogs subjected to lethal degrees of hemorrhagic or endotoxin shock. There is a marked increase in the weight of the splanchnic viscera and both gross and microscopic evidence of congestion, edema and focal hemorrhage. Most impressive are the widespread foci of hemorrhagic necrosis in the intestinal mucosa. These changes have suggested that the effects of shock on the gastrointestinal tract might be a major lethal factor. Originally, hepatosplanchnic congestion was held to be responsible for the mucosal lesions. However, when provision was made for decompression of the portal system by the prior construction of a portacaval shunt,

little if any improvement was noted in the dog's response to shock. In particular, the hemorrhagic mucosal lesions still occurred.[56] On the other hand, Lillehei found that these lesions did not occur and that survival was improved if the superior mesenteric artery was selectively perfused during the shock period with oxygenated blood at normal pressures.[99] This implies that these lesions were the result of poor inflow ito the splanchnic bed rather than obstructed outflow. Since similar lesions were observed after toxic doses of epinephrine, it was surmised that prolonged vasoconstriction in the splanchnic bed was responsible.

Subsequently, Bounous et al. showed that these mucosal lesions could be prevented by giving a trypsin inhibitor or by prior ligation of the pancreatic duct.[19] They demonstrated that the mucous covering of the intestinal villi disappeared and that biosynthesis of mucin in the mucosal cells ceased during the course of hemorrhagic shock.[20] These findings suggest the possibility that, in protracted shock, either because of focal ischemia or because the high energy requirements of mucin production cannot be met, there is a loss of the protective mucous covering and the intestinal villi have no defense against intraluminal trypsin. The result is widespread hemorrhagic necrosis of the mucosa.

Darin et al. have been able to prevent these lesions in an endotoxin shock preparation by exclusion of the small intestine from the gastrointestinal stream.[50] However, pursuing this further, they found that neither diversion of pancreatic nor biliary drainage was as effective in preventing the mucosal lesions as total gastrectomy or subtotal gastrectomy with vagotomy. They also point out that all animals died regardless of the presence or absence of the intestinal lesion. Unfortunately, they used a dose of endotoxin that produced 100 per cent mortality in the controls, so that a "supralethal" dose may have obscured some degree of benefit from the prevention of hemorrhagic necrosis. Gurd et al. have also been able to prevent this lesion by hypertonic glucose instilled intraluminally.[30] This was thought to provide an available energy substrate in the face of shock.

In considering the significance of these

intestinal lesions, it must be kept in mind that they are *not* an outstanding characteristic of primate shock. However, in spite of this reservation, one cannot dismiss the possible importance of the gastrointestinal effects of shock in the human. It is still possible that a breakdown in the gastrointestinal barrier against bacteria and exogenous toxins could occur in humans without the association of the striking hemorrhagic mucosal lesions seen in dogs. This point has been made convincingly by recent studies of the back diffusion of hydrogen ion through the gastric mucosa following the ingestion of alcohol and certain drugs (e.g., aspirin, indomethacin) and following shock. As pointed out by Silen, this invisible but striking breakdown in the gastric mucosal barrier to back diffusion of hydrogen ion, combined with a concomitant release of pepsin against a background of focal ischemic necrosis, may be the common mechanism for the erosive gastritis and stress ulcers that occur under these circumstances and that, unlike the hemorrhagic enteritis of canine shock, have a very real and serious clinical counterpart.[153]

Endotoxin and Septic Shock

For many years investigators have studied experimental preparations in which shock was produced by injections of a high molecular weight phospholipid-polysaccharide-protein complex derived from the cell wall of certain gram-negative bacteria, particularly *E. coli*. This substance, called endotoxin, is generally thought to be responsible for the state of shock occasionally seen with certain clinical infections. The basis for endotoxin shock is still thought to be a hypersensitivity reaction or an accelerated Schwartzman's phenomenon. For example, the California hagfish shows no tissue response to injected antigen and is completely resistant to the lethal effects of endotoxin. The same bacteria that possess this endotoxin are commonly responsible for these infections, and the injection of this endotoxin mimics many of the changes seen clinically. Some have taken exception to this conclusion, pointing out that human septic shock is nearly always associated with a bacteremia and that certain hemodynamic parameters, particularly peripheral vascular resistance,

do not consistently follow the pattern observed after endotoxin injection. However, these difference may be explained by species differences in response to endotoxin, superimposition of endotoxemia on the dynamic picture of a systemic infection rather than the normal baseline of experimental studies and, finally, the variable release pattern of endotoxin in clinical infections compared with the single lethal dose usually used experimentally.

Using the labeled microsphere method, the author has recently shown that the hemodynamic and regional blood flow patterns, produced by a continuous infusion of *E. coli* and by an identical dose of endotoxin from the same bacteria at progressive stages of shock, were qualitatively indistinguishable from each other,[143] proving that endotoxin alone will reproduce the hemodynamic events of bacteremic shock.

The Effects of Shock on Bacterial Defense Mechanisms. There seems to be little doubt that the body's bacterial defense mechanisms are profoundly impaired in shock. Impressive laboratory evidence of this has nurtured the idea that an overwhelming endotoxemia is the essence of irreversible shock regardless of the participating cause. However, until recently, the mechanisms themselves have not been studied in detail.

Olledart and Mansberger have presented evidence indicating that this impairment is due to a combination of reduced opsonization, decreased contact time between the bacterium and the phagocyte and reduced phagocytic ability.[123]

Complement, which is a complex system of at least six components, sensitizes the bacterium and facilitates contact between it and the natural antibody. This process, called opsonization, appears to injure the bacterium and render it less resistant to phagocytosis. Contact between the sensitized bacteria and phagocytes takes place largely in the reticuloendothelial system, the greater portion of which lies in hepatosplanchnic viscera, which in turn are particularly poorly perfused in shock. Not only does this circulatory impairment afford less opportunity for the reticuloendothelial system to make contact with bacteria but the phagocytic cells themselves are damaged. These authors also noted that all three phases of antibacterial activity were even further impaired by transfusions of homologous (ACD) bank blood.

Pagano and Mersheimer have studied the immunologic response to shock.[125] They found a fall in complement, and elevation of lysosome enzymes in the serum, the formation of substances that increase capillary permeability and the appearance of an abnormal toxic immunoprotein which suggested that an autologous immunotoxic reaction occurs. They point out that soluble antigen antibody complexes, which utilize complement in forming this abnormal immunoprotein, are found in old nonfrozen serum, which may explain Olledart's observation on the effects of blood transfusion.

Conceding that the antibacterial defense mechanisms are significantly impaired in these and other experimental shock models, one cannot freely extrapolate these observations to the clinical counterpart since, as Zweifach has pointed out, marked species differences exist in bacterial flora, sensitivity to bacterial products, the target organ in endotoxemia, functional capacities of the reticuloendothelial system, opsonizing ability and the ability to develop tolerance.[185]

Hemodynamic Changes in Endotoxin and Septic Shock. After the injection of endotoxin there is a sudden fall in blood pressure. In a dog there is a moderate drop in plasma volume with a marked decrease in venous return. Although the heart is not immune to the effects of endotoxin, most of the circulatory changes appear to be related to peripheral effects. The decrease in venous return is due primarily to pooling in the hepatosplanchnic bed. This is caused by constriction of hepatic vein sphincters from histamine released by endotoxin. Wide species variations in the regional distribution of histamine and in the development of hepatic vein sphincters partly explain species variations in the hemodynamic responses to the injection of endotoxin. However, most of the other species differences appear to be quantitative rather than qualitative. Thomas et al. have shown that injections of viable washed *E. coli* and injections of *E. coli* endotoxin each produce similar hemodynamic responses (to each other) in dogs and in monkeys.[170] The author[143] has shown this to be true for regional blood flow patterns as well.

After the initial hypotensive response to endotoxin injection, the blood pressure is returned toward normal by the pressor effect of released catecholamines. Then, depending on the lethality of the dose given, it will either be maintained or gradually decline again as the animal sinks into a state of profound and lethal shock, which is virtually indistinguishable from the refractory stages of shock from hemorrhage or other causes. The intense vasoconstriction wanes as catecholamine activity is overshadowed by the effects of histamine and vasoactive polypeptides.[169] Vasomotor tone collapses with peripheral pooling, loss of effective circulating blood volume and increased capillary permeability and loss of fluid into the extravascular space. That some of this vasomotor collapse may be intrinsic, secondary to damage to vascular smooth muscle, is suggested by the electron microscopic studies of Ashford.[4]

It has previously been mentioned that the hepatosplanchnic pooling that characterizes the canine response to endotoxin is comparatively insignificant in the monkey.[176] In addition, the marked increase in peripheral resistance observed in the dog is not found in the cat or monkey. These species differences have been used to explain dissimilarities between experimental endotoxin shock preparations and the clinical picture of septic shock. However, there is even a disagreement about what hemodynamic changes are characteristic of septic shock in the human. Originally, clinical septic shock was thought to be a problem of vasomotor collapse with peripheral pooling of blood. Udhoji and Weil, in a careful hemodynamic study of six patients, suggested that this was due not to arteriolar dilatation but to failure of venous return secondary to changes in the venous or capacitance sphincters.[172] On the other hand, most of the patients studied by Thal and Wilson showed a normal blood volume and decreased peripheral resistance but an increased cardiac index.[168] It is apparent that the hemodynamic picture is quite variable. This may be the result of differences in the state of the circulation imposed by the underlying infection prior to the onset of septic shock. Siegel and Del Guercio's study has documented the correlation of this variability with cardiac output and the degree of pulmonary and systemic arteriovenous "shunting" with many patients exhibiting a syndrome of high output circulatory failure.[152]

MacLean et al. described four different groups of septic shock patients by arbitrarily separating 56 consecutive cases according to whether they had a high or low central venous pressure (CVP) and whether they were alkalotic or acidotic.[104] Half the patients fell into Group 1 with a high CVP and a normal or high pH. Twenty-four of these survived their shock episode. The patients in this group were thought to represent the typical early septic shock picture, characterized by hyperventilation and respiratory alkalosis and a high CVP, high cardiac index, and low peripheral resistance with warm, dry skin in the face of hypotension, oliguria and lactacidemia. In the second group of 11 patients with a high CVP and acidosis, only one survived. These patients showed the same hyperdynamic circulatory state but were thought to have become acidotic, because even their increased cardiac output was insufficient to meet the increased circulatory demands of their septic state. Pulmonary edema was a prominent additional feature in this group, and it did not respond to conventional therapy. In Group 3, there were 10 patients with a low CVP and a normal or high pH. Nine of these were resuscitated from shock. These patients were relatively hypovolemic and responded to intravenous fluids. The fourth group were acidotic with a low CVP and all seven died. The authors suggested that the variable patterns described in previous studies of septic shock were related to two factors, the relative ability of the heart to meet the increased circulatory demands placed on it and the patient's state of hydration or blood volume. Half of the patients who died were unable to raise their cardiac outputs. The authors suggested that the other half who died in spite of a supranormal cardiac output must have succumbed for one of three reasons: (1) their cardiac output was still not sufficient to meet the increased needs of the body, (2) enough oxygen and metabolites were not reaching the vital tissues because of arteriovenous shunting or (3) there was a failure of tissue utilization of the oxygen and nutrients delivered to it because of deteriorization or death of the cells.

Siegel et al. reported similar findings in comparing a series of septic shock patients with those suffering from other forms of shock.[151] They pointed out that all patients in septic shock, regardless of cause or bacterial etiology, have a significantly decreased vascular tone as compared to nonseptic shock patients. That is, at a given systemic flow rate, the vascular resistance is less in septic shock than in other forms of shock, a relationship that holds true over the entire range of cardiac outputs. They also noted signs of anaerobic metabolism in spite of high cardiac outputs. Patients with septic shocks showed a different pattern of effectiveness of their oxygen transport mechanisms in that oxygen consumption varied independently of cardiac index. The hyperdynamic or high output failure patients with septic shock exhibited very inefficient oxygen extraction. To achieve a normal oxygen consumption, they required two to four times the cardiac output needed by normal patients. Those patients with septic shock and a small cardiac output had oxygen transport patterns that were similar to those of nonseptic shock patients. Finally, every patient they studied with septic shock had a diminished ventricular function relationship, in that the relationship between stroke work and venous pressure was decreased. The high cardiac output cases obviously had a better ventricular function than those with low cardiac output, but the eventual incidence of myocardial failure was equal in both groups.

The Endotoxin Theory of Irreversible Shock. The possibility that overwhelming endotoxemia might be the final common denominator in irreversible shock, regardless of the precipitating factor, has been suggested by Fine.[134] Attention was initially attracted to this possibility by the strikingly similar pathologic changes in the hepatosplanchnic bed in dogs subjected to hemorrhagic shock and those given lethal injections of endotoxin. Since the splanchnic viscera represent a major interface of bacterial growth with the body's defense mechanisms, it was suggested that, in severe shock of any origin, the reticuloendothelial system — which normally detoxifies any endotoxin that might be absorbed from bacteria in the gut — may be rendered ineffective, resulting in an overwhelming endotoxemia. Evidence was presented in support of this contention. The toxicity of blood taken from animals suffering from irreversible hemorrhagic shock suggested a transferable factor. It was shown that there was a decreased tolerance to hemorrhage after blockade of the reticuloendothelial system, and that increased tolerance could be achieved by multiple sublethal doses of endotoxin. Experiments in the same laboratory showed that sterilization of the gut gave a significant degree of protection against the lethality of hemorrhagic shock. Finally, support can be drawn from the growing evidence that the body's antibacterial defense mechanisms are greatly impaired in hemorrhagic shock[123] and from the demonstration of Bounous and associates of the breakdown of the integrity of the mucosal barrier of the gut in shock.[19, 20]

Nevertheless, formidable barriers were raised against the acceptance of this theory. First, both Lillehei and Simeone failed to confirm whether or not there was a protective effect of gut sterilization against the lethality of hemorrhagic shock.[99, 154] Secondly, McNulty and Linares showed that germ-free rats were no more tolerant of hemorrhagic shock than littermates reared in a contaminated environment.[106] In rebuttal, Fine has dismissed the failure of others to confirm his observations on the benefit of gut sterilization as the result of technical differences. He points out that even germ-free animals eat food that has ample quantities of dead bacteria in it. Furthermore, workers in his laboratory feel they have been able to detect circulating endotoxin in hemorrhagic shock by indirect assay. Although some workers have confirmed these findings in dogs, others have not. There have been no confirmatory studies in primates. Specifically, Herman et al.[78] conducted serial assays for endotoxin on portal, right atrial and aortic blood samples in awake restrained baboons who were either resuscitated or allowed to remain hypotensive until death. Endotoxemia was found to be infrequent and was no more frequent in portal than in systemic blood; there was no difference in frequency in preshock, early shock or late shock samples. Finally the author,[140] in studying the hemodynamic and regional blood flow patterns at three equivalent stages of endotoxin and hemorrhagic shock in monkeys, found that while the early stages were strikingly different from each other, by the late terminal stage the hemodynamic and regional blood flow patterns were identical. However, more importantly, the final pattern bore no resemblance to that seen in the earlier stages of either endotoxin or hemorrhagic shock, suggesting that some common vasoactive humoral factor or factors not present in significant amounts earlier in shock predominated at this final stage.

As this controversy continues without clear-cut victory for either side, much valuable information is being gained about the effects of endotoxin. Evidence has been presented that many of the effects of endotoxin may be mediated through the nervous system. Penner and Bernheim found that one twentieth of the intravenous lethal dose would be fatal if injected into the third ventricle.[128]

There is also evidence that the lethal effects of endotoxin are largely due to a direct action on the cell. Simeone feels that, in endotoxin shock, tissue damage occurs at the outset in contradistinction to other types of shock, in which it occurs as the late effect of inadequate tissue perfusion.[155] Thal et al. feel that endotoxin might interfere directly with the intracellular enzyme systems involved in aerobic metabolism.[167] Bell and Schloerb have shown a relatively greater fall in intracellular pH in endotoxin shock than in hemorrhagic shock.[13] Rush has even noted acidosis following doses of endotoxin so small that hypotension was not provoked.[139] More will be said of the effects of endotoxin on the cell later in this chapter.

Vasoactive Substances in Shock

The control of flow through the peripheral circulation in shock is a complex process. Peripheral resistance reflects the summation of intrinsic, neural and humoral vasomotor adjustment to changes in cardiac output and blood volume. It is difficult if not impossible to isolate their relative contributions. This difficulty is exemplified by attempts to separate the effects of the sympathetic neurohumoral axis that are mediated by catecholamines released from the adrenal medulla from those of the sympathetic nerve endings. If a sympathectomy is done, the sensitivity of effector sites to centrally released catecholamines is heightened. If the adrenals are removed, cortical as well as medullary function is eliminated.

Equally difficult is the attempt to estimate the relative contributions of vasoactive humoral agents in shock. This is compounded by species variations in both sensitivity to these substances and the pattern of end organ response. Understandably, the study of vasoactive substances in human shock has been limited.

Peripheral blood levels of these substances do not necessarily reflect their activity. A substance may be released, exert its effects locally and be quickly degraded without attaining a significant elevation in its peripheral level. On the other hand, the action of one of these substances may be blocked by drugs or other agents so that their effect may be minimal in spite of high circulating levels.

Some vasoactive substances, such as epinephrine and serotonin, can produce different, even opposite, effects at different dosage levels or in the face of differences in existing vasomotor tone. Furthermore, many of these agents act on the same receptor site. Finally, one must also consider the influence of background factors, such as pH, the concentration of certain electrolytes and the sensitivity of the end organ.

These limitations should be kept in mind during the following discussion of the effects of these vasoactive agents in shock.

Catecholamines. Properly defined, catecholamines are any low molecular weight substances combining a catechol nucleus and an amine group, but the term is usually reserved for dopamine and its metabolic end products, norepinephrine and epinephrine. They are synthesized in the brain, in the chromaffin cells of the adrenal medulla and at sympathetic nerve endings from tyrosine. In addition to tissues that can synthesize catecholamine, many other tissues are capable of removing it from the circulation and storing it. The synthesis, release, breakdown and degradation of catecholamines as well as other pertinent details of their metabolism have been fully reviewed by Wurtman.[183]

The actions of the catecholamines are variable. Attempts have been made to organize their effects in terms of alpha and beta receptors. These may not be receptors in the usual physiologic sense but rather key enzymatic processes. Sutherland and Rall have presented evidence suggesting that the beta receptor may be the cyclizing enzyme that catalyzes the conversion of ATP to cyclic 3,5-adenosine monophosphate (3,5-AMP), a key reaction in the hormonal control of certain energy systems.

Epinephrine appears to act predominantly on the beta receptor when given in small doses, whereas at higher doses, its alpha effects predominate. Norepinephrine also has both alpha and beta effects, although the alpha effects predominate at all doses. The most important expression of alpha activity is the excitation of smooth muscle, particularly vascular smooth muscle. Beta stimulation, on the other hand, produces an inotropic and chronotropic effect on the heart, a mobilization of glucose from glycogen stores and free fatty acid from adipose tissue, a release of ACTH and relaxation of smooth muscle. Thus, the overall hemodynamic effects of catecholamine release depend on the relative levels of epinephrine and norepinephrine. When the alphamimetic effects predominate, there is an increased arteriolar tone, venous pooling and bradycardia, whereas the betamimetic effects lead to decreased arteriolar constriction and an increase in heart rate and stroke volume. These usually act in combination, and the differences in end organ sensitivity to each provide a selective hemodynamic response.

Thus, the usual effects of combined catecholamine activity are an increase in blood flow to the heart, brain and striated muscle and a decrease in the flow to the skin, splanchnic viscera and kidney, just what one would expect from the "flight or fight" function of the sympathetic nervous system. In hemorrhagic shock, the regional blood flow pattern is thought to be influenced by catecholamine release, but it differs slightly from that described above in that flow to striated muscle is diminished and splanchnic vasoconstriction is partly compensated for by an increased distribution of cardiac output through the hepatic artery.

In experimental shock preparations, high catecholamine levels are found in the blood. Since high doses of norepinephrine can produce pathologic changes identical to those seen with lethal degrees of endotoxin or hemorrhagic shock, some have contended that it is the excessive and prolonged catecholamine activity that causes the irreversible effects of shock. Although the deleterious effects of excessive catecholamine activity are not challenged, most feel that inadequate tissue perfusion of any cause will lead to the same end result. Furthermore, alpha blocking agents given in the refractory stages of shock are not protective. Indeed, late in hemorrhagic shock there appears to be a profound loss of vasomotor tone[141] and, in endotoxin shock at least, 80 per cent of the vasoactivity at the stage appears to be derived from histamine and vasoactive polypeptides.[93] The central point in this debate is whether catecholamine activity is physiologic and reversible or excessive and self-perpetuating. On this there is no general agreement.

Histamine. In 1912 Dale and Richards discovered that histamine was a vasodilator that increased tissue permeability and, when given to cats in large doses, produced severe hypotension.[42] When the experiments of Cannon and Bayliss shortly after this suggested a toxemic basis for traumatic shock, histamine became a prime suspect.[27] The initial hypotensive episode that follows the injection of endotoxin in dogs has been shown to be due to hepatosplanchnic pooling secondary to the effect of histamine on hepatic vein sphincters. It can be mimicked by histamine injection, prevented by prior histamine depletion, and blocked by Dibenzyline administration.[80]

Thal and his associates have studied the pattern of histamine activity after both endotoxin and exotoxin injection.[93] After the initial peak there is a secondary rise late in the course of the shock, at which time histamine and vasoactive polypeptides contribute most of the total vasoactivity. Thal has also shown that endotoxin releases histamine in vivo and, if first incubated with blood or tissue homogenates, releases it in vitro as well. He found the tissues that liberate the largest amount of histamine are the liver, pancreas and upper small intestine and that greater amounts of histamine are released after portal injections of endotoxin than after systemic injections. Hepatectomy and evisceration experiments suggest that the initial peak of histamine is caused by release mainly from the hepatosplanchnic bed, whereas the terminal rise results from slower biosynthesis in other tissues. Schayer's experiments have suggested to him that the local synthesis of histamine by histidine decarboxylase may, in balance with the catecholamines, exert a controlling influence on the microcirculation.[144]

The loss of arteriolar resistance, increased capillary permeability and persistent venous sphincter tone, which are thought to be characteristic of the late stages of shock in the dog, have been explained by some as indicating a predominance of histamine over catecholamines at this point. Thal's assays of histamine and catecholamine activity injection are compatible with this contention. The work of Visscher and associates suggests that the increased capillary permeability from histamine may be the result of postcapillary venular spasm alone.[175] However, it must be remembered that this impression of histamine's effect on the venous outflow sphincters has been derived mainly from canine experiments. As shown by Brockman and Vasko and Waldhausen et al., these changes are much less marked in subhuman primates.[23, 176] Histamine stores in primates also differ in amount (less) and pattern of distribution from dogs. Thus, while the role of histamine in human shock is still unsettled, its importance appears to be waning.

Serotonin. 5-Hydroxytryptamine, or serotonin, is widely distributed throughout the body and is particularly abundant in the brain, upper small intestine, platelets and mast cells. Elevations in circulating serotonin levels have been demonstrated in both experimental and clinical shock studies. Serotonin is capable of amphibaric effects. It may raise or lower the blood pressure under different circumstances, usually acting in opposition to the existing direction of change. Its contribution to total vasoactivity in the canine endotoxin shock studies of Thal was definitely less than histamine. One of the areas in which serotonin has been suspected of contributing most to the pathogenesis of shock is the pulmonary circulation. Serotonin greatly increases pulmonary vascular resistance and, unlike a similar response to histamine, this is independent of any bronchoconstrictive effects.[115] It has been suggested that the *drop* in peripheral resistance and the narrowing of arteriovenous oxygen differences seen late in shock may represent the opening of arteriovenous shunts secondary to serotonin release, similar to the effect described in the carcinoid flush.[14]

However, the evidence that serotonin exerts a *significant* systemic hemodynamic effect in shock is not substantial. Nevertheless, at a local level, the release of serotonin from injured platelets may play an important role in the clotting and constriction of injured vessels. In addition, the tendency for platelet aggregation after trauma may be the result of serotonin release.[165]

Vasoactive Polypeptides. Recent years have witnessed a growing interest in certain plasma polypeptides possessing powerful vasoactive properties. This began with Werle's work on a hypotensive proteolytic substance derived from the pancreas.[181] This substance, called kallikrein, was first thought to exert its effect directly, but further research has established that it activated polypeptides from their precursors in the plasma or the pancreas, probably through another enzyme system, the kinases. Trypsin and other proteolytic enzymes also appear capable of activating these kinin peptides and, in turn, along with kallikrein, these proteases may be activated by Hageman factor, plasmin and possibly endotoxin. With the uncovering of this complex system of interacting enzymes, there has been a renewed interest in the pathogenesis of shock resulting from pancreatitis and endotoxemia.

The best known of the kinin peptides is bradykinin, a nonapeptide whose amino acid sequence has been determined. It is known to produce vasodilation, smooth muscle relaxation, increased capillary permeability, leukocytic infiltration and pain, all of which are interrelated, suggesting that bradykinin may be the mediator of the local inflammatory response and an important factor in local microcirculatory control in other situations. In comparative tests it is a more potent universal vasodilator than histamine.

Bradykinin release has been detected in both experimental and clinical shock studies.[90, 94] In hemorrhagic shock, bradykininogen levels rose initially and then fell below control levels.[45] Kobold, Thal and associates have compared the relative contributions of vasoactive polypeptides and catecholamines, histamine and serotonin to total vasoactivity at different stages of endotoxin shock using a strip of ox carotid.[94] Their studies suggest that these vasoactive polypeptides, along with histamine, contribute heavily late in shock.

The hyperdynamic circulatory state seen in early septic shock and in the late refractory stages of shock of other etiologies is compatible with, and suggestive of, the systemic effects of kinins on the circulation. However, the role of these peptides in the pathogenesis of these shock states has been generally downgraded because their supposed short half-life had relegated them, in the thinking of most investigators, to only a local humoral role. And yet, the demonstration that the hypotensive reponse to intravenous bradykinin in the rat was only one fiftieth that of an aortic injection[54] led to the realization that the apparent minor systemic effect of intravenous bradykinin and its presumed short half-life are due to its extremely effective (90 to 98 per cent) breakdown during passage through the lungs by a system of pulmonary kininases suspected of being located in the pinocytotic vesicles directly under the pulmonary capillary endothelium.[129]

The enzymes in these vesicles are depleted in the lungs of animals subjected to shock and it is known that the pulmonary kininase system is subject to tachyphylaxis and can be overwhelmed by larger doses of bradykinin.[14] Acute pulmonary edema can be produced in normal rats by this means. Furthermore, the electron microscopic appearance of tissues perfused with kinins is not unlike that demonstrated for shock lung, with opening up of the septa between endothelial cells, pouring out of plasma and large protein molecules into the interstitial space, and other such effects.[166] Bradykinin is more powerful than either histamine or serotonin in producing these tissue changes. Finally, the demonstrated protection from "shock lung" by hilar cross-clamping during shock[182] and the sparing of the downstream lung of two lungs perfused in series from a similar pulmonary lesion produced by extracorporeal perfusion with autologous blood[159] could be blamed equally well on circulating humoral substances as on microemboli or fat emboli.

It has been demonstrated in experimental shock that lysosomal disruption occurs and lysosomal products have been revealed in the peripheral circulation in both experimental and clinical shock.[102, 135] Kinin-forming enzymes in the tissues are lysosomal in origin with optimal activity in the lower pH range seen in shock, whereas kinin inhibitors or kininases are less efficient at these pH's. These factors suggest the possibility that significant amounts of vasoactive polypeptides may be released during shock and eventually may not only contribute significantly to the pathogenesis of shock lung but, having overwhelmed or bypassed the pulmonary kininase system, may reach the systemic arterial circulation in increasing amounts and contribute to the hyperdynamic circulatory failure that characterizes refractory stages of some types of clinical shock. At the moment this is merely conjecture or at best circumstantial evidence that must await proper clinical investigation.

Another vasoactive polypeptide, apparently unrelated to the kinins, has recently been brought to the forefront of shock research. It is called MDF, or myocardial depressant factor. Although a similar substance was identified earlier by Brandt et al. as a vasodepressor factor following declamping shock, its role in the pathogenesis of shock has been mainly elaborated by the work of Lefer and his associates.[96] Brand and Lefer originally identified this substance in the plasma of cats after severe hemorrhagic shock. Plasma samples were shown to decrease the developed tension of isolated cat papillary muscles, and this has remained the basis for its bioassay. High activities of plasma cathepsinlike substances appearing in the blood prior to increased levels of MDF suggested that the appearance of MDF may be related to enzymatic cleavage of plasma proteins by proteases. MDF has since been found in the plasma of animals subjected to hemorrhagic shock, pancreatitis, endotoxin shock, splanchnic ischemia and cardiogenic shock. Lovett et al. studied the plasma of 24 patients for the myocardial depressant factor; 14 of the patients were in severe shock and 10 were controls.[102] A significantly higher plasma MDF level and lysosomal enzyme activities were present in the plas-

ma of patients with circulatory shock. In 10 of 14 there was evidence of impaired myocardial function at the time the specimen was obtained.

In spite of this suggested information, the relative importance of MDF in the pathogenesis of irreversible shock has not been established, particularly since in many other similar shock preparations in other laboratories, alterations in myocardial contractility have not been considered a significant finding. Greenfield et al. performed cross-circulation experiments between normal isolated hearts in dogs in terminal shock, 18 to 21 hours after administration of endotoxin.[66] The cross-circulation was carried out for a period of 3 hours and compared to control animals studied similarly but without endotoxin administration. Isometric cardiac performance (measured by intraventricular balloon distention) was *not* impaired in the endotoxin group, which actually showed consistently better time-tension curves and pressure work than control animals. No alteration in force-velocity curves was noted in either group. Increases in both oxygen uptake and pressure work in the endotoxin group indicated no changes in calculated myocardial efficiency. The conclusion of these investigators was that no deleterious effect on the normal heart perfused with blood from a dog in terminal endotoxin shock could be demonstrated to substantiate the primary role suggested for the myocardial depressant factor.

More damning has been the report by one of Lefer's former co-workers that plasma MDF has been identified as salt and represents an artifact of the bioassay system, and that its depressant activity plays no significant role in shock.[177] However, Lefer and Inge[95] reported that MDF was eluted *prior* to salt in the Biogel P–2 column, and that the amount of salt required to produce the negative inotropic effect reported for MDF would be 450 mEq/l. Following this, Lefer's laboratory claims to have not only identified but also synthesized MDF. Nevertheless, the inability to show myocardial depressant activity late in shock in intact hearts with experimental preparations which were specifically designed to detect it suggests to the authors that the significance of MDF may have been unwittingly magnified by the sensitivity of the bioassay method employed to detect it.

Angiotensin. Angiotensin is a potent vasoactive octapeptide formed by the action of the renal protease renin on the plasma precursor angiotensinogen. Its hemodynamic effects are essentially the reverse of bradykinin. It is a more potent and universal vasoconstrictor than norepinephrine. Evidence from human and animal studies suggests that angiotensin increases vascular resistance by constricting artiolar sphincters, without the degree of postcapillary resistance seen with norepinephrine.[101] Thus, it has been suggested that angiotensin reduces capillary hydrostatic pressure and allows rather than retards transcapillary plasma refilling. This impression that angiotensin may support the blood pressure more physiologically has led to its evaluation as a therapeutic agent for hypotensive states with conflicting conclusions that may eventually be resolved by establishment of proper dosage levels.

At present, there is not enough information to allow firm conclusions to be drawn about the natural or therapeutic role angiotensin plays in various shock states. Its relationship to aldosterone production has been discussed earlier in this chapter.

Prostaglandins. Prostaglandins are a family of structurally related, hormone-like substances with extremely powerful activity effecting a wide range of physiological processes. Many of the prostaglandins have marked hemodynamic effects, and it is understandable that they are suspected of playing a role in the pathogenesis of refractory shock. Prostaglandin concentrations (PGE_2 and PGF_{2a}) have been found to be elevated above basal levels in both hemorrhagic and endotoxin shock, and in the absence of evidence of their decreased degradation they are presumed to reflect increased synthesis or release.[55] The renal prostaglandin, PGA, is a potent vasodilator and has been shown to decrease peripheral resistance and cardiac output.[126] Indomethacin, also a prostaglandin inhibitor, has been shown to ameliorate aortic declamping shock. Nevertheless, all data that have been gathered to date have been such suggestive but flimsy bits of circumstantial evidence that, at the moment, there is no proof that their action is anything other than physiologic in facilitating the actions of hormones and nerves at the common interface of the cell membrane.

The Effects of Shock on the Cell and on Metabolism

As stated earlier, the decreased arteriovenous oxygen differences that characterize the hyperdynamic circulatory failure of late shock could be due to a circulatory system driven beyond the perfusion demands of the tissues, opening of arteriovenous shunts, abnormalities in oxygen transport, or the inability of dead, dying or deranged cells to utilize oxygen. There is a growing conviction that the latter is the case, and in the final analysis, mortality is determined at a cellular level. More is implied by this than simply an equation of cellular death with its summation or the death of the whole organism. Rather it is felt, and from a therapeutic standpoint hoped, that some discrete form of cellular damage or dysfunction is *primarily* responsible for the refractory state that develops in protracted shock. This view is most plausible for endotoxin shock, in which, as outlined in the preceding section, there is evidence for a direct, early toxic effect on the cell.

If the functional and structural integrity of the cell is to be maintained, it must be able to generate energy. This requires access to both oxygen and nutrients. Most of the energy generated by the cell is captured in the terminal phosphate bond ($\sim p$) of adenosine triphosphate (ATP), although considerable storage capacity is provided by the transfer of this terminal phosphate bond to creatinine. Ninety per cent of the $\sim p$ is generated aerobically and captured by a most efficient energy trapping system, a chain of flavoproteins and cytochrome oxidases called the "respiratory enzymes." At each level $\sim p$'s are generated until the two hydrogen atoms are finally united with oxygen to form water. Essentially, all the energy captured by this system is derived from the reactions of the Krebs cycle into which acetyl CoA (the two-carbon unit of carbohydrate), fat and protein breakdown are fed. This highly organized process operates wholly within the mitochondria and in the presence of oxygen.

The cell performs many functions on its

own behalf that require this energy. The sodium ion pump that maintains membrane potential and permeability and the active transport of certain substances across the cell membrane and between the cytoplasm and the mitochondria and other components of cell ultrastructure are prime examples of this. In addition, the survival of the organism as a whole depends on such specialized, energy-dependent, cellular functions as the contraction of cardiac, smooth and striated muscle, the transmission of nerve impulses, the metabolic activity of hepatic cells, the refining of urine by the kidney's countercurrent multiplier sodium pump system and the production of mucin, surfactant and various exocrine and endocrine substances.

The importance of continued energy production by the cell seems obvious. If the hallmark of metabolism following trauma is an increased metabolic rate and catabolism, shock places added demands on the organism by interfering with the metabolic pathways that are most propitious for meeting such energy demands. However, this does not necessarily mean that energy depletion is *the* critical factor in the outcome of shock.

The natural suspect as the main cause for the breakdown in cellular metabolism is, of course, an inadequate oxygen supply to the cell. If oxygen is no longer available to accept the hydrogen atoms at the end of the respiratory enzyme chain, this system will grind to a halt, forcing the cell to utilize anaerobic pathways, which are a rather limited source of energy. Anaerobic metabolism produces only 2 moles of ATP for every mole of glucose, compared to 38 moles of ATP generated by complete passage through aerobic pathways. Although a switch to anaerobic metabolism is characteristic of shock states, the explanation seems to be more complex than the unavailability of oxygen. Oxygen consumption appears to be normal until the terminal phase of shock and, although oxygen availability may be reduced, some oxygen must be available to the tissues.

Nevertheless, a switch to anaerobic glycolysis does occur relatively early in shock. Shumer has shown, by studying the relative amounts of ^{14}C-labeled glucose that appeared downstream in metabolic intermediates, that a metabolic block appeared

in shocked animals between pyruvate and acetyl CoA.[149] However, the failure of hyperbaric oxygen therapy at this point in shock would also suggest that cellular dysfunction has occurred that prevents utilization of oxygen.[84]

It has been suggested that the *acidosis that develops during shock has an adverse effect on cell function.* As shock deepens and the cell turns more and more to anaerobic glycolysis, pyruvate is converted to lactate rather than being processed through the Krebs cycle. Huckabee has shown that the excess accumulation of lactate is a fairly sensitive index of cellular hypoxia, a phenomenon long known by the name of "oxygen debt."[83] However, this metabolic acidosis is initially compensated for by hyperventilation so that the pH of *peripheral arterial blood* may even suggest an alkalosis. Studies of combat casualties in Vietnam[31, 32] and civilian clinical investigations[9] have indicated that in healthy young subjects (and when hemorrhage is not too rapid or hypotension too prolonged) acidosis is *not* a regular accompaniment of shock. In fact, hyperventilation will usually have caused some degree of alkalosis. Recent primate shock studies,[141] in contrast to earlier canine studies, have shown that periods of hemorrhagic hypotension, sufficiently profound and prolonged to be lethal, may not be associated with acidosis until the terminal phase. Nevertheless, even in these situations the venous pH is usually quite low, suggesting a masked, concomitant metabolic acidosis.

To a degree, acidosis has a homeostatic value. It facilitates the release of oxygen and the uptake of carbon dioxide in the tissues, increases the coagulability of blood, and results in increases in respiratory rate, cerebral circulation and arterial pressure.

However, *profound* degrees of acidosis have been shown to decrease myocardial contractility, to decrease the vasomotor response to humoral agents, and, in dogs, to produce a constriction of venous (capacitance) sphincters. More telling may be its effects inside the cell. It may interfere with cellular metabolism if the pH is lowered beyond the optimum range of key intracellular enzymes.

Some experiments have shown beneficial effects in shock from buffering therapy, using sodium bicarbonate or the buffer amine, trishydroxymethanolamine. Like most therapeutic measures claiming success in the treatment of experimental shock, this benefit is not significant once a stage of recognizable "irreversibility" has been reached. However, buffering seems to result in improved urinary output[121] and an amelioration of clotting abnormalities in shocked animals[142] and, in combination with increased oxygen delivery, to improve survival.[108]

It has been known since Claude Bernard's experimental observations in 1877 that the blood sugar became elevated in shock. This was eventually attributed to the hepatic glycogen mobilization effect of catecholamine release, although Carey's work suggests that the initial hyperglycemia is not simply an epinephrine effect.[40] After an initial increase, probably from the release of preformed insulin, the insulin response to this hyperglycemia appears to be depressed, probably as a result of severely reduced pancreatic blood flow. Coran's studies suggest that the hypotensive baboon is both physiologically and immunochemically insulin-deficient.[34] On the other hand, in milder degrees of shock, as in volunteers to hemorrhage by Skillman, insulin production may even be increased.[157] In any event, in late shock hypoglycemia intervenes and is characteristic of the terminal state. However, infusions of hypertonic glucose at *this* stage of shock have no effect on the outcome or even the hemodynamic picture.

Glucose makes a relatively greater contribution to total body energy in shock and trauma, but, as in the normotensive state, fatty acids still constitute the main circulating energy source. Like glucose, fatty acids are mobilized and released in response to epinephrine. It would appear from Drucker's work that the changes in the peripheral levels of glucose and fatty acids in response to hemorrhagic shock depend on the rapidity and depth of the hemorrhage.[52] With slow hemorrhage, plasma-free fatty acids increased intially and then decreased later as hyperglycemia developed. However, if the volume loss was rapid enough, hyperglycemia occurred early and free fatty acids decreased. As pointed out by Cahill, a labile protein pool exists and provides the body requirements for glucose when glycogen stores are depleted.[47] But all protein, in contrast to fats, exists in the body for a purpose, so there is no expendable depot of nitrogen.

Once the essential nutrients become unavailable and the cell's energy stores are depleted, the cell is forced, in a sense, to turn on itself for other sources of energy. Steinberg has shown that cells may survive for up to 2 hours with no external source of nutrients.[161] However, in doing so, they penalize themselves, since *structural phospholipids* are one of the major components depleted by this effort.

Loss of the structural integrity of the cell membrane and ultrastructure has important consequences beyond those of increased permeability. The mitochondrial apparatus may not be able to function if the intricate structural and spatial arrangements of its enzyme network are disrupted, preventing enzymes involved in a chain of related biochemical reactions from "getting together." Structural changes in the mitochondria have been demonstrated by electron microscopic techniques in the tissues of animals subjected to shock or hypoxia.[5, 164] Others have reported only mitochondrial swelling, but even this may interfere with function. Thus, it is possible that the configurational templates that are felt to be so vital for molecular synthesis might be disrupted and the maintenance of ion gradients and the active transport of substances vital to cell life are no longer possible.

Disruption of the limiting membranes of the *lysosomes* inside the cell is one of the more interesting recent proposals. These subcellular structures are thought to play a protective role by isolating the cell from essential but potentially destructive enzymes such as proteases, esterases, hydrolases and phosphatases. The works of DeDuve have drawn attention to this possibility, and indeed the lysosomal apparatus has been considered the cell's "suicide sac."[43] Lysosomes appear to be disrupted when the cell is subjected to anoxic injury, and the appearance of proteolytic enzymes in the peripheral circulation in certain shock states may be a reflection of this. Their release may in turn activate the kinase system, with the release of vasoactive polypeptides and the initiation of intravascular clotting.

Mela et al. have observed lysosomal derangements following endotoxin injection.[111] Lefer et al. have shown increased cathepsin-like activity in association with increased myocardial depressant factor in shock.[96] On the other hand, Shumer could not show lysosomal enzymes in circulating blood after hemorrhagic shock.[150]

Janoff et al. have shown that graded injury (drum shock), and Weissmann and Thomas that steroids may increase the resistance of lysosomes to rupture.[85, 180] The acquired tolerance to shock and the beneficial effects of steroids may have some foundation in these observations.

The question has been raised whether, in

shock, there is a weak link in the chain of intracellular enzymes that support cell life or whether the abnormal metabolism simply reflects a summation of effects. At the moment, there is no answer to this question. Some have even suggested that cellular metabolism is not intrinsically abnormal but reflects only inadequate tissue perfusion. McShan et al. in 1945 and LePage found decreases in tissue levels of high energy phosphate compounds and energy-yielding substrates in rats subjected to drum shock and to hemorrhagic shock.[97, 98, 107] However, Rosenbaum et al. found that the decreases in high energy phosphate compounds in the liver of bled dogs did not

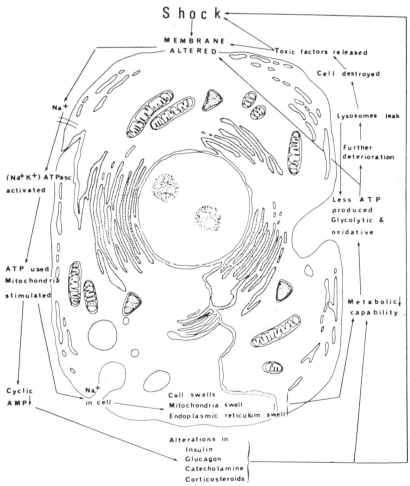

Figure 3–3. Baue's hypothesis for progressive deterioration of cell function with shock or inadequate circulation.[11] (From Baue, A. E., Chaudry, I. H., Wurth, M. A., and Sayeed, M. M.: Cellular alterations with shock and ischemia. Angiology 25:31, 1944.)

correlate with their response to reinfusion.[138]

Strawitz and Hift[163] subjected dogs to hemorrhagic shock and found mitochondrial abnormalities, specifically, the capacity for oxidative phosphorylation, in the heart, liver and kidney. However, in vitro studies, such as these, must be interpreted with caution because the mitochondrial preparation may not reflect in vivo function. This is because these organelles are again placed in an optimum environment and significant distortions in spatial relationships of related enzymes may be masked by the preparation process that breaks up the mitochondria so that that function possible through random association is measured.

Recent investigations by Baue et al. have demonstrated a partial uncoupling of ATP-dependent and ATP-yielding reactions.[10] Liver mitochondria of shocked animals had a decreased ability to resynthesize ATP from ADP, particularly with DPN-linked substrates, such as alphaketoglutarate. These changes were revised by volume restoration and appeared to correlate with changes in the cation content (increased sodium and decreased potassium and bound magnesium) of the mitochondria. Increased activity of the transport enzyme sodium and potassium ATP-ase was also found. This finding fit well with changes in cell membrane potential in shock reported by others and was thought to indicate that the cell membrane might be the initial weak point in the functional disintegration of the cell. In fact, Baue[11] has proposed a hypothesis of progressive cellular injury in shock (Fig. 3–3).

The uniform finding of decreased ATP levels in shock and the critical role of ATP in metabolism and cellular respiration has led many to attempt to correct this deficit. Chaudry and Baue have championed this approach and have shown that, in in vitro preparations, ATP-MgC1 is capable of reversing several of the metabolic deficits associated with shock.[28, 29] This form of therapy remains experimental, and the mainstay of therapy for the metabolic consequences of shock remains, as it should, an all-out attack on the primary cause of shock, with the restoration of circulating blood volume, vascular tone and cardiac output.

REFERENCES

1. Alexander, R. S.: Venomotor tone in hemorrhage and shock. Circ. Res. 3:181, 1955.
2. Allison, S. P., Hinton, P., and Chamberlain, W. J.: Intravenous glucose tolerance, insulin, and free fatty acid levels in burned patients. Lancet 2:1113, 1968.
3. Aoki, T. T., Muller, W. A., Brennan, M. F., and Cahill, G. F., Jr.: Effect of glucagon on amino acid nitrogen metabolism in fasting man. Metabolism 23:805, 1974.
4. Ashford, T.: A lesion in vascular smooth muscle in shock and its response to corticosteroid: Electron microscopic study. (Paper presented before the American Surgical Association, March, 1966.) Ann. Surg. 164:575, 1966.
5. Ashford, T. P., and Burdette, W. J.: Response of the isolated perfused hepatic parenchyma to hypoxia. Ann. Surg. 162:191, 1965.
6. Attar, S., Kirby, W. H., Jr., Masaitis, C., Mansberger, A. R., Jr., and Crowley, R. A., Coagulation changes in clinical shock: I. Effect of hemorrhagic shock on clotting time in humans. Ann. Surg. 164:34, 1966.
7. Bains, J. W., Crawford, D. T., and Ketchman, A. S.: Effect of chronic anemia on wound tensile strength: Correlation with blood volume, total red blood cell volume and proteins. Ann. Surg. 164:243, 1966.
8. Bartter, F. C., Biglieri, E. G., Pronove, P., and Delea, C. S., Effect of changes in intravascular volume on aldosterone secretion in man. In Muller, A. F., and O'Connor, C. M. (eds.): International Symposium on Aldosterone. Boston, Little, Brown & Co., 1958, p. 100.
9. Bassin, R., Vladek, B. C., Kark, A. E., and Shoemaker, W. C.: Rapid and slow hemorrhage in man. Ann. Surg. 173:325, 1970.
10. Baue, A. E., and Sayeed, M. M.: Alterations in the functional capacity of mitochondria in hemorrhagic shock. Surgery 68:40, 1970.
11. Baue, A. E., Chaudry, I. H., Wurth, M. A., and Sayeed, M. M.: Cellular alterations with shock and ischemia. Angiology 25:31, 1974. p. 31–41
12. Baue, A. E., Wurth, M. A., and Sayeed, M. M.: The dynamics of altered ATP-dependent and ATP-yielding cell processes in shock. Surgery 72:94, 1972.
13. Bell, D. J., and Schloerb, R. R.: Cellular response to endotoxin and hemorrhagic shock. Surgery 60:69, 1966.
14. Biron, P.: Pulmonary extraction of bradykinin and eledoisin. Rev. Can. Biol. 27:75, 1968.
15. Bjork, V. I., Intouti, F., and Norlung, S.: Correlation between sludge in the conjunctiva and the mesentery. Ann. Surg. 159:428, 1964.
16. Blackburn, G. L., Flah, J. P., Clowes, G. H. A., O'Donnell, T. F., and Hensle, T. E.: Protein sparing therapy during periods of starvation with sepsis or trauma. Ann. Surg. 177:588, 1973.
17. Blalock, A.: Experimental shock: The cause of

the low blood pressure produced by muscle injury. Arch. Surg. *20*:959, 1930.

18. Blalock, A.: Acute circulatory failure as exemplified by shock and hemorrhage. Surg. Gynecol. Obstet. *58*:551, 1934.

19. Bounous, G., McArdle, A. H., Hampson, L. G., and Gurd, F. N.: The cessation of intestinal mucus production as a pathogenic factor in irreversible shock. Surg. Forum *16*:11, 1965.

20. Bounous, G., McArdle, A. H., Hodges, D. M., Hampson, L. G., and Gurd, F. N.: Biosynthesis of intestinal mucin in shock: Relationship to tryptic hemorrhagic enteritis and permeability to curare. Ann. Surg. *164*:13, 1966.

21. Boyd, D. R., and Mansberger, A. R.: Serum water and osmolal changes in hemorrhagic shock; an experimental and clinical study. Ann. Surg. *34*:744, 1968.

22. Boyland, J. W., and Asheur, E.: Depletion and restoration of medullary osmotic gradient in dog kidney. Arch. Ges. Physiol. *276*:99, 1962.

23. Brockman, S. K., and Vasko, J. S.: Hemodynamics in endotoxin shock. Surg. Forum *17*:17, 1966.

24. Burke, J. F.: Identification of the sources of staphylococcus contaminating the surgical wound during operation. Ann. Surg. *158*:898, 1963.

25. Bywaters, E. G. L.: ischemic muscle necrosis. J.A.M.A. *124*:1103, 1944.

26. Cannon, W. B.: Traumatic Shock, New York, D. Appleton and Co., 1923.

27. Cannon, W. B., and Bayliss, W. M.: Muscle injury in relation to shock. Report of Shock Committee, March, 1919. No. 26, 19–23, cited by Blalock (reference 10).

28. Chaudry, I. H., Sayeed, M. M., and Bave, A. E.: The effect of adenosine triphosphate magnesium chloride administration and shock. Surgery *75*:220, 1974.

29. Chaudry, I. H., Sayeed, M. M., and Bave, A. E.: Depletion and restoration of tissue ATP in hemorrhagic shock. Arch. Surg. *108*:208, 1974.

30. Chiu, C. J., Scott, H. J., Gurd, F. N.: Intestinal mucosal lesion in low-flow states: II. The protective effect of intraluminal glucosa as energy substrate. Arch. Surg. *101*:484, 1970.

31. Cloutier, C. T., Lowery, B. D., and Carey, L. C.: Acid-base disturbances in hemorrhagic shock. Arch. Surg. *98*:551, 1969.

32. Collins, J. A., Simmons, R. L., James, R. M., Bredenberg, C. E., Anderson, R. W., and Heistercamp, C. A.: Acid-base status of seriously wounded combat casualties: I. Before treatment. Ann. Surg. *171*:595, 1970.

33. Cope, O., and Litwin, S. B.: Contribution of lymphatic system to replenishment of plasma volume following hemorrhage. Ann. Surg. *156*:655, 1962.

34. Coran, A. G., Cryer, P. E., Horwitz, D. L., and Herman, C. M.: Fat and carbohydrate metabolism during hemorrhagic shock in the unanesthetized baboon. Surg. Forum *22*:9, 1971.

35. Cournand, A., Riley, A. R., Bradley, S. E., Breed, E. S., Noble, R. P., Lawson, H. D., Griegersen, M. I., and Richards, D. W.: Studies of the circulation in clinical shock. Surgery *13*:964, 1943.

36. Crile, G. W., and Lower, W. E.: Anoci-Association. Philadelphia, W. B. Saunders Co., 1914.

37. Crowell, J. W.: Cardiac deterioration as the cause of irreversibility in shock. *In* Mills, L. C., and Moyer, J. H. (eds.): Shock and Hypotension. The Twelfth Hahnemann Symposium. New York, Grune & Stratton, 1965.

38. Crowell, J. W., and Houston, B.: The effect of acidity on blood coagulation. Am. J. Physiol. *201*:379, 1961.

39. Cunningham, J. N., Jr., Shires, G. T., and Wagner, Y.: Cellular transplant defects in hemorrhagic shock. Surgery *70*:215, 1971.

40. Curtin, R. A., Sapira, J. D., Danon, A., and Carey, L. C.: Comparison of exogenous and endogenous epinephrine on hyperglycemia in unanesthetized pigs. Surg. Forum *22*:85, 1971.

41. Cuthbertson, D. P.: Observations of the disturbance of metabolism produced by injury to the limbs. Q. J. Med. *1*:233, 1932.

42. Dale, H. H., and Richards, A. N.: Vasodilatory actions of histamine and other substances. J. Physiol. *52*:110, 1918.

43. DeDuve, C.: Lysosomes: A New Group of Cytoplasmic Particles. Subcellular Particles. New York, The Ronald Press Co., 1959.

44. Dillinger, M. R., and Gardner, B.: Newer aspects of the carcinoid spectrum. Surg. Gynecol. Obstet. *123*:1335, 1966.

45. Diniz, C. R., and Carvalho, I. F.: Micromethod for determination of bradykinogen under several conditions. Ann. N. Y. Acad. Sci. *104*:77, 1963.

46. Douglas, D. M.: The healing of aponeurotic incisions, Br. J. Surg. *40*:79, 1952.

47. Drucker, W. R.: What's new in shock and metabolism. Surg. Gynec. Obstet. *132*:234, 1971.

48. DuBois, E.: Basal metabolism in health and disease. New York, Lea & Febiger, 1924.

49. Dunphy, J. E., and Jackson, D. S.: Practical aspects of experimental studies in the care of the primary closed wound. Am. J. Surg. *104*:273, 1962.

50. Evans, W. E., Shore, R., and Darin, J. C.: Studies in endotoxin shock. II. Relationship of the pancreas and gastric secretion. Paper presented before the 27th Annual Meeting of the Society of University Surgeons, February 10, 1966.

51. Exton, J. H., Friedmann, N., Wong, E. H., et al.: Interaction of glucocorticoids with glucagon and epinephrine in the control of gluconeogenesis and glycogenolysis in the liver and of lipolysis in adipose tissue. J. Biol. Chem. *247*:3579, 1972.

52. Farago, G., Levene, R. A., Lau, T. S., and Drucker, W. R.: Availability of lipid for energy metabolism during hypovolemia. Surg. Forum 22:7, 1971.

53. Farrell, G. L.: Physiological factors which influence secretion of aldosterone. Recent Progr. Hormone Res. 15:275, 1959.

54. Ferreira, S. H., and Vane, J. R.: The disappearance of bradykinin and eledoisin in the circulation and vascular beds of cats. Br. J. Pharm. 30:417, 1967.

55. Flynn, J. T., and Lefer, A. M.: Prostaglandin metabolism during circulatory shock. Biochim. Biophys. Acta 497:775, 1977.

56. Frank, H. A., Glotzer, P., Jacob, S. W., and Fine, J.: Hemorrhagic shock in Eck fistula dogs. Am. J. Physiol. 167:508, 1951.

57. Fulks, R. M., Li, J. B., and Goldberg, A. L.: Effects of insulin, glucose, and amino acids on protein turnover in rat diaphragm. J. Biol. Chem. 250:290, 1975.

58. Fulton, R. L.: Adsorption of sodium and water by collagen during hemorrhagic shock. Ann. Surg. 172:861, 1970.

59. Gallie, B. L., Koven, I. H., Lo, S. F., Taubenfligel, V., and Drucker, W. R.: Correction of interstitial diffusion defect in hemorrhagic shock by balanced salt solution. Surg. Forum 22:21, 1971.

60. Gamble, J. L.: Physiologic information gained from studies on the life raft ration. Harvey Lectures 42:247, 1947.

61. Gann, D. S.: Endocrine control of plasma protein and volume. Surg. Clin. North Am. 56:1135, 1976.

62. Ganong, W. F., and Mulrow, P. J.: Role of kidney in adrenocortical response to hemorrhage in hypophysectomized dogs. Endocrinology 70:182, 1962.

63. Goetz, R. H., Selmonosky, C. A., and State, D.: Effect of amine buffer tris (hydroxylmethyl) amino methane (THAM) on renal blood flow during hemorrhagic shock. Surg. Gynecol. Obstet. 117:715, 1963.

64. Goldberg, A. L., and Obessey, R.: Oxidation of amino acids by diaphragms from fed and fasted rats. Am. J. Physiol. 6:1384, 1972.

65. Grant, R. T., and Reeves, E. B.: Observations on the general effects of injury in man. Med. Res. Council, Spec. Rep. Ser. No. 277. London, His Majesty's Stationery Office, 1941.

66. Greenfield, L. J., McCardy, J. R., Hinshaw, L. B., and Elkins, R. C.: Preservation of myocardial function during cross-circulation in terminal endotoxin shock. Surgery 72:111, 1972.

67. Gross, S. D.: System of Surgery, 1850. Cited by Mann, F. C.: Bull. Johns Hopkins Hosp. 25:205, 1914.

68. Gump, F. E., Long, C. L., Geiger, J. W., and Kinney, J. M.: The significance of altered gluconeogenesis in surgical catabolism. J. Trauma 15(8):704, 1975.

69. Guyton, A. C., and Lindsay, A. W.: Effect of elevated left arterial pressure and decreased plasma protein concentration on the development of pulmonary edema. Circ. Res. 7:649, 1959.

70. Guyton, A. C., Taylor, E., Granger, H. J., and Gibson, W. H.: Regulation of interstitial fluid volume and pressure. Adv. Exp. Med. Biol. 33:111, 1973.

71. Haljamäe, H.: "Hidden" cellular electrolyte responses to hemorrhagic shock and their significance. Rev. Surg. 27:315, 1970.

72. Hardaway, R. M.: Intravascular coagulation in irreversible shock. In Mills, L. C., and Moyer, J. H. (eds.): Shock and Hypotension. The Twelfth Hahnemann Symposium, New York, Grune & Stratton, 1965.

73. Hardaway, R. M., Chun, B., and Rutherford, R. B.: Histologic evidence of disseminated intravascular coagulation in clinical shock. Vasc. Dis. 2:254, 1965.

74. Hardaway, R. M., Johnson, D. G., Elovitz, M. J., Houcin, D. N., Jenkins, E. B., Burns, J. W., and Jackson, D. R.: Studies on the fibrinogen replacement rate in dogs. Ann. Surg. 160:835, 1964.

75. Harkins, H. M.: Wound healing. In Allen, J. G., Harkins, H. M., Moyer, J. H., and Rhoads, J. E. (eds.): Surgery Principles and Practice. Philadelphia, J. B. Lippincott Co., 1957.

76. Henderson, Y.: Acapnia and shock. Am. J. Physiol. 24:66, 1909.

77. Henry, J. N., McArdle, A. H., and Bounous, G., et al.: The effect of experimental hemorrhagic shock on pulmonary alveolar surfactant. J. Trauma 7:691, 1967.

78. Herman, C. M., Kraft, A. R., Smith, K. R., Artnak, E. J., Chisholm, F. C., Dickson, L. G., McKee, E. E., Jr., Homer, L. D., and Levin, J.: The relationship to circulating endogenous endotoxin to hemorrhagic shock in the baboon. Ann. Surg. 179:910, 1974.

79. Hewson, W.: In Gulliver, G. (ed.): The Work of William Hewson, F.R.S. London, Sydenham Society, 1846, p. 46.

80. Hinshaw, L. B., Brake, C. M., and Emerson, T. E.: Biochemical and pathologic alterations in endotoxin shock. In Mills, L. C., and Moyer, J. H., (eds.): Shock and Hypotension. The Twelfth Hahnemann Symposium. New York, Grune & Stratton, 1965.

81. Hopkinson, B. R., Borden, J. R., Heyden, W. C., and Schenk, W. G.: Interstitial fluid pressure changes during hemorrhage and blood replacement with and without hypotension. Surgery 64:68, 1968.

82. Howard, J. E. (ed.): Battle Casualties in Korea. Washington, D.C., U.S. Government Printing Office, 1955.

83. Huckabee, N. E.: The relationship of pyruvate and lactate during anaerobic metabolism. J. Clin. Invest. 37:264, 1958.

84. Jacobson, Y. G., DeFalco, A. J., Mundth, E. D., and Keller, M. A.: Hyperbaric oxygen in the therapy of experimental shock. Surg. Forum 16:15, 1965.

85. Janoff, A., Weismann, G., Zweifach, B. W., and Thomas, L.: Pathogenesis of experimental shock: IV. Studies on lysosomes in normal and tolerant animals subjected to lethal trauma and endotoxemia. J. Exp. Med. 116:451, 1962.

86. Jenkins, M. T., Jones, R. F., Wilson, B., and

Moyer, C.: Congestion atelectasis; complications of intravenous infusions of fluids. Ann. Surg. *132*:327, 1950.

87. Johnston, I. D. A., Ross, H., Welborn, T. A., and Wright, A. D.: The effect of trauma on glucose tolerance and the serum levels of insulin and growth hormone in combined injuries and shock. *In* Schmidt, B., and Tloren, L. (eds.): Proceedings of the Symposium on Combined Injuries and Shock. Oppsola, 1967, p. 127.

88. Jordan, G. L., Jr., Fischer, E. P., and LeFrak, E. A.: Glucose metabolism in traumatic shock in the human. Ann. Surg. *175*:685, 1972.

89. Kaihara, S., Rutherford, R. B., Schwentker, E. P., et al.: The distribution of cardiac output of experimental hemorrhagic shock in dogs. J. Appl. Physiol. *27*:218–222, 1969.

90. Kalfus, L., and Thal, A. P.: Plasma kinin and kininase in various forms of shock. Fed. Proc. (Part I) *23*:539, 1964.

91. Kinney, J. D., Duke, J. H., Long, C. L., and Gump, F. E.: Carbohydrate and nitrogen metabolism after injury. J. Clin. Pathol. *23*(Suppl. 4): 65, 1970.

92. Knisely, M. H., Eliot, T. S., and Bloch, E. H.: Sludged blood in traumatic shock. Arch. Surg. *51*:220, 1945.

93. Kobald, E. E., Lobell, R., Katz, W., and Thal, A. P.: Chemical mediators released by endotoxin. Surg. Gynecol. Obstet. *118*:807, 1964.

94. Kobald, E. E., Lucas, R., and Thal, A. P.: Chemical mediators in clinical septic shock. Surg. Forum *14*:16, 1964.

95. Lefer, A. M., and Inge, T. F., Jr.: Differentiation of a myocardial depressant factor present in shock plasma from known plasma peptides and salts. Proc. Soc. Exp. Biol. Med. *142*:429, 1973.

96. Lefer, A. M., and Martin, J.: Relationship of plasma peptides to the depressant factor in hemorrhagic shock. Circ. Res. *26*:59, 1970.

97. LePage, G. A.: Biologic energy transformations during shock as shown by their tissue analyses. Am. J. Physiol. *146*:267, 1946.

98. LePage, G. A.: The effects of hemorrhage on tissue metabolites. Am. J. Physiol. *147*:446, 1946.

99. Lillehei, R. C.: The intestinal factor in irreversible hemorrhagic shock. Surgery *42*:1043, 1957.

100. Lillehei, R. C., Longerbeam, J. K., Block, J. H., and Manax, W. G.: The nature of irreversible shock. Experimental and clinical observations. Ann. Surg. *160*:682, 1964.

101. Lister, J., McNeil, L. F., Marshal, V. C., Pizak, L. F., Dagher, F. J., and Moore, F. D.: Transcapillary refilling after hemorrhage in normal man: Basal rates and volumes; effect of norepinephrine. Ann. Surg. *158*:698, 1963.

102. Lovett, W. L., Wangensteen, S. L., Glenn, T. M., and Lefer, A. M.: Presence of a myocardial depressant factor in patients in circulatory shock. Surgery *70*:223, 1971.

103. MacLean, L. D., Duff, J. H., Scott, H. M., and Derftz, D. J.: Treatment of shock in man based on hemodynamic diagnosis. Surg. Gynecol. Obstet. *120*:1, 1965.

104. MacLean, L. D., Mulligan, W. G., McLean, A. P. H., and Duff, J. H.: Patterns of septic shock in man — A detailed study of 56 patients. Ann. Surg. *166*:543, 1967.

105. McMichael, J.: The oxygen supply of the liver. Q. J. Exp. Physiol. *27*:73, 1937.

106. McNulty, W. P., Jr., and Linares, R.: Hemorrhagic shock of germfree rats. Am. J. Physiol. *198*:141, 1960.

107. McShan, W. H., Potter, V. R., Goldman, A., Shipley, E. G., and Meyer, R. K.: Biologic energy transformation during shock as shown by blood chemistry. Am. J. Physiol. *145*:93, 1945.

108. Manger, W. M., Nahas, G. G., Hassam, D., Habif, D. V., and Papper, E. M.: Effect of pH control and increased O_2 delivery on the course of hemorrhagic shock. Ann. Surg. *156*:503, 1962.

109. Marks, L. J., King, D. W., Kingsbury, P. F., Boyett, J. E., and Dell, E. S.: Physiologic role of the adrenal cortex in the maintenance of plasma volume following hemorrhage of surgical operation. Surgery *58*:510, 1965.

110. Mathews, R. E., and Douglas, G. J.: Sulphur-35 measurements of functional and total extracellular fluid in dogs with hemorrhagic shock. Surg. Forum *20*:3, 1969.

111. Mela, L. M., Miller, L. D., and Nicholas, G. G.: Influence of cellular acidosis and altered cation concentrations on shock-induced mitochondrial damage. Surgery *72*:102, 1972.

112. Moore, F. D.: Metabolic Care of the Surgical Patient. Philadelphia, W. B. Saunders Co., 1960.

113. Moore, F. D.: The effects of hemorrhage on body composition. N. Engl. J. Med. *273*:567, 1965.

114. Moore, F. D., and Ball, M. R.: The Metabolic Response to Surgery. American Lecture Series, No. 132. Springfield, Ill., Charles C Thomas, 1952.

115. Moore, T. C., Normel, L., and Eiseman, B.: Effect of histamine and serotonin on blood flow and tracheal resistance in the isolated perfused lung. Surgery *57*:730, 1965.

116. Morris, R.: Personal communication.

117. Moyer, C. A., and Butcher, H. R.: Burns, Shock and Plasma Volume Regulation. St. Louis, C. V. Mosby Co., 1967.

118. Moyer, C. A., Margraf, H. W., and Monafo, W. W.: Burn shock and extravascular sodium deficiency. Treatment with Ringer's solution with lactate. Arch. Surg. *90*:799, 1965.

119. Nayman, J.: Effect of renal failure on wound healing in dog's response to hemodialysis following uremia induced by uranium nitrate. Ann. Surg. *164*:227, 1966.

120. Neill, S. A., Gaisford, W. D., and Zuidema, G. D.: A comparative anatomic study of the hepatic veins in the dog, monkey and human. Surg. Gynecol. Obstet. *116*:451, 1963.

121. Nelson, R. M., Poulson, A. M., Lyman, J. H., and Henry, J. W.: Evaluation of tris (hydroxymethyl) aminomethane (THAM) in experimental hemorrhagic shock. Surgery *54*:86, 1963.

122. O'Connell, R. C., Morgan, A. P., Aoki, T. T., Ball, M. R., and Moore, F. D.: Nitrogen conservation in starvation: Graded response to intravenal glucose. J. Clin. Endocrinol. Metab. 59:555, 1974.

123. Olledart, R., and Mansberger, A. R.: The effect of hypovolemic shock on bacterial defense. Am. J. Surg. 110:302, 1965.

124. Owen, O. E., and Cahill, G. F.: Metabolic effects of exogenous glucocorticoids in fasted man. J. Clin. Invest. 35:62, 1973.

125. Pagano, V. P., and Mersheimer, W. L.: Immunochemical changes observed with shock. Surg. Forum 16:45, 1965.

126. Parker, J., Jelks, G., and Emerson, T., Jr.: Cardiovascular effects of prostaglandin A. in the dog. Fed. Proc. 1979. In press.

127. Parsons, E., and Phemister, D. B.: Hemorrhage and "shock" in traumatized limbs: Experimental study. Surg. Gynecol. Obstet. 51:196, 1930.

128. Penner, A., and Bernheim, A. I.: Studies in the pathogenesis of experimental dysentery intoxication. J. Exp. Med. 111:145, 1960.

129. Piper, P. J., and Vane, J. R.: Release of additional factors in anaphylaxis and its antagonism by anti-inflammatory drugs. Nature 223:29, 1969.

130. Pirkle, J. C., and Gann, D. S.: Restitution of blood volume after hemorrhage: Role of the adrenal cortex. Am. J. Physiol. 230:1683, 1976.

131. Porte, D., Graber, A. L., Kuzuya, T., and Williams, R. H.: The effect of epinephrine on immuno-reactive insulin levels in man. J. Clin. Invest. 45:228, 1966.

132. Porte, D.: A receptor mechanism for the inhibition of insulin release by epinephrine in man. J. Clin. Invest. 46:86, 1967.

133. Pozefsky, T., Felig, P., Tobin, J. D., Soeldner, J. S., and Cahill, G. F.: Amino acid balance across tissues of the forearm in postabsorptive man. J. Clin. Invest. 48:2273, 1969.

134. Ravin, H. A., and Fine, J.: Current concepts and controversies on traumatic shock. Progr. Surg. 3:102, 1963.

135. Reich, T., Dierolf, B. M., and Reynolds, B. M.: Plasma cathepsin-like acid proteinase activity during hemorrhagic shock. J. Surg. Res. 5:116, 1965.

136. Rhoads, J. E., and Howard, J. M.: The chemistry of trauma. Springfield, Ill., Charles C Thomas, Publishers, 1963.

137. Robb, H. J.: The role of micro-embolism in the production of irreversible shock. Ann. Surg. 158:685, 1963.

138. Rosenbaum, D. K., Frank, E. D., Rutenburg, A. M., and Frank, H. A.: High energy phosphate content of liver tissue in experimental hemorrhagic shock. Am. J. Physiol. 188:86, 1957.

139. Rush, B. J.: Discussion of Bell, D. J., and Schloerb, P. R.: Cellular response to endotoxin and hemorrhagic shock. Surgery 60:69, 1966.

140. Rutherford, R. B., Balis, J. V., Trow, R. S., and Graves, G. M.: Comparison of hemodynamic and regional blood flow changes at equivalent stages of endotoxin and hemorrhagic shock. J. Trauma 16:886, 1976.

141. Rutherford, R. B., and Trow, R. S.: The pathophysiology of irreversible hemorrhagic shock in monkeys. J. Surg. Res. 14:538, 1973.

142. Rutherford, R. B., West, R. L., and Hardaway, R. M.: Coagulation changes during experimental hemorrhagic shock. Ann. Surg. 164:203, 1966.

143. Rutherford, R. B., Trow, R. S., and Monaghan, T. D.: Comparison of hemodynamic and regional blood flow changes at equivalent stages of E. coli bacteremic and endotoxin shock in monkeys. (In press, 1979.)

144. Schayer, R. W.: Relationship of stress-induced histidine decarboxylase activity in histamine synthesis to circulatory homeostasis and shock. Science 131:226, 1960.

145. Selkurt, E. E.: Renal blood flow and renal clearances during hemorrhage and shock. In Block, K. D.: Shock Pathogencsis and Therapy. Berlin, Springer-Verlag, 1962, p. 445.

146. Sherry, S.: Homeostatic mechanisms and proteolysis in shock. Fed. Proc. (Suppl.):9:209, 1961.

147. Shires, G. T., Brown, F. T., Canizaro, P. C., and Somerville, N.: Distributional changes in extracellular fluid hemorrhagic shock. Surg. Forum 11:115, 1960.

148. Shires, G. T., Carrico, C. J., and Cohn, D.: The role of the extracellular fluid in shock. In Hershey, S. (ed.): Shock, Boston, Little, Brown & Co., 1964.

149. Shumer, W.: Localization of the energy pathway block in shock. Surgery 64:55, 1968.

150. Shumer, W., Kapica, S. K., Teng, Ta-Lee: Validity of the hysosomal therapy of oligemic shock. Arch. Surg. 99:325, 1969.

151. Siegel, J. H., Goldwyn, R. M., and Friedman, H. P.: Pattern and process in the evolution of human septic shock. Surgery 70:232, 1971.

152. Siegel, J. J., and Del Guercio, L. R. M.: The high cardiac output syndrome and ventricular failure — A problem in surgical management. (Paper presented before the Halsted Society, Baltimore, Maryland, September 16, 1966.)

153. Silen, W.: Horizons in gastrointestinal research. Surgery 72:91, 1972.

154. Simeone, F. A.: Shock, trauma and the surgeon. Ann. Surg. 158:759, 1963.

155. Simeone, F.: Discussion of Rosenberg, J. C., and Rush, B. J.: Basic biochemical difference in endotoxin and hemorrhagic shock. Surg. Forum 16:23, 1965.

156. Simmons, R. L., Collins, J. A., Heistercamp, C. A., et al.: Coagulation disorders in combat casualties. Ann. Surg. 169:455, 1969.

157. Skillman, J. J., and Moore, F. O.: Volume regulatory and endocrine relationships after blood loss in man. Ann. N.Y. Acad. Sci. 150:639, 1968.

158. Slonim, M., and Stahl, W. M.: Sodium and water content of connective versus cellular tissue following hemorrhage. Surg. Forum 19:53, 1968.

159. Spencer, F. C.: Personal communication.

160. Stahl, T. H.: Pressure-flow factors in the renal excretory response to hemorrhage. Surg. Forum 16:23, 1965.

161. Steinberg, D.: Paper presented at The Conferences on Energy Metabolism and Body Fuel Utilization, Boston, Massachusetts, July 13, 1966.

162. Steward, J. M.: Peptide Hormones. In Cain, C. K. (ed.): Annual Reports in Medicinal Chemistry, 1969.

163. Strawitz, J. G., and Hift, H. L.: The structure and function of mitochondria in irreversible hemorrhagic shock. Proc. Soc. Exper. Biol. Med. 91:641, 1956.

164. Strawitz, J. G., and Hift, H.: Subcellular changes in hemorrhagic shock. In Mills, L. C., and Moyer, J. H. (eds.): Shock and Hypotension. The Twelfth Hahnemann Symposium. New York, Grune & Stratton, 1965.

165. Swank, R. L., Hissen, W., and Bergentz, S. E.: 5-Hydroxytryptamine and aggregation of blood elements after trauma. Surg. Gynecol. Obstet. 119:779, 1964.

166. Teplitz, C.: The ultrastructural basis for pulmonary pathophysiology following trauma. Pathogenesis of pulmonary edema. J. Trauma 8:700, 1968.

167. Thal, A. P.: Discussion of Rosenberg, J. C., and Rush, B. J.: Basic biochemical difference in endotoxin and hemorrhagic shock. Surg. Forum 16:23, 1965.

168. Thal, A. P., and Wilson, R. F.: Curr. Probl. Surg. September, 1965.

169. Thal, A. P., Wilson, R. F., Kalfuss, L., and Andre, J.: The role of metabolic and humoral factors in irreversible shock. In Mills, L. C., and Moyer, J. H., (eds.): Shock and Hypotension. The Twelfth Hahnemann Symposium, New York, Grune & Stratton, 1965.

170. Thomas, C. S., Jr., Melly, M. A., Koenig, M. G., et al.: The hemodynamic effects of viable gram-negative organisms. Surg. Gynecol. Obstet. 128:753, 1969.

171. Udenfriend, S.: Formation of hydroxyproline in collagen. Science 152:1335, 1966.

172. Udhoji, V. N., and Weil, M. H.: Hemodynamic and metabolic studies on shock associated with bacteremia. Ann. Intern. Med. 62:966, 1965.

173. Unger, R. H.: Glucagon and the insulin: glucagon molar ration in diabetes and other catabolic illness. Diabetes 20:834, 1971.

174. Valeri, C. R.: Viability and function of preserved red cells. N. Engl. J. Med. 284:81, 1971.

175. Visscher, M. D., Haddy, F. J., and Stephen, G.: Physiology and pharmacology of lung edema. Pharmacol. Rev. 8:389, 1956.

176. Waldhausen, J. A., Abel, F. L., and Selkurt, E. E.: Splanchnic blood flow in the monkey during hemorrhagic shock. Surg. Forum 15:7, 1964.

177. Wangensteen, S. L., Ramey, W. G., Ferguson, W. W., and Starling, J. R.: Plasma myocardial depressant activity (shock factor) identified as salt in the cat papillary muscle bioassay system. J. Trauma 13:181, 1973.

178. Warner, W. A.: Release of free fatty acids following trauma. J. Trauma 9:692, 1969.

179. Weidner, M. G., Albrecht, M., and Clowes, G. H.: Relationship of myocardial function to survival after oligemic hypotension. Surgery 55:73, 1964.

180. Weismann, G., and Thomas, L.: Studies on lysosomes: I. Effects of endotoxin, exotoxin tolerance, and cortisone on release of enzymes from granular fraction of rabbit fever. J. Exp. Med. 116:433, 1962.

181. Werle, E.: Kallikrein, Kallidin and Related Substances: Polypeptides Which Affect Smooth Muscles and Blood Vessels. New York, Pergamon Press, 1960.

182. Willwerth, B. M., Crawford, F. A., Young, W. G., Jr., et al.: The role of functional demand on the development of pulmonary lesions during hemorrhagic shock. J. Thorac. Cardiovasc. Surg. 54:658, 1967.

183. Wurtman, R. J.: Catecholamines. N. Engl. J. Med. Medical Progress Series. Boston, Little, Brown & Co., 1966.

184. Wyler, F., Forsyth, R. P., Nies, A. S., Neutze, J. M., and Melmon, K. L.: Endotoxin induced regional circulatory changes in the unanesthetized monkey. Circ. Res. 24:777, 1969.

185. Zweifach, B. W.: Aspects of comparative physiology of laboratory animals relative to the problems of experimental shock. Fed. Proc. (Suppl.) 9:18, 1961.

CHAPTER 4

THE TREATMENT OF SHOCK

Donald D. Trunkey, M.D.
George F. Sheldon, M.D.
John A. Collins, M.D.

INTRODUCTION

There are few conditions in clinical medicine more demanding than the prompt recognition and treatment of traumatic injury. Unrecognized or inadequately treated traumatic shock may cause immediate or delayed mortality and morbidity. The attending physician is truly "under the gun" because his diagnostic decisions and therapeutic interventions must be both rapid and correct. His immediate concern encompasses the function and integrity of all the vital organs and systems as well as a number of immediately life-threatening injury patterns. His view must be broad yet detailed, and the most important decisions must often be made primarily on the basis of examination of the patient, without time for laboratory or radiologic confirmation. There are very few parallel situations in modern medicine.

In the past decade a number of new concepts and improvements in the resuscitation of the injured patient have been introduced. Some involve in-hospital diagnosis and treatment, but others are related to resuscitation of the victim at the scene of the accident and his rapid transportation to a prepared medical facility. The use of the 911 telephone number to gain immediate access to emergency medical services, the use of paramedics and better designed and equipped ambulances that allow shock to be treated in the field, and the introduction of new devices such as the esophageal airway and the MAST trousers or G-suit all have contributed to the fact that many more critically injured victims are now arriving alive at hospital emergency departments. Finally, while fewer advances have been made in hospital emergency departments themselves during this period, the problems and their solutions have been more clearly defined (see Chapter 27). It is to be hoped that these improvements along with long awaited improvements in the overall EMS system, such as the categorization of hospitals according to their therapeutic capabilities and the regional distribution of trauma care according to such considerations, will contribute to further major improvements in trauma care.

In Chapter 3 the different clinical types of shock were categorized as hypovolemic, cardiogenic, or vasogenic. In this chapter we will emphasize the treatment of *traumatic* shock, which is a combination of hypovolemic shock and tissue injury or destruction. This is not meant to imply that shock due to sepsis or cardiac factors does not occur following trauma. Rather, it is an effort to emphasize the type of shock that is most common and most critical in dealing with the injured. Therefore, we will discuss cardiogenic shock and septic shock only as they affect the trauma victim.

CAUSES OF SHOCK IN ACUTELY INJURED PATIENTS

By far the commonest cause of shock or circulatory collapse in injured patients is blood loss. Often this is evident from examination of the patient, but appearances may be deceiving. In some instances a history carefully extracted from witnesses or the ambulance personnel will reveal that considerable blood loss occurred at the scene of the accident or en route from it. However, the patient who arrives with a face and shirt covered with blood from a scalp laceration and accompanied by distraught or hysterical family members may attract the attention of the entire waiting room. Most of the time he has lost less than one tenth the amount of blood lost by the patient with a fractured femur who arrives quietly on a stretcher without a drop of blood on him.

Many guidelines and rules of thumb have been devised for estimating the blood loss with "typical" injuries, but the variations in individual patients are too great to make them of much use. An awareness of the potential magnitude of hidden blood loss can be gained from simple geometry (Fig. 4–1). If a thigh of average dimensions is considered to be a cylinder for computation purposes, an increase of only 1 centimeter in the radius of that thigh represents a net gain of 2 liters in volume. If the increase in the radius is 2 centimeters, the volume gain is 4.5 liters

over normal. In the acutely injured patient, immediate changes in dimensions are due largely to bleeding into injured tissues. Even the relatively small upper arm can contain a significant amount of extravasated blood. It should also be pointed out that when a limb such as the thigh has a fracture of its main support bone (femur), the extremity loses its cylindrical shape and assumes a more spherical shape. Again geometry indicates that the volume of a sphere is much more than that of a cylinder.

If the injury is in the abdomen the situation may be particularly misleading because the length of the abdominal cavity can and does change in an unapparent manner when the diaphragm is raised. In fact, this may be the dominant dimensional change soon after abdominal injury. If we consider concurrent and equal changes in both the radius and the length of our typical abdominal "cylinder" (Fig. 4–2), a gain of 1 centimeter represents a volume change of 2.9 liters; a gain of 2 centimeters represents a volume change of 6.1 liters. Changes of this magnitude are not usually evident externally. Abdominal swelling in an injured patient may also be due to the accumulation of air in the gastrointestinal tract and the sequestration of predominantly extracellular fluid in the enteric lumen and/or the peritoneal space. Nevertheless, a briskly bleeding intra-abdominal vessel can quickly fill the abdominal cylinder before these other contents can add to the dimensional changes, and a patient can exsanguinate into the peritoneal cavity without any dramatic change in abdominal dimensions or appearance. *Therefore, it can be a tragic blunder to assume that*

Figure 4–1. Injured thigh considered as a cylinder for computational purposes: change in volume (= blood loss) corresponding to changes in radius.

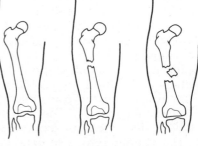

AVERAGE DIMENSIONS: 40 cm. length, 8 cm. radius	40 cm. length, 9 cm. radius	40 cm. length, 10 cm. radius
VOLUME CHANGE – Normal	+ 2.1 liters	+ 4.5 liters

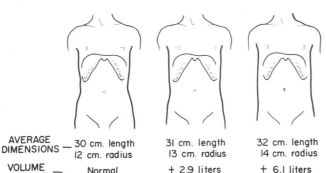

AVERAGE
DIMENSIONS — 30 cm. length   31 cm. length   32 cm. length
              12 cm. radius   13 cm. radius   14 cm. radius

VOLUME
CHANGE —   Normal   + 2.9 liters   + 6.1 liters

Figure 4–2. Injured abdomen considered as a cylinder for computational purposes: change in volume corresponding to changes in length and radius. Change in length occurs as raising of the diaphragms and thus remains inapparent to external examination. Exsanguination can occur with minimal change in external appearance.

because the abdomen is not distended, hypotension is not due to intra-abdominal bleeding.

The cranial vault, because of its fixed volume, is not considered an important site for sequestration of hidden blood. Each hemithorax, on the other hand, may contain 2 to 3 liters of blood, a fact that emphasizes the importance of physican examination and x-ray of the chest even in the most critically injured patient. The pelvis is also notorious as a locus of hidden blood loss, particularly if the bleeding is retroperitoneal. Six to eight units of whole blood can easily be sequestrated in the pelvis without externally visible signs. Any sizeable area can, of course, "hide" lost blood, including retroperitoneal areas, the buttocks and the shoulder girdle. The problems of estimating blood loss in the injured patient are further complicated by the nonlinear relationship between the signs and symptoms of hypovolemia and the volume of blood lost; this relationship will be considered later.

Specific types of injury may result in losses of fluid other than blood. Burns are the best example of an injury in which extracellular type filling and plasma are lost in very large amounts, producing profound shock in the extensively burned individual. Crush injuries can produce losses of all three types of fluid. In a situation that has fortunately become rare, tight tourniquets left on limbs long enough can result in rapid sequestration of plasma and extracellular fluid in the ischemic limb after release of the tourniquet. However, "tourniquet shock" is not uncommon and will be discussed subsequently. It is rare to see venous return so extensively interrupted at the time of injury that it produces massive fluid sequestration in the hind

quarter, but this can be a life-threatening complication of acute iliofemoral thrombosis. Whatever the mechanism of injury, the presence of extravasated blood in body cavities or in soft tissues evokes an inflammatory response that is accompanied by the sequestration of extracellular fluid in varying amounts. With time, then, both blood that is "shed internally" and the responses of the tissues to the injuring force can cause additional volume losses in the form of extracellular fluid that may well exceed the volume of the original blood loss.

The acutely injured patient may be hypotensive for reasons other than blood loss. In this regard, one must consider all of the factors that influence cardiac output. Cardiac output is the product of heart rate and stroke volume. If one examines these contributing components as they relate to the injured patient (see Table 4–1), the patient can be more sensibly approached from a physiologic viewpoint.[74] *Heart rate* (bradycardia or tachycardia) is rarely a

TABLE 4–1. Mechanisms of Reserve to Severe Stress

Heart rate

Stroke volume
  preload
  afterload
  contractility

Distribution of regional blood flow

Oxygen transport mechanisms
  blood hemoglobin concentration
  oxygen extraction, diffusion
    and tissue oxygen levels
  anaerobic metabolism
  temperature
  ventilation

cause of shock in the trauma victim, the single exception being the patient with severe head injury and brain stem involvement. In such a patient, a profound bradycardia may occur. Treatment in these situations is usually futile because of the extensiveness of the brain injury. *Stroke volume* is determined by preload, afterload and contractility. The most common preload factor contributing to shock is volume, which has already been discussed. However, shock may be due to other preload factors, the most important ones being pericardial tamponade and tension pneumothorax. In both instances the venous return to the heart has been impaired.

Pericardial tamponade is most important because it may be rapidly lethal yet can be promptly treated in the emergency department. The usual signs — distant heart sounds, paradoxical pulse, narrow pulse pressure, distended neck veins and large globular heart shadow on x-ray — are of very limited value in the acutely injured patient, and concomitant blood loss may mask some of the circulatory signs. Heart sounds can be hard to evaluate in a noisy emergency department and in the presence of associated injuries; thus, absence of any or all of the above signs does not rule out tamponade. It must be considered in the differential diagnosis in all hypotensive patients who are known to have sustained a penetrating or significant blunt injury to the chest. The key to detection in the seriously injured patient is accurate determination and monitoring of the central venous pressure. The concurrence of an elevated or even high normal central venous pressure and systemic hypotension in a patient with chest trauma mandates serious consideration of pericardial tamponade.

Tension pneumothorax may also be a cause of "preload" cardiogenic shock. In this syndrome the hemithorax becomes overdistended with air, causing collapse of the lung and a shift of the mediastinum to the opposite hemithorax. This shift in the mediastinum causes compression and distortion of the great veins and impedes venous return to the heart. Compression of the lungs and their low pressure vascular system also adds significantly to this damming up of blood in the central circulation. If it develops quickly enough, if it occurs in the presence of concomitant volume

loss, or if it occurs in children whose mediastinum is less firm, tension pneumothorax can quickly produce death (see Chapter 13). Signs that aid in differentiating this condition from other preload causes of shock include shift of the trachea to the contralateral side, percussion tympany and decreased breath sounds on the ipsilateral side. If there is a strong suspicion of this diagnosis it is better to insert a chest tube or a thoracocentesis needle than to wait for more obvious signs or radiographic confirmation.

Afterload causes of cardiogenic shock are rare in the emergency department. This type of shock may exist in regard to the right ventricle following pulmonary embolism, and confirmation of this diagnosis should be pursued by EKG, radionuclide scanning of the lungs, and/or pulmonary arteriography. Afterload causes involving the left ventricle are limited to those rare patients in whom head injury causes acute hypertension, an event thought to be due to the so-called Cushing reflex. When it does occur it is most often seen in young individuals, and systolic pressures as high as 300 torr may be recorded.

The most common cause of poor contractility leading to acute cardiac failure is myocardial infarction. This is a prime example of why one must not assume that shock is invariably due to hypovolemia in an injured patient. Myocardial infarction may have occurred prior to the accident and in fact may have caused the accident. An increasingly common finding in blunt trauma victims, particularly motor vehicle accident victims, is myocardial contusion.[71] This is associated with steering wheel or dashboard injuries to the sternum. It is impossible in some situations to differentiate between myocardial infarct and myocardial contusion. Arrhythmias are common following this injury and are the predominant cause of early death. However, although cardiogenic shock is rare with uncomplicated cardiac contusion, it may occur in alcoholics, in older patients with limited cardiac reserve, and in patients who have received certain pharmacologic agents — most importantly, an anesthetic agent used to allow repair of other injuries.

Other factors contributing to contractility changes following trauma are less well defined and include the so-called toxic factors.[19] For example, Lefer and his associates have described a myocardial depressant factor (MDF) in the blood of animals and man following hemorrhage, burns and sepsis.[75] These humoral factors, which are more likely to appear in the later stages of trauma and shock, may be particularly deleterious in this setting, since one of the most common compensatory mechanisms for decreased oxygen transport is an increased cardiac output.

An acute spinal cord injury can cause hypotension by the same mechanism as spinal anesthesia — i.e., the sudden removal of the neural control of vasomotor tone in much of the vascular system. This is usually well tolerated unless central aortic pressure drops markedly or unless there has been significant associated blood loss. It is surprising how easy it is to overlook temporarily a spinal cord injury when other more attention-getting injuries are present. Needless to say, intact motor and sensory responses can be quickly and easily determined even in injured legs. Although spinal injuries can cause hypotension, it is a good policy *never* to consider a *head injury* as the cause of hypotension or shock. While it is true that the head, scalp and face have a rich blood supply and that blood loss from injuries to these structures can be severe, this should be clinically evident. Intracranial bleeding and brain injury do *not* cause hypotension except terminally when there is decompensation or compression of the medullary centers. The usual response to increased intracranial pressure is peripheral vasoconstriction and a rising blood pressure. Hemorrhage may, of course, mask this response. Nevertheless, the occurrence of hypotension in a patient with a serious head injury necessitates a careful search for *other* causes. If the central venous pressure is low and other evidence indicates hypovolemia, blood loss must be assumed and its source found. In this regard the abdomen is difficult to evaluate in head injury patients. Thus, if no other site of blood loss is found, objective evidence must be sought to diagnose or rule out intra-abdominal bleeding (e.g., paracentesis with peritoneal lavage — see Chapter 14).

Certain "tissue factors" may contribute to the overall end result of traumatic shock. There are major changes in the co-

TABLE 4–2. Etiology of Stress to Myocardium

Preload
    loss of plasma volume
        (trauma, operations, etc.)
    neurogenic or toxic venodilation
    cardiac tamponade
    tension pneumothorax

Afterload
    right ventricle
        (pulmonary embolus)
    left ventricle
        (head injury)

Contractility
    myocardial infarct
    cardiac surgery
    sustained shock
        (MDF, endotoxin, Ca^{++})

agulation mechanisms that may cause a hypercoagulable state with consumption of clotting factors. This is aggravated by the so-called "tourniquet" effect that is caused by stasis and sludging in the microcirculation during the shock period. With the onset of resuscitation, a "declamping" type of shock similar to that occurring during aortic surgery may then develop, aggravating the original shock insult. As these clotting by-products and metabolites and possibly toxic factors from anoxic cells are returned to the circulation they contribute to increased capillary permeability and further interstitial fluid losses. Another similar contributing factor may be that of continuing tissue injury, as exemplified by unsplinted fractures.

THE EXTRACELLULAR RESPONSES TO HEMORRHAGE IN MAN

A great deal of experimental work has been done on the circulatory, metabolic and endocrine responses to hemorrhage, but much of the work in animals is of limited value because of species differences and the use of anesthesia (see Chapter 3). However, there have been several studies in humans, in both injured patients and normal volunteers.[8, 15, 20, 23, 30, 31, 41, 43, 50, 53, 58, 62, 68, 72, 78, 83, 92, 97, 102, 108, 117, 120, 125, 127, 129, 132, 146, 150] The following brief and oversimplified version of the sequence of events that follows blood loss is based on

TABLE 4–3. Composite of Reported Responses to Hemorrhage in Man*

BLOOD LOSS	VASCULAR RESPONSE	ENDOCRINE RESPONSE	METABOLIC RESPONSE	SIGNS AND SYMPTOMS
Minimal (15%)	Contraction of great veins; recruitment of ECF	Slight	Slight	Usually transient
Moderate (30%)	All of above. Arteriolar constriction with reduced flow to skin and muscle. Decreased cardiac output; narrow pulse pressure; tachycardia.	Increase in aldosterone, ADH, growth hormone. Variable increase in cortisol, catecholamines. No increase in insulin.	Increased glycolysis and mild hyperglycemia. Increased lipolysis and free fatty acid levels. Small increase in lactate levels. Hyperventilation with alkalemia. Oxygen consumption may be increased. Decreased urinary sodium and volume.	Thirst, orthostatic hypotension, apprehension, weakness, pallor, cool skin.
Severe (45%)	All of above. Cardiac output less than 50% normal. Hypotension. Most of remaining cardiac output to heart and brain.	All of above. Marked increase in catecholamines.	Severe lactic acidosis. Severe oliguria. Mixed venous pO_2 approaching 20 mm. Hg or less.	Air hunger. Deteriorating state of consciousness.

*Note: individual variation is most marked at the 15 per cent hemorrhage level.

such studies (see Table 4–3 and Figure 4–3).

The initial response to blood loss is contraction of the great veins, the "capacitance" system. This response is both intrinsic and under neural control and results in a smaller vascular space in which the resulting decreased blood volume can still serve adequately with little change needed elsewhere in the system. It is therefore a very efficient response, similar to an internal transfusion. However, it can only buffer the loss of about 10 per cent of the normal blood volume. At the same time some inflow of extracellular fluid to the vascular space begins. However, cardiac output and oxygen consumption do not change, and the endocrine and metabolic changes are minimal.

At about 15 to 20 per cent of blood volume loss, more extensive adjustments occur. The compensatory ability of the venous capacitance system has been exceeded. The ability of the extracellular space to replenish plasma volume is still intact, assuming a normally nourished and hydrated individual, but this takes hours to exert its effect. Triggered by atrial and arterial wall receptors, sympathetic stimulation of the heart results in tachycardia, which moves the heart to a new work-pressure relationship in which a higher output is achieved for a given filling pressure. This involves more work by the heart muscle, requiring coronary dilation and an increased fraction of the cardiac output diverted to the heart itself. Blood flow to skin and muscle may be reduced by sympathetically mediated arteriolar constriction. Endocrine responses become more evident, and aldosterone and antidiuretic hormone levels are increased, resulting in salt

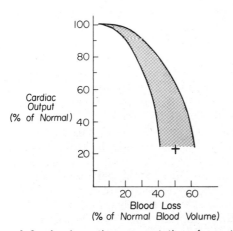

Figure 4–3. A schematic representation of reported changes in cardiac output corresponding to acute changes in blood volume. A considerable range of response is indicated. Data are least complete at the largest volume losses. Sources are cited in the text.

and water retention and a lower urinary output. Blood sugar and free fatty acid levels will rise, oxygen consumption will increase and lactate levels may rise slightly as anaerobic metabolic pathways begin to be utilized. Hyperventilation will begin, resulting in alkalemia. With this amount of blood loss cardiac output begins to decrease, and systolic blood pressure and central venous pressure fall. The patient may experience thirst, weakness and some apprehension. He will begin to look pale and his skin will be cool. If he moves or sits up he may exhibit orthostatic hypotension and become light-headed and nauseated or may even lose consciousness. This amount of blood loss (15 to 20 per cent) also has the greatest individual variation of response, varying from partial decompensation and a clinical picture of severe shock in some patients to a deceptively normal appearance in others. This latter situation is treacherous because decompensation may occur suddenly with relatively small further losses, and it will almost certainly occur if the patient is given general anesthesia without some form of effective volume replacement.

At a 30 per cent loss of blood volume, practically all patients will exhibit some if not most of the signs and symptoms of shock: thirst, pallor, cool skin, severe orthostatic hypotension, tachycardia, oliguria and a systolic blood pressure of below 100 mm. Hg even when supine. Cardiac output is significantly reduced despite the institution of perfusion priorities by selective regional arteriolar constriction. Blood flow to the viscera is maintained at the expense of the carcass, and even the distribution of visceral flow is altered to protect the heart and brain. Renal blood flow decreases as renal vascular resistance increases. The endocrine responses become more marked, and lactic acid levels are significantly elevated.

If blood loss continues, all of the compensatory responses are exceeded and blood flow to the heart and brain decreases. Air hunger is marked, and the patient will lose consciousness. Metabolic acidosis becomes profound as blood flow to the liver falls below a critical level. A blood volume of 50 per cent of normal cannot be tolerated for long. Even with a 50 per cent loss that has been stopped, expansion of plasma volume from endogenous

sources alone may not occur in time. When central aortic pressure falls below the level at which coronary perfusion can be maintained, cardiac output falls, resulting in a further fall in central aortic pressure (the adrenergic neural and humoral responses, already at maximum levels, cannot increase further to maintain pressure), which in turn causes a further fall in coronary perfusion. Once this vicious circle is entered, death rapidly ensues.

This "classic" pathophysiological interpretation of hemorrhagic shock as a circulatory phenomenon is incomplete. A prolonged, severe reduction of peripheral and visceral blood flow will also lead to a number of serious decompensations or breakdowns in various organs and systems that are distinct from the circulatory decompensation; these have been described in the previous chapter.

TREATMENT

Traumatic shock is an acute emergency that takes precedence over all other conditions except respiratory failure or ventilatory arrest. Assessment and treatment are often simultaneous. For purposes of the initial discussion of treatment we will assume that the patient is critically injured and that heroic measures are required. Lesser degrees of injury will allow more time for assessment and judgment in regard to treatment. Also, traumatic shock allows inadequate delivery of oxygen and substrate to the tissues, and therefore we will consider all possible means of increasing oxygen transport to the microcirculation.

Initial Assessment. The priorities for resuscitation and treatment are listed in Table 4–4. To assign these priorities the condition of the patient must first be assessed. Quickly undress the patient entirely; roll him from side to side to check for posterior wounds. Feel the extremities to ascertain peripheral perfusion, and simultaneously check the neck veins. If the patient's extremities are cool and pale (indicating shock) and the neck veins are distended, one can assume a cardiogenic etiology such as tension pneumothorax, pericardial tamponade, or myocardial contusion. If, however, the patient has signs of shock and the neck veins are flat, hypovo-

TABLE 4–4. Treatment Priorities in Traumatic Shock

1. Establish airway

2. Ensure cardiovascular function —
   pump
   volume

3. Arrest hemorrhage

4. Check for neurological injuries

5. Splint fractures

6. Make definitive diagnosis

lemia should be assumed until proven otherwise.

Airway. After this initial assessment, which should take less than a few moments, ventilatory exchange should be assessed. Obvious ventilatory arrest should be treated immediately with either mouth-to-mouth resuscitation or the use of a bag and mask. It is not necessary to intubate immediately a patient who has sustained ventilatory arrest. This may take more than a few seconds and precious time will have been lost during the attempt. In the great majority of cases a bag and mask or the mouth-to-mouth technique is all that is necessary for the initial resuscitation. Stridor and suprasternal or intercostal retraction indicate airway obstruction. If these are observed, quickly clear the airway and remove all secretions and foreign material, including vomitus and blood, from the mouth and posterior pharynx. *Adequate suction is invaluable.* Hold up the patient's chin, pull out his tongue or force the mandible forward by pressure behind the angle of the jaw to prevent soft tissue obstruction of the hypopharnyx. An oropharyngeal or nasopharyngeal airway in the unconscious patient is useful. In patients with extensive soft tissue injury or facial fractures, clamping the tongue with a towel clip and pulling it forward may at least partially relieve the soft tissue obstruction. Tracheal intubation with an endotracheal or nasotracheal tube may be required immediately in some instances but usually can be delayed until resuscitation has progressed and specific indications for intubation are present. Tracheostomy as an emergency procedure is rarely indicated but may be necessary if there is an upper airway injury or foreign body ob-

struction. Other indications include blast injuries to the face or other severe maxillofacial injuries or a combination of head and cervical spine injuries in which the hyperextension required for intubation is contraindicated. If respiratory distress is due to other causes, maintain a clear airway, treat the underlying cause, and, if possible, increase the level of inspired oxygen.

Cardiovascular Factors. Once oxygen has been brought in from the ambient air to pulmonary alevoli it is necessary to insure that it reaches the most critical organs, the heart and brain. This requires a functioning heart and adequate blood volume. During the initial assessment we attempt to differentiate between cardiac or pump failure and volume deficiency. If the primary problem appears to be inadequate cardiac action, the cause must be rapidly discovered. Tension pneumothorax may be ruled out quickly simply by feeling for the trachea above the suprasternal notch. If this is deviated to one side or the other, a tube thoracostomy should be performed immediately in the side opposite the deviation. A large bore needle inserted into the side of the deviation will also have dramatic results in relieving a tension pneumothorax. This treatment, however, is temporary and must be followed by tube thoracostomy. *Do not wait* for radiographic confirmation of a pneumothorax in a critically ill patient. If pneumothorax is suspected, proceed immediately to tube thoracostomy.

If tension pneumothorax has been ruled out, the next step is elimination of cardiac tamponade and myocardial contusion or infarct. If the patient is not in extremis, tamponade can be diagnosed by measuring the central venous pressure line and/or by performing a diagnostic (and therapeutic) pericardiocentesis. An 18- or 20-gauge spinal needle is inserted precutaneously at a 45-degree angle beneath the xiphoid and is directed toward the left shoulder. Attachment of the precordial lead of an EKG apparatus will aid in determining that the needle has entered the pericardial space; as the needle contacts the epicardial surface, there will be an inversion of the QRS wave, confirming that the needle is in the pericardial sac and not the ventricular cavity. Aspiration of blood in this position should have a dramatic therapeutic effect as well as obvious diagnostic implications.

If the patient is in extremis, one should not bother with these measures but should make an immediate left anterior thoracotomy through the fourth or fifth intercostal space (usually the intercostal space directly beneath the left nipple). Skin preparation is preferred but not mandatory. A single long incision should be made from the sternal border towards the mid-axillary line. Once the chest has been entered, one or two costal cartilages may be divided using heavy (i.e., bandage) scissors just lateral to the sternal margin to avoid the internal mammary vessels. A chest retractor is then inserted and opened, and the pericardium is inspected. If it is bulging, a vertical pericardiotomy is made on its anterior lateral aspect, just anterior to the phrenic nerve. The evaluation of clotted and unclotted blood will often result in dramatic improvement. Often there is a gushing of blood from the pericardial cavity with each systolic contraction. Digital control of the cardiac wound is all that is necessary until definitive repair can be carried out in the operating room. Myocardial defects larger than one digit are usually not compatible with survival, and such patients rarely reach an emergency department alive.

Other indications for emergency thoracotomy include cardiac arrest from exsanguinating hemorrhage and suspected air embolism. It is impossible to resuscitate by closed chest massage the empty heart of a patient who has suffered a cardiac arrest from hypovolemic shock. In addition to the advantages of directly massaging the heart, the descending thoracic aorta may be clamped, and what little circulating volume is left can be diverted primarily to the heart and brain. *Air embolism* is a rare cause of circulatory collapse in the emergency department and is even more difficult to diagnose.[137] Left-sided air embolism should be suspected in patients with penetrating wounds of either side of the chest who present with shock and focal neurological findings. Another diagnostic sign includes aspiration of air or froth when arterial blood is withdrawn for blood gas analysis. In such cases, the suspected hemithorax should be opened immediately, and the hilum of the lung should be clamped with a vascular clamp to mini-

mize the air inoculum. Excess air can then be aspirated from the heart (see later discussion).

PUMP FAILURE.   Patients with "pump failure" secondary to myocardial contusion or infarction should be treated like any patient who has had a myocardial infarct. Arrhythmias are common early and may require administration of lidocaine and occasionally atropine, depending on the specific arrhythmia. In most instances of myocardial contusion, left ventricular failure is minimal, and treatment can be conservative, consisting of oxygen to relieve hypoxemia and the judicious use of diuretics if fluid retention is noted. With more severe left ventricular failure more aggressive treatment with cardiac drugs should be considered, but this should be preceded by hemodynamic monitoring of the arterial pressure, pulmonary arterial wedge pressure and cardiac output. The stroke work index can be computed from these measurements, and rational therapy can be given on the basis of the specific hemodynamic abnormality found.

Hypotension is often the first sign that cardiac injury may be more severe than is suggested by slight dyspnea and pulmonary rales. If the left ventricular filling pressure is low (less than 12 torr) and cardiac output is normal despite the low arterial pressure, hypovolemia is the most probable cause of the hypotension; it should be treated by increments of volume replacement beginning with 100 ml. of saline or balanced salt solution. Right sided air embolism following trauma is usually seen with penetrating neck wounds, which should be quickly covered by an impervious material and the patient placed in the left lateral position. Thoracotomy may be required for resuscitation. If the cardiac output does not increase as the left ventricular filling pressure increases to 15 to 20 torr, further volume replacement should be stopped to prevent pulmonary edema, which may occur abruptly.

If the only hemodynamic abnormality is a raised left ventricular filling pressure and the blood pressure and output are maintained normally, more vigorous diuresis should be attempted with large doses of furosemide. Excessive diuresis must be avoided because the patient may then become hypovolemic, particularly if there are associated injuries. Some patients with acute myocardial contusion or myocardial infarction may have hypotension with impaired tissue perfusion caused primarily by failure of compensatory peripheral vasoconstriction, with no substantial change in cardiac filling pressures or output. These patients often respond with a rise in arterial pressure to sympathomimeticamines (epinephrine and dopamine), which simulate the beta-adrenergic receptors. These drugs should be infused at a slow rate to avoid tachycardia, a marked increase in blood pressure or ventricular arrhythmias. The goal is to maintain the blood pressure without increasing stroke work or provoking arrhythmias.

When cardiac dysfunction is more severe, with reduced cardiac output, increased left ventricular filling (above 20 torr), and arterial blood pressures at or above 90 torr, vasodilator therapy to reduce the afterload on the heart should be begun cautiously while the hemodynamic result is monitored. Drugs such as sodium nitroprusside, phentolamine or nitroglycerine given by intravenous drip decrease the impedance to left ventricular ejection. Reduced left ventricular volume and filling pressure may improve the left ventricular stroke work, decrease myocardial oxygen consumption and thereby improve perfusion to the brain, kidney and heart. Vasodilator therapy cannot be used if there is a significant reduction in arterial pressure because it may aggravate the situation. Therefore, efforts should be made to raise the arterial pressure to about 100 torr before vasodilator therapy is used. If this is not possible with vasopressors without worsening the left ventricular filling pressure and aggravating the cardiac failure, aortic balloon counter pulsation may be used to provide a temporary circulatory assist. It must be stressed that isolated myocardial contusion or infarction is an uncommon cause of hypotension following trauma. More commonly associated injuries cause the hypotension on the basis of hypovolemia. Therefore, the treatments for myocardial contusion and infarct described above *should be used only when hypovolemia has either been treated or ruled out.*

VOLUME REPLACEMENT. If the original assessment of the patient reveals that the patient is in shock and the neck veins are flat, hypovolemia must be assumed.

Successful treatment depends on rapidly gaining major access to the vascular space by the insertion of one or more venous catheters. The number of catheters will depend on the severity of shock. A cutdown on the long saphenous vein at the ankle is the surest and quickest way to gain access. A cutdown on the basilic vein in the antecubital space is also desirable so that central venous pressure monitoring can be achieved. Percutaneous insertion of central venous catheters via the subclavian or internal jugular veins is not usually recommended for treatment of hypovolemic shock because the great veins will be collapsed and the chances of complications, such as pneumothorax, are greatly increased. In extenuating circumstances, such as resuscitation by a single physician, percutaneous femoral vein catheterization may provide rapid access to the circulation without the risk of such serious complications. All catheters inserted percutaneously or by cutdown should be of large caliber.

In these circumstances the primary goal is to restore adequate plasma volume. The types of fluids to be used will be discussed in greater detail in a following section, but in general, during the first 24 hours, it is advisable to use primarily balanced salt solution and whole blood. In mild or moderate shock it makes little difference what type of intravenous fluid is used — balanced salt solution, normal saline, plasma or plasma products. Cost and availability may be the prime factors in determining which is preferable. However, in *severe* shock the type of fluid used *is* important! This statement is based on the premise that in severe traumatic shock endothelial permeability may be increased, not only in the area of injury but systemically. Thus, if the endothelium is altered by the shock insult, a "capillary leak" occurs, and the choice of type of fluid administered should be based on physiologic principles (Starling's forces)[64, 65] (see later discussion).

As soon as fluid replacement has been properly initiated, monitoring of the effects of this resuscitative effort is invaluable because fluid replacement should be governed by physiologic principles and not determined by fixed formulas.[63] The best indices for successful resuscitation are atrial filling pressures and urinary output. The central venous pressure is all that is necessary for monitoring the resuscitation of most trauma patients. Although the monitoring of left atrial filling pressures is ideal, it is quite impractical in most emergency department situations. Of course, true left atrial pressure is only rarely measured; instead, the pulmonary arterial wedge pressure obtained by a Swan-Ganz catheter is monitored as a direct reflection of left atrial pressure. This measurement should be made in patients who are critically injured, particularly in the postoperative period, in patients who have antecedent diseases such as congestive heart failure and chronic obstructive pulmonary disease, and in some patients who require mechanical ventilatory support. In mild or moderate shock atrial filling pressures of up to 25 torr are readily tolerated. In patients with severe shock in whom the capillary leak syndrome has occurred, atrial filling pressures must be kept at or near normal (3 to 8 torr). Higher filling pressures will simply increase the formation of interstitial edema.

The urethra must be catheterized in all patients with traumatic shock so that urine output can be carefully monitored. Urine output of greater than 0.5 ml./kg./hr. indicates an adequate renal and presumably visceral blood flow. Other evidences of adequate volume restoration include a clear sensorium and the return of color, warmth and prompt capillary filling to the extremities. It is useful to monitor the arterial blood gases. They may reveal unsuspected hypoxemia, which, if uncorrected, will impair the delivery of oxygen that is so essential in traumatic shock. Significant metabolic acidosis (base deficit) indicates profound or prolonged shock or the presence of some other complicating factor such as diabetic ketoacidosis. The absence of significant lowering of the arterial pH does not mean that significant blood loss or circulatory insufficiency has not occurred. It is clear that metabolic acidosis is a relatively late development in injured patients and that the arterial pH does not correlate well with the clinical situation soon after injury[39] at least in part because a respiratory alkalosis compensates for the metabolic acidosis by the time the returning venous blood has passed through the lungs. For this reason, sampling the central venous pO_2 can provide a more sensitive index of the circulatory status. A mixed venous pO_2 ($\bar{v} pO_2$) of below 25 torr indicates a severe circulatory insufficiency in which barely enough oxygen is being supplied to maintain life. A $\bar{v} pO_2$ of greater than 40 torr generally indicates that the circulatory system is adequately meeting its demands. Serial monitoring is valuable because a rising $\bar{v} pO_2$ indicates an improving circulatory status, whereas a falling $\bar{v} pO_2$ is cause for concern. The central venous catheter usually samples blood from the superior vena cava, which under conditions of stress yields somewhat higher pO_2 values than mixed venous blood, but the above relationships remain the same.[66]

By following the above parameters, the adequacy of one's resuscitative efforts may be objectively gauged. If atrial filling pressure and urine output are both elevated, too much intravenous fluid is being administered and the rate of infusion should be promptly decreased. On the other hand, if atrial filling pressure and urine output are decreased, more fluid volume is required. A common finding is increased atrial filling pressure and decreased urine output. In this situation measurement of the cardiac output is very useful. If the cardiac output is high in this setting, it usually means that renal function is decreased, and an osmotic diuretic (such as 12.5 to 25 grams of mannitol) may be helpful. This may be followed by a gradual infusion of an additional 50 grams of mannitol, until a urine output in the range of 0.5 mg./kg./hr. is achieved. However, in the presence of continued anuria or severe oliguria, the maximum dose of mannitol should be 75 to 100 grams. If there is no response to mannitol and blood volume restoration has been adequate, a chemical diuretic such as furosemide may be cautiously administered. Because these compounds may cause systemic vasodilation as well as redistribution of blood flow within the kidney, only small intravenous doses, such as 10 to 20 mg. should be given.

On the other hand, if the cardiac output is low when atrial filling pressures are high and urine output is low, decreased myocardial contractility must be suspected. In the absence of a myocardial contusion or infarction, an inotropic agent is indicated, the most widely used being dopamine, isoproterenol and 10 per cent calcium chloride. Dopamine hydrochloride (200 mg. in 500 ml. of sodium injection USP; 400 μg./per ml.) is given initially at a rate of 2.5 micrograms per kilogram per minute. These doses stimulate both the dopanergic receptors (which increase the renal blood flow and urine output) and the beta-adrenergic cardiac receptors (which increase cardiac output). Higher doses (i.e., above 20 μg./kg./min.) stimulate the alpha receptors, which causes systemic vasoconstriction and reverses the renal vasodilation seen at lower doses. Isoproterenol, a beta-adrenergic stimulator, increases cardiac output by its action on the myocardial contraction mechanism and produces peripheral vasodilation. One should administer 1 to 2 milligrams in 500 milliliters of 5 per cent dextrose and water intravenously. Because of its inotropic effect, this drug is associated with an increased incidence of cardiac arrhythmia. Therefore, its use is not advised if the cardiac rate is above 100 to 200 per minute. Calcium chloride (10 ml. of a 10 per cent solution) may be administered directly intravenously over a 2 to 3 minute period, provided there is continuous cardiac monitoring for arrhythmia. Although this may provide an instant and impressive inotropic response, it is usually short-lived, and repeated doses are required. Measurement of ionized calcium levels is valuable in such situations because calcium chloride may have specific therapeutic value following massive transfusions when citrate toxicity may be causing myocardial depression.[25]

As stated earlier, resuscitation efforts during the first 24 hours should consist primarily of infusions of balanced salt solution and whole blood. During the second 24 hours, after the capillaries have regained their integrity, the patient needs enough water to replace sensible and insensible losses and colloid solutions to maintain the serum albumin and the hematocrit at near normal levels. The patients' needs for salt will be minimal since they will be mobilizing interstitial and intracellular fluid.

Hemorrhage. When there is ongoing hemorrhage, every effort to control it must be taken. External bleeding can be controlled in most instances by the application of direct pressure. Rarely, a tourniquet will be necessary for wounds of the extremities usually when a traumatic amputation has occurred. Pelvic and abdominal bleeding may be temporarily controlled using the MAST suit.[10] This three-compartment pressure suit can be inflated to 80 torr, but its safety and the allowable duration of inflation have not been completely determined. Removal of the suit may prove hazardous, particularly if the suit has been applied in the "field" and the patient arrives without having received intravenous fluids. Therefore, two large caliber intravenous catheters should be inserted prior to deflation, and each of the compartments should be deflated separately with concomitant restoration of volume. The opportunity for definitive operative intervention must be available at the time the G-suit is deflated.

Internal hemorrhage may or may not have ceased by the time the patient arrives in the emergency department. The administration of two liters of crystalloid solution may be used as an arbitrary index of the patient's status. If after the rapid administration of this volume, the patient's vital signs are normal or near normal, continued resuscitation and definitive diagnosis may then be carried out. If, on the other hand, the patient's response is inadequate or his condition is unstable and continues to deteriorate, *immediate operative intervention is usually indicated.* The only necessary diagnostic maneuver in this situation is a chest radiograph to rule out significant blood loss within the thoracic cavity. At this point laparotomy becomes a resuscitative measure, since it is carried out under the assumption that there is a massive, uncontrolled internal hemorrhage requiring direct surgical control.

BLOOD VOLUME RESTORATION: HEMOTHERAPY (TABLE 4–5). Modern surgery, including trauma surgery, is not possible without the availability of adequate supplies of blood. Hospitals should survey their transfusion practices regularly and determine the appropriate number of units of blood that need to be routinely available for emergencies.

Surgical patients usually receive blood tranfusions for the restoration of red cell mass or whole blood volume. In the stable preoperative patient, a blood transfusion to normalize the red cell mass is optimally performed by using packed red blood cells. In the patient with major hemor-

TABLE 4–5. Component Hemotherapy

COMPONENT	ADVANTAGES/DISADVANTAGES	PATIENT'S CONDITION
Packed red blood cells	Less citrate, sodium, antibodies, antigen	Anemia without hypovolemia
Frozen red blood cells	Long storage, expense, less hepatitis	Anemia
Reconstituted whole blood	Permits component use from donation	Hypovolemia
Platelet-rich plasma	Minimal centrifugation	Thrombocytopenia
Platelet concentrates	High centrifugation allows low volume transfusion	
Fresh frozen plasma	All clotting factors	Multiple coagulation defects
Platelet poor plasma	Many coagulation factors, normal oncotic pressure	Certain clotting defects, hypovolemia
Single donor plasma		
Cryoprecipitate (anti-hemophilic concentrate)	Storage, high concentration of clotting factors per protein	Hemophilia

rhage, however, whole blood is the best choice because the viscosity of packed red cells precludes rapid transfusion.

The amount of blood that is administered should be governed by the clinical situation and by the amount and kind of other intravenous fluid replacement. The guidelines for volume restoration have been described previously. Ideally, in the severely traumatized patient, the hematocrit should be kept at or near 30 per cent since this effects a compromise between the desired levels of viscosity and oxygen-carrying capacity. Autotransfusion is a useful and occasionally life-saving practice that makes it possible for patients to receive autologous blood with minimal delay. Moreover, blood donated by the recipient is the safest blood that can be administered to him. Emergency autotransfusion can be performed using various types of commercially available equipment or cardiopulmonary bypass pumps. The simplest method of autotransfusion involves the collection of blood from chest tube drainage — if hemothorax is present — into receptacles containing citrate anticoagulant; this mixture can then be directly infused into the recipient. Autotransfusion using commercial or other autotransfusion apparatus is of definite clinical value, but coagulopathies frequently develop with reinfusion of large quantities of autotransfused blood. Autotransfusion is particularly useful when difficulty is encountered in obtaining compatible blood.

The pronounced changes that occur in liquid blood during storage do not necessarily cause metabolic defects after transfusion. Stored blood is intrinsically acid and hyperkalemic. When it is transfused, citrate and lactate, the normal intermediary metabolites in blood, are rapidly metabolized. Citrate, in fact, yields bicarbonate, which results in post-transfusion metabolic alkalosis. Metabolic alkalosis, in the metabolic mileu of sodium retention after injury, contributes to potassium excretion, so the use of hyperkalemic stored blood in this clinical setting seldom presents a problem.

Deterioration of the primary glycolytic intermediate 2,3-diphosphoglycerate (2,3 DPG) in red cells in liquid-preserved blood results in blood with a high affinity of hemoglobin for oxygen administered to patients. The potentially deleterious effects of administering high affinity whole blood to a hypoxic, hypotensive patient have not been definitely established. It is clear that within 12 to 24 hours after receiving 2,3-DPG–deficient blood, mobilization of inorganic phosphate and other metabolic processes results in normalization of 2,3-DPG values.

Hypothermia is a frequent side effect of receiving blood stored at 4° C. Cold patients are less able to metabolize acid and potassium, and hypothermia increases the affinity of hemoglobin for oxygen, a defect that adds to low 2,3-DPG values and post-transfusion alkalosis. Therefore, blood should be administered through blood warmers. Unfortunately, currently available commercial blood warmers are frequently unable to return the temperature of blood to normal when rapid blood volume restitution is necessary.

The citrate anticoagulant in liquid preserved blood will bind ionized calcium in the recipient and is a potential cause of cardiac arrhythmia. Normothermic adults, however, can metabolize the citrate of one unit of blood every 5 minutes without requiring calcium administration. Calcium, however, is a useful inotropic agent, and lacking a reliable electrode to measure ionized calcium current, management in massive transfusion calls for the administration of 14.5 mEq. of calcium for every 5 units of blood if that amount of transfusion occurs in less than 30 minutes. On the other hand, it should be pointed out that *hyper*calcemia is potentially lethal, and calcium should be administered cautiously with EKG monitoring.

Defective hemostasis occurs with massive transfusion. The exact cause of transfusion coagulopathy is incompletely defined. The labile factors (Factors V and VIII) are the only hemostatic factors that decay significantly during liquid preservation of blood. Moreover, in the patient who has been hemodynamically resuscitated, Factor VIII levels will actually be higher than normal because of the accelerated manufacture of Factor VIII by the liver. Therefore, Factor V is the only clotting factor that is significantly lowered in massive blood transfusion. Fresh frozen plasma provides the necessary clotting components, but its effectiveness in transfusion-related bleeding is not firmly established.

More importantly, all blood routinely dispensed from the blood bank should be assumed to lack functioning platelets. Platelets lose their ability to aggregate in cold storage, and preservatives do not maintain platelet viability beyond 72 hours. In addition, most blood banks with component programs routinely remove the platelets from the donated unit. For these reasons, it should be assumed that blood received by routine order contains no platelets. In massive blood transfusions the quantity and functions of platelets in the recipient are roughly proportional to the number of units of blood administered. In general, it is advisable to administer platelet concentrates or "packs" whenever 10 units of blood have been administered in less than 1 hour.

COMPLICATIONS OF TRANSFUSION. Complications of blood transfusion are common and are potentially fatal. Blood is the most dangerous drug used by most physicians. Infectious complications of transfusion—i.e., transmission of syphilis, malaria, bacteria and viruses—are infrequent with current blood banking practices. Hepatitis, however, remains a problem. Blood products carry a hepatitis risk that is proportional to the number of donors contributing to the pool. The recent multiplicity of assays for hepatitis has greatly reduced the potential risk of dispensing blood from hepatitis carriers. New assays for hepatitis have recently shown that most hepatitis that follows transfusion in the United States is not hepatitis B or any other known virus and may represent an unidentified hepatocellular virus. The true risk of hepatitis is unknown because there are many subclinical cases. Most states now require blood to be provided by volunteer donors, which has greatly improved the quality of the donor pool.

Because transfusions are grafts, they may cause isoimmunization against HLA antigen, platelet antigens and red cell antigens. The commonest source of immunologic mismatch, however, is the administration of blood to the wrong recipient. When a significant amount of mismatched blood is administered, massive hemolysis with renal failure and death occurs. A variety of less serious transfusion reactions can occur, but these should be assessed by established criteria.

Early hemolysis is usually the result of incorrect identification of blood specimens. Clinical symptoms are usually chills, fever, back pains, circulatory collapse or hemorrhage. Delayed hemolysis occurs from several days to 4 weeks after transfusion and is manifest as anemia or mild jaundice. Leukocyte antigens are the probable cause of many febrile reactions that are adequately treated with antihistamines. Reactions to transfusions of proteins (especially IgA) are frequently severe and may be hemolytic in nature. Incompatibilities result in antibodies that may cause early or late thrombocytopenia.

Transfusion reactions should be managed according to fundamental principles. The most important requirement is to stop the transfusion but maintain an intravenous infusion to keep the patient well hydrated. A specimen of plasma and urine should be sent to the laboratory to be examined for hemoglobin, which implies hemolysis. The blood and tube used in the transfusion should be saved for investigation as to appropriateness of the cross match, Rh compatibility and Coombs' test. Laboratory identification should be carefully checked and cultures should be done. If a severe reaction has occurred renal function should be evaluated, and the patient should be protected by administration of mannitol and bicarbonate. Subsequent transfusions may be accomplished with great difficulty if the patient has been isoimmunized, and for this reason the patient should receive washed red cells.

Neurological Injuries. The fourth priority in resuscitation is evaluation and treatment of neurological injuries. This is discussed in greater detail in Chapter 8, but it is important for the attending physician to be able to assess the patient for central nervous system injury by frequent brief neurological examinations, including evaluation of the state of consciousness, cranial nerve function, rectal tone and peripheral reflexes, gross skin sensation and motor function.

Fractures. Although occupying last priority, the splinting of all fractures and reduction of dislocations should not be ignored or unduly delayed. The patient should be palpated carefully from head to foot, and all joints should be moved cautiously, exerting gentle pressure on the spine, chest and pelvis. Pain, swelling, deformity crepitus and limitation of motion are the classic signs of fracture and dislocation. Prompt splinting of all fractures is important to prevent further soft tissue injury, neurovascular damage and even continuing hemorrhage, for it has been estimated that as much as 1 liter of blood lost by hemorrhage can be prevented by early use of the Thomas splint.

Failures of Resuscitation: Multiple Organ Failure. Resuscitation can fail if the injury sustained is incompatible with survival. This is not really a failure of resuscitation but rather a reflection of our current therapeutic limitations. Brain injury is the common cause of this situation, but extensive destruction of any of the "vital" organs can also be responsible. In a recent autopsy study of trauma victims, almost 50 per cent of deaths were due to brain injury, but 35 per cent were due to hemorrhage.[141] Of the latter group, most died of either single or multiple organ failure. In fact, multiple organ failure following resuscitation and treatment of traumatic shock now seems to be the major barrier to salvaging these patients. In spite of articles emphasizing the statistical importance of a particular organ or system, most of these patients die of multisystem failure. In some patients a single event or organ failure has clearly led to failure of other organs, but this type of analysis is usually missing in statistics that are focused primarily on one or another system.

Circulatory failure has received by far the most attention in experimental work with hemorrhagic shock in laboratory animals. The concept of "irreversible shock" arose from work in which animals died in shock long after all their shed blood had been restored.[147]

However, patients resuscitated from traumatic shock rarely exhibit a pure form of cardiogenic shock. In fact, several groups of clinical investigators have tried to abolish the concept as being potentially harmful in the clinical context.[15, 68, 132] This issue is closely linked to the role of the heart in persistent circulatory failure. The heart is potentially vulnerable because of a number of peculiarities in its oxygen supply. Because it normally extracts almost all of the available oxygen from its blood supply, leaving very little reserve, increased demands must be met by increases in coronary blood flow. Coronary blood flow in turn is dependent on central aortic *diastolic* pressure and on the ability of the coronary vessels to dilate. Since most of the coronary blood flow occurs during diastole, the total fraction of time the heart spends in diastole significantly influences coronary flow. Most physiologic consequences of severe hemorrhage challenge this system: diastolic pressure falls, the work demands on the heart increase and a higher fraction of time is spent in systole. These events place a critical demand on the coronary vessels to dilate, and this constitutes one of the weak links in the patient's defenses against hemorrhage.

In animal models, although there is evidence on both sides, it seems clear that the heart retains enough reserve function to prevent death, and the prime causes of low cardiac output are impaired venous return and decreased coronary flow.[56, 91, 106, 111, 121] Most instances of persistent volume-resistant circulatory failure observed by the authors have occurred in patients with arteriosclerotic coronary disease who have been subjected to prolonged hypotension. These patients apparently died from acute heart failure, although this was not corroborated by left atrial pressure measurements. This situation also occurs, albeit rarely, in younger patients, but almost always in these patients it is accompanied by clotting abnormalities and renal/pulmonary failure.

Recent work has indicated the existence of a specific "shock factor" that becomes manifest following burn, sepsis or trauma.[75] This myocardial depressant factor (MDF) leads to decreased contractility and subsequent low cardiac output. However, the existence of this factor remains controversial.[61] Conceivably this kind of cardiac failure is not due to circulating humoral factors but is the result of a failure in excitation-contraction coupling due to electrolyte abnormalities or changes in myocardial compliance.[103]

The clotting system can deteriorate to the point of allowing diffuse, uncontrollable bleeding as a consequence of shock but only after very severe blood loss — i.e., almost never with losses of less than 30 per cent unless a mismatched blood transfusion is involved. In addition to the bleeding diathesis that can occur after massive transfusions of bank blood, abnormal bleeding can result from a consumptive coagulopathy known as disseminated intravascular coagulation (DIC). This is a well-documented sequela of hemorrhage in animals.[57, 87] In man the situation is complicated by the effects of injury which involve the probable release of tissue thromboplastins and local platelet sequestration, but well-documented cases have occurred after hemorrhage alone. The most common setting for DIC, however, is in the patient who develops post-injury sepsis. When serious pathologic bleeding develops, prognosis is poor. Heparin and clotting factor replacements may improve clotting factor levels in the circulation, but renal, pulmonary and circulatory failure is the usual consequence, and death occurs within 24 hours. Against this background, the clinician must differentiate "medical" from "surgical" bleeding. As several wise observers have commented, the most common and significant clotting deficit in injured patients is silk, a principle that should always be kept in mind, but when pathologic bleeding occurs it is usually obvious, even to the skeptic.

Renal failure is one of the best known causes of resuscitative failure in injured patients. It became recognized as an entity in its own right during World War II, and its pathophysiology was further elucidated during the Korean War. Since then it has been further defined by the recognition of a variety of forms and by the impact of hemodialysis. Unfortunately, hemodialysis is far more successful in treating renal failure in patients with medical diseases than in trauma victims. Renal failure after major injury still carries a very high mortality, essentially unchanged from that in the Korean War.[17, 96, 110, 151] The causes and mechanisms are still debated. Tubular precipitation with mechanical blockage, uncontrolled back diffusion of urine, renal tubular toxin, ischemic damage due to prolonged vasoconstriction or shunting of blood away from the cortex, interstitial edema sufficient to cause mechanical obstruction and disseminated intravascular coagulation are among the factors that have been suggested as causes of acute renal failure following injury. No single animal model has duplicated the antecedent clinical setting and the pathologic picture found in patients. Renal failure sometimes follows apparently moderate degrees of hemorrhage and injury, and its cause is then particularly puzzling. Some investigators have implied that resuscitation and the injudicious use of certain agents set the stage for acute tubular necrosis.[60, 81] The incidence of post-traumatic renal failure in Vietnam was much less than had been expected, and many clinicians feel that this was due to the aggressive use of crystalloid solutions and prevention of hypovolemia. Clearly, the reduction in delay between wounding and treatment was also an important factor.

Pulmonary failure continues to be a topic of considerable interest and concern; it is discussed in detail in Chapter 6. Although our ability to handle this form of organ failure has improved dramatically in the past few years, it still contributes significantly to mortality and morbidity following injury. The recognition of ventilatory failure is now much easier because of the widespread use of blood gas analysis. Formerly, unexpected deaths and "cardiac arrests" were often undoubtedly the result of unrecognized and hence untreated ventilatory failure.

The important principle that follows from these observations is that routine arterial blood gas analysis is advisable in the seriously injured patient. The frequency of sampling should be determined by the status of the patient but should be more frequent in the more seriously ill and in those with conditions that carry an extra risk of pulmonary impairment. Use of oxygen therapy should not be indiscriminate, since oxygen itself is potentially damaging to alveoli; the inspired oxygen tension should be no higher than is necessary for nearly complete saturation of hemoglobin with oxygen. Since an arterial pO_2 of 70 torr usually signifies 90 per cent saturation or better, there is little to be gained by increasing the inspired oxygen concentration to raise the pO_2 above this level. In addition, oxygen that is delivered without adequate humidification can seriously impair the clearing of bronchial secretions. Once hypoxemia is detected, however, it should be treated promptly and to the extent necessary. There is probably more damage done by delaying the use of ventilatory assistance than by overaggressive intervention. Indirect evidence indicates that early and correct ventilatory assistance can prevent more serious pulmonary insufficiency a day or two later. This complex of problems appears to be much more easily halted and reversed in its early stages.

There are many well-documented causes of hypoxemia in injured patients. These have been reviewed elsewhere.[36, 46, 93] The effects of severe hemorrhage on pulmonary function are also rather well documented.[38] Gas exchange is well maintained during hemorrhage. The ratio of dead space to tidal ventilation increases as reduced pulmonary blood flow occurs mainly through dependent parts of the lungs under the influence of gravity, while ventilation of the upper parts continues. After reinfusion of shed blood there is a variable amount of congestion, interstitial edema, leukocyte and platelet aggregation and loss of compliance. But gas exchange remains intact in most cases, and these changes do not progress but rather improve during the days following resuscitation. The degree of change may be related to the type of fluid used for resuscitation. Severe hemorrhage and resuscitation, then, do affect the lungs in a detrimental way, but a progressive or delayed onset pulmonary insufficiency has been so difficult to reproduce experimentally that there is a growing conviction that ventilatory failure in patients after resuscitation is due to other causes, most commonly post-injury sepsis.[48, 67] See Chapter 6 for more detailed discussion.

With the possible exception of CNS deterioration, sepsis is the most common cause of organ failure following injury. Causes of sepsis include prolonged hypoperfusion, inappropriate resuscitation, injudicious use of drugs such as antibiotics and steroids, inadequate debridement and splinting, poor aseptic technique and, last but not least, failure of the immune system. It is this last category — failure of the immune system — that may lead to other organ failures after the development of sepsis. The immune system is made up of immunocompetent cells, including the thymus-derived (T) cells, bone marrow-derived (B) cells and accessory (A) cells or macrophages. This immune system is very tightly regulated, and insults such as burns or trauma may upset its delicate balance. Recent evidence shows that there is a predominance of T suppressor cells and/or inhibitory A cells that subsequently leads to immune depression and sets the stage for sepsis in the post-injury state.[9] Several factors may contribute to this immune depression, including splenectomy and the inappropriate or injudicious use of various drugs. Antibiotics and steroids have been shown to have a deleterious effect on the immune system, but the mechanisms are beyond the scope of this chapter. Factors such as age, nutrition and diabetes are also important contributors to this immune depression. Those factors over which the surgeon may have direct influence include the removal of necrotic tissue from the wound, removal of foreign bodies, use of appropriate sutures, evacuation of hematomas, and closure of dead space. Clearly, the frontier of better trauma management today lies in reducing the incidence of post-injury sepsis and infection. Progress here holds the key to reducing the incidence of post-injury organ failure.

Stress ulceration is a cause of resuscitative failure that usually follows other complications, in particular, sepsis. Recent investigations indicate that the mucosal barriers in the stomach may be impaired after serious injury, thereby explaining the paradoxically low free acid content found in the stomachs of patients at high risk of acute ulcerative complications as well as the somewhat peculiar pattern of distribution of these ulcers.

In summary, seriously injured patients who reach a hospital alive but do not survive die for a variety of reasons. Some have injuries incompatible with life, and little can be done for them. Most such injuries are in the category of CNS damage. Some patients have associated disease that seriously impairs the capacity of certain vital systems to withstand the stress of hemorrhage and injury. Most will have identifiable failures in various organs or systems, including the renal, pulmonary, clotting, hepatic, gastrointestinal and immune systems. Circulatory failure usually occurs because coronary disease combined with high work demands will not allow adequate coronary perfusion at low pressures. In light of all these considerations, reducing the *delay* between injury and treatment and insuring satisfactory *initial* management can be expected to do more to decrease mortality and morbidity than any immediately foreseeable scientific development.

REFERENCES

1. Alexander, J. W., Dionigi, R., and Meakins, J. L.: Periodic variation in the antibacterial function of human neutrophils and its relationship to sepsis. Ann. Surg. *173*:206, 1971.
2. Alexander, J. W., and Meakins, J. L.: Natural defense mechanisms in clinical sepsis. J. Surg. Res. *11*:148, 1971.
3. Alexander, J. W., and Moncrief, J. A.: Alterations of the immune response following severe thermal injury. Arch. Surg. *93*:75, 1966.
4. Alho, A.: Lysosomal functions in circulatory shock. Ann. Clin. Gyn. Fenn. *60*:159, 1971.
5. Altemeier, W. A.: The significance of infection in trauma. Bull. Am. Coll. Surg. *57*(1 Feb.):7, 1972.
6. Altemeier, W. A., Fullen, W. D., and McDonough, J. J.: Sepsis and gastrointestinal bleeding. Ann. Surg. *175*:759, 1972.
7. Altura, B. M., and Hershey, S. G.: Sequential changes in reticuloendothelial system function after acute hemorrhage. Proc. Soc. Exp. Biol. Med. *139*:935, 1972.
8. Anderson, R. W., Simmons, R. L., Collins, J. A., Bredenberg, C. E., James, P. M., and Levitsky, S.: Plasma volume and sulfate spaces in acute combat casualties. Surg. Gynec. Obstet. *128*:719, 1969.
9. Baker, C., and Miller, C.: Suppressor cells in burn patients' leukocytes. Proc. Am. Burn Assn. p. 55, 1978.
10. Batalden, D. J., Wichstrom, P., Ruez, E., and Gustilo, R.: Value of the G suit in patients with severe pelvic fracture: Controlling hemorrhagic shock. Arch. Surg. *109*:326, 1974.
11. Baue, A. E., Chaudry, I. H., Wurth, M. A., and Sayeed, M. M.: Cellular alterations with shock and ischemia. Angiology *25*:(1):31, 1974.
12. Baue, A. E., and Sayeed, M. M.: Alterations in the functional capacity of mitochondria in hemorrhagic shock. Surgery *68*:40, 1970.
13. Baxter, C. R., Canizaro, P. C., Carrico, C. J., and Shires, G. T.: Fluid resuscitation of hemorrhagic shock. Postgrad. Med. *48*:95, 1970.
14. Bayliss, W. M.: Intravenous injection in wound shock. London, Longman, Green and Co., 1918.
15. Beecher, H. K., Burnett, C. H., Shapiro, S. L., Sunione, F. A., Smith, L. D., Sullivan, E. R., and Mallory, T. B.: The physiologic effects of wounds. Medical Dept., U.S. Army: Surgery in World War II. Office of the Surgeon General, Department of the Army, Washington, D.C., 1952.
16. Bell, M. L., Herman, A. H., Smith, E. E., Egdahl, R. H., and Rutenberg, A. M.: Role of lysosomal instability in the development of refractory shock. Surgery *70*:341. 1971.
17. Berne, T. V., and Barbour, B. H.: Acute renal failure in general surgical patients. Arch. Surg. *102*:594, 1971.
18. Boyan, C. P., and Howland, W. S.: Blood temperature: A critical factor in massive transfusion. Anesthesiology *22*:559, 1961.
19. Brand, E. D., and Lefer, A. M.: Myocardial depressant factor in plasma from cats in irreversible post-oligemic shock. Proc. Soc. Exp. Biol. Med. *122*:200, 1966.
20. Bull, J. P.: Circulatory responses to blood loss and injury. Progr. Surg. *4*:35, 1964.
21. Bunker, J. P.: Metabolic effects of blood transfusion. Anesthesiology *22*:446, 1966.

22. Bunker, J. P., Stetson, J. B., Coe, R. C., Grillo, H. C., and Murphy, A. J.: Citric acid intoxication. J.A.M.A. *157*:1361, 1955.

23. Cannon, W. B.: Traumatic shock. New York, D. Appleton and Co., 1923.

24. Carey, L. C., Cloutier, C. T., and Lowery, B. D.: The use of balanced electrolyte solution for resuscitation. *In* Fox, C. L., Jr., and Nahas, G. G. (eds.): Body fluid replacement in the surgical patient. New York, Grune & Stratton, 1970.

25. Carpenter, M. A., Trunkey, D., and Holcroft, J.: Ionized calcium and magnesium in the baboon: Hemorrhagic shock and resuscitation. Circ. Shock *5*:163, 1978.

26. Champion, H. R., Jones, R. T., Trump, B. F., Decker, R., Wilson, S., Migniski, M., and Gill, W.: A clinicopathologic study of hepatic dysfunction following shock. Surg. Gynec. Obstet. *142*:657, 1976.

27. Chaudry, I. H., Sayeed, M. M., and Baue, A. E.: Effect of adenosine triphosphate-magnesium chloride administration in shock. Surgery 75:220, 1974.

28. Chien, S., Usami, S., and Gregersen, M. I.: Effects of plasma expanders on blood viscosity. *In* Fox, C. L., Jr., and Nahas, G. G. (eds.): Body fluid replacement in the surgical patient. New York, Grune & Stratton, 1970.

29. Chinitz, J. L., Kim, K. E., Onesti, G., and Swartz, C.: Pathophysiology and prevention of dextran-40-induced anuria. J. Lab. Clin. Med. 77:76, 1971.

30. Chute, A. L., Cleghorn, R. A., and Lathe, G. A.: Reports of No. 1 research unit, Vol. 2. Ottawa, Proceedings of the 8th Meeting of the Association of Canadian Army Medical Research, 1945.

31. Clarke, R., Topley, E., and Flear, C. T. G.: Assessment of blood loss in civilian trauma. Lancet *1*:629, 1955.

32. Cleland, J., Pluth, J. R., Tauxe, W. N., and Kirklin, J. W.: Blood volumes and body fluid compartment changes soon after closed and open intracardiac surgery. J. Thorac. Cardiovasc. Surg. 52:698, 1966.

33. Cloutier, C. T., Lowery, B. D., and Carey, L. C.: Acid-base disturbances in hemorrhagic shock. Arch. Surg. 98:551, 1969.

34. Cohnen, G.: Changes in immunoglobulin levels after surgical trauma. J. Trauma *12*:249, 1972.

35. Collins, J. A.: First six months' activities. Walter Reed Army Institute of Research, Surgical Research Team, Vietnamese Office of the Surgeon General, Department of the Army, Washington, D.C., 1967.

36. Collins, J. A.: The causes of progressive pulmonary insufficiency in surgical patients. J. Surg. Res. 9:685, 1969.

37. Collins, J. A.: Fluid replacement in trauma. *In* Ballinger, W. F., and Drapanas, R. (eds.): Practice of Surgery: Current Review. St. Louis, C. V. Mosby Co., 1972.

38. Collins, J. A., Braitberg, A., and Butcher, H. R.: Changes in lung and body weight and lung water content in rats treated for hemorrhage with various fluids. Surgery 73:401, 1973.

39. Collins, J. A., Simmons, R. L., James, P. M., Bredenberg, C. E., Anderson, R. W., and Heisterkamp, C. A.: The acid-base status of seriously wounded combat casualties: I. Before treatment. Ann. Surg. *171*:595, 1970.

40. Collins, J. A., Simmons, R. L., James, P. M., Bredenberg, C. E., Anderson, R. W., and Heisterkamp, C. A.: Acid-base status of seriously wounded combat casualties: II. Resuscitation with stored blood. Ann. Surg. *173*:6, 1971.

41. Cournand, A., Riley, R. L., Bradley, S. E., Breed, E. S., Noble, R. P., Lausen, H. D., Gregersen, M. I., and Richards, D. W.: Studies of the circulation in clinical shock. Surgery *13*:964, 1963.

42. Crowell, J. W., and Smith, E. E.: Determinant of the optimal hematocrit. J. Appl. Physiol. 22:501, 1967.

43. Doty, D. B., Moseley, R. V., and Simmons, R. L.: Sequential changes in blood volume after injury and transfusion. Surg. Gynec. Obstet. *130*:801, 1970.

44. Drucker, W. R., Holden, W. D., Kingsbury, B., Hofmann, N., and Graham, L.: Metabolic aspects of hemorrhagic shock. II. Metabolic studies on the need for erythrocytes in the treatment of hypovolemia due to hemorrhage. J. Trauma 2:567, 1962.

45. Earley, L. E.: Pathogenesis of oliguric acute renal failure. N. Engl. J. Med. *282*:1370,

46. Eiseman, B., and Ashbaugh, D. G.: Pulmonary effects of nonthoracic trauma. J. Trauma 8:625, 1968.

47. Eiseman, B., and Heyman, R. L.: Stress ulcers — a continuing challenge. N. Engl. J. Med. *282*:372, 1970.

48. Fulton, R. L., and Jones, C.: The cause of posttraumatic pulmonary insufficiency in man. Surg. Gynec. Obstet. *140*:179, 1975.

49. Gaar, K. A., Jr., Taylor, A. E., Owens, L. J., and Guyton, A. C.: Effect of capillary pressure and plasma protein on development of pulmonary edema. Am. J. Physiol. *213*:79, 1967.

50. Gauer, O. H., Henry, J. P., and Sieker, H. O.: Changes in central venous pressure after moderate hemorrhage and transfusion in man. Circ. Res. *4*:79, 1956.

51. Gollub, S., Schechter, D. C., Schaefer, C., Svigals, R., and Bailey, C. P.: Absolute hemodilution cardiopulmonary bypass: Free water distribution and protein mobilization in body compartments. Am. Heart J. 78:626, 1969.

52. Grady, G. F., Bennett, A. J. E., et al.: Risk of post-transfusion hepatitis in the United States: A prospective cooperative study. J.A.M.A. *220*:692, 1972.

53. Grant, R. T., and Reeve, E. B.: Observations on the general effects of injury in man. Special Report Series, Medical Research Council (London) No. 277, 1951.

54. Gump, F. E., Butler, H., and Kinney, J. M.: Oxygen transport and consumption during acute hemorrhage. Ann. Surg. *168*:54, 1968.

55. Gump, F. E., Kinney, J. M., Iles, M., and Long,

C. C.: Duration and significance of large fluid loads administered for circulatory support. J. Trauma 10:431, 1970.

56. Guyton, A. C., and Crowell, J. W.: Dynamics of the heart in shock. Fed. Proc. 20:51, 1961.

57. Hardaway, R. M.: Syndromes of Disseminated Intravascular Coagulation. Springfield, Ill., Charles C Thomas, Publishers, 1966.

58. Hardaway, R. M., James, P. M., Anderson, R. W., Bredenberg, C. E., and West, R. L.: Intensive study and treatment of shock in man. J.A.M.A. 13:199, 1967.

59. Hardaway, R. M., Johnson, D. G., Houchin, D. N., Jenkins, E. B., Burnes, J. W., and Jackson, D. R.: The influence of extracorporeal handling of blood on hemorrhagic shock in dogs. Exp. Med. Surg. 23:28, 1965.

60. Hayes, D. F., Werner, M. H., Rosenberg, I. K., Lucas, C. E., Westreich, M., and Bradley, V.: Effects of traumatic hypovolemic shock on renal function. J. Surg. Res. 16:490, 1974.

61. Hinshaw, L. B.: Role of the heart in the pathogenesis of endotoxin shock. J. Surg. Res. 17:134, 1974.

62. Hopkins, R. W., Sabga, G., Penn, I., and Simeone, F. A.: Hemodynamic aspects of hemorrhagic and septic shock. J.A.M.A. 191:127, 1965.

63. Holcroft, J. W., Trunkey, D., and Carpenter, M. A.: Excessive fluid administration in resuscitating baboons from hemorrhagic shock and an assessment of the thermodye technique for measuring extravascular lung water. Am. J. Surg. 135:412, 1978.

64. Holcroft, J. W., and Trunkey, D. D.: Pulmonary extravasation of albumin during and after hemorrhagic shock in baboons. J. Surg. Res. 18:91, 1975.

65. Holcroft, J. W., and Trunkey, D. D.: Extravascular lung water following hemorrhagic shock in the baboon: Comparison between resuscitation with Ringer's lactate and plasmanate. Ann. Surg. 180:408, 1974.

66. Horovitz, J. H., Carrico, C. J., and Shires, G. T.: Venous sampling sites for pulmonary shunt determinations in the injured patient. J. Trauma 11:911, 1971.

67. Horovitz, J. M., Carrico, C. J., and Shires, G. T.: Pulmonary response to major surgery. Arch. Surg. 108:319, 1974.

68. Howard, J. M. (ed.): Battle Casualties in Korea: Studies of the Surgical Research Team. Washington, D.C., Army Medical Service School, Walter Reed Army Medical Center, 1960.

69. Hutchin, P., Terzi, R. G., Hollandsworth, L. C., Johnson, G., and Peters, R. M.: The influence of intravenous fluid administration on postoperative urinary water and electrolyte excretion in thoracic surgical patients. Ann. Surg. 170:813, 1969.

70. Jannoff, A., Weissmann, G., Zweifach, B. W., and Thomas, L.: Pathogenesis of experimental shock. IV. Studies on lysosomes in normal and tolerant animals subjected to lethal trauma and endotoxemia. J. Exp. Med. 116:451, 1962.

71. Jones, J. W., Hewitt, R. L., and Drapanas, T.:

Cardiac contusion: A capricious syndrome. Ann. Surg. 181:567, 1975.

72. Keith, N. M.: Blood volume changes in wound shock and primary hemorrhage. Medical Research Council, Report No. 9, Special Report Series No. 27. London, His Majesty's Stationery Office, 1919, p. 5

73. Kendrick, D. B..: Medical Department, United States Army, Blood Program in World War II. Washington D.C., Office of the Surgeon General, 1964.

74. Kirklin, J. W., and Archie, J. P.: The cardiovascular subsystem in surgical patients. Surg. Gynec. Obstet. 139:17, 1974.

75. Lefer, A. M.: Blood-borne humoral factors in the pathophysiology of circulatory shock. Circ. Res. 32:129, 1973.

76. Levine, O. R., Mellins, R. B., Senior, R. M., and Fishman, A. P.: The application of Starling's law of capillary exchange to the lungs. J. Clin. Invest. 46:934, 1969.

77. Levinsky, N. C.: Pathophysiology of acute renal failure. N. Engl. J. Med. 296:1453, 1977.

78. Lister, J., McNeill, I. F., Marshall, V. C., Plzak, L. F., Jr., Dagher, F. J., and Moore, F. D.: Transcapillary refilling after hemorrhage in normal man: Basal rates and volumes; effect of norepinephrine. Ann. Surg. 158:698, 1963.

79. Lowery, B. D., Cloutier, C. T., and Carey, L. C.: Blood gas determinations in the severely wounded in hemorrhagic shock. Arch. Surg. 99:330, 1969.

80. Lucas, C E., Sugawa, C., Riddle, J., Rector, F., Rosenberg, B., and Walt, A. J.: Natural history and surgical dilemma of "stress" gastric bleeding. Arch. Surg. 102:266, 1971.

81. Lucas, C. E., Zito, J. G., Carter, K. M., Cortez, A., and Stebner, C.: Questionable value of furosemide in preventing renal failure. Surgery 82:314, 1977.

82. MacLean, L. D.: Blood volume versus central venous pressure in shock. Surg. Gynec. Obstet. 118:594, 1964.

83. MacLean, L. D., Duff, J. H., Scott, H. M., and Peretz, D. L.: Treatment of shock in man based on hemodynamic diagnosis. Surg. Gynec. Obstet. 120:1, 1965.

84. Mailloux, L., Swartz, C. D., Capizzi, R., Kim, K. E., Onesti, G., Ramirez, O., and Brest, A. N.: Acute renal failure after administration of low-molecular-weight dextran. N. Engl. J. Med. 277:1113, 1967.

85. McArdle, A. H., Chiu, C., and Hinchey, E. J.: Cyclic AMP response to epinephrine and shock. Arch. Surg. 110:316, 1975.

86. McConn, R., and Derrick, J. B.: The respiratory function of blood: Transfusion and blood storage. Anesthesiology 36:119, 1972.

87. McKay, D. G.: Disseminated Intravascular Coagulation. New York, (Hoeber) Harper, 1964.

88. McNamara, J. J., Molot, M. D., and Stremple, J. F.: Screen filtration pressure in combat casualties. Ann. Surg. 172:334, 1970.

89. Mela, L. M., Miller, L. D., and Nicholas, G. G.: Influence of cellular acidosis and altered cation concentrations on shock-induced mitochondrial damage. Surgery 72:102, 1972.

90. Middleton, E. S., Mathews, R., and Shires, G. T.: Radiosulphate as a measure of the extracellular fluid in acute hemorrhagic shock. Ann. Surg. *170*:174, 1969.
91. Miller, R. P., Robbins, T. O., Tong, M. J., et al.: Coagulation defects associated with massive blood transfusions. Ann. Surg. *174*:794, 1971.
92. Monroe, R. G., Gamble, W. J., LaFarge, C. G., Aquilar, S. R., and Goldblatt, A.: A comparison of the effect of hemorrhage and infused catecholamines on ventricular performance, coronary flow, and myocardial oxygen consumption. J. Pharmacol. Exper. Therap. *153*:455, 1966.
93. Moore, F. D., Dagher, F. J., Boyden, C. M., Lee, C. J., and Lyons, J. H.: Hemorrhage in normal man: I. Distribution and dispersal of saline infusions following acute blood loss — clinical kinetics of blood volume support. Ann. Surg. *163*:485, 1966.
94. Moore, F. D., Lyons, J. H., Pierce, E. C., Morgan, A. P., Drinker, P. A., MacArthur, J. D., and Dammin, G. J.: Post-traumatic pulmonary insufficiency. Philadelphia, W. B. Saunders Co., 1969.
95. Moseley, R. V., and Doty, D. B.: Changes in the filtration characteristics of stored blood. Ann. Surg. *171*:329, 1970.
96. Moss, G.: Fluid distribution in prevention of hypovolemic shock. Arch. Surg. 98:281, 1969.
97. Muehrcke, R. C.: Acute Renal Failure: Diagnosis and Management. St. Louis, C. V. Mosby Co., 1969.
98. Northfield, T. C., and Smith, T.: Physiologic significance of central venous pressure in patients with hemorrhage. Surg. Gynec. Obstet. 35:267, 1972.
99. Ollodart, R., and Mansberger, A. R.: The effect of hypovolemic shock on bacterial defense. Am. J. Surg. *110*:302, 1965.
100. Pardy, B. J., and Dudley, H. A. F.: Comparison of pulmonary artery pressures and mixed venous oxygen tension with other indices in acute hemorrhage: An experimental study. Br. J. Surg. *64*:1, 1977.
101. Polimeni, P., and Page, E.: Magnesium in heart muscle. Circ. Res. 33:367, 1973.
102. Pruitt, B. A., Foley, F. D., and Moncrief, J. A.: Curling's ulcer: A clinical-pathology study of 323 cases. Ann. Surg. *172*:523, 1970.
103. Pruitt, B. A., Moncrief, J. A., and Mason, A. D.: Efficacy of buffered saline as the sole replacement fluid following acute measured hemorrhage in man. J. Trauma 7:767, 1967.
104. Raffa, J., and Trunkey, D.: Myocardial depression in acute thermal injury. J. Trauma *18*:90, 1978.
105. Randall, H. T.: Fluid, electrolyte, and acid-base balance. Surg. Clin. North Am. 56(5):1019, 1976.
106. Ranney, H. M.: Clinically important variants of human hemoglobin. N. Engl. J. Med. 282:144, 1970.
107. Regan, T. J., LaForce, F. M., Teres, D., Block, J., and Hellems, H. K.: Contribution of left ventricle and small bowel in irreversible hemorrhagic shock. Am. J. Physiol. *208*:938, 1965.
108. Robbins, R., Idjadi, F., Stahl, W. M., and Essiet, G.: Studies of gastric secretion in stressed patients. Ann. Surg. *175*:555, 1972.
109. Robertson, O. H., and Bock, A. V.: Memorandum on blood volume after hemorrhage. Medical Research Council, Report No. 6, Special Report Series No. 25. London, His Majesty's Stationery Office, 1918, p. 226.
110. Robinson, G. A., Butcher, R. W., and Sutherland, E. W. (eds.): Cyclic AMP. New York, Academic Press, 1971.
111. Rosenberg, I. K., Gupta, S. L., Lucas, C. E., Khan, A. A., and Rosenberg, B. F.: Renal insufficiency after trauma and sepsis. Arch. Surg. *103*:175, 1971.
112. Rothe, C. F.: Heart failure and fluid loss in hemorrhagic shock. Fed. Proc. 29:1854, 1970.
113. Rush, B. F., and Stewart, R. A.: More liberal use of a plasma expander: Impact on a hospital blood bank. N. Engl. J. Med. *280*:1202, 1969.
114. Rush, B. F., and Wilder, R. J.: Mortality and renal tubular necrosis in hemorrhagic shock in dogs: The effect of blood handling. Surg. Forum *14*:1, 1963.
115. Schildt, B. D., and Low, H.: Relationship between trauma, plasma corticosterone and reticuloendothelial function in anaesthetized mice. Acta Endocrinol. 67:141, 1971.
116. Scott, R., and Crosby, W. H.: Changes in coagulation mechanism following wounding and resuscitation with stored blood; a study of battle casualties in Korea. Blood 9:609, 1954.
117. Sheldon, G. F., Lim, R. C., and Blaisdell, F. W.: The use of fresh blood in critically injured patients. J. Trauma *15*:670, 1975.
118. Shenkin, R. A., Cheney, R. H., Govons, S. R., Hardy, J. D., Fletcher, A. G., Jr., and Starr, I.: On the diagnosis of hemorrhage in man: A study of volunteers bled large amounts. Am. J. Med. Sci. *208*:421, 1944.
119. Shields, C. E., Dennis, L. H., Eichelberger, J. W., and Conrad, M. E.: The rapid infusion of large quantities of ACD adenine solution into humans. Transfusion 7:133, 1967.
120. Shires, G. T., Canizaro, P. C.: Fluid resuscitation in the severely injured. Surg. Clin. North Am. 53(6):1341, 1973.
121. Shires, G. T., Cohn, D., Carrico, J., and Lightfoot, S.: Fluid therapy in hemorrhagic shock. Arch. Surg. 88:688, 1964.
122. Siegel, H. W., and Downing, S. E.: Contributions of coronary perfusion pressure, metabolic acidosis and adrenergic factors to the reduction of myocardial contractility during hemorrhagic shock in the cat. Circ. Res. 27:875, 1970.
123. Silberman, H.: Renal failure and the surgeon. Surg. Gynec. Obstet. *144*:775, 1977.
124. Simmons, R. L., Collins, J. A., Heisterkamp, C. A., Mills, D. E., Anderson, R., and Phillips, L. L.: Coagulation disorders in combat casualties. II. Effects of massive transfusion. Ann. Surg. *169*:462, 1969.

125. Simmons, R. L., Heisterkamp, C. A., Moseley, R. V., and Doty, D. B.: Post-resuscitative blood volumes in combat casualties. Surg. Gynec. Obstet. *128*:1193, 1969.
126. Skillman, J. J., Awwad, H. K., and Moore, F. D.: Plasma protein kinetics of the early trans-capillary refill after hemorrhage in man. Surg. Gynec. Obstet. *125*:983, 1967.
127. Skillman, J. J., Gould, S. A., Chung, R. S., and Silen, W.: The gastric mucosal barrier: clinical and experimental studies in critically ill and normal man, and in the rabbit. Ann. Surg. *174*:911, 1971.
128. Skillman, J. J., Hedley-White, J., and Pallotta, J. A.: Cardiorespiratory, metabolic and endocrine changes after hemorrhage in man. Ann. Surg. *174*:911, 1971.
129. Skillman, J. J., Lauler, D. P., Hickler, R. B., Lyons, J. H., Olson, J. E., Ball, M. R., and Moore, F. D.: Hemorrhage in normal man — effect on renin, cortisol, aldosterone and urine composition. Ann. Surg. *166*:865, 1967.
130. Skillman, J. J., Olson, J. E., Lyons, J. H. and Moore, F. D.: The hemodynamic effect of acute blood loss in normal man, with observations on the effect of the Valsalva maneuver and breath holding. Ann. Surg. *166*:713, 1967.
131. Smith, E. E., and Crowell, J. W.: Influence of hematocrit ratio on survival of unacclimatized dogs at simulated high altitude. Am. J. Physiol. *205*:1172, 1963.
132. Smith, L. L., Hamlin, J. T., Walker, W. F., and Moore, F. D.: Metabolic and endocrinologic changes in acute and chronic hypotension in man. Metabolism 8:862, 1959.
133. Smith, L. L., and Moore, F. D.: Refractory hypotension in man — is this irreversible shock? N. Engl. J. Med. *267*:734, 1962.
134. Stahl, W. M., and Stone, A. M.: Prophylactic diuresis with ethacrynic acid for prevention of postoperative renal failure. Ann. Surg. *172*:361, 1970.
135. Stremple, J. F., Molot, M. D., McNamara, J. J., Mori, H., and Glass, G. B.: Post-traumatic gastric bleeding. Arch. Surg. *105*:177, 1972.
136. Sugerman, H. J., Davidson, D. T., Vibul, S., et al.: The basis of defective oxygen delivery from stored blood. Surg. Gynec. Obstet. *131*:733, 1970.
137. Takaori, M., and Safar, P.: Treatment of massive hemorrhage with colloid and crystalloid solutions. J.A.M.A. *199*:297, 1967.
138. Thal, A. P., Brown, E. B., Hermreck, A. S., and Bell, H. H.: Shock: A Physiologic Basis for Treatment. Chicago, Year Book Medical Publishers, 1971.
139. Thomas, A. N., and Stephens, B. G.: Air embolism: A cause of morbidity and death after penetrating chest trauma. J. Trauma *14*:633, 1974.
140. Trunkey, D., Carpenter, M. A., and Holcroft, J.: Ionized calcium and magnesium: The effect of septic shock in the baboon. J. Trauma *18*:166, 1978.
141. Trunkey, D., Holcroft, J. W., and Carpenter, M. A.: Monitoring resuscitation of primates from hemorrhagic and septic shock. J. Am. Coll. Emergency Physicians, 5:249, 1976.
142. Trunkey, D. D., and Lim, R. C.: Analysis of 425 consecutive victims of trauma: An autopsy study. J. Am. Coll. Emergency Physicians 3:368, 1974.
143. Valeri, C. R.: Viability and function of preserved red cells. N. Engl. J. Med. *284*:81, 1971.
144. Valeri, C. R., and Collins, F. B.: The physiologic effect of transfusing preserved red cells with low 2,3-diphospho-glycerate and high affinity for oxygen. Vox Sang. *20*:329, 1971
145. Valtis, D. J., and Kennedy, A. C.: Defective gas transport function of stored red blood cells. Lancet *1*:119, 1954.
146. Veith, F. J., Hagstrom, J. W. C., Panossian, A., Nehlsen, S. L., and Wilson, J. W.: Pulmonary microcirculatory response to shock, transfusion, and pump-oxygenator procedures: A unified mechanism underlying pulmonary damage. Surgery *64*:95, 1968.
147. Warren, J. V., Brannon, E. S., Stead, E. A., Jr., and Merrill, A. J.: The effect of venesection and the pooling of blood in the extremities on the atrial pressure and cardiac output in normal subjects with observations on acute circulatory collapse in three instances. J. Clin. Invest. *24*:337, 1945.
148. Wiggers, C. J.: Physiology of Shock. New York, Commonwealth Fund, 1950.
149. Williams, A. D., Mandell, G. L., and Lefer, A. M.: Phagocytosis and bactericidal activity of leucocytes in hemorrhagic shock. Infect. Immun. 2:345, 1970.
150. Wilson, R. F., Mammen, E., and Walt, A. J.: Eight years of experience with massive blood transfusions. J. Trauma *11*:275, 1971.
151. Wilson, R. F., Sarver, E., and Birks, R.: Central venous pressure and blood volume determinations in clinical shock. Surg. Gynec. Obstet. *132*:631, 1971.
152. Zimmerman, J. E.: Respiratory failure complicating post-traumatic acute renal failure: Etiology, clinical features and management. Ann. Surg. *174*:12, 1971.

CHAPTER 5

ANESTHETIC MANAGEMENT OF THE TRAUMA VICTIM

William D. Owens, M.D.
Milton L. Cobb, M.D.

INTRODUCTION

Trauma usually presents a special challenge to the anesthetist because of the multifaceted pathophysiological problems involved. This challenge can be met with management directed toward prevention of renal failure. The therapeutic measures commonly utilized to prevent renal failure are essentially the same as those used to combat cardiovascular collapse, hepatic failure and further CNS damage. This mode of management often temporarily compromises respiratory function but does so in a manner that can be successfully treated when the other physiological systems are stabilized. Regardless of the approach chosen, the anesthetist should always be prepared for the worst; if and when it occurs, he or she will be prepared.

PREOPERATIVE ANESTHETIC MANAGEMENT

In cases of trauma all too often the medical team is impressed by the grossly evident lesion and forgets to check for the more subtle, often more serious, injuries. Preoperative anesthetic management needs to be thorough but expeditious. For

this reason a systematic evaluation is required.

Knowledge of the medical history of the patient and the cause of trauma is imperative. Pre-existing disease can be present in all age groups. Endocrine dysfunction and coronary insufficiency are just two examples of such disease that may alter the planning of anesthetic management or the course of the anesthetic. The same caution applies to any prescribed medication — the ingestion of psychotropic drugs and/or alcohol not only may precipitate the original accident but also may make an otherwise safe anesthetic a catastrophe.

Knowledge of the cause of the trauma — a high speed automobile accident, a 10-foot fall, a lawn mower accident, for example — is very helpful in evaluating the physical state of the patient. Obviously, one would be more suspicious of a contused lung following an automobile accident than when a lawnmower has amputated the patient's toes. The details of the type and severity of the accident can be the essential clue to discovery of the unsuspected injury.

The physical examination of the trauma victim should include the cardiovascular, respiratory and central nervous systems whether or not they appear to have been traumatized. A quick overview of the extent and nature of the injuries is necessary before a more detailed physical examination is carried out. Larkin and Moylan[15] have suggested an order of injury priorities. Highest priority is assigned to cervical spine injuries, respiratory impairment, cardiovascular insufficiency and severe external injuries. Also of high priority but slightly lower on the list are intraperitoneal injuries, retroperitoneal injuries, craniocerebral and spinal cord injuries and severe burns. This list can be used as a systematic check list in the physical examination. Gallagher and Civetta[8] suggest a slightly different approach but one that is equally valid and useful.

The state of consciousness, both at the time of injury and in the preoperative phase, is an important indication of serious head and central nervous system injury. The pupillary size *of each eye* and its reaction to light should be noted. The possibility of papilledema, which may indicate increased intracranial pressure, should be investigated preoperatively.

Assessment of respiratory status starts with the evaluation of the upper airway, which should be free of obstruction. The presence of an obstructed airway or respiratory impairment is cause for treatment before taking a history or doing a complete physical examination. Oral or nasal airways should be utilized or endotracheal intubation accomplished immediately. We cannot overstress that one of the highest priority items is the respiratory system.

Paradoxical movement of the chest wall indicates two or more rib fractures — a flail chest. This suggests a need for endotracheal intubation, mechanical ventilation and/or end-expired pressure. Contusion of the lung may be present even when rib fractures are absent. The physician should be aware of the signs of blunt trauma to the chest wall that may be suggested from the history or by bruises or scratches. Oxygenation, as determined by arterial blood gases, may still be normal during the initial evaluation, as it takes several hours for impaired oxygenation to be fully manifest.[7]

Pneumothorax or hemothorax or both should be suspected whenever there is chest trauma. Since the physical assessment is often misleading, a roentgenographic examination should be obtained immediately or aspiration of the chest cavity effected as a diagnostic test. Treatment usually consists of a properly functioning chest tube or tubes.

Assessment of the cardiovascular status starts with blood volume. Look for external hemorrhage. Internal hemorrhage is often more subtle, but large volume losses will be present in patients with a fractured pelvis, fractured femur or retroperitoneal injuries. Blood pressure in itself is not a sufficient guide. A compensatory tachycardia and/or vasoconstriction will often maintain a normal blood pressure. Observe signals of poor perfusion such as vasospasm, low urine output, and cold extremities, among many other things. Volume replacement is mandatory and should be immediate in the blood loss victim. Preoperative volume resuscitation is dependent on having several large bore intravenous lines available. A cutdown at the ankle or antecubital area can be done quickly without interfering with the other aspects of the examination or treatment. One of the most common mistakes in the preoperative and intraoperative phases of management is having an inadequate number and size of volume replacement routes.

Pericardial contusion and tamponade, as well as myocardial infarct, should be suspected if there is lack of response to adequate treatment of shock. Beware of distended neck veins and a paradoxical pulse. Interpret a 12-lead electrocardiogram. Immediate relief of a tamponade is mandatory.

A cardiac arrest, regardless of etiology, requires prompt recognition and treatment. Personnel should be certified in basic life support and advanced life support techniques. They should be knowledgeable about airway management, countershock, arrhythmias and proper use of adjuvant drugs. They should be thoroughly familiar with the standards for emergency cardiac care of the American Heart Association* as discussed in Chapter 2.

Skeletal injuries are common with trauma. To the anesthetist, the status of the cervical spine is important preoperatively. Evaluation for the possibility of a cervical

---

*Standards for Emergency Cardiac Care in Advanced Life Support Units (including hospital emergency departments), 1976. Available from the American Heart Association.

spine fracture must be completed prior to manipulation of the neck. This may indicate the need for a "blind" nasotracheal intubation rather than laryngoscopy and orotracheal intubation.

Maxillofacial injuries often compromise the airway either mechanically or through aspiration of blood. The extent and type of injury will dictate the type of airway management: nasotracheal intubation, orotracheal intubation or tracheostomy.

As can be perceived, examination and treatment often proceed simultaneously. Preoperative anesthetic management requires a team approach utilizing anesthesia, surgical and nursing personnel. It is important that communication among team members be at its best. Documentation of findings and treatment in the preoperative phase will help solve many puzzles during the operative and postoperative phases of treatment.

Monitoring

Reliable monitoring begins in the preoperative period and extends into postoperative care in the intensive care unit. Invasive monitoring is often necessary and should be followed by aggressive therapy as guided by the findings. Monitoring is a guide to the degree of physiological embarrassment of blood volume, cardiac status, vascular resistance, acid-base status, respiratory status and pulmonary vascular status. Obviously, the kind and degree of monitoring will depend on the extent of physiological derangement secondary to trauma in the individual case, as well as on pre-existing conditions.

Electrocardiogram. This indicator of cardiac electrical activity should be used in all patients requiring anesthesia — not just trauma patients. From the ECG we can detect heart rate, conduction defects, dysrhythmias and ischemic patterns. Obviously, however, it is only as reliable as the interpreter of the signs — the anesthetist. It is also dependent on lead placement. Preferably bipolar electrodes should be used with the exploring electrode over the left ventricle.[2] This will provide better detection of left ventricular ischemic changes.

Blood Pressure. Blood pressure is usually determined by indirect methods employing a stethoscope and blood pressure cuff. This auscultatory method is of limited value in the traumatized patient, especially when he is vasoconstricted or in shock. Another important limitation is its intermittent nature — it is usually only taken every 3 to 5 minutes. More sophistication in blood pressure detection is obtained with the use of a Doppler apparatus, which is particularly useful in the pediatric patient but has the same limitation of intermittency.

Significant physiological disturbances mandate direct arterial pressure measurements that are displayed through a transducer to an oscilloscope and perhaps also on a paper write-out. This technique provides a means of determining beat-to-beat changes in the arterial pressure and pressure wave forms. This configuration of the pressure curve can provide qualitative but not quantitative information about stroke volume and peripheral vascular resistance. Availability of blood for arterial blood gases and other laboratory tests is another important indication for direct arterial monitoring.

Almost any artery can be used for cannulation, but the radial artery, ulnar artery and dorsalis pedis artery are generally used because they are more accessible and have a lower incidence of thrombosis. Before cannulation, one should check the patency of the radial or ulnar artery by a modified Allen's test.[18] Return of color after blanching the great toe nail while occluding the dorsalis pedis artery indicates satisfactory collateral flow to the foot.

The incidence of thrombosis is related to the size and type of catheter used. The lowest incidence of thrombosis in adults occurs with the use of a 20-gauge Teflon nonradiopaque nontapered catheter over a needle.[1] The occurrence of thrombosis and embolization also depends on the method of flushing with heparinized solutions.[16] A continuous flush technique is preferable.

Central Venous Pressure. A central venous pressure catheter will enable the physician to detect major abnormalities in right ventricular function and blood volume only when there is no disparity between the right and left ventricles. To be useful, documentation of the catheter location (by chest x-ray) is mandatory, and any interpretation must be made in conjunction with the arterial presure. Other uses of a central venous catheter include aspiration of air when an air embolus occurs, sampling of blood, hyperalimentation and injection of dye for dye-dilution cardiac output studies.

Pulmonary Artery Pressure. The balloon-tipped, flow-directed pulmonary artery catheter has added a major dimension to monitoring the critically ill and traumatized patient. Right heart catheterization, which provides information about independent function of the right and left ventricles as well as the pulmonary vascular tree, is now available in the emergency room, in the operating room, and at the bedside. Proper insertion and interpretation of the pulmonary artery catheter remove the element of uncertainty from the treatment and provide accurate physiologic data that justify the intervention modality.

The independence of the right and left ventricles and the disparity of ventricular function in the critically ill patient have been well documented.[6] Indications for pulmonary artery catheterization include:

1. Suspicion of right and/or left ventricular dysfunction.
2. Pulmonary hypertension.
3. Management of volume replacement.
4. Shunt calculations.
5. Cardiac output determinations.

The insertion and maintenance of the pulmonary artery catheter are not without morbidity. Even though the incidence is low, the complications can be major: arterial puncture, infarcted pulmonary parenchyma, dysrhythmias, knotted catheters, and sepsis. Before using the pulmonary artery catheter, one should be thoroughly familiar with the technique and interpretations. A review of the pathophysiology and diagnosis of cardiac abnormalities in the perioperative period is given in Chapter 3.[14]

Cardiac Output. Since the delivery of oxygenated blood to tissue is the determining factor for viability, cardiac output is a much more meaningful guide than the arterial pressure per se. However, cardiac output must be interpreted in light of other events, such as the anesthetic agent used or other pharmacologic treatments. Although total flow may remain normal, each anesthetic agent and vasodilating agent has its peculiarities in directing or diverting flow to individual types of tissue.

The determination of cardiac output can be achieved by either the dye-dilution technique or the thermodilution technique. The dye-dilution method is cumbersome and technically more difficult to perform, but when done with meticulous care it is probably more accurate. The thermodilution cardiac output determination is somewhat easier to perform and can be repeated at very short intervals; it has been shown to have good correlation with the dye-dilution technique[9] and the more direct method using the Fick principle.[4]

Regardless of the method used, the cardiac output can provide data that can be used to assess myocardial contractility and peripheral vascular resistance. It can provide information about the effectiveness of our pharmacologic interventions, advantageous or deleterious, and it can often be a guide to a specific type of intervention: inotropic support, vasopressor therapy, vasodilator therapy, volume replacement, or a combination of these.

Arterial Blood Gases. In trauma patients, the interpretation of arterial blood gases (ABG's) should not be limited to assessing the adequacy of ventilation and oxygenation. ABG's also can be used, in whole or in part, for calculation of other parameters such as left to right shunt and ratio of dead space to tidal volume (V_D/V_T). They are essential for determining the acid-base status, which may be used as an indicator of degree of perfusion.

Normal arterial blood gas determinations immediately after trauma often induce a false sense of security. For example, lung contusion is a progressive lesion and may not result in abnormal ABG's for several hours after injury. Furthermore, each of the cardiovascular or respiratory interventions used may influence the quality of ventilation, arterial oxygenation, and tissue oxygenation. For these reasons, frequent sampling of arterial blood gases after major trauma is urged.

Urine. Acute renal failure cannot be reversed. Therefore, monitoring of urine output and urine content is vitally important. Besides serving as an inelegant guide to renal perfusion, urine output can also be an aid, although a poor one, to volume replacement. An appropriate goal would be 0.5 to 1 ml. of urine output per kilogram of body weight per hour. This type of monitoring requires an indwelling bladder drainage system (e.g., a transurethral or suprapubic catheter).

The urine sodium level helps to distinguish between prerenal oliguria and acute renal failure. A urine sodium level of less than 20 mEq./l implies prerenal oliguria, whereas a sodium level of greater than 40 mEq./l suggests acute renal failure. The urine/plasma creatinine ratio is also helpful in this regard; prerenal oliguria has a ratio of greater than 40 to 1, whereas acute renal failure is characterized by a ratio of less than 10 to 1. Acute renal failure may be manifest by a urine/plasma osmolality ratio of less than 1.1 to 1 due to impairment of concentrating mechanisms. In prerenal failure the ratio is greater than 2 to 1. Determination of the urine potassium will serve as a guide to the amount of potassium necessary for replacement therapy.

A note of caution is necessary. Following diuretic therapy, the useful information obtained from measurements of urine electrolytes and osmolarity is considerably limited. Since loop diuretics (e.g., furosemide and ethacrynic acid) interfere with sodium reabsorption and urine concentrating mechanisms, a 6- to 12-hour delay is imperative before diagnostic information becomes practical again. However, measurement of urine electrolytes is valuable as a guide to electrolyte replacment therapy.

Temperature. Hypothermia can often be a problem in the preoperative and intraoperative phases of management. This is especially true in patients with massive trauma who have had rapid volume replacement and a great amount of exposed surface area. Hypothermia, when severe and uncontrolled, will have deleterious effects on the heart and will antagonize the action of muscle relaxants. In addition, the rewarming process requires a 200 to 400 per cent increase in oxygen delivery to the tissues. Prevention of hypothermia is accomplished by warming fluids and blood and keeping the environment warm.

Hyperthermia may herald the onset of sepsis or malignant hyperthermia. Immediate therapy is warranted. If sepsis is suspected, appropriate antibiotics and cooling are initiated after obtaining blood specimens for culture. Recognition and treatment of malignant hyperthermia present

special problems, and the reader is referred to a recent review.[12]

Temperature monitoring should be directed toward obtaining a "core" temperature. This can be accomplished with tympanic membrane, esophageal, nasopharyngeal or rectal temperature probes, whichever is appropriate for the individual patient.

Neurological Monitoring. Some of the earliest and most readily available techniques for monitoring intracranial pressures include observation of eye movement and pupillary size and reaction to light. Of course, much of this reaction is lost when the patient is anesthetized with a general anesthetic. Preoperative eye examinations followed by monitoring during regional or "monitor only" anesthesia are quite helpful. When there is a high degree of suspicion for increased intracranial pressure, it may be necessary to monitor intracranial pressure continuously with indwelling pressure sensing devices.

GENERAL PRINCIPLES OF OPERATIVE ANESTHETIC MANAGEMENT

Anesthetic techniques used in trauma patients are basically not unlike those used for any other patient. Three areas, however, require additional consideration when planning the anesthetic approach. First, airway management must be considered, especially if injury to the craniofacial area has occurred or if neck trauma has occurred. A LeFort III fracture involving massive facial trauma, for example, may require a tracheostomy under local anesthesia before any further steps can be safely undertaken. Blind awake nasotracheal intubation under topical anesthesia in the patient with a cervical spine fracture or fracture-dislocation is an alternative if tracheostomy is not elected. Second, blood and extracellular fluid volume must be rapidly assessed. The effects of any proposed anesthetic agents or techniques on myocardial contractility, heart rate, stroke volume, systemic and pulmonary vascular resistance, and regional blood flow must be considered in relation to the volume assessments. Third, the trauma patient must be assumed to have a full stomach. As a result, a special approach to securing the airway is necessary if a general anesthetic is to be employed, since significant morbidity and mortality are associated with aspiration of gastric contents.

Whether one chooses local, regional, or general anesthesia, the factors mentioned above must enter into the decision-making process. Although there may be few data that dictate absolutely a certain anesthetic approach, there are relatively strong contraindications to particular approaches in specific situations. These can best be considered in relation to various anesthetic techniques.

Local Anesthesia

Obviously, less physiological disturbance to the trauma patient will result when a properly administered local anesthetic is used than from the use of either regional or general anesthesia. Therefore, one should always consider whether the operative procedure, particularly if it is superficial and limited in extent, can be done with least overall risk under local anesthesia. A number of adjunctive sedative and tranquilizing drugs are available that, when knowledgeably administered, are capable of producing a quiet cooperative patient, provided pain is abolished by a local anesthetic. This, of course, requires careful assessment of the patient's emotional stability as well as an ability to maintain a soothing conversation with the patient who may remain awake. The inebriated, combative patient is certainly no candidate for local anesthesia alone, unless one believes the risk of heavy sedation to be less than the risk of general anesthesia. "Heavy sedation" with multiple hypnotics, sedatives, and/or narcotics sometimes approaches the CNS sedation of general anesthesia.

Major procedures can rarely be done with a local anesthetic alone, except in the moribund patient. The moribund patient is probably exactly the patient who needs no anesthetic but rather endotracheal intubation and maximal ventilatory and circulatory support. It is in such cases that, as empathetic physicians overly concerned with pain relief, we have perhaps been guilty of "misguided humanitarianism."

Regional Anesthesia

Procedures on the extremities lend themselves especially well to regional anesthetic techniques. Subarachnoid block or extradural (epidural or caudal) block with local anesthetic agents may be indicated occasionally. However, one must use particular caution to avoid these techniques when hypovolemia is present. Reduced peripheral resistance from sympathetic blockade together with a reduced circulating blood volume may combine to produce disastrous hypotension refractory to vasoconstriction. If blood loss has been minimal and is expected to be slight in association with the surgical procedure, then subarachnoid or epidural block may be cautiously employed. Ordinary precautions must also be observed. These include avoiding this anesthetic technique if peripheral nerve damage is already present or if cord damage or closed head injury is suspected. The level of sensory blockade should be carefully controlled, remembering that with subarachnoid or extradural block the sympathetic blockade is two to six dermatomes higher than the sensory level. Because of the large volumes of drug required for caudal or epidural anesthesia, the circulation is also affected by absorption of the anesthetic agent and by epinephrine, if it is added to the anesthetic solution.[3] This may be tolerated satisfactorily by the young, previously healthy patient who, after all, is more frequently involved in trauma. The older patient with coronary artery disease or underlying hypertensive cardiovascular disease, whose hypertension may now be masked by hypovolemia, cannot be expected to tolerate further hypotension without serious sequelae.

Peripheral nerve blocks have much more to recommend them in that the sympathectomy produced by the block is much more restricted in terms of the circulatory bed affected. Circulatory effects from absorbed local anesthetic agent and incorporated vasoconstrictors still must be considered. However, since the remaining unblocked portion of the circulatory bed is able to react in compensation, significant hypotension is rather unlikely and is far more responsive to stimulation with a drug such as ephedrine. An interscalene block[14] can be accomplished without abducting the arm and is especially useful for upper extremity trauma. This is an obvious advantage when an upper extremity fracture or a shoulder dislocation is present. Lower extremity blocks can be done if trauma to a single lower extremity has occurred. A recently described block,[19] consisting of a single injection of local anesthetic agent to produce a lumbar plexus block, can be performed with the patient supine. Combined with a sciatic nerve block, this will allow almost any surgical procedure on a lower extremity. The same thing may also be accomplished with a combined lumbosacral plexus block.

Although wrist blocks for hand procedures or ankle blocks for foot procedures can be done, they are unsatisfactory if an extremity tourniquet is to be used. An intravenous regional block of the upper extremity is compatible with tourniquet use, since performance of the block itself requires a tourniquet. However, this block is not useful for a procedure requiring more than 60 to 90 minutes, including skin and open wound surgical prep time.

The biggest advantage of local or regional blocks occurs in the patient with both an extremity injury and a question of closed head injury or abdominal injury. In such a patient, continuous assessment of these unresolved problems can occur while the extremity injury is being repaired without having to await the patient's emergence from a general anesthetic.

General Anesthesia

In considering general anesthesia for the trauma patient, the most important issues are securing the airway and maintaining adequate organ perfusion with oxygenated blood. Although these are extreme generalizations, little else in the anesthetic management will be of consequence unless they are given top priority. The best means of securing the airway will depend in part on the patient's level of consciousness at the time he arrives in the operating room, or wherever his preanesthetic care begins. Other determining factors include site of trauma (e.g., orofacial, neck, airway), age, presence of abdominal distention, and degree of cardiopulmonary dysfunction secondary to the trauma. One must always assume that the trauma patient has a full stomach. The controversy over how the airway should be secured is not resolved. Some would introduce an endotracheal tube with the patient awake, with or without topical anesthesia. Others would use a sequence of preoxygenation, rapid intravenous induction followed by an intravenous rapidly acting relaxant, application of cricoid pressure (Sellick maneuver), and rapid introduction of a cuffed endotracheal tube. There are appropriate situations for both approaches.[10] However, we see no place for airway management of the trauma patient with general anesthesia without either an endotracheal tube or tracheostomy. One occasionally hears an argument in favor of using intravenous ketamine for a brief procedure in a trauma patient without securing the airway. Experience has proved that regurgitation and aspiration do occur in such circumstances, and the technique is to be condemned.

Specific Rules of General Anesthetic Management

Induction. Induction of anesthesia in the traumatized hypovolemic patient has been significantly altered by the introduction of ketamine into clinical practice. Because of the lack of cardiovascular depression with ketamine, the frequently alarming hypotension produced by thiopental in the marginally compensated patient who is not completely "fluid resuscitated" can be avoided. Given in a dose range of 2 mg./kg., ketamine rapidly produces unconsciousness. If thiopental is chosen for induction instead, it must be recognized that with a reduced circulating blood volume, the percentage of the cardiac output perfusing the heart and brain will be greater, so that both less pentothal will be required to produce unconsciousness and more cardiovascular depression will be seen with a lower dose. In the acutely intoxicated patient less pentothal is required, since the patient's state of consciousness is already altered by his ethanol "premedication."

As previously stated, we believe that tracheal intubation should be a sine qua non for general anesthesia in the trauma patient. If the patient arrives in the operating room with an endotracheal tube in place, its position and patency must be ascertained and not assumed. If an endotracheal tube was not placed with the patient awake, it should be rapidly introduced following intravenous induction, with the aid of an appropriate rapidly acting muscle relaxant. Succinylcholine is most often used in this situation. Pretreatment with a nondepolarizing muscle relaxant is often employed to minimize the rise in intragastric pressure from muscle fasciculations and the accompanying increased risk of regurgitation and aspiration. Cricoid pressure should be applied from the time consciousness is lost until endotracheal intubation is successful. Although fasciculations after administration of succinylcholine can be diminished or abolished by the pretreatment, one must be aware of several caveats. For optimal effects, the nondepolarizing relaxant (curare 3 to 4.5 mg., gallamine triethiodide 20 mg., or pancuronium bromide 2.0 mg.) must be given intravenously approximately 3 minutes prior to administration of succinylcholine. In addition, the dose of succinylcholine must be increased by 50 per cent to produce the same degree of relaxation usually associated with a dose of 1 mg./kg. IV. Further, the time from IV succinylcholine administration to production of profound relaxation will be slightly prolonged. Finally, even when all these techniques are followed, an occasional patient will cough or retch during introduction of the endotracheal tube.

As an alternative to succinylcholine, if careful evaluation of the airway indicates no likelihood of difficulty in exposing the larynx, pancuronium can be used for relaxation for intubation. If that choice is made, pancuronium can be given immediately prior to the induction drug, so that within 60 to 90 seconds after administration of the induction drug, adequate relaxation for intubation should be present. A benefit of this approach is that relaxation can be continued with pancuronium. However, a major disadvantage accompanies this technique — if the airway assessment is in error and endotracheal intubation cannot be accomplished, rapid tracheostomy may have to be performed.

Regardless of the method chosen for intubation, it is just as important to protect the patient's airway at the end of the procedure as at the beginning. The use of elaborate precautions at the beginning of the anesthetic will be to no avail if the endotracheal tube is removed prior to the return of protective airway reflexes, thereby permitting aspiration of gastric contents that are often regurgitated as emergence from anesthesia occurs. The physician must avoid lulling himself into the belief that he can completely empty the stomach with a nasogastric tube.

Maintenance. As previously stated, a major goal in providing anesthesia is to avoid renal failure associated with further cardiovascular depression. Therefore, the potent inhalation agents, if used, must be used in the least effective concentrations. Often they will be tolerated only intermittently. These agents, particularly halothane and enflurane, offer advantages in some situations, however. Since they are potent, they can be used without nitrous oxide, thus allowing a high concentration of oxygen to be delivered. When significant pulmonary dysfunction either antedates or accompanies the trauma, adequate oxygenation may be possible only with high inspired oxygen concentrations. Another advantage has been claimed for halothane that one would expect to apply to enflurane — namely, that it adds another dimension to intravascular volume assessment during the anesthetic and operative event. This assessment will be briefly discussed because it addresses a crucial issue — the importance of organ perfusion rather than arterial pressure per se.

The traumatized but incompletely "fluid-resuscitated" patient may maintain a normal or near-normal arterial pressure by peripheral vasoconstriction. This compensatory mechanism may result in marked reduction of regional blood flow to splanchnic organs and, of more immediate importance, may reduce renal blood flow to an inadequate level. In turn, this may result in acute renal failure or at least in severely impaired renal function. We often find it extremely difficult in the anesthetized patient to assess whether the administration of fluid and blood is adequate on the basis of blood pressure, pulse rate, and urine output. Because of the importance of restoring adequate intravascular volume and organ perfusion, the value of an easily performed means of assessment is obvious. Some have proposed using halothane to produce a readily reversible vasodilation, once adequate fluids have been given, to return arterial blood pressure to the normal range. If a precipitous fall in blood pressure occurs with the myocardial depression and vasodilation produced by low concentrations of halothane, one could then assume that additional volume is indicated. In that case, one would either discontinue halothane or sharply reduce its concentration, rapidly administer more fluids, and then reintroduce halothane to re-evaluate whether still more blood and/or fluids were needed. Others prefer to use low concentrations of halothane or enflurane, accepting some degree of hypotension and assuming that perfusion will be enhanced by reducing vasoconstriction. There is opposition to both of these approaches among other groups, who prefer a technique that incorporates nitrous oxide, oxygen, intravenous narcotic, and intravenous relaxant. The rationale underlying this approach is the avoidance of vasodilators and myocardial depressants so that changes in pulse rate and blood pressure more nearly reflect intravascular volume and myocardial function.

The paucity of data relating to the effects of various anesthetic agents on perfusion of different organs in man in the hypovolemic state makes it impossible to point to one or another anesthetic technique as the best. Continued success in managing trauma patients with all these combinations leads one to conclude that each choice has merit and when used *properly*, this technical aspect is not the most crucial part of the management of anesthesia for the trauma patient.

Volume Replacement. Many controversies about blood, blood product, and fluid administration to the trauma patient remain unsettled. No brief discussion could begin to address the disagreements about concepts and research methods. It is our present intent only to express our viewpoint, based on what we believe to be careful studies backed up by extensive clinical experience.

In our view, the methods proposed by Shires and associates,[5, 10, 11] both as to type and quantity of balanced electrolyte solutions that should be administered to the traumatized patient, are appropriate for intraoperative use. Many times fluid resuscitation must of necessity be incomplete when the traumatized patient arrives in the operating suite. Therefore, the princi-

ples used in initial resuscitation logically extend to the point at which fluid and blood replacement is deemed to be adequate, as indicated by properly interpreted, appropriate monitoring techniques. In short, fluid administration usually consists of both dextrose-containing and plain lactated Ringer's solution in addition to appropriate amounts of whole blood or blood components. These should be given in quantities needed to restore blood pressure to a range presumed to be normal for the patient and to provide a urine output of approximately one ml./kg./hr. The rationale underlying this approach as well as the details of its application have recently been extensively reviewed.[5] Briefly, the concept, supported by both experimental data and clinical experience, is that a reduction in the functional extracellular fluid (ECF) volume accompanies hemorrhagic shock. This functional ECF deficit appears to arise both from sequestration of ECF in injured tissues ("third-space losses") and from changes in the distribution of a significant portion of the ECF from extracellular spaces to intracellular space. Such distributional shifts may be secondary to alterations in cell membrane function that accompany severe shock. The clinical significance of this concept is that repair of these functional ECF deficits can be achieved by administering sufficient quantities of balanced salt solutions in addition to blood. While we admit that this approach can be and has been overdone, we also submit that the same is true of any approach and that good judgment is, therefore, a requirement. Although fluid overload to the point of pulmonary edema can occur, it can be relatively easily treated provided renal function remains intact.

By itself, fluid overload does not appear to be capable of producing adult respiratory distress syndrome.[13] By the same token, if pulmonary contusion is suspected or if preexisting organic heart disease or impaired renal function is present, it would be injudicious to administer fluids rapidly without also monitoring extensively and invasively. In other words, when the risk imposed by the possibility of fluid overload is high, one should use appropriate monitoring techniques to optimize volume in a situation that is subject to rapid change. The result of being hesitant to give adequate fluid volumes can well be renal damage. Renal failure combined with other critically injured organ systems is associated with an inordinately high mortality rate.

In recent years, because of both donor selection difficulties and blood storage problems, there has been increased awareness that whole blood should be used on a very limited basis. When massive transfusions (greater than one and one half times the patient's blood volume) are necessitated intraoperatively in the trauma patient, it is difficult as a practical matter to rapidly administer blood components separately. It is true that packed cells can be diluted with saline for administration, but whole blood is far more convenient to administer when a massive transfusion is necessary. If large quantities of whole blood are administered rapidly, most would agree that fine screen filtration should be employed.[17] Although it has not been conclusively demonstrated that ultrafiltration affects morbidity or mortality, it seems beneficial intuitively to prevent accumulation (in the pulmonary vascular bed) of debris from large quantities of transfused blood. Other major considerations during massive transfusions[17] include warming the blood to body temperature prior to infusion, monitoring coagulation factors so that coagulopathies can be treated properly and early, and monitoring pH and serum-ionized calcium to determine whether sodium bicarbonate or calcium chloride is needed and in what quantities.

As mentioned previously, the use of individual blood components is rapidly replacing whole blood. When infusing large quantities of packed red blood cells, it must be remembered that crystalloid fluids, such as lactated Ringer's solution, should be given concurrently in amounts that will supply the volume of plasma normally accompanying the administered red blood cells. This must be given in addition to any other balanced electrolyte solution administered. Otherwise, one soon finds that volume replacement is inadequate and that blood viscosity is increased, further adding to decreased capillary perfusion. Fresh frozen plasma and platelet concentrations should be given when indicated. Frequently, these must be given empirically because laboratory facilities that provide rapid coagulation status results are lacking. Another complication occasionally seen in the patient receiving massive blood transfusions is disseminated intravascular coagulation (DIC). If DIC is strongly suspected, the major consideration should be rapid establishment of the diagnosis. Only with a confirmed diagnosis of DIC should one give heparin to a patient who is already bleeding. It must also be remembered that in the anesthetized patient, persistent ooze may be the first evidence of a transfusion reaction. Despite many exotic possibilities that may account for persistent bleeding, one must not forget that an open vessel is still the most likely cause, even in the traumatized patient! When there is an unligated open vessel, no amount of component therapy is likely to be beneficial until closure of the vessel is effected.

INTRAOPERATIVE EMERGENCIES IN THE TRAUMA PATIENT

Hypotension

Blood loss in excess of replaced volume is almost always the reason for a falling blood pressure in the trauma paient on the operating table. The diagnosis is most easily made when one has a plan by which blood loss can be continually re-evaluated and an accurate record can be made of the quantity and type of fluid and blood administered. If in doubt, the question can usually be answered by administering a fluid challenge of 500 to 1000 ml. of a balanced electrolyte solution. If the blood pressure rapidly responds to this approach, one can, for practical purposes, assume at least a 10 per cent deficit in intravascular volume that needs to be replaced with blood. If, however, there is no response to the fluid challenge, the cause of the hypotension may be a problem either with the pump (cardiogenic shock) or with vascular resistance (neurogenic or septic shock).

Clues suggesting myocardial dysfunction include evidence of trauma to the anterior chest, electrocardiographic indications of myocardial ischemia or infarction, dysrhythmias, and evidence of either left or right ventricular failure if a pulmonary artery catheter is in place. Blunt trauma to the chest can produce myocardial contusion resulting in an ECG picture similar to that of acute myocardial infarction. Appropriate therapy would include an inotropic agent such as dopamine, treatment of dysrhythmias that might be present, and cautious fluid administration. If cardiac tamponade is the cause, pericardiocentesis should be performed immediately.

When myocardial function is normal but hypotension persists in the face of evidence of adequate peripheral perfusion, one can proceed on the assumption that vascular resistance is inappropriately low and use volume replacement to achieve adequate vascular filling. In addition, continuing concealed blood loss must be considered (e.g., hemothorax or retroperitoneal hematoma).

In general, vasoconstrictors have extremely limited usefulness in the hypotensive anesthetized trauma patient. In the patient with a volume deficit, vasoconstrictors decrease perfusion in the microcirculation and thus result in further deterioration in organ function. If afterload is increased by increased peripheral resistance secondary to vasoactive drugs while myocardial contractility is decreased, further myocardial dysfunction may result. Although one often hears the argument that one "buys time" in this situation by increasing coronary filling, it is now known that most of the vasoconstrictors increase myocardial oxygen consumption more than they increase myocardial oxygenation.

Hypertension

In the older patient, essential hypertension may have existed prior to trauma, although frequently the history is either not sought or not obtained. In such a patient, hypertension would be expected. In patients with closed head injury, increasing intracranial pressure, which would be accompanied by bradycardia rather than by tachycardia, must be considered. Endocrine disorders must also be considered in the differential diagnosis, with pheochromocytoma and thyrotoxicosis being possibilities.

Tension Pneumothorax

Lung puncture by a fractured rib or by a missile or pointed weapon may produce a small pneumothorax. Traumatic rupture of the trachea or a bronchus could result from blunt chest trauma. If positive pressure ventilation is then initiated, especially while employing nitrous oxide in the anesthetic management, a rapidly expanding tension pneumothorax may result. This may be heralded by wheezing, hypotension, tachycardia, diminished breath sounds on the affected side, cyanosis, and/or decreased lung compliance. Because of the potential for progression to cardiac arrest from unrecognized and untreated tension pneumothorax, especially during positive pressure ventilation, a high index of suspicion is necessary, as is needle aspiration of the chest followed by tube thoracostomy when indicated.

Fat Embolism

Although the classic fat embolism syndrome is rarely seen preoperatively, hypoxia may begin to occur during the stage of operative and anesthetic management. Again, recognition of the setting in which fat embolism would be likely is essential. If it is considered likely, monitoring of arterial blood gases would then be the appropriate means of insuring that hypoxia did not occur intraoperatively. Evidence of fat embolization to the lungs includes bronchospasm, wheezing, tachypnea and cyanosis, all of which are nonspecific but raise the index of suspicion.

Respiratory Dysfunction

If clinical evidence of pulmonary injury is present, an arterial cannula to monitor blood gases should be inserted so that therapeutic measures may be initiated intraoperatively. Common injuries in which this maneuver is indicated include flail chest, contused lung, sepsis, fat embolization and aspiration of gastric contents.[13] Only by monitoring arterial pressures and blood gases can one deliver the most appropriate inspired oxygen concentration, adjust the level of alveolar ventilation for maintenance of normocarbia, and adjust the level of end-expiratory pressure for adequate oxygenation at the least toxic inspired oxygen concentration. In short, there is no reason why prophylactic and therapeutic pulmonary intensive care cannot begin intraoperatively. Even though the mechanical ventilators best suited for use in situations characterized by low pulmonary compliance and pathological levels of shunting are generally not present in the operating room, equipment for maintaining graded levels of end-expiratory pressure is commercially available.

SUMMARY

Anesthetic management of the trauma victim should not be an isolated event but a significant component of the continuum of care if one is to provide the best chance of successful recovery for the victim. Its primary objective is to salvage a live individual with intact renal function. This is accomplished by preoperative and intraoperative management directed toward the establishment and maintenance of a normal physiological state. The pathway to this stabilization is multifaceted and encumbered with controversy. Regardless of the specific techniques utilized, the approach must be systematic and preplanned but flexible. Constant awareness of potential catastrophes and attention to detail are mandatory. One should be thoroughly familiar with invasive monitoring techniques and their interpretation. Above all, be prepared for the worst! Only then can the necessary therapy be instituted appropriately and without undue delay.

REFERENCES

1. Bedford, R. F.: Percutaneous radial-artery cannulation—increased safety using Teflon catheters. Anesthesiology 42:219–222, 1975.
2. Blackburn, H., Taylor, H. L., Okamoto, N. et al.: Standardization of the exercise electrocardiogram. A systematic comparison of chest lead configurations employed for monitoring during exercise. In Karsonen, M. J., and Barry, A. J. (eds.): Physical Activity and the Heart. Springfield, Ill., Charles C Thomas, Publisher, p. 101, 1967.
3. Bonica, J. J. (ed.): Regional Anesthesia: Recent Advances and Current Status. Philadelphia, F. A. Davis Company, 1971.
4. Branthwaite, M. A., and Bradley, R. D.: Measurement of cardiac output by thermodilution in man. J. Appl. Physiol. 24:434–438, 1968.
5. Carrico, C. J., Canizaro, P. C., and Shires, G. T.: Fluid resuscitation following injury: rationale for the use of balanced salt solutions. Crit. Care Med. 4:46–54, 1976.
6. Civetta, J. M., Gabel, J. C., and Laver, M. B.: Disparate ventricular function in surgical patients. Surg. Forum 22:136, 1971.
7. Fulton, R. L., and Peter, E. T.: The progressive nature of pulmonary contusion. Surgery 67:499–586, 1970.
8. Gallagher, T. J., and Civetta, J. M.: The multiple trauma patient: Assessment and anesthesia. In Brunner, E. A. (ed.): Current Problems in Anesthesia and Critical Care Medicine. Chicago, Year Book Medical Publishers, Inc., 1977.
9. Ganz, W., Donoso, R., Mateus, I. S., et al.: A new technique for measurement of cardiac output by thermodilution in man. Am. J. Cardiol. 27:392–396, 1971.
10. Giesecke, A. H. (ed.): Anesthesia for the Surgery of Trauma. Philadelphia, F. A. Davis Company, 1976.
11. Giesecke, A. H., and Beyer, C. W.: Perioperative fluid management. In Brunner, E. A. (ed.): Current Problems in Anesthesia and Critical Care Medicine. Chicago, Year Book Medical Publishers, Inc., 1977.
12. Henschel, E. O. (ed.): Malignant Hyperthermia: Current Concepts. New York, Appleton-Century-Crofts, 1977.
13. Horovitz, J. H., Carrico, C. J., and Shires, G. T.: Pulmonary response to major injury. Arch. Surg. 108:349–355, 1974.
14. Lappas, D. G., Powell, W. M. J., and Daggest, W.: Cardiac dysfunction in the perioperative period: Pathophysiology, diagnosis and treatment. Anesthesiology 47:117–137, 1977.
15. Larkin, J., and Moylan, J.: Priorities in management of trauma victims. Crit. Care Med. 3:192–195, 1975.
16. Lowenstein, E., Little, J. W., and Lo, H. H.: Prevention of cerebral embolization from flushing radial artery cannulas. N. Engl. J. Med. 285:1414–1415, 1971.
17. Miller, R. D.: Complications of massive blood transfusions. Anesthesiology 39:82–93, 1973.
18. Ryan, J. F., Raines, J., Dalton, B. C., et al.: Arterial dynamics of radial artery cannulation. Anesth. Analg. 52:1017–1025, 1973.
19. Winnie, A. P.: Regional anesthesia. Surg. Clin. North Am. 55:861–892, 1975.

CHAPTER 6

POST-TRAUMATIC PULMONARY INSUFFICIENCY

John A. Collins, M.D.

INTRODUCTION

A small but significant number of patients develop pulmonary insufficiency after major injury. In some, the causes are readily apparent, but often they are obscure. A number of theories of the pathophysiology of post-traumatic pulmonary insufficiency have been advanced, some of which have been very helpful in understanding and treating the disease, but others have been confusing at best. By focusing on the more obscure possibilities, there has been a tendency to lose sight of the considerable amount of knowledge dealing with post-traumatic pulmonary insufficiency that is reasonably well established. In this chapter we will attempt to deal with the known and the obscure in a balanced manner.

A number of recent reviews have dealt with this overall clinical problem each with a somewhat different orientation and point of view. Since no one chapter can do justice to this subject, the reader is advised to consult these references for completeness.[24, 31, 45, 145, 166, 193, 229, 267]

The incidence of post-traumatic pulmonary insufficiency is difficult to define. If the end point of definition is the need for mechanical ventilatory assistance, then the incidence is moderately high in patients with direct injury to the chest and its contents, and very high if the chest is crushed. If the thoracic cage is not injured

primarily and special circumstances such as inhalation of fumes or aspiration of blood are not present, the overall incidence is probably 1 or 2 per cent of patients hospitalized for injury. This was probably (but not clearly) the incidence for combat casualties in Vietnam under similar circumstances. It seems to be rather common opinion that the incidence may be less than it was about 10 years ago.[146, 266] The mortality definitely seems to be lower. Even that may not be a precise statement: Death from hypoxia is no longer common in such patients, but injured patients are still dying with pulmonary insufficiency. Treatment has improved sufficiently to maintain many patients in the viable range of oxygenation, but the progression of sepsis and failure of other organ systems still lead to death in a moderate number of patients with major post-traumatic pulmonary insufficiency of seemingly obscure cause. The disease is less likely to be the primary cause of death but is now recognized as part of a broader problem that is still significantly lethal.

Many clinical series indicate that in the absence of a recognizable specific cause, post-traumatic pulmonary insufficiency is most often associated with systemic sepsis. In this setting it is very often part of multiple-system failure. The concordance of failure of a number of major organ systems seems to increase lethality almost linearly.

When both renal and pulmonary failure occur after a major septic complication, mortality may well approach or exceed 90 per cent. The problem here is no longer the pulmonary failure itself, which must still be properly managed, but the setting of an almost totally failing patient in whom each further setback diminishes the chances for survival. If there is a single obscure syndrome that applies to the post-traumatic patient, it is this specter of multiple-system failure that often begins with major infection.

In addition to this most recently recognized manifestation of the systemic nature of traumatic injury, however, there are many specific causes of pulmonary failure that appear in every series of injured patients, plus a small group that does not neatly fit anyone's preconceived ideas.

Prolonged ventilatory disability in an injured patient with pre-existing chronic respiratory insufficiency is easy to understand, very likely to occur, and very difficult to treat. We will not deal with it further in this chapter. Respiratory insufficiency that accompanies direct injury to the chest may not be as simple as it first appears and will be discussed briefly here, even though there is a special chapter on thoracic injuries (Chapter 13). The prolonged pulmonary parenchymal disease that occasionally occurs in patients without pre-existing pulmonary disease, without direct injury to the lungs, and without obvious cause has received the most attention recently. Because so much uncertainty and some controversy surround this entity, it will receive the greatest attention in this chapter.

We will discuss the principles of treatment on the assumption that the reader has a moderately well-developed base in pulmonary physiology and some familiarity with modern ventilatory equipment. If review is necessary in these areas, several recent publications are recommended.[110, 193, 229, 267]

DIRECT THORACIC INJURY

Direct injury to the chest is an obvious situation in which pulmonary insufficiency might be expected to develop. It was also the first entity in which a linkage to pulmonary insufficiency was recognized, and indeed the management of thoracic injuries, especially penetrating thoracic injuries, is prominent in the history of surgery as a distinct specialty.[143] Thoracic injuries are dealt with in Chapter 13, so only a few comments pertinent to ventilatory support and postresuscitative pulmonary insufficiency will be made here.

Contusion is a characteristic response of the thinly supported, richly perfused pulmonary parenchyma to a wide variety of blunt and penetrating injuries. It is one of, if not the most important single component of direct mechanical injury to the chest. Some experimental and clinical data suggest that contusion produces a disproportionately large shunt, which results in severe hypoxemia that is resistant to the administration of supplemental oxygen. There is good evidence that the extent of contusion and the degree of shunting after standardized injuries in animals can be limited by the use of positive pressure ventilation.[176, 215] This prophylactic benefit is time-dependent and becomes progressively less apparent with increasing intervals from injury to institution of treatment. Many physicians favor the early and frequent use of mechanical ventilatory support in patients with severe mechanical thoracic injuries. There is, however, a contrary proposal. Trinkle and associates[260] have proposed a regimen utilizing minimal mechanical ventilatory support, restriction of fluids, and prophylactic use of steroids. This regimen is based on experience with a series of patients that was acknowledged not to be controlled; also, it is not clear if fluid management was similar in the two groups.[260] More recently, these investigators have reported use of mechanical ventilation in half of their patients with serious thoracic injuries. Most surgeons treating thoracic injuries probably still prefer the more frequent use of mechanical ventilatory support, more liberal use of fluids to avoid hypovolemia, and avoidance of steroids with their added septic hazard.

The roentgenographic changes in pulmonary contusion characteristically lag behind the changes in lung compliance and in oxygenation, both during development of the lesion and during recovery. Extensive use of salt water without "colloid" (plasma-specific osmotic substances) worsens the hypoxemia after contusion in experimental models.[83, 205, 215] Contused areas of the lung seem to clear inhaled bacteria much more slowly than noninjured areas.[206] This is not a surprising finding, but it does re-emphasize the need for meticulous aseptic technique in handling the airway in such patients.

The concept of the "flail chest" as an injury in which paradoxical motion of the chest wall causes the main functional defect is mechanistically attractive. It is well known and seemingly widely accepted. Clinical or experimental proof that such a mechanism is important is singularly lacking, however.[152] A great advance in the treatment of patients with crushing chest injuries occurred when the various means of external support of the chest wall, based on the above mechanical theory of pathophysiology, were exchanged for the use of volume-cycled ventilators and controlled ventilation.[14] Even with the relative crude piston ventilators then used, the results were demonstrably better. This was attributed to "internal pneumatic splinting" of the defective chest wall. Subsequently, abundant experimental work and clinical observation have strongly suggested that the important lesion in crushing injuries is the contusion of the underlying pulmonary parenchyma, not the defects in the chest wall. The clinical, radiological, and functional course of patients with these injuries has been well documented.[70, 86, 88, 117, 200, 211, 224]

Patients with penetrating injuries of the chest usually have lesser degrees of pulmonary parenchymal injury because so little of the energy of the missile is transmitted to the lung. If the missile has very high energy and an irregular or tumbling profile, however, extensive damage can be done.[76] Associated injuries to the abdomen or major vessels in the chest or the disruptions of the thoracic cage are often more important than the injury to the lung itself. Nevertheless, especially with missile injuries, hypoxemia, decreased compliance, increased work of breathing, secondary infection, atelectasis, and many other factors may remain prominent parts of the clinical problem for prolonged periods. During the recent war in Vietnam a large number of patients had penetrating missile injuries of the chest in the era of blood gas analysis and volume-cycled ventilatory support. Several series of such patients have been reported in some detail.[168, 196, 232, 233] Tables 6-1 and 6-2 are taken from the reports by Simmons et al.[232, 233] They provide interesting data on the severity of hypoxemia after wounding in relation to contusion, pneumothorax and the apparent energy of the wounding missile. The same group reported a change in arterial pO_2 after pulmonary re-expansion by insertion of chest tubes on arrival at the hospital. In 17 patients with an initial arterial pO_2 of above 80 mm. Hg, re-expansion was associated with a mean decrease of 5 mm. Hg in arterial pO_2 probably as a result of further pain and splinting resulting from the tubes. In 20 more seriously injured patients with an initial pO_2 of below 80 mm. Hg, re-expansion was associated with improvement of less than 5 mm. Hg (62.5 to 67.2 mm. Hg) in mean arterial pO_2. This is not to imply that re-expansion of the lung is

TABLE 6–1.   Distribution of Patients by Per Cent within Groups According to Range of Arterial pO_2 on Admission, Breathing Room Air*

pO_2 (MM. HG)	PNEUMOTHORAX (73)	NO PNEUMOTHORAX (14)	CONTUSION (51)	NO CONTUSION (26)	HIGH VELOCITY (19)	LOW VELOCITY (69)
> 100	3	14	4	8	—	6
80–99	26	57	22	58	10	36
60–79	48	29	51	27	47	45
40–59	22	—	24	4	42	12
< 40	1	—	—	4	—	1
	p = 0.05		p = 0.01		p = 0.02	

*All patients had penetrating wounds of the chest; number of patients in each group in parentheses. Data adapted from Simmons et al.[232]

TABLE 6–2.   Distribution of Patients by Per cent Within Groups According to Lowest Arterial pO$_2$ BreatHing Room Air During Convalescence*

LOWEST CONVALESCENT pO$_2$ (MM. HG)	CHEST ONLY		CHEST AND ABDOMEN		ALL	
	Contusion (36)	No contusion (9)	Contusion (19)	No contusion (12)	Contusion (55)	No contusion (21)
> 80	19	22	—	17	13	19
70–79	14	67	11	50	13	57
60–69	19	11	37	25	25	19
50–59	22	—	37	8	27	5
40–49	17	—	15	—	16	—
30–39	8	—	—	—	5	—
	p = 0.05		p = 0.001		p = 0.01	

*Numbers of patients are in parentheses. Data adapted from Simmons et al.[233]

unimportant in the management of patients with thoracic injuries but rather that when such patients are hypoxemic before re-expansion they will probably remain so after re-expansion. Again, contusion of the underlying pulmonary parenchyma is probably the cause of the hypoxemia not a limited pneumothorax.

NONTHORACIC INJURY

Early after a major monthoracic injury the patient may exhibit very little evidence of respiratory difficulty, but after one or a few days dyspnea appears, signalling a falling compliance. The condition may then progress to worsening hypoxia and a rising arterial carbon dioxide tension concomitant with a radiological appearance of diffuse or fluffy bilateral pulmonary infiltrates. After some initial improvement following intubation, progressively worsening hypoxemia may again appear, requiring mechanical ventilatory assistance, high inspired concentrations of oxygen, positive end expiratory pressure, and a variety of specific treatments related to the underlying cause of the pulmonary problems. The main therapeutic problem is that of maintaining oxygenation. The main pathophysiological problem is probably increased pulmonary vascular permeability.

The clinical picture has been nicely summarized by Moore and associates[166] and has been extensively discussed in a number of subsequently published reviews.[24, 31, 45, 145, 193, 267] Several groups have reviewed the pathological changes in patients who have died of the syndrome;[142, 181, 201, 253] others have reviewed the temporal sequence of structural changes in the lungs of injured patients.[23, 112]

Remote Infection

In those series in which sufficient data are given, the most prominent element contributing to progressive, indirect pulmonary injury appears to be sepsis, especially septic peritonitis.[45] Examples of such occurrences after hemorrhage alone are relatively rare. The most detailed study comparing and contrasting subsequent pulmonary function in patients sustaining severe hemorrhage versus those with major infection is that of Clowes and co-workers.[42] This study demonstrated striking differences in pulmonary function between the two groups. The only patients in the hemorrhagic group who developed pulmonary insufficiency were those who became infected. As more groups examine their experiences, the evidence linking pulmonary insufficiency with systemic sepsis in man and minimizing the clinical association with hemorrhage alone becomes more compelling.

A cause and effect relationship between gram-negative sepsis and pulmonary insufficiency is well supported by an abundance of laboratory observations.[41, 44] Most mammalian species react to the injection of endotoxin or of gram-negative bacteria with increased pulmonary vascular resistance, bronchoconstriction, increased extravascular lung water and protein, increased shunting, and indirect and ultrastructural evidence of increased pulmonary capillary permeability. The characteristic pattern is one of damage to the pulmonary capillary endothelium with increased leakage of fluids and protein.[28] Theses findings are compatible with the observed clinical changes.

The temporal sequence that is observed clinically suggests that the lungs can withstand these multiple challenges initially but that self-defense (and perhaps defense of the systemic circulation) breaks down as the onslaught continues. Clearly, the best thing the physician can do for the patient's lungs in these circumstances is to control the remote infection. Abundant and still accumulating clinical evidence indicates that infection may be the factor that determines survival in these patients. The relationship is so compelling that several authors have proposed that the appearance of progressive pulmonary insufficiency after injury and without apparent cause should prompt a vigorous search for hidden infection, including exploration or re-exploration of the abdomen if infection there is a feasible complication of the injury.

Pulmonary Infection

The lower airway must remain sterile in order to function properly, but it is constantly exposed to bacteria. In addition, the lungs are the main filter for bloodborne material and bear the brunt of bacteremic episodes. The pulmonary defense mechanisms are fairly complex and are still incompletely defined.[175] The key elements appear to be the pulmonary alveolar macrophages, which are very metabolically active and efficient phagocytic cells.[43, 175] The ability of the lungs to clear and kill inhaled bacteria is adversely affected by serious injury,[63] hemorrhage,[72, 213] aspiration,[172] hypoxia,[43] cigarette smoke, high concentrations of oxygen, and adrenocorticosteroid hormones,[94, 173] among other things.[43] In addition, the lungs probably share in the suppression of systemic antibacterial defenses that result from anesthesia and operation.[240] *Pseudomonas* organisms may be particularly difficult to sterilize in the airway.[243]

The bacterial challenge to the lower airway is increased in injured patients by such factors as intubation, retained secretions, and aspiration. The oropharyngeal flora of sick hospitalized patients converts to a predominantly gram-negative pattern within a few days.[92, 120, 212] Administration of antibiotics is not necessary for the change to occur.[121, 212] Gram-negative pneumonia may occur primarily in patients whose upper airways have been first colonized by gram-negative bacteria.[121]

Most available evidence indicates that the gram-negative bacteria that colonize the lungs of sick postoperative patients arise from the patients themselves,[160, 241] although there are contrary data and opinions.[128] This is an important point in practical terms because it bears on the question of isolation of such patients. If infection occurs mainly from endogenous sources, isolation not only would be futile but would interfere with frequent contact with the patient by the physician and nursing staff. If sepsis is easily transmissible through the air, however, isolation is mandatory. The evidence on this point in patients with gram-negative pneumonia is not clear, and the important question of the degree of formal isolation that should be enforced is still unsettled. This uncertainty, however, must never be translated into sloppiness in technique. On the contrary, the proper care of the airway of a seriously injured patient requires compulsive attention to sterile technique in handling, hand washing after each contact with the patient, proper disposal of contaminated materials and set protocols for sterilizing and monitoring the sterility of equipment, among other techniques. It is only the formal isolation that implies ease of airborne contamination that is in doubt. Contamination by direct contact is not only possible, it is inevitable if the proper precautions are not taken.[15, 69, 97, 105, 186, 190]

Once gram-negative tracheitis or pneumonia is established, dissemination throughout the entire lower airway may occur via ventilatory equipment. Use of elongated tubing that is a common pathway for inspiration and expiration (increased dead space) may be particularly harmful in redisseminating *Pseudomonas*.[15, 105] There are better ways of controlling carbon dioxide levels than by increasing dead space. The topical characteristics of secondary gram-negative pneumonia in sick hospitalized patients are so striking that "topical" use of antimicrobial agents has been tried.[73, 96, 131, 133] Adding the proper antibiotic, usually an aminoglycoside, to a nebulization device in the ventilatory equipment will delay the appearance of gram-negative organisms in the airway and may well improve the results of treatment with systemic antibiotics. After prolonged use in an individual patient or with routine use in all patients, resistant organisms appear; they assume increasingly aggressive characteristics and may rapidly colonize all patients admitted to the unit. More selective and intermittent use of nebulized antibiotics seems to avoid this problem and may be a useful maneuver in very highly susceptible patients. Further controlled trials seem worthwhile. Another interesting approach, which needs further evaluation, is active immunization against *Pseudomonas*.[192]

Bacteremic gram-negative pneumonias occur primarily in patients with significantly impaired antimicrobial defenses and carry a very high mortality.[119] There have been no studies on the effect of brief intermittent bacteremias (such as might occur in the patient with multiple indwelling catheters) on the ability of the lungs to handle an inhaled bacterial challenge.

The diagnosis of gram-negative pneumonia can be very difficult to make in a patient already ill with pulmonary complications. Fever, leukocytosis, pulmonary infiltrates and hypoxemia may be due to other causes. Proper interpretation of tracheal cultures in such a patient is very difficult.[191] Most such patients will soon show gram-negative organisms in the tracheal aspirate, especially if intubated. Untimely use of antibiotics will probably do more harm than good, but even this is not proven. Distinguishing colonization from bronchopneumonia is a practical problem that is faced almost daily in every active intensive care unit but is still very difficult to solve.

Superimposed pulmonary infection, usually gram-negative and most often *Pseudomonas*, is often the final terminal event in those who died of postraumatic pulmonary insufficiency.[13] It is rarely the primary problem, but the superimposition of further loss of pulmonary function and an added septic burden may prove insurmountable. Few patients who die of acute respiratory distress after injury die with sterile lower airways. Pulmonary sepsis is a complication of complications, occurring in damaged lungs in a compromised host.

Thrombosis and Pulmonary Embolism

In recent years there has been a great expansion of our knowledge of the incidence and natural history of deep venous thrombosis in the legs following major operations and injury.[124, 236] Similar data on pulmonary embolism have not accrued, but since deep venous thrombosis in the legs is the most common event leading to post-traumatic pulmonary embolism, the information obtained has been pertinent.

The factors predisposing the patient toward deep venous thrombosis are those commonly associated with pulmonary embolism: congestive heart failure, certain malignancies, severe trauma, prolonged bed rest, obesity and a prior history of deep venous disease or of pulmonary embolism. Surprising, fully 50 per cent of newly formed clots begin forming during the operation itself; most of the rest begin within a few days afterward. Understandably, there are no similar studies on what happens immediately after accidental injury, but a similar pattern would not be surprising. Most postoperative deep venous clots are asymptomatic; nearly half the patients with signs and symptoms suggesting thrombophlebitis in the calf do not have venous clots. In most circumstances, low doses of heparin are effective in preventing postoperative deep venous thrombosis except when a clot is already present before operation.[124] Various mechanical maneuvers may also be effective. Again, detailed studies in the immediate post-traumatic state are lacking. With pre-existing clots, fully anticoagulating doses of heparin are required. Continuous intravenous administration of heparin seems to be safer and is at least as effective as the older practice of intermittent doses.[218] Heparin itself can cause thrombocytopenia in a significant percentage of patients.[203]

Pulmonary emboli in man lyse spontaneously at a significant but somewhat unpredictable rate.[50] Heparin usually prevents recurrent embolizaton but may do little to alter the rate of resolution of existing emboli. The newer fibrinolysins derived from bacterial or human sources significantly hasten the resolution of pulmonary emboli and of peripheral deep venous clots.[82] They carry a very significant risk of hemorrhage in early postoperative or post-traumatic patients, however, and also when used concurrently with heparin. These products have recently been approved for clinical use in the United States. Various mechanical devices inserted into the inferior vena cava transvenously appear to be effective in preventing recurrent embolization in high-risk patients who are unacceptable for or failures of treatment with heparin.[95, 164] The rate of complications of insertion decreases sharply with the experience of the technician.

Pulmonary embolization is much more common in post-traumatic patients than is clinically apparent.[23, 71, 142, 167, 174] The degree is often fairly small, but occasionally inapparent recurrent embolization, contributes significantly to pulmonary dysfunction in sick surgical patients. The clinical picture of hypoxemia, bilateral pulmonary infiltrates and fever can mimic that of many other entities. The diagnosis can be difficult to establish. In spite of heightened awareness, plain roentgenograms of the chest remain rather inaccurate.[141] Scintiscanning is often of little diagnostic value in such patients.[174] Pulmonary arteriography is necessary to establish the diagnosis. The treatment involves either anticoagulation with heparin or interruption of the inferior vena cava. The use of fibrinolytic agents in the first week after major injury seems very hazardous. There are insufficient data to establish the risks and benefits of prophylactic low dose heparin in seriously injured patients.

Disseminated Intravascular Coagulation and Platelet Sequestration

Disseminated intravascular coagulation (DIC) and an interesting variant, microembolization or sequestration of leukocytes and platelets, have been proposed as possible mechanisms of pulmonary dysfunction in septic or injured patients. DIC has been implicated on the basis of numerous studies of DIC induced in animals[103, 113, 123, 217] and on the frequent coincidence of respiratory failure and some evidence of DIC in patients.[163, 217] Our experience has been that few patients with acute pulmonary insufficiency exhibit either DIC or notable clotting abnormalities, but that many patients who exhibit postoperative or post-traumatic DIC develop significant pulmonary insufficiency. Laterman et al.[137] and Manwaring et al.[154] have recently presented evidence that human fibrinolytic fragment D, which is a major component of fibrin split products found in burn patients, causes florid pulmonary insufficiency when infused into rabbits. It is hoped that these studies can be extended to primates. Intrapulmonary hemorrhage is a rather common but often overlooked complication of DIC that can cause fatal pulmonary insufficiency.[207] There is an interesting reverse relationship; The lungs may play an important role in regulating fribrinolysis.[158] The effect of acute parenchymal pulmonary disease on fibrinolysis is unknown. Instances of apparently localized intravascular coagulation in one lung have been reported.[280] A pathogenetic role for microembolization or sequestration of platelets or leukocytes is less well supported. A considerable amount of experimental work has yielded often contradictory results, but certain findings are fairly consistent. Platelets and serotonin sequester in the lungs after soft tissue injury, hemorrhage, endotoxemia or bacteremia. The primary functional effect seems to be bronchoconstriction, which is probably related to the local release of serotonin. There is often little effect on oxygenation. In studies, white cells often sequester in the lungs along with platelets, especially after endotoxemia or bacteremia. The sequestration of platelets in the lung is usually viewed as a potentially damaging event,[180, 246, 255] but there is contrary evidence as well.[134] If the sequestration is due to interaction with already damaged vascular endothelium, it may well be protective.[273]

In contrast to the many studies in animals, there have been very few pertinent studies in patients. Two very recent such studies overshadow much of the preceding experimental work.[60, 107, 108] Except in the septic patients in one of these series, changes in platelet count, even when measured across the lungs, did not correlate with measurements of pulmonary function. In neither group could the observed sequestration in the lungs account for the degree of thrombocytopenia present. This finding was also noted in another study of platelet kinetics in patients in acute ventilatory failure; in these there was thrombocytopenia and increased platelet turnover but no sequestration in the lungs. Sequestration of the platelets in the liver and spleen was prominent.[223]

There are many causes of postoperative, post-traumatic pulmonary insufficiency, and these studies do not rule out an effect of platelet or leukocyte aggregation or of DIC for some of these, but sepsis and hemorrhage have been high on the list of conditions for which such a pathogenetic mechanism has been proposed. Many more careful prospective studies, such as these in defined groups of patients in which the proposed mechanism — DIC, platelet or leukocyte sequestration — is contrasted against the supposed effects, are needed before these relationships can be defined. It is not known whether minidoses of heparin can prevent post-traumatic DIC or sequestration of platelets, but it seems doubtful. Before accepting the hazards of full anticoagulation in recently injured patients, better evidence of an important role for these conditions is required.

Anesthesia and Operation

A series of challenges to pulmonary function is involved in general anesthesia, a major operation or injury to the trunk.[138, 189] Some of these have been well documented but tend to be forgotten when new or exotic causes of pulmonary impairment are sought.

The effects of premedication and general anesthesia on pulmonary function have recently been reviewed in some detail.[155] The postoperative effects of narcotics on patients are still not well documented, however. Differences in doses, routes of administration, age and clinical status are all significant.

The various agents used for general anesthesia all suppress ventilation when deep planes of anesthesia are induced. Almost all agents significantly depress myocardial function and have varying effects on peripheral vascular tone. The reduction of oxygen consumption that occurs with general anesthesia alone is rather small.

Hypothermia, especially with neuromuscular paralysis, is very effective in reducing oxygen consumption. Periodic passive hyperinflation of the lungs during general anesthesia prevents a significant and progressive fall in arterial oxygenation that would otherwise occur, especially in patients with tidal volumes of less than 8 ml./kg. body weight. This probably represents a tendency to closure of terminal airways and perhaps concomitant or subsequent alveolar collapse, especially if highly absorbable gas is "trapped" behind the closed airways. There are marked changes in lung compliance during general anesthesia, but much of this is due to the lower functional residual capacity that occurs with recumbency and relaxation.

These effects persist into the early postoperative period but only for a matter of hours. The occurrence and degree of postoperative pulmonary impairment is dominated by such factors as location of incision, obesity, duration of operation, pre-existing pulmonary disease and perhaps even "personality."

The influence of the incision on postoperative pulmonary impairment dramatically demonstrates the importance of pain and splinting. Churchill in 1927 first demonstrated the differential effect of upper abdominal incisions on pulmonary function (vital capacity).[36] Many observations utilizing a variety of measurements have since reaffirmed the detrimental effects of incisions near the diaphragm. In some instances, upper laparotomies were more detrimental than thoracotomies. Most studies show decreases in vital capacity, functional residual capacity, compliance and arterial oxygen tension, a restrictive pattern in timed expiratory studies, and a shift toward frequent shallow breathing with an absence of deep breaths. All of these changes are worse with upper abdominal incisions and least or absent with peripheral incisions.

The previously mentioned study of the relationship between transfusion and hypoxemia in combat casualties in Vietnam yielded, in addition, a large body of data on the effect of the site of the wound on pre- and postoperative arterial oxygen tension (Table 6–3).[47] Almost all of these casualities were operated upon on the day of injury, but this is characteristic of most seriously injured patients. The differences between those with peripheral injury and those with thoracic injury were as expected. The minimal degree of hypoxemia in the severely injured patients with peripheral injury is noteworthy. The degree of hypoxemia in patients with abdominal injuries was less than expected, but Lowe and his co-workers have reported similar data.[146] These patients, of course, were all vigorously healthy young adults at the time of injury. The pattern would most likely to be somewhat different in an older population.

There is general (but not unanimous) agreement that several variables clearly increase the risk of postoperative, post-traumatic pulmonary complications. Pre-existing pulmonary disease is one of the most significant, leading to at least a two- to threefold increase in postoperative pulmonary complications. Even seemingly minor upper respiratory infections have been found to increase risk greatly. Smoking is similarly a high risk factor, and much of the data concerning smoking is included in the groups of patients classified as having preoperative pulmonary disease. Obesity seems to be a moderate risk factor. The location of the incision has already been discussed. The type of incision (especially horizontal versus vertical) has been found to be both significant and not significant, but one of the best controlled studies showed less respiratory impairment in massively obese patients explored through transverse as opposed to vertical abdominal incisions.[263] Age is a debatable risk factor, as much of the increased difficulty can be attributed to associated diseases rather than to age itself. The duration of the operation is probably important, at least for prolonged (over 3- to 4-hour) procedures. Sex is probably not significant; the several studies that showed more impairment in men usually did not correct smoking. Surprisingly, the type of agent used for anesthesia made little or no difference, and the incidence of delayed postoperative pulmonary complications was no less after regional than after general inhalation anesthesia. Because there may be differences relating to individual anesthesiologists, however, technique is probably somewhat significant. A number of more recent studies further confirm this pattern of findings[6, 8, 231, 283] and have added the first demonstration of the importance of

personality traits in the patient,[51] something well known to practicing surgeons.

A number of practices or devices designed to promote deep breathing postoperatively have been successful in reducing pulmonary complications after elective operations.[18, 159, 262] "Intermittent positive pressure breathing" as commonly dispensed is not one of these, and it should be specifically singled out because although it is commonly used, it is at best worthless and often wasteful of money and at worst harmful (promoting sepsis, meteorism and failure to handle adequately pulmonary problems). Some of the most effective maneuvers include careful use of narcotics, regional anesthesia for relief of postoperative pain, and preoperative chest physical therapy (although this last requires several days preoperatively to achieve full effectiveness). Simple and inexpensive incentive deep breathing devices may be effective.[56]

Various other factors may contribute to pulmonary impairment during or after operation. Anesthetic gases as commonly used are almost totally dry. This is demonstrably harmful and probably accounts for some of the harmful effects of prolonged anesthesia.[81, 268] Recumbency produces an instantaneous decrease in functional residual capacity.[9] Several studies have indicated that there is a modest fall in arterial oxygenation with prolonged bed rest, but a recent study found no change after 48 hours of recumbency by normal volunteers.[259]

The pattern of findings confirmed in many studies over a 40-year period is rather clear and consistent. There are changes in pulmonary function induced by anesthesia and by narcotic drugs, but even more marked and prolonged changes result from operative wounds. These changes suggest that diaphragmatic motion is hindered by pain, producing an altered pattern of breathing, changes in various lung volumes and a restrictive functional pattern, all of which contribute to airway closure and alvolar collapse. Some clearly defined factors make this more likely to happen, and various maneuvers can minimize the occurrence, extent and duration of these changes. These changes unquestionably contribute in a major way to the development of more severe forms of pulmonary insufficiency, at least by allowing certain complications to occur more easily, if not contributing directly to whatever causes the severe impairment.

Aspiration Pneumonitis

The true incidence of aspiration pneumonitis is almost impossible to define. The mortality after clinically diagnosed aspiration remains surprisingly high, mostly because of the type of patients who aspirate.[16, 32]

A number of studies have documented the predictable occurrence of "silent" regurgitation during general anesthesia and have identified several factors leading to a higher risk of aspiration: operations on the abdomen or oropharynx, the presence of nasogastric tubes (doubles the incidence), tracheostomy and perhaps the anesthetic agent. Much of this aspiration produces little in the way of clinical disease and probably represents primarily an increased bacterial challenge to the lower airway.

Aspiration pneumonitis is a more complex disease than it appears. The most serious threats to function and survival are probably drowning, chemical damage, bacterial contamination and mechanical obstruction of the airway. Failure to distinguish between these various components makes some clinical reports and experimental studies difficult to evaluate. Drowning is straightforward. It obviously requires a grossly distended stomach and hence is associated with injury soon after eating or drinking or, in the postoperative patient, with improper intragastric feeding by tube, forced oral intake or severe ileus. The treatment is immediate suctioning of the airway, intubation and mechanical ventilatory support, and safely emptying the stomach to prevent recurrence. It is much more likely to happen in obtunded or unconscious patients.

Chemical damage is usually caused by the low pH of the aspirate and is probably a combined acid-peptic lesion. It is difficult to determine how frequently this form of aspiration occurs, but since it requires an empty stomach it probably does not occur frequently. In the absence of better data, it seems likely that this form of aspiration has received far more attention than it deserves. If there is a role for steroids in

patients who have aspirated, it is only in this highly acid form of aspiration, and even then there is some contrary evidence.[34, 68] The incidence of late infection is not clear but is probably increased by using steroids. If significant aspiration is thought to have occurred, and especially if impairment of oxygenation has been documented, early use of mechanical ventilatory assistance will probably be beneficial.[26, 33, 34, 68, 80]

Most sizable aspirations that occur clinically involve either recently ingested food or obstructed intestinal contents; occasionally purulent material is involved. The goal should be to remove mechanically obstructing material and to control bacterial contamination. If particles are observed in the mouth or returned in the tracheal aspirate, bronchoscopic examination and removal of remaining particles should be undertaken quickly. Removal of particles is more cumbersome with the fiberoptic devices, but the initial examination is easier and can demonstrate the extent of the problem and the need for rigid bronchoscopy. Bacterial contamination is especially likely with aspiration of obstructing intestinal contents, and with either food or obstructing contents, late infection is probably the leading cause of death. The range of bacterial flora is very broad and nonspecific following aspiration, and the use of antibiotics prophylactically is of uncertain value.[5, 17, 144] Aspiration by hospitalized patients tends to result in more gram-negative and staphylococcal infections, whereas anaerobic organisms predominate in out-of-hospital aspiration. The role of early ventilatory support in this latter group of patients is not as well established. These forms of aspiration need more experimental study.

Aspiration of blood produces a particularly intense inflammatory response. This usually occurs with endobronchial bleeding, which is fortunately not often great or prolonged after accidental or violent trauma, even with direct injury to the lungs. The supine position, drug- or injury-induced stupor and nasogastric tubes all greatly increase the chances of aspiration in the patient vomiting or regurgitating blood. Repeated hematemesis is probably usually associated with significant aspiration of blood, and this accounts for much of the pulmonary impairment in such patients. Effective therapy for aspiration of blood is largely preventive.

The available data indicate that aspiration is underestimated in incidence and extent and that the favorite form among investigators (acid aspiration) is not the main problem clinically. Early use of positive pressure ventilation and of bronchoscopy seems very beneficial in some forms, the role of prophylactic antibiotics is not settled, and the value of steroids is limited or nonexistent.

Vasoactive Materials

The lungs receive the entire cardiac output. All venous blood passes through the pulmonary capillary bed before reaching the systemic circulation, coming in contact with a huge endothelial surface area. This is a unique situation, and it is not surprising that the lungs have been found to be metabolically and hormonally very active. This activity is still under investigation, but a certain pattern of biological activity is already evident.[78, 89, 216, 256]

The lungs are of prime importance in determining the activity of many circulating vasoactive substances. The vasoactive amines and the prostaglandins are selectively inactivated. Among peptides, angiotensin I is almost completely converted to angiotensin II, bradykinin is 95 to 99 per cent inactivated, and there is evidence of activity against gastrin and insulin. In some of these processes, specific enzymes have been identified on are suspected to be on the luminal surface of the endothelial cells. For the prostaglandins, there is probably a transport mechanism that determines the specificity. The structural alterations occur within the endothelial cells. Norepinephrine and 5-hydroxytryptamine are also selectively transported intracellularly for further processing. It is likely, and in some cases it has been established, that these energy-dependent processes are altered by temperature, oxygen supply and perhaps availability of fuel substrate.

In addition to inactivating or changing a variety of vasoactive materials, normal lungs release stored or rapidly synthesized vasoactive material in response to various stimuli. This function is only beginning to be clarified, but it is probable that prostaglandins of the E and F families are released in response to alveolar hypoxia, pulmonary embolism, overinflation and overventilation (hypocarbia). Histamine is present in large amounts in the lungs and is released after certain stimuli. Paradoxically, the lungs are capable of generating kinins rapidly. Many of the substances associated with anaphylaxis may be released primarily from the lungs. It has been speculated that release of vasoactive substances in response to elevated end inspiratory pressure mediates the myocardial depression that might accompany such treatment.

A variety of drugs alter some of this activity. Hypothermia probably affects the mechanisms involving 5-hydroxytryptamine (5-HT) and norepinephrine. Various vasoactive materials alter the activity against other agents arriving simultaneously. The effects of systemic or local hypoperfusion have not been studied, but ischemia or hypoxia do alter oxygen consumption and uptake of glucose by the lung, so significant effects on the metabolism of vasoactive agents would not be surprising. All of the inactivating mechanisms probably can be overwhelmed by rapid sustained rates of delivery.

The lungs, and specifically the pulmonary vascular bed, are an important part of the control mechanism for systemic circulatory homeostasis and for the systemic manifestations of the response to the inflammation. The pulmonary vascular bed is obviously and grossly damaged in many of the conditions grouped together as "acute respiratory distress." There has been very little documentation of what this does to the homeostatic mechanisms, but the possibility is very great, almost compelling, that alterations in the metabolic activity of the lungs contributes significantly to the abnormalities observed. Elevated kinin levels have been found in the peripheral blood of septic patients in ventilatory failure.[179] A sustained hyperdynamic circulatory state and evidence of agglutination and sequestration of platelets, for example, are prominent accompanying features of respiratory failure in many patients. The hyperdynamic circulatory state might in turn contribute ventilatory failure by elevating the pulmonary capillary pressure in nondamaged areas or by forcing pulmonary capillary flow through already damaged vascular beds.

Systemic agglutination of platelets resulting from elevated levels of 5-HT in the systemic circulation would cause sequestration of platelet clumps primarily in the pulmonary vascular bed. Other examples of vicious circles and systemic circulatory havoc are not difficult to imagine. The fact that some forms of respiratory failure characteristically occur in patients with major inflammatory conditions elsewhere in the body lends further credence to these speculations. This may be one of the most important areas for current investigation in the entire field of acute respiratory distress.

Oxygen Toxicity

Oxygen toxicity is now a well-recognized hazard of the treatment of hypoxemia. Many excellent reviews of the subject are available.[38, 106, 226, 277] The changes induced by high inspired concentrations of oxygen are dependent on both length of time of exposure and concentration of inspired oxygen; changes occur rather rapidly when 100 per cent oxygen is inspired. These changes can be fatal. Animals with hypoxemia may be somewhat less susceptible,[276] but this has been challenged.[162] The control settings on the older style of ventilators are often inaccurate for the percentage of oxygen supplied to the patient; periodic checks of the inspired oxygen concentrations from these ventilators should be made with specially designed and calibrated instruments.

When more than 50 per cent inspired oxygen is required to maintain arterial oxygenation, other maneuvers must be considered (diuresis, positive end expiratory pressure, bronchoscopy, etc.) depending on the circumstances. An arterial oxygen tension of above 70 mm. Hg adds little in the way of arterial oxygen content, and the added risks of high oxygen concentrations in the lungs are clearly not acceptable. The practice of measuring arterial blood oxygen tension after breathing 100 per cent oxygen for 20 minutes is rather popular. There is evidence that in sick surgical patients the intrapulmonary shunt can increase during this period.[156, 249] Even though some of this increase is due to the redistribution of blood flow, which reverses when the inspired oxygen concentration is lowered, some of it seems to be due to atelectasis. Since this maneuver adds no unique information and in fact usually requires an additional analysis of arterial blood to confirm the proper long range setting of the ventilator, its continued wide use does not seem wise.

It is ironic that the lung is so resistant to hypoxia and so sensitive to hyperoxia. There is still accumulating evidence that indicates how destructive hyperoxia is to the metabolic processes of the lung. Most clinicians are now very well aware of this problem and allow for it in the day-to-day management of patients in respiratory failure. The true incidence of oxygen-mediated damage to the lungs of sick surgical patients is unknown. Some clinicians minimize its importance, and it is clearly hazardous to err on the side of using too little supplemental oxygen. Often oxygen is used without properly considering all the elements of the oxygen-delivering system, however, and an awareness of its dangers is necessary in order to provide the best care for the injured patient.

Fat Embolism

Fat embolism is a less common but often overlooked cause of ventilatory failure in injured patients. It can mimic other forms of ventilatory distress quite closely. The clinical onset usually occurs one to several days after injury. The presentation is one of progressively worsening hypoxemia, sometimes with disproportionate deterioration of mental status. The roentgenographic picture is that of generalized bilateral fluffy infiltrates progressing to nearly complete opacification. Death occurs from hypoxemia, and at autopsy the lungs are very heavy and congested. Microscopically, there is hemorrhagic infiltration and consolidation with small skip areas of nearly normal architecture. Fat is not seen unless a stain for it is used, and it may be mostly gone by the time the patient dies. Other factors such as aspiration, bacterial pneumonitis, thromboembolism, oxygen toxicity and fluid overloading may be superimposed, but fat embolism alone can cause death from ventilatory insufficiency.

The diagnosis of fat embolism is rather nonspecific. Fat occurs in the sputum and urine of normal or minimally injured patients and may be absent in patients with severe fat embolism. Changes in circulating lipase appear not to correlate with the disease at all, and circulating lipids change in a nonspecific manner. Typical changes in the retina and characteristic petechiae suggest but do not establish the diagnosis. A significantly elevated alveolar-arterial gradient for oxygen is present in nearly all clinically significant instances. The nonspecific roentgenographic changes already described usually lag behind the changes in oxygenation of the blood.

The clinical incidence of fat embolism is very hard to estimate because of the difficulty in establishing a firm diagnosis and the degree to which it mimics other pulmonary problems that occur in injured patients. The true incidence is probably not greater than 10 to 20 per cent of adult patients with major long bone fractures. The term "incidence" needs some definition, because embolic fat can be found in the lungs of most patients with long bone fractures or indeed in most patients after major orthopedic procedures. It is likely that there is a continuum extending from the subclinical event, which is never detected unless death occurs early from some other cause and a specific search is made for it, all the way to massive fatal embolization of fat and marrow to the lungs, brain, heart and kidneys. The milder forms are more common.

The nature and especially the cause of post-traumatic fat embolism have been the subject of controversy and confusion. This is unfortunate because there is in fact little evidence to support the exotic interpretations of the disease that have been popular in recent years. There is much that is known. By far the most common clinical setting is the patient with major fractures, especially of the femur, tibia and axial skeleton. The more fractures and the larger the bones involved, the greater the incidence of fat embolism. No other disease, including those diseases associated with lipemia, bears such a relationship. Almost all the nonfracture settings in which fat embolism has occurred with some regularity involve direct mechanical disruption of depot fat or bone marrow: sickle cell crisis, Caisson's disease and fatty liver. The low incidence of fat embolism in children is noteworthy. The incidence rises sharply in children with conditions in

which the normally cellular marrow is replaced with fat. All of this is compelling evidence in favor of the "classic" theory of fat embolism — namely, that direct mechanical injury results in entrance of depot fat into the venous circulation with embolization to the lungs.

Less extensive but reasonably firm data from animals and man indicate that embolization of fat continues from the injured part for several days after injury and that motion of the injured parts increases and prolongs this continued embolization. Embolization of bone marrow proper seems to occur primarily at the time of injury.

The histologic and perhaps also the functional changes occurring are very time-dependent and somewhat organ-dependent. Fat embolism in the lungs is initially bland but is later associated with hemorrhagic consolidation as the neutral fat disappears. In organs with less lipase activity, especially the renal glomeruli, the fat remains with little tissue reaction or destruction until mechanically traverses the endothelium and basement membrane into the lumen of the nephron or until it is swept back into the venous circualtion to be trapped in the lungs. These observations suggest that more than simple mechanical embolization is involved in the lungs. Local breakdown with release of unbound fatty acids in high local concentrations would be destructive to the regional pulmonary capillaries, thereby leading to all the observed structural, clinical and functional changes. It is an attractive hypothesis.

The treatment of fat embolism is also a subject of some controversy, reflecting various theories of etiology and pathophysiology. The problems of assessing treatment have been magnified by the uncertainities of the clinical diagnosis and the lack of a suitable experimental model. Heparin has been proposed because of its anticoagulant properties, assuming that DIC plays a prominent role. This strikes us as hazardous therapy in acutely injured patients who usually exhibit a changing mental status. Heparin has also been proposed in lower doses because it activates a circulating lipase. It is not known if this would accelerate lysis of embolic fat, and if it did, it is not clear whether this would be beneficial, especially in the lungs. Experimentally, heparin has usually increased the mortality in animals after they have been injected with neutral fat. Ethanol has been proposed, originally because of its ability to dissolve fat (a ridiculous proposal), and later because it inhibits formation of lipase. Again, the effect of this drug on embolic fat is not known, and the pharmacologic side effects of ethanol are significant. One occasionally hears of simultaneous adminstration of heparin and ethanol; the rationale for this is completely obscure. Steroids have received support on the basis of bolus injections of oleic acid (highly artifactitious) in experimental models and uncontrolled clinical trials. It is conceivable that some benefit might result, but certainly there is an increased risk of other complications. Only controlled clinical trials can answer the questions about treatment for this disorder.

There is, however, a rational basis for treating fat embolism that most students of the disease accept. First, the fractures should be immobilized as early and as effectively as possible. This may require skeletal traction, narcosis or even neuromuscular blocking agents (the latter two obviously require mechanical ventilatory assistance). Second, the pulmonary complications should be treated by appropriate methods. This requires detection of the hypoxemia; frequent sampling of arterial blood should be routine when a diagnosis of fat embolism is being considered. Many patients will require mechanical ventilatory assistance; they may do better if they receive such assistance early rather than late, but this is not certain. Their ventilatory management is no different from that of most hypoxemia postoperative or posttraumatic patients. The variety of proposed "specific" drugs, only a few of which were mentioned above, are almost certainly useless at best, and may often be harmful. With modern ventilatory management, mortality should be less than 10 per cent in those patients with with a firm clinical diagnosis. It is important to realize that sudden dramatic improvement is quite common. This can easily convince the uninformed that some "specific" drug or remedy has been marvelously effective. Controlled trials are mandatory to evaluate such drugs. Neurological recovery was formerly thought to be complete in survivors, but this is probably not always true and is further reason for early diagnosis and treatment.

Head Injury

Intracranial injury is often accompanied by pulmonary edema.[66, 235, 247] The effect is probably produced by massive shifts of blood volume centrally following peripheral vasoconstriction.[21, 35, 65, 67] Many of the changes that occur in experimental models can be prevented or reversed with sympathetic blockade. It is possible that direct, neurally induced changes in pulmonary vascular compliance also contribute to edema.[251] Fibrin in parts of the central nervous system may induce similar changes.[219] A nonrandomized clinical study suggests that steroids may be effective in reducing the pulmonary dysfunction that follows head injury;[3] it is not clear from the report whether this dysfunction is due to effects on intracranial pressure, pulmonary vasculature or renal fluid balance. The well-known relationship between cerebral injury and pulmonary edema has recently been extended to include the cerebral hypoxia that accompanies hemorrhage as a cause of post-traumatic respiratory failure.[169] As noted in the next section of this chapter on Hemorrhage and Resuscitation, the relationship between blood loss and pulmonary dysfunction is tenuous at best. Efforts by other groups to produce pulmonary changes on the basis of cerebral hypoxia have been unsuccessful[126] or mixed.[49] Patients who are rendered unconscious or obtunded by their injuries are also more likely to aspirate, as noted earlier. This increases the association of head injury with pulmonary dysfunction but by a totally different mechanism.

Burns

Severely burned patients often develop pulmonary complications that are occasionally the primary cause of death.[149, 197] The early complications are related to direct injury of the lungs by noxious gases, but there are also effects on the pulmonary vascular bed that result from obscure causes.[54] The later complications are related to sepsis. Older patients are prone to left ventricular failure because of the initially large fluid shifts and the sustained high cardiac outputs that accompany the large unhealed wounds. Some of the ventilatory patterns after major burns can be adversely effected by treatment; sulfamylon is an inhibitor of carbonic anhydrase and increases the work of maintaining carbon dioxide balance.[188] Simultaneous ventilation-perfusion lung scans may allow earlier definition of the extent of inhalation injury.[4] Fiberoptic bronchoscopy allows direct serial observation of the tracheobronchial tree.[188]

Currently, there is little that can be done for most patients with pulmonary insufficiency that develops early after major burns apart from nonspecific ventilatory support. Steroids have been proposed for this condition[64] but have showed no apparent benefit in a controlled study in burned patients[139] and in an experimental model using nitrogen tetroxide.[272] Aerosolized gentamicin was also apparently ineffective in the clinical study.

Malnutrition

Protein-caloric malnutrition may precede or follow serious injury.[165] Septic complications or large unhealed wounds are powerful stimuli to the catabolic response, so the nutritional reserves of even previously well-nourished patients can become depleted rapidly if significant complications occur during recovery from injury. Although the relationship between malnutrition and disease is a very complex field, it is known that malnutrition may impair a variety of antimicrobial defenses. Acute starvation in mice impairs ability to clear inhaled bacteria.[94] Very little is known about the effects of starvation or, conversely, of nutritional supplementation on host defenses after a major injury with ongoing complications. Since sepsis is one of the main clinical accompaniments (and perhaps causes) of post-traumatic pulmonary insufficiency, these questions are pertinent and important. In addition, there may be a depression of the hypoxic ventilatory drive after relatively short-term starvation in normal subjects.[55]

In the catabolic response to injury and infection, working muscles tend to be spared. If the respiratory muscles are kept at rest through the use of mechanical ventilatory assistance during a period of prolonged catabolism, as is often the case, marked wasting of the ventilatory muscles may occur. This is a particularly dangerous situation because the requirements for work in breathing are increased by the usual lingering decreased pulmonary compliance and the often persistent increased ventilatory demands of fever or large healing wounds. The course of such a patient is deceptive but lethal. Initially the patient seems well, but exhaustion of the respiratory motors occurs at an accelerating rate. Retention of carbon dioxide occurs, and when the retained carbon dioxide reaches narcotic levels, a vicious circle begins and rapidly leads to death. Restlessness or agitation along the way may be treated by narcotic drugs, which will hasten the lethal end. Early after discontinuing mechanical ventilatory support, arterial blood gases typically are acceptable and may remain so for several hours. A false sense of security in the physician contributes to a tragic outcome. This sad sequence of events undoubtedly led to some of the unexpected deaths that formerly occurred in these patients. Greater awareness of this danger plus the use of intermittent mandatory ventilation (IMV) and measurements of maximum inspiratory force before discontinuing ventilatory support have helped greatly. There is a strong feeling that better nutritional support of the patient when he is on the mechanical ventilator also significantly reduces the hazards of discontinuation.

Miscellaneous

Anemia has been proposed as a factor contributing to the development of postresuscitative pulmonary changes,[170] but the study was improperly controlled: The control dogs should have been bled and reinfused at the same interval before the study as were the anemic dogs. Preventing or reversing the acidosis that develops in dogs during hemorrhage reduces the very high pulmonary vascular resistance that also develops in this species.[130, 151, 230] Maintaining carbon dioxide concentration near normal improved compliance in bled dogs[184] and improved oxygenation in severely hypoxemic patients.[183] Excessive beta-adrenergic stimulation has also been proposed as a cause, but this has not been confirmed by others. Severe metabolic alkalosis depresses ventilation in man and presumably can also lead to the complications of sustained hypoventilation and increase the difficulties and hazards of discontinuing mechanical ventilatory support.[93, 245, 261]

HEMORRHAGE AND RESUSCITATION

There is potentially a very strong relationship among hemorrhage, the treatment for hemorrhage and post-traumatic pulmonary insufficiency. Hemorrhage is a common accompaniment of serious injury. There is some evidence that severe hemorrhage may damage the lungs. The types and quantities of fluids that are used to restore the circulation could induce fluid overloading and pulmonary edema if misused. If the lungs have indeed been damaged by hemorrhage, this would occur more easily. Some authors believe strongly in such a chain of events, but proving the existence of the various links and assigning quantitative values to the various factors has proved to be extremely difficult. Although there are seemingly contradicting data on many points, a considerable amount is known, but the effects of hemorrhage and of resuscitation should be considered together for obvious reasons (see also Chapter 4).

Hemorrhage

The relationship between hemorrhage and pulmonary insufficiency has been reviewed elsewhere.[46, 145] The degree to which hemorrhage induces deterioration of pulmonary structure and function is not clear, and clinical evidence supporting such a relationship is rather thin, as noted previously. Pulmonary insufficiency is not a common event after hemorrhage alone or after the hypovolemic shock of cholera. Most experimental efforts to demonstrate significant pulmonary insufficiency after hemorrhage alone have been unsuccessful. Morphologic changes of varying degrees have been reported, mostly in dogs. Lung compliance and shunting usually improve during hemorrhage, as pulmonary blood volume and extravascular lung water content decrease. Following treatment, there have been varying and usually unimpressive decreases in compliance and very little, if any, impairment of oxygenation. Only a few experimental studies have extended into the postresuscitative period and have involved treatment of the animals in a manner similar to that used in clinical practice, and few have systematically compared different treatment regimens. Treatments that most effectively support survival may be associated with the least alteration in pulmonary structure and function.[46]

There are at least two studies that do imitate some clinical circumstances. Kim et al. reported hypoxemia in dogs after very prolonged periods of hypovolemia followed by resuscitation.[129] The hypoxemia seemed to occur preterminally, however. More recently, Rutherford et al. reported hypoxemia in primates who had hemorrhaged to varying degrees and were then resuscitated according to monitoring criteria currently in use clinically.[214] There may well have been an element of fluid overloading in these animals, as the authors noted systemic vasodilatation. This probably led to excessive administration of fluids by pursuing certain goals of systemic and central venous pressure on a protocol basis that mimicked clinical practice. This model may support a direct causal link between hypoperfusion and pulmonary insufficiency, but it may implicate current resuscitative practices even more. Studies in primates using different protocols for treatment have yielded little or no evidence of pulmonary insufficiency.[85]

One of the simplest explanations for any damage that does occur to the lungs as a result of hemorrhage is hypoperfusion. The lungs are rather unique, however, in that they are able to tolerate total ischemia for several hours with surprisingly little detrimental effect, provided alveolar ventilation is maintained.[25] Even static inflation with nitrogen is largely protective. An atelectatic lung, however, tolerates ischemia rather poorly. Hemorrhage plus contusion may be worse than either condition alone.[260]

Studies on pulmonary capillary permeability during and after hemorrhage have yielded mixed results. The contradictory data in primates are discussed in the following section. Studies in sheep[53] and dogs[116] failed to demonstrate increased permeability to protein when the animals were in treated or untreated hemorrhagic shock, but other studies in dogs produced evidence of a greatly increased leak.[178] Two kinds of intermediate findings have also been reported in hemorrhaged dogs. One study reported increased flow of fluid and accelerated migration of molecular markers of less than 20,000 daltons,[75] while another discerned two populations of animals, one that developed a leak (high mortality) and one that did not (low mortality).[178] Anderson and De Vries studied the pulmonary lymphatic drainage in dogs and found that they could produce either result after hemorrhage;[119] the critical variable was the microvascular driving pressure. Perhaps this could explain the surprising and contradictory data on the effects of infused albumin on primate lungs after hemorrhage (discussed later). Staub has questioned the validity of some of the assumptions used in collecting pulmonary lymph in many of these studies, however.[244] Berman reported marked changes in permeability after extensive transfusion in rats, but this will be discussed later (p. 131).[22]

The earlier finding of Henry et al.[111] that hemorrhagic shock in dogs led to alterations in the metabolic patterns of pulmonary tissue has been confirmed in rats by measuring oxygen consumption by the pulmonary tissue itself with and without added glucose.[209] Other studies of pulmonary cellular function after hemorrhage have been less impressive.[220] This is a very interesting line of investigation that should be pursued further: What are the temporal sequences, how does treatment alter these changes, and how do the changes after hemorrhage compare with those after similar periods of ischemia without systemic hypotension?

The evidence relating hemorrhage to pulmonary dysfunction has not changed appreciably in recent years with the single exception just noted. With several contradictory experimental results remaining unexplained, it appears that severe hemorrhage does induce some deterioration of pulmonary structure and function but that this is not marked and is not progressive. The details of treatment may well have more to do with subsequent functional changes than the hemorrhage itself. How much this degree of damage facilitates the development of other pulmonary complications remains an important but unanswered question.

There are some aspects of severe hemorrhage in man that alter pulmonary function indirectly. Many, perhaps most, patients with repeated hematemesis aspirate significant amounts of blood. This is a prominent cause of posthemorrhagic pulmonary dysfunction, which is sometimes labeled "shock lung." Hemorrhagic shock in the elderly, whatever the cause, is more likely to damage the left ventricle because of the

increasing incidence of coronary arteriosclerosis with age. Thus, patients with ruptured abdominal aortic aneurysms show a high incidence of left ventricular dysfunction after operation.[271] Measurement of pulmonary arterial wedge pressures helps to define this population, as the central venous pressure may initially be deceptively normal. There is mounting evidence that left ventricular damage may be quite common after severe hemorrhage, even if the coronary vessels are normal.[11] This would contribute to the development of pulmonary edema directly and would reduce the safety margin for the administration of fluids. Based on experience with patients after myocardial infarctions, it is likely that some form of mechanical assistance to the left ventricle, such as intra-aortic balloon pumping, might help some of these patients through hazardous postoperative periods.

Resuscitation

There is an almost self-evident link between the treatment of hemorrhage and the subsequent development of pulmonary insufficiency. Defining this relationship in anything like precise terms, however, has proved to be unexpectedly difficult. There are several mechanisms whereby resuscitation might cause or facilitate the development of pulmonary insufficiency: damaging the lungs with the infused fluid (especially blood), overloading the circulation, or diluting the plasma-specific osmotic activity. Each of these mechanisms will be considered in turn, although there is considerable overlapping among them.

Massive Transfusion

Many heavily transfused patients develop pulmonary insufficiency. Some investigators believe there might be a causal relationship between transfusion and pulmonary insufficiency, and there are a number of reasons why this might be so. Perhaps the most likely is circulatory overloading leading to pulmonary edema. This is likely to occur when blood loss and transfusion occur rapidly, with rapid changes in blood volume, in patients with pre-existing cardiac disease, but it can also occur in younger patients. Such occurrences are not the result of the transfused blood itself.

Immunological reactions to certain protein fractions of transfused blood can cause pulmonary edema without circulatory overloading, but this is very unusual.[278] There is provocative older evidence that certain plasma proteins become altered during storage. Such changes may play a role in the pulmonary insufficiency that occurs after cardiopulmonary bypass when blood is used to prime the "pump."[185] It is not clear whether this can occur with the usual methods of transfusion. The plasticizer that leaches from the plastic bag into stored blood has been implicated in altered pulmonary capillary permeability in experimental animals,[22] but others have found no evidence of such alterations in other species.[161] Microembolization has received the most attention recently as a possible cause of post-transfusion pulmonary insufficiency. Microaggregates accumulate throughout the period of storage and easily pass through the standard transfusion filters. There are contradictory results on the subsequent development of pulmonary insufficiency from clinical studies on the effect of using fine filters during extensive transfusion.[202, 210, 264] Experimentally, the relationship can be demonstrated in dogs but not in primates.[157, 210, 257] Since stored blood is cold, acidotic and hyperkalemic, it might damage the pulmonary microcirculation if transfused rapidly directly into the right atrium.

Studies on civilian casualties using fine filters yielded contradictory results as noted. Studies on combat casualties in Vietnam on whether there was a relationship between transfusion and hypoxemia also yielded contradictory results. We reexamined this question using data on combat casualties studied by the first three U.S. Army Surgical Research Teams in Vietnam.[47] Data from nontransfused casualties are also included and indicate the degree of hypoxemia that occurs early in the postoperative period with various kinds of wounds (Table 6–3). As seen in the table, the location of the wound strongly affected the mean arterial oxygen tensions before

TABLE 6–3. Arterial Oxygen Tension Studies of Combat Casualties (Breathing Room Air)*

NUMBER OF TRANSFUSION UNITS (MEAN)	PRE	DAY 1	DAY 2	DAY 3
Peripheral injury				
Not transfused	83 (18) ±11	77 (18) ±15	80 (18) ±14	78 (6) ±12
1–5 (3.2)	87 (24) ±15	85 (24) ±13	84 (21) ±10	82 (11) ±12
6–10 (7.9)	88 (12) ±14	77 (12) ±11	80 (12) ±14	76 (7) ±6
>10 (24.5)	87 (18) ±18	75 (16) ±16	77 (17) ±17	80 (13) ±11
Abdominal injury				
Not transfused	81 (9) ±15	79 (8) ±18	78 (9) ±13	75 (4) ±18
1–5 (3.2)	86 (16) ±14	78 (16) ±15	78 (14) ±10	72 (12) ±11
6–10 (7.8)	85 (10) ±13	76 (10) ±17	81 (7) ±11	82 (9) ±13
>10 (25.2)	87 (10) ±8	76 (10) ±20	72 (10) ±20	72 (9) ±21
Thoracic injury				
Not transfused	72 (24) ±21	72 (24) ±14	77 (15) ±14	73 (16) ±16
1–5 (3)	70 (31) ±15	71 (26) ±17	70 (27) ±15	71 (26) ±16
6–10 (7.9)	71 (14) ±22	63 (14) ±13	64 (14) ±10	69 (13) ±13
>10 (21.4)	72 (13) ±16	59 (12) ±14	59 (12) ±17	65 (12) ±17

* Studied before and at least 2 of the first 3 postoperative days, according to type of injury and volume of blood transfused. From Collins et al.[47]

Mean ± SD (N).

and after wounding in these casualties. In the patients with peripheral injuries only, there was no relationship between transfusion and hypoxemia, and there was minimal hypoxemia even in patients receiving very large volumes of transfused blood. In patients with abdominal injuries, there was greater hypoxemia and a suggestive relationship to large volumes of transfusion. In patients with thoracic injuries there was clearly greater hypoxemia in the most heavily transfused patients and intermediate levels of hypoxemia in those receiving moderately large transfusions.

This pattern of findings can be interpreted either way. In those with thoracic injuries, there was an obvious relationship between transfusion and hypoxemia that was proportional to the extent of transfusion. As these patients were already hypoxemic from their injuries, it could be argued that the effects of transfusion alone were subliminal and therefore only appeared in the patients who were already hypoxemic from other causes. It seems unlikely, however, that such an effect could be so marked in the group with thoracic injuries and completely absent in those with peripheral injuries. We considered it more likely that both hypoxemia and transfusion were related to the degree of injury. In other words, they were coincidentally connected, not directly causally connected. The most heavily transfused patients had the most severe injuries. When the lungs were involved, this degree of injury was reflected in greater postoperative hypoxemia as well as the need for more blood in transfusion.

In this simple attempt to answer a seemingly simple question it became apparent that the system is far from simple. The "perfect" study, in fact, cannot be done because the most massively injured patients cannot now be treated without transfusions. An approach could be made if washed red cells and fresh frozen plasma were compared with stored blood. Some, but not all, of the potential causes of pulmonary insufficiency in transfused blood could thus be eliminated in one group. In the absence of such a study, we believe that the available evidence indicates that factors other than the blood used for transfusion contribute to the postresuscitative pulmonary insufficiency often seen in seriously injured, massively transfused patients. It would be a serious mistake indeed to delay or limit transfusion in a rapidly bleeding patient in the mistaken notion that more harm than good might result. More seriously injured patients die of the blood they don't receive than from the blood they do receive.

Fluid Overload and Plasma-Specific Osmotic Activity

Several recent publications review the mechanisms for maintaining an appropriate content and distribution of fluids in the lungs, the effects of alterations in plasma-oncotic pressure and in capillary hydrostatic pressure, and the impact of alterations in pulmonary capillary permeability.[27, 77, 208, 244] These articles can provide the physiological principles needed to understand what may be happening in some of the very complex clinical situations discussed in this section.

The "traditional wisdom" in treating hemorrhage has been that a greater than normal blood volume is required for adequate resuscitation from severe hypotension. Measurements of blood volume in apparently well-resuscitated, stable patients following severe hemorrhage, however, have almost always shown less than the predicted normal blood volumes for at least the first day, with (often) greater than normal blood volumes by the third day. This pattern has been very consistent in studies on severely injured combat casualties,[57, 58, 195] even when central venous pressure was included as a guide for fluid replacement.[234] Data in reports on postoperative civilian patients have often been obscured by the inclusion of septic patients, who usually require and develop blood volumes greater than normal. When data on hemorrhage alone can be extracted, however, a pattern similar to that reported in combat casualties is apparent,[274] again even when central venous pressure is included as a criterion for adequate replacement of blood loss.[30, 177, 275]

This pattern suggests that there may be a fixed contraction of the capacitance system (great veins) following severe blood loss.[7, 39] The classic study on the relationship of blood volume to central venous pressure showed no evidence of such a phenomenon but was performed on normal volunteers in the supine position who were bled less than 15 per cent of expected blood volume.[87] Simmons et al., in their study on combat casualties, looked especially at this possibility.[234] They found that the degree of "undertransfusion" despite clinical stability and normal central venous pressure was directly related to the amount of blood lost at injury. Of great interest is the fact that four of these casualties developed pulmonary edema when measured blood volumes were at predicted normal or less. It appears that the pulmonary artery may also participate in the loss of vascular compliance that occurs in the response to stress.[251] Earlier studies showing that blood volumes after resuscitation were less than normal were taken as evidence of clinical error in managing the patient. It may be that persistent contraction of the capacitance and pulmonary arterial systems, plus some impairment of left ventricular function, make the severely hemorrhaged patient much more susceptible to overtransfusion.

Although there is some disagreement on details, it is clear that overloading the circulation produces pulmonary edema by elevating capillary hydrostatic pressure. This form of edema is associated with a prominent leak of protein along with fluid. Dilution of plasma-specific osmotic pressure allows edema to form at lower hydrostatic pressures. Such edema usually begins in the pulmonary interstitial space but can extend to alveolar flooding with increased capillary permeability. The earliest practical way of detecting interstitial edema is probably through changes in compliance.[100, 254] Interstitial pulmonary edema clearly need not cause shunting,[46, 109] but if alveolar flooding occurs, shunting is inevitable. Even before alveolar flooding develops, the effects of interstitial edema on the closing of terminal airways could conceivably lead to atelectasis and shunting.[104]

The fact that excessive retention of salt and water results in pulmonary edema is neither new nor surprising. Fatal pulmonary edema can be produced by extensive infusions of salt water in animals with normal central venous pressures; clinical examples of the same phenomenon have been too common.[122] An important component of the clinical situation may be the ability of the patient to excrete the excess quantities of salt and water after resuscitation.[2, 98, 147]

The role of the concentration of albumin in plasma in the genesis of pulmonary edema and respiratory failure after resuscitation is one of the most controversial areas in the entire field of resuscitation from hemorrhage. There are at least two main opposing arguments: (1) plasma-specific osmotic pressure (colloid osmotic pressure, or COP) should be kept near normal during resuscitation to minimize the risk of pulmonary edema, and (2) abundant use of simple salt solutions without supplemental albumin ("crystalloid") poses no threat to pulmonary function. Recently, another provocative concept has been developed and offered—namely, that use of supplemental albumin may in fact increase the risk of postresuscitative pulmonary insufficiency.

The conservative position, favoring preservation of near normal COP, has firm theoretical and some experimental and clinical support. Ironically, the isolated, perfused lung has proved to be one of the easiest organs in which to demonstrate Starling's principles of fluid exchange across capillary membranes. Reducing the COP of the perfusate allows pulmonary edema to occur at lower perfusion pressures.[84, 102, 140] Adding albumin to the resuscitative regimen of primates treated for hemorrhagic shock minimized the amount of fluid that accumulated in the lungs, but there is disagreement on this point (see below, p. 135).[85] A similar study in dogs did not measure lung water content.[90] Another dealt with hemodilution with saline; accumulation of fluid in the lungs could be partly reversed by giving albumin.[48]

Evidence from clinical studies is confirmatory. Elective hemodilution preoperatively with salt solutions produced greater impairment of oxygenation than when colloid was used, but the studies were not simultaneous.[135] Giordano et al. and Skillman et al. reported improved oxygenation in patients on ventilatory support who were given albumin and diuretics.[91, 238] Patients on mechanical ventilators may retain fluids excessively, however. An earlier study showed significant improvement in pulmonary function in some injured patients from the use of diuretics alone.[79] I know of no such study in which patients were given albumin alone. Skillman et al. later reported a prospective, controlled study in which patients undergoing operations on the abdominal aorta were given salt water either alone or with supplemental albumin.[239] Those given the supplemental albumin had less impairment of oxygenation postoperatively. The patients were treated by a predetermined protocol, however, and not on the basis of clinical signs and measured pressures. In addition, the method for measuring oxygenation was one that is influenced by changes in mixed venous oxygen tension, which was not measured.

Rackow et al. and Weil et al. have reported findings that are very similar: COP correlates inversely with survival in patients in ventilatory failure and is very low in patients with noncardiogenic pulmonary edema.[199, 269] Chest roentgenograms were rated independently, and a correlation was found between low COP and radiologic evidence of pulmonary edema. Interestingly, measured intrapulmonary "shunt" did not correlate with COP or with the radiologic changes. All patients on ventilators with a COP of less than half normal died, while those with a COP of 75 per cent of normal or above survived. Other studies have indicated similar patterns.[2, 74, 91, 98, 101, 150, 237, 238] The trouble with many of these studies is that although they document concurrence, they don't necessarily indicate cause. It is likely that dying patients have a low COP from a variety of causes, including sequestration in infected areas, failure of synthesis and occasionally widespread loss of capillary integrity. What is needed is a controlled study showing that death can be prevented or ventilatory failure reversed by the administration of albumin. A "clean" study of this type has not yet been reported.

The argument that abundant salt solution can be administered without causing pulmonary edema has considerable experimental and clinical support. A large number of experimental studies document the efficacy of salt solutions in replacing up to half the expected blood volume in patients with acute hemorrhages.[46, 145] With greater hemorrhages, the need for red blood cells overrides the issue of the need to restore COP. If normal animals are deliberately overloaded with salt solutions, very large excesses are needed to produce pulmonary edema. A number of investigators are finding that it is very difficult to produce pulmonary edema in intact animals solely by lowering COP. Most of these studies have not yet been published. Even when COP is lowered and large amounts of salt water are infused, a surprisingly large amount of fluid can be sequestered in nonpulmonary sites, especially the skin, fat and muscle, thus protecting the lungs.[182]

The clinical evidence largely supports this position. To begin with, it is difficult to produce severely lower COP in previously healthy subjects. The study by the U.S. Navy Surgical Research Team in Vietnam demonstrated this point very well: There was little difference in total protein levels 24 hours after resuscitation in groups treated with or without supplemental albumin.[40] Recently, a number of prospective studies have compared albumin-rich and albumin-poor treatment regimens and have studied pulmonary function in detail. Lowe et al. found no differences between the two groups.[146] It is noteworthy, however, that the difference in total protein concentration between the two groups was rather small, as in the Navy study, and that the total protein (and presumably COP) in the nonalbumin group was not greatly depressed. It is also interesting that there was very little postresuscitative pulmonary insufficiency in either group in this study of 141 seriously injured patients. A similar prospective study by Virgilio et al. duplicated many of the conditions of the Skillman study but also calculated "shunt," which eliminated the effect of varying mixed venous oxygen tensions, and treated all patients according to vital signs and measured pressures.[265] Pulmonary capillary wedge pressure was monitored very closely. There were no differences between the two groups. COP was reduced below the level in the Lowe study but was still above half normal. In this study, even when pulmonary capillary wedge pressure exceeded COP, pulmonary edema was not evidence as long as the wedge pressure was not elevated. Weil's group has claimed this difference is critically important in avoiding pulmonary edema.[198] There are a number of similar studies now in press, but to the author's knowledge, all match this pattern except those noted below. These studies, if they can be summarized, showed little difference between patients treated with and those treated without supplemental albumin, but either COP was not drastically lowered or pulmonary capillary wedge pressures was very carefully monitored and kept well within normal ranges.

Finally, there is the interesting question of whether supplemental albumin might make a pulmonary lesion worse. Theoretically, if the capillary membrane becomes permeable to albumin, no effect on fluid exchange would be expected from administering albumin. In fact, the higher concentrations produced in the interstitial or intra-alveolar fluid might delay recovery, but this concept is unproven. Furthermore, the pulmonary interstitial fluid is normally relatively rich in albumin, so that there is a lower intravascular-extravascular gradient than in most organs studied. The pulmonary lymphatics seem to play an important role in protecting the lungs from becoming overloaded with fluid.[244] Early flooding of the interstitial space with protein-poor filtrate might lower the concentration of albumin in the interstitial fluid by a washout effect and thus be partly protective. Gump et al. and Smith et al. have documented that the lungs of surgical patients dying with ventilatory insufficiency have several times the normal amount of albumin, but clearly this represents advanced disease.[99, 242] Teplitz has suggested, on the basis of ultrastructural studies of patients dying with post-traumatic pulmonary insufficiency, that the capillary lesions are skip lesions, in which there are normal-appearing areas interspersed with areas of obvious damage.[253] If these normal areas are keeping the patient alive, they should be protected from pulmonary edema if possible. Furthermore, the real questions about the use of albumin arise early in the process of resuscitation, when there is little evidence of pulmonary vascular injury.

The possibility that a paradoxically harmful effect may occur from administering albumin during resuscitation is based almost entirely on experimental observations. Collins et al. found increased fluid in the lungs of rats treated for hemorrhage with plasma compared to those treated with simple electrolyte solutions.[46] These rats were treated by protocol, not by measured pressures, although rather small volumes of fluid were used by modern criteria. Plasma was used as the protein solution, and there is provocative older evidence that plasma components become denatured during storage and may be detrimental. Schloerb

et al. found more fluid in the lungs of rats when they were overloaded with albumin (human) than with salt solutions in equal volume, but this is what one would expect from the plasma volume-expanding properties of these fluids.[221] Holcroft and Trunkey and Moss et al. found increased early after resuscitation in the lungs of baboons treated for hemorrhage with protein solution compared to those treated with lactated Ringer's solution.[114, 115, 171] Both studies unfortunately used human protein. Moss recently reported that the ultrastructural changes occurring in baboon lungs were the same after resuscitation with baboon albumin as with human albumin, but the results of the full study are still being awaited.[29] Holcroft and Trunkey used human plasma protein fraction, in which about 15 per cent of the protein is alpha and beta globulin. These preparations contain variable and sometimes considerable levels of bradykinin. Recently these protein fractions have been associated in man, with cardiovascular collapse, which may be due to very high levels of prekallikrein activator.[10] This might trigger extensive activation of the kinin system in a "primed" recipient; hemorrhage might be such a prime. One hopes that future studies in valuable animals such as baboons will use species-specific albumin. As they now stand, the results are not clearly interpretable.

Most published and to-be-published clinical studies comparing albumin-supplemented with albumin-free regimens do *not* show increased pulmonary complications from the use of albumin, with one exception. Lucas et al. reported that injured patients treated with albumin had much greater dependency on mechanical ventilatory support than those treated with saline.[148] This study has several features that must be noted, however. Plasma volumes were nearly 10 per cent greater in the albumin-treated group, and both central venous pressures (15.4 vs. 8.4) and pulmonary capillary wedge pressures (11.2 vs. 5.5) were also significantly higher. The plasma albumin concentration in the "albumin-poor" group was 3 grams per 100 ml.; in the albumin-treated group it was 4.5 grams per 100 ml. Thus no group was notably hypoalbuminemic, and the treated group had remarkably high concentrations for seriously injured patients. All patients in fact received considerable amounts of albumin in blood and fresh frozen plasma; in addition, the "albumin" group apparently received 900 grams over the first 6 days! If anything, what this study shows is that it is possible to give too much albumin to an injured patient. This is not a facetious statement. There are states of congenital hypoalbuminemia and even analbuminemia, with reasonable duration of survival. To this author's knowledge, there are no documented instances of spontaneous, sustained hyperalbuminemia. As ·with many substances, albumin should be considered as potentially dangerous in excess. One of the interesting facets of the Lucas study, in fact, was the finding of impaired renal excretion of salt and water in these overloaded patients. There is growing experimental evidence indicating that the concentration of albumin in the plasma has an important effect on renal function. One of the built-in protections against fluid overload, in fact, may be a greater ease of renal excretion of excessive amounts of salt and water in the presence of acute dilutional hypoalbuminemia.

It is difficult to summarize such a controversial area. The evidence seems clear that a lower COP allows pulmonary edema to occur more easily but that without elevation of perfusion pressure, pulmonary edema is difficult to produce simply by lowering COP. A reasonable position seems to be that if one is going to lower COP during resuscitation, pulmonary perfusion pressure should be monitored and elevation of left atrial pressure should be avoided. There is currently no clinical evidence that adding albumin is harmful, except for one study in which excessive amounts of albumin and salt solutions apparently were used. In practical terms, there may well be a threshold COP above which little is gained by administering albumin, but below which there is increasing risk of pulmonary edema.[225] Some investigators estimate this threshold at a COP somewhat above half normal, or concentrations of albumin somewhere around 25 grams per liter. Even in patients with leaking pulmonary capillaries, the proper use of albumin remains obscure because of the possibility that the leaking may not be uniform throughout the pulmonary vascular bed. As noted before, the available experimental evidence indicates that use of salt solutions alone increased edema in areas of

pulmonary contusion, but there are not many studies on this point. The ability of the patient to excrete salt and water in the urine if needed can be an important variable.

TREATMENT AND OUTCOME

One of the highly beneficial advances in respiratory therapy in recent years has been the use of positive end expiratory pressure (PEEP). The exact mechanisms involved are debatable (increasing the functional residual capacity, preventing terminal expiratory closure of airways, forcing open collapsed airways, hydraulically driving fluid out of the interstitium back into the circulation, externally compressing the left ventricle, etc.), but in many sick patients moderate levels of PEEP allow adequate arterial oxygenation at lower levels of inspired concentration of oxygen.[110, 187, 193, 194] The degree of benefit obtained in injured patients may vary with the cause of the pulmonary insufficiency. PEEP may also hasten the resolution of pulmonary edema, although there is some contrary evidence on this point.

The use of PEEP brings with it several disadvantages, however. Pneumothorax is more likely to occur, even in the absence of prior mechanical injury to the lungs, and tension pneumothorax can develop very rapidly. With very high levels of PEEP, multiple episodes of pneumothorax are likely. It is almost certain that penetrating injuries of the lungs greatly increase the chances for developing pneumothorax or tension pneumothorax from even moderate levels of PEEP. PEEP decreases cardiac output, especially at high levels of PEEP. This effect is pronounced if the patient is also hypovolemic;[282] it was thought to be due to impaired venous return and/or compression of the pulmonary vasculature, but there is recent evidence of depressed myocardial contractility, which may be mediated by something released from the stretched or compressed pulmonary parenchyma.[153] Whatever the cause, PEEP can be dangerous in patients with hypovolemia. In patients with head injury, PEEP may increase intracranial pressure, decrease cerebral perfusion, and perhaps contribute to neurological deterioration.[228] If monitoring of intracranial pressure is not available, PEEP must be used very cautiously in patients with significant head injuries. High levels of PEEP may paradoxically increase pulmonary interstitial edema, at least in experimental models.[258] PEEP can also cause pulmonary capillary wedge pressure measurements to deviate significantly from left atrial measurements. This is particularly unfortunate because the avoidance of hypovolemia is very important if more than minimal levels of PEEP are used, although this effect may be practically important only at high levels of PEEP.[52]

Because of the adverse cardiovascular effects that may occur, frequent measurements of cardiac output may be necessary to manage some patients properly. The development of thermal dilutional methods of measuring cardiac output has made possible frequent measurements by specially trained nursing personnel and has improved the care of these patients. If the method is not available or the proper catheter has not been inserted, serial measurements of mixed venous pO_2 can be quite helpful. A declining mixed venous pO_2, especially if below 35 mm. Hg, indicates insufficient supply of oxygen to the body cell mass. If this decline has occurred during a period when PEEP has been increased but all other variables seem stable, there is a strong implication that the higher levels of PEEP have impaired oxygen delivery by impairing cardiac output. This may even occur in the presence of a rising arterial pO_2. In such circumstances, the mixed pO_2 is a far better indicator of the adequacy of oxygen delivery. A lower arterial pO_2, if accomplished by lowering PEEP and if accompanied by improved perfusion, may be associated with better oxygenation of the patient. Mixed venous pO_2 can be a valuable monitoring device during unstable periods in patients with complex disorders of oxygen delivery. It is probably not used often enough.

Despite the potential disadvantages of PEEP, it is used very extensively in the management of patients with post-traumatic pulmonary insufficiency. It has significantly improved the care of many such patients and has probably tipped the balance in favor of survival in a significant number. Nevertheless, it must be used with caution and awareness of the potential problems. Hypovolemia, significant head injury and penetrating wounds of the lung are conditions that particularly mandate great caution in the use of PEEP in injured patients.

The optimal level of PEEP varies in different patients and at different times in the same patient.[250] Tidal volume also alters the effect of PEEP on compliance.[248] Very high levels are sometimes necessary and produce surprisingly good long-term results.[59, 61] Several methods are used to determine the optimal level of PEEP. One can vary PEEP over a reasonable range, 5 to 15 or 20 cm. water, and measure arterial blood gases after 15 to 20 minutes at each level. The value that gives the highest arterial pO_2 or the lowest pressure that gives an equivalent pO_2 is chosen. As discussed above, either cardiac output or mixed venous pO_2 should also be measured to be sure that oxygen delivery is being improved along with arterial pO_2. Another method is to measure static compliance at different levels of PEEP and choose the level that yields the highest compliance, on the assumption that this will also yield the best oxygenation.[250] This assumption may not always be correct, however.[252] The best approach is one of cautious use of a potentially beneficial but also potentially harmful method of treatment. The lowest level that allows adequate oxygenation at concentrations of inspired oxygen of 50 per cent or less is probably best. Levels above 10 cm. water require care in selection and very close monitoring of the patient. Continuous positive airway pressure may produce some of the same beneficial effects with fewer risks[222] but is appropriate only for less seriously ill patients, and if pressures are raised sufficiently, cardiac output may not only decline but also the patient may rapidly become fatigued.[270]

The process of discontinuing mechanical ventilatory assistance is a demonstrably stressful one for the patient.[127] There are many published criteria, ranging from simple to elaborate, on which decisions of how and when to discontinue mechanical ventilatory support can be based; some of the important principles are: individualize for each patient, follow the patiently closely and well beyond the first few apparently successful hours, consider the work required of the patient in relation to the work that he can sustain, and err on the side of continuing ventilatory support if there is real doubt. Unsuccessful attempts at discontinuation seem to prolong subsequent disability, but this is obviously a very difficult thing to prove.

Intermittent mandatory ventilation (IMV) is a technological device that allows the patient to remain attached to the ventilator and spontaneously breathe the specific ventilator-blended inspiratory mixture, with continuous positive expiratory pressure if desired, yet the machine will deliver predetermined volumes of inspiratory gas at chosen intervals, typically a few times per minute.[62] The result can be a gradual decrease in the work performed by the machine and a concomitant increase in the work performed by the patient, while retaining the safety of mechanical support sufficient to preserve life if the patient fails while no one is observing. In addition, the periodic breaths of air delivered by the machine minimize the atelectasis that often occurs in patients who breathe rapidly and shallowly after coming off ventilatory support. IMV is a relatively simple concept and is delivered by relatively inexpensive modifications of existing ventilators, but it has almost certainly significantly reduced the hazards of discontinuing ventilatory support.

Other technical advances in ventilators in recent years have also greatly improved the care of patients in ventilatory failure. Reliable control of the concentration of oxygen over a continuous range, ability to control inspiratory and expiratory pressures, durations and flow rates, better humidification, more reliable mechanical operation, improved alarm systems, built-in spirometers and pressure gauges continuously displaying the important data are examples of advances that have become generally available in the last 10 years. More important than the machines, however, have been the improvements that have occurred in organization, nursing care and education of physicians. Most such patients are now cared for in specially designated units with specially trained personnel in a high nurse/patient ratio, with expert advice quickly available.

Monitoring of pulmonary capillary wedge pressure has a definite role in managing some patients in or at high risk of developing ventilatory failure. There are surgical patients in whom there is a significant and important difference between wedge pressure and central venous pressure.[37, 204, 271] Serious mistakes in management can be made by relying on the latter.

It is also true, however, that most patients being treated for hypovolemia do not require the added risk or the added expense of such monitoring. Unstable circulation, very extensive hemorrhage and blood replacement, failure to respond as expected, known or suspected left ventricular dysfunction, unexplained worsening pulmonary insufficiency, and COP near or below half normal are some of the situations in which measuring and monitoring wedge pressures may well be necessary for proper management of the injured patient.

Percutaneous on-line monitoring of pO_2 is being attempted with specially designed electrode devices. In some circumstances these seem to work very well. If clinical trials indicate that they are accurate, speedy, and practical, such devices could greatly improve the monitoring of the patient in pulmonary insufficiency. Unfortunately, they are very expensive in their current form.

There is some disagreement on the long-term outlook for patients who develop severe post-traumatic pulmonary insufficiency. Studies on autopsy material indicate that fibrosis and vascular obliteration may be prominent features of the disease. Studies on survivors up to one year later, however, indicate surprisingly little persistent functional pulmonary impairment.[59, 61, 132, 136, 279] These differences may well reflect fundamental differences between survivors and nonsurvivors. As indicated earlier, however, death from post-traumatic pulmonary insufficiency has become unusual. A defeatist attitude is certainly not warranted in this disease. Some believe the incidence of it is decreasing.[266] There are no provable causes for this, but greater care and sophistication in the use of resuscitative fluids, better awareness of the disease and better monitoring for early detection, and perhaps earlier use of ventilatory support have probably helped.

REFERENCES

1. Aarseth, P., Karlsen, J., and Bo, G.: Effects of catecholamine-infusions and hypoxia on pulmonary blood volume and extravascular lung water content in cats. Acta Physiol. Scand., 95:34–40, 1975.
2. Abrams, J. S., Deane, R. S., and Davis, J. H.: Adverse effects of salt and water retention on pulmonary function in patients with

multiple trauma. J. Trauma, 13:788–798, 1973.

3. Abrams, J. S., Deane, R. S., and Davis, J. H.: Pulmonary function in patients with multiple trauma and associated severe head injury. J. Trauma, 16:543–549, 1976.

4. Agee, R. N., Long, J. M., Hunt, J. L., Petroff, P. A., Lull, F. J., Mason, A. D., and Pruitt, B. A.: Use of ¹³³ xenon in the early diagnosis of inhalation injury. J. Trauma, 16:218–224, 1976.

5. Aldrete, J. A., Liem, S. T., and Carrow, D. J.: Pulmonary aerobic bacterial flora after aspiration pneumonitis. J. Trauma, 15:1014–1020, 1975.

6. Alexander, J. I., Horton, P. W., Millar, W. T., Parikh, R. K., and Spence, A. A.: The effect of upper abdominal surgery on the relationship of airway closing point to end tidal position. Clin. Sci., 43:137–141, 1972.

7. Alexander, R. S.: Venomotor tone in hemorrhage and shock. Circ. Res., 3:181–190, 1955.

8. Ali, J., Weisel, R. D., Layung, A. B., Kripke, B. J., and Hechtman, H. B.: Consequences of postoperative alterations in respiratory mechanics. Am. J. Surg., 128:376–382, 1974.

9. Altschule, M. D.: The significance of changes in the lung volume and its subdivisions during and after abdominal operation. Anesthesiology, 4:385–391, 1943.

10. Alving, B. M., Hojima, Y., Pisano, J. J., Mason, B. L., Buckingham, R. E., Mozen, M. M., and Finlayson, J. S.: Hypotension and Hageman-factor fragments in plasma protein fraction. N. Engl. J. Med., 299:66–70, 1978.

11. Alyono, D., Ring, W. S., and Anderson, R. W.: The effects of hemorrhagic shock on the diastolic properties of the left ventricle in the conscious dog. Surgery, 83:691–698, 1979.

12. Anderson, R. W., and De Vries, W. C.: Transvascular fluid and protein dynamics in the lung following hemorrhagic shock. J. Surg. Res., 20:281–290, 1976.

13. Ashbaugh, D. G., and Petty, T. L.: Sepsis complicating the acute respiratory distress syndrome. Surg. Gynec. Obstet., 135:865–869, 1972.

14. Avery, E. E., Mörch, E. T., and Benson, D. W.: Critically crushed chests: A new method of treatment with continuous mechanical hyperventilation to produce alkalotic apnea and internal pneumatic stabilization. J. Thorac. Surg., 33:291–311, 1956.

15. Babington, P. C., Baker, A. B., and Johnston, H. H.: Retrograde spread of organisms from ventilator to patient via the expiratory limb. Lancet, 1:61–62, 1971.

16. Bartlett, J. G., and Gorbach, S. L.: The triple threat of aspiration pneumonia. Chest, 68:560–566, 1975.

17. Bartlett, J. G., Gorbach, S. L., and Finegold, S. M.: The bacteriology of aspiration pneumonia. Am. J. Med., 56:202–207, 1974.

18. Bartlett, R. H., Brennan, M. L., Gazzaniga, A. B., and Hanson, E. L.: Studies on the pathogenesis and prevention of postoperative pulmonary complications. Surg. Gynec., Obstet., 137:925–933, 1973.

19. Beck, J. P., and Collins, J. A.: Theoretical and clinical aspects of post-traumatic fat embolism syndrome. American Academy of Orthopedic Surgeons, Instructional Course Lectures, 22:38–87, 1973.

20. Berk, J. L., Hagen, J. F., Koo, R., and Maly, G.: Pulmonary insufficiency produced by isoproterenol. Surg. Gynec. Obstet., 143:725–726, 1976.

21. Berman, I. R., and Ducker, T. B.: Pulmonary, somatic and splanchnic circulatory responses to increased intracranial pressure. Ann. Surg., 169:210–216, 1969.

22. Berman, I. R., Iliescu, H., and Stachura, I.: Pulmonary effects of blood container materials. Surg. Forum, 28:182, 1977.

23. Blaisdell, F. W.: Pathophysiology of the respiratory distress syndrome. Arch. Sug., 108:44–49, 1974.

24. Blaisdell, F. W., and Schlobohm, R. M.: The respiratory distress syndrome: A review. Surgery, 74:251–262, 1973.

25. Blumenstock, D. A., Hechtman, H. B., and Collins, J. A.: Preservation of the canine lung. J. Thorac. Cardiovasc. Surg., 44:771–775, 1962.

26. Booth, D. J., Zuidema, G. D., and Cameron, J. L.: Aspiration penumonia: Pulmonary arteriography after experimental aspiration. J. Surg. Res., 12:48–52, 1972.

27. Bredenberg, C. E.: Acute respiratory distress. Surg. Clin. North Am., 54:1043–1066, 1974.

28. Brigham, K. L., Woolverton, W. C., Blake, L. H., and Staub, N. C.: Increased sheep lung permeability caused by Pseudomonas bacteremia. J. Clin. Invest., 54:792–804, 1974.

29. Brinkman, R., Moss, G. S., Sehgal, L., Newson, R., and Da Gupta, T. K.: Effects of infusion of human vs. baboon serum albumin on pulmonary interstitium. Surg. Forum, 27:180–182, 1976.

30. Brisman, R., Parks, L. C., and Benson, D. W.: Pitfalls in the clinical use of central venous pressure. Arch. Surg., 95:902–907, 1967.

31. Campbell, G. S.: Respiratory failure in surgical patients. Curr. Probl. Surg., 13:1–67, 1976.

32. Cameron, J. L., Mitchell, W. II., and Zuidema, G. D.: Aspiration pneumonia: Clinical outcome following documented aspiration. Arch. Surg., 106:49–52, 1973.

33. Cameron, J. L., Sebar, J., Anderson, R. P., and Zuidema, G. D.: Aspiration pneumonia: Results of treatment by positive pressure ventilation in dogs. J. Surg. Res., 8:447–457, 1968.

34. Chapman, R. L., Downs, J. B., Modell, J. II., and Hood, C. I.: The ineffectiveness of steroid therapy in treating aspiration of hydrochloric acid. Arch. Surg., 108:858–861, 1974.

35. Chen, H. I., Sun, S. C., and Chai, C. Y.: Pulmonary edema and hemorrhage resulting from cerebral compression. Am. J. Physiol., 224:223–229, 1973.

36. Churchill, E. D., and McNeil, D.: The reduction in vital capacity following operation. Surg. Gynec. Obstet., 44:483–488, 1927.

37. Civetta, J. M., and Gabel, J. C.: "Pseudocardiogenic" pulmonary edema. J. Trauma, 15:143–149, 1975.

38. Clark, J. M., and Lambertsen, C. J.: Pulmonary

oxygen toxicity: a review. Pharmacol. Rev. 23:37–133, 1971.

39. Cleland, J., Pluth, J. R., Tauxe, W. N., and Kirklin, J. W.: Blood volumes and body fluid compartment changes soon after closed and open intracardiac surgery. J. Thorac. Cardiovasc. Surg., 52:698–705, 1966.

40. Cloutier, C. T., Lowery, B. D., and Carey, L. C.: The effect of hemodilutional resuscitation on serum protein levels in hemorrhagic shock. J. Trauma, 9:514–521, 1969.

41. Clowes, G. H.: Pulmonary abnormalities in sepsis. Surg. Clin. North Am., 54:993–1013, 1974.

42. Clowes, G. H., Hirsch, E., Williams, L., Kwasnik, E., O'Donnell, T. F., Cuevas, P., Sani, V. K., Moradi, I., Farizan, M., Sarovis, C., Stone, M., and Kuffler, J.: Septic lung and shock lung in man. Ann. Surg., 181:681–692, 1975.

43. Cohen, A. B., and Cline, M. J.: Human alveolar macrophage isolation, cultivation and morphological and functional characteristics. J. Clin. Invest., 50:1390–1398, 1971.

44. Collins, J. A.: The causes of progressive pulmonary insufficiency in surgical patients. J. Surg. Res., 9:685–704, 1969.

45. Collins, J. A.: The acute respiratory distress syndrome. Adv. Surgery, 11:171–225, 1977.

46. Collins, J. A., Braitberg, A., and Butcher, H. R.: Changes in lung and body weight and lung water content in rats treated for hemorrhage with various fluids. Surgery, 73:401–411, 1973.

47. Collins, J. A., James, P. M., Bredenberg, C. E., Anderson, R. W., Heisterkamp, C. A., and Simmons, R. L.: The relationship between transfusion and hypoxemia in combat casualties. Ann. Surg., 188:513–520, 1978.

48. Cooper, J. D., Marder, M., and Lowenstein, E.: Lung water accumulation with acute hemodilution in dogs. J. Thorac. Cardiovasc. Surg., 69:957–965, 1975.

49. Crockard, H. A., Clark, J., Warnock, M. L., Chung, A. M., and Hanlon, K.: The significance of pulmonary changes associated with cerebral perfusion with hypoxic blood in monkeys. Surgery, 82:588–598, 1977.

50. Dalen, J. E., Banas, J. S., Brooks, H. L., Evans, G. L., Paraskos, J. A., and Dexter, L.: Resolution rate of acute pulmonary embolism in man. N. Engl. J. Med., 280:1194–1199, 1969.

51. Dalrymple, D. G., Panbrook, G. D., and Steel, D. F.: Factors predisposing to postoperative pain and pulmonary complications. Br. J. Anaesthesiol., 45:589–598, 1973.

52. Davison, R., Parker, M., and Harrison, R. A.: The validity of determinations of pulmonary wedge pressure during mechanical ventilation. Chest, 73:352–355, 1978.

53. Demling, R. H., Selinger, S. L., Bland, R. D., and Staub, N. S.: Effect of acute hemorrhagic shock on pulmonary microvascular fluid filtration and protein permeability in sheep. Surgery, 77:512–519, 1975.

54. Demling, R. H., Will, J. A., and Belzer, F. O.: Effect of major thermal injury on the pulmonary microcirculation. Surgery, 83:746–751, 1978.

55. Dockel, R. C., Zwilbich, C. W., Scoggin, C. H., Kryger, M., and Weil, J. V.: Clinical semistarvation: Depression of hypoxia ventilatory response. N. Engl. J. Med., 295:358–361, 1976.

56. Dohi, S., and Gold, M. I.: Comparison of two methods of postoperative respiratory care. Chest, 73:592–595, 1978.

57. Doty, D. B., Hulfnagel, H. V., and Moseley, R. V.: The distribution of body fluids following hemorrhage and resuscitation in combat casualties. Surg. Gynec. Obstet., 130:453–458, 1970.

58. Doty, D. B., Moseley, R. V., and Simmons, R. L.: Sequential changes in blood volume after injury and transfusion. Surg. Gynec. Obstet., 130:801–805, 1970.

59. Douglas, M. E., and Downs, J. B.: Pulmonary function following severe acute respiratory failure and high levels of positive end-expiratory pressure. Chest, 71:18–23, 1977.

60. Douglas, M. E., Downs, J. B., Dannemiller, F. J., and Hodges, M. R.: Acute respiratory failure and intravascular coagulation. Surg. Gynec. Obstet., 143:555–560, 1976.

61. Downs, J. B., and Olsen, G. N.: Pulmonary function following adult respiratory distress syndrome. Chest, 65:92–23, 1974.

62. Downs, J. B., Perkins, H. M., and Modell, J. H.: Intermittent mandatory ventilation: An evaluation. Arch. Surg., 109:519–523, 1974.

63. Dressler, D. P., and Skornik, W. A.: Pulmonary bacterial susceptibility in the burned rat. Ann. Surg., 180:221–227, 1974.

64. Dressler, D. P., Skornik, W. A., and Kupersmith, S.: Corticosteroid treatment of experimental smoke inhalation. Ann. Surg., 183:46–52, 1976.

65. Droste, P. L., and Beckman, D. L.: Pulmonary effects of prolonged sympathetic stimulation. Proc. Soc. Exp. Biol. Med., 146:352–353, 1974.

66. Ducker, T. B.: Increased intra-cranial pressure and pulmonary edema. 1. Clinical study of eleven patients. J. Neurosurg., 28:112–117, 1968.

67. Ducker, T. B., Simmons, R. L., and Anderson, R. W.: Increased intracranial pressure and pulmonary edema. III. The effect of increased intracranial pressure on the cardiovascular hemodynamics of chimpanzees. J. Neurosurg., 29:475–483, 1968.

68. Dudley, W. R., and Marshall, B. E.: Steroid treatment for acid-aspiration pneumonitis. Anesthesiology, 40:136–141, 1974.

69. Dyer, E. D., and Peterson, D. E.: How far do bacteria travel from the exhalation valve of IPPB equipment? Anesthesiol. Analges., 51:516–519, 1972.

70. Ebert, P. A.: Physiologic principles in the management of the crushed-chest syndrome. Monographs Surg. Sci., 4:69–94, 1967.

71. Eeles, G. H., and Sevitt, S.: Microthrombosis in injured and burned patients. J. Pathol. Bact., 93:275–293, 1967.

72. Esrig, B. C., and Fulton, F. L.: Sepsis, resuscitation, hemorrhagic shock and "schock lung": An experimental correlation. Ann. Surg., 182:218–227, 1975.

73. Feeley, T. W., du Moulin, G. C., Hedley-Whyte, J., Bushnell, L. S., Gilbert, J. P., and Feingold, D. S.: Aerosol polymyxin and pneumonia in seriously ill patients. N. Engl. J. Med., 293:471–475, 1975.

74. Finley, R. J., Holliday, R. L., Lefcoe, M., and Duff, J. H.: Pulmonary edema in patients with sepsis. Surg. Gynec. Obstet., 140:851–857, 1975.

75. Fischer, P., Millen, J. E., and Glauser, F. L.: The pulmonary alveolar capillary membrane during hemorrhagic hypotension in dogs. Surg. Synec. Obstet., 146:383–386, 1978.

76. Fischer, R. F., Geiger, J. P., and Guernsey, J. M.: Pulmonary resections for severe pulmonary contusions secondary to high-velocity missile wounds. J. Trauma, 14:293–302, 1974.

77. Fishman, A. P.: Pulmonary edema: The water-exchanging function of the lung. Circulation, 46:390–408, 1972.

78. Fishman, A. P., and Pietra, G. P.: Handling of bioactive materials by the lung. N. Engl. J. Med., 291:884–890, 953–959, 1974.

79. Fleming, W. H., and Bowen, J. C.: The use of diuretics in the treatment of early wet lung syndrome. Ann. Surg., 175:505–509, 1972.

80. Flint, L., Gosdin, G., and Carrico, C. J.: Evaluation of ventilatory therapy for acid aspiration. Surgery, 78:492–498, 1975.

81. Fonkalsrud, E. W., Sanchez, M., Higashyima, I., and Arima, E.: A comparative study of the effects of dry vs. humidified ventilation on canine lungs. Surgery, 78:373–380, 1975.

82. Fratantoni, J. C., Ness, P., and Simon T. L.: Thrombolytic therapy: Current status. N. Engl. J. Med., 293:1073–1078, 1975.

83. Fulton, R. L., and Peter, E. T.: Compositional and histologic effects of fluid therapy following pulmonary contusion. J. Trauma, 14:783–790, 1974.

84. Gaar, K. A. J., Taylor, A. E., and Owens, L. J.: Effect of capillary pressure and plasma protein on development of pulmonary edema. Am. J. Physiol., 213:79–82, 1967.

85. Gaisford, W. D., Pandey, N., and Jensen, C. G.: Pulmonary changes in treated hemorrhagic shock. II. Ringer's lactate solution versus colloid infusion. Am. J. Surg., 124:738–743, 1972.

86. Garzon, A. A., Seltzer, B., and Karlson, K. E.: Physiopathology of crushed chest injuries. Ann. Surg., 168:128–136, 1968.

87. Gauer, D. H., Henry, J. P., and Sieker, H. O.: Changes in central venous pressure after moderate hemorrhage and transfusion in man. Circ. Res., 4:79–84, 1956.

88. Gibbons, J., James, O., and Quail, A.: Management of 130 cases of chest injury with respiratory failure. Br. J. Anaesthesiol., 45:1130–1135, 1973.

89. Gillis, C. N.: Metabolism of vasoactive hormones by lung. Anesthesiology, 39:626–632, 1973.

90. Giordano, J. M., Campbell, D. A., and Joseph, W. L.: The effect of intravenously administered albumin on dogs with pulmonary interstitial edema. Surg. Gynec. Obstet., 137:593–596, 1973.

91. Giordano, J. M., Joseph, W. L., Klingemaier, C. H., and Adkins, P. C.: The management of interstitial pulmonary edema. Significance of hypoproteinemia. J. Thorac. Cardiovasc. Surg., 64:739–746, 1972.

92. Glover, J. L., and Jolly, L.: Gram-negative colonization of the respiratory tract in postoperative patients. Am. J. Med. Sci., 261:24–26, 1971.

93. Goldring, R. M., Cannon, P. J., Heinemann, H. O., and Fishman, A. P.: Respiratory adjustment to chronic metabolic alkalosis in man. J. Clin. Invest., 47:188–202, 1968.

94. Green, G. M., and Kass, E. H.: Factors influencing the clearance of bacteria in the lung. J. Clin. Invest., 43:766–769, 1964.

95. Greenfield, L. J., McCurdy, J. R., Brown, P. P., and Elkins, R. C.: A new intracaval filter permitting continued flow and resolution of emboli. Surgery, 73:599–606, 1973.

96. Greenfield, S., Teres, D., Bushnell, L. S., Hedley-Whyte, J., and Feingold, D. S.: Prevention of gram-negative bacillary pneumonia using aerosol polymixin as prophylaxis. I. Effect on colonization pattern of the upper respiratory tract of seriously ill patients. J. Clin. Invest., 52:2935–2940, 1973.

97. Grieble, H. G., Colton, F. R., Bird, T. J., Toigo, A., and Griffith, L. G.: Fine-particle humidifiers: Source of *Pseudomonas aeruginosa* infections in a respiratory-disease unit. N. Engl. J. Med., 282:531–534, 1970.

98. Gump, F. E., Kinney, J. M., Iles, M., and Long, C. G.: Duration and significance of large fluid loads administered for circulatory support. J. Trauma, 10:431–439, 1970.

99. Gump, F. E., Mashima, Y., Ferenczy, A., and Kinney, J. M.: Pre- and postmortem studies of lung fluids and electrolytes. J. Trauma, 11:474–482, 1971.

100. Gump, F. E., Zikria, B. A., and Mashima, Y.: The effect of interstitial edema on pulmonary function in the dog. J. Trauma, 12:764–770, 1972.

101. Gutierrez, V. S., Berman, I. R., Soloway, H. B., and Hamit, H. F.: Relationship of hypoproteinemia and prolonged mechanical ventilation to the development of pulmonary insufficiency in shock. Ann. Surg., 171:385–393, 1970.

102. Guyton, A. C., and Lindsay, A. W.: Effect of elevated left atrial pressure and decreased plasma protein concentration on the development of pulmonary edema. Circ. Res., 7:649–657, 1959.

103. Hardaway, R. M.: Disseminated intravascular coagulation as a possible cause of acute respiratory failure. Surg. Gynec. Obstet., 137:419–423, 1973.

104. Harken, A. H., and O'Connor, N. E.: The influence of clinically undetectable pulmonary edema on small airway closure in the dog. Ann. Sug., 184:183–188, 1976.

105. Harris, T. H., Ramon, T. K., Richards, W. J., Covert, S. V., Blake, J. A., and Accurso, J.: An evaluation of bacteriologic contamination of ventilator humidifying systems. Chest, 63:922–925, 1973.

106. Haugaard, N.: Cellular mechanisms of oxygen toxicity. Physiol. Rev., 48:311–373, 1968.

107. Hechtman, H. B., Lonergan, E. A., and Shepro, D.: Platelet and leukocyte lung interactions in patients with respiratory failure. Surgery, 83:155–163, 1978.

108. Hechtman, H. B., Lonergan, E. A., Staunton, P. B., Dennis, R. C., and Shepro, D.: Pulmonary entrapment of platelets during acute respiratory failure. Surgery, 83:277–283, 1978.

109. Hechtman, H. E., Weisel, R. D., Vito, L., Ali, J., and Berger, R. L.: The independence of pulmonary shunting and pulmonary edema. Surgery, 74:300–306, 1973.

110. Hedley-Whyte, J., Burgess, G. E., Feeley, T. W., and Miller, M. G.: Applied Physiology of Respiratory Care. Boston, Little, Brown and Company, 1976.

111. Henry, J. N., McArdle, A. H., Buonous, G., Hampson, L. G., Scott, H. J., and Gurd, F. N.: The effect of experimental hemorrhagic shock on pulmonary alveolar surfactant. J. Trauma, 7:691–726, 1967.

112. Hill, J. D., Ratliff, J. C., and Parrott, J. C.: Pulmonary pathology in acute respiratory insufficiency: Lung biopsy as a diagnostic tool. J. Thorac. Cardiovasc. Surg., 71:64–71, 1976.

113. Hoie, J., and Schenk, W. G.: Pulmonary hemodynamics and function in acute experimental disseminated intravascular coagulation. J. Trauma, 13:887–894, 1973.

114. Holcroft, J. W., and Trunkey, D. D.: Extravascular lung water following hemorrhagic shock in the baboon: Comparison between resuscitation with Ringer's lactate and plasmanate. Ann. Surg., 180:408–417, 1974.

115. Holcroft, J. W., Trunkey, D. D., and Lim, R. C.: Further analysis of lung water in baboons resuscitated from hemorrhagic shock. J. Surg. Res., 20:291–297, 1976.

116. Horovitz, J. H., and Carrico, C. J.: Lung colloid permeability in hemorrhagic shock. Surg. Foru, 23:6–7, 1972.

117. Howell, J. F., Crawford, E. S., and Jordan, G. L.: The flail chest: An analysis of 100 patients. Am. J. Surg., 106:628–635, 1963.

118. Hunt, J. L., Agee, R. N., and Pruitt, B. A.: Fiberoptic Bronchoscopy in acute inhalation injury. J. Trauma, 15:641–649, 1975.

119. Iannini, P. B., Claffey, T., and Quintiliani, R.: Bacteremic Pseudomonas pneumonia. J. A. M. A., 230:558–561, 1974.

120. Johanson, W. G., Pierce, A. K., and Sanford, J. P.: Changing pharyngeal bacterial flora of hospitalized patients. N. Eng. J. Med., 281:1137–1140, 1969.

121. Johanson, W. G., Pierce, A. K., Sanford, J. P., and Thomas, G. D.: Nosocomial respiratory infections with gram-negative bacilli: The significance of colonization of the respiratory tract. Ann. Intern. Med., 77:701–714, 1972.

122. Johnson, G., and Lambert, J.: Responses to the rapid intravenous administration of an overload of fluid and electrolytes in dogs. Ann. Surg., 167:561–567, 1965.

123. Josephson, S., Swedenborg, J., and Dahlgren, S. E.: Delayed lung lesion in dogs after thrombin-induced disseminated intravascular coagulation. Acta Chir. Scand., 140:431–435, 1974.

124. Kakkar, V. V.: Prevention of fatal postoperative pulmonary embolism by low doses of heparin: An international multicentre trial. Lancet, 2:45–51, 1975.

125. Kakkar, V. V., Howe, C. T., Nicolaides, A. N., Renney, J. T., and Clarke, M. B.: Deep vein thrombosis — is there a "high risk" group? Am. J. Surg., 120:527–530, 1970.

126. Kasajima, K., Wax, S. D., and Webb, W. W.: Cerebral hypotension and shock lung syndrome. J. Thorac. Cardiovasc. Surg., 67:969–975, 1974.

127. Kennedy, S. K., Weintraub, R. M., and Skillman, J. J.: Cardiorespiratory and sympathoadrenal responses during weaning from controlled ventilation. Surgery, 82:233–240, 1977.

128. Khanam, T., Branthwaite, M. A., English, I. C., and Preutis, J. J.: The control of pulmonary sepsis in intensive therapy units. Anaesthesiology, 28:17–28, 1973.

129. Kim, S. I., Desai, J. M., and Shoemaker, W. C.: Sequential respiratory changes in an experimental hemorrhagic shock preparation designed to simulate clinical shock. Ann. Surg., 170:166–173, 1969.

130. Kim, S. I., and Shoemaker, W. C.: Role of the acidosis in the development of increased pulmonary vascular resistance and shock lung in experimental hemorrhagic shock. Surgery, 73:723–729, 1973.

131. Klastersky, J., Hensgens, C., Noterman, J., Mouawad, E., and Meunier-Carpentier, F.: Endotracheal antibiotics for the prevention of tracheobronchial infections in tracheotomized unconscious patients: A comparative study of gentamicin and aminosidin-polymyxin B combination. Chest, 68:302–306, 1975.

132. Klein, J. J., van Haeringen, J. R., Sluiter, H. J., Holloway, R., and Peset, R.: Pulmonary function after recovery from the adult respiratory distress syndrome. Chest, 69:350–354, 1976.

133. Klick, J. M., du Moulin, G. C., Hedley-Whyte, J., Teres, D., Bushnell, L. S., and Feingold, D. S.: Prevention of gram-negative bacillary pneumonia using polymixin aerosol as prophylaxis. II. Effect on the incidence of pneumonia in seriously ill patients. J. Clin. Invest., 55:514–519, 1975.

134. Kux, M., Coalson, J. J., Massion, W. H., and Guenter, C. A.: Pulmonary effects of E. coli endotoxin: Role of leukocytes and platelets. Ann. Surg., 175:26–34, 1972.

135. Laks, H., O'Connor, N. E., Anderson, W., and Pilon, R. N.: Crystalloid versus colloid hemodilution in man. Surg. Gynec. Obstet., 142:506–512, 1976.

136. Lakshiminarayan, S., Stanford, R. E., and Petty, T. L.: Prognosis after recovery from adult respiratory distress syndrome. Am. Rev. Resp. Dis., 113:7–16, 1976.

137. Laterman, A., Manwaring, D., and Curreri, P. W.: The role of fibrinogen degradation products in the pathogenesis of the respiratory distress syndrome. Surgery, 82:703–709, 1977.

138. Latimer, R. G., Dickman, M., Day, W. C., Gunn, M. L., and Schmidt, C. D.: Ventilatory patterns and pulmonary complications after

upper abdominal surgery determined by preoperative and postoperative computerized spirometry and blood gas analysis. Am. J. Surg., *122*:622–632, 1971.

139. Levine, B. A., Petroff, P. A., Slade, C. L., and Pruitt, B. A.: Prospective trials of dexamethasone and aerosolized gentamicin in the treatment of inhalation injury in the burned patient. J. Trauma, *18*:188–193, 1978.

140. Levine, O. R., Mellins, R. B., and Fishman, A. P.: Quantitative assessment of pulmonary edema. Circ. Res., *17*:414–426, 1965.

141. Liebman, P. R., Philips, E., Weisel, R., Ali, J., and Hechtman, H. B.: Limitations of portable roentgenography of the chest in patients with acute respiratory failure. Surg. Gynec. Obstet., *146*:705–708, 1978.

142. Lindquist, O., Rammer, L., and Saldeen, T.: Pulmonary insufficiency, microembolism and fibrinolysis inhibition in a post-traumatic autopsy material. Acta Chir. Scand., *138*:545–549, 1972.

143. Lindskog, G.: Some historical aspects of thoracic trauma. J. Thorac. Cardiovasc. Surg., *42*:1–11, 1961.

144. Lorber, B., and Swenson, R. M.: Bacteriology of aspiration pneumonia. Ann. Intern. Med., *81*:329–331, 1974.

145. Lowe, R. J., and Moss, G. S.: Pulmonary failure after trauma. *In* Nyhus, L. M. (ed.): Surgery Annual, Vol. 8. 1976, pp. 63–90.

146. Lowe, R. J., Moss, G. S., Jilek, J., and Levine, H. D.: Crystalloid vs. colloid in the etiology of pulmonary failure after trauma: A randomized trial in man. Surgery, *81*:376–683, 1977.

147. Lucas, C. E., Ledgerwood, A. M., Shier, M. R., and Bradley, V. E.: The renal factor in the post-traumatic "fluid overload" syndrome. J. Trauma, *17*:667–676, 1977.

148. Lucas, C. E., Weaver, D., Higgins, R. F., Ledgerwood, A. M., Johnson, S. D., and Bowman, D. L.: Effects of albumin versus non-albumin resuscitation on plasma volume and renal excretory function. J. Trauma, *18*:564–570, 1978.

149. Luce, E. A., Su, C. T., and Hoopes, J. E.: Alveolar-arterial oxygen gradient in the burn patient. J. Trauma, *16*:212–217, 1976.

150. Lundsgaard-Hansen, P.: Oncotic deficit and albumin treatment. *In* Proceedings of Workshop on Albumin. (HEW Publication No. 76–295.) Washington, D.C., U. S. Government Printing Office, 1976, pp. 242–252.

151. Malik, A. B.: The role of metabolic acidosis in the pulmonary vascular response to hemorrhage and shock. J. Trauma, *18*:108–114., 1978.

152. Maloney, J. V., Schmutzer, K. J., and Raschlke, E.: Paradoxical respiration and "Pendelluft." J. Thorac. Cardiovasc. Surg., *41*:291–298, 1961.

153. Manny, J., Grindlinger, G., Mäthé, A. A., and Hechtman, H. B.: Positive end-expiratory pressure, lung stretch, and decreased myocardial contractility. Surgery, *84*:127–133, 1978.

154. Manwaring, D., Thorning, D., and Curreri, P. W.: Mechanisms of acute pulmonary dysfunction induced by fibrinogen degradation product D. Surgery, *84*:45–54, 1978.

155. Marshall, B. E., and Wyche, M. Q.: Hypoxemia during and after anesthesia. Anesthesiology, *37*:178–209, 1972.

156. McAslan, T. C., Chiu, J. M., Turney, S. Z., and Cowley, R. A.: Influence of inhalation of 100% oxygen on intrapulmonary shunt in severely traumatized patients. J. Trauma, *13*:811–821, 1973.

157. McDarral, J., and McNamara, J. J.: Pulmonary and systemic effects of stored vs. fresh blood in traumatized, shocked baboons. Surg. Forum, *27*:178–179, 1976.

158. Menon, I. S., Weightman, D., and Dewar, H. A.: The role of the lung in blood fibrinolysis. Clin. Sci., *36*:427–433, 1969.

159. Meyers, J. R., Lembeck, L., O'Kane, H., and Baue, A. B.: Changes in functional residual capacity of the lung after operation. Arch. Surg., *110*:576–583, 1975.

160. Michel-Briand, Y., Michel-Briand, C., Vieu, J. F., and Le Bras, Y.: Infections pulmonaires graves à Pseudomonas aeruginosa dans un service de réanimation, à propos de dix cas: Etudes épidémiologiques et dépistage systématique chez 623 malades. Presse Méd., 79:2103–2108, 1971.

161. Miller, L. W., Collins, J. A., Sherman, L., and Ladenson, J.: Massive transfusion in swine. Surg. Forum, *28*:21–23, 1977.

162. Miller, W. W., Waldhausen, J. A., and Rashkind, W. J.: Comparison of oxygen poisoning of the lung in cyanotic and acyanotic dogs. N. Engl. J. Med., *282*:943–947, 1970.

163. Milligan, G. F., MacDonald, J. A., Millon, A., and Ledingham, I. M.: Pulmonary and hematologic disturbances during septic shock. Surg. Gynec. Obstet., *138*:43–49, 1974.

164. Mobin-Uddin, K., Collard, G. M., Bolooki, H., Robinson, R., Michie, D., and Jude, J. R.: Transvenous caval interruption with umbrella filter. N. Engl. J. Med., *286*:55–58, 1972.

165. Moore, F. D., and Brennan, M. F.: Surgical injury: Body composition, protein metabolism and neuroendocrinology. *In* Ballinger, W. F., et al. (eds.): Manual of Surgical Nutrition, American College of Surgeons. Philadelphia, W. B. Saunders Company, 1975, pp. 169–222.

166. Moore, F. D., Lyons, J. H., Pierce, E. C., Morgan, A. P., Drinker, P. A., MacArthur, J. D., and Dammin, G. J.: Post-Traumatic Pulmonary Insufficiency. Philadelphia, W. B. Saunders Company, 1969.

167. Moseley, R. V., and Doty, D. B.: Death associated with multiple pulmonary emboli soon after battle injury. Am. Surg., *171*:336–346, 1970.

168. Moseley, R. V., Doty, D. B., and Pruitt, B. A.: Physiologic changes following chest injury in combat casualties. Surg. Gynec. Obstet., *129*:233–242, 1969.

169. Moss, G. S., Staunton, C., and Stein, A. A.: The centrineurogenic etiology of the acute respiratory distress syndrome: Universal, species independent phenomenon. Am. J. Surg., *126*:37–41, 1973.

170. Moss, G. S., and Stein, A. A.: Shock Lung — anemia as a predisposing factor. Am. J. Surg., *126*:419–420, 1973.

171. Moss, G. S., Siegel, D. C., Cochin, A., and Fres-

quez, V.: Effects of saline and colloid solutions on pulmonary function in hemorrhagic shock. Surg. Gynec. Obstet., *183*:53–58, 1971.

172. Mullane, J. F., Huber, G. L., Popvic, N. A., Wilfong, R. G., Bielke, S. R., O'Connel, D. M., and La Force, F. M.: Aspiration of blood and pulmonary host defense mechanisms. Ann. Surg., *180*:236–242, 1974.

173. Mullane, J. F., La Force, F. M., O'Connell, D. M., and Huber, G. L.: Acute blood loss and pulmonary host defense mechanisms in the rat. J. Surg. Res., *14*:228–234, 1973.

174. Neuhaus, N., Bentz, R. D., and Way, J. G.: Pulmonary embolism in respiratory failure. Chest, *73*:460–465, 1978.

175. Newhouse, M., J. Sanchis, and J. Bienenstock. Lung defense mechanisms. New Engl. J. Med. *295*:990–998, 1045–1052, 1976.

176. Nichols, R. T., Pearce, H. J., and Greenfield, L. J.: Effects of experimental pulmonary contusion on respiratory exchange and lung mechanics. Arch. Surg., *96*:723–730, 1968.

177. Northfield, T. C., and Smith, T.: Physiologic significance of central venous pressure in patients with hemorrhage. Surg. Gynec. Obstet., *135*:267–270, 1972.

178. Northrup, W. F., and Humphrey, E. W.: The effect of hemorrhagic shock on pulmonary vascular permeability to plasma proteins. Surgery, 83:264–273, 1978.

179. O'Connell, T. F., Clowes, G. H., Talamo, R. C., and Colman, R. W.: Kinin activation in the blood of patients with sepsis. Surg. Gynec. Obstet., *143*:539–545, 1976.

180. Olsson, P., Swedenborg, and Lindquist, O.: Effects of slow defibrinogenation on the canine lung. J. Trauma, *14*:325–329, 1974.

181. Orell, S. R.: Lung pathology in respiratory distress following shock in the adult. Acta Path. Microbiol. Scand., *79A*:65–76, 1971.

182. Pappova, E., Bachmeier, W., Crevoisier, J. L., Kollar, J., Kollar, M., Tobler, P., Zahler, H. W., Zaugg, D., and Lundsgaard-Hansen, P.: Acute hypoproteinemic fluid overload: Its determinants, distribution, and treatment with concentrated albumin and diuretics. Vox Sang., *33*:307–317, 1977.

183. Park, M. I., Alvarez, C., and Hampson, L. G.: The influence of normalization of CO_2 tension with positive end-expiratory pressure ventilation on severe hypoxemia. J. Surg. Res., *22*:435–441, 1977.

184. Patterson, R. W., and Sullivan, S. F.: The interrelationship between lung compliance and airway carbon dioxide concentration during hemorrhagic shock. J. Trauma, *13*:283–244, 1973.

185. Pennock, J. L., Pierce, W. S., and Waldhausen, J. A.: The management of the lungs during cardiopulmonary bypass. Surg. Gynec. Obstet., *145*:917–927, 1977.

186. Perea, E. J., Criado, A., Moreno, M., and Avello, F.: Mechanical ventilators as vehicles of infection. Acta Anaesthesiol. Scand., *19*:180–186, 1975.

187. Perel, A., Olschvang, D., Simerl, D., Katzenelson, R., and Cotev, S.: The variable effect of PEEP in acute respiratory failure associated with multiple trauma. J. Trauma, *18*:218–220, 1978.

188. Petroff, P. A., Hander, E. W., and Mason, A. D.: Ventilatory patterns following burn injury and effect of sulfamylon. J. Trauma, *15*:650–656, 1975.

189. Pierce, A. K., and Robertson, J.: Pulmonary complications of general surgery. Ann. Rev. Med., *28*:211–221, 1977.

190. Pierce, A. K., Sanford, J. P., Thomas, G. D., and Leonard, J. S.: Long-term evaluation of decontamination of inhalation-therapy equipment and the occurrence of necrotizing pneumonia. N. Engl. J. Med., *282*:528–530, 1970.

191. Polk, H. C.: Quantitative tracheal cultures in surgical patients requiring mechanical ventilatory assistance. Surgery, *78*:485–491, 1975.

192. Polk, H. C., Borden, S., and Aldrete, J. A.: Prevention of Pseudomonas respiratory infection in a surgical intensive care unit. Ann. Surg., *177*:607–615, 1973.

193. Pontoppidan, H., Geffin, B., and Lowenstein E.: Acute Respiratory Failure in the Adult. Boston, Little, Brown and Company, 1973.

194. Powers, S. R.: The use of positive end-expiratory pressure (PEEP) for respiratory support. Surg. Clin. North Am., *54*:1125–1136, 1974.

195. Prentice, T. C., Olney, J. M., Artz, C. P., and Howard, J. M.: Studies of blood volume and transfusion therapy in the Korean battle casualty. Surg. Gynec. Obstet., *99*:542–554, 1954.

196. Proctor, H. J., Ballantine, T. V., Broussard, N. D., and Hirsch, E. A.: An analysis of pulmonary function following penetrating pulmonary injury with recommendations for therapy. Surgery, *68*:92–98, 1970.

197. Pruitt, B. A., Erickson, D. R., and Morris, A.: Progressive pulmonary insufficiency and other pulmonary complications of thermal injury. J. Trauma, *15*:369–379, 1975.

198. Puri, V. K., Freund, U., Carlson, R. W., and Weil, M. H.: Colloid osmotic and pulmonary wedge pressures in acute respiratory failure following hemorrhage. Surg. Gynec. Obstet., *147*:537–540, 1978.

199. Rackow, E., Feir, A., and Leppo, J.: Colloid osmotic pressure as a prognostic indicator in critically ill patients. Chest, *70*:429, 1976 (abstr.).

200. Relihan, M., and Litevin, M. S.: Morbidity and mortality associated with flail chest injury: A review of 85 cases. J. Trauma, *13*:663–671, 1973.

201. Remmele, W., and Goebel, U.: Zur pathologischen Anatomie des Kreislaufschocks beim Menschen. V. Pathomorphologie der Schocklunge. Klin. Wochenschr., *51*:25–36, 1973.

202. Reull, G. J., Greenburg, S. D., Lefrak, E. A., McCollum, W. B., Beall, A. C., and Jordan, G. L.: Prevention of post-traumatic pulmonary insufficiency: Fine screen filtration of blood. Arch. Surg., *106*:386–394, 1973.

203. Rhodes, G., Dixon, R., and Silver, D.: Heparin induced thrombocytopenia with thrombotic and hemorrhagic manifestations. Surg. Gynec. Obstet., *136*:409–416, 1973.

204. Rice, C. L., Hobelman, C. F., John, D. A., Smith, D. E., Malley, J. D., Commack, B. F.,

James, D. R., Peters, R. M., and Virgilio, R. W.: Central venous pressure or pulmonary capillary wedge pressure as the determinant of fluid replacement in aortic surgery. Surgery, 84:437–449, 1978.

205. Richardson, J. D., Franz, J. L., Grover, F. L., and Trinkle, J. K.: Pulmonary contusion and hemorrhage: Crystalloid versus colloid replacement. J. Surg. Res., 16:330–336, 1974.

206. Richardson, J. D., Woods, D., Johanson, W. G., and Trinkle, J. K.: Lung bacterial clearance following pulmonary contusion. Surgery (In press, 1979).

207. Robboy, S. J., Minna, J. D., Colman, R. W., Birndorf, N. I., and Lopas, H.: Pulmonary hemorrhage syndrome as a manifestation of disseminated intravascular coagulation: Analysis of ten cases. Chest, 63:718–721, 1973.

208. Robin, E. D., Cross, C. E., and Zelis, R.: Pulmonary edema. N. Engl. J. Med., 288:239, 246, 292–304, 1973.

209. Rohatgi, P., Tauber, I., and Massaro, D.: Hemorrhagic hypotension and the lung: In vitro respiration. Am. Rev. Resp. Dis., 113:763–767, 1976.

210. Rosario, M. D., Rumsey, E. W., Arakaki, G., Tanque, R. E., McDanal, J., and McNamara, J. J.: Blood microaggregates and ultrafilters. J. Trauma, 18:498–506, 1978.

211. Roscher, R., Bittner, R., and Stockmann, U.: Pulmonary contusion. Arch. Surg., 109:508–510, 1974.

212. Rose, H. D., and Babcock, J. B.: Colonization of intensive care unit patients with gram-negative bacilli. Am. J. Epidemiol., 101:495–501, 1975.

213. Roth, R. R., Mullane, J. F., Huber, F. L., Phelps, T. D., and Wilfong, R. G.: Blood loss and factors affecting pulmonary antibacterial defenses. J. Surg. Res., 17:36–42, 1974.

214. Rutherford, R. B., Arora, S., Fleming, P. W., Monaghan, T., and Lowenstein, D. H.: Delayed onset pulmonary insufficiency in primates resuscitated from hemorrhagic shock. J. Trauma (In press, 1979).

215. Rutherford, R. B., and Valenta, J.: An experimental study of "traumatic wet lung." J. Trauma, 11:146–166, 1971.

216. Said, S. E.: Endocrine role of the lung in disease. Am. J. Med., 57:453–465, 1974.

217. Saldeen, T.: The microembolism syndrome. Microvasc. Res., 11:227–259, 1976.

218. Salzman, E. W., Deykin, D., Shapiro, R. M., and Rosenberg, R.: Management of heparin therapy: Controlled prospective trial. N. Engl. J. Med., 292:1046–1050, 1975.

219. Sarnoff, S. J., and Sarnoff, L. C.: Neurohemodynamics of pulmonary edema. II. The role of sympathetic pathways in the evaluation of pulmonary and systemic vascular pressure following the intracisternal injection of fibrin. Circulation, 6:51–62, 1952.

220. Sayeed, M. M., Chaudry, I. H., and Baue, A. E.: Na⁺–K⁺ transport and adenosine nucleotides in the lung in hemorrhagic shock. Surgery, 77:395–402, 1975.

221. Schloerb, P. R., Hunt, P. T., Plummer, J. A., Cage, G. K.: Pulmonary edema after replacement of blood loss by electrolyte solution. Surg. Gynec. Obstet., 135:893–896, 1972.

222. Schmidt, G. B., O'Neill, W. W., Kotb, K., Hwang, K. K., Bennett, E. J., and Bombeck, C. T.: Continuous positive airway pressure in the prophylaxis of the adult respiratory distress syndrome. Surg. Gynec. Obstet., 143:615–618, 1976.

223. Schneider, R. C., Carvalho, A., Bloom, S., and Zapol, W. M.: Platelet kinetics in severe acute respiratory failure. Am. Rev. Resp. Dis., 113(Suppl.): 135, 1976 (abstr.).

224. Schramel, R. J., Tyler, J., Kirkpatrick, J. L., Ziskind, M. M., and Creech, O.: Studies of respiratory function after thoracic injuries. J. Trauma, 3:206–216, 1963.

225. Schüpbach, P., Pappova, E., Schilt, W., Kollar, J., Kollar, M., Sipos, P., and Vucic, D.: Perfusate oncotic pressure during cardiopulmonary bypass. Vox Sang., 35:332–344, 1978.

226. Senior, R. M., Wessler, S., and Avioli, L. V.: Pulmonary oxygen toxicity. J.A.M.A., 217:1373–1377, 1971.

227. Sevitt, S.: Fat Embolism. London, Butterworth, 1962.

228. Shapiro, H. M., and Marshall, L. F.: Intracranial pressure responses to PEEP in head-injured patients. J. Trauma, 18:254–256, 1978.

229. Shoemaker, W. C., (ed.): The Lung in the Critically Ill Patient: Pathophysiology and Therapy of Acute Respiratory Failure. Baltimore, The Williams & Wilkins Company, 1976.

230. Shubrooks, S. J., Schneider, B., Dabin, H., and Turino, G. M.: Acidosis and pulmonary hemodynamics in hemorrhagic shock. Am. J. Physiol., 225:225–229, 1973.

231. Siler, J. N., Rosenber, H., Mull, T. D., Kaplan, J. A., Bardin H., and Marshall, B. F.: Hypoxemia after upper abdominal surgery: Comparison of venous admixture and ventilation/perfusion inequality components, using a digital computer. Ann. Surg., 179:149–155, 1974.

232. Simmons, R. L., Heisterkamp, C. A., Collins, J. A., Genslar, S., and Martin, A. M.: Respiratory insufficiency in combat casualties: III. Arterial hypoxemia after wounding. Ann. Surg., 170:45–52, 1969.

233. Simmons, R. L., Heisterkamp, C. A., Collins, J. A., Bredenberg, C. E., Mills, D. E., and Martin, A. M.: Respiratory insufficiency in combat casualties: IV. Hypoxemia during convalescence. Ann. Surg., 170:53–62, 1969.

234. Simmons, R. L., Heisterkamp, C. A., and Doty, D. B.: Postresuscitative blood volumes in combat casualtes. Surg. Gynec. Obstet.: 128:1193–1201, 1969.

235. Simmons, R. L., Martin, A. M., Heisterkamp, C. A., and Ducker, T. B.: Respiratory insufficiency in combat casualties. II. Pulmonary edema following head injury. Ann. Surg., 170:39–44, 1969.

236. Skillman, J. J.: Postoperative deep vein thrombosis and pulmonary embolism: A selective review and personal viewpoint. Surgery, 75:114–122, 1974.

237. Skillman, J. J., Bushnell, L. S., and Hedley-

Whyte, J.: Peritonitis and respiratory failure after abdominal operations. Ann. Surg., 170:122–127, 1969.

238. Skillman, J. J., Parikh, B. M., and Tanenbaum, B. J.: Pulmonary arteriovenous admixture: Improvement with albumin and diuresis. Am. J. Surg., 119:440–447, 1970.

239. Skillman, J. J., Restall, D. S., and Salzman, E. W.: Randomized trial of albumin vs. electrolyte solutions during abdominal aortic operations. Surgery, 78:291–303, 1975.

240. Slade, M. S., Simmons, R. L., Yunis, E., and Greenburg, L. J.: Immunodepression after major surgery in normal patients. Surgery, 78:363–372, 1975.

241. Smith, H. B., and Tuffnell, P. G.: Pseudomonas aeruginosa in respiratory illness: Endogenous or exogenous? Canad. Anesthesiol. Soc. J., 516–521, 1970.

242. Smith, P. C., Frank, H. A., Kasdon, E. J., Dearborn, E. C., and Skillman, J. J.: Albumin uptake by skin, skeletal muscle and lung in living and dying patients. Ann. Surg., 187:31–37, 1978.

243. Southern, P. M., Mays, B. B., Pierce, A. K., and Sanford, J. P.: Pulmonary clearance of Pseudomonas aeruginosa. J. Lab. Clin. Med., 76:548–559, 1970.

244. Staub, N. C.: Pulmonary edema. Physiol. Rev., 54:678–812, 1974.

245. Steer, M. L., Cloeren, S. E., Bushnell, L. S., and Skillman, J. J.: Metabolic alkalosis and respiratory failure in critically ill patients. Surgery, 72:408–413, 1972

246. Stein, M., and Thomas, D. P.: Role of platelets in the acute pulmonary responses to endotoxin. J. Appl. Physiol., 23:47–52, 1967.

247. Sugimoto, T., Katsurada, K., Yamada, R., Ogawa, M., Minami, T., and Onji, Y.: Posttraumatische respiratorische Insuffizienz bei Kopfverletzten. Anaesthesist, 23:263–267, 1974.

248. Suter, P. M., Fairley, H. B., and Isenberg, M. D.: Effect of tidal volume and positive end-expiratory pressure on compliance during mechanical ventilation. Chest, 73:158–162, 1978.

249. Suter, P. M., Fairley, H. B., and Schlobohm, R. M.: Shunt, lung volume and perfusion during short periods of ventilation with oxygen. Anesthesiology, 43:617–627, 1975.

250. Suter, P. M., Fairley, H. B., and Isenberg, M. D.: Optimum end-expiratory airway pressure in patients with acute pulmonary failure. N. Engl. J. Med., 292:284–298, 1975.

251. Szidon, J. P., and Fishman, A. P.: Participation of pulmonary circulation in the defense reaction. Am. J. Physiol., 220:364–370, 1971.

252. Tenaillon, A., Labrousse, J., Gateau, O., and Lissac, J.: Optimal positive end-expiratory pressure and static lung compliance. N. Engl. J. Med., 299:774–775, 1978.

253. Teplitz, C.: The core pathobiology and integrated medical science of adult acute respiratory insufficiency. Surg. Clin. North Am., 56:909–1133, 1976.

254. Terzi, R. G., and Peters, R. M.: The effect of large fluid loads on lung mechanics and work. Ann. Thorac. Surg., 6:16–24, 1968.

255. Thomas, D., Stein, M., Tanabe, G., Rege, V.,

and Wessler, S.: Mechanism of bronchoconstriction produced by thromboemboli in dogs. Am. J. Physiol., 206:1207–1212, 1964.

256. Tierney, D. F.: Lung metabolism and biochemistry. Ann. Rev. Physiol., 36:209–231, 1974.

257. Tobey, R. E., Kopriva, C. J., Homer, L. D., Solis, R. T., Dickson, L. G., and Herman, C. M.: Pulmonary gas exchange following hemorrhagic shock and massive blood transfusion in the baboon. Ann. Surg., 179:316–321, 1974.

258. Toung, T. J. K., Saharia, P., Mitzner, W. A., Pennott, S., and Cameron, J. L.: The beneficial and harmful effects of positive end-expiratory pressure. Surg. Gynec. Obstet.: 147:518–524, 1978.

259. Trimble, C., Smith, D. E., Cook, T. I., and Trummer, M. J.: The effect of supine bed rest upon alveolar-arterial oxygen gradients and intrapulmonary shunting in normal man. J. Thorac. Cardiovasc. Surg., 63:873–879, 1972.

260. Trinkle, J. K., Richarrdson, J. D., and Frenz, J. L.: Management of flail chest without mechanical ventilation. Ann. Thorac. Surg., 19:355–363, 1975.

261. Tuller, M. A., and Mehdi, F.: Compensatory hypoventilation and hypercapnia in primary metabolic alkalosis: Report of 3 cases. Am. J. Med., 50:281–290, 1971.

262. Van de Water, J. M., Watring, W. G., Linton, L. A., Murphy, M., and Byron, R. L.: Prevention of postoperative pulmonary complications. Surg. Gynec. Obstet., 135:229–233, 1972.

263. Vaughan, R. W., and Wise, L.: Choice of abdominal operative incision in the obese patient: A study using blood gas measurements. Ann. Surg., 181:829–835, 1975.

264. Virgilio, R.: A prospective controlled study on the effect of the use of fine filters on postoperative pulmonary function in heavily transfused patients. Presented at the U. S. Army Medical R & D Command Symposium on Microaggregates, Letterman Army Medical Center, June, 1977.

265. Virgilio, R. W., Smith, D. E., Rice, C. L., Hobelmann, C. L., Zarins, C. K., James, D. R., and Peters, R. M.: Effect of colloid osmotic pressure and pulmonary capillary wedge pressure on intrapulmonary shunt. Surg. Forum, 27:168–170, 1976.

266. Walker, L., and Eiseman, B.: The changing pattern of post-traumatic respiratory distress syndrome. Ann. Surg., 181:693–697, 1975.

267. Webb, W. R. (ed): Symposium on pulmonary problems in surgery. Surg. Clin. North Am., 54:941–1224, 1974.

268. Weeks, D. B.: Humidification during anesthesia. N.Y. State J. Med., 75:1216–1218, 1975.

269. Weil, M. H., Henning, R. J., Morisetta, M., and Michaels, S.: Relationship between colloid osmotic pressure and pulmonary artery wedge pressure in patients with acute cardiorespiratory failure. Am. J. Med., 64:643–650, 1978.

270. Weinstein, M. E., Rice, C. L., Peters, R. M., and

Virgilio, R. W.: Hemodynamic and respiratory response to varying gradients between end-expiratory pressure and end-inspiratory pressure in patients breathing on continuous positive airway pressure. J. Trauma, *18*:231–235, 1978.

271. Weisel, R. D., Dennis, R. C., Manny, J., Mannick, J. A., Vabri, C. R., and Hechtman, H. B.: Adverse effects of transfusion therapy during abdominal aortic aneurysmectomy. Surgery, *83*:682–690, 1978.

272. Welch, G. W., Lull, R. J., Petroff, P. A., Hander, E. W., McLeod, C. G., and Clayton, W. H.: The use of steroids in inhalation injury. Surg. Gynec. Obstet., *145*:539–544, 1977.

273. White, M. K., Shepro, D., and Hechtman, H. B.: Pulmonary function and platelet-lung interaction. J. Appl. Physiol., *34*:697–703, 1973.

274. Williams, J. A., Grable, E., Frank, H. A., and Fine, J.: Blood loss and plasma volume shifts during and following major surgical operations. Ann. Surg., *156*:648–654, 1962.

275. Wilson, R. F., Sarver, E., and Birks, R.: Central venous pressure and blood volume determinations in clinical shock. Surg. Gynec. Obstet.: *132*:631–636, 1971.

276. Winter, P. M., Gupta, R. K., Michalski, A. H., and Lanphier, E. H.: Modification of hyperbaric oxygen toxicity by experimental venous admixture. J. Appl. Physiol., *23*:954–963, 1967.

277. Winter, P. M., and Smith, G.: The toxicity of oxygen. Anesthesiology, *37*:210–241, 1972.

278. Wolf, C. F., and Canale, V. C.: Fatal pulmonary hypersensitivity reaction to HL-A incompatible blood transfusion: Report of a case and review of the literature. Transfusion, *16*:135–140, 1976.

279. Yernault, J. C., Englert, M., Sergysels, R., and DeCosta, A.: Pulmonary mechanics and diffusion after "shock lung." Thorax, *30*:252–257, 1975.

280. Zapol, W. J.: Post-traumatic respiratory distress (CPC). N. Engl. J. Med., *296*:1279–1287, 1977.

281. Zapol, W. M., Kobayashi, K., Snider, M. T., Greene, R., and Laver, M. B.: Vascular obstruction causes pulmonary hypertension in severe acute respiratory failure. Chest, *71*:306–307, 1977.

282. Zarins, C. K., Virgilio, R. W., Smith, D. E., and Peters, R. M.: The effect of vascular volume on positive end-expiratory pressure-induced cardiac output depression and wedge-left atrial pressure discrepancy. J. Surg. Res., *23*:348–360, 1977.

283. Zikria, B. A., Spencer, J. L., Kinney, J. M., and Broell, J. R.: Alterations in ventilatory function and breathing patterns following surgical trauma. Ann. Surg., *179*:1–7, 1974.

CHAPTER 7

ACUTE RENAL FAILURE IN THE SURGICAL PATIENT

Edward E. Etheredge, M.D., Ph.D.
Keith A. Hruska, M.D.

INTRODUCTION

Acute renal failure is a term used to describe a host of diseases and clinical syndromes that are characterized by an abrupt and usually reversible impairment of renal excretory function that is frequently accompanied by oliguria. Of the various acute renal dysfunctional states associated with trauma and surgical therapy, the form that will be considered at greatest length in this discussion has been called, historically, "acute tubular necrosis." This designation is considered by many investigators to be a misnomer, since the forms of acute renal failure included under this heading do not uniformly manifest necrosis of tubular epithelial cells. Others prefer the designation "acute vasomotor nephropathy" because it reflects an emphasis on alternate mechanisms for the intrinsic dysfunction of the kidney. In this chapter we will utilize the term "acute renal failure" generically to describe intrinsic renal dysfunction without special emphasis on mechanisms unless indicated. Prerenal and postrenal forms of renal failure are other causes of acute renal dysfunction and usually oliguria in the surgical patient, and these will be discussed in terms of their differentiation from acute renal failure.

A classification of the prerenal, renal and postrenal forms of acute renal failure that may be found commonly in the surgical patient is shown in Table 7–1.

CLINICAL SETTING

The syndrome of acute renal failure presents variably, with several etiologies acting through some independent and some common pathophysiological mechanisms, and cannot be dissected precisely for definition in an epidemiological sense. It is difficult to ascertain the true incidence of acute renal failure within the diversity of surgical and trauma-related conditions. Nevertheless, the experiential data of collected patient series permit some clinical generalizations about the syndrome.

Shires[102] estimates that the incidence of acute renal failure following elective operations is less than 1 per cent, although moderate to severe acute renal failure was detected in 7 per cent of postoperative cardiac surgery patients[3] and 13 per cent of a series of aneurysmectomy patients, many of whom had ruptured aneurysms;[40] some degree of renal dysfunction was detected in 40 per cent of patients with ruptured aortic aneurysms.[43] In a series of 125 postoperative acute renal failure patients requiring dialysis, 38 per cent had had intra-

TABLE 7–1. Major Forms of Acute Renal Failure Associated With Trauma and Surgery

I. Prerenal
   A. Hypovolemia
      1. Burns
      2. GI losses
      3. Hemorrhage
      4. Sequestration (burns, peritonitis, operatively related third space)
   B. Cardiovascular failure
      1. Myocardial failure
         a. Infarction, tamponade
      2. Vascular pooling
         a. Sepsis, severe acidosis
II. Acute tubular necrosis
   A. Postischemic. All causes of prerenal azotemia (see I above), especially postoperatively
   B. Nephrotoxic
      1. Antibiotics, aminoglycosides, cephalosporins, anesthetics, neomycin, polymyxin B, Bacitracin
   C. Heme pigments
      1. Intravascular hemolysis — transfusion reactions, sepsis
      2. Rhabdomyolysis and myoglobinuria — trauma, coma, seizures, crush syndrome, electric shock, burns
III. Postrenal
   A. Obstruction — trauma, retroperitoneal hemorrhage, surgical accidents
   B. Rupture of bladder
IV. Miscellaneous
   A. Vascular obstruction — thrombosis, embolism, aneurysm
   B. Primary renal diseases — glomerulonephritis, hypertension, vasculitis, others
   C. Nephrotoxic (interstitial nephritis) — penicillins, diagnostic pyelography and angiography, Dextran therapy, mannitol therapy

abdominal operations, 39 per cent had had cardiovascular operations, 14 per cent had sustained traumatic injury and 9 per cent had had urologic operations.[86] Advanced age and pre-existing renal disease are consistently identified as predisposing factors to acute renal failure of various causes in the surgical patient.

Acute volume depletion may be followed by acute renal failure that demonstrates both tubular necrosis and the arteriolar vasoconstriction of the vasomotor nephropathy type. Gastrointestinal hemorrhage, sepsis, burns and trauma are leading causes of this form of acute renal failure. Gram-negative septicemia, with or without documented hypotension, undoubtedly causes a high proportion of acute renal failure cases in a surgical population,[51] and disseminated intravascular coagulation (DIC) is, of itself, associated with acute renal failure.[65, 95] A rarer form of acute renal failure has been described in association with visceral suppuration.[14] This is glomerular in origin and is characterized by diffuse proliferative and crescentic glomerulonephritis; it probably has an immune basis. Such a mechanism has also been suggested as a cause of the acute renal failures seen with other nonsurgical conditions such as subacute bacterial endocarditis. Specific surgical diseases such as suppurative cholangitis have a high rate of association with acute renal failure.[21]

Acute renal failure from nephrotoxic agents has become significant in the surgical patient. There are multiple drug-related syndromes that alter renal function, and these have been reviewed recently.[15] Since infectious complications are common following massive trauma and operative procedures, antibiotics are frequently required, and many of these are nephrotoxic.[105] Drug-induced nephrotoxicity is not uncommon, although in the trauma victim who has experienced shock, anesthesia, operations, transfusions and sepsis, it is frequently difficult to separate drug-induced nephrotoxicity from acute renal failure of other causes. Undoubtedly, the intrinsic toxicity of many compounds is potentiated by other drugs such as diuretics and the effects of dehydration or hypotension and sepsis. The aminoglycoside antibiotics, including gentamicin, kanamycin, neomycin, streptomycin, tobramycin and amikacin, are widely used in the treatment of serious gram-negative infections and are well known to be nephrotoxic. These antibiotics, as well as cephaloridine, amphotericin B, polymyxin B, colistimethate, tetracyclines and sulfonamides, cause acute renal failure by proximal tubular necrosis. The incidence of acute renal failure in patients treated with gentamicin alone is 2 to 6.5 per cent.[49, 105, 122] Most cases of drug-induced nephrotoxicity are nonoliguric, although oliguric acute renal failure has been reported following combination treatment with tobramycin and cephalothin[114] and with gentamicin and clindamycin.[29] Gary and colleagues[61] noted the absence of oliguria in gentamicin-associated acute renal failure, but others[105] characterize this condition as an oliguric acute renal failure. There are numerous scattered reports of acute renal failure, both oliguric and nonoliguric, in association with gentamicin used in combination with cephalothin.[23, 30, 50] The potentiation of gentamicin nephrotoxicity by cephalothin has been disproved and proved in animal models, but it seems likely that the potentiation is real.

Penicillins, including penicillin G, ampicillin, methicillin and nafcillin, may cause acute renal failure from acute interstitial nephritis, and a similar syndrome may be caused by rifampin, sulfonamides, furosemide and cephalothin.[15] This nonoliguric renal failure gradually begins 7 to 14 days after exposure to the drug, may present with gross and microscopic hematuria and may be associated with fever, cutaneous rash and peripheral eosinophilia. This condition is thought to result from a humoral immune response directed against tubular basement membrane antigen.

The anesthetic agent methoxyflurane is also potentially nephrotoxic and may potentiate the nephrotoxicity of other drugs such as antibiotics. Methoxyflurane-induced acute renal failure may be oliguric or nonoliguric. Acute renal failure may be precipitated by radiologic contrast agents, especially in the diabetic and the dehydrated patient.[5, 45, 62] Diabetic patients with serum creatinine levels of 5 mg./dl. or greater are at extreme risk. Another form of nephrotoxic acute renal failure seen in the surgical patient is caused by the toxic biologic pigments hemoglobin and myoglobin. Hemolytic reactions caused by mismatched transfusions, burns, snake bites[35] and insect stings[36] liberate free hemoglobin, and rhabdomyolysis caused by crush injuries, prolonged ischemia to a limb, or exercise will release toxic myoglobin.

In a large clinical series of acute renal failure patients, most had had an operation and 62 per cent had documented hypotension, which was most commonly induced by gastrointestinal hemorrhage.[7] A similar incidence of hypotension was documented in battle casualty patients sustaining acute renal failure.[81] The occurrence of hypotension and the use of nephrotoxic antibiotics are common associations in surgical patients who sustain renal failure.[19] However, the disconcerting fact remains that frequently neither hypotension nor any other associated causal factor can be identified in surgical patients with acute renal failure.

Nonoliguric acute renal failure has become the commonest form of this disease,[101] constituting 53 per cent of patients in a large clinical series;[7] it was even found in 42 per cent of patients in a series of battle casualties who suffered acute renal failure.[81] This prevalence of nonoliguric acute renal failure has been due, in large part, to recent increases in the use of the aminoglycoside antibiotics. Patients with acute nonoliguric renal failure are less likely to require dialysis[25, 81] and are reported by some[25] to have an improved prognosis, but this is not the uniform experience, as reported mortality rates for acute nonoliguric renal failure after surgery or trauma range from 33 to 82 per cent.[13, 81, 118] For patients who survive, the duration of acute renal failure from diagnosis to onset of recovery averages 11 to 13 days.[11, 25, 86] Abnormal renal function of the nonoliguric variety persists an average of 24 days,[25] but the duration of oliguria may vary from 24 hours to over 90 days. Subtle abnormalities may persist much longer than this. The longer the duration of oliguria, the poorer the prognosis for return to adequate renal function. There are scattered reports[103] of complete or partial recovery from renal failure after prolonged oliguria (30 days or more), but this is uncommon. Kidney biopsy may be necessary for diagnosis in selected cases of prolonged oliguria. In patients who survive acute renal failure, the function that returns is usually sufficient to sustain the patient without dialysis, but some patients may survive with moderate to severe chronic renal failure, and some may require chronic hemodialysis.[86]

In spite of significant advances in medical and surgical care, including hemodialysis, the mortality rate from acute renal failure in surgical patients remains very high. In patients who died, the mean duration of acute renal failure until time of death was 8.5 ± 0.8 days.[11] In large clinical series of surgical patients with acute renal failure, the mortality rate is about 60 per cent or more.[11, 28, 71, 86] Acute renal failure following aortic aneurysmectomy carries a 61 per cent mortality;[40] following operations for ruptured aneurysms it has a 95 per cent mortality;[113] following major cardiovascular operations in which dialysis is required there is a 74 per cent mortality;[32] and after major cardiac operations it carries 88.8 per cent mortality.[3] While the requirement for dialysis indirectly indicates the severity of acute renal failure, there is a surprisingly high mortality even in patients who do not require dialysis for their renal conditions. Baek et al.[11] reported a 65 per cent mortality rate for dialyzed patients and a 58 per cent mortality rate for nondialzyed patients. In addition, these investigators noted that 39 per cent of patients who were nonoliguric on the day of diagnosis died, whereas 71 per cent of patients who were oliguric on the day of diagnosis died.

It has been observed consistently that medical or surgical conditions in patients with acute renal failure are more likely to cause the patient's death than the renal failure itself. In fact, death related directly to the uremic complications of acute renal failure has become uncommon since the widespread application of modern techniques of medical and surgical management. Sepsis is clearly the leading cause of death following post-traumatic or post-surgical acute renal failure, accounting for at least 25 per cent of the deaths.[11, 28, 30, 77, 85] Kennedy et al.[71] identified four major factors that have an adverse influence on the prognosis of patients with acute renal failure, namely: age, infection, surgical gastrointestinal lesions and gastrointestinal hemorrhage. The requirement for prolonged mechanical ventilation is another detrimental factor. Jaundice in conjunction with acute renal failure is associated with a 90 per cent mortality, and upper gastrointestinal hemorrhage occurring during acute renal failure is associated with a mortality of 80 per cent.[41,44]

PATHOPHYSIOLOGY OF ACUTE RENAL FAILURE

Acute renal failure following shock, sepsis and major trauma is characterized by oliguria in 80 to 90 per cent of cases. Although the pathophysiological mechanisms that result in oliguria following these insults have been exhaustively sought for the past 20 to 30 years, extensive investigation with experimental models of acute renal failure[91] and limited studies in

TABLE 7-2.   Pathophysiologic Mechanisms of Oliguria

I. Decreased formation of glomerular ultrafiltrate
  A. Decreased formation of glomerular ultrafiltrate
    1. Afferent arteriolar vasoconstriction
    2. Endothelial swelling
  B. Altered glomerular permeability
  C. Increased intratubular hydrostatic pressure
    1. Tubular obstruction from cellular debris or casts
II. Passive back-flow of glomerular ultrafiltrate
    1. Tubular necrosis

human subjects have not yet clearly elucidated these mechanisms.

Historically, three mechanisms of oliguria have been considered, and great controversy has centered upon the potential role of each mechanism in any one form of acute renal failure. The three classic mechanisms of oliguria are (1) renal tubular obstruction, (2) passive backflow of glomerular filtrate and (3) preglomerular arteriolar vasoconstriction with subsequent decreased glomerular plasma flow. A more recent classification of the proposed mechanisms of oliguria based on the forces determining glomerular ultrafiltration and incorporating the classic mechanisms is shown in Table 7-2. The purpose of this section will be to relate the proposed pathophysiological mechanisms of oliguria to the acute renal failure observed in various experimental models and, when possible, to correlate the oliguria observed in the experimental models with the human counterpart. The goal is thus to increase our understanding of the oliguria of human renal failure and of the possible pathophysiological mechanisms involved in its production, maintenance and recovery. The unexpected logic of oliguria in acute renal failure has been thoughtfully presented in a recent review.[112]

Experimental Models of Acute Renal Failure

The models of acute renal failure that have been investigated and are related to the oliguria of trauma-related acute renal failure in the human are listed in Table 7-3. The renal injury resulting in clinical acute renal failure must be considered within the framework of the temporal course of the disease. Thus, as shown in

TABLE 7–3. Models of Experimental Renal Failure With Possible Relationships to Human Syndromes

EXPERIMENTAL MODEL	POSSIBLE HUMAN COUNTERPARTS

Nephrotoxic models
    Uranyl nitrate
    Mercury chloride
	Aminoglycosides, endotoxemia

Circulatory alterations
    Renal artery clamp
    Renal arterial vasoconstriction
	Hypotension

Mixed
    Glycerol
    Hemoglobinemia
	Myohemoglobinuria, crush syndrome

Table 7–4, there is an initiating event that induces renal dysfunction, which eventually reaches a plateau or maintenance stage, and finally recovery of renal function occurs. The role of each potential mechanism of oliguria in a clinical syndrome must be considered in the framework of the phases of acute renal failure.

One of the prototypical forms of experimental nephrotoxic renal failure is caused in rats or dogs by the injection of uranyl nitrate in doses ranging from 5 to 10 mg./kg. Flamenbaum and associates[52, 53] have investigated in depth uranyl nitrate-induced acute renal failure in the rat. Their studies during the early initiation phase of renal dysfunction failed to demonstrate increased intratubular hydrostatic pressure or intratubular casts, the experimental findings indicative of significant tubular obstruction. Ultrastructural studies utilizing scanning electron microscopy revealed no abnormalities of glomerular ul-

TABLE 7–4. Phases of Acute Renal Failure

INITIATION PHASE

The time from the pathologic event to the clinical appearance of renal failure

MAINTENANCE PHASE

The time during which established renal failure is stable or continuing to worsen
1. Oliguric
2. Nonoliguric

RECOVERY PHASE

The time characterized by improving renal function
1. Early — diuretic stage with still impaired function
2. Late — stable renal function

trastructure that would suggest altered glomerular permeability in the first 6 hours after injection of uranyl nitrate. Similar values were also demonstrated for single nephron filtration rate at varying distances from the renal glomerulus, and lissamine green microinjected into the proximal tubule appeared in the distal tubules. Thus, significant back-leak of glomerular ultrafiltrate was ruled out. Using the radioactive xenon washout technique, abnormalities of renal hemodynamics were observed that were similar to those that have been seen after clinical human acute renal failure of diverse etiology.[69, 70, 94] Marked diminution of proximal tubular sodium reabsorption and increased delivery of sodium to the distal tubule were also observed.

These results led the authors to exclude primary roles for elevated tubular hydrostatic pressure, altered glomerular permeability and cell swelling in the genesis of the decreased glomerular filtration rate seen early after uranyl nitrate injection. Rather, these authors proposed that uranyl nitrate decreased proximal tubular sodium and chloride transport, leading to increased distal tubular sodium delivery. The latter stimulated the juxtaglomerular apparatus to increase intrarenal renin production and angiotensin generation, which led to increased anteriolar tone and decreased glomerular plasma flow. Thus these authors and others[112] suggest that tubuloglomerular feedback may be the mechanism responsible for the pathogenesis of renal dysfunction characteristic of the initiation phase of uranyl nitrate-induced acute renal failure. The evidence in support of this hypothesis is still incomplete, but Schwartz and Flamenbaum[99] have demonstrated that uranyl nitrate has a direct effect on active sodium chloride transport without alterations in membrane electrical resistance in the urinary bladder of the fresh water turtle. They also demonstrated increased juxtaglomerular apparatus renin activity and plasma renin activity.

The same authors have also investigated the maintenance phase of renal dysfunction following uranyl nitrate administration. They demonstrated that 24 to 48 hours following administration of uranyl nitrate distortion of epithelial cells appeared with swelling and broadening of the foot processes. These results are similar to those reported by Stein et al.,[107] who also found abnormalities in the epithelial cells of the glomerulus. These authors and Blantz[22] also demonstrated a lack of significant change in total renal blood flow 48 hours following administration of uranyl nitrate and a marked decrease in urine output, with a decrease in total kidney filtration rate to less than 1 per cent of the normal value. However, there was only a 40 per cent decrease in single nephron filtration rate and a decrease in recovery of microinjected inulin compared to control animals. These data were taken to indicate that increased permeability to water and solute across tubular basement membranes was involved in the disparity between the determinations of single nephron and total kidney filtration rate. Both authors concluded that maintenance of acute renal failure in the nephrotoxic model of uranyl nitrate was contributed both by leakage of filtrate across damaged tubular basement membranes and a modest fall in glomerular filtration rate due to decreased glomerular permeability.

Although the scope and the purpose of this chapter do not allow in-depth descriptions of the pathophysiological mechanisms responsible for oliguria in each of the experimental models listed in Table 7–2, the above description of the uranyl nitrate model serves to point out the extent of the current investigation into the pathophysiology of oliguria. It also emphasizes the fact that in recent years the classic concepts of tubular obstruction and back-leak of glomerular filtrate have come to be challenged as the sole mechanisms of oliguria. Mercury chloride ($HgCl_2$) has been shown

to share generally similar pathophysiologic mechanisms that are now ascribed to uranyl nitrate-induced forms of acute renal failure in the rat.[20, 56]

Variable alterations in renal plasma flow present one of the major drawbacks of nephrotoxic ischemic and glycerol-myohemaglobinuric forms of murine acute renal failure in the attempt to relate these to human clinical forms. Numerous studies of the renal blood flow in these models of acute renal failure have been made, the most recent of which[37] demonstrates that only in glycerol-induced myohemaglobinuria was there sufficient fall in cortical blood flow to account for oliguria and that this decrease in cortical blood flow was short-lived and returned to normal by 24 hours. Blood flow was normal at all times following mercury chloride injection except for early minimal depression following one-half hour of total bilateral renal occlusion, but it was again normal at 24 hours. In contrast, human studies all indicate a 50 to 70 per cent fall in renal blood flow. Angiographic studies demonstrate marked attenuation of the preglomerular vascular tree. If this effect is sufficient to decrease glomerular capillary pressure below that needed to sustain adequate filtration, then decreased renal plasma flow is a major explanation of oliguria in human acute renal failure. However, recent studies by Hollenberg[68] and Ladgeford and Winkler[78] have shown that renal cortical blood flow in human acute renal failure can be brought toward normal by infusions of vasodilator agents with no demonstrable change in glomerular filtration rate or increase in urine output.

Considering the drawbacks of the nephrotoxic models of acute renal failure, the models of ischemic renal failure due to renal arterial clamping or renal arterial norepinephrine infusion seem to be more attractively related to human postischemic renal failure. However, currently there is great controversy concerning the pathogenetic mechanisms of oliguria in these experimental models. Arendhorst et al.[110] studied oliguric renal failure in rats, beginning 1 hour after unilateral main renal artery clamping. For the first 3 hours they observed tubules dilated with proteinacious debris in medullary areas, decreases of 50 per cent in total renal blood flow, a twofold increase in renal vascular resistance, and a very slow transit of dye that rarely reached distal tubular sites. Measured intratubular pressures were markedly increased and glomerular capillary pressure was normal. The authors concluded that in the induction phase of ischemic renal failure oliguria was due to tubular obstruction.

These authors used animals, which were studied for 24 hours following unilateral renal ischemia, to represent the maintenance phase of acute renal failure. They demonstrated collapsed tubules with very little flow of microinjected dye. Intratubular pressures were decreased, as were glomerular capillary pressures. Renal blood flow was decreased by 50 per cent. They concluded that oliguria in the maintenance phase of ischemic injury was due to vasomotor changes similar to those observed in nephrotoxic forms of acute renal failure. However, covert tubular obstruction and back-leak of glomerular filtrate was present when rats were expanded with saline. This maneuver resulted in a return of renal blood flow to normal, a decrease in renal vascular resistance and an increase in glomerular capillary pressure to normal. When intratubular pressure returned to normal, however, no urine output occurred, and observable loss of a microinjected dye was seen across proximal tubular epithelial cells. In the recovery phase of ischemic injury-induced oliguria the authors observed a persistent mild decrease in renal blood flow and increased renal vascular resistance. At this stage intratubular pressures were normal, but there was wider variation in the tubular pressure profile than in normal pressure profiles. There was also an increased heterogeneity of glomerular capillary pressures.

Stein and Sorkin,[107] using a similar model of unilateral renal ischemia that they studied at 3 hours following induction of the ischemia, observed normal intratubular pressure, complete recovery of microinjected inulin and a normal glomerular permeability. However, there was decreased glomerular capillary plasma flow because of increased preglomerular vasoconstriction, which is in agreement with the results of Daugharty and colleagues.[42] These authors also observed a decrease in total renal blood flow following 48 hours of norepinephrine injection into unilateral

renal arteries. This decrease in renal blood flow is reversed to normal by loading with Ringer's solution, but again, urine output did not occur and the tubules remained collapsed. In contrast to the Arendhorst study,[6] these authors proposed that the oliguria was related to ultrastructural abnormalities observed within the renal glomerulus. They demonstrated loss of the normal foot process structures of glomerular epithelial cells, suggesting changes in glomerular permeability. Thus, despite the attractiveness of a relationship of these post-ischemic animal models to human studies, the pathogenesis of oliguria in these models remains controversial.

Another model of experimental acute renal failure, glycerol-induced myohemoglobinuria, is attractive because of its relationship to a human form of acute renal failure. The relation of this form of acute renal failure to human rhabdomyolysis, myoglobinuria and the crush syndrome appears to be fairly well established, especially in view of the fact that parenterally administered glycerol has caused human acute renal failure.[66] Some authors have listed glycerol-induced acute renal failure as a form of ischemic acute tubular necrosis. However, the types of tubular malfunction and morphologic alterations, produced by ischemic clamping of the vascular tree differ from those seen in glycerol-induced acute tubular necrosis.[93] The initial events in rats following glycerol injection are decreased cardiac output, decreased renal blood flow, myohemoglobinuria and tissue injury. The presence of myohemoglobinuria in the setting of circulatory insufficiency suggests that these substances may be toxic to ischemic kidneys only, since the injection of hemoglobin or of myoglobin into normal rats or human subjects has not caused tubular malfunction.

In the experimental setting the oliguria of glycerol-induced acute renal failure in the rat is characterized in the induction phase by normal intratubular pressures, significant decreases in renal plasma flow and total renal blood flow, a redistribution of renal blood flow to deeper structures and cortical ischemia. Suzuki and Mostofie[108] demonstrated no evidence of tubular back-leak of inulin, only minor transient cellular abnormalities of the glomerulus on scanning electron microscopy, and subcellular histological abnormalities of the tubular cells. Thus, at least in the generation phase of acute renal failure, glycerol-induced myohemoglobinuria seems clearly to be established as a cause of oliguria due to diminished formation of glomerular filtrate resulting from decreased glomerular capillary hydrostatic pressure from apparent arteriolar vasoconstriction.

The glycerol-induced myohemoglobinuria model is of further interest because protection can be given against the deleterious renal effects of glycerol by volume expansion with saline, mannitol or furosemide diuresis and prostaglandin inhibition. Volume expansion and mannitol diuresis have been shown to be protective not only in glycerol-induced myohemoglobinuria but also in other forms of experimental acute renal failure.[57, 60, 82, 89, 108] These effects have been variously reported to be due to an increase in cardiac out-

put, an increase in plasma volume, an increase in renal blood flow, a decrease in renal vascular resistance, decreased renin release and finally, increased tissue oxygen tension.

The renin-angiotensin system was first suggested to play a role in the pathogenesis of acute renal failure by Goomaghtigh. Additional work by numerous subsequent authors has produced support for the postulate that increased plasma renin activity seen in acute renal failure is related to the pathogenesis of oliguria. The primary support for this suggestion stems from experimental studies that demonstrate that chronic salt loading almost completely protects against the development of renal cortical ischemia and filtration failure in various models of acute renal failure[54, 55] while simultaneously blocking renin production. The mechanisms proposed to explain the protective action of the saline loading have been the intrarenal depletion

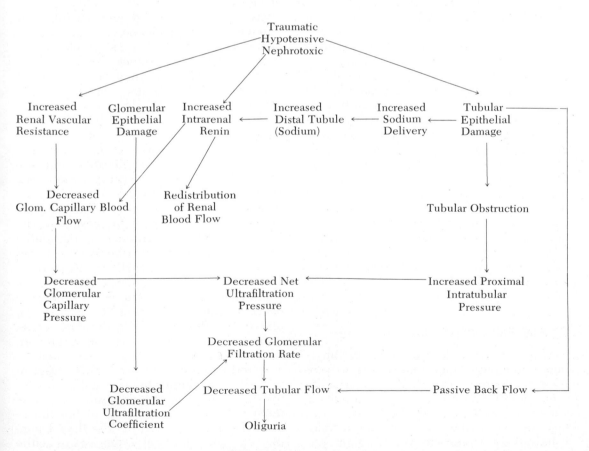

Figure 7–1. *Renal injury.*

of renin and the suppression of plasma renin activity. Flamenbaum's studies with potassium chloride suppression of plasma renin activity seemed to establish excellent correlation between the degree of renin suppression and protection against the development of acute renal failure. However, the use of renin blocking agents and angiotensin antagonists, as well as immunization against renin, have failed to give protection against the development of acute renal failure.[55, 92, 115] These studies seem to indicate that the protection against the development of acute renal failure after chronic saline loading may not be related to the suppression of the renin-angiotensin system. Of interest in this regard is the observation that indomethacin, an inhibitor of prostaglandin synthesis, increases the severity of acute renal failure produced by glycerol.[115] This may suggest that the effect of chronic saline loading is mediated through alterations in the myogenic tone of the renal vasculature that lead to persistent decreases in renal resistance. Indomethacin and decreased prostaglandin synthesis, which lead to an increase in renal resistance prior to the induction of acute renal failure, promote this severity of lesion. This is especially important in models of ischemic renal failure because indomethacin has no effect in mercury chloride-induced renal failure.[72]

In summary, the pathogenetic mechanisms that have been involved in the production of oliguria in experimental models of acute renal failure are portrayed in Figure 7–1. Although no one pathogenetic mechanism can be given the major role in the production of oliguria, in most of the models, especially those that seem to relate best to human acute renal failure, there is a prominent decrease in glomerular capillary pressure due to arteriolar vasoconstriction that is a part of their oliguric mechanism.

Clinical Pathophysiology

Although our understanding of the aberrant renal physiology that serves to produce the clinical manifestations of acute renal failure is incomplete, enough is known or can be surmised to provide details of the pathophysiological mechanisms of the fluid and electrolyte abnormalities seen in acute renal failure. As a consequence of the renal dysfunction, there is a disruption of those major processes that insure a constant composition and volume of body water and electrolytes and excrete the catabolic end-products of protein breakdown. The consequences of this renal dysfunction must be understood in a pathophysiological sense in order to diagnose the disease and manage the patient, and especially to exclude other forms of acute renal dysfunction such as prerenal azotemia or postrenal failure due to urinary obstruction.

The most prominent effects of filtration failure are the retention of catabolic end-products, mainly creatinine, urea, uric acid and certain electrolytes. Creatinine, an end-product of muscle metabolism, is handled by the kidneys essentially through glomerular filtration and urinary excretion. There is no evidence of creatinine reabsorption except across damaged tubular epithelium; however, at very low glomerular filtration rates, creatinine secretion becomes an important additional mechanism of creatinine clearance. This causes overestimation of the glomerular filtration rate when creatine clearance is considered to be equivalent to the glomerular filtration rate and that clearance rate is less than 15 ml./min. The rise in serum creatinine that occurs in acute renal failure can be considered a direct reflection of decreasing rates of glomerular filtration. Thus, the daily rise in serum creatinine is approximate to the daily production rate minus the residual glomerular filtration and urinary excretion. In this setting, serum creatinine will rise 1 to 1.5 mg./dl./day in patients with near cessation of glomerular filtration. In settings of increased or decreased creatinine production the daily rise in serum creatinine due to acute renal failure will vary. For instance, in myohemoglobinuria due to crush injury or traumatic rhabdomyolysis the rise in the production rate of serum creatinine is markedly accelerated, and the daily creatinine increments can be much greater than 1.5 mg./dl./day. Also, when creatinine production is decreased, as in patients with decreased muscle mass and cirrhosis, the daily rise in serum creatinine as acute renal failure supervenes, as in the hepatorenal syndrome, will be less than 1 mg. per day with comparable degrees of acute renal failure.

Urea, an end-product of protein metabolism, is also handled by glomerular filtration and is retained in disease states associated with decreases in glomerular filtration rates. However, in contrast to creatinine, urea is partially reabsorbed. Thus, in catabolic states associated with dehydration, the daily rises in urea can be much greater than those of creatinine, since both increased urea production and enhanced urea reabsorption are contributing to the observed increments in plasma urea. This is a hallmark not only of prerenal azotemia but also of acute renal failure when tissue catabolism is accelerated. In this setting, the normal blood urea nitrogen to creatinine ratio, which is 10–15, quickly becomes distorted as urea concentrations rise much more rapidly than creatinine concentrations. The increased urea to creatinine ratios in the plasma reflect the degrees of tissue catabolism when these substances are used to follow patients with acute renal failure.

Actual estimations of glomerular filtration rate by urea and creatinine clearance rates may be useful in patients with acute renal failure. In oliguric acute renal failure, patients manifest creatinine clearance rates of less than 2 ml./min. However, patients with nonoliguric acute renal failure may have creatinine clearance rates of 2 to 10 ml./min. The nonoliguric patient with less severe impairment of glomerular filtration rate is much easier to manage in terms of fluid and electrolyte balance because he has significant residual renal function. This is probably the major reason why the prognosis of nonoliguric acute tubular necrosis may be better than that of the oliguric variety.

The renal handling of creatinine and, to some degree, of urea can also be used in a diagnostic sense to differentiate the various forms of acute renal dysfunction. This will be considered in greater detail in the section on diagnosis. However, the physiological basis of altered ratios of urine to plasma (U/P) creatinine or urea in acute renal failure is severely deranged reabsorption of salt and water. Urine tends to resemble a plasma ultrafiltrate in its concentration of water and solute, and this is reflected in a reduction of the urine to plasma concentration ratios of creatinine and urea.

Uric acid, the end-product of purine metabolism, is also retained in acute renal failure. Uric acid is handled in the kidney both by glomerular filtration and tubular reabsorption and secretion. Therefore, the relationship between increasing plasma uric acid and decreasing glomerular filtration rate is less direct than the relationship between plasma creatinine and glomerular filtration rate. In most forms of acute renal failure, serious rises in plasma uric acid are infrequent, and plasma concentrations of uric acid from 8 to 12 mg./dl. are the rule. In certain forms of tubular necrosis, especially those associated with rhabdomyolysis or extreme tissue catabolism, extremely high levels of uric acid can be seen. The retention of uric acid becomes a threat owing to the potential for crystallization of uric acid in tubular lumina. Practically, a level of uric acid greater than 13 mg./dl. should be considered to merit treatment by urinary alkalinization in those patients with sufficient residual urinary volume and glomerular filtration rate. In patients with severe oliguria, dialysis for control of uric acid levels may need to be considered.

In the recovery phase of acute renal failure, an increase in urine output is often observed before a measurable increase in glomerular filtration rate can be detected. This is due simply to a return of glomerular filtration in a few nephrons that do not as yet have reconstituted tubular function. The urine in this setting continues to show high fractional excretion rates of water and solute. Thus, the observed increase in urinary volume occurs without an increase in urea or creatinine clearance, and plasma levels of urea and creatinine continue to rise at the same rate seen during the oliguric phase. Part of the increase in urinary volume may be osmotically driven at this state, especially in patients who are not being aggressively dialyzed. However, once the number of nephrons returning to the functioning population increases to a degree sufficient to increase measurably the glomerular filtration rate, then the daily rises in creatinine and urea levels in the plasma diminish. In the predialysis era, the onset of significant recovery of acute renal failure often was heralded by a severe diuresis due to the excretion of retained metabolites such as urea. However, the use of dialysis in the routine management of patients during the oliguric phase of acute renal failure has markedly decreased the incidence of this osmotic diuresis in the early recovery phase.

In a normal individual, insensible water loss by vaporization from the skin and lungs is 12 ml./kg. body weight, or about 850 ml./day in a 70 kg. man. This is predominantly a water loss with few accompanying electrolytes. It is modified by rates of respiration, fever, the ambient temperature, and sweating. In the absence of water intake, insensible water loss will be partially compensated by endogenous water of oxidation formed from the catabolism of body fat and protein (1.07 ml. of water per gram of fat; 0.41 ml. of water per gram of protein). The water of oxidation made available in this manner is ordinarily about 300 ml./day, or about one third of the insensible loss, and must be considered as intake in calculations of the water balance. In oliguric patients with acute renal failure, numerous events usually result in a relatively large excess of body water, as verified by measurements of total body water. The catabolism of both fat and protein is usually markedly increased, and the utilization of fat in a patient with acute renal failure or in the postoperative or traumatic injury patient may be twice normal amount. These patients, therefore, produce far more endogenous water from oxidation than does a normal individual. This must be considered as water intake. Unfortunately, despite increased endogenous water production, excessive administration of fluids remains common in the management of acute renal failure. As a result of increased intake of both water and salt, both intracellular and extracellular volume expansion may occur and are often seen in patients with acute renal failure.

The majority of patients with acute renal failure exhibit some degree of hyponatremia. This decrease in sodium concentration is almost invariably secondary to dilution from excessive intake or administration of sodium free fluids and is increased by the increased production of endogenous water. Moderate hyponatremia per se is usually asymptomatic. However, since sodium is a major determinant of extracellular osmolality, enough water may be shifted intracellularly in response to osmotic demand to cause the signs and symptoms of water intoxication when the serum sodium concentration is markedly reduced (below 120 mEq./l.).

Urinary sodium concentrations reflect the disordered reabsorptive processes of solute by the acutely damaged tubular epithelium. Thus, high urinary concentrations of sodium are delivered from the proximal tubule to the distal parts of the nephron and usually appear in the urine. Urinary sodium concentrations in established oliguric acute renal failure usually are greater than 40 mEq./l., even in the face of vascular volume contraction of moderate degree. The increased distal tubular concentration of sodium may be important in maintaining the vasoconstrictive process that occurs in human acute renal failure. As discussed below, the high urinary sodium concentration may be used diagnostically.

Just as urinary sodium concentrations are reflective of abnormalities in solute handling in acute renal failure, isosthenuria is reflective of disordered water handling by the damaged nephron. Urinary water may be divided into two moieties: (1) that volume necessary to excrete all the urinary solutes in isosmotic proportions and (2) that urinary volume freed from solute during the urinary diluting process. These two moieties are referred to as the osmolar clearance (C_{osm}) and the free water clearance (C_{H_2O}) respectively. Thus, determination of urinary osmolality and plasma osmolality allows the determination of osmolar clearance, the formula for which is $C_{osm} = U_{osm} \times V/P_{osm}$, where U_{osm} equals urinary osmolality, V equals urinary flow in ml./min., and P_{osm} equals plasma osmolality. When U_{osm} is hypertonic to plasma the ratio of U_{osm} to P_{osm} will exceed 1, and therefore the $U_{osm}/P_{osm} \times V$ will exceed urinary volume. Thus: urinary volume (V) = $C_{osm} + C_{H_2O}$, and by rearranging, $C_{H_2O} = V - C_{osm}$. The free water clearance will have a negative value when the urine is hypertonic and a positive value when the urine is hypotonic. The generation of negative free water clearance values requires sodium chloride reabsorption in the ascending limb. Since this process is markedly deranged in acute tubular necrosis, so is the generation of negative free water clearance, and negative free water clearances move from a negative value toward zero. This may be used diagnostically as discussed below.

Potassium intoxication is one of the major causes of death in patients with acute renal failure. The marked reduction of urinary potassium excretion results from disruption of the process of tubular secretion of potassium into tubular fluid. This, in the presence of continuing breakdown of muscle protein, results in potassium accumulation in the extracellular fluid. This process is accelerated by catabolism, trauma and infection and by negative caloric balance and depletion of carbohydrate depots. Blood transfusions and the hemolysis of transfusion reactions also contribute to potassium intoxication. In the majority of patients with acute renal failure, significant hyperkalemia develops during the oliguric phase. This may become life-threatening in approximately one third of the cases in the absence of specific preventive therapy. The management of hyperkalemia is discussed in depth in a later section.

Acute renal failure is also complicated by the occurrence of metabolic acidosis. The metabolism of ingested foods and increased breakdown of body tissue, chiefly protein, in the face of renal shutdown results in the rapid accumulation of nonvolatile acids, chiefly sulfuric, phosphoric and organic acids. This increase in extracellular hydrogen ion is partly buffered by serum bicarbonate. Elevations of these acids contribute to the concentration of "undetermined anions," and therefore the metabolic acidosis of acute renal failure is typically an anion-gap acidosis. The metabolic acidosis may occasionally become severe and may be associated with the deep, labored, slow respirations known as Kussmaul's respirations. This degree of metabolic acidosis requires aggressive therapy.

The retention of phosphoric acids causes plasma phosphorus levels to rise, and this is usually accompanied by hypocalcemia. This hypocalcemia of acute renal failure rarely causes tetany, since the concomitant acidosis increases the proportion of ionized free calcium. However, if the metabolic acidosis is corrected rapidly, tetany may result from the reduced free calcium concentration. The hyperphosphatemia and hypocalcemia of acute renal failure causes increased production of parathyroid hormone. However, this increased rate of parathyroid secretion is in-

effective in correcting hypocalcemia. Thus, some degree of parathyroid resistance to parathyroid hormone action and changes in vitamin D metabolism are present in acute renal failure.

Serum magnesium also increases progressively during the oliguric phase of acute renal failure and decreases during the diuretic phase. Hypomagnesemia will occasionally be noted in the late recovery phase of acute renal failure. The hypermagnesemia seen in the early acute phase of acute tubular necrosis is rarely sufficient to cause a magnesium intoxication with central nervous system or cardiac depression. This has been seen but usually occurs only when serum magnesium levels reach 7 to 8 mEq./l. These levels are seldom reached during acute renal failure.

PRESENTATION AND DIAGNOSIS OF ACUTE RENAL FAILURE

Acute renal failure associated with trauma or surgery often occurs within the framework of complicated multiorgan damage or dysfunction. In the patient with massive trauma, circulatory stabilization may not be achievable in the emergency department, and immediate operative intervention may be necessary to control ongoing blood loss. When the patient has been stabilized, frequently after an operation of several hours' duration, individual organ function must be assessed.

Catheter drainage of the urinary bladder is an integral part of the management scheme for the victim of significant trauma and a mandatory maneuver for the patient with shock, blunt or penetrating abdominal injuries or major long bone fractures and pelvic injuries. Catheter drainage decompresses the bladder for diagnostic peritoneal lavage, provides indirect evidence of the integrity of the lower urinary tract, can be used for cystograms if necessary, and provides the first urine specimen for examination. If blood is present in the bladder specimen, it should alert the physician to the possibility of direct injury to the genitourinary tract. From this point on, including any intraoperative period, the hourly determination of urine output may be helpful in assessing the adequacy of extracellular volume or in showing the first signs of oliguria.

Although the presentation of acute renal failure may vary inconstantly according to the type and severity of the precipitating injury, oliguria, practically defined as a urine volume of less than 400 ml./day or 10 to 20 ml./hour, is a sign of renal dysfunction and requires differential maneuvers to define its etiology. Oliguria per se is not necessarily a sign of acute renal failure but may simply represent initially the normal physiological response to a decrease in renal blood flow that accompanies reduction in extracellular water, as with dehydration; alternatively, it may represent a more profound alteration to the circulating blood volume such as occurs with hemorrhage or a decreased cardiac output. These prerenal conditions are common causes of oliguria. Resuscitation of a patient from hypovolemic shock may not necessarily result in correction of oliguria. On the other hand, the persistence of oliguria does not guarantee a diagnosis of acute renal failure. Assessment of overall fluid and blood volume status is difficult, especially following major injury or extensive operations and their attendant fluid management. Under these circumstances, apparent normovolemia may be contradicted by a low urine output, and here spot urine samples and blood samples should be submitted for chemical determinations, as discussed below. Apparent normovolemia and adequate cardiovascular function should be confirmed by adequate blood pressure, pulse rate, pulse pressure, central venous pressure and pulmonary capillary wedge pressure measurements. A chest roentgenogram should be obtained, and chest auscultation should be performed to detect rales or gallop rhythms.

Oliguria in the surgical patient most commonly results from inadequate fluid or blood replacement, and when this seems likely, volume expansion may be both diagnostic and therapeutic. An acute expansion of the circulating blood volume by about 10 per cent or 500 ml. in 15 minutes would·be appropriate for a 70 kg. man. Fluids such as normal saline (0.9 per cent saline) should be used. If there is little or no response this maneuver can be repeated, provided there have been no significant changes in other measurements that indicate impending fluid overload. The fluid challenge is a common diagnostic maneuver, but it must be utilized with extreme caution in the older patient.

Clinical experience and certain physiological data suggest that mannitol administration may influence the course of early renal dysfunction by changing intrarenal distribution of blood flow and perhaps preventing established acute renal failure. Similar claims have been made for furosemide,[8, 31, 48, 58, 73, 87] but currently these have not been established. When oliguria persists after restoration of blood volume and correction of hypotension, and initial urine samples have been submitted for appropriate chemical determinations, 50 to 100 ml. of 25 per cent mannitol (12.5 to 25 gm.) may be given intravenously over 10 to 20 minutes. Others have recommended the use of 40 to 80 mg. of furosemide as an initial dose that is doubled every 30 minutes until either diuresis is produced or several hundred milligrams have been administered. Large intravenous doses of mannitol may cause rapid expansion of the blood volume because of its osmotic effect; it too should be given with caution in the older patient. Ototoxicity has also been reported in association with large doses of furosemide, and, as noted elsewhere, large doses of this diuretic are thought to potentiate the nephrotoxicity of certain antibiotics. A few patients will respond to these diuretics even though they have suffered considerable renal damage. They have severe nonoliguric renal failure, and the physician must not be misled by the diuretic-induced response.

Just as prerenal causes of oliguria must be excluded, so should direct injury or mechanical factors (postrenal failure) be excluded. For the patient with blunt or penetrating abdominal or pelvic injuries that require an operation, intraoperative assessment of kidney size, presence of perirenal or retroperitoneal hematomas and bladder integrity should be made. In other postoperative patients presenting with acute renal dysfunction, severe oliguria and especially anuria should raise the possibility of ureteral injury or ligation, provided the bladder has been drained by catheter. The medical history and pertinent operative reports should be reviewed. Even in established cases of acute renal failure, intravenous urography and nephrotomography are useful.[33, 84, 100] In addition, renal sonography can also be used to determine dilatation of the renal collecting systems. Similarly, radioisotope renograms and renal perfusion scans are rapid and useful techniques for establishing the presence of blood flow to both kidneys and can occasionally detect obstruction. Less frequently, retrograde pyelograms or bulb ureterograms may be necessary to exclude obstruction. Common causes of urinary obstruction, such as renal stones and prostatism, may occur in the surgical patient and be completely unrelated to the surgical illness.

Laboratory Determinations

An unremarkable urinary sediment and normal urinary chemistries from the bladder urine should not mislead the clinician to think that renal damage has not occurred. Re-evaluation of the urinary sediment and urinary chemistry is especially important following resuscitation from shock and/or surgical procedures. This is especially true in the patient in whom oliguria persists in spite of clinically adequate restoration of circulatory function. If there has been direct injury to the genitourinary tract the value of the urinary sediment examination may be obscured. In prerenal azotemia, the sediment is usually unremarkable except for the presence of a few hyaline and finely granular casts. In acute renal failure, the sediment may show low-grade, microscopic hematuria, coarsely granular casts that usually include tubular epithelial cells, free epithelial cells and modest proteinuria. Darkly colored urine showing strong reactivity to benzidine or to dipsticks that detect blood, in the absence of significant hematuria, indicates either hemoglobinuria or myoglobinuria. In a clinical setting in which significant muscle injury from

crush or ischemia is suspected, a negative benzidine test should be followed by serum creatinine phosphokinase and uric acid determinations. Should either of these values be markedly elevated, one should begin the alkalinizing regimen (see later discussion) until the result of the urinary myoglobin determination is returned.

Oliguria does not necessarily occur in immediate proximity to the precipitating injury but may evolve over a period of several to many hours. It is in this clinical setting that urine and blood chemical determinations are most useful in differentiating etiologies. Table 7–5 summarizes useful diagnostic values in oliguric conditions. It should be cautioned that there may be some overlap in these values between the two types of renal dysfunction but that discrimination is usually possible on the basis of one or more of these determinations.

In prerenal dysfunction significant concentrating capacity is retained, and the urine specific gravity and urine osmolality will be high. The urinary/plasma (U/P) osmolal ratio will be greater than 1.5 and the free water clearance may approach −100 ml./hr. Both the U/P urea ratio and the U/P creatinine ratio will be elevated, but because filtered urea is partially reabsorbed, the U/P creatinine ratio is considered a more reliable index. In prerenal dysfunction there is a marked tendency for sodium retention, and therefore the urinary sodium valve is usually very low.

In contrast, acute renal failure is characterized by a loss of concentrating ability, and this is reflected in a fixed specific gravity equivalent to that of plasma, a low urine osmolality and a U/P osmolal ratio that, if less than 1.1, is highly diagnostic of acute renal failure. Similarly, free water clearance may move from a highly negative

TABLE 7–5. **Diagnostic Values in Oliguric Conditions**

	PRERENAL DYSFUNCTION	ACUTE RENAL FAILURE
Specific gravity	> 1.020	1.010–1.012
Urine Na+	< 20 mEq./l.	> 30 mEq./l.
U Na/(U/P creatinine ratio)	< 1.5	>1.98
Urine osmolality	> 400	< 400 mOsm./kg.
U/P osmolal ratio	> 1.5	< 1.1
Free H$_2$O clearance	< − 25 ml./hr.	− 15 to + 25 ml./hr.
U/P creatinine ratio	> 30	< 15
U/P urea ratio	> 10	≤ 5

value toward zero or an actual positive value. The U/P creatinine ratio falls and when it is below 15, it is highly diagnostic of acute renal failure. As mentioned, the U/P urea ratio is less reliable, but when it falls to 5 or below, it too has significant diagnostic importance. For the U/P urea ratio, intermediate values of 8 to 10 may be seen with evolving renal dysfunction; Baxter[12] reported that the U/P urea ratio commonly ranges from 8 to 15 following operation. He has noted that when acute renal failure is suspected, the administration of 1000 ml. of crystalloid solution is a useful diagnostic test — it will alter the ratio in the direction of normal but will not change it or will decrease it when acute renal failure is present. Baek et al.[9] described studies of osmolar and free water clearance in a series of 15 patients who developed acute renal failure following hypotension or hypoxia. As the renal failure became manifest, there was a decline is osmolar clearance, which averaged less than 40 ml./hr. 3 days prior to conclusive diagnosis of acute renal failure. In addition, there was an earlier appearance of free water clearances that approached zero. This range of -15 ml./hr. to $+15$ ml./hr. was seen in 11 of 13 patients at 72 or more hours preceding established diagnosis of acute renal failure, in 13 of 14 patients 48 hours before and in all 15 patients at the time of definitive diagnosis.

In seven patients who experienced an episode of shock there followed a period of marked positive free water clearance, averaging $+ 85$ ml./hr.; only one patient developed a picture of acute renal failure. In those patients with free water clearances near zero, there was virtually no response to intravenous furosemide, either in urine volume or in free water clearance. These authors suggested using furosemide as a confirmatory test.

Handa and Morrin[67] studied 10 patients with acute renal failure and 13 patients with prerenal dysfunction. In the group with established acute renal failure, the mean urinary sodium concentration was 51.4 ± 9.48 mEq./l. and the mean U/P creatinine ratio was 11.1 ± 1.12; in the group with prerenal failure, the mean urinary sodium concentration was 14 ± 4.2 mEq./l., and the mean U/P creatinine ratio was 42.5 ± 11.5. In spite of striking differences between these values for the two groups,

these authors noted significant overlap in values when individual patients were considered. They therefore created the "renal failure ratio," in which the urinary sodium concentration is divided by the U/P creatinine ratio. The value of this ratio is largely dependent on the fraction of filtered sodium excreted. When this ratio was applied, statistically significant differences were defined between the two patient groups.

Although the oliguria of an acute phase may show a modest response to expansion of extracellular volume, this does not guarantee the absence of significant renal injury that may become manifest by a progressive fall in urine volume and biochemical evidence of progressive azotemia over the succeeding few days. In this setting it is common for the acute trauma victim to have undergone massive fluid and blood therapy during resuscitation, anesthesia and extensive surgical procedures, and the gradually declining urine output may provoke excessive fluid administration, resulting in mild electrolyte imbalances and significant fluid overload. Similarly, nonoliguric acute renal failure presents with progressive azotemia or, all too frequently, pulmonary edema, unfortunately surprising the physician who has been satisfied with a numerically adequate urine volume. Retrospective scrutiny frequently discloses subtle evidence of renal dysfunction that, coupled with enthusiastic fluid administration, appears as mild hyponatremia, dependent edema and progressive weight gain.

Hemoglobinuria or myoglobinuria may be recognized in spite of normal or reduced urine volumes. There is increasingly good evidence that the renal dysfunction caused by these pigments is preventable by aggressive therapy if applied early. This condition should be immediately treated with an alkalinizing solution of mannitol and sodium bicarbonate (25 gm. mannitol; 2 ampules (89 mEq.) sodium bicarbonate in a liter of 5 per cent dextrose), which should be infused rapidly if the patient's volume status allows this or at 200 to 300 ml./hr. If there is a relative diuretic response, this solution can be used to replace quantitatively the urine output and can be continued until the urine is free of visible pigment. If there is no increase in urine volume, renal damage is likely, and the infusion should be limited to 1 liter. Since this pigment nephropathy is largely preventable by early aggressive therapy, the physician should have a high index of suspicion when caring for patients who have sustained crush or ischemic injury and patients in whom a transfusion-related hemolysis is suspected.

INITIAL MANAGEMENT

Maintaining Fluid, Electrolyte and Acid-Base Balance

The initial fluid and electrolyte therapy for the patient with acute renal failure may vary considerably according to the phase of the surgical disease and its therapy as well as the stage of the renal dysfunction. Resuscitation from massive trauma, hemorrhage or sepsis is directed toward restoration of adequacy of circulating blood volume and correction of hypotension. This therapy is guided by the patient's blood pressure, pulse, central venous pressure or pulmonary capillary wedge pressure, hematocrit and urine output. These fundamental guidelines pertain again when the patient with established acute renal failure, especially the oliguric variety, sustains a common complication such as gastrointestinal hemorrhage and septic shock and again requires colloid and crystalloid fluid resuscitation. The loss of urine output as a useful indicator of tissue perfusion does not change the validity of the interrelationships of other estimates of adequate blood volume and cardiac performance.

Following stabilization of such patients in a euvolemic state, anticipation of potential or impending renal dysfunction is mandatory and should elicit early diagnostic maneuvers, as previously described. Patients who have sustained acute renal failure require a cautious and thoughtful assessment of their fluid and electrolyte requirements. Accurate daily weights should be consistent with intake and output records. Progressive weight gain is expected acutely as fluids are administered to compensate for sequestration of body fluids in the area of injury, the surgical "third space" that accompanies burns, soft tissue trauma, inflammation and the like. Unless the process is a continuing one, sequestration is usually complete by 36 to 48 hours; after that, the semistarved, catabolic patient is expected to lose about 0.5

per cent or more of his body weight daily. After resuscitation many patients are overloaded with both salt and water, and early volume restriction is most important. While insensible water loss may normally be as high as 800 to 1000 ml./day, it is practical to underreplace this loss acutely to make allowances for the contribution of endogenous water as oxidation; this endogenous water may be strikingly increased by trauma, infection, fever and immobilization from 150 to 200 ml./day to 800 to 1000 ml./day. In addition, reabsorption of the "third space" fluid, which has been likened to an "autotransfusion," may cause serious overload, and this phenomenon should be anticipated in calculating approximate fluid requirements. In the absence of fluid overload and large specific ion losses from the gastrointestinal tract, additional administration of fluids and electrolytes is fundamentally restricted to quantitative replacement of water and sodium chloride losses. Potassium-containing solutions should be routinely avoided except under unusual circumstances. These patients may be remarkably unstable, and small fluid volumes may push the patient from hypotension to congestive heart failure. Mild congestive heart failure should be treated with digitalis and fluid restriction, but severe cardiovascular overload and pulmonary edema may require phlebotomy or urgent dialysis since most acute renal failure patients will not respond to diuretics. These gravely ill patients are frequently elderly, require mechanical ventilation, have relative or absolute hypotension in the face of congestive heart failure and require sensitive orchestration of multiple therapeutic modalities. Digitalis, pressors such as dopamine, and manipulation of mechanical ventilation dynamics such as determined by the PEEP (positive end-expiratory pressure) -compliance curve may be required to stabilize the patient. The pulmonary capillary wedge pressure determination is a most useful adjunct in the management of these patients.

The metabolic acidosis of acute renal failure is generally well tolerated by the patient, especially if dialysis is being employed. However, complications such as hemorrhage or sepsis that lead to hypovolemia and decreased tissue perfusion may contribute to a profound acidosis that, with hyperkalemia, may be rapidly fatal. Arterial blood pH, in addition to arterial blood gases, should be determined at frequent intervals. While progressive or severe acidosis (arterial pH 7.25 or lower) may be treated temporarily with intravenous sodium bicarbonate, restitution of normotension and normal tissue perfusion must be the primary therapeutic effort. For approximation of the intravenous dose of sodium bicarbonate, the bicarbonate deficit can be estimated using the body bicarbonate space as 40 per cent of the body weight. Approximately one third to one half of the calculated deficit may be replaced by rapid infusion of 7.5 per cent sodium bicarbonate (44.5 mEq./ampule). Treatment of acidosis in the presence of hypokalemia may lead to serious cardiac arrhythmias.

Hyperkalemia is a significant threat to life in the acutely ill patient with acute renal failure, and an aggressive management policy must be instituted early in the course of therapy. Hyperkalemia may be induced or worsened by the use of banked whole blood, by hemolytic reactions, devitalized tissue, retroperitoneal hematoma, gastrointestinal hemorrhage and potassium-containing drugs. Electrocardiographic monitoring is required and will usually show characteristic changes of hyperkalemia when the serum potassium is about 6.5 mEq./l. or higher. High peaked T waves, especially in the precordial leads, and prolongation of the P-R interval are the early characteristic signs that may be followed, as the potassium level rises, by loss of T waves, widening of the QRS complex, S-T depression and then profound QRS complex widening. The myocardial effects of hyperkalemia are potentiated by hyponatremia and counteracted by relative hypercalcemia. This effect of calcium forms the basis of the emergency medical management of profound hyperkalemia. For serum potassium levels of 7.0 mEq./l. or higher or electrocardiographic evidence of severe myocardial toxicity, intravenous calcium must be used under continuous electrocardiographic monitoring. Calcium gluconate (10 per cent solution) should be administered as a 5 to 10 ml. intravenous dose infused over 2 to 5 minutes. This dose may be repeated in about 5 minutes if electrocardiographic manifestations of hyperkalemic toxicity persist. If the patient has received digitalis, calcium infusion is contraindicated except under the direst of circumstances. Hyperkalemia may temporarily be treated by dextrose-insulin infusions, employing one unit of regular insulin per 2 gm. of dextrose infused. Since volume constraints are usual, we employ 50 ml. of 50 per cent dextrose administered over a 2- to 5-minute period. While sodium bicarbonate infusion can be used alone, its simultaneous use with glucose and insulin is preferred. Sodium bicarbonate, 7.5 per cent (44.5 mEq. in 50 ml. volume), can be infused rapidly, and the dose may be repeated at frequent intervals, especially if hypoperfusion and profound acidosis exist concurrently with the hyperkalemia. These therapeutic maneuvers are only temporary in effect, and a favorable therapeutic response must not mislead the physician. Hyperkalemia can recur with sometimes alarming rapidity. Only the use of cation-exchange resins and dialysis will remove excess potassium from the body. For the surgical patient with acute renal failure, the use of exchange resins may be impossible because of gastrointestinal dysfunction. In such a situation, temporizing pharmacologic management of hyperkalemia must be accompanied by preparations for dialytic treatment. For the most stable patient, especially in the interdialytic period, the use of cation exchange resins is effective. Polystyrene sulfonate (Kayexalate, Winthrop) exchanges approximately 1.7 to 2.5 mEq. sodium for 1 mEq. of potassium and removes approximately 1 mEq. of potassium per gram of resin. For oral administration, 20 to 50 grams of resin is dissolved in 100 to 200 ml. of 20 per cent sorbitol; this dose may be repeated every 3 to 4 hours for four to six doses. Administered orally, this preparation may cause considerable abdominal cramping and diarrhea, and integrity of the gastrointestinal tract is therefore an obvious requirement for its use. In addition, Kayexalate may be used as a retention enema, employing 50 gm. of resin and sorbitol in 200 to 300 ml. volumes. Its usefulness is limited by the ability of the patient to retain the enema for at least 30 to 60 minutes, although occasionally a balloon catheter may help accomplish this. If retention of the edema is achieved, it can be repeated several times. Although the resin is an effective means of removing potassium, it does so relatively slowly and may be quantitatively insufficient to manage the seriously hyperkalemic patient.

Frequent determinations of serum potassium, even at hourly intervals, are required to prevent this commonly lethal complication.

Sodium rich fluids are routinely employed in resuscitation from hypovolemia, and this usually causes considerable salt loading. Following stabilization of the patient, salt restriction is the rule. Unless the patient is expected to sequester a large volume of sodium-rich fluid in a surgical third space, only quantitative replacement of measured losses such as those from the gastrointestinal tract should be given. Normalization of serum sodium and chloride is usually achieved with dialysis, provided a quantitative replacement regimen is employed to deal with measured losses.

PERIOPERATIVE MANAGEMENT

One or more operative procedures may be necessary in the patient with established acute renal failure. A rational plan of management should be followed carefully to avoid certain common preventable complications.

Pre- and Postoperative Dialysis

Ideally, a well-controlled hemodialysis should be performed on the day prior to a scheduled operation. For the patient who has been a victim of massive trauma or who has experienced an unexpected complication such as massive gastrointestinal hemorrhage, this scheduled dialysis may not be possible. An anticipatory reaction to a pending crisis may allow a comparatively brief but effective hemodialysis treatment that may forestall the development of serious intraoperative metabolic complications such as hyperkalemia. Besides the requirement for reduction of azotemia, the hemodialysis treatment should be directed toward restoration of a euvolemic state. Ultrafiltration can be used to correct relative or absolute water excesses but should not be overly vigorous, since excessive ultrafiltration may lead to a contracted blood volume and a tendency for profound hypotension in association with the autonomic blockade of anesthesia. The intradialytic use of albumin is a useful maneuver to maintain adequacy of the plasma volume while allowing a net water loss through ultrafiltration. The patient's behavior during dialysis, especially muscle cramps, seizures, and/or hypotension requiring large volumes of saline and albumin for maintenance of blood pressure, should alert the surgeon and his anesthesiologist to the possibility that troublesome hypotension may accompany induction of anesthesia.

Correction of anemia is best accomplished during hemodialysis, since the threat of volume overload is minimal, as is the possibility of induced hyperkalemia from blood products. The use of frozen blood products not only minimizes the risk of transmission of hepatitis but minimizes the potassium load that is attendant on transfusion.

The catabolic stress following major trauma or operations may cause a significant acidosis and rapidly progressive hyperkalemia in the patient with acute renal failure. Several hours of dialysis against a zero potassium bath may be necessary, although this must be done with caution if the patient has received digitalis preparations. A serum potassium determination obtained at the conclusion of a hemodialysis treatment is not adequate proof that hyperkalemia is controlled, since some patients show a remarkable reaccumulation of serum potassium. A serum potassium value obtained 4 to 6 hours after hemodialysis will be an important indicator of the progression of hyperkalemia and will indicate the frequency with which this value must be repeated and perhaps treated. A serum potassium value immediately preceding an operation should ideally range from 3.5 to 5.0 mEq./l. Serum potassium values that are above this upper limit may require intraoperative medical management. It should be noted that the depolarizing muscle relaxant succinylcholine causes a rapid increase in serum potassium in normal and uremic subjects.[104] Although the increase is generally small, 0.5 mEq./l. of potassium,[75] it may cause hyperkalemic patients to suffer cardiac arrest. The pharmacology of various muscle relaxants in renal failure has been recently reviewed.[104] Hemorrhage that requires transfusions or sepsis may significantly alter the serum potassium level and may require intensive medical management as outlined, even following vigorous hemodialysis or in anticipation of the next. It is occasionally necessary to take the patient directly from the operating room to the hemodialysis facility. For the patient who has sustained trauma or operation or for whom an urgent operation is planned, hemodialysis should be conducted under regional heparinization.

Intraoperative Fluid and Electrolyte Management

Normal saline solutions alternated with 5 per cent dextrose and normal saline solutions are the fluids of choice for intraoperative administration. Potassium-containing solutions such as Ringer's lactate should, for the most part, be avoided. If significant acidosis and normal to high serum potassium values are present, then 5 per cent dextrose in half normal saline to which one ampule (44 mEq.) sodium bicarbonate has been added may be used or alternated with the normal saline solutions. If the preoperative serum potassium value is high, intraoperative medical management must be employed and the response determined by hourly serum potassium determinations. If insulin is used intraoperatively, blood glucose concentrations must be measured and hypoglycemia avoided. The rate of fluid administration depends, in part, on the type of operation and its duration. If the patient is oliguric, quantitative replacement of urine output is inconsequential, but in the patient with high output renal failure it may be necessary to account for urine output in calculating the intraoperative requirements. Crystalloid fluid administration at 5 to 10 ml./kg. of body weight/hr. may be necessary during the intraoperative period for major abdominal operations. Obviously these rates are estimates and may require modification in the presence of signs suggesting volume overload or volume contraction. Replacement of blood loss in the patient with a relatively contracted red cell mass should be quantitative. The pulmonary capillary wedge pressure measurement should be more commonly employed intraoperatively.

In spite of rigorous regional heparinization techniques employed during hemodialysis, relative differences in heparin and protamine metabolism may occur, manifesting as a "heparin rebound." The uremic patient has well-defined coagulation defects, most specifically reduced platelet adhesiveness.[47] Either or both of these phenomena may be associated with diffuse intraoperative bleeding. Heparin "re-

bound" anticoagulation can be identified by a prolonged partial thromboplastin time and can be corrected with small intravenous doses of protamine sulfate (not to exceed 50 mg. protamine sulfate in a 10-minute period). If there is unusual bleeding in the absence of a readily demonstrable coagulation defect, as in practice seems to be rather common, intravenous administration of fresh frozen plasma seems clinically useful although of unproven merit.

POSTOPERATIVE MANAGEMENT

In the acute renal failure patient it may be assumed for practical purposes that measured and calculated losses are quantitatively replaced, whereas the anticipated third space loss must be estimated, based on the usual parameters of blood pressure, pulse, central venous pressure and the like. Fluid and electrolyte replacement should account for an insensible loss of 10 to 12 ml./kg. of body weight/day in addition to the urine output and other measurable losses, such as that from nasogastric suction. Provision must be made for sequestration of plasma according to the type of operation and disease process. This estimated volume may be frighteningly high in the functionally anephric patient who has extensive peritonitis, small bowel obstruction or pancreatitis. The fluid loss to the surgical third space, to the lumen of the bowel in obstruction or in peritonitis is protein-rich, containing 30 to 50 gm./l. Replacement of this protein sequestration may be accomplished by the administration of albumin, 12.5 to 25 gm. every 4 to 6 hours. One of two ml./kg. body weight/hour is not an uncommon rate for anticipation of loss to the surgical third space. Again, potassium-containing solutions are usually avoided. In planning fluid management, one must anticipate eventual reabsorption of the third-space fluid, usually after 36 to 48 hours, and be prepared to reduce intravenous fluid volumes to avoid serious volume overload. Too, the usually inconsequential production of endogenous water may be substantially increased by sepsis or massive trauma and must be accounted for in planning fluid balance.

Medical management of hyperkalemia is more problematic in the postoperative patient in whom the use of oral cationic exchange resins may be contraindicated or inadvisable and in whom the use of retention enemas of the cationic exchange resin type is ineffective. The use of insulin, sugar and sodium bicarbonate is only a temporary measure with limited effectiveness, and rapid escape from its effects is usual. Early hemodialysis may be required, although when possible it is desirable to wait at least 24 hours following a major operative procedure before beginning the next hemodialysis treatment. Again, hemodialysis with strict regional heparinization techniques may be necessary immediately or soon after any operative procedure. Careful intradialytic monitoring of Lee-White clotting times followed by determination of partial thromboplastin time 4 to 6 hours after dialysis may prevent serious hemorrhage in the operative site. In contrast to the chronic hemodialysis patient who is relatively stable in the interdialytic period, the post-traumatic or postoperative acute renal failure patient may be notoriously unstable and must be followed most carefully to avoid progressive acidosis and life-threatening hyperkalemia.

DIURETIC PHASE MANAGEMENT

After the usual 10- to 14-day period of oliguria in oliguric acute renal failure, the patient commonly begins the diuretic phase with gradual incremental changes in urine output, but the diuresis may start abruptly and be profound. While the diuretic phase heralds recovery, it must be remembered that approximately 25 per cent of the deaths occur during this phase. Renal function is still abnormal and strict attention must be paid to fluid and electrolyte balance during this phase. The striking water and salt losses that occur usually require quantitative replacement, even parenterally. Serious volume contraction can occur rapidly. Daily weights and blood chemistries must be obtained, strict intake and output records maintained, and urinary sodium and potassium losses quantitated. Natruresis is usual and may exceed 300 to 400 mEq./day. Kaliuresis may also occur and require quantitative replacement to prevent serious hypokalemia. Hypercalcemia has been reported during this phase.[125] As renal function returns to normal, urine volumes begin to decline. If polyuria persists longer than 5 to 6 days after the onset of the diuretic phase, one should consider the possibility that the diuresis is now promoted by excessive volume expansion. Careful reduction of fluid and salt administration should be initiated while weights, output, blood pressure, pulse and serum and urine electrolytes are monitored.

Should the patient in the diuretic phase of acute renal failure require an operation, the fundamental guidelines presented earlier apply to his management. For major procedures catheter drainage of the bladder is probably mandatory; quantitative replacement of the urine volume may be necessary. Potassium excretion may be impaired, so potassium loading can still cause lethal hyperkalemia.

DIALYTIC THERAPY IN ACUTE RENAL FAILURE

The widespread availability of intermittent hemodialysis therapy for acute renal failure in the early 1950's had an immediate effect on the outcome of trauma-related acute renal failure.[111] The mortality rate prior to the advent of hemodialysis was 80 to 90 per cent, but with the availability of intermittent dialytic therapy, mortality dropped immediately to around 50 to 60 per cent. However, since 1955, there was relatively little improvement in the mortality rates from acute renal failure until a further improvement in survival was recently reported in association with intensive dialytic therapy combined with hyperalimentation. A controlled evaluation of prophylactic dialysis in post-traumatic acute renal failure was recently reported by Conger.[39] The patients in the study were divided into two groups; the first group was dialyzed daily and the second was dialyzed intermittently only when the BUN approached 150 mg./dl. or when there was another indication for dialysis. Five of eight patients in the intensely dialyzed group survived, compared to two of eight in the control group. The incidence of sepsis appeared to be higher in the control group. While this study is problematic because of its small size, it suggests that dialysis, in and of itself, may play a role in decreasing the incidences of sepsis and gastrointestinal hemorrhage in acute renal failure.

From 1955 to 1977 most of the clinical studies on the efficacy of dialytic therapy have compared current experience with acute renal failure with that of the past. They generally have concluded that despite the initial drop in mortality of acute renal failure associated with the advent of dialysis, the continuing high mortality rate was due to an absence of an effect of dialysis therapy on sepsis. Further, they concluded that this complication has become the major cause leading to death in a patient with acute renal failure. The second leading cause of mortality, gastrointestinal hemorrhage, may be more responsive to aggressive dialysis.[74] In recent years the use of parenteral hyperalimentation has been combined with frequent, usually daily, hemodialysis in patients with acute renal failure following severe trauma. Preliminary reports suggest that this mode of therapy has been effective in decreasing the incidence of sepsis and improving mortality rates.[2]

The major therapeutic goals of intermittent dialytic therapy in acute renal failure can be categorized as follows: control of azotemia and establishment of sodium and water balance, potassium balance, acid-base balance, and calcium-phosphorus balance. The severity of the abnormalities varies considerably in acute renal failure, as does the presence or absence of the other manifestations of the uremic syndrome. These and other clinical parameters must be considered together to reach the most appropriate application of dialysis therapy.

Control of Azotemia

The control of azotemia is generally based on control of serum urea concentrations in spite of the lack of a well-defined experimental relationship between urea concentration and the complications of uremia. However, urea concentrations indirectly reflect the degree of catabolism in post-traumatic acute renal failure. On the basis of clinical experience, the general recommendation is to maintain the blood urea nitrogen below 80 mg./dl., and thus the duration and frequency of dialysis should be sufficient to achieve this level.

Owing to the degree of tissue injury sometimes seen in association with post-traumatic renal failure, the initial dialysis treatment is often performed in the presence of extremely high blood urea nitrogen levels, and because of this there is an in-

creased incidence of post-dialysis disequilibrium syndrome. Although the pathogenesis of dialysis disequilibrium is not clear, it is probably related to an increase in idiogenic osmols produced in the central nervous system in association with rapid removal of urea from extracellular fluid and correction of the metabolic acidosis. Therefore, care must be taken during the first dialysis treatment to reduce urea concentrations at a slower rate than might normally be accomplished. Generally, a reduction of urea concentration by 40 to 50 per cent with the first dialysis is a safe recommendation.

Control of Sodium and Water Balance

There is tremendous variability among patients in terms of the degree of fluid overload that occurs and the need for ultrafiltration during intermittent dialytic therapy for acute renal failure. It is important to establish the amount of ultrafiltration required for optimal control of vascular volume and also the degree of ultrafiltration that the patient can tolerate. This latter parameter varies directly with the patient's circulatory status. Frequently, hypotensive patients require hemodialysis in the setting of acute renal failure, and they obviously cannot tolerate ultrafiltration. The judicious use of vasopressor agents, salt-poor albumin, and/or packed red cell transfusions, depending upon the overall clinical assessment of circulating blood volume, may be beneficial in maintaining or controlling sodium and water balance.

Control of Hyperkalemia

The most common acute life-threatening problem to be controlled by dialysis is hyperkalemia. Although less common, hypokalemia, especially in patients on digitalis therapy, may also need to be controlled during dialysis. The removal rate of potassium by the dialyzer must be closely tailored to the clinical situation and should be discussed prior to institution of dialysis therapy. In cases of severe trauma the rate of tissue catabolism is such that a reduction in plasma potassium by dialysis will be followed shortly by rapid increases in plasma potassium. In such a patient, only prolonged and frequent dialytic therapy can control potassium levels. In addition, in the intervals between dialytic therapy, temporary measures may still be required to control potassium balance. When hyperalimentation is combined with dialytic therapy for acute renal failure, potassium depletion may occasionally occur and will tend to inhibit the stimulation of protein anabolism. Therefore, careful monitoring of potassium levels in the late maintenance phase of acute renal failure is very important.

Control of Acid-Base Homeostasis

Acetate rather than bicarbonate is generally added to the dialysis fluid for the correction of metabolic acid-base disturbances. However, in patients with sepsis or patients with an unstable circulatory status, the ability to metabolize acetate is diminished, and in these instances substitution with bicarbonate is required for correction of the acidosis. In patients with large gastrointestinal losses of hydrogen ions due to nasogastric suction, the high endogenous bicarbonate generation rate may contribute to a severe metabolic alkalosis. In these patients a low bicarbonate or relatively low acetate dialysate is required to correct the alkalitic abnormality. Generally, however, dialysis therapy with short interdialytic intervals controls the acidosis associated with acute renal failure.

Control of Calcium and Phosphorus Balance

Finally, dialysis therapy is of limited help in controlling the hyperphosphatemia and hypocalcemia associated with acute renal failure. Appropriate phosphate-binder therapy is needed to gain effective control of hyperphosphatemia in patients who are able to eat. In patients with rhabdomyolysis or severe crush syndrome, where tissue breakdown is extremely rapid, daily dialysis may be required to maintain phosphorus and uric acid levels within tolerable ranges.

Dialysis therapy has altered the frequency and severity of uremic symptomatology in association with acute renal failure. Uremic pericarditis associated with acute renal failure or severe metabolic encephalopathies is less frequently seen in present-day

medicine. However, the occurrence of these complications of renal failure must be kept in mind, as must the less severe uremic features of pruritus, peripheral neuropathy and gastrointestinal ulcerations. All these problems may complicate acute renal failure in individual patients and are variously responsive to intermittent dialytic therapy.

Peritoneal Dialysis

Peritoneal dialysis may be a useful part of the dialytic therapy of patients with acute renal failure. This is especially true when there is no available hemodialysis or when the institution of dialysis has been delayed. In the latter case, the patient with pronounced azotemia may be at special risk for development of the dialysis disequilibrium syndrome. In this setting the inherent slowness of peritoneal dialysis may dictate its choice as the first dialysis treatment. Peritoneal dialysis is not contraindicated in patients who have sustained abdominal trauma or who are in the immediate postoperative period[116] and is favored by some for patients with acute renal failure and intraabdominal sepsis.[85] Peritoneal dialysis has been performed successfully in such patients without necessarily increasing risk of infection, peritonitis or failure of the wound to heal. The technique of peritoneal dialysis, while not especially complicated, is best performed by someone trained in its use but can be performed with relative safety by any physician who follows the description of the techniques of peritoneal dialysis that have been published. In general, hypertonic dialysis solutions are rarely indicated, since adequate fluid removal can almost always be obtained by using the 1.5 per cent dialysis solutions. The increased rate of fluid removal induced by the hypertonic dialysis solutions has not been shown to be necessary, since the concomitant increase in hyperosmolar status significantly complicates the use of these solutions.

The complications of peritoneal dialysis are largely iatrogenic, usually from placement of the catheter, and include bowel or bladder perforation. Such complications may be especially common in patients who have had abdominal surgery or abdominal trauma but may be avoided by intraoperative placement of the catheter. The treatment of peritonitis may be aided by antibiotics instilled with the dialysate. Transperitoneal absorption of antibiotics will occur, and serum concentrations of potentially nephrotoxic drugs should be assayed. In addition, the use of the new Tenckhoff catheters makes possible the repeated use of peritoneal dialysis if it is required for management of the patient. Compared to hemodialysis, peritoneal dialysis has definite disadvantages in the management of patients with trauma-related or surgery-related acute renal failure. These include a prolonged time for adequate therapeutic effect to be obtained and an accentuated protein loss that further complicates the catabolic state associated with acute renal failure. Thus, in the most common situation hemodialysis is the appropriate mode of maintaining the patient during the maintenance phase of acute renal failure.

DIETARY MANAGEMENT OF ACUTE RENAL FAILURE PATIENTS

Malnutrition contributes significantly to the morbidity and mortality of the victim of acute, profound injury or major operative procedure, since enteral feeding is frequently impossible for prolonged periods of time. The imposition of acute renal dysfunction compounds the problem of dietary management, since in general there is a reduction or loss of the capacity to excrete water, electrolytes and especially the nitrogenous metabolites of an accelerated catabolic phase. Independent advances in dietary management of patients with profound surgical illnesses and of patients with chronic renal failure[120] have converged to provide definition of certain basic principles that can be applied in the management of the surgical patient with acute renal failure. This topic has been reviewed by Able[1] and Chapman et al.[34]

For the surgical patient with acute renal failure, optimal dietary therapy must (1) provide sufficient calories to reverse the loss of lean body mass through protein catabolism; (2) provide essential substrates, including nitrogenous compounds and vitamins, to induce net protein anabolism; (3) stabilize or reduce the rate of urea produc-

tion; and (4) minimize electrolyte and metabolite abnormalities.

Early studies recognized the "protein-sparing" effects of dietary carbohydrates, and a high carbohydrate content has been the foundation of most subsequently developed diets. Meeting this caloric requirement is problematic in itself since the acutely ill, hypercatabolic patient may require 50 kilocalories per kilogram of body weight per day or more. Carbohydrate and fat-rich diets were generally unsuccessful in chronic renal failure patients, and furthermore, additions of even small amounts of protein caused an increase in endogenous urea production. The elegant studies of Rose and his colleagues defined certain amino acids as essential and others as nonessential and quantitated the daily requirements of the essential amino acids in normal volunteers.[10, 97, 98] This definition of the minimal requirement of essential amino acids led to the clinical dietary studies of Giordano,[63] who devised a high-carbohydrate, low-protein diet composed of proteins of "high biologic value" (high essential amino acid content) for uremic patients. He concluded, on the basis of an observed decrease in azotemia in spite of a positive nitrogen balance, that urea and other nitrogenous compounds were being utilized for protein synthesis. Similar observations, based on a high-carbohydrate, protein-deficient diet with either essential amino acids alone or proteins of high biologic value, were made by Giovannetti and Maggiore.[64] Numerous other studies documented a reduced rate of blood urea nitrogen when renal failure patients were treated with the Giordano-Giovannetti type diet. This has been interpreted to show that urea nitrogen is reutilized for synthesis of nonessential amino acids following enzymatic hydrolysis of urea by bacteria in the gut. While this undoubtedly occurs, it now appears, in light of recent experiments,[6, 88, 117, 119] that reutilization of urea nitrogen is quantitatively insignificant. Nevertheless, these studies conclusively proved that administration of sufficient calories, usually in the form of carbohydrates and fats combined with a minimal amount of essential amino acids, could reverse established catabolism and in a few cases slow progression of renal disease and provide a positive nitrogen balance and a general improvement in overall health.

Both the oral diets and the parenteral diets developed subsequently contain essential amino acids in quantities and proportions that were defined for normal volunteers. However, it has been shown that the requirements for essential amino acids are twice as high in the chronic renal failure patient as in the normal individual,[17] and the actual requirement for amino acids in acute renal failure has not been determined. There are recognized abnormalities in the plasma amino acid pattern in acute and chronic renal failure patients, and other abnormalities are now being recognized in the quantitatively important intracellular free amino acid pool. Specific differences in the plasma amino acid pattern and intracellular free amino acid pool have been identified for chronic uremic patients as compared to starved, catabolic postoperative patients.[17] Furthermore, hemodialysis removes amino acids,[126] and peritoneal dialysis removes amino acids and up to 50 to 60 grams of protein per day.[18] The superimposition of acute renal failure on the patient with starvation and postoperative catabolism adds to the complexity of the problem, which presently has no clear definition. It seems likely, based on several studies, that histidine behaves as an essential amino acid in the uremic state,[17, 59] and in addition, its specific metabolism may also be altered, since abnormally high plasma concentrations of 1- and 3-methylhistidine have been identified in uremic patients.[38] Histidine probably should be included with the eight essential amino acids in parenteral hyperalimentation and is currently available in an oral, high calorie, essential amino acid supplement preparation (see later, p. 173).

The concepts that culminated in an oral diet of the Giovannetti-Maggiore type led to the creation of a parenteral preparation composed of hypertonic glucose and essential l-amino acids, again in the proportions and concentrations required for normal subjects. This parenteral hyperalimentation solution was administered to surgical patients with acute renal failure,[46, 123] and weight gain, wound healing and positive nitrogen balance were achieved in these patients. Able and colleagues,[2] in a prospective double blind clinical trial, evaluat-

ed the efficacy of intravenous hyperalimentation in the treatment of acute renal failure patients, most of whom were postoperative. In this study, parenteral administration of hypertonic glucose and essential l-amino acids was compared with the use of hypertonic glucose alone. Twenty-one of 28 patients receiving this renal failure fluid recovered from acute renal failure compared to 11 of 25 who received glucose alone, and this difference was statistically significant. The salutary effects of hyperalimentation were apparent in the higher survival rate in the higher risk patients who had sustained severe complications of acute renal failure such as gastrointestinal hemorrhage and generalized sepsis. It was suggested that recovery from acute renal failure was hastened by the use of renal failure fluid in hyperalimentation, and the authors interpreted the data to show that survival was improved because of the overall duration of renal dysfunction. Baek et al.[10] studied 129 consecutive postoperative patients with acute renal failure and treated approximately half with hypertonic glucose alone and the other half with hypertonic glucose plus essential l-amino acids. The use of the amino acids solution was associated with a lower mortality and morbidity rate in patients who required dialysis as well as those who did not. While the group of patients receiving the glucose and amino acid infusion had a lesser incidence of hyperkalemia and hyperosmolality, these patients did not show a stabilization of blood urea nitrogen. This was probably related to the use of a protein hydrolysate as a source of amino acids. These hydrolysates contain a significant quantity of nonessential amino acids and peptides, and these contribute significantly to the nitrogenous load whose excretion is impaired. This underscores the value of using crystalline essential amino acids in the parenteral hyperalimentation fluid when these become generally available.

In a small blind-controlled study, Leonard et al.[80] could not show an increased survival rate of patients with acute renal failure treated with essential l-amino acids and hypertonic glucose compared to a group treated with hypertonic glucose alone. In addition, there were no significant differences between the serum potassium and phosphate concentrations of the two groups. The mortality of patients with acute renal failure did not seem to be improved in an uncontrolled, collected series of patients from 18 independent medical centers, but again there was confirmation that electrolyte management was improved and that the rate of rise of the blood urea nitrogen was significantly reduced by the use of hyperalimentation solutions employing dextrose and amino acids.[106] In a series of anephric, postsurgical patients Briggs et al.[24] showed a striking decrease in total body urea in those patients who had parenteral hyperalimentation with hypertonic dextrose and amino acids compared to the group treated with hypertonic dextrose alone.

Although the fluid restriction that is usually required for a stabilized, oliguric acute renal failure patient has been considered an impediment to effective hyperalimentation, it should be remembered that insensible losses are usually greater than expected and all other measured losses such as urine and gastrointestinal secretions can be replaced volumetrically by the thoughtful use of hyperalimentation solutions. The electrolyte content of the hyperalimentation solution should be dictated by the measured losses of electrolytes and by frequent determinations of blood chemistry. It should be noted that effective hyperalimentation, even in the patient with acute renal failure, may cause a reduction in the serum potassium and serum phosphate, and both electrolytes may be required as additives to the hyperalimentation regimen. Post-trauma and postoperative patients may have a decreased glucose tolerance, and uremic patients have a decreased glucose tolerance[76] and abnormalities of fat metabolism. Although both conditions are improved with dialysis, they are not eliminated. Abel[1] recommends an initial infusion rate of approximately 14 gm. of glucose per hour (30 ml./hr. of 47 per cent glucose solution) and recommends the use of regular insulin, 15 units/l. of solution, added directly to the intravenous solution should hyperglycemia persist at the minimal infusion rates. Higher concentrations of insulin may be added, depending on the individual patient response. Blood glucose concentration should be determined every 6 hours during the first few days of hyperalimentation and longer, according to the patient's response.

There is a limited experience with intravenous fat emulsion for parenteral dietary therapy in acute and chronic renal failure patients,[79] but neither the renal dysfunction nor its associated disordered fat metabolism is a contraindication to its use. As commercially available the preparation is isotonic, can be infused by a peripheral vein and is an acceptably concentrated source of calories (1.2 kilocal./ml. as 10 per cent emulsion). It can be used effectively in conjunction with each hemodialysis treatment in which, during the last 30 to 60 minutes of treatment, a liter of the intravenous fat emulsion can be infused and the patient simultaneously diafiltrated to remove approximately half the infused volume. This infusion is quantitatively complete since the fat emulsion is not removed from the blood by dialysis. Intravenous fat emulsion can be used as part of a total parenteral nutrition regimen, especially when volume restriction is not a major requirement or when relative or absolute glucose intolerance is a problem. Hypophosphatemia is less likely to occur in regimens employing fat emulsions, since a substantial amount of phosphate is available from the metabolism of the component phospholipids.

Vitamin supplements are especially important for the acute renal failure patient who requires dialysis because water soluble vitamins are lost in the dialysis process. Vitamins of the B complex, including pyridoxine, and ascorbic and folic acids are required and can be given intravenously or orally.

Central venous cannulation of parenteral hyperalimentation has well-identified risks and is not necessary in the acute renal failure patient who is undergoing dialysis by means of the Scribner shunt. Parenteral hyperalimentation solutions can be infused directly into the shunt adapted by a T-connector, and this is best accomplished by a constant infusion pump. Strict aseptic technique is mandatory. The Scribner shunt should suffice for most acute renal failure patients, although in a selected few the shunt described by Broviac and colleagues[26, 27] may be advantageous if parenteral hyperalimentation is required for a substantially longer period than hemodialysis. Should a central venous line be required, a percutaneous subclavian venous cannulation should probably not be performed on the side ipsilateral to a forearm Scribner shunt.

When the gastrointestinal function of the patient with acute renal failure is not severely impaired, it is possible to provide an adequate diet without the use of parenteral alimentation. There is a high calorie, essential amino acid supplement (Amin-Aid, McGaw) that provides 654 nonprotein kilocalories and the minimal adult requirement of essential amino acids plus histidine in 340 ml. volume. Since the product is very well absorbed proximally it can occasionally be used even in patients with enterocutaneous fistulae. The product has an insignificant cation content, but it is hyperosmolar (1125 mOsm./kg.). It should be administered initially in a more dilute form until patient tolerance increases; the most efficient administration is by continuous drip through an infant feeding tube, bypassing problems of palatability and minimizing the hyperosmolality effects such as nausea, sweating and diarrhea.

In the stabilized patient whose acute renal failure remains unresolved and who continues to require dialysis, normal gastrointestinal function will allow the use of a diet akin to that used by the chronic renal failure patients. This palatable diet allows about one gram of protein per kilogram of body weight and one milliequivalent of potassium per kilogram of body weight, up to 70 grams of protein per day and about 60 milliequivalents of potassium per day, although these quantities must be adjusted according to the response of the individual patient. A 4-gram sodium chloride restriction is usual, but frequently a greater restriction is required. Dietary phosphorus is usually restricted, and phosphate binders (basic aluminum carbonate or aluminum hydroxide) are coadministered with meals to reduce adsorption of phosphorus. A more stringent diet may be required for the patient for whom hemodialysis is no longer a frequent or necessary occurrence but in whom renal failure has not been totally reversed.

It seems likely that hyperalimentation should be considered for the surgical patient or trauma victim who sustains acute renal failure, although there have been few well-controlled studies to confirm its influence on the mortality rate of the disease. Anticipation of prolonged gastrointestinal dysfunction should cause the physician to consider specific nutritional support as an early maneuver rather than a late one. Since the average time of death follows the diagnosis of acute renal failure by only 8 days, it is obvious that early nutritional support is mandatory if its benefits are to be realized. It is logical that the improved nutrition and improved metabolic conditions will contribute to a reduction in morbidity and mortality, and these benefits probably outweigh the recognized complications of hyperalimentation by any of the several forms.

Keys to Drug Management

Many drugs and their active metabolites are excreted primarily by the kidneys. Loss of some or all renal function requires quantitative adjustment of dosages of these medications. Quantitative adjustments in drug dosage have a twofold purpose: (1) avoidance of toxic accumulation and (2) assurance of therapeutic concentrations. This adjustment must reflect the fact that hemodialysis and, to a lesser degree, peritoneal dialysis remove certain drugs with an efficiency that is inversely related, in part, to drug-protein binding. It should be emphasized that therapeutic generalizations from one drug to another within a general class (e.g., the penicillins) are unwise and potentially dangerous. For example, since oxacillin and dicloxacillin are removed in insignificant amounts by hemodialysis, an extra postdialysis dose of these drugs is unnecessary for maintenance of therapeutic levels; however, ampicillin and carbenicillin are removed by hemodialysis, and therefore an extra dose is required. This "booster" dose is especially important for medications whose interdose intervals are quite prolonged because of severe renal dysfunction. Similarly, hemodialysis may remove a drug such as cefazolin that is not significantly affected by peritoneal dialysis.

It is beyond the scope of this chapter to detail administration of the many drugs that may be required by surgical patients with acute renal failure. Instead, guidelines are presented for some commonly used drug classes, and specific recommendations are given for certain management situations. It is imperative for the clinician to study the specific pharmacologic factors of any drug administered to a patient with renal failure.

The reader is referred to the recent extraordinary review of guidelines for drug therapy in renal failure by Bennett et al.[16]

Antibiotics. This may be the most common class of drugs employed in the surgical patient with acute renal failure, and excellent reviews of the subject exist.[1, 16, 124] Of the antibiotics commonly employed for serious surgical infection, only oxacillin, cloxacillin, dicloxacillin, nafcillin, doxycycline, erythromycin, clindamycin and chloramphenicol are administered without dosage or interval change in patients with severe renal dysfunction. Other antibiotics, such as the aminoglycosides, must be adjusted by dose reduction, interdose interval prolongation or both, and formulas and nomograms are available for some drugs.

Gentamicin is the hallmark drug of the aminoglycoside antibiotics; it has been studied extensively, and its characteristics provide insightful information about the class of drugs in general. Although the prevention of nephrotoxicity is extremely important, the use of this class of antibiotic requires thought to be effective. Noone et al.[90] showed that 30 per cent of patients receiving the recommended dose of gentamicin (3 mg./kg./day) did not get peak levels of higher than 3 μg./ml., an inadequate level to combat severe infections. This exemplifies the problem with the use of gentamicin and other aminoglycosides —namely, that there may be an unpredictable variation in serum levels in patients despite the use of conventional dosage schedules. Riff and Jackson[96] showed, for example, that red cell volume affects the serum concentration of gentamicin so that peak levels of the drug vary inversely with the hematocrit. Progressive anemia developing independently during the course of gentamicin therapy may result in toxic serum levels of the drug. In addition, gentamicin serum concentrations may be lower in febrile patients than in afebrile patients of the same body weight given the same dose of drug. In order to provide therapeutic levels of the antibiotic and at the same time prevent toxic accumulation, it is most important to monitor serum levels of these drugs when possible. Since about 70 per cent of gentamicin and the other aminoglycosides is excreted in the urine, impairment of renal function requires adjustment of the drug dosage. Even modest reductions in renal function re-

quire appropriate changes in the dosage schedule. Published guidelines for dosage alterations are only guidelines, and appropriateness of therapy must be monitored by serum concentration assays. This caveat is especially important in the patient with established acute renal failure who requires aminoglycoside antibiotics. If the patient has a measurable creatinine clearance, then drug dosage may be altered by the usual guidelines employing the clearance value and/or the serum creatinine. If the patient is undergoing hemodialysis and requires the use of an aminoglycoside antibiotic, a loading dose followed by interval administration is used. For gentamicin, the usual loading dose is 1.7 mg./kg. of body weight followed by a dose of 1 to 1.5 mg./kg. body weight after each dialysis treatment. For the hypercatabolic patient who requires daily dialysis, this dosage will probably require reduction, since an 8-hour hemodialysis treatment will remove only approximately 50 per cent of the administered gentamicin, and toxic accumulation can occur in spite of hemodialysis.

Gentamicin and other aminoglycosides, used singly or in combination with other drugs, have sufficient nephrotoxic potential to warrant careful monitoring of the patient. Since many patients with drug-induced nephrotoxicity are nonoliguric, it is mandatory to follow the guidelines utilizing the serum creatinine value as well as to monitor urine output. In this type of patient a slight rise in serum creatinine, even within the normal range, should be viewed with suspicion, and renal function should be assessed with creatinine clearances as well. It should be remembered that, among other side effects of these antibiotics, ototoxicity is prominent and is perhaps more common in patients with compromised renal function. The nephrotoxicity of these antibiotics is generally thought to be potentiated by advanced patient age, pre-existing renal disease, dehydration, prolonged administration of the drug, coexistent use of potent diuretics and concurrent use of other potentially neurotoxic and/or nephrotoxic drugs.

It must be remembered that some antibiotic preparations have a significant cation content. The potassium salt of penicillin contains 1.7 mEq./million units, and the sodium content of carbenicillin is 4.7 mEq./gram of antibiotic. A sodium salt of penicillin G is available for patients with potassium intolerance.

Antihypertensives. Hypertension can be a complication of acute renal failure or a pre-existing condition in the older victim of acute renal failure. Modest hypertension, except in the presence of congestive heart failure, is well tolerated and usually responds to restitution of the relatively normal fluid-salt balance achieved by dialysis. Acute exacerbations of hypertension may be commonly seen in the immediate postoperative period as the cardiodepressant and vasodilatory effects of anesthesia abate. The agitated patient who complains of pain can be treated with small (5 mg.) repeated intravenous doses of meperidine (watch for respiratory depression), and frequently the blood pressure falls as an analgesic and sedative effect is achieved. Persistent hypertension may be treated with hydralazine, 5 to 20 mg., intravenously; this dose (up to 20 mg.) may be repeated in 30 to 60 minutes. This drug should be used with caution in the patient with coronary artery disease, since there is a reflex tachycardia and increased cardiac work, and angina pectoris or myocardial infarction may be precipitated. Hypotension induced by hydralazine should be treated with norepinephrine. Maintenance doses may require a prolonged interval with severe renal failure.

An occasional transplant recipient, salt- and water-loaded but with an anuric kidney, or other postoperative acute renal failure patients may experience severe hypertension (systolic 180 mm. Hg or more; diastolic, 120 mm. Hg or more) and prove to be unresponsive to hydralazine. In such patients diazoxide, 300 mg., should be given as a bolus intravenously in less than 30 seconds. Its effects usually reach maximum extent by 5 minutes, and the patient should be continuously monitored. The dose can be repeated after 30 minutes if the response is unsatisfactory. The hypotensive effect of this drug may be striking or minimal, however, and the unpredictability of response and relative lack of control cause us to prefer continuous intravenous titration with sodium nitroprusside for management of severe hypertension. Sodium nitroprusside, used in a solution of 100 μg./ml of 5 per cent dextrose and water, the only solvent, is used in titration to bring the blood pressure to acceptable levels. Higher

concentrations may be used if fluid restriction is necessary. Thiocyanate, an active metabolite, is toxic, and prolonged use of nitroprusside in the patient with acute renal failure must be accompanied by assays of blood thiocyanate that should not exceed 10 mg./dl. This ion is dialyzable and this drug can be used effectively and safely in acute renal failure patients. The drug effect begins rapidly and is immediately lost with discontinuance of the drug. Nitroprusside is photosensitive, and any preparations must have a protective coating such as aluminum foil and may not be used for more than 4 hours before replacement with a fresh solution.

Alpha-methyl dopamine is usually given orally in three divided doses up to a total of 3 gm./day. It may be administered parenterally in a similar dose. Although theoretically the dose should be reduced in patients with severe renal failure, the blood pressure response, balanced against postural hypotension, is the best practical guide to the administration of this drug. Its antihypertensive effects are slow, and therefore it is inadequate for treatment of severe hypertension. The drug is effective, but postural hypotension is not rare; it is commonly used with orally administered hydralazine (200 to 400 mg./day in divided doses).

A few patients with normal or high renin levels will respond to oral doses of propranolol, a beta-adrenergic blocking agent. This drug is relatively contraindicated in the presence of congestive heart failure but is useful for coadministration with hydralazine, since some cardiac effects of hydralazine are blocked by propranolol. Propranolol, 10 to 80 mg., is given orally four times daily, with a smaller dose used in patients with severe renal dysfunction.

Cardiac Drugs. Digitalis preparations may be required for treatment of congestive heart failure. A baseline electrocardiogram is mandatory, as is a current serum potassium value. We prefer digoxin for oral or parenteral use. When the clinical situation allows it, the slow oral route is recommended for digitalization. The loading dose is theoretically the same for patients with normal or impaired renal function when this cardiac glycoside is given intravenously, but it should be somewhat lower if the slow oral route is used in the patient with renal failure. The average oral digitalizing dose for patients with normal renal function is 1.25 to 1.5 mg., given in divided doses over 12 to 24 hours. The average intravenous digitalizing dose is 0.75 to 1.25 mg., given as 0.5 mg. intravenously and in 0.125 to 0.25 mg. increments every 2 to 4 hours until digitalization has been achieved. For the patient with no renal function and dialysis, the maintenance dose of digoxin, 0.125 mg., is given every other day, orally or intravenously, on the interdialysis day. For the patient with impaired renal function, the *daily* maintenance dose of digoxin is calculated by the formula:[121] desired body content of digoxin (DBCD) = 0.1 to 0.2 mg./kg. × body weight.

The maintenance dose of digoxin = 14 + 0.2 × C_{Cr} (ml./min.) × DBCD, where an 80 kg. man with a creatinine clearance (C_{Cr}) of 15 ml./min. will have a desired body content of digoxin of 0.8 mg. (80 kg. × 0.1 mg./kg.) and will require a daily maintenance dose of digoxin of 0.136 mg. These and other formulas are guidelines only. It is most important to measure serum digoxin concentrations in these patients.

Lidocaine, given by continuous intravenous drip or as intermittent boluses, can be used to treat cardiac arrhythmias without modification of dose. Procainamide can be used acutely in standard dosage for treatment of major arrhythmias but must be administered at somewhat prolonged intervals for maintenance; no modification is necessary for quinidine sulfate. The propranolol dosage is modified only in maintenance doses.

Sedatives and Analgesics. Diazepam is generally used without dosage adjustment and is useful both for its tranquilizer and anticonvulsant effects. Morphine sulfate, meperidine, codeine, pentazocine and prophoxyphene are also used in standard dosage. Recently, however, an active metabolite of meperidine, normeperidine, has been shown to accumulate and cause seizures,[109] and a drug-related encephalopathy has been described for diazepam and flurazepam. These syndromes are probably caused by active, minor metabolites produced by the liver that accumulate to toxic levels in the absence of renal excretion.

Antacids. Magnesium-containing antacids are contraindicated in acute and chronic renal failure unless hyperalimenta-

tion has fortuitously induced hypomagnesemia. The aluminum-based antacids, acting also as dietary phosphate binders, are generally well tolerated, although a recently described, potentially lethal syndrome of dyspraxia and multifocal seizures[83] may be due to aluminum toxicity.[4]

SUMMARY

Acute renal failure is a catastrophic complication in the surgical patient, but it is a potentially reversible condition. Aggressive surgical and medical therapy is required, and great diligence must be exercised by the physicians responsible for the care of these patients. Only with the best application of contemporary techniques of patient management can we hope to reduce the unacceptable mortality of this complication.

REFERENCES

1. Abel, R. M.: Parenteral nutrition in the treatment of renal failure. *In* Fischer, J. E. (ed.): Total Parenteral Nutrition. Boston, Little, Brown and Company, 1976, p. 143.
2. Abel, R. M., Beck, C. H., Abbott, W. M., Ryan, J. A., Barnett, G. O., and Fischer, J. E.: Improved survival from acute renal failure after treatment with intravenous essential l-amino acids and glucose. N. Engl. J. Med., 228:695, 1973.
3. Abel, R. M., Buckley, M. H., Austen, W. G., Barnett, G. O., Beck, C. H., and Fischer, J. E.: Etiology, incidence, prognosis of renal failure following cardiac operations. J. Thorac. Cardiovasc. Surg., 71:323, 1976.
4. Alfrey, A. C., LeGendre, G. R., and Kaehny, W. D.: The dialysis encephalopathy syndrome; possible aluminum intoxication. N. Engl. J. Med., 294:184, 1976.
5. Ansari, Z., and Baldwin, D. S.: Acute renal failure due to radio-contrast agents. Nephron, 17:28, 1976.
6. Arendshorst, W. J., Finn, W. F., and Gottschalk, C. W.: Micropuncture study of acute renal failure following temporary renal ischemia in the rat. Kidney Int., (Suppl.) 10:S100, 1976.
7. Baek, S. M., Brown, R. S., and Shoemaker, W. C.: Early prediction of acute renal failure and recovery: I. Sequential measurements of free water clearance. Ann. Surg., 177:253, 1973.
8. Baek, S. M., Brown, R. S., and Shoemaker, W. C.: Early prediction of acute renal failure and recovery: II. Renal function response to furosemide. Ann. Surg., 178:605, 1973.
9. Baek, S., Makabali, G. G., Brown, R. S., and

Shoemaker, W. C.: Freewater clearance patterns as predictors and therapeutic guides in acute renal failure. Surgery, 77:632, 1975.

10. Baek, S., Makabali, G. G., Bryan-Brown, C. W., Kusek, J., and Shoemaker, W. C.: The influence of parenteral nutrition on the course of acute renal failure. Surg. Gynecol. Obstet., 141:405, 1975.

11. Baek, S., Makabali, G. G., and Shoemaker, W. C.: Clinical determinants of survival from postoperative renal failure. Surg. Gynecol. Obstet., 140:685, 1975.

12. Baxter, C. R.: Acute renal failure. In Shires, G. T. (ed.): Care of the Trauma Patient. New York, McGraw-Hill Book Company, 1966, p. 578.

13. Baxter, C. R., Zedlitz, W. H., and Shires, G. T.: High output acute renal failure complicating traumatic injury. J. Trauma, 4:567, 1964.

14. Beaufils, M., Morel-Maroger, L., Sraer, J. D., Kanfer, A., Kourilsky, O., and Richet, G.: Acute renal failure of glomerular origin during visceral abscesses. N. Engl. J. Med., 295:185, 1976.

15. Bennett, W. M., Plamp, C., and Porter, G. A.: Drug-related syndromes in clinical nephrology. Ann. Intern. Med., 87:582, 1977.

16. Bennett, W. M., Singer, I., Golper, T., Feig, P., and Coggins, C. J.: Guidelines for drug therapy in renal failure. Ann. Intern. Med., 86:754, 1977.

17. Bergstrom, J., Furst, P., Noree, L. O., and Vinnars, E.: Intracellular free amino acids in uremic patients as influenced by amino acid supply. Kidney Int., (Suppl.) 7:S345, 1975.

18. Berlyne, G. M., Lee, H. A., Giordano, C., de Pascale, C., and Esposito, R.: Aminoacid loss in peritoneal dialysis. Lancet, 1:1339, 1967.

19. Berne, T. V., and Barbour, B. H.: Acute renal failure in general surgical patients. Arch. Surg., 102:594, 1971.

20. Biber, T. U. L., Mylle, M., Baines, A. D., Gottschalk, C. W., Oliver, J. R., and MacDowell, M. C.: A study by micropuncture and microdissection of acute renal damage in rats. Am. J. Med., 44:664, 1968.

21. Bismuth, H., Kuntziger, H., and Corlette, M. B.: Cholangitis with acute renal failure: Priorities in therapeutics. Ann. Surg., 181:881, 1975.

22. Blantz, R. C.: The mechanism of acute renal failure after uranyl nitrate. J. Clin. Invest., 55:621, 1975.

23. Bobrow, S. N., Jaffe, E., and Young, R. C.: Anuria and acute tubular necrosis associated with gentamicin and cephalothin. J.A.M.A., 222:1546, 1972.

24. Briggs, W. A., Kaminski, M. V., Kyle, R. W., Light, J. A., and Yeager, H. C.: Hyperalimentation in anephrics. Acta Chir. Scand., Suppl. 466:100, 1976.

25. Brooks, D. H., and Schulhoff, J. W.: Acute nonoliguric renal failure in the postoperative patient. Crit. Care Med., 4:193, 1976.

26. Broviac, J. W., Cole, J. J., and Scribner, B. H.: A silicone rubber atrial catheter for prolonged parenteral alimentation. Surg. Gynecol. Obstet., 136:602, 1973.

27. Broviac, J. W., and Scribner, B. H.: Prolonged parenteral nutrition in the home. Surg. Gynecol. Obstet., 139:24, 1974.

28. Brown, C. B., Cameron, J. S., Ogg, C. S., Bewick, M., and Stott, M. B.: Established acute renal failure following surgical operations. In Friedman, E. A., and Eliahou, H. E. (eds.): Proceedings, Acute Renal Failure Conference, Washington D.C. (DHEW Publication #NIH 74–608.) Washington, D.C., U. S. Government Printing Office, 1973, p. 187.

29. Butkus, D. E., de Torrente, A., and Terman, D. S.: Renal failure following gentamicin in combination with clindamycin. Nephron, 17:307, 1976.

30. Cabanillas, F., Burgos, R. C., Rodriguez, R. C., and Baldizon, C.: Nephrotoxicity of combined cephalothin-gentamicin regimen. Arch. Intern. Med., 135:850, 1975.

31. Cantarovich, F., Fernandez, J. C., Locatelli, A., Loredo, J. P., and Cristhot, J.: Furosemide in high doses in the treatment of acute renal failure. Postgrad. Med. J., 47 (Suppl.):13, 1971.

32. Casali, R., Simmons, R. L., Najarian, J. S., von Haritizsch, B., Buselmeier, T. J., and Kjellstrand, C. M.: Acute renal insufficiency complicating major cardiovascular surgery. Ann. Surg., 181:370, 1975.

33. Cattell, W. R., and Fry, I. K.: Urography in acute renal failure. Am. Heart J., 90:124, 1975.

34. Chapman, A., Loirat, P., Beaufils, F., Rohan, J., and David, R.: Nutritional problems in patients with acute renal failure. Adv. Nephrol., 6:321, 1976.

35. Chugh, K. S., Aikat, B. K., Sharma, B. K., Dash, S. C., Mathew, M. T., and Das, K. C.: Acute renal failure following snakebite. Am. J. Trop. Med. Hyg., 24:692, 1975.

36. Chugh, K. S., Sharma, B. K., and Singhal, P. C.: Acute renal failure following hornet stings. J. Trop. Med. Hyg., 79:42, 1976.

37. Churchill, S., Zarlengo, M. D., Carvalho, J. S., Gottlieb, M. N., and Oken, D. E.: Normal renocortical blood flow in experimental acute renal failure. Kidney Int., 11:246, 1977.

38. Condon, J. R., and Asatoor, A. M.: Amino acid metabolism in uraemic patients. Clin. Chim. Acta, 32:333, 1971.

39. Conger, J. D.: A controlled evaluation of prophylactic dialysis in post-traumatic acute renal failure. J. Trauma, 15:1056, 1975.

40. Couch, N. P., Lane, F. C., and Crane, C.: Management and mortality in resection of abdominal aortic aneurysms. Am. J. Surg., 119:408, 1970.

41. Danielson, R. A.: Differential diagnosis and treatment of oliguria in post-traumatic and postoperative patients. Surg. Clin. North Am., 55:697, 1975.

42. Daugharty, T. M., Ueki, I. F., Mercer, P. F., and Brenner, B. M.: Dynamics of glomerular ultrafiltration in the rat. V. Response to ischemic injury. J. Clin. Invest., 53:105, 1974.

43. David, E., and Bernatz, P. E.: Diagnosis and management of ruptured abdominal aortic aneurysm. Postgrad. Med. J., 49:123, 1971.

44. Dawson, J. L.: Renal failure in obstructive jaun-

dice — clinical aspects. Postgrad. Med. J., 51:510, 1975.

45. Diaz-Buxo, J. A., Wagoner, R. D., Hattery, R. R., and Palumbo, P. J.: Acute renal failure after excretory urography in diabetic patients. Ann. Intern. Med., 83:155, 1975.
46. Dudrick, S. J., Steiger, E., and Long, J. M.: Renal failure in surgical patients; treatment with intravenous essential amino acids and hypertonic glucose. Surgery, 68:180, 1970.
47. Eknoyan, G., Wacksman, S. J., Glueck, H. I., and Will, J. J.: Platelet function in renal failure. N. Engl. J. Med., 280:677, 1969.
48. Epstein, M., Schneider, N. S., and Befeler, B.: Effect of intrarenal hemodynamics in acute renal failure. Am. J. Med., 58:510, 1975.
49. Falco, F. G., Smith, H. M., and Arcieri, G. M.: Nephrotoxicity of aminoglycosides and gentamicin. J. Infect. Dis., 119:406, 1969.
50. Fillastre, J. P., and Kleinknecht, D.: Acute renal failure associated with cephalosporin therapy. Am. Heart J., 89:809, 1975.
51. Fischer, R. P., and Polk, H. C.: Changing etiologic patterns of renal insufficiency in surgical patients. Surg. Gynecol. Obstet., 140:85, 1975.
52. Flamenbaum, W.: Pathophysiology of acute renal failure. In Kurtzman, N. A., and Martinez-Maldonado, M. (eds.): Springfield, Ill., Charles C Thomas, 1977, p. 795.
53. Flamenbaum, W., Hamburger, R. J., Huddleston, M. L., Kaufman, J., McNeil, J. S., Schwartz, J. H., and Nagle, R.: The initiation phase of experimental acute renal failure: An evolution of uranyl nitrate-induced acute renal failure in the rat. Kidney Int. (Suppl.), 6:S115, 1976.
54. Flamenbaum, W., Kotchen, T. A., Nagle, R., and McNeil, J. S.: Effect of potassium on the renin-angiotensin system and $HgCl_2$-induced acute renal failure. Am. J. Physiol., 224:305, 1973.
55. Flamenbaum, W., Kotchen, T. A., and Oken, D. E.: Effect of renin immunization on mercuric chloride and glycerol-induced renal-failure. Kidney Int., 1:406, 1972.
56. Flamenbaum, W., McDonald, F. D., DiBona, G. F., and Oken, D. E.: Micropuncture study of renal tubular factors in low dose mercury poisoning. Nephron, 8:221, 1971.
57. Fojas, J. E., and Schmid, H. E.: Renin release, renal autoregulation and sodium excretion in the dog. Am. J. Physiol., 219:464, 1970.
58. Fries, D., Pozet, N., Dubois, N., and Traeger, J.: The use of large doses of furosemide in acute renal failure. Postgrad. Med. J., 47 (Suppl.):18, 1971.
59. Furst, P.: N15 Studies in severe renal failure: II. Evidence for the essentiality of histidine. Scand. J. Clin. Lab. Invest., 30:307, 1972.
60. Gagnon, J. A., Murphy, G. P., and Teschan, P. E.: Renal function in the normotensive and hypotensive dog during hypertonic mannitol and dextrose infusions. J. Surg. Res., 4:468, 1964.
61. Gary, N. E., Buzzeo, L., Salaki, J., and Eisinger, R. P.: Gentamicin-associated acute renal failure. Arch. Intern. Med., 136:1101, 1976.
62. Gleysteen, J. J., Aldrete, J. S., and Rutsky, E. A.: Cholegraphy-induced acute renal failure: Its relation to subsequent surgical therapy. South. Med. J., 69:173, 1976.
63. Giordano, C.: Use of exogenous and endogenous urea for protein synthesis in normal and uremic subjects. J. Lab. Clin. Med., 62:231, 1963.
64. Giovannetti, S., and Maggiore, Q.: A low-nitrogen diet with proteins of high biological value for severe chronic uraemia. Lancet, 1:1000, 1964.
65. Gotta, A. W., Murray, D., Sullivan, C. A., and Seaman, J.: Post-operative renal failure caused by disseminated intravascular coagulation. Can. Anaesth. Soc. J., 22:149, 1975.
66. Hägnevik, K., Gordon, E., Lins, L. E., Wilhelmsson, S., and Forster, D.: Glycerol-induced haemolysis with haemoglobinuria and acute renal failure. Report of three cases. Lancet, 1:75, 1974.
67. Handa, S. P., and Morrin, P. A. F.: Diagnostic indices in acute renal failure. Can. Med. Assn. J., 96:78, 1967.
68. Hollenberg, N. K., and Adam, D. F.: Vascular factors in the pathogenesis of acute renal failure in man. In Friedman, E. A., and Eliahous, H. E. (eds.): Proceedings: Acute Renal Failure Conference, State University of New York, Downstate Medical Center, Brooklyn, 1973. (HEW Publication No. NIH 74–608. Washington, D.C., U.S. Government Printing Office, 1973, p. 209.
69. Hollenberg, N. K., Adams, D. F., Oken, D. E., Abrams, H. L., and Merrill, J. P.: Acute renal failure due to nephrotoxins. N. Engl. J. Med., 282:1329, 1970.
70. Hollenberg, N. K., Epstein, M., Rosen, S. M., Basch, R. I., Oken, D. E., and Merrill, J. P.: Acute oliguric renal failure in man: Evidence for preferential renal cortical ischemia. Medicine, 47:455, 1968.
71. Kennedy, A. C., Burton, J. A., Luke, R. G., Briggs, J. D., Lindsay, R. M., Allison, M. E. M., and Edward, N.: Factors affecting the prognosis in acute renal failure. A survey of 251 cases. Q. J. Med., 42:73, 1973.
72. Kirschenbaum, M. A., White, N., Stein, J. H., and Ferris, T.: Redistribution of renal cortical blood flow during inhibition of prostaglandin synthesis. Am. J. Physiol., 227:801, 1974.
73. Kleinknecht, D., Ganeval, D., Gonzalez-Duque, L. A., and Fermanian, J.: Furosemide in acute oliguric renal failure: A controlled trial. Nephron, 17:51, 1976.
74. Kleinknecht, D., Jungers, P., Chanard, J., Barbanel, C., and Ganeval, D.: Uremic and nonuremic complications in acute renal failure: Evaluation of early and frequent dialysis on prognosis. Kidney Int., 1:190, 1972.
75. Koide, M., and Waud, B. E.: Serum potassium concentration after succinylcholine in patients with renal failure. Anesthesiology, 36:142, 1972.
76. Kokot, F., and Kuska, J.: The endocrine system in patients with acute renal insufficiency. Kidney Int. (Suppl.), 6:S26, 1976.
77. Kornhall, S.: Acute renal failure in surgical dis-

ease with special regard to neglected complications. A retrospective study of 298 cases treated during the period 1960–1968. Acta Chir. Scand. (Suppl.), *419*:3, 1971.

78. Ladefoged, J., and Winkler K.: Hemodynamics in acute renal failure: The effect of hypotension induced by dihydralazine on renal blood flow, mean circulation time for plasma, and renal vascular volume in patients with acute oliguric renal failure. Scand. J. Clin. Lab. Invest., *26*:83, 1970.
79. Lee, H. A., Sharpstone, P., and Ames, A. C.: Parenteral nutrition in renal failure. Postgrad. Med. J., *43*:81, 1967.
80. Leonard, C. D., Luke, R. G., and Siegel, R. R.: Parenteral essential amino acids in acute renal failure. Urology, *6*:154, 1975.
81. Lordon, R. E., and Burton, J. R.: Post-traumatic renal failure in military personnel in Southeast Asia. Experience at Clark USAF Hospital, Republic of the Philippines, Am. J. Med., *53*:137, 1972.
82. Lucas, C. E., and Read, R. C.: Red cell crenation and the renal hemodynamic effect of mannitol. Surgery, *59*:408, 1966.
83. Mahurkar, S. D., Dhar, S. K., Salta, R., Meyers, L., Smith, E. C., and Dunea, G.: Dialysis dementia. Lancet, *1*:1412, 1973.
84. Mamdani, B. H., Mehta, P. K., Mahurkar, S. D., Sassoon, H., and Dunea, G.: High dose bolus urography: A superior technique in advanced renal failure. J.A.M.A., *234*:1054, 1975.
85. Matas, A. J., Payne, W. D., Simmons, R. L., Buselmeier, T. J., and Kjellstrand, C. M.: Acute renal failure following blunt civilian trauma. Ann. Surg., *185*:301, 1977.
86. Merino, G. E., Buselmeier, T. J., and Kjellstrand, C. M.: Postoperative chronic renal failure: A new syndrome. Ann. Surg., *182*:37, 1975.
87. Minuth, A. N., Terrell, J. B., and Suki, W. N.: Acute renal failure: A study of the course and prognosis of 104 patients and of the role of furosemide. Am. J. Sci., *271*:317, 1976.
88. Mitch, W. E., Lietman, P. S., and Walser, M.: Effects of oral neomycin and kanamycin in chronic uremic patients: I. Urea metabolism. Kidney Int., *11*:116, 1977.
89. Murphy, G. P., and Gagnon, J. A.: Renal alterations in dogs during renal arterial constriction, hemorrhagic hypotension and osmotic diuresis. J. Surg. Res., *5*:11, 1965.
90. Noone, P., Parsons, T. M. C., Pattison, J. R., Slack, R. C. B., Garfield-Davies, D., and Hughes, K.: Experience in monitoring gentamicin therapy during treatment of serious gram-negative sepsis. Br. Med. J., *1*:477, 1974.
91. Oken, D. E.: Local mechanisms in the pathogenesis of acute renal failure. Kidney Int. (Suppl.), *6*:S94, 1976.
92. Powell-Jackson, I. D., Macgregor, J., Brown, J. J., Lever, A. F., and Robertson, I. S.: The effect of angiotensin II antisera and synthetic inhibitors of the renin-angiotensin system on glycerol-induced acute renal failure in the rat. *In* Friedman, E. A., and Eliahou, H. E. (eds.): Proceedings, Acute Renal Failure Conference, Washington, D.C. (HEW Publication #NIH 74–608.) Washington, D. C., U. S. Government Printing Office, 1973. p. 281.
93. Preuss, H. G., Tourkantonis, A., Hsu, C. H., Shim, P. S., Barzyk, P., Tio, F., and Schreiner, G. E.: Early events in various forms of experimental acute tubular necrosis in rats. Lab. Invest., *32*:286, 1975.
94. Reubi, F. C., and Vorburger, C.: Renal hemodynamics in acute renal failure after shock in man. Kidney Int. (Suppl.), *10*:137, 1976.
95. Ribes, E. A., Domenech, J. C., Nicolas, J. M. M., and Gaspar, M. L.: Risk of acute renal failure associated with disseminated intravascular coagulation. Br. Med. J., *3*:745, 1975.
96. Riff, L. J., and Jackson, G.G.: Pharmacology of gentamicin in man. J. Infect. Dis., *124* (Suppl.):98, 1971.
97. Rose, W. C., and Wixom, R. L.: The amino acid requirements of man. XVI. The role of the nitrogen intake. J. Biol. Chem., *217*:997, 1955.
98. Rose, W. C., Wixom, R. L., Lockhart, H. B., and Lambert, G. F.: The amino acid requirements of man. XV: The valine requirements; summary and final observations. J. Biol. Chem., *217*:987, 1955.
99. Schwartz, J. H., and Flamenbaum, W.: Uranyl nitrate and $HgCl_2$-induced alterations in ion transport, Kidney Int. (Suppl.), *10*:123, 1976.
100. Sherwood, T.: Radiology in renal failure. Contrib. Nephrol., *5*:63, 1977.
101. Shires, G. T., and Baxter, C. R.: Acute renal insufficiency complicating surgery and trauma. *In* Artz, C. P., and Hardy, J. D. (eds.): Management of Surgical Complications, 3d ed. Philadelphia, W. B. Saunders Company, 1975, p. 83.
102. Shires, G. T., Carrico, C. J., and Canizaro, P. C.: Renal Responses. Philadelphia, W. B. Saunders Company, 1973.
103. Siegler, R. L., and Bloomer, H. A.: Acute renal failure with prolonged oliguria: Account of five cases. J.A.M.A., *225*:133, 1973.
104. Silberman, H.: Renal failure and the surgeon. Surg. Gynecol. Obstet., *144*:775, 1977.
105. Silverblatt, F. J.: Antibiotic nephrotoxicity: A review of pathogenesis and prevention. Urol. Clin. North Am., *2*:557, 1975.
106. Sofio, C., and Nicora, R.: High calorie essential amino acid parenteral therapy in acute renal failure. Acta Chir. Scand. (Suppl. *466*), 98, 1976.
107. Stein, J. H., and Sorkin, M. I.: Pathophysiology of a vasomotor and nephrotoxic model of acute renal failure in the dog. Kidney Int. (Suppl.) *10*:86, 1976.
108. Suzuki, T., and Mostofi, F. K.: Electron microscopic studies of acute tubular necrosis; early changes in the glomeruli of the rat kidney after subcutaneous injection of glycerin. Lab. Invest., *23*:8, 1970.
109. Szeto, H. H., Inturrisi, C. E., Houde, R., Saal, S., Cheigh, J., and Reidenberg, M. M.: Accumulation of normeperidine, an active metabolite of meperidine, in patients with renal failure or cancer. Ann. Intern. Med., *86*:738, 1977.

110. Tanner, G. A., Sloan, K. L., and Sophasan, S.: The effects of renal artery occlusion on kidney function in the rat. Kidney Int., 4:377, 1973.

111. Teschan, P. E., Baxter, C. R., O'Brien, T. F., Freyhof, J. N., and Hall, W. H.: Prophylactic hemodialysis in the treatment of acute renal failure. Ann. Intern. Med., 53:992, 1960.

112. Thurau, K., and Boylan, J. W.: Acute renal success: Unexpected logic of oliguria in acute renal failure. Am. J. Med., 61:308, 1976.

113. Tilney, N. L., Bailey, G. L., and Morgan, A. P.: Sequential system failure after rupture of abdominal aortic aneurysms: An unresolved problem in postoperative care. Ann. Surg., 178:117, 1973.

114. Tobias, J. S., Whitehouse, J. M., and Wrigley, P. F. M.: Severe renal dysfunction after tobramycin/cephalothin therapy. Lancet, 1:425, 1976.

115. Torres, V. E., Strong, C. G., Romero, J. C., and Wilson, D. M.: Indomethacin enhancement of glycerol-induced acute renal failure in rabbits. Kidney Int., 7:170, 1975.

116. Tzamaloukas, A. H., Garella, S., and Chazan, J. A.: Peritoneal dialysis for acute renal failure after major abdominal surgery. Arch. Surg., 106:639, 1973.

117. Varcoe, R., Halliday, D., Carson, E. R., Richards, P., and Tavill, A. S.: Efficiency of utilization of urea nitrogen for albumin synthesis by chronically uraemic and normal man. Clin. Sci. Mol. Med., 48:379, 1975.

118. Vertel, R. M., and Knochel, J. P.: Nonoliguric acute renal failure. J.A.M.A., 200:598, 1967.

119. Walser, M.: Urea metabolism in chronic renal failure. J. Clin. Invest., 53:1385, 1974.

120. Walser, M., and Mitch, W.: Dietary management of renal failure. Kidney, 10:13, 1977.

121. Weiss, E. S., and Weiss, A. N.: Congestive heart failure. In Boedeker, E. C., and Dauber, J. H. (eds.): Manual of Medical Therapeutics. Boston, Little, Brown and Company, 1974. p. 101.

122. Wilfert, J. N., Burke, J. P., Bloomer, H. A., and Smith C. B.: Renal insufficiency associated with gentamicin therapy. J. Infect. Dis., 124 Suppl.:148, 1971.

123. Wilmore, D. W., and Dudrick, S. J.: Treatment of acute renal failure with intravenous essential L-amino acids. Arch. Surg., 99:669, 1969.

124. Winter, R. E.: Antibiotic management in renal failure. Urol. Clin. North Am., 3:353, 1976.

125. Wysenbeek, A., Goldsmidt, Z., Nemesh, L., and Rosenfeld, J. B.: Hypercalcemia during the polyuric stage of acute renal failure. Israel J. Med. Sci., 12:1316, 1976.

126. Young, G. A., and Parsons, F. M.: Amino nitrogen loss during haemodialysis, its dietary significance and replacement. Clin. Sci., 31:299, 1966.

CHAPTER 8

INJURIES OF THE HEAD AND SPINAL CORD

A. Earl Walker, M.D.
Charles D. Ray, M.D.
Edward R. Laws, Jr., M.D.
George B. Udvarhelyi, M.D.
J. Donald McQueen, M.D.
Perry Black, M.D.

INTRODUCTION

A. Earl Walker, M.D.

When hand-to-hand combat was common, the head apparently was recognized as a vulnerable target. Helmets — often bulky, heavy and obviously uncomfortable — are depicted in the graphic records of early ages. Although the uniform of the warrior has changed greatly, the use of protective headgear has remained a symbol of the profession. When gunpowder was introduced, the larger parts of the body became easy targets for balls and bullets, but the head still required a helmet of some type.

The importance of head injury in early times is further documented by the emphasis placed upon it in ancient medical and surgical manuscripts. Breasted's papyrus devoted a section to head wounds. Hippocrates likewise has a book *Of Injuries of the Head*. In Roman and Byzantine manuscripts a prominent place is given to discussion of these wounds. In the Middle Ages the surgical treatment of head injuries apparently fell into disrepute, perhaps because treatment by trephination of such injuries increased rather than decreased their morbidity and mortality.

In later centuries, as modern warfare developed high-velocity arms that could mortally wound an individual with an injury of the chest or of the abdomen, the head was no longer the prime target of the soldier. However, in recent years the frequency and seriousness of head injuries have again come to the fore. Not open warfare but accidents, especially traffic, have subjected the head to trauma.

In most countries of the world, accidents are the number one cause of death in young people. During 1976, more people in the United States between the ages of 1 and 44 years died of accidents than from any other cause. These injuries do not all involve the central nervous system, but over 60 per cent affect the head and, in the category of fatal accidents, this percentage is over 85. These figures are about the same for all populous countries of the world, although in underdeveloped lands where vehicular traffic is light and slow, falls or assaults are more common causes of head injury.

For some years in the United States, the toll of traffic accidents was steadily increasing. With the threatened oil and gas shortage and the imposition of a national speed limit of 55 miles an hour, traffic accidents and deaths precipitously declined after 1973. But as law enforcement became lax, drivers, all too frequently under the influence of alcohol, ignored the law, began to drive faster and traffic accidents started to rise.

Safety measures in the design of cars and the construction of roads have advanced, but not to the extent that they have in industry. Because of the vested interest of industrial firms in their workers, preventive measures for the protection of the employees have been adopted. On the other hand, although a great number of safety measures have been suggested for the regulation of automobiles and their use, relatively few have been put into practice.

The magnitude of the accident problem is difficult to define accurately because of the lack of precise figures. Automobile collisions causing a certain amount of damage must be reported, but many car accidents do not involve a second party. Falls and injuries in the home are rarely brought to the attention of the accident prevention bureaus, yet they constitute about one third of all accidents. It has been estimated that each year one person in 200 will require medical care for a head injury. At the present time, approximately 1 per cent of the entire working community is disabled on any one day as the result of a head injury.

The problem concerns not only the safety divisions of the bureaus of traffic and roads but is of serious moment to the medical profession since trauma constitutes one of the major conditions with which physicians must contend. This problem is of particular interest to the general practitioner because he is usually the first to see

the person with a head injury, and what he does in the first few hours may be the difference between life and death or permanent disability. Accordingly, it is imperative that practitioners and house officers serving in emergency treatment rooms be well informed about the emergency treatment of head injuries.

Fortunately, house officers are now taught that a respiratory toilet and treatment of shock are primary considerations. Unquestionably, the immediate attention to pulmonary ventilation, intratracheal intubation if necessary and administration of oxygen to comatose patients may be lifesaving, or at least "brain-saving."

As more and more hospitals improve their diagnostic and therapeutic facilities in the emergency department, the initial care of the injured person is bettered. However, in comatose patients unable to cooperate in an examination, the diagnosis of spinal cord injuries often remains unsuspected, especially if the patient has a head injury. If the sequelae of spinal cord injuries are to be lessened, physicians in the emergency room must be alert to the possibility of a spine injury in every head-injured traffic victim. To suspect such an injury and to use neck traction (even if it later proves unnecessary) until a diagnosis can be established is not a high price to pay for the prevention of a paraplegia.

The role of the general surgeon and the emergency department surgeon in such cases is of extreme importance. By the time a specialist in neurological surgery is called and sees the patient, the patient's fate is often decided. Bleeding into the intracranial cavity, an important factor in acute head injuries, is an extremely common cause of death and is thought to occur in almost 50 per cent of individuals who have prolonged periods of unconsciousness following a head injury. Studies by medical examiners in a number of different countries have indicated that intracranial hemorrhage is a cause of death in approximately 35 to 50 per cent of patients who come to autopsy following head injury.

Modern advances have revolutionized the care of these comatose head-injured patients. For now, it is possible by simple means to tell which of the 50 per cent have the blood clot. After the initial cardiopulmonary resuscitation, intubation and treatment for shock, the comatose patient is taken for a computerized tomogram which, without additional risk and little delay, allows the physician to diagnose intracerebral hemorrhage, cerebral contusion or cerebral edema. Thus, the appropriate treatment may be initiated early by a specialist called by the primary physician, who no longer hesitates to bring in a consultant because of the fear that he may be unnecessarily disturbing his colleague.

The following sections dealing with specific aspects of head and spinal cord injury are, for the reasons mentioned, written for the general surgeon and house officer rather than for the neurosurgical specialist.

CRANIOCEREBRAL INJURY: CLASSIFICATION, PHYSICAL MECHANISM AND UNDERLYING PATHOLOGY

Edward R. Laws, Jr., M.D.
Charles D. Ray, M.D.

Head injuries account for approximately three fourths of all injuries sustained in automobile accidents. Since a knowledge of the tolerance of the nervous system to various stresses is essential in the prevention of injury and subsequent damage, a great deal of study and experimentation has dealt with the nature of injuries produced by various types of trauma. In order to reduce the likelihood of death from head injuries, the surgeon must have an adequate working knowledge of the mechanisms and consequences of craniocerebral trauma to aid in the diagnosis and treatment of brain injury.

Since the brain is an endoskeletal organ lying within a "closed-box cavity," injuries and their consequences must be considered somewhat differently from trauma inflicted elsewhere on the body. Other than direct destruction of brain substance, the most important physical mechanism to be considered is the *development of pressure*. As pressure rises and the brain substance is compressed, secondary phenomena occur which may lead to death. As one learns in medicine, there are relatively few *true* emergencies. However, an expanding lesion within the cranial cavity requires prompt diagnosis and surgical relief to avert death.

ANATOMICAL CONSIDERATIONS

Injuries of the head involve more than just the brain. The *scalp* acts as a protective covering for the head and is able by deformation and stretching to absorb and cushion a certain proportion of the energy impacted to the head. Injuries to the scalp may produce (1) a contusion or bruise; (2) a laceration; (3) hemorrhage which may be copious, or if the bleeding is confined, a subgaleal hematoma.

The *skull* provides the brain with more substantial and more rigid protection. Injuries to the skull may produce (1) transient deformation and distortion of the skull transmitted to the brain substance; and (2) fracture, either linear or fragmentary, with simple separation of the edges or depression of both cranial tables. Depressed fractures are usually quite fragmentary and may also be communicating ("compound"), with associated injury of the underlying dura and brain.

The *meninges* contain the thin layer of cerebrospinal fluid which covers the surface of the brain and acts to a certain extent as a hydraulic shock-absorber. Injury to the meninges may produce (1) a tear, as may be associated with a fracture; (2) hemorrhage, which may occur from disruption of a meningeal artery or injury to a dural sinus — these hemorrhages may develop and elaborate in the epidural space or the subdural space; or (3) cerebrospinal fluid leak.

Injuries to the *brain* are far more complex: (1) superficial trauma to the cortex and its blood vessels usually produces only mild focal effects, dependent upon the area of brain involved; (2) subcortical injuries produce more widespread effects upon neurological function; (3) deep or central injuries may result from shearing forces that disrupt and distort brain substance. These last injuries may be produced either by the initial injury or by subsequent transtentorial herniation of the brain; such injuries rarely allow satisfactory survival.

THE MECHANICS OF CRANIOCEREBRAL TRAUMA

At the moment of initial impact and for the immediate period that follows, head trauma is a problem in pure physics. By definition, the injury is produced by a mechanical or physical change of the head with respect to its environment. There have been numerous investigations of pathophysiological changes in the brain subsequent to trauma, and the problem is still not settled.

Table 8–1 gives a resume of various studies regarding the physics and pathophysiology of head injury. Several concepts are presented in this summary.

When an object is in motion, any sudden change in this motion will be expressed as an acceleration or deceleration. It has been shown[47] that when the head is struck and its velocity is changed to about 1.7 meters per second, or roughly 38 miles per

hour, a positive pressure of about one atmosphere will develop at the percussed side of the brain-skull interface and, simultaneously, a *minus* one atmosphere pressure develops at the opposite pole. Thus vacuum (minus one atmosphere) produces transient cavitation (gas bubble formation) within the brain substance and probably is a significant contributing factor in so-called contrecoup injuries. A second major result of force is produced by a sliding or rotary motion of the brain substance within the cranial vault. This has been demonstrated experimentally[35] using a transparent plastic skullcap on monkeys. The internal landmarks of the skull are not uniform and show definite prominences. Along with the semirigid falx and tentorium, these structures may "trap" the brain during its rotation, and certain areas will show the greatest damage when a complex force is applied to the skull. Such factors, presented in Table 8–1 under the column marked shear-strain, have been well described.[19]

It is less the velocity of the impact force than the momentum imparted to the head and brain that dictates the type and degree of injury. It is this momentum that suddenly changes the position of the head and also of the brain relative to the skull. It is known that most blows and falls result in complex movements involving both linear and rotary changes in brain position. Rotary shear-strains produce the most damaging effects.

As indicated in Figure 8–1, a severe fall injury results in considerable damage to the brain. The head is in motion and is brought to a sudden standstill as it encounters a solid object. This is essentially the set of circumstances in which the head strikes a dashboard or windshield during a head-on automobile collision. In such instances, sudden deceleration of the head produces a sliding forward of the brain within the cranial vault, resulting in abrupt negative pressure on the opposite pole of the brain. Rotary shear-strain will add significantly to the injury and lead to laceration in areas of relative anatomical entrapment. It has been emphasized that, regardless of the direction of the blow, the frontal and temporal lobes will receive greater contusion and laceration than the remainder of the cortical substance.[5]

TABLE 8–1. Physics and "Typical" Pathology of Head Injury

| | INJURY | | | | RESULTS | | | | | |
| | | | | | Damage to: | | | | | |
Type	Impact Velocity	Forces* Momentum	Velocity Imparted† (Change)	Shear-strain‡	Scalp	Bone	Vessels	Brain	Stem	Clinical Effects
Stab	Low	Low	Small	Linear+	++	+	+	Local, mild	0	Specific, mild
Gunshot§	High	Low	Small	Linear+	++	++	Deep+++	Specific, variable	0	Specific, variable
Crush	Very low	Very low	0	Linear+	+++	++++	+	Diffuse, mild	0	General, mild
Blow, mild	Low	Low	Small	Linear+ Rotary+	+	+	+	Local, mild	+	General, moderate
Blow, severe	Mod.	High	Large	Linear++ Rotary+++	++	+++	++	Contrecoup	+++	General, moderate to severe
Fall, mild	Low	High	Large	Linear++ Rotary+++	+	+	++	Contrecoup	++	General, moderate to severe
Fall, severe	Low	Very large	Very large	Linear+++ Rotary++++	+++	+++	Surface+++	Diffuse, severe	++++	General, severe

*Impact forces are for moving object striking head (producing acceleration) or for head in motion striking object (producing deceleration).

†Velocity change for skull and brain relative to velocity before impact.

‡Shear-strain force is movement of brain relative to skull.

§Variability of injuries associated with gunshot wounds precludes exact rules. Extent of damage is predominantly dependent on the impact velocity (kinetic energy) of the bullet.

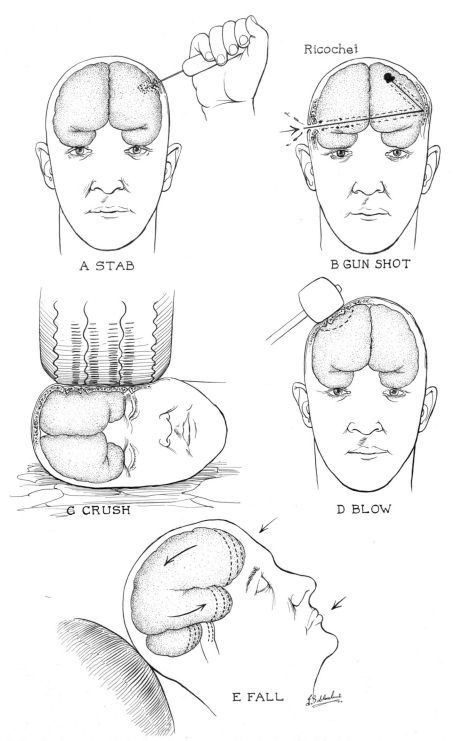

Figure 8–1. *Common types of craniocerebral injuries and means by which they are often inflicted.*

As the brain slides inside the cranial vault, traction occurs, with rupture of small vessels perforating the brain substance. Many of the consequences of head injury are the result of disruption of these vessels, rather than the direct effect of physical forces on brain substance. Some of the cranial nerves are especially vulnerable to traction injuries as the brain moves in the skull, particularly the first, second, third and eighth nerves.

When the skull itself has been bent or distorted, injuries to the brain are usually more superficial. This gives rise to the seeming paradox that one patient who has a depressed skull fracture may show little clinical change, yet another patient with no fracture at all may exhibit profound unconsciousness.

It is the velocity of the injuring object that will determine the type of skull fracture produced. Linear fractures are usually produced by low-velocity injuries and depressed fractures by higher velocities.

A static type of crush injury to the head, unless it is so extensive that it disrupts or avulses neural structures, usually produces no unconsciousness, and the prognosis is quite good. Small children whose heads have been run over by automobiles will often make remarkably good recoveries. In marked contrast, a fall or a blow such as a boxer's uppercut imparts high momentum, produces a sudden change in velocity and causes a complex rotation of the head, resulting in far greater damage than if the blow had been applied in a more linear manner.

The most severely damaging blow commonly encountered occurs in sudden deceleration injuries, as when the head strikes the dashboard of a car. The patient may remain unconscious for a matter of days or months. This unconsciousness, however, is rarely the result of direct cortical brain damage alone but rather is due to changes within the brainstem. Nearly one third of the patients sustaining such brainstem injuries die instantly. Of those who survive approximately one half die at a later date. Most of these patients simply never wake up.

No matter what the mechanism of head injury, the possibility of an associated cervical spine injury must be kept in mind.

CAUSES OF DEATH: A CLASSIFICATION

In trauma to the central nervous system death may be attributed to the following factors:

Immediate Causes

1. Direct brain surgery (especially vital brainstem centers).
2. Indirect brain injury
   a. Vascular
      (1) vasospasm with ischemia.
      (2) vascular disruption with hemorrhage (subarachnoid, epidural, subdural, intracerebral).
      (3) vascular occlusion; arterial or venous.
      (4) loss of autoregulation.
   b. Compressive
      (1) cerebral edema.
      (2) intracranial hematoma.
   c. Systemic effects
      (1) massive sympathetic discharge causing fulminant pulmonary edema.
3. Extracerebral causes
   a. Hemorrhage, cardiogenic shock.
   b. Respiratory obstruction, respiratory arrest, pulmonary edema.
   c. Air embolism to the cerebral circulation.
   d. Cardiac arrhythmia, cardiac failure.

Delayed Causes

1. Direct brain injury.
2. Indirect brain injury.
3. Infection within the cranium, meningitis or abscess (depressed communicating fracture, cerebrospinal fluid leak).
4. Systemic causes: fluids, electrolytes, metabolites.
5. Respiratory factors.
6. Fat embolism.
7. Systemic infection, toxins.

COMPLICATIONS IN THE MANAGEMENT OF THE UNCONSCIOUS PATIENT

The following are some of the difficulties which may occur following head injury:

1. Airway (aspiration, obstruction, atelectasis).

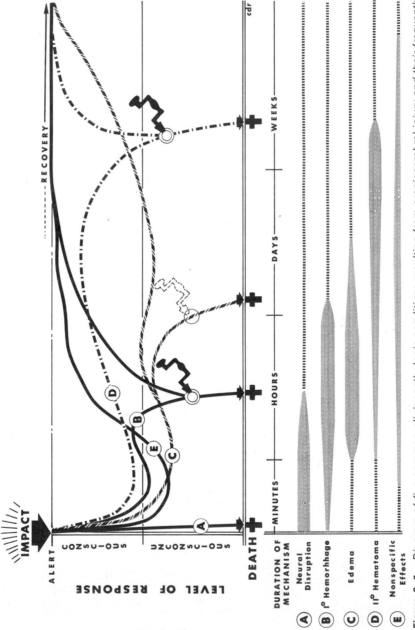

Figure 8–2. Diagram of five common clinicopathologic conditions resulting from craniocerebral injury and their frequently observed sequence of events.

2. Fluid and electrolytes (inappropriate ADH secretion, "cerebral salt wasting").

3. Infections (central nervous system, respiratory, urinary, open fractures, decubitus ulcers).

4. Gastrointestinal distention.

5. Bladder distention.

6. Agonal (Cushing) ulceration and hemorrhage from the gastrointestinal tract.

7. Hormonal stress reactions.

8. Seizures.

9. "Vegetative" phenomena (management of abnormal respiration, blood pressure and temperature).

10. Metabolic (acid-base problems, usually a combination of metabolic acidosis and respiratory alkalosis).

11. Abnormalities in cerebrospinal fluid flow and absorption (hydrocephalus, either acute high-pressure or more chronic low-pressure syndromes).

CONSEQUENCES OF HEAD INJURY

It is important to present a generalized classification of the series of events that are usually seen in association with various pathological entities.

In Figure 8–2 the time sequence of five clinicopathological results of head injury are shown: (A) a disruption of vital centers leading promptly to death; (B) an acute epidural hematoma with compression of underlying brain; (C) contusion of brain

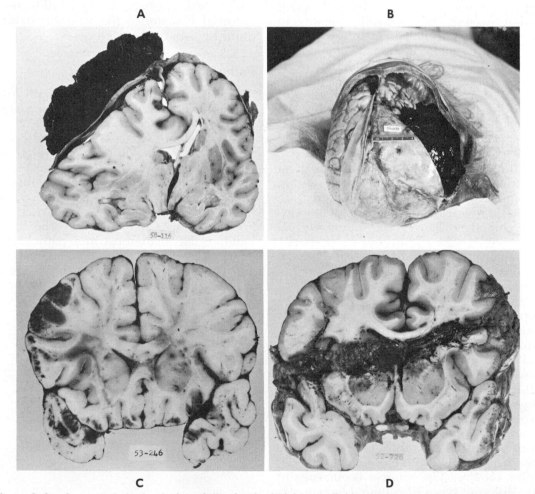

Figure 8–3. Gross pathologic changes following brain injury. A, Epidural hematoma. Note displacement of intact dura and underlying brain. B, Subdural hematoma. Note firm organization of the clot. C, Cortical contusions. Note principal involvement of crests of convolutions. D, Gunshot wound. Changes due to widespread contusions are also seen. (Courtesy of Dr. Richard Lindenberg.)

substance with subsequent formation of edema; (D) a chronic subdural hematoma that produces compression as the trapped blood undergoes autolysis, absorbs fluid and expands; and (E) simple traumatic unconsciousness without specific pathological changes. The time base shown is roughly logarithmic. Below the time base are given approximate durations of the mechanisms responsible for the effects seen in each clinical condition. Probabilities are also implicated; e.g., death within the first few days following injury is probably due to compression from edema, which exhibits its maximum effects within a few hours to a few days.

Progressive expanding lesions within the skull, whether hematomas or cerebral edema, eventually produce *transtentorial herniation of the brain* (Fig. 8–3). The sequence of events is fairly classical, and if uninterrupted, leads to death. Alteration in the state of consciousness is usually the earliest sign of herniation. Unilateral expanding lesions will produce hemiparesis either from compression of cortex (contralateral weakness) or from compression of the opposite cerebral peduncle against the edge of the tentorium (ipsilateral weakness). Herniation of the medial temporal lobe compresses the third cranial nerve, leading to dilatation of the ipsilateral pupil. As herniation causes brainstem compression and intracranial pressure rises, bradycardia develops and the systolic blood pressure rises (unless the patient is in a state of cardiovascular shock). Ultimately, brainstem reflexes (corneal, "doll's eyes," caloric) are lost and respiratory irregularity develops.

Subdural hematomas fall into three types: acute, subacute and chronic. This classification is primarily based on the time between injury and the onset of clinical signs; namely, less than 24 hours, up to a week or two and those appearing thereafter. Not so obvious, however, are the degrees of severity associated with different types. About 60 per cent of patients with acute subdural hematoma, about 20 per cent of those with subacute and about 10 per cent of those with chronic will die despite surgery. The relative occurrence of the different types of subdural hematomas is about the reverse of these mortality rates; i.e., 20 per cent are acute, 30 per cent subacute and 50 per cent chronic.

When the mechanism of compression is contusion with edema, the patient may show a gradual decline in responsiveness within a few hours. As indicated in Figure 8–2, surgery, if performed for decompression, is generally of little value; if other methods of reducing intracranial pressure (see later discussion of therapy) are unrewarding, death may ensue.

Most cases of epidural hematoma are of a rather violent origin (head-on collision, motorcycle accident) and the patients die abruptly. Further, most epidural hematomas are associated with bleeding from the middle meningeal artery, seldom occur bilaterally and are rarely seen without a fracture (except in the very young). Most have homolateral dilation of the pupil and contralateral body weakness or paralysis. Although less than 2 per cent of all patients with significant head injuries will have an epidural hematoma, the mortality rate is quite high in unoperated cases.

Pathological Changes

Classically, injuries to the brain substance have been classified as *concussion, contusion* and *laceration*.

Concussion. Concussion implies a traumatic event resulting from a relatively minor injury process and is manifested by a transient loss or change in consciousness from which the patient will make a relatively quick and satisfactory recovery.

Contusion. Contusion, on the other hand, is an anatomical and pathological change that can be found on a microscopic and macrocellular level in brain tissue (Fig. 8–4). There is a bruising of the brain

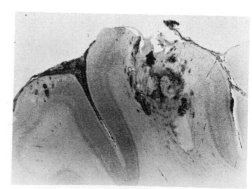

Figure 8–4. *Microscopic changes in cortical contusion. The lesion is essentially wedge-shaped, involving hemorrhagic necrosis of both gray and white matter. (Courtesy of Dr. Richard Lindenberg.)*

substance that results in an injury to vessels and a consequent diapedesis of red blood cells.

Laceration. Laceration of brain substance may result from open or closed fractures. It is a tearing of the substance of the brain and may be produced by a sudden movement of the brain against a relatively fixed intracranial landmark.

Delayed Effects. Most studies, and for that matter actual clinical observation on patients with head injuries, show that the delayed effects of injury are the more problematic. Without any question the most important aspect of delayed response to injury is swelling of the brain, or edema, which may occur even in the absence of hemorrhage. It can be shown experimentally that even minor injury to the brain may lead to generalized swelling lasting perhaps for days or weeks. Intensive electron microscopic studies and histochemical preparations show an actual change in the blood-brain barrier that subsequently permits fluid leakage from the vessels into the brain substance. These changes apparently occur on a molecular basis. Cerebral edema localizes in the glial cells, myelin sheaths and intercellular spaces.

An important pathophysiological consequence of severe head injury is a loss of autoregulation of the circulation of the brain. Under normal circumstances, the cerebral blood vessels automatically adjust caliber and flow rate to keep cerebral perfusion relatively constant despite wide variations in systemic blood pressure. After trauma, this capacity for regulation may be lost, and, if systemic blood pressure rises in response to increasing intracranial pressure, the hydrostatic pressure in the arterial side of the cerebral circulation will also rise, producing more hydrostatic edema and creating a vicious circle which will have a fatal outcome unless terminated.

Another vicious circle may occur when the intracranial pressure rises to a level which compresses and obstructs the major venous outflow from the brain, particularly the vein of Galen and the sigmoid sinuses. This increases both cerebral venous and intracranial pressures and may become rapidly fatal.

A report on nearly 1400 cases of brain injuries from blunt forces that had resulted in death (collected from a forensic series over a period of 10 years)[10] showed that nearly half of the accidents were the result of falls. About one fourth were traffic accidents involving pedestrians; in less than 10 per cent the victim was a passenger or driver of a car. Over one half of the patients died within 24 hours, and one fourth survived from one day to one week.

Over one third of the patients died in spite of cranial operation. Seventy per cent had skull fractures, with the smallest number of fractures occurring in children under 10 years of age. It is interesting to note that approximately one fourth of these patients died from epidural hematomas, yet only a small percentage of the *treatable* patients arriving at the emergency treatment room will have epidural hemorrhages. Obviously, most patients with such bleeding never reach medical hands. Two thirds of the patients had subdural bleeding, of whom less than half had skull fractures. Massive subarachnoid hemorrhage was the most frequent finding in all deaths. Table 8–2 gives a summary of causes of death.

From this work we may draw some important conclusions: Secondary lesions of the mid-brain and pons appear to be the most frequent factors leading to death (respiratory collapse) from head injuries. Such secondary lesions may develop within a matter of minutes and may explain why acute subdural hematomas bear such a poor prognosis. Particularly notable is the fact that massive subarachnoid hemorrhages of a fatal nature may occur without obvious contusion of the brain. Com-

TABLE 8–2. Cause of Death Following Blunt Head Injuries*

(1367)	PER CENT
Concussion of vital centers (leading to acute dysfunction without morphologic changes)	6
Contusion of vital areas	8
Secondary involvement of vital areas by edema	25
Secondary involvement of vital areas by hemorrhage and necrosis	24
Meningitis	2
Severe generalized body injuries	11
Disease related or unrelated to the injuries	24

*Based on information in Freytag, E.: Arch. Pathol. 75:402–413, 1963.

monly, brain surface contusions are associated with contusions of deep structures.

Final Outcome

A brief note on follow-up of patients with severe head injuries gives one additional insight into the overall problem. Although a majority have some persistent difficulties, those who survive the immediate accident and subsequent few days or weeks rarely die as a direct consequence of the head injury. The listing of *delayed* causes and complications given previously presents the more common factors.

After the patient has recovered from the acute clinical phases of head injury, the following signs, which represent management problems for the patient and his family, may be present. Miller and Stern[30] report the more common sequelae as amnesia, dyspraxia, dysphasia and dysgnosia (i.e., changes in memory, difficulty in performing practical tasks, difficulty with speech and with recognition of objects). There may be paresis or paralysis of a mixed or unilateral type, usually accompanied by spasticity. Most patients with spastic paresis will show an unexpectedly good recovery. Cranial nerve changes may persist, especially anosmia, as may visual changes such as double vision and discoordinate eye movements, decrease in hearing, ataxia and vertigo. Perhaps the most sensitive and reliable index of severity of injury for cases without signs of focal damage (such as a depressed fracture of intracranial hemorrhage) is post-traumatic amnesia. The duration of amnesia increases both with the severity of the injury and with the patient's age at time of injury. Indeed, the persistence of most clinical sequelae of head injury increases with age.

About 20 per cent of the patients will have some persistent psychiatric or behavioral problems and a similar number will show epilepsy. In most cases, the epileptic seizures begin within two years following the injury, and most of these patients are still subject to seizures after five years. Persistent headache, visual disturbance and vestibular dysfunction comprise a post-traumatic syndrome which may be troublesome for long periods of time after the injury. Approximately half the patients will not show any loss of occupational capabilities, about one third will not be able to perform as satisfactorily on the job, and 10 per cent or more will be totally disabled. Reports of long-term follow-up of patients with severe head injuries indicate that the outcome has generally been more favorable than had been expected or predicted from earlier studies. Such a favorable outcome is doubtless related to an improvement in immediate and subsequent medical care.

REFERENCES

1. Braakman, R.: Depressed skull fracture: Data, treatment, and follow-up in 225 consecutive cases. J. Neurol. Neurosurg. Psychiatry, 35:395–402, 1972.
2. Caveness, W. F., and Walker, A. E.: Head Injury. Philadelphia, J. B. Lippincott Co., 1966.
3. Courville, C. B.: The mechanism of coupcontrecoup injuries of the brain. Bull. Los Angeles Neurol. Soc. 15:72, 1950.
4. Davis, D., Bohlman, H., Walker, A. E., Fisher, R., and Robinson, R.: The pathological findings in fatal craniospinal injuries. J. Neurosurg. 34:603–613, 1971.
5. Denny-Brown, D., and Russell, W. R.: Experimental cerebral concussion. Brain. 64:93–164, 1941.
6. Echlin, F., and Sordillo, S. V.: Acute, subacute and chronic subdural hematoma. J.A.M.A. 161:1345–1350, 1956.
7. Edberg, S., Reiker, J., and Angrist, A.: Study of impact pressure and acceleration in plastic skull models. J. Lab. Invest. L2:1305, 1963.
8. Feiring, E. H.: Brock's Injuries of the Brain and Spinal Cord. (2nd Ed.) New York, Springer Publishing Co., 1974.
9. Foltz, E. L., Jenkner, F. L., and Ward, A. A., Jr.: Experimental cerebral concussion. J. Neurosurg. 10:342–352, 1953.
10. Foltz, E. L., and Schmidt, R. P.: The role of the reticular formation in the coma of head injury. J. Neurosurg. 13:145–154, 1956.
11. Ford, L. E., and McLaurin, R. L.: Mechanisms of extradural hematomas. J. Neurosurg. 20:760–769, 1963.
12. Freytag, E.: Autopsy findings in head injuries from blunt forces. Statistical evaluation of 1,367 cases. Arch. Pathol. 75:215, 1963.
13. Freytag, E.: Autopsy findings in head injuries from firearms. Arch. Pathol. 75:215, 1963.
14. Goodman, J. M., and Kalsbeck, J.: Outcome of self-inflicted gunshot wounds of the head. J. Trauma 5:636, 1965.
15. Graf, C. J., and Rossi, N. P.: Pulmonary edema and the central nervous system: A clinicopathological study. Surg. Neurol. 4:319–325, 1975.
16. Gurdjian, E. S.: Recent advances in the study of the mechanism of impact injury of the head. A summary. Clin. Neurosurg. 19:1–42, 1972.

17. Gurdjian, E. S.: Head Injury from Antiquity to the Present with Special References to Penetrating Head Wounds. Springfield, Ill.: Charles C Thomas Co., 1973.
18. Gurdjian, E. S.: Impact Head Injury: Mechanistic, Clinical and Preventive Correlations. Springfield, Ill., Charles C Thomas Co., 1975.
19. Gurdjian, E. S., Hodgson, V. R., Thomas, L. M., and Patrick, L. M.: Significance of relative movements of scalp, skull and intracranial contents during impact injury of the head. J. Neurosurg. 29:70–72, 1968.
20. Gurdjian, E. S., and Lissner, H. R.: Photoelastic confirmation of the presence of shear strains at the craniospinal junction in closed head injury. J. Neurosurg. 18:58–60, 1961.
21. Gurdjian, E. S., Lissner, H. R., and Latimer, F. R., et al.: Quantitative determination of acceleration and intracranial pressure in experimental head injury. Preliminary report. Neurology (Minneap.) 3:417–423, 1953.
22. Gurdjian, E. S., Lissner, H. R., and Webster, J. E., et al.: Studies of experimental concussion; relation of physiologic effect to time duration of intracranial pressure increase at impact. Neurology (Minneap.) 4:674–681, 1954.
23. Gurdjian, E. S., Webster, J. E., and Lissner, H. R.: Observations on the mechanism of brain concussion, contusion and laceration. Surg. Gynecol. Obstet. 101:680–690, 1955.
24. Hammon, W. M.: Analysis of 2187 consecutive penetrating wounds of the brain from Vietnam. J. Neurosurg. 34:127–131, 1971.
25. Hendrick, E. B., Harwood-Nash, D. C. F., and Hudson, A. R.: Head injuries in children: A survey of 4465 consecutive cases at the Hospital for Sick Children, Toronto, Canada. Clin. Neurosurg. 11:46–65, 1964.
26. Hodgson, V. R., Gurdjian, E. S., and Thomas, L. M.: Experimental skull deformation and brain displacement demonstrated by flash x-ray technique. J. Neurosurg. 25:549–552, 1966.
27. Holbourn, A. H. S.: Mechanics of head injuries. Lancet 2:438, 1943.
28. Jennett, B.: Assessment of the severity of head injury. J. Neurol. Neurosurg. Psychiatry, 39:647–655, 1976.
29. Jennett, B., Graham, D. I., and Adams, H., et al.: Ischemic brain damage after fatal blunt head injury. In McDowell, F. H., Brennan, R. W. (eds.): Cerebral Vascular Disease, Eighth Conference. New York, Grune and Stratton, 1973, pp. 163–170.
30. Johnston, I. H., Johnston, J. A., and Jennett, B.: Intracranial pressure changes following head injury. Lancet 2:433–436, 1970.
31. Langfitt, T. W., Tannenbaum, H. M., and Kassell, N. F.: The etiology of acute brain swelling following experimental head injury. J. Neurosurg. 24:47–56, 1966.
32. Lidvall, H. F., Linderoth, B., and Norlin, B.: Causes of the postconcussional syndrome. Acta Neurol. Scand. 50, Suppl. 56, 1974.
33. Lindenberg, R., and Freytag, E.: The mechanism of cerebral contusions. A pathologic-anatomic study. Arch. Pathol. 69:440, 1960.
34. Marshall, W. J. S., Jackson, J. L. F., and Langfitt, T. W.: Brain swelling caused by trauma and arterial hypertension. Hemodynamic aspects. Arch. Neurol. 21:545–553, 1969.
35. McLaurin, R. L., and Helmer, F.: The syndrome of temporal lobe contusion. J. Neurosurg. 23:296–303, 1965.
36. Miller, H., and Stern, G.: Long-term prognosis of severe head injury. Lancet 1:225, 1965.
37. Mitchell, D. E., and Adams, J. H.: Primary focal impact damage to the brainstem in blunt head injuries. Does it exist? Lancet 2:215–218, 1973.
38. Nilsson, B., Ponten, U., and Voigt, G.: Experimental head injury in the rat. Part 1: Mechanics, pathophysiology and morphology in an impact acceleration trauma model. J. Neurosurg. 47:241–251, 1977.
39. Nilsson, B., and Ponten, U.: Experimental head injury in the rat. Part 2: Regional brain energy metabolism in concussive trauma. J. Neurosurg. 47:252–261, 1977.
40. Nilsson, B., and Nordstrom, C. H.: Experimental head injury in the rat. Part 3: Cerebral blood flow and oxygen consumption after concussive impact acceleration. J. Neurosurg. 47:262–273, 1977.
41. Ommaya, A. K., and Gennarelli, T. A.: Cerebral concussion and traumatic unconsciousness. Correlation of experimental and clinical observations on blunt head injuries. Brain 97:633–654, 1974.
42. Ommaya, A. K., Rockoff, S. D., and Baldwin, M.: Experimental concussion. A first report. J. Neurosurg. 21:249–265, 1964.
43. Oppenheimer, D. R.: Microscopic lesions in the brain following head injury. J. Neurol. Neurosurg. Psychiatry 31:299–306, 1968.
44. Preston, F. E., Malia, R. G., Sworn, J. J., Timperley, W. R., and Blackburn, E. K.: Disseminated intravascular coagulation as a consequence of cerebral damage. J. Neurol. Neurosurg. Psychiatry, 37:241–248, 1974.
45. Pudenz, R. H., and Shelden, C. H.: The lucite calvarium — A method for direct observation of the brain; cranial trauma and brain movement. J. Neurosurg. 3:487, 1946.
46. Rand, C. W.: Histological changes in the human brain consequent to head injuries. Clin. Neurosurg. 3:59–103, 1957.
47. Reivich, M., Marshall, W. J. S., and Kassell, N. F.: Loss of autoregulation produced by cerebral trauma. In Brock, M., Fieschi, C., Ingvar, D. H., et al. (eds.): Cerebral Blood Flow. New York, Springer-Verlag, 1969, pp. 205–208.
48. Rockoff, S. D., and Ommaya, A. K.: Experimental head trauma: Cerebral angiographic observation in early post-traumatic period. Am. J. Roentgenol. 91:1026, 1964.
49. Rowbotham, G. F.: Acute Injuries of the Head; Their Diagnosis, Treatment, Complications, and Sequels. London, E. & S. Livingston, Ltd., Fourth Ed., 1964.
50. Russell, W. R.: Cerebral involvement in head injury. Brain 55:549, 1932.
51. Schneider, R. C.: Head and Neck Injuries in Football: Mechanisms, Treatment and Prevention. Baltimore, The Williams & Wilkins Co., 1973.

52. Scott, W. W.: Physiology of concussion. Arch. Neurol. Psychiatry 43:270–283, 1940.
53. Sellier, K., and Unterharnscheidt, F.: Mechanik det Gewaltenwirkung auf dem Schaedel. Excerpta Medica 93:55, 1963.
54. Shatsky, S. A., Evans, D. E., Miller, F., et al.: High-speed angiography of experimental head injury. J. Neurosurg. 41:523–530, 1974.
55. Smith, D. R., Ducker, T. B., and Kempe, L. G.: Experimental in vivo microcirculatory dynamics in brain trauma. J. Neurosurg. 30:664–672, 1969.
56. Strich, S. J.: Shearing of nerve fibres as a cause of brain damage due to head injury. A pathological study of twenty cases. Lancet 2:443–448, 1961.
57. Symon, L.: An experimental study of traumatic cerebral spasm. J. Neurol. Neurosurg. Psychiatry 30:497–505, 1967.
58. Symonds, C.: Concussion and its sequelae. Lancet 1:1–5, 1962.
59. Tindall, G. T., Patton, J. M., Dunion, J. J., and O'Brien, M. S.: Monitoring of patients with head injuries. Clin. Neurosurg. 22:332–363, 1975.
60. Unterharnscheidt, F.: About boxing: Review of historical and medical aspects. Texas Rep. Biol. Med. 28:421–495, 1970.
61. Walker, A. E.: Posttraumatic Epilepsy. Springfield, Ill., Charles C Thomas, 1949.
62. Walker, A. E.: The acute head injury: A multidisciplinary problem. Neurologia Medio-Disurgia. 9:7–20, 1968.
63. Walker, A. E., and Jablon, S.: A follow-up study of head wounds in World War II. VA Medical Monograph. Washington, D.C., U.S. Government Printing Office, 1961.
64. Walker, A. E., Kollros, J. J., and Case, T. J.: The physiological basis of concussion. J. Neurosurg. 1:103–116, 1944.
65. Ward, A. A., Jr.: The physiology of concussion. Clin. Neurosurg. 12:95–111, 1966.
66. Wilkins, R. H.: Intracranial vascular spasm in head injuries. In Vinken, P. J., Bruyn, G. W., and Braakman, R.: Handbook of Clinical Neurology. Amsterdam, North-Holland, 23:163–197, 1975.
67. Woodhall, G.: Acute cerebral injuries: Analysis of temperature, pulse, and respiration curves. Arch. Surg. 33:560, 1936.
68. Wurtman, R. J., and Zervas, N. T.: Monoamine neurotransmitters and the pathophysiology of stroke and central nervous system trauma. J. Neurosurg. 40:34–36, 1974.
69. Zervas, N. T., Lavyne, M. H., and Negoro, M.: Neurotransmitters and the normal and ischemic cerebral circulation. N. Engl. J. Med. 293:812–816, 1975.

THE DIAGNOSIS OF CRANIOCEREBRAL INJURIES

George B. Udvarhelyi, M.D.

In civilian practice a majority of the patients brought into hospital emergency rooms with craniocerebral trauma have injuries of the closed type. By definition, in closed head injuries the brain and its coverings have not been penetrated by any missile and there is no evidence of compound fracture of the skull with subsequent exteriorization of the brain. In cases of compound fractures of the skull, the injury is usually apparent to the layman who may be present at the time of the injury and to the physician who receives the injured patient. The real diagnostic difficulty in closed head injuries lies in the correct and timely recognition of intracranial damage.

In the past seven years considerable progress has been made in the understanding of the pathophysiology of craniocerebral trauma, which in turn has provided for a sound assessment of the unconscious patient.[19, 34, 45]

Effective collaboration with biomedical engineering has provided for the practical application of new techniques in monitoring patients with head injuries[10, 11, 26, 33, 41, 47, 49] and improved the diagnostic accuracy in selecting cases for appropriate surgical intervention. Critical surveys measured the outcome of severe head injuries, putting the various efforts of the past decade into proper perspective.[4-6, 21]

From the diagnostic point of view, the introduction of computerized axial tomography (CT scan) has revolutionized and significantly improved the management of patients with craniocerebral injuries.[2, 28, 35] It is a noninvasive technique that can be done in less than two minutes' time. Its accuracy is superior to all previous neuroradiological diagnostic procedures. The interested reader is advised to consult the original communications.[1, 3, 16, 32] The principle is simple: The computed tomogram represents a mathematical reconstruction of computer assisted absorption density measurements of tomographic cuts of the brain obtained in the axial projection. The equipment is relatively expensive, but the investment seems to be mandatory for any hospital which receives head injured patients. The experience of the past five years in many centers in Europe and in the United States has shown that most of the previously recommended diagnostic procedures have been replaced by the CT scan. Therefore a revision of our previous recommendations is mandatory.

However, technical advances should not replace, but supplement, clinical judgment.

THE IMPORTANCE OF A CAREFUL HISTORY

Even in cases that represent an extreme surgical emergency, clear-cut information about the type and mode of injury has great practical value. Eyewitness descriptions of the accident should be carefully evaluated. If the patient has already been seen by a physician before arriving at the emergency treatment room of the hospital, the doctor's findings, if known, should be meticulously recorded.

Injuries to the central nervous system may be manifested in various ways. In general, any moderately severe head injury will cause some interruption of the normal function of the central nervous system. In most instances this is not specific; von Monakow[27] called the effect of any sudden impact on the structure of the brain "diaschisis." In moderate-to-severe head injuries, loss of consciousness at the outset is the rule. Since the subsequent prognosis for recovery depends partly on the length of the period of unconsciousness, reliable information on this is very helpful.

In addition to the immediate derangement of the function of the brain as a whole, local damage to various parts of the brain or its coverings may occur at the time of the head injury. Such local damage may be masked in the beginning by the immediate generalized effect of the injury. However, quite often it is possible to detect symptoms that indicate motor weakness of one side of the body or of individual limbs, brainstem involvement, pupillary disturbances and faulty coordination of the eye movements, and so forth. Changes in vital signs (pulse rate, blood pressure, respiration and temperature) also occur. Slowing of pulse and respiration coupled with elevation of blood pressure and temperature indicates increasing severity of head injury.[53] It should be emphasized, however, that concomitant injuries to other systems often complicate the clinical picture. Their recognition at the time of the injury is important in choosing an intelligent plan for step-by-step management of the patient.

Although the causal relationship between the injury and subsequent brain damage can usually be established, the examiner must also consider the possibility of pre-existing disease processes, such as diabetes, hypertension, renal insufficiency or a severe heart condition, since these may worsen as a result of the head injury. Occasionally, head injuries produce bleeding from a congenital vascular malformation, aneurysm or tumor; therefore, relevant data about the patient's status prior to the injury may be of great help in arriving at the right diagnosis. It is also important to investigate the possibility of concomitant injury to the cervical spine, a not uncommon occurrence when there are severe head injuries (Fig. 8–5).

GENERAL EXAMINATION

Careful examination should be performed to determine the existence of injuries to other organs and systems. The acute head injury is a multidisciplinary

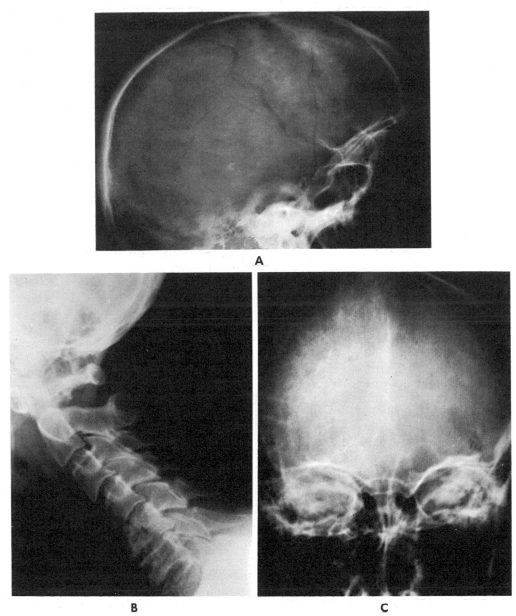

A

B   C

Figure 8-5. A, *Radiograph of the skull, lateral view. Irregular, linear fracture, running through the middle meningeal vascular groove. B, Radiograph of the cervical spine (lateral view) of the same patient, showing compression-fracture with multiple dislocations at C5-C6 and C7. C, Right carotid angiogram, anteroposterior view, capillary phase. An epidural hematoma of considerable size is demonstrated as an avascular area between the internal table and cerebral cortex over the right hemisphere.*

problem. Respiratory, cardiovascular and abdominal implications, metabolic disturbances, wounds of the accessory cranial sinuses, complicating injuries of the cervical spine and limb fractures form the most essential parts of a broad spectrum. Judgment in assigning priorities within a cooperative team is essential to handle such complex situations. These aspects are discussed in detail in other sections of the book. Inspection of the whole body after removal of all clothing is mandatory. The recognition and immediate treatment of shock should precede other system evaluations and treatment of the head injury. If there are signs of aspiration or choking, immediate intubation or tracheostomy and clearing of the airway must be undertaken before further examination of the patient.

The patient with a head injury should be placed immediately on a special "head chart" regimen, with frequent recordings of pulse rate, blood pressure, respiratory rate and temperature. It is important to remain alert to the possibility of progressive signs that may be caused by gradual increase of intracranial pressure, even in the presence of concomitant and apparently severe injuries to the extremities or to other organ systems. Oversight in this regard can have a tragic result if dangerous but remediable hemorrhages such as an epidural hematoma are overlooked because of concentrated efforts to deal with a compound fracture of a femur or a pneumohemothorax.

Careful examination of the scalp, head, face and neck should precede special neurological tests. Abrasions, contusions, subcutaneous hematomas and lacerations should be recorded. Gentle palpation of the head may reveal the existence of subcutaneous hematomas or fractures of the calvaria. Palpation must be done with care, however; in some instances of skull fracture, brain substance may be extruded through a torn dura, and undue pressure on dislocated bone fragments may cause further neurological damage.

Hematomas in the periorbital and perinasal areas, or along the neck musculature, are suggestive of possible underlying and more profound damage. Cerebrospinal fluid leak through the nose (rhinorrhea) or through the ear (otorrhea) should be recognized at an early stage of the examination. Fractures of the skull base, quite often not recognizable on routine x-ray examination, may produce "hematomas-at-distance," which usually occur around the eye, in the eyelids, over the mastoid processes or behind the eardrum (hemotympanum).

Concomitant involvement of some of the cranial nerves with close anatomical relationship to the base of the skull may be present. The most common are loss of smell (olfactory nerve), abducens palsy, peripheral facial weakness or hearing loss. These clinical findings, together with the presence of rhinorrhea or otorrhea, are highly suggestive of basal skull fracture, even in the absence of radiographic confirmation.

If, after thorough search, doubt exists about the presence or the extent of hematomas or lacerations in the area of the scalp covered by hair, the entire head should be shaved to permit a more complete and reliable assessment at the time of the first inspection.

NEUROLOGICAL EXAMINATION

It is outside the scope of this chapter to describe the various stages of a complete neurological examination. Most physicians who are not regularly engaged in diagnosis of neurological diseases have an understandable but unfounded aversion to assessment of disorders within the central nervous system. It is, however, usually not necessary to apply the rigorous rules of a highly specialized neurological evaluation to reach a correct diagnosis. As Klingler[20] has pointed out, the following aspects should be covered in evaluating the condition of a patient with head injury who is admitted to the emergency room:

1. Assessment of the level of consciousness.

2. Assessment of posture and movements (motor system), including reflexes.

3. Evaluation of eye movements and pupils.

4. Evaluation of gross focal neurological deficit.

Assessment of the Level of Consciousness

A clear definition of unconsciousness is still debatable. Russell states: "The state of full consciousness is that in which any occurrence in which the patient is actively or passively concerned, makes an impression on the memory, and can be subsequently called to mind. Any state of consciousness less than this is to be regarded as a grade of unconsciousness."[38, 39]

Symonds[42, 43] points out, however, that the only practicable criterion of "recovery of consciousness" is awareness of external environment and accessibility, as proposed by Mapother.[24] The terms coma, semicoma, stupor, lethargy and drowsiness have been used with various connotations in the past. For practical purposes, an operational description is more valuable. According to Rowbotham,[36] the depth of con-

TABLE 8–3. Glasgow Coma Scale*

1974 SCALE	1977 SCALE
Eye opening	Eye opening
Spontaneous	Spontaneous
To speech	To speech
To pain	To pain
None	None
Best verbal response	Verbal response
Orientated	Orientated
Confused	Confused conversation
Inappropriate	Inappropriate words
Incomprehensible	Incomprehensible sounds
None	Nil
Best motor response	Best motor response
Obeying	Obeys
Localizing	Localizes
Flexing	Withdraws
Extending	Abnormal flexion
None	Extensor response
	Nil

*From Langfitt, T. W.: J. Neurosurg. 48:675, 1978.

sciousness may be judged by the reactions of the patient to external stimuli, on various levels.

TABLE 8–4. Additional Data to Be Recorded in Head-injured Patients*

Age
Sex
Cause of injury
Associated injuries/shock/hypoxemia
Medical complications (e.g., alcohol, congestive failure)
Time from injury to admission to hospital
Time from onset of coma to admission to study (6 hrs)
Lucid interval
Presence of mass lesion†
Vital signs (blood pressure, heart rate, temperature, intracranial pressure)
Management
  Steroids
  Intubation/ventilation/pharmacological paralysis
  Continuous measurement of intracranial pressure
  Hypertonic solutions
  Hyperventilation
  Hypothermia
  Barbiturates

*From Langfitt, T. W.: J. Neurosurg. 48:677, 1978.
†A set of criteria for assessing head injuries by CT scan should be developed.

Therefore, based on the experience of various head injury centers, it has been proposed lately[21] to adopt a practical "coma scale" developed at the Glasgow Head-injury Center[19, 45] (Table 8–3). This should allow a more descriptive evaluation of the condition of the head-injured patient. Initially a list of additional data should be recorded so that an intelligent comparison of head-injured patients can be achieved[21] (Table 8–4).

Assessment of the level of consciousness at the time of arrival at the emergency room should always be considered in the light of the information obtained by the history. If the patient was unconscious for only a short period of time, with a subsequent relatively lucid interval followed by progressive clouding of consciousness again, the possibility of an increasing hematoma inside the intracranial cavity, usually extradural in location, is the best working diagnosis. If the patient was found only mildly confused at the time of injury, but during the following hours a gradual decrease in the level of consciousness occurred, progressive shift of the intracranial contents can be assumed, caused either by increasing edema or by collection of blood in the subdural space or in the cerebral parenchyma. On the other hand, if the level of consciousness shows definite evidence of clearing, the patient probably is on the way to recovery from the initial derangement of cerebral function and will not need surgical intervention. Only about 10 to 15 per cent of patients who suffer from head injury will require operation.

From the practical point of view it should be emphasized that, in evaluation of the involvement of consciousness, the "time profile" is important. Evidence of progressive deterioration should alert the examining surgeon to the possible need for immediate action. These patients may require special diagnostic studies or, in cases of extreme emergency, immediate exploration. Unnecessary delay in diagnosis and treatment may result in irreversible secondary damage to the brainstem from massive herniation of the cerebral hemisphere and pressing of the brainstem against the sharp edge of the tentorium or from secondary vascular compression inside the tentorial notch (Fig. 8–6).

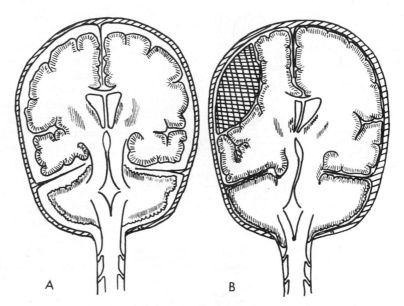

Figure 8-6. Schematic diagrams of craniospinal contents contrasting A (normal CSF pathways) with B (brain compression by supratentorial mass lesion). In B, note obliteration of the cranial subarachnoid space, reduction in size of the lateral ventricle on the side of the lesion, and examples of subfalcial, tentorial, and tonsillar herniation, with distortion and downward displacement of brainstem.

Assessment of Posture and Motor Function

Complete flaccidity of all limbs and a flaccid jaw are usually exhibited when the patient is still in the initial state of severe shock. If such general flaccidity persists, the prognosis is poor.

The term "decerebrate rigidity" is used to describe the signs that generally indicate severe injury to the brainstem, usually below the red nucleus. The patient shows extensor rigidity of all four limbs, with adduction and rotation of the upper extremities on painful stimuli. The ankles are generally plantar flexed, the hips and knees are fully extended. Passive movements are difficult to elicit, and severe spasm usually is present. No reflexes can be elicited. In extreme cases, in addition to the rigidity of the extremities, opisthotonus can also be found. This situation is compatible with primary brainstem injury, although occasionally a rapidly developing hematoma can cause similar postural changes, indicating additional secondary damage to the stem.

The most common motor sign is evidence of a hemiparesis or hemiplegia. Only occasionally is a monoparesis present. In a comatose patient the hemiplegic limbs can usually be recognized by their decreased tone, the muscles taking the position determined by gravity. The lower extremity is externally rotated, the foot is slightly dropped and turned outward.

When elevated by the examiner, the arm or leg is usually hypotonic, especially in the early period after the injury. By use of painful stimuli (a pinprick or pinch) some movement of the limb may be elicited and the degree of paretic involvement assessed. If, in addition to the hemiparetic syndrome, contralateral involvement of one or several cranial nerves is present, the diagnosis of localized brainstem injury can be made, the clinical picture being that of "alternating hemiplegia."

In a few instances, when the lesion is below the vestibular nuclei, marked spasm of the flexor muscles occurs, causing acute flexion of the limbs and body (Fig. 8–7).

The motor weakness usually also involves the muscles of the face. In moderate disturbance of consciousness that produces various degrees of confusion, some information may be obtainable from the patient about any sensory involvement, including visual fields. If a combination of motor, sensory and hemianoptic visual-field defects is present, the lesion is in all probability in the region of the internal capsule and indicates an intracerebral hematoma or severe interruption of the fiber tracts at this level.

If the patient also has signs and symptoms indicating poverty or slowness of purposeful movements, various degrees of tremor or rigidity, concomitant involvement of the subcortical nuclei can be assumed.

The reflexes may be hyperactive, and

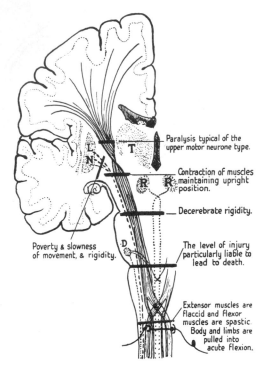

Figure 8-7. The pyramidal and extrapyramidal pathways. According to the level of interruption of these pathways different nervous phenomena ensue. This is one of the main reasons why the clinical pictures in head injuries are so variable. LN, Lenticular nucleus; T, optic thalamus; R, red nucleus; D, Deiters' nucleus.

pathological reflexes may be present. However, in most cases the patients are not seen until a few hours after the acute injury, at which time these reflex changes may not be manifest.

Evaluation of Eye Movements and the Pupils

Eye Deviation. Conjugate deviation of both eyes toward the paralyzed side indicates a lesion of the frontal adversive fields. Spontaneous nystagmus may be present from damage to the cerebellum or the vestibular connections. Skew deviation of the eyes occurs in injuries to the brainstem. Frequently, uncoordinated movements of the eyes, without fixation, can be observed on careful observation, another sign of severe brainstem involvement. Local damage to the orbit or to the eye muscles can also be responsible for deviation of the eyes from the axis. A common finding in severe head injuries is involvement of the third or sixth cranial

nerves, and recognition of this is highly important. Since the third cranial nerve innervates all the eye muscles except the superior oblique and the external rectus, paralysis of the third nerve will result in an external deviation of the eye, with slight downward rotation. If there is complete interruption of third nerve function, the pupil will also be dilated and fixed. If the sixth cranial nerve is involved alone, pupillary reaction will not be involved; but the eye will be deviated inward by the other intact muscles innervated by the third and fourth cranial nerves.

Pupillary Reaction. The examination of the pupils is of great importance. If one pupil is dilated and fixed from the very beginning of the injury, this generally means either direct trauma to the third nerve or a very sudden increase of intracranial pressure, as can occur in intraventricular hemorrhage. However, if the pupils were noted to have been of the same size just after the injury, but during the subsequent hours one pupil starts to dilate, a progressive lesion is present that requires immediate diagnosis and treatment. Since the third cranial nerve can be damaged at any point in its entire course from the upper brainstem to the eye bulb, the exact clinical significance of the involvement of the third nerve can be more correctly evaluated if it is considered together with the changes in the level of consciousness.

If the patient is fully awake and oriented, third nerve involvement generally means damage to this nerve in the orbit, in the superior orbital fissure or in the cavernous sinus. If, however, the level of consciousness is definitely involved, or the patient is in a coma, third nerve involvement by compression through a transtentorial herniation is more likely. Rapid progressive involvement of the third cranial nerve requires immediate measures; no time should be wasted with unnecessary diagnostic studies, since the probability of an epidural or acute subdural hematoma is high. Frequent careful observation of the pupillary size and reactions and the position of the eyes is mandatory; these should be checked as frequently as possible, with the recording of the vital signs.

A very small, nonreactive pupil in a patient who is in coma or semicoma is generally indicative of primary involvement of the brainstem. This is also the case if sudden changes in the pupillary size are noted within a relatively short period of time. Sudden pupillary constriction, or sudden dilation of one or both pupils in irregular fashion, is a severe sign and generally indicates a poor prognosis. The consensual reaction of the pupils should also be investigated. Occasionally, a pupil does not react to direct stimulus by light because the optic nerve is damaged; however, good contraction can be elicited when light is thrown into the opposite eye. This means that the damage is in the afferent part of the reflex arc (the optic nerve) and not in the efferent limb (third cranial nerve).

Fundus Examination. Examination of the "eyegrounds" (fundus) may be of some value, although development of significant papilledema within a few hours of cerebral injury is infrequent. The presence of hemorrhages, especially subhyaloid hemorrhages, is indicative of severe head injury with subarachnoid bleeding. A warning should be given to avoid drugs such as homatropine to dilate the pupils for a better view of the eyegrounds. Paralysis of the iris constrictor muscles by miotics prevents careful observation of the pupillary reaction for signs of progressive involvement of the third cranial nerve.

Focal Neurological Deficit. Certain focal neurological deficits can be established even by surgeons or residents who are not familiar with the intricacies of detailed neurological examination. The possible presence of aphasia should be checked if the patient is fully conscious or only mildly confused. *Expressive aphasia* is an inability to formulate words because of lesions of the dominant hemisphere, mostly in the area of the third frontal convolution or within the insular region affecting the intercortical connections of the various speech centers. *Receptive aphasia* is an inability to understand spoken or written words; this indicates a more posterior lesion of the dominant hemisphere, in the neighborhood of the angular gyrus in the lower parietal area. (It is important for the examiner to distinguish between an aphasic patient and one who has a severe degree of confusion or is in semicoma.)

Marked parietal damage in either hemisphere may result in various degrees of apraxia, a condition in which the patient is not able to use the contralateral limbs; this should not be confused with the presence of hemiparesis or hemiplegia. Extrapyramidal motor disorder may be present and indicates focal involvement of the basal ganglia. Marked ataxia of the peripheral type (as manifested in the finger-nose or knee-heel test), or of the more central type (as manifested in truncal ataxia or inability to walk), may indicate involvement of the cerebellum or its connections.

Occasionally, damage to the lower cranial nerves can be established; the patient may show inability to swallow, difficulty of phonation from involvement of the vocal cords and weakness of the sternocleidomastoid and trapezius muscles from injury to the eleventh cranial nerve. Deviation of the tongue and the uvula indicates injury of the twelfth cranial nerve. In cooperating patients, the finding of complete homonymous hemianopsia (or occasionally quadrant hemianopsia) can provide strong evidence that the lesion is located in the optic radiation, either in the posterior limb of the internal capsule or in the temporal lobe near the occipital cortex.

A focal seizure discharge occurs infrequently but may be of diagnostic value in locating a lesion. However, it should be emphasized that postictal involvement of the corresponding contralateral limbs should not be misinterpreted as indicating permanent hemiparesis or hemiplegia. Focal, or occasionally generalized, epileptic discharges may be observed starting a few hours after the head injury. This generally indicates that the lesions — from cerebral concussion or laceration, mostly related to compound fractures or penetrating injuries to the brain — are located in the area of the motor strip or in its immediate vicinity. The more marked participation of one limb (leg versus arm) or even the face may facilitate a more exact focal diagnosis.

SPECIAL DIAGNOSTIC AIDS

Various special diagnostic methods were described in the past to assess more accurately the type and site of head injury and its intracranial complications. The introduction of the CT scan has radically changed the course of action in selecting these methods. Most of them became obsolete; they are time-consuming and with low return of accurate information, compared with the advantages of computerized axial tomography. In most cases, plain x-rays of the skull and echoencephalography are indicated as first choice, followed immediately by the CT scan. The previously mentioned limited use of radioactive brain scan, rheoencephalography and electroencephalography[15, 51] proved to be of no practical value in the study of acutely head injured patients. Air injections (pneumoencephalography or ventriculography) belong entirely to the past;[37] of the so-called invasive methods, cerebral angiography is still practiced if a CT scan is not available, and will be discussed in some detail.

X-ray Examination. Routine x-ray examination of the skull should be performed after the general and neurological examinations have excluded the possibility of cervical spine fracture, dislocation of the atlanto-occipital joint (with or without fracture of the odontoid process) and other conditions in which any excessive movements, including the necessary flexion or extension of the head to obtain the desired quality of radiography, are contraindicated. The routine films should include:[12]

ANTEROPOSTERIOR VIEW. This should be taken with the patient lying face up on the radiography table, with the orbitomeatal line perpendicular to the table and the tube inclined 25 degrees caudally.

HALF-AXIAL VIEW. (Towne's projection.) This is made with a 35-degree inclination of the tube caudally (using the same position of patient as previously).

POSTEROANTERIOR VIEW. The patient is in the face-down position with the tube inclined 25 degrees caudally, and the orbitomeatal line perpendicular to the table.

LATERAL VIEWS. Right and left lateral views are taken with the patient in the supine, brow-up position and with the central beam horizontal, entering a point approximately 1 cm. above the external auditory meatus.

BASAL VIEWS. If the clinical and neurological examinations indicate a possible *basal skull fracture*, a basal view (and possibly oblique views of the petrous pyramids) should be obtained. The recognition of a basal fracture on the routine films, including the basal and oblique views, is occasionally very difficult; probably in a majority of cases such a fracture cannot be seen on the radiograph obtained in the emergency room. On the other hand, the presence of a skull fracture (or even several fractures) does not necessarily indicate the exact severity of a head injury; multiple linear fractures may be present without any significant neurological involvement. However, the recognition of linear fractures has significance, especially if there is indication that the fracture line is crossing some of the important vascular channels,

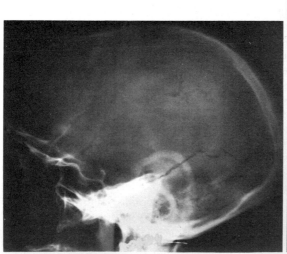 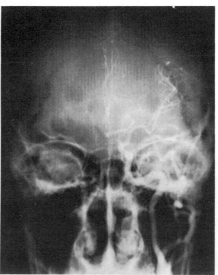

Figure 8–8. A, *Radiograph of the skull, lateral view. Temporo-occipital linear fracture, crossing ramifications of the middle meningeal vessels. B, Left carotid angiogram, anteroposterior view, showing elevation and inward displacement of the middle cerebral artery and mild shift of the anterior cerebral artery, caused by an extradural hematoma originating underneath the fracture line.*

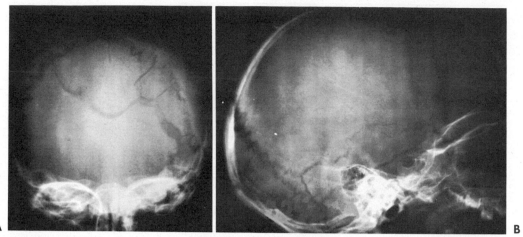

Figure 8-9. *Radiograph of the skull (A, anteroposterior view; B, lateral view), showing multiple linear fractures and widening of the suture lines.*

particularly the middle meningeal artery or its ramifications, or some of the large venous sinuses (Figs. 8–5; 8–8 to 8–10).

The recognition of a *depressed fracture* has more importance (Fig. 8–11). If there is radiographic evidence of depressed fracture that shows displacement more than 4 mm. in depth, surgical intervention (elevation of the fracture) is probably indicated, even in the absence of neurological deficit or altered consciousness, especially if the site is a so-called "low threshold" area of the cerebral cortex (precentral or temporal). If the fracture is depressed over one of the large sinuses, in general it is safer *not* to elevate it, except in the presence of an ongoing severe hemorrhage, when the sinus has to be repaired.

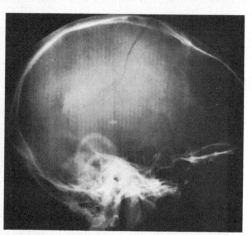

Figure 8-10. *Radiograph of the skull, lateral view. Linear fracture line can be seen crossing the superior longitudinal sinus. Pineal gland is calcified but not displaced.*

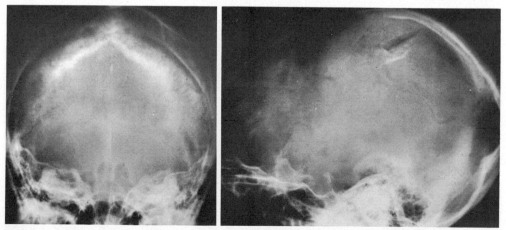

Figure 8-11. *Radiograph of the skull (A, anteroposterior view; B, lateral view), showing a healed depressed fracture which has not been surgically elevated. This patient developed focal seizures starting 8 months after the injury.*

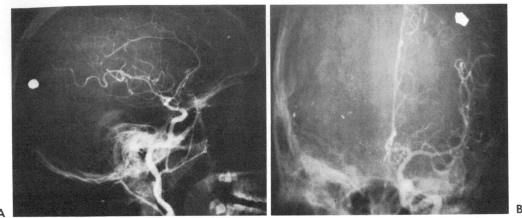

Figure 8–12. *Left carotid angiogram (A, lateral view; B, anteroposterior view) in a patient who received a gun-shot injury. The bullet can be seen in the occipital region. Although the posterior cerebral artery is not visu-alized, no displacement can be seen in the course of the other intracranial vessels. The trajectory of the bullet can be recognized; the entrance was in the right frontal region.*

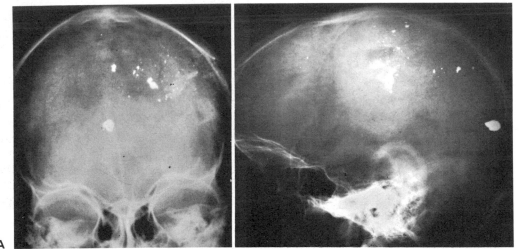

Figure 8–13. *Radiograph of the skull (A, anteroposterior view; B, lateral view), showing multiple fragmenta-tion and the final lodgment of a high-velocity bullet with entrance in the left parietal area.*

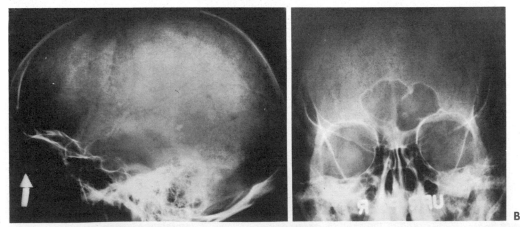

Figure 8–14. *Radiograph of the skull (A, lateral view; B, posteroanterior view) showing displacement of the calcified pineal gland from right to left and inferoposteriorly by a proven subdural hematoma.*

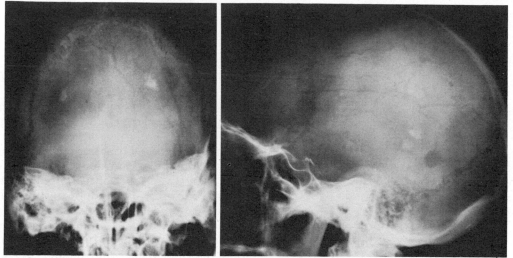

Figure 8–15. *Radiograph of the skull (A, anteroposterior view; B, lateral view), showing calcified choroid plexus bilaterally. The right one is displaced downward and posteriorly by a subdural hematoma.*

The importance of skull radiographs in cases of *compound fracture* is evident. The same is true of *penetrating injuries* from missiles. The location of the bullet, the assessment of the trajectory and the possibility of concomitant injuries to the sinuses should be evaluated on the basis of the appropriate radiographs (Figs. 8–12 and 8–13). Plain radiographs of the skull may be of significant value in assessing the presence of a *space-occupying lesion* inside the cranial cavity. Since the pineal gland is calcified in about 70 per cent of the population beyond the age of 20, displacement of the calcified pineal gland indicates the pres-

ence of a space-occupying lesion, in the form of localized or diffuse cerebral edema or epidural or subdural hematomas (Fig. 8–14). Occasionally, displacement of a calcified choroid plexus may be of some value also (Fig. 8–15).

Plain skull radiographs may show the presence of a pre-existing abnormality inside the cranial cavity. As mentioned before, head injuries may occur as a result of decompensation and sudden hemorrhage into such lesions. Increased vascular grooves on one side of the skull may be of importance on the x-rays. Similarly, abnormal intracranial calcifications in a tumor, or

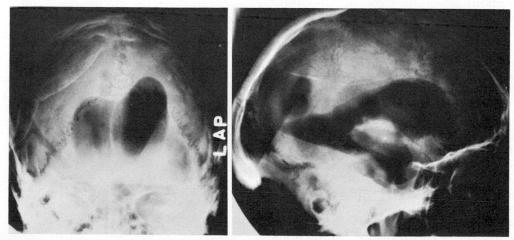

Figure 8–16. *Ventriculogram, anteroposterior (A) and lateral views (B), showing displacement of the ventricular system by a large subdural hematoma. This patient underwent a craniectomy of the posterior fossa years before, when an astrocytoma of the cerebellum was removed. The calcification of the membrane of the subdural hematoma can clearly be seen in both views.*

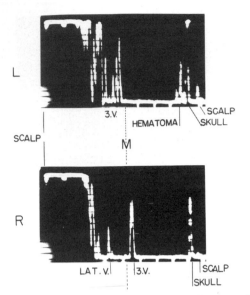

Figure 8–17. *Echoencephalograph tracing from the left and right temporal region, showing a significant displacement of the midline echo (third ventricle) by a large hematoma.*

occasionally in a chronic hematoma, will help to establish the correct diagnosis (Fig. 8–16). Separations of the sutures or increased digital markings of the internal table are indicative of pre-existing increased intracranial pressure (see Fig. 8–9). In a few instances, fractures through the frontal sinuses may result in communication with the subarachnoid space or the ventricular system, and the x-rays will show air in the subarachnoid space or inside the ventricular cavity.

Occasionally, in addition to the routine projections, tangential views may be useful to visualize small linear fractures or minimal depressed fractures in the cranial vault. Such views are generally obtained on an elective basis and are not a routine procedure in emergency room situations.[18, 25]

Echoencephalography. Since the introduction of ultrasonic techniques by Leksell,[22] several reports have been published about the use of echoencephalography in acute head injuries.[11, 23, 40, 48] The method used varies in different treatment centers. The apparatus is basically an ultrasound generator and receiver, displaying the echoes on an oscilloscope, with a camera attachment for permanent recording. A 2.25 MG transducer with a 10 mm. barium titanate crystal is most frequently used.

The examination should be made with a constant intensity of ultrasound. The pa-

tient is placed on his back, if possible, and the head is kept motionless. The region of the skull to be investigated is moistened with water or lubricating jelly before the transducer is applied; the transducer's face is in apposition to the scalp and the shaft is at right angles to the sagittal plane. To detect the midline echo, the optimal place for application of the transducer is 4 to 5 cm. above (and slightly in front of) the external auditory meatus. The temporal placement of the transducer can demonstrate a midline shift (Fig. 8–17) or a temporal hematoma (Fig. 8–18). Placement in the frontal, parietal and occipital regions confirms the midline shift and can be used to check ventricular asymmetry. Important observations can be made from echoes reflected from the subarachnoid space, the inner or outer tables of the skull, the subcutaneous tissue and the scalp surface on the side opposite the transducer.

Uematsu and Walker[48] commented on the great practical significance of this diagnostic tool. In patients with acute head injury, echograms may detect within a few minutes' time the presence of an epidural hematoma (Fig. 8–17) or an intracerebral hematoma (Fig. 8–18). The finding of a midline shift is important of itself, as it gives accurate information about the extent of the space-occupying lesion (hematoma, rapid increase in cerebral edema, subdural collection) in the involved hemisphere. The accuracy of the midline shift is about 98 per cent according to a report by White and Blanchard.[52] Children with head injuries

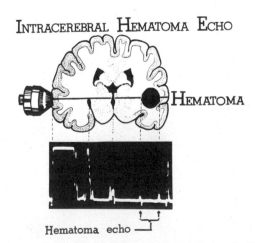

Figure 8–18. *Schematic representation of the placement of the transducer and a small intracerebral hematoma. The tracing below shows the corresponding echogram.*

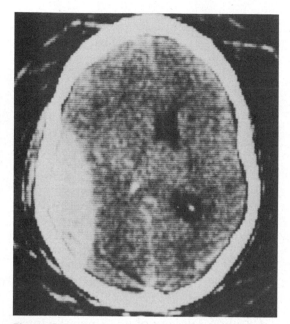

Figure 8–19. *CT scan showing a huge left-sided subdural hematoma. The high density indicates fresh blood. Note the marked displacement of the ventricular system from left to right. The patient, a 65 year old man, was hit by a car and struck the pavement with his head. Although confused, he was able to answer questions in the emergency department. Within 90 minutes, he lapsed into coma, developed a right-sided hemiplegia and dilated left pupil. The acute subdural collection was successfully drained.*

are particularly suitable for echoencephalographic studies because of the ease with which ultrasound is transmitted through the thin skull. Repeated echoencephalography and repeat neurological examination can be used as a reliable combination to establish the progression or regression of a lesion caused by acute head injury.

Lumbar puncture, even if it is performed properly, may cause sudden herniation of the medial temporal lobe into the tentorial notch, or the cerebellar tonsils into the foramen magnum, causing sudden death or irreversible brainstem damage. For this reason, lumbar puncture is not only of little diagnostic value but generally contraindicated in head-injured patients. The information obtained from the examination of the cerebrospinal fluid does not justify the risk of lumbar puncture.[31]

Computerized Axial Tomography. The initial description of the system of Hounsfield appeared in 1973[16] together with the first reports of its clinical application.[1, 2, 32] Within 18 months a large number of communications confirmed its usefulness and

safety.[2, 3, 28] Textbooks and comparative studies with other neuroradiological procedures followed the initial reports.[29, 35]

Its application in head injured patients was somewhat limited in the beginning, as the study required a completely immobilized subject. Movement produces serious artifacts, which in turn interfere with the correct interpretation of the findings. Sedation in acute head injury patients is contraindicated. However, technical progress was such that within a few years the time required for the examination was cut from the original 20 minutes to 20 seconds, making the use of the CT scan acceptable and reliable in diagnosing correctly acute head injuries.

The presence of blood in the epidural and subdural spaces, in the cerebral parenchyma or in the ventricles can easily be diagnosed (Figs. 8–19 to 8–23). The shift of the intracranial structures (ventricles, falx)

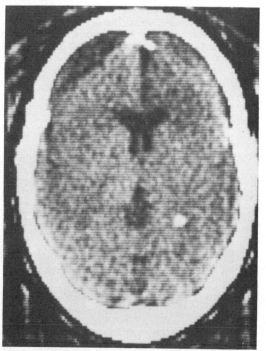

Figure 8–20. *CT scan showing a subacute left-sided frontal subdural collection. Note the difference in density from that of Fig. 8–19, indicating liquefaction of the content. The ventricular system shows practically no shift. The patient, a 54 year old man, was involved in a fight two weeks previously, when he was hit on the left side of the head. Prior to his hospital visit he had had two epileptic seizures. The subdural collection gradually disappeared; the patient was placed on anticonvulsant medication. No operation was necessary.*

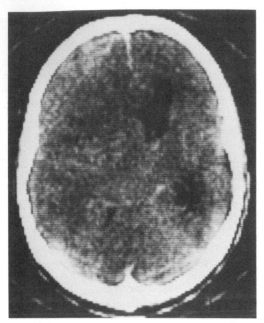

Figure 8–21. *CT scan showing a huge subdural collection (subacute hematoma) with severe shift of the ventricular system from left to right (note herniation under the falx). The patient, a 46 year old man, was involved in a car accident. The accident occurred a few days previously, but the patient was placed in a small hospital until signs of deterioration prompted his transfer. At transfer, he was barely responsive to painful stimuli. The subdural hematoma was successfully removed.*

can clearly be appreciated (Figs. 8–19 and 8–21). The presence of intracerebellar hemorrhage, a condition always difficult to diagnose in the past, can be easily confirmed (Fig. 8–24). Liquified subdural or intradural hematomas lose density and after two to three weeks they may become isodense with the normal cerebral tissue. But even in these cases, the persistent edema and the shift of the ventricles will help to establish the correct diagnosis (Fig. 8–21). Concomitant injuries (intracerebral and intraventricular hematomas) (Fig. 8–25) or pre-existing conditions (Fig. 8–26) can be precisely diagnosed.

Another advantage of the technique is that consequential studies will show decrease (Fig. 8–27) or increase of the subdural or intracerebral hematomas, guiding the surgeon in regard to possible reintervention.

Cerebral Angiography. Since the introduction of cerebral angiography by Moniz in 1927, many reports have emphasized its value in indicating the presence and exact location of space-occupying lesions in acute and chronic head injuries.[8, 9, 13, 14, 30, 44, 46] However, the introduction of CT scanning almost eliminated the use of this invasive technique, with a

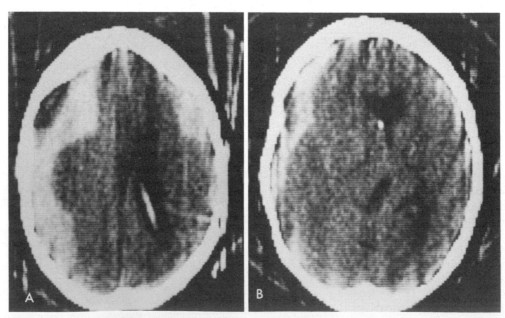

Figure 8–22. *CT scan in a higher (A) and lower (B) cut, showing a huge, left-sided, irregularly shaped subdural hematoma and a smaller right-sided collection. Again, the high density indicates the presence of fresh blood.*

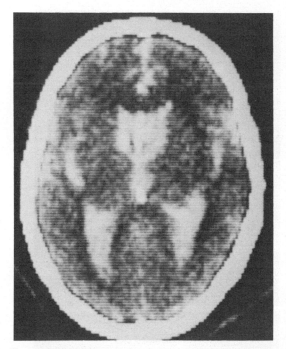

Figure 8-23. CT scan showing the outline of the ventricular system with fresh blood and the presence of bilateral small subdural collections. The patient, a 64 year old woman, was found unconscious in the street and died shortly after this scan was obtained.

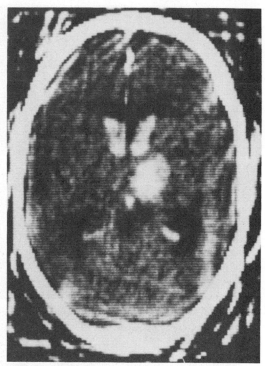

Figure 8-25. CT scan of a thalamic hemorrhage with intraventricular fresh blood in the frontal horns.

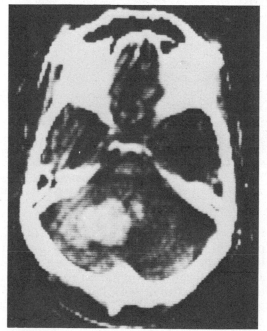

Figure 8-24. CT scan showing the presence of a huge intracerebellar hematoma on the left side, mainly in the cerebellar hemisphere, although fresh blood can be observed in the cavity of the fourth ventricle. The patient was in a deep coma on arrival at the hospital and died before surgical evacuation could be undertaken.

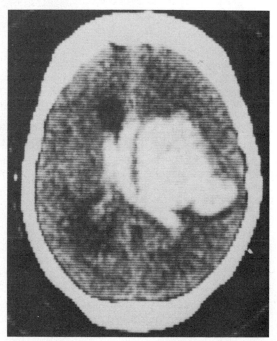

Figure 8-26. CT scan showing massive intracerebral (right central) and intraventricular hemorrhage of recent onset in a 22 year old woman who had had a minor fall. She was found to have a large arteriovenous malformation.

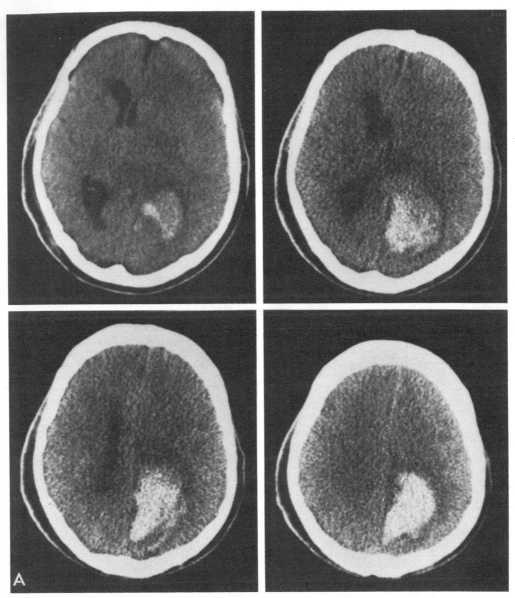

Figure 8–27. A, CT scan showing the presence of an intracerebral and intraventricular hemorrhage 6 hours after a minor accident in a hypertensive 69 year old man. Note the marked shift of the ventricular system from right to left.

low but undesirable complication rate. If a scanner is not available, cerebral angiography is still the most reliable method of diagnosis in expert hands. Cerebral angiography can be performed by subcutaneous puncture of the common carotid arteries, of the brachial artery (retrograde injection) or by transfemoral catheterization. The last technique is the most reliable one, and gives the most informative angiographic pictures with the smallest amount of dye injected. Its performance requires a well-trained neuroradiological team. It is still

time-consuming. Generally 50 per cent Hypaque or 60 per cent Renografin is used. At least three films should be taken in the anteroposterior position and three films in the lateral position. A biplane serial angiograph requires only one injection; simultaneous anteroposterior and lateral views can be obtained, showing the vascular structure in two planes at the same time.

The arterial phase of the cerebral angiography may reveal a displacement of the anterior cerebral artery across the midline, indicating a space-occupying lesion (Fig.

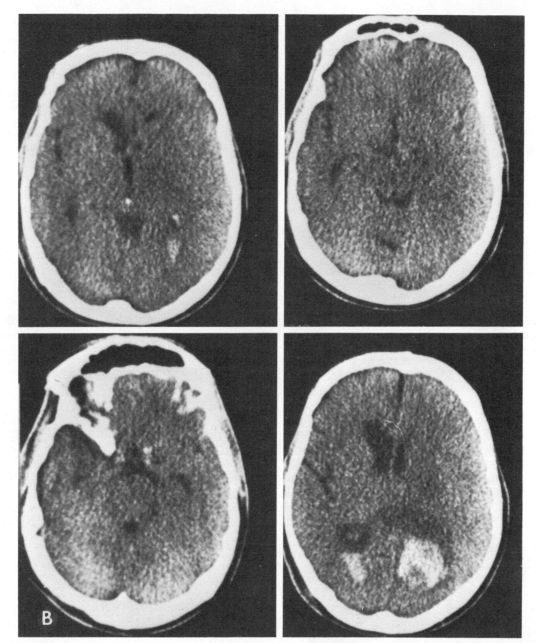

Figure 8–27. B, Forty-eight hours later the shift is much less. The intraventricular blood can be detected in the left occipital horn also. There is no evidence of subdural or extradural collection.

8–28). The cause may be increased cerebral edema, an intracerebral hematoma (Fig. 8–32) or a subdural or extradural hematoma (Fig. 8–28). The capillary phase is more diagnostic for subdural and extradural blood collections. The small arterioles and capillaries usually extend to the internal table since they are lying on the surface of the brain substance just beneath the dura. If there is any collection of blood between the cerebral cortex and the dura mater (sub-dural hematoma) or between the dura and the internal table (extradural hematoma), displacement of the capillary blush can be visualized in the anteroposterior view (Figs. 8–28 and 8–29). In the lateral views the detection of subdural or extradural collection is much more difficult, although occasionally displacement of the capillary shadow in the anterior fossa and in the anterior portion of the temporal fossa can be detected in the form of an avascular area.

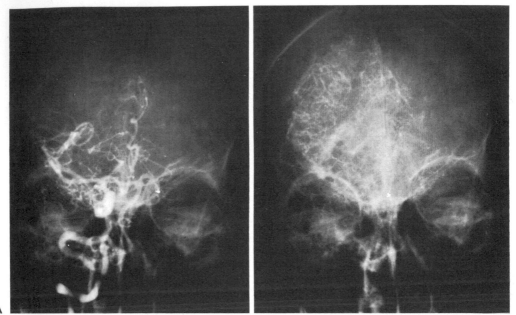

A

B

Figure 8–28.   *Percutaneous right retrograde brachial angiogram. A, anteroposterior view, early arterial phase, showing displacement of the anterior cerebral artery from left to right with concomitant shift of the posterior cerebral and middle cerebral arteries. B, anteroposterior view, capillary phase, indicating clearly the avascular area between the internal table and the cerebral cortex, which corresponds to a large collection of subdural hematoma.*

Bilateral subdural collections can be detected by angiography, not by displacement of the large vessels, because they remain in their normal position, but by the meniscus-like avascular shadows over both hemispheres in the capillary phase (Fig. 8–30).

The venous phase of the angiograms may show an obstruction of the venous sinuses by fracture fragments. Displacement of the

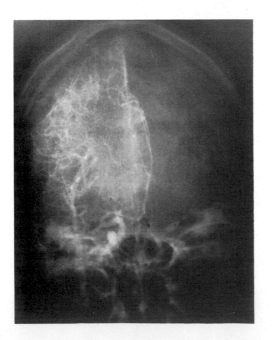

Figure 8–29.   *Right carotid angiogram, anteroposterior view, late arterial, early capillary phase. Marked shift and bowing of the anterior cerebral artery is present. The extent of the subdural hematoma can be assessed by the avascular zone over the right convexity.*

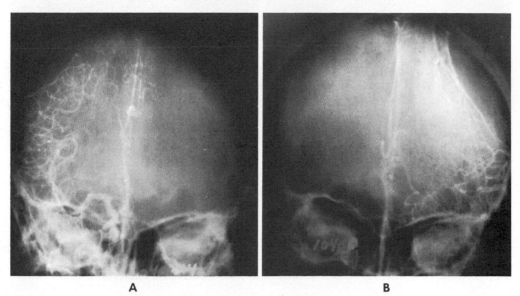

Figure 8–30. Right carotid angiogram, late arterial phase, anteroposterior view (A), and left carotid angiogram, capillary phase, anteroposterior view (B), showing the presence of a large subdural hematoma (left) and a smaller one (right). Note: There is only a minimal shift of the anterior cerebral artery from left to right.

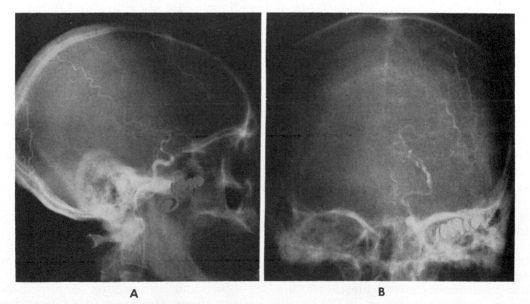

Figure 8–31. Right carotid angiogram (A, lateral view; B, anteroposterior view), showing severe narrowing of the internal carotid artery at its penetration of the dura. Only a small amount of dye entered the markedly displaced middle cerebral artery. The patient harbored a huge (250 ml.) subdural hematoma and demonstrated signs of extremely severe increased intracranial pressure.

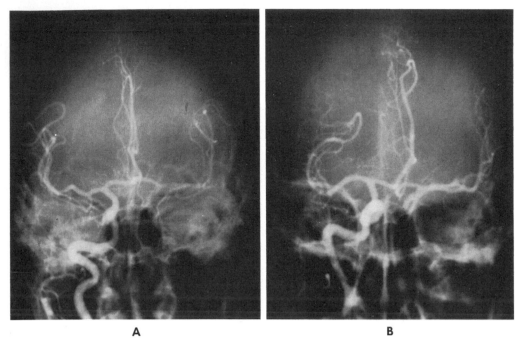

A   **B**

Figure 8–32.   *Right carotid angiogram with simultaneous compression of the left carotid artery in the neck in a patient with a deep intracerebral hematoma (A). Note the increased distance between the right middle and anterior cerebral arteries. Similar investigation (right carotid angiogram with simultaneous compression of the contralateral carotid artery) in a patient with a large subdural hematoma (B). Note the marked shift of both vessels, anterior and middle cerebral arteries, from right to left. The Sylvian point is depressed in B in contrast with A.*

deep cerebral veins, and occasional shift of the bridging veins, may indicate posteriorly placed intracerebral hematomas. Occasionally, cerebral angiography may reveal partial or complete occlusion of the carotid artery as it penetrates the dura (Fig. 8–31).

Angiography should be performed only in those treatment centers in which these procedures are done on a routine basis; otherwise, in patients with acute head injuries with a possible extradural hematoma and rapid clinical deterioration, valuable time may be wasted in trying to perform an angiography inexpertly, perhaps in the middle of the night, with insufficiently trained technical personnel or by residents who do not do this type of diagnostic study routinely. On the other hand, if well-trained personnel are available, the routine cerebral angiography generally can be obtained within 20 to 30 minutes, a reasonable proposition even in the acute situations. However, the value of angiography is greater in the detection of subacute and chronic hematomas. The availability of CT scanning puts cerebral angiography in sec-

ond place. Its use is justified if and when the CT scanner is not available or is not functioning.

Widening of the distance between the anterior and middle cerebral arteries in the anteroposterior view suggests the possibility of a deep intracranial clot (Fig. 8–32). Elevation of the middle cerebral artery indicates the presence of a hematoma in the temporal lobe (Fig. 8–33). In patients in whom the head injury resulted from a sudden hemorrhage, angiography is also of value in establishing the possibility of a pre-existing arteriovenous malformation, intracranial aneurysm or, occasionally, intracerebral tumor.

Electroencephalography.   The value of electroencephalography in head injuries was emphasized first by Williams and Gibbs,[51] and later reports confirmed their observations. However, its value in acute head injuries became negligible; but in severe head injuries with clinical evidence of deep coma, the biological activity of the brain may be so much reduced that the EEG will show only a "flat record." Although recovery from such conditions is extremely rare, care should be taken before a conclusion of "cerebral death" is reached.

SUMMARY AND CONCLUSIONS

In spite of the remarkable progress in diagnostic techniques, the accurate management of acute head injury patients still depends on clinical judgment. In a few cases the sequence of events is so rapid that no time can be lost in performing special diagnostic studies. If the neurological status suggests rapid deterioration, simple twist-drill burr holes[7] may be of considerable value. Through the twist-hole openings, needles can be introduced into the epidural and subdural spaces or into the brain substance, relieving the rapidly increasing pressure caused by the extradural,

subdural or intracerebral collection of blood. Such procedures are lifesaving. The most expedient method in such cases, however, is to take the patient into the operating room, place six routine burr holes over the cerebral hemispheres and two over the cerebellar hemispheres, confirm the presumed diagnosis and, at the same time, drain the hematomas.

As mentioned before, the CT scan will confirm the presence of posterior fossa hematomas, a condition often not diagnosed in the past. However, in the absence of a CT scanner, the routine placement of burr holes over the posterior fossa will ensure the proper diagnosis and treatment.

The remarkable progress in our diagnostic techniques, the sophistication of intracranial pressure measurements and the development of complex monitoring provide a better outcome for severely head-injured

A

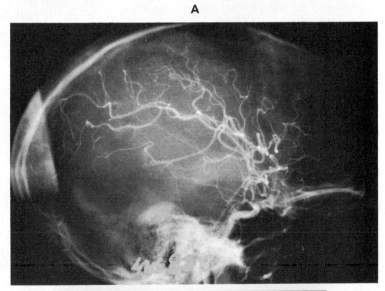

Figure 8–33. Left carotid angiogram, lateral (A) and anteroposterior (B) views. The middle cerebral artery is elevated, with upward bowing. Severe spasm can be observed in the internal carotid and anterior cerebral arteries. The patient had a large intratemporal hematoma.

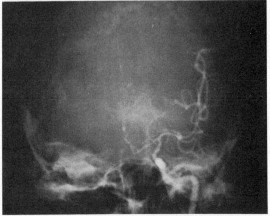

B

TABLE 8–5. Algorithm for Cerebral Death*

The patient, normothermic and normotensive,† must be comatose, apneic and without cephalic reflexes.

and

The case must meet the conditions specified in A, B, or C.

A.
  1. This state must be present for at least 3 days.

or

B.
  1. The primary condition must be known to be an irreparable lesion of the brain.
  2. The patient, by appropriate examinations, must be shown to have for at least 30 minutes:
      (a) electrocerebral silence in the EEG

or

      (b) absence of cerebral blood flow‡

or

      (c) no cerebral metabolism§

or

C.
  1. The primary condition, not a known irreparable lesion of the brain, has not responded to appropriate treatment.
  2. The patient's EEG must be isoelectric for 2 days

or

at least 6 hours after the ictus, the EEG must be isoelectric for 30 minutes and either there must be no evidence of cerebral blood flow, or no cerebral metabolism for 30 minutes.

---

*From Walker, A. E.: Cerebral Death.

†The rectal temperature should be above 90° F (32° C) and the systolic blood pressure should be above 80 mm. Hg, for hypothermia and hypopiesia may so depress cerebral activity that areflexia and ECS result; if these vital functions cannot be restored to a normal level, cerebral death may be declared on the basis of the other criteria and the absence of cerebral blood flow for 30 minutes.

‡This may be determined by quantitative measurements of CSF, four-vessel angiography, isotopic angiography, bolus passage of isotopes intravenously injected or demonstration of the absence of a midline echo.

§A $CMRO_2$ level below 1 ml./gm./min., or an $AVDO_2$ of less than 2 vols. per cent, or a lactic acid level greater than 6 mEq./L.

patients.[5, 6, 41, 47, 49] Therefore, after the initial clinical evaluation, if the patient shows signs of a relative stabilization, transportation with the care of appropriately trained nursing personnel to one of the nearest head injury centers or acute neurosurgical units is recommended. On the other hand, patients whose condition is unstable, patients in shock and patients with rapidly increasing neurological deficit or deteriorating level of consciousness should be treated immediately along the guidelines outlined previously. The specific surgical techniques are discussed elsewhere in this book.

As patients with severe, irreversible head injury comprise a large number of organ donors, the question of cerebral death should be briefly discussed. It has been the object of continuing studies in many countries; a clear representation of the development of the concept and its practical application can be found in Walker's recent monograph.[50] An algorithm for cerebral death has been prepared (Table 8–5).

The state of the cerebral circulation complements the clinical impression of brain death in several respects. First, these techniques offer a means of establishing brain death without knowledge of the causative factor — whether it be an irreparable cerebral lesion or exogenous intoxication — because a half hour's cessation of cerebral blood flow from any cause predicates a dead brain. Secondly, because a long wait for laboratory determinations is unnecessary, an early diagnosis of brain death provides a large number of more viable donor organs for transplantation.

REFERENCES

1. Ambrose, J.: Computerized transverse axial scanning (tomography): Part 2. Clinical Application. Br. J. Radiol. 46:1023–1047, 1973.
2. Baker, H. L., et al.: Computer assisted tomography of the head: An early evaluation. Mayo Clin. Proc. 49:17–27, 1974.
3. Baker, H. L., Jr., et al.: Computerized transaxial tomography in neuro-ophthalmology. Am. J. Ophthalmol. 78:285–294, 1974.
4. Becker, D. P., et al.: The outcome from severe head injury with early diagnosis and intensive management. J. Neurosurg. 47:491–502, 1977.
5. Britt, R. H., and Hamilton, R. D.: Large decompressive craniotomy in the treatment of acute subdural hematoma. Neurosurgery 2:195–200, 1978.
6. Bruce, D. A., et al.: Outcome following severe head injuries in children. J. Neurosurg. 48:679–688, 1978.
7. Burton, C., and Blacker, H. M.: A compact hand drill for emergency brain decompression. J. Trauma 5:643, 1965.
8. Carton, C. A.: Cerebral Angiography in the Management of Head Trauma. Springfield, Ill., Charles C Thomas, 1959.
9. Cronqvist, S., and Kohler, R.: Angiography in epidural haematomas. Acta Radiol. 1:42, 1963.

10. Enevoldsen, E. M., and Jensen, F. T.: Autoregulation and CO_2 responses of cerebral blood flow in patients with acute severe head injury. J. Neurosurg. *48*:689–703, 1978.

11. Gobiet, W.: Monitoring of intracranial pressure in patients with severe head injury. A review of 100 cases. Neurochirurgia *20*:35–47, 1977.

12. Gryspeerdt, G. L.: Radiology of acute head injuries. *In* Rowbotham, G. F.: Acute injuries of the Head. (4th Ed.) Baltimore, The Williams & Wilkins Co., 1964, pp. 361–407.

13. Hancock, D. O.: Angiography in acute head injuries. Lancet *2*:745, 1961.

14. Hirsch, J. R., David, M., and Borne, G.: An angiographic sign of extradural hematomas. Neurochirurgia *5*:91, 1962.

15. Hoefer, P. F. A.: The electroencephalogram in cases of head injury. *In* Brock, S.: Injuries of the Brain and Spinal Cord and Their Coverings. New York, Springer Publishing Co., 1960, pp. 707–732.

16. Hounsfield, G. N.: Computerized transverse axial scanning (tomography): Part 1. Description of system. Br. J. Radiol. *46*:1010–1022, 1973.

17. Jefferson, A., and Hill, A. I.: Echoencephalography. *In* Progress in Neurological Surgery. (Vol. 1.) Chicago, Year Book Medical Publishers, Inc., 1966, pp. 64–93.

18. Jefferson, A., and Lewtas, N.: Value of tomography and subdural pneumography in subfrontal fractures. Acta Radiol. *1*:118, 1963.

19. Jennett, B., and Bond, M.: Assessment of outcome after severe brain damage. A practical scale. Lancet *1*:480–484, 1975.

20. Klingler, M.: Das Schädelhirntrauma. Leitfaden der Diagnostik und Therapie. Stuttgart, G. Thieme Verlag, 1968.

21. Langfitt, T. W.: Measuring the outcome from head injuries. J. Neurosurg. *48*:673–678, 1978.

22. Leksell, L.: Echoencephalography. I. Detection of intracranial complications following head injury. Acta Chir. Scand. *110*:301, 1955.

23. Leksell, L.: Echoencephalography. II. Midline echo from the pineal body as an index of pineal displacement. Acta Chir. Scand. *115*:255, 1958.

24. Mapother, E.: Mental symptoms associated with head injury: The psychiatric aspect. Br. Med. J. *2*:1055, 1937.

25. Mayer, E. G.: Schädelröntgenologie. Berlin, Springer Verlag, 1959, pp. 173–191.

26. Miller, J. D., et al.: Significance of intracranial hypertension in severe head injury. J. Neurosurg. *47*:503–516, 1977.

27. Monakow, C. von: Die Lokalisierung in das Grosshirn und der Abbau der Funktion durch kortikale Herde. Wiesbaden, Ed. Bergman, 1914.

28. New, P. F. J., et al.: Computerized axial tomography with the EMI scanner. Radiology *110*:109–123, 1974.

29. New, P. F. J., and Scott, W. R.: Computer Tomography of the Brain and Orbit (EMI Scanning). Baltimore, The Williams and Wilkins Co., 1975.

30. Norman, O.: Angiographic differentiation between acute and chronic subdural and extradural haematomas. Acta Radiol. *46*:371, 1956.

31. Paterson, J. H.: Some observations on the cerebrospinal fluid in closed head injuries. J. Neurol. Psychiatry *6*:87, 1948.

32. Perry, B. J., and Bridges, C.: Computerized transverse axial scanning (tomography): Part 3. Radiation dose consideration. Br. J. Radiol. *46*:1048–1051, 1973.

33. Pevsner, P. H., Bhushan, C., Ottesen, O. E., and Walker, A. E.: Cerebral blood-flow and oxygen consumption. An on-line technique. Johns Hopkins Med. J. *128*:134–140, 1971.

34. Posner, J. B.: Clinical evaluation of the unconscious patient. Clin. Neurosurg. *22*:281–301, 1975.

35. Ramsey, R. G.: Computer tomography of the brain, with clinical angiographic and radionucleic correlation. No. 9. *In* Advanced Services in Diagnostic Radiology. Philadelphia, W. B. Saunders Co., 1977.

36. Rowbotham, G. F.: Acute Injuries of the Head. (4th Ed.) Baltimore, The Williams & Wilkins Co., 1964.

37. Ruggiero, G.: L'Encéphalographie Fractionnée. Paris, Masson & Cie, Ed. Librairie de L'Académie de Médecine, 1957.

38. Russell, W. R.: Discussion of the diagnosis and treatment of acute head injuries. Proc. Roy. Soc. Med. *25*:751, 1932.

39. Russell, W. R.: Cerebral involvement in head injury. Brain *55*:549, 1932.

40. Schiefer, W.: Die Echo-Enzephalographie diagnostischer Möglichkeiten. Dtsch Med. Wochenschr. *89*:1394, 1964.

41. Simeone, F. A., et al.: The neurosurgical intensive care unit of the future. Clin. Neurosurg. *22*:422–431, 1975.

42. Symonds, C. P.: The effects of injury upon the brain. Lancet *7*:820, 1932.

43. Symonds, C. P.: Assessment of symptoms following head injury. Guy's Hosp. Rep. *51*:461, 1937.

44. Taveras, J. M., and Wood, E. H.: Diagnostic Neuroradiology. Baltimore, The Williams & Wilkins Co., 1964.

45. Teasdale, G., and Jennett, B.: Assessment of coma and impaired consciousness. A practical scale. Lancet *2*:81–84, 1974.

46. Thomson, J. L. G.: Arteriography in head injuries. J. Fac. Radiologists *14*:339, 1961.

47. Tindall, G. T., et al.: Monitoring of patients with head injuries. Clin. Neurosurg. *22*:332–363, 1975.

48. Uematsu, S., and Walker, A. E.: A Manual of Echoencephalography. Baltimore, The Williams & Wilkins Co., 1971.

49. VanderArk, G. D.: Cardiovascular monitoring in neurosurgery. Clin. Neurosurg. *22*:462–475, 1975.

50. Walker, A. E.: Cerebral death. Professional Information Library, 1977.

51. Williams, D., and Gibbs, F. A.: Electroencephalography in clinical neurology: its value in routine diagnosis. Arch. Neurol. Psychiatry *41*:519, 1939.

52. White, D. N., and Blanchard, J. B.: Studies in ultrasonic echoencephalography. IV. Results of an averaging technique to localize the cerebral midline structure. Neurology *15*:1041, 1965.

53. Woodhall, G.: Acute cerebral injuries: Analysis of temperature, pulse, and respiration curves. Arch. Surg. *33*:560, 1936.

THE TREATMENT OF CRANIOCEREBRAL INJURIES

J. Donald McQueen, M.D.

MANAGEMENT IN THE EMERGENCY DEPARTMENT

Data from the work of Caveness[2] suggests that craniocerebral injuries accounted for 8 million cases and 13.7 per cent of all trauma for this country in the year 1974. Serious injuries were found in 1.9 million cases or 3.2 per cent of the total (after contusions and lacerations of the face, neck and scalp were excluded).

Certain aspects of symptomatic treatment are handled before decisions are made on neurosurgical interventions. These include respiratory insufficiency and shock.

Initially, attention is directed to the maintenance of a free airway. The collar is loosened, the mouth is searched for loosened teeth or foreign material and the pharynx is suctioned assiduously. Obstruction from a lax, mislocated tongue is common in the unconscious patient. Bronchial secretions are not cleared and may form excessively as a result of upper brainstem stimulation. Occasionally, frank pulmonary edema ensues. It is therefore wise to consider tracheal intubation for patients in whom tongue traction or positioning and the use of an airway fail to alleviate respiratory obstruction. This is perhaps the single most important decision in the management of these patients; the lowered mortality rates during the past two decades may be traced to this rather than to the use of specific operative techniques or the use of such adjuncts as hypothermia or intravenous hypertonic fluids. Clinically it is often difficult to be sure of the exact contribution of upper airway obstruction to brain swelling; the profound deterioration after aspiration is usually clear, and vomitus and blood are commonly demonstrated in the lungs of head injury victims on postmortem examination. Therefore, equal consideration should be given to the aspiration of gastric contents, and a nasogastric tube should be retained in this group of patients. This problem is especially common in intoxicated individuals.

With acute head trauma, signs of shock point to associated injuries. Sustained neurogenic shock is an entity with spinal cord injury but not with brain injury except in terminal states. Occasionally, a large extradural hematoma will induce incipient shock in an infant because of a disproportionately large head, the adaptability of the brain and the compliance of the skull. The blood pressure levels are usually normal even in this instance, and the diagnosis is made primarily from the combination of pallor and listlessness. However, this is an exception and extracranial trauma must be assumed in the presence of established shock. It should be stressed, as well, that a normotensive state may reflect a combination of intracranial hypertension plus pre-existing systemic hypotension, or, alternately, intracranial hypertension and blood loss.

About one third of patients with serious head trauma have other significant injuries. Fractures of the long bones and facial bones, abdominal and chest injuries are relatively common. These diagnoses are often difficult to make in the unconscious patient. A retroperitoneal hematoma, in particular, may be hard to discern in this circumstance. In general, the arrest of hemorrhage from a ruptured spleen or liver will be given priority over neurosurgical procedures, although trephine openings may be placed at the time of the laparotomy. General anesthesia is not contraindicated with acute head injury; however, great emphasis should be placed on the avoidance of hypercarbia and the use of an agent such as halothane since the consequent cerebral vasodilation may not be tolerated in a crowded cranium. Similarly, adequate oxygen therapy and deft tracheal intubations and extubations should be stressed.

Concurrent chest and head injuries constitute a particularly unfavorable combination because of the possible aggravation of brain injury by hypoxemia and hypercarbia. Here again, respiratory control is the prime consideration; present-day management, especially with the use of respirators, has greatly improved the prognosis of patients in this group.

With all of these injuries, one or more cannulae are placed in appropriate veins, blood is withdrawn for matching, intravenous fluids are started, a Foley catheter is inserted and blood is replaced. Vasoconstrictors are used very sparingly in order not to mask hemorrhage.

Special effort is required in obtaining the details of the history of these patients because of obvious problems in communication. Knowledge of the previous status of the patient is important in many ways; for example, the prior blood pressure levels should be known since temporarily induced neurogenic hypertension is common with head trauma. A record of cerebrovascular disease may suggest the cause of the injury; one of alcoholism may aid in recognition of a subdural collection. Similarly, an accurate description of the accident may help in locating a depressed fracture, in diagnosing suspected transorbital or infratentorial damage and in mapping sites of contrecoup injury. Information on the sequence of events after the impact is most important. A progressive deterioration of the state of consciousness, with or without a lucid interval, is an indication for neurosurgical intervention. The longterm use of anticoagulants should be determined because of the added risk of intracranial hematoma formation, and patients with trivial head trauma who are receiving such agents should be detained or followed closely. These are elementary points; however, they should be stressed since the search for pertinent information in the accident room is commonly deficient.

Certain fundamental clinical findings that bear on neurosurgical interventions are noted here. The essentials are: depression of the level of consciousness, slowing of the pulse, pupillary changes, loss of muscle power, reflex alterations and local changes about the head. A deterioration in the state of consciousness is always the pre-eminent sign and is seldom misleading, although patients with chronic subdural hematomas and other long-standing lesions may become more responsive from time to time as the brain accommodates to the mass. When there is a known head injury, the prime indications for burr-hole

explorations are: (1) deep coma, (2) a progressive lowering of awareness or (3) a lucid interval. With the exclusion of hopeless high-velocity missile injuries, explorations should be carried out quickly if the depression of the level of consciousness is sustained and reaches the point where only limited reactions to painful stimuli remain. This exigency is uncommon, and a period of close observation is usually possible. CT scanning and/or arteriography should be strongly considered and completed with proper indications and when time permits.

A fixed, dilated pupil is a reliable sign. Misjudgments may occur because of orbital trauma, and transient pupillary changes may be associated with irritation of the frontal eye fields and with seizures. The third nerve is stretched by displaced medial temporal lobe structures which are thrust down by a hematoma or with brain swelling. This process usually occurs bilaterally, and fortuitously, there may be greater involvement on the opposite side in about 20 per cent of cases.

Slowing of the pulse rate is a helpful sign in the diagnosis of an intracranial hematoma, but it is not reliable as an isolated finding since it is often found without brain compression. The presence of a heart block or intraocular hypertension should be considered.

Hemipareses and reflex changes are valuable localizing findings, although an expanding lesion may be on the same side as the motor loss. Here, the brainstem is displaced so that the contralateral motor fibers are impinged upon the sharp, tentorial edge. Changes in motor power and tone per se are not indications for trephinations and occur commonly with contusions.

Twist drill openings are placed infrequently in the accident room because of the danger of missing significant collections of clotted blood which are unable to pass through small-bore needles. However, such openings are placed in a few instances. One example is that of the unresponsive patient with a suspected massive intraventricular hemorrhage.

The patterns of intravenous fluid administration in the emergency room vary greatly because of the coexistence of other factors such as shock. Infusions of 5 per cent glucose in distilled water are given for serious injuries. They are administered slowly (in the absence of shock) because of the common, trauma-induced augmentation of antidiuretic hormone secretion. It is wise to draw early and repeated blood samples for electrolyte levels. The detection of hyponatremia is of particular importance, and, with care, fluid administration may be regulated so as to avoid iatrogenic water intoxication.

Hypertonic mannitol (or a non-osmotic agent such as furosemide) is commonly used for the alleviation of brain swelling; except in extreme circumstances its use before explorations (or definitive CT scanning or angiography) is contraindicated because of the facilitated expansion of intracranial hematomas.

Hyperventilation is frequently utilized with severe injuries and will be discussed later.

The corticosteroid derivatives are used very commonly at the present time but are reserved for serious injuries in which the outcome is in question and those causing such states as persistent unresponsiveness and decerebration. If corticosteroid injections are to be given, they should be used soon after the initial evaluation in the accident room or held for later use in patients with regressions. Methylprednisolone compounds are popular; the dosage of dexamethasone is 10 mg. immediately and 4 mg. every 6 hours, either intravenously or intramuscularly.

There are three types of open head wounds: blunt injuries with compound depressed fractures and high- and low-velocity penetrating wounds. All patients with injuries in the first category should be taken promptly to the operating room; initially, the wound is inspected but is not thoroughly irrigated. Routine skull films are obtained and a snug head bandage is applied.

Many injuries from high-velocity missiles are irrecoverable. For example, in a study by Goodman and Kalsbeck[4] 70 per cent of the self-inflicted gunshot wounds were fatal. The force that is expended in the brain varies as the square of the velocity (or the cube at very high speeds) and is sufficient per se to burst the skull. In addition, the bullet commonly traverses the skull and often ricochets about with added damage. These victims arrive in the accident room in deep coma with fixed and dilated pupils. Roentgenograms are made to demonstrate the missile path but specific therapy should be withheld.

Often bullets are slowed or deflected by bone and skirt the brain or enter it at low velocity. In these instances patients may display varied cranial nerve palsies and/or limited brain damage. Adequate antibiotic therapy is instituted; operative intervention is delayed when the major objective is missile removal but is prompt in other instances. Other low-velocity injuries include trauma from perforating knife and fan blades, ice picks, rods and shafts. Patients suffering this type of trauma are taken directly to the operating room, where the undisturbed penetrating object is "prepped" in the field.

OPERATIVE MANAGEMENT

Operative procedures may be divided into four main groups of explorations and are directed to: (1) hematoma evacuation, (2) elevation of depressed bone, (3) debridement of brain, or (4) frontal or temporal lobectomies for unrelieved brain swelling.

Intracranial hematomas are usually evacuated through trephine openings or craniotomy defects. The latter approach is particularly useful for acute and subacute subdural hematomas since clotted blood is inadequately removed through the standard one half-inch trephine opening. A CT scan is very helpful in placing the craniotomy flaps. Craniotomies may also be required for the late removal of subdural membranes. This occurs in only a few instances (and after simpler measures have failed).

The head is fully shaved in the anesthetic room, and a second search is made for local signs of trauma. Subgaleal hematomas are of particular importance when located over fractures since this fluid may constitute drainage from an extradural collection.

General anesthesia is preferred over local blocks in most cases because of the necessity of immobilizing the head during operative procedures. Anesthesia is induced with Pentothal in such a way that struggling is minimized and cerebrospinal fluid pressures are not unduly elevated. The patient may then be curarized, intu-

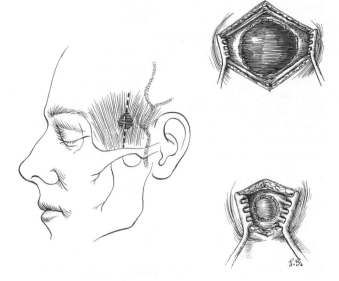

Figure 8–34. *Trephine openings. The site of the common temporal opening is shown to the left. This defect is enlarged to the size of a silver dollar, as noted in the upper right. The smaller frontal or parietal opening is depicted in the lower right diagram.*

bated and ventilated with nitrous oxide and oxygen. Nitrous oxide may be eliminated in some cases; halothane and ether should be avoided since they induce vasodilatation and hence augment intracranial crowding. The trachea is intubated, as coughing or other airway obstruction will intensify brain swelling and displace intracranial contents through dural openings.

The patient is placed on a headrest for routine trephinations. This supports the head and exposes the vault so that bilateral burr holes may be readily placed in frontal, temporal and parietal regions. The shoulders are supported on pads and the head of the table is elevated a few degrees. The vertical position is not used since shock may be a concomitant problem. Adhesive surgical drapes are valuable because immoderate amounts of irrigation fluids are often used.

Burr hole placements were commonly made bilaterally in the past; many of these may be omitted now because of the current usage of CT scanning and improved angiographic techniques.

The initial trephine opening is often placed in the temporal region (Fig. 8–34) — especially when an extradural hematoma is suspected. However, the actual choice will depend on many factors, including the results of diagnostic studies and the position of fracture lines.

The temporal incision extends vertically above the zygomatic arch over a distance of 2.5 inches. Branches of the superficial

temporal artery are cauterized and Weitlander self-retaining retractors are inserted to expose bone down to the level of the floor of the middle fossa. A cone-shaped opening is drilled through the bone with a McKenzie perforator and is enlarged to a hole of five eighths-inch diameter with a burr. The instruments are shown in Figure 8–35; they should be fashioned from steel that has high degrees of ductility and strength. Motorized units including a perforator such as the Smith drill may be used; however, the important points are the quality of the metal and the sharpness of the cutting edge rather than the choice between individual perforators. The tem-

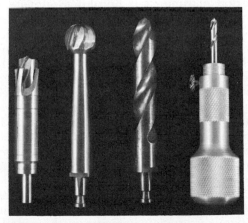

Figure 8–35. *Instruments for burr-hole and twist-drill explorations in acute head trauma. From left to right these are: a motor-driven Smith perforator, a burr, a McKenzie perforator and a small hand drill.*

poral hole is routinely enlarged to the size of a silver dollar. This is done because of the necessity for explorations beneath the temporal lobe and because of the opportunities for small, muscle-protected decompressions and limited temporal lobe resections. The temporal squama is very thin; it is rongeured rapidly and then waxed. Small, self-retaining mastoid retractors are used for the frontal and parietal openings, which are usually not enlarged.

Extradural hematomas are readily apparent as the perforator exposes black clot in breaking through the inner table. The torn middle meningeal vessel is nearly always marked by a fracture, which is commonly linear. It is wise to expose all of the collection with a craniectomy before aspirating deep portions of clot. The meningeal vessel is cauterized at the site of the rent and extensively along its course. It is necessary, on occasion, to follow the artery down to the base of the skull and to insert a small cottonoid sliver into the foramen spinosum with a right-angle hook. Numerous other areas are cauterized because of the secondary oozing that occurs as the hematoma lifts the dura mater from bone.

According to Gurdjian and Thomas,[5] varied combinations of extradural, subdural or parenchymatous hematomas may be expected in about 17 per cent of cases. The dura mater is therefore opened transversely near the base to rule out a concomitant subdural collection and to inspect the temporal lobe. If this lobe is significantly displaced and remains so over a reasonable period of time, it is helpful to elevate it with a flat brain spatula and then to tease the herniated medical temporal lobe structures back from the tentorial notch. Fine silk sutures are used to close the dura mater and to tack it to the bony edges. An extradural catheter drain is placed. Since the worldwide mortality rate from extradural hematomas remains significant, it is worthwhile stressing the dispatch that is required in all phases of their management. The lesion is depicted in Figure 8–36.

To evacuate a subdural hematoma, the darkened dura mater is thoroughly cauterized; a cruciate incision is then made with a small hook and knife. The opening should be wide enough to avoid the dangers of incising or inadvertently tear-

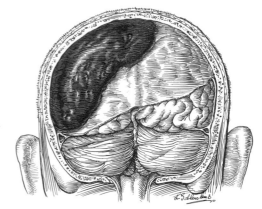

Figure 8–36. *A massive extradural hematoma that was first uncovered by the medical examiner.*

ing the cortical veins that are turgid under states of intracranial hypertension. Membranes are present around chronic subdural hematomas, and the dural incision must be deep enough to nick the exterior covering. The contents — black liquefied blood and clot — are released under raised pressure and are expelled with the respiratory and vascular pulsations of the brain. A catheter is introduced between two holes for saline irrigations. In an adult, it is usually not necessary to turn a craniotomy flap to remove the residual clot or membrane, although there are exceptions as noted earlier. The cortex sometimes remains sunken after these evacuations and may not return to its normal position. Some neurosurgeons attempt to expedite this return by directly inflating the ventricular system with saline or mock CSF, although it is not certain that the expansion persists after the added saline has been absorbed.

Massive chronic subdural hematomas of the aged present special problems and many of the results are unsatisfactory. It is helpful to consider the use of local anesthesia and the placement of a single twist-drill or a standard or enlarged trephine opening for this group. The fluid is removed slowly in order to minimize sudden shifts of intracranial structures. Repeat taps are required or a drain may be used an an alternative.

In these chronic lesions, the significant space-occupying component is the hematoma; in an acute subdural hemorrhage, the clot is relatively unimportant, but the underlying laceration and edema are significant. Exceptionally, the brain may not be lacerated and, with luck, torn bridging temporal veins may be isolated. The bleeding is then controlled by tamponade, cautery and the application of silver clips. An acute subdural hematoma is shown in Figure 8–37.

An intracerebral hematoma will often be located by arteriography or, more clearly, by a CT scan. Sometimes the diagnosis is made when a temporal clot ruptures through the cortex during a subdural exploration. In all these instances a blunt ventricular needle is passed into the hematoma cavity for gradual drainage, and a dime-sized cortical window is then made to sluice away the larger clots. Excellent results are obtained in treating these lesions if they are well contained and if they are polar.

Unfortunately, brain swelling is the major finding in many instances. Some neurosurgeons perform large craniotomies to provide decompression. Bifrontal bone flaps may be removed or bony openings provided over one hemisphere (and sometimes both). A remarkable release of constricted brain is obtained. Unfortunately, the overall results have not justified common use of this procedure and its efficacy remains debatable.

Similarly, the so-called internal decompression, which in practice constitutes a partial temporal or frontal lobe resection, is sometimes performed. When edematous cerebral tissue pouts from all burr holes, one has a reasonable indication of substan-

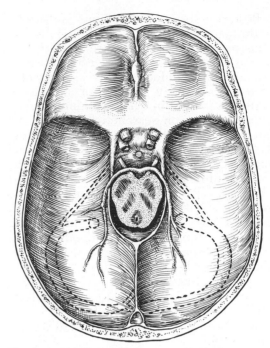

Figure 8–38. The incisura tentorii. Transtentorial herniations may occur from above or below to cause circulatory embarrassment in the distribution of the midline perforating vessels. The brainstem may be displaced against the sharp tentorial edge; the posterior cerebral artery may be kinked over it. Anterior herniations press on the third nerve to induce the common pupillary dilatation.

tial, generalized brain swelling; little chance of gain is offered with these extirpations. Contrarily, striking improvement often follows the use of these limited resections when the fullness is largely limited to one lobe. Here again, the CT scan is most helpful. On *a priori* grounds, a section of the tentorium should give relief from the pressure effects that are so devastating to the upper brainstem with generalized brain swelling. Unfortunately, it is difficult to reach the edge of the tentorium when such a section is needed because of swelling of the temporal and occipital lobes. Conversely, when ready access is possible, the procedure may be unnecessary. The crucial area for transtentorial herniations is indicated in Figure 8–38.

Excessive brain needling is often demonstrated on postmortem examination. In general, it is best to restrict these taps to single punctures of zones that are indicated by diagnostic films or that lie under cortical swellings that bulge disproportionately.

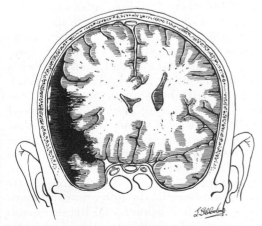

Figure 8–37. An acute subdural hematoma. Note the laceration and swelling of the brain and the subfalcial herniation.

Posterior fossa trephinations are rarely performed. Indications include (1) a venous sinus-traversing fracture of the occipital squama in association with a substantial neurologic defect, (2) the existence of a blood dyscrasia or the use of anticoagulants in a patient in whom subdural hematomas have been searched for and ruled out supratentorially, and (3) local cerebellar and lower cranial nerve signs. Fortunately CT scanning resolves many of the posterior fossa problems. It is necessary to place the patient in the cerebellar or Gardner headrest and to prep and drape anew. Either a long midline incision or two small longitudinal paramedian incisions may be used; in either case, the muscle is quickly split to bone, and self-retaining retractors are placed. A cerebellar extension is added to the Hudson brace. Hematomas occur in the same extra- and subdural compartments and within the cerebellum.

Exploration for depressed fractures is carried out without delay if the injury is compound. A few cases are dismissed because of insignificant depressions; the remainder are operated upon within a period of about 24 hours. Tangential skull films and CT scans are considered for problem cases; the latter technique is of special value when indriven bony fragments are suspected. If there is no laceration, a skin flap is preferred rather than a linear incision. The sunken bone may be elevated in several ways. It is often easy to retrieve the depressed pieces of bone with a rongeur after inserting this instrument through a small hole that has been nibbled in the margin of the intact bone. Sometimes the impinging fragments can be grasped directly or elevated with a dissector that is introduced from an adjacent burr hole. The bone may be retained if reasonable stability can be achieved. However, bony defects usually remain and cranioplasties are required. These may be carried out immediately if there is no contamination but are more frequently performed as secondary procedures. If the dura mater is intact, it is opened only with specific indications.

Although all debridements should be done fastidiously, special care is required for those of the brain since the penalties that accrue from the retention of devitalized brain tissue, bony spicules and other foreign material are severe and include the formation of abscesses and the establishment of epileptogenic foci.

The scalp edges are trimmed and the pericranial tissues are washed with saline. The bone edges are rongeured in the case of a limited injury; a craniotomy flap is opened for an extensive one. Arterial dural bleeding is arrested with the cautery; hemorrhage from rents in venous sinuses is controlled with fingertip pressure over pledgets of absorbable gelatin or cellulose. Attempts are made to completely remove the devitalized brain, using suction and excessive amounts of warm saline. Particular attention is given to the retrieval of all bony fragments. The venous oozing in the depth of these resections is usually handled with gentle tamponade from a loose, cotton "fish." Dural defects are always closed, usually with grafts of pericranial tissue. Fascia lata may be used, but plastic materials should be avoided. Local antibiotics are not instilled and drains are not placed. Fine wire or plastic suture material is used throughout. The results of this procedure are usually quite satisfactory, and it is perhaps worthwhile to emphasize the painstaking effort that should be expended in the case of such patients because of the focal nature of their injuries.

EARLY MANAGEMENT IN THE INTENSIVE CARE UNIT

An endotracheal tube may be retained for several days if needed for airway problems. Careful and frequent suctioning is carried out via a sterile catheter to remove stationary and excessive secretions. A tracheostomy is carried out later if required.

Intracranial pressure monitoring is useful in the management of many patients with severe head injury. The use of CT scanning will help in patient selection since brain swelling and/or transtentorial herniation may be demonstrated. Similarly, the presence of significant swelling at the end of an operative procedure or the clinical diagnosis of transtentorial herniation may prompt use of this technique. Its application permits the detection and analysis of sustained intracranial hypertension and permits the judicious use of osmotic agents or artificial ventilation. It sometimes provides unexpected indications for changes in head posture or tracheal suctioning.

Intraventricular pressures may be measured with a catheter. Alternately, subdural or extradural pressures may be detected. Physiological pressure transducers are used — preferably in conjunction with paper recording in order to provide a continuous tracing. Isolated, extradural sensors are under current development. This latter application is very promising since these sensors are used with telemetry to eliminate the need for transcutaneous connections.

Oxygen therapy is valuable if there is any suspicion of ischemia of the brain; carbon dioxide inhalations augment cerebral blood flow but are not used because of the attendant vasodilation in normal brain. In the absence of shock, the head of the bed is elevated 20 to 30 degrees to facilitate venous drainage.

Fluids are given parenterally at first and via a stomach tube after four to five days if the patient cannot swallow. When there is established brain swelling, the fluid intake is usually restricted for several days. During this time, approximately 1500–2000 ml. is given to an adult; the acute amount is based, in part, on the results of electrolyte determinations. In general, two thirds is administered as 5 per cent glucose in distilled water, and the remainder as isotonic saline. Detailed fluid balance sheets are kept and include repeated serum and urine electrolyte values.

Hypertonic intravenous infusions are often used to accomplish a more abrupt and drastic dehydration. Because of the osmotic effect, these agents induce a temporary fall in intracranial pressures and a decrease in brain bulk, as shown in the classic study of Weed and McKibben.[5] There is also a possible long-term benefit from the loss of water with the diuresis and a possible detrimental action as cerebrospinal fluid pressures rise secondarily. Mannitol is currently popular and in comparison with urea offers a relatively long relaxation period (and minimal rebound) because of its nonpenetrating characteristics. It is given quickly in a 20 per cent solution in a dosage range of 1–2 gm. per kg. It may be used occasionally after operations (or diagnostic procedures) when the patient worsens suddenly — as with decerebration or pupillary dilatation or when measured intracranial pressures rise precipitously during pressure waves. Insertion of a Foley catheter is mandatory. Furosemide with a dosage of 20–40 mg. may be used as an alternative as noted previously.

General hypothermia was first used for head injury problems by Fay[3]; however, the technique did not become popular until Bigelow et al.[1] demonstrated the specific depression of metabolism during cooling. A cooling blanket is used, and its temperature is conveniently regulated within a range of one to two degrees by a temperature controller and a rectal temperature probe. If the temperature is lowered more than a few degrees below the normal level, shivering and restlessness are provoked; these add serious problems in management and although they can be influenced by Phenergan, they are usually incompletely suppressed unless the patient is curarized. There is also an increased incidence of pulmonary infection in the lower temperature range (30 to 32° C.) because of depressed ciliary action in the tracheobronchial tree. Because of these drawbacks and the fact that cooling is usually instituted sometime after the injury, this measure is usually reserved for combating hyperthermia and holding temperatures at or a little below the normal level.

The use of corticosteroid derivatives is continued for severe injuries (and in the absence of gastric problems). Their initial or continued dosage will have to be reevaluated in the intensive care unit. An antacid regimen should be employed and the dosage should be tapered as quickly as possible.

The use of controlled respiration and hyperventilation is popular for the treatment of high, sustained intracranial hypertension as demonstrated with the use of a pressure monitor or when marked brain swelling is depicted on a CT scan. This technique is a substitute for the usage of wide bony decompressions (and some lobectomies). Hyperventilation is maintained through the retained endotracheal tube and $PACo_2$ values are held in the range of 26–28 torr. Intermittent curarization is often necessary and barbiturate coma therapy is popular in the presence of high pressure rises.

Excessive motor activity is frequently a

major problem in the recovery room. A minor degree of restlessness is common and requires only restraint. Agitation is found less frequently and is often inadequately controlled. Paraldehyde is the drug of choice, but its use should be restricted so that the patient's condition is not jeopardized by loss of the opportunity to follow changes in the state of consciousness. The adult dosage is 10 ml., which is given via a gastric tube or as a small retention enema. If initially ineffective, the dose may be repeated with caution; as in the management of status epilepticus, large amounts may be tolerated. Diazepam may be used as an alternative.

Seizure activity in the recovery room is relatively uncommon with acute head injury, but it should be anticipated when gross brain damage is established. Diphenylhydantoin sodium is used with an adult dosage of 100 mg., given 2–3 times a day. The actual dosage will depend on the use of other drugs.

Serial blood gas determinations are mandatory in patients with depressed responsiveness and particularly those who require respiratory support.

Fat embolism with complications from intracranial deposits or pulmonary lesions with secondary cerebral effects should be considered in all patients with major injuries. Chest roentgenogram, cryostat frozen secretions of clotted blood, blood gas studies and the search for petechial hemorrhages are stressed. Positive findings add special indications for steroid therapy as well as particular care in ventilation.

Fortunately this entity is now seen much less commonly than previously.

The finding of cerebrospinal fluid rhinorrhea or otorrhea is not uncommon in the acute trauma setting. These are associated with anterior and posterior basal skull fractures respectively and are treated conservatively with antibiotic coverage in nearly all instances. In very rare circumstances, an open (and usually missile-induced) wound will prompt use of spinal drainage, cerebrospinal fluid shunting (or transposition of a living muscle flap for otorrhea). Later, another more common and well-defined group of patients will return with meningitis or recurrent cerebrospinal fluid rhinorrhea and require anterior fossa dural repair.

REFERENCES

1 Bigelow, W. G., Lindsay, W. K., Harrison, R. C., Gordon, R. A., and Greenwood, W. F.: Oxygen transport and utilization in dogs at low body temperatures. Am. J. Physiol. *160*:125, 1950.
2. Caveness, W. F.: Epilepsy, a product of trauma in our time. Epilepsia *17*:207–215, 1976.
3. Fay, T.: Observations on generalized refrigeration in cases of severe cerebral trauma. Res. Publ. Ass. Res. Nerv. Ment. Dis. *24*:611, 1945.
4. Goodman, J. M., and Kalsbeck, J.: Outcome of self-inflicted gunshot wounds of the head. J. Trauma *5*:636, 1965.
5. Gurdjian, E. S., and Thomas, L. M.: Organization of Services for the Treatment of Acute Head Injury in Community and Industrial Practice. Presented at the Third International Congress of Neurological Surgery, Copenhagen, August 1965.
6. Weed, L. H., and McKibben, P. S.: Pressure changes in the cerebrospinal fluid following intravenous injection of solutions of various concentrations. Am. J. Physiol. *48*:512, 1919.

INJURIES OF THE SPINE AND SPINAL CORD: MANAGEMENT IN THE ACUTE PHASE

Perry Black, M.D., C.M.

Few nonfatal injuries match the devastating physical and psychological disability caused by severe spinal cord trauma. With improved techniques in management over the past half century, there has been a steady decline in the mortality and morbidity of those who survive the initial injury. The question of the indications for surgical exploration of closed spinal wounds continues to be a controversial subject among neurosurgeons. There is considerable agreement, however, regarding those aspects of patient care that relate to protection against increase in the neural damage, the prevention of complications and the promotion of an optimistic attitude toward rehabilitation. Careful attention to several relatively simple principles in management can sometimes convert a potentially serious outcome into a gratifying result. What is done in the first few hours after spinal injury — at the scene of injury, transportation to hospital and management in the emergency department — can be more important than all subsequent efforts. Although many patients face the grim prospect of permanent paraplegia or quadriplegia, much progress has been made in the social and economic rehabilitation of these patients to happy, useful lives.

This survey outlines various mechanisms of injury and principles of management with emphasis on the acute period.

MECHANISMS OF INJURY

Spinal trauma in civilian practice is generally of the *closed* variety and results from traffic accidents and falls. *Open* wounds due to missiles predominate among battle casualties, but are not uncommon in civilian life. The critical factor in spinal trauma is damage to the neural contents of the spinal canal; the vertebral injury itself is secondary. Consideration in long-term management must also be given, however, to restoration of vertebral column function; this consists of a delicate balance between mobility and stability of the neck and trunk, as well as protection of the neural contents. A knowledge of the mechanics of the injury in each patient is helpful in evaluating the extent of the trauma and may influence management and prognosis.

Closed Injuries

The regions of the vertebral column that allow the greatest mobility are also characterized by relative instability. Their muscular and articular supports are insufficient to resist violent forces. Although all portions of the spine are subject to injury, the junctional region between the rigid thoracic spine and the lower three cervical vertebrae is the most vulnerable. The thoracic spine is infrequently subject to closed injury by virtue of its minimal motion and its

support by the rib cage. The thoracolumbar junction, however, allows free movement and is consequently a common site of injury. The lower lumbar region, which is quite flexible, is similarly affected near its junction with the fixed sacrum.

Hyperflexion Injuries. Most closed spinal injuries are the result of *indirect* violence that produces extreme movement of a portion of the spine beyond its normal range. To illustrate, a dive into shallow water, or sudden deceleration in a head-on auto collision, causes extreme neck *flexion*, which is the most common mechanism of serious spinal injury (Figs. 8–39 to 8–41). The wedging force on adjacent vertebrae may crush one of the bodies, and bone fragments may be driven posteriorly into the spinal canal. Depending on the direction and intensity of the forces, there may be associated fracture of the pedicles or laminae. The fracture may be further complicated by forward dislocation of the upper vertebrae on the lower, if the powerful posterior longitudinal ligament or the articular ligaments are torn. Disruption of the intervertebral disc may result in extrusion into the spinal canal. The extent to which the deranged spine encroaches upon the canal determines the degree to which the cord is compressed. Adjacent nerve roots may be similarly compromised within the intervertebral foramina. The suddenness and force of the impact contribute to the severity of the injury.

Hyperextension Injuries. In cervical extension injuries, the spinal cord may be stretched against the forward bulging ligamenta flava, which may contuse the dorsal columns. In extreme cases, posterior dislocation occurs (Fig. 8–40). Older individuals are particularly prone to cord injury during hyperextension (e.g., under anesthesia or in a fall, striking the forehead or chin) because of pre-existing thickening of the ligamenta flava and narrowing of the spinal canal by osteoarthritic spurs. The cord is "squeezed" between the wrinkled ligamentum flavum posteriorly and the spurs anteriorly. The main stress in such an injury is in the center of the cord, resulting in the *syndrome of acute central cervical cord injury*,[23] the clinical features of which are described under "Pathophysiology of the Neural Lesion." The syndrome may also be produced by insufficiency of the blood supply to the cervical cord in hyperextension

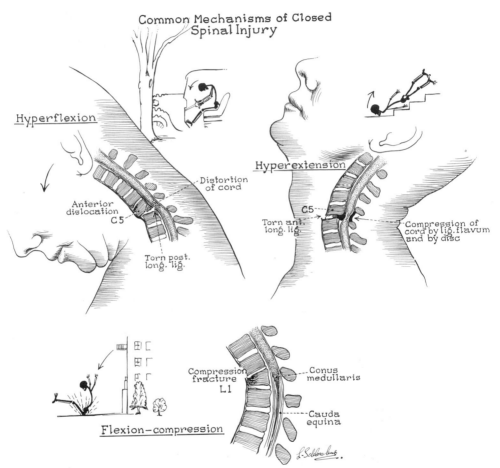

Figure 8–39. *Schematic illustrations of closed spinal injury mechanisms. The cervical hyperflexion and hyperextension diagrams represent a composite of possible factors, any number of which may occur in a particular case.*

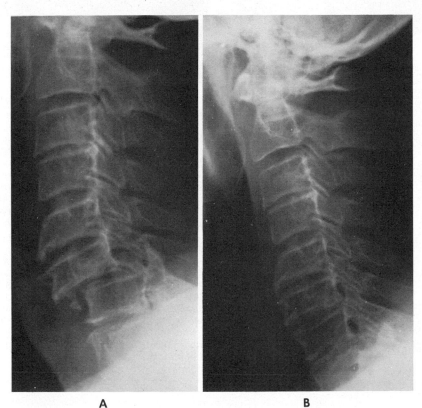

A   B

Figure 8–40.   A, *Lateral radiograph of cervical spine after hyperflexion injury, showing fracture at C6–7 with forward dislocation. Encroachment of spinal canal resulted in severe cord compression with paraplegia and partial involvement of upper extremities. B, Radiograph of same patient after closed reduction had been achieved by skeletal cervical traction with tongs. If fracture site is stable, traction may be maintained for 6 to 8 weeks of stabilization until spontaneous fusion occurs. Although, as often occurs in severe spinal cord injuries, this patient did not recover neurological function, it is important to avoid additional neural injury that might jeopardize the patient's few remaining capabilities.*

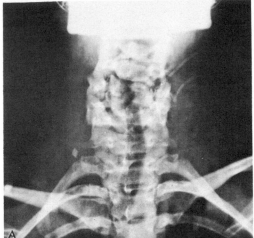

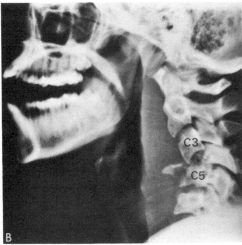

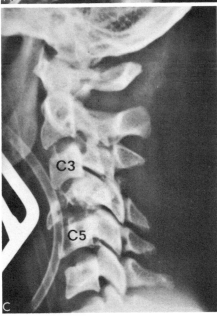

Figure 8–41. Cervical spine radiographs of 17 year old girl with severe hyperflexion fracture dislocation sustained in auto crash. A, Anteroposterior view. Note disruption of vertebral elements at C3, 4 and 5. B, Lateral view showing complete shattering of C4 vertebral body and angulation of spine. Note prevertebral swelling due to hematoma formation; in retropharyngeal area, such hematomas can obstruct the airway. C, Lateral view after closed reduction by means of skeletal traction with tongs. The patient was immediately quadriplegic, with motor and sensory level at C4. There was respiratory embarrassment with right diaphragmatic paralysis owing to partial involvement of phrenic outflow; tracheostomy and respirator were necessary for 6 weeks. Two months after injury, anterior and posterior fusions (in two stages) were performed because of likelihood of instability associated with the severe disruption of the bony and ligamentous spinal elements. Despite permanence of the quadriplegia, some rehabilitation proved possible.

injuries.[25] These two mechanisms — contusion and vascular insufficiency — illustrate how serious cord injury can occur without fracture or dislocation; the possibility of transient, spontaneously reduced dislocation should also be borne in mind.

Dislocations. Dislocations are usually associated with fractures. Displacement into the spinal canal occasionally occurs without producing spinal cord injury. This is explained by the fact that the cord occupies approximately half the spinal canal; the cord may thus be spared. This observation accounts for the survival of some patients with atlantoaxial dislocation, which is often fatal because of compression of the vital cardiac and respiratory centers in the medulla oblongata.

Acceleration ("Whiplash") Injuries of the Neck. Varying degrees of cervical injury may occur when the head suddenly accelerates in relation to the trunk, as in the so-called *whiplash* injury of rear-end automobile collisions. The extension component of the recoil or oscillating neck motion is the significant mechanism in these injuries,[17] which are usually milder than those that result from a direct impact on the head. The large majority of cases involve a noncomplicated "sprain," consisting of an overstretching of cervical muscles and ligaments. Occasionally, there is associated disc or nerve root injury, subluxation due to stretching or tearing of ligaments, or fracture.[9] Symptoms such as blurring of vision, vertigo, tinnitus and nystagmus have been ascribed to vertebral-artery spasm or cervical sympathetic irritation, but the evidence for this viewpoint remains controversial.[17] Some authorities believe that mild brain injury (with transient unconsciousness) can occur in whiplash injuries as a result of acceleration-deceleration of the brain, despite the absence of a direct blow to the head.[11, 19]

Falls. Falls from a height, with the patient landing on the feet or buttocks, can cause compression fractures of the lower

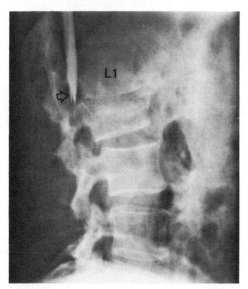

Figure 8–42. Lateral myelogram of lumbar region in middle-aged man who fell down flight of stairs, landing on buttocks. Note compression fracture of L2 vertebral body with bone fragment displaced backward into spinal canal. Compression of conus medullaris and cauda equina caused immediate loss of bladder function (retention) and moderate paraparesis with motor and sensory level at L1. On lumbar puncture, there was an inadequate flow of cerebrospinal fluid, suggesting a manometric block. Contrast medium for myelogram was introduced into spinal subarachnoid space via cisternal puncture. Film shows failure of contrast medium to flow below L2, despite upright position of the patient. Since major defect at level of block (arrow) was ventral (anterior to conus and cauda equina), surgical decompression and fusion were carried out by an anterolateral approach. The patient regained bladder function in 1 month and virtually full use of legs within 6 months, with minimal residual spasticity. This case illustrates that prognosis for eventual recovery is often good, if, on initial examination, some neurological function is preserved below level of injury.

thoracic and lumbar regions (Figs. 8–39 and 8–42). Consideration should be given to the possibility that an apparent traumatic compression fracture may be *pathological* in nature; the differential diagnosis includes osteoporosis, neoplasm (myeloma or metastasis most likely) and osteomyelitis. Dislocation in the lower vertebral column is less common than in the cervical spine because of less mobility and greater muscular and ligamentous support in this region.

Combined Craniospinal Injuries. Injuries of the spine are often associated with injuries to other parts of the body, especially in high-speed traffic accidents. Multiple injuries may include one or more of the following: fractured long bones, head, chest, pelvis and abdomen. Since the cervical spine serves as a fulcrum for the relatively heavy head, it is not surprising that injuries of head and neck are commonly associated.[7, 12] Direct impact injuries on the *vertex* of the head — as in falls from a height or blocking with the head in football — represent one serious and often fatal type of combined brain and cord injury. Schneider et al. have postulated that the severe impact force on the vertex causes the brain to herniate through the tentorial notch and foramen magnum, resulting in massive cerebral edema.[24] The force is also transmitted to the medulla and upper cervical spine. There may be associated vascular insufficiency due to compression of the vertebral arteries by the occipital condyles against the laminae of the atlas. An additional stress is said to occur at the cervicomedullary junction, owing to the disparity between the relatively mobile brain and the limited mobility of the upper cervical cord which is held by the dentate ligaments.

Open (Penetrating) Injuries

Missile Injuries. Bullet and shrapnel wounds of the spine may injure the cord by direct penetration into the spinal canal (Fig. 8–43). Complete cord transection is more apt to occur by this mechanism than by indirect closed injury. The missile impact may also drive bone fragments into the cord or nerve roots. A high-velocity bullet may produce transient or permanent paralysis, presumably as the result of a pressure wave in the wake of its passage in proximity

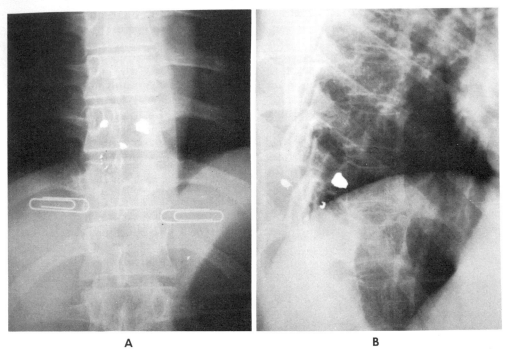

A   B

Figure 8–43.   *Anteroposterior (A) and lateral (B) radiographs of thoracic spine showing bullet injury at level of T10 and T11. The missile entered from the back and fragments are seen lying within the spinal canal. Paper-clip markers were attached to the patient's skin to aid in localization for subsequent surgical exploration. In general, penetrating injuries of the spinal canal should be explored early for debridement. Priority is, however, given to associated penetrating injuries of the chest or abdomen that may be more immediately life-threatening.*

to, but without penetrating, the spinal cord. A similar shock-wave phenomenon occurs in cord injury as the result of a nearby explosive blast in which there is no demonstrable vertebral or gross neural damage.

The missile trajectory may be estimated by inspection of the wounds of entrance and exit combined with roentgenographic evidence of the location of metallic fragments. If the missile lodges on the same side of the midline as the wound of entry, it may be inferred that the missile did not pass through the spinal canal. The bullet may initially strike a rib, then ricochet along the rib curvature and finally penetrate the spinal canal via the intervertebral foramen. Through-and-through perforation of the spinal canal and cord has probably occurred when the sites of entry and of exit are on opposite sides of the midline.

By comparison with closed injuries, spinal trauma due to missiles is often more destructive of the spinal cord but less disruptive of the ligaments supporting the spine. For this reason, there is less tendency to dislocation.

Stab Injuries.   Stab wounds of the spine are fairly common in civilian life. These injuries frequently occur in the thoracic region. They may be associated with a nondisplaced fracture of the neural arch, or the tip of the weapon may slip between adjacent neural arches. Classically, half the cord is traumatized, resulting in the Brown-Séquard hemisection syndrome.

PATHOPHYSIOLOGY OF THE NEURAL LESION

Transient Traumatic Paralysis, Contusion and Laceration

Cord injuries range in severity from transient physiological interruption to the permanent paralysis of anatomical cord transection. *Transient traumatic paralysis* is recommended as a substitute for the term "spinal concussion," which has vague connotations. The temporary paralysis from which the patient recovers fully may be accompanied by edema or ischemia of several cord segments. *Contusion* follows a blunt impact against the cord and is characterized by petechiae, edema and focal cellular and tract destruction at one or more segments. Healing is by gliosis, and partial return of function is possible. *Laceration* of the cord is commonly the result of penetrating injuries but may also follow fracture-dislocation. In extreme cases, there is total structural transection of the cord.

Hemorrhage

Bleeding may occur in the epidural and subdural spaces in the spinal canal as well as in the substance of the cord. Whereas epi- and subdural hematoma are frequent causes of brain compression in head injury, extramedullary bleeding in the spinal canal rarely causes serious cord compression. Subarachnoid bleeding may cause meningeal irritation (headache, stiff neck, fever). Blood in either the cranial or spinal *subarachnoid* space, however, does *not* accumulate locally to compress the brain or cord. On the other hand, hemorrhage into the cord itself is of major consequence, owing to local destruction of neural tissue and not to the loss of blood-volume, which is negligible. The extravasation, which may vary in degree from petechiae to frank hematoma at the site of injury, is usually confined to the central gray matter. Proximal and distal extension of the bleeding, hours or days after the injury, may account

for the progression of neurological deficit that occurs in some cases. Thrombosis of damaged blood vessels may also contribute to an advancing deficit.

The *syndrome of acute central cervical cord injury*[23] is often associated with central cord hemorrhage and variable surrounding edema. The striking feature of the syndrome is the greater motor impairment of the upper limbs as compared with the lower. This disparity is explained by the proximity to the damaged corticospinal (pyramidal) motor fibers destined for the upper limbs (Fig. 8–44). The more peripherally situated lower limb fibers tend to suffer less damage. Bladder dysfunction and varying degrees of sensory loss also occur. Partial motor and sensory recovery may ensue spontaneously (without surgical intervention) as the edema subsides, but recovery is limited by the extent to which the central cord has been permanently damaged.

Cord Compression

The effects of compression are those of mechanical distortion of the neural tissues combined with local cord ischemia and contusion. The cord can withstand gradual compression over a period of days or weeks, as in the case of slow-growing tumors, but acute compression is tolerated poorly. It has been shown in animal ex-

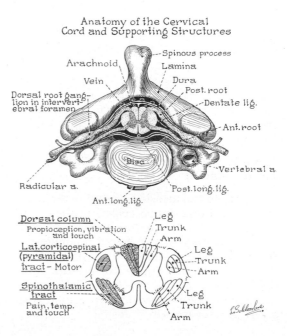

Figure 8–44. Upper, *Anatomical relationships of the sixth cervical vertebra viewed from above.* Lower, *Outline of the major motor and sensory tracts in the white matter of the cervical spinal cord.*

periments that, if recovery of function is to occur, severe compression of sudden onset must be relieved in minutes.[27] The neurological loss associated with *mild* compression can be reversed, provided the pressure on the cord is removed within two hours. The conus medullaris and the nerve roots of the cauda equina can tolerate longer periods of compression. Unfortunately, in clinical practice, decompression is often impossible within these time limits. Experience has shown, however, that partial recovery from *incomplete* lesions caused by acute compressive forces can occur if surgical decompression is performed even days or weeks after the onset.

It is sometimes possible to determine from the clinical examination and radiographs whether the compression is mainly anterior or posterior. This will determine the surgical approach in decompressing the cord. *Anterior (ventral) cord compression* is suspected when there is motor paralysis and loss of spinothalamic tract function (pain and temperature sense) below the level of the lesion, with preservation of dorsal column sensation (touch, position, vibration) (Fig. 8–45). Anterior cord compression is particularly apt to be associated with a "tear-drop" fracture of a vertebral body in cervical flexion injuries; the anterior fragment slides forward while the posterior vertebral fragment impinges against the anterior cord. Similar compression may result from a ruptured disc, but since the radiolucent disc cannot be demonstrated by plain radiographs, the diagnosis in this case must be made on clinical grounds or by myelography.

Loss of dorsal column sensation, with preservation of other sensory or motor functions, would suggest *posterior cord compression* or contusion (Fig. 8–45).

Vascular Insufficiency of the Cord and Brainstem

The vertebral arteries ascend in the neck via the foramina transversaria of the cervical spine and enter the posterior fossa at the lateral margins of the foramen magnum. Before uniting to form the basilar artery, they each give off a posterior inferior cerebellar artery and a branch which passes caudally to become the anterior spinal artery. The latter unpaired vessel is joined by

collaterals (radicular arteries which accompany the nerve roots) from the subclavian, intercostal and lumbar arteries. Collateral supply is poorest in the upper three cervical segments, at T4 and at L1; the capability of compensation for vascular insufficiency in these three zones is therefore deficient.

Fractures or dislocations of the spine or contusions of the cord may impair the local blood supply as a result of direct compression; alternatively, spasm or thrombosis may follow arterial contusion.[25] In the cervical region, bilateral injury of the vertebral arteries, in their foramina or at the craniocervical junction, may cause ischemia in the distribution of the anterior spinal artery. The resulting neurological disability may be reversible or permanent. In cases *without* fracture or dislocation, it is difficult to determine whether a neurological deficit is secondary to direct contusion of the cord or to vertebral artery insufficiency; either of these may occur in cervical hyperextension injuries *with or without dislocation*.

Vertebral insufficiency, with reduced flow to the posterior inferior cerebellar arteries or to the basilar artery, may produce brainstem dysfunction. Symptoms include nausea, dizziness, nystagmus, dysarthria, blurred vision and impaired consciousness (which may vary in individual cases from confusion to coma). These vascular manifestations are, however, difficult to distinguish from brainstem contusion or compression.

Spinal Shock

A state of "spinal shock" immediately follows cord injury and consists of a relative loss of motor, sensory and reflex function in those parts of the body innervated by the cord distal to the lesion. Bladder and rectal function are also interrupted. This acute phase may subside within days but commonly persists for three weeks or longer. If the pathological lesion is not severe, normal cord function is at least partially restored as the shock phase recedes. In severe, irreparable lesions, spinal shock is replaced by a state of hyperactive and pathological spinal reflexes, but the sensory loss and the paralysis of voluntary motor function continues. Because all cord lesions initially exhibit some degree of spinal shock, it is not possible to distinguish clinically in the acute phase between an anatomical and a physiological lesion. Hence, it is important to assume the possibility of recovery until proved otherwise.

Regeneration

Damage to the neural cells and tracts of the cord is reversible if the injury is of mild degree. When the damage is beyond the limit of tolerance, the involved cord tissue degenerates and is replaced by glial scarring. Regeneration of nervous tissue cannot occur to any practical degree in the brain and spinal cord in man. For this reason, surgical approximation of the severed ends of a structurally divided cord is futile. Sensory roots may be considered part of the central nervous system because their cell bodies lie distally in the dorsal root ganglia in the intervertebral foramina (Fig. 8–45). By contrast, motor roots, originating in the anterior horn cells, are theoretically comparable to peripheral nerves in regenerative capacity. This applies to clean cuts which do not greatly distort the fiber pattern, but effective regeneration does not generally follow approximation of torn or shredded nerve roots.[6]

Prognosis

In cases with or without continued cord compression, immediate *complete* loss of function below the level of the lesion is usually an ill omen for neurological recovery if the total loss persists longer than 24 hours. The presence of some voluntary motor function — perhaps only a flicker of movement — often signifies that, barring complications, the patient may eventually walk unaided. Complete motor loss with some initial preservation of sensation is less promising, carrying a 50 to 60 per cent chance of useful motor recovery; motor control may begin to appear days to months following injury. Some authors, however, have observed that the distinction between motor and sensory preservation immediately after injury is of little prognostic value.[28] Central lesions of the cord, referred to as the *syndrome of acute central cervical cord injury*,[23] are associated with greater motor deficit in the upper than in the lower limbs and carry a better prognosis for recovery than injuries that affect equally both the upper and lower extremities (see also other references in this chapter to the central cord syndrome).

Although some fortunate patients with physiologically incomplete lesions may show gratifying return of function in a relatively short time, the recovery process is generally slow; a plateau of maximal recovery may not be reached until about two years after injury. As in brain injuries, the prognosis for spinal cord trauma is better in younger individuals. The outlook for both survival and recovery of function declines for each decade beyond the age of 40.

In a series of 494 cases of spinal cord injury at the University of Maryland Baltimore, 55 per cent of the patients had initially complete sensory-motor paralysis.[22] Two thirds of the patients with initially complete lesions had involvement of the cervical cord and one third the thoracic cord. Mortality of patients with complete cervical lesions after one year was 35 per cent, and 8 per cent for those with complete thoracic cord injuries. About 9 per cent of those presenting with initially complete cervical or thoracic lesions ultimately showed significant recovery, but only 2.5 per cent were regarded as functionally normal or near normal.

The gross appearance of the spinal cord at the time of surgical exploration is often of little prognostic value. Only if the cord is anatomically transected or is severely contused can a definite prediction of permanent paralysis be made. However, a cord grossly normal on the surface may conceal serious intramedullary destruction with a correspondingly poor prognosis.

The electrophysiological technique of "cortical evoked response" has recently been employed in some spinal injury centers for early prediction of eventual physiological conduction in a damaged spinal cord. A favorable prognosis is tentatively suggested if an electrical stimulus applied to the skin overlying a peripheral nerve in the leg evokes a scalp EEG response. A satisfactory response implies electrical conduction across the injured portion of the cord. An advantage of this method of testing cord conduction is that it is noninvasive and can be repeated at intervals to monitor recovery.

FIRST AID AT THE SCENE OF ACCIDENT

Recognition of Injury

Spinal trauma is suspected if the patient has any difficulty in moving the lower extremities on command. Similar motor difficulty in the upper limbs indicates cervical cord involvement. The presence of a sensory level on pinprick testing confirms the suspicion of cord or nerve root injury. The patient may complain of local pain in the neck or back. Gentle palpation by sliding the fingers along the spine (without moving the patient) may reveal gross deformity or tenderness. When spinal injury is suspected, special precautions are taken in handling the patient, even in the absence of motor or sensory loss. In the management of an *unconscious* accident victim, consideration is given to the possibility that both head injury and cervical spine trauma have occurred. A bruised forehead or facial lacerations suggest the possibility of a hyperextension injury of the neck. Penetrating spinal injuries are easily identified by inspection and by the accompanying neurological signs. The open wounds are covered with a sterile dressing. Fractures of long bones are splinted in the usual manner.

Respiration

In all patients immediate attention is directed to the airway. Patients with injuries to the upper half of the cervical cord are subjected to respiratory embarrassment because neural control of both the intercostal muscles and the diaphragm is impaired. (The diaphragm is innervated by the phrenic nerve which is derived from the third, fourth and fifth cervical cord segments.) In lower cervical injuries, the intercostal muscles are paralyzed, but the diaphragm remains functional. Airway obstruction due to secretions is cleared by suction, if the apparatus is available. Provision of a pharyngeal airway for unconscious patients is helpful. If a skilled person is available at the scene of the accident, introduction of an endotracheal tube (avoiding hyperextending the neck) or an emergency tracheostomy with assisted respiration can be lifesaving in cases of high cervical cord injury. Narcotics for pain

or restlessness are avoided in cervical cord injury in view of their respiratory depressant effect.

Artertial Hypotension

Unless there is blood loss from other injuries, hypotension after spinal injury is usually due to vasodilatation. If this occurs, venous return to the heart may be increased by elevating the legs.

Oxygen Administration

Lactate accumulates at the site of spinal cord injury, reflecting local ischemia.[16] Cord lactate is also increased in response to anoxia, although the spinal cord is more resistant to anoxia than cerebral tissue. Administration of oxygen (preferably humidified, to prevent drying of the tracheobronchial lining) may therefore have some protective effect on the injured cord, especially if there is respiratory embarrassment or hypotension.

Extrication of Victim from Vehicle or Water

It is more important to initiate resuscitation and to safeguard alignment of the spine than to rush in moving the patient to an ambulance, especially if there is no immediate danger from hazards such as fire or fumes. The cardinal principle in moving a patient with suspected spinal injury is prevention of any spinal motion that can further damage the cord or nerve roots. The neck should be the single most important consideration in the mechanics of removing an injured person from a car or other confined space. The head and neck must be supported at all times, whether the patient is conscious or unconscious. One rescue worker firmly grasps the head and applies longitudinal traction to bring the head and neck into neutral position, while other rescue personnel ease the trunk and extremities out of the vehicle. Alternatively, before moving the patient out of the vehicle, a "spinal board" or any makeshift board may be slid behind the patient's head and back, after which straps are applied so as to fix the head and trunk to the board.[8]

In rescuing a diving accident victim with a suspected spinal injury from the water, float the victim onto his back into shallow water. If necessary, give mouth-to-mouth resuscitation, avoiding neck extension. Place a board (such as a door, surf board, or ironing board) under the victim by sliding it under the water and letting it float up. As an additional precaution to prevent his sliding or rolling when he is lifted out of the water, use any available material to strap the body and head to the board.[11]

Transfer to Stretcher

In transfer of a patient from the ground to a stretcher, and if he is not already on a rigid board, he is lifted "like a log" with spinal alignment maintained by several persons. The individual most responsible for the transfer exerts firm, steady traction on the head and neck (Fig. 8–45A). The patient is placed *supine* on the stretcher, and sandbags are placed on either side of the head to prevent rotation. Canvas halter traction for temporary neck immobilization during transport is desirable. A commercially available constant-tension spring attached to the halter and stretcher is ideal for maintaining immobilization. Alternatively, a 5-lb. weight may be suspended from a rope

which is hung over the end of the stretcher (Fig. 8–45B). If a standard head halter is not available, a makeshift emergency neck traction sling can be made at the scene of the accident from a piece of cloth (Fig. 8–46). If a traction device is not feasible, a soft collar (felt, sponge rubber, or a towel) gently placed around the neck is another reasonable method of emergency splinting. As a last resort, sandbags or other heavy objects placed on each side of the neck will provide some protective neck stability. Immobilization of the neck is, of course, not necessary in thoracolumbar injuries. However, if there is any doubt regarding the exact level of spinal injury, the safe approach is to handle the patient as a cervical injury.

Transport to a Hospital

An attendant should accompany the patient in the ambulance during the trip to the hospital, with constant attention to the airway (suction as necessary) and to maintenance of neck stability. A record should be kept, for subsequent reporting to the receiving hospital, of the patient's neurologi-

A

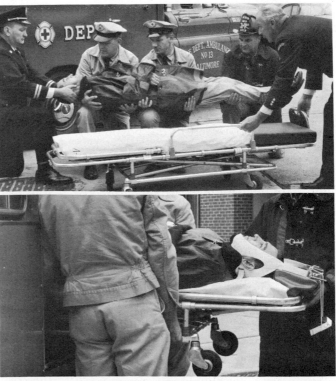

Figure 8–45. A, Method of lifting patient with injury of cervical spine, illustrating the maintenance of spinal alignment to prevent further damage to the spinal cord or nerve roots. Steady traction is applied to the head and neck, which is held in neutral position. This technique is employed even if there is only slight suspicion of spinal injury. B, Canvas halter traction (or emergency sling shown in Figure 8–46) for temporary immobilization during transport. A 5-lb. weight (shown in photo), or a constant tension spring, is attached. (Courtesy of Ambulance Service, Baltimore Fire Dept.)

B

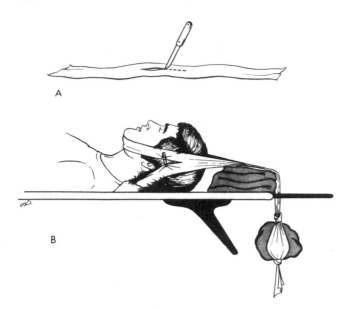

Figure 8–46. A, *Makeshift emergency neck-traction sling, which can be made at the scene of the accident, from a muslin sling, bandage roll or other heavy piece of cloth about 4 feet long and 6 inches wide; a 10-inch longitudinal slit is cut in the middle for the head to slide through (Lewin, 1930).* B, *The slit is held snugly with a safety pin above each ear to prevent slipping off the occiput. The free ends are tied to a 3- to 5-lb. weight for traction.*

cal status, including observations of motor or sensory involvement of the extremities and any indication of worsening. Oxygen is given by mask or resuscitator (Ambu) bag at a flow rate of approximately 4 liters per minute. If possible, an intravenous line is started for circulatory support. Coldness and wetness should be prevented and the patient reassured.

If the trip to the hospital will be longer than several hours, an indwelling urethral catheter is introduced to prevent the irreparable damage of an overdistended flaccid bladder. The catheter is allowed to drain freely.

Protection of the denervated skin against the development of decubitus ulcers begins during transport to the hospital. A smooth, dry sheet is used on the stretcher; bony pressure points such as sacrum and heels are padded. The sheet may be used later to lift the patient on arrival at the hospital.

When possible, the hospital is notified in advance of the patient's arrival. In this way, necessary personnel (neurosurgeon, orthopedic surgeon, anesthesiologist, radiology staff) and equipment (e.g., respirator, canvas head halter, tongs for cervical traction, Stryker turning frame) may be prepared for service when the patient arrives.

Transfer to Another Hospital

Summary notes should accompany a patient being transferred from one hospital to another. The notes should include time and nature of injury, neurological status with emphasis on changes since first examination, associated injuries, medications administered and course of vital signs (level of consciousness, respiration, pulse, blood pressure). Before transfer, temporary neck immobilization should be applied (if this was not already done at the scene of the accident), an intravenous infusion started and an indwelling urethral catheter inserted. In patients with depressed level of consciousness or impaired respiratory function, a pharyngeal airway, endotracheal tube or tracheostomy should be added.

Balance Between Speed and Caution

Ambulance personnel are the first major link in the chain of care for the seriously injured patient. They are frequently faced with difficult emergency situations requiring judgment and ingenuity. There can be no question that speed is important in getting the patient to the hospital so that definitive care can begin. An extra few minutes, however, in preparing the patient for transport can help to prevent unnecessary complications. This includes removal of the victim from the site of the accident with particular attention to the spine, cautious transfer to the stretcher, assurance of the airway, splinting of limb fractures and administration of intravenous fluids where indicated. The same principles apply equally in cases where speedy transportation by airplane or helicopter is available.

MANAGEMENT IN HOSPITAL IN THE ACUTE PHASE

Immediate Care

On arrival in hospital, the patient is transferred to a portable lightweight x-ray penetrable lifter to which cervical traction can be attached.* The vital signs are checked, and appropriate resuscitation is promptly instituted. Adequacy of respiration is determined. Endotracheal intubation to permit suctioning is performed when there is doubt of the patient's ability to cough up secretions or when mechanically assisted respiration is necessary to prevent hypoxia. During endotracheal intubation, care is taken to avoid neck hyperextension which might further traumatize the cervical cord; angulation of the neck can be minimized by displacing the mandible forward with upward pressure on the rami. In the hands of an experienced person, the blind nasotracheal method avoids the risk of neck extension.[12] Tracheostomy may be considered later if it is clear that prolonged endotracheal intubation will be necessary.

Following cord injury, the blood pressure may drop temporarily to the lower normal range because of loss of sympathetic vasomotor tone. This may be corrected by elevation of the legs; blood replacement is unnecessary since there has been no loss of volume. The absence of tachycardia helps to distinguish the hypotension of "spinal shock" from that of "surgical shock." If the blood pressure is unduly low, and particularly if this is associated with tachycardia, falling hematocrit, or low

urinary output, suspicion is aroused of hemorrhage from concomitant injury within the thorax, abdomen or long bones.

After the patient's vital processes have been stabilized, a rapid evaluation is made of the total situation. The patient's clothes are removed carefully, avoiding spinal motion, nothing is removed over the head and clothing not easily removable is cut. The spinal lesion is identified in broad terms and a cursory examination of other systems is carried out to identify quickly any associated trauma. Specialty consultations are requested as indicated, and decisions are made regarding priority in the management of the various problems. Apart from cardiorespiratory difficulty in high cervical trauma, cord injury itself is not generally immediately life-threatening. Priority is given, therefore, to any cerebral, thoracic or abdominal injuries, the delayed treatment of which may endanger survival. It is often feasible for separate surgical teams to perform procedures simultaneously.

When cervical spine trauma is evident or suspected, halter traction is applied if this has not already been done as a first-aid measure at the scene of accident. The patient is asked to void to test micturition. If paraplegia is present, an indwelling urethral catheter is inserted and the volume of residual urine noted.

Use of Corticosteroids

Trials in laboratory animal models suggest slight benefit from the intramuscular administration of corticosteroids for 1–2 weeks.[2] Although no controlled trials have been reported thus far in human spinal cord injury, use of these agents seems warranted. If corticosteroids are employed, following is a suggested regimen: methylprednisolone sodium succinate (Solu-Medrol) 125 mg., *or* dexamethasone sodium phosphate (Decadron) given intravenously as a push dose, and continued every 6 hours by the intramuscular or oral route for 1 week (methylprednisolone 30 mg., or dexamethasone 6 mg.), then tapered over the next week. Corticosteroids reduce secretion of gastric mucoprotein and may thereby increase the risk of stress ulceration[5]; the risk may be minimized by the use of antacids and anticholinergic agents. The use of corticosteroids may be

---

*Lying on this lifter, the patient may be safely transferred from one stretcher to another or to an x-ray table without disturbing the traction or spinal alignment. To further minimize handling the patient, it would be desirable for such lifters to be employed in ambulances and exchanged with a similar lifter on arrival in hospital. Such exchangeable lifters, known as "unilitters," have been installed in ambulances and in a number of emergency rooms of local hospitals in San Antonio, Texas.[29] The unilitter may be made economically of plywood covered by a foam-rubber pad and the entire litter enclosed in vinyl plastic.

contraindicated in patients with a past history of gastrointestinal ulceration.

Detailed Clinical Evaluation

Having attended to the patient's immediate needs, the physician carries out a thorough general physical and neurological examination. A search is made for associated injuries, including head trauma. A brief description from the patient or from witnesses of the circumstances surrounding the accident may indicate the mechanism of injury. A distinction can sometimes be made between a physiologically complete or an incomplete lesion on the basis of the rate of onset of the neurological deficit. If power and sensation were completely lost immediately, then the outlook for recovery is not so favorable as in cases in which the functional loss occurred over a period of minutes or hours. Progressive neurological loss may reflect continued or increasing cord compression which may be remedied by traction (in cervical injuries) or by surgical decompression. Progressive loss, however, may also result from extension of intramedullary edema or hemorrhage or from local cord ischemia. Enquiry is made regarding previous illnesses, such as diabetes, coronary insufficiency or epilepsy, since they may affect the general care of the patient.

The neurological examination at this time is recorded as a baseline for all subsequent examinations in assessing progression or regression of the functional deficit. Ideally, the same examiner carries out the serial evaluations. In addition to localizing the site of the lesion by the sensory and motor level, the examiner checks all sensory modalities throughout the affected dermatomes, including the perineum, in search of islands of residual sensation (Fig. 8–47). Motor function is similarly tested, since preservation of even minimal voluntary motor or sensory function has favorable prognostic significance (see also section on "Prognosis" in this chapter). The level of the motor loss, except in thoracic injuries, is a somewhat more reliable indicator of the cord segment involved than is the sensory level. Paralysis is flaccid in character during the phase of spinal shock. Some spasticity often appears later in the chronic convalescent phase. Pathological reflexes, such as the extensor plan-

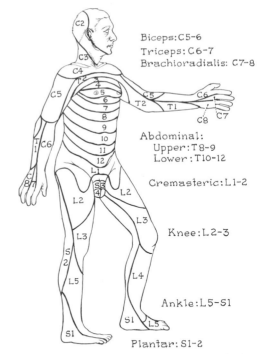

Figure 8–47. *Sensory dermatomes and spinal cord segmental reflex innervation. This is helpful in localizing area and level of cord injury.*

tar response (Babinski), signify damage to the pyramidal tract in either or both the brain and spinal cord. In the acute phase, all reflexes below the level of cord injury are usually absent, and even the Babinski response may not appear until the spinal shock recedes. Priapism is also occasionally seen during the acute period.

The brachial plexus is derived from segments C5 to T1. Thus, if the arms as well as the legs are paralyzed (quadriplegia), the cord lesion is situated at or above the C5 segment. When some function is retained in the upper limbs, the segmental level is determined by the specific muscle groups, reflexes and dermatomes affected.

If the upper limbs are spared, the lesion lies below T1. A sensory level on the chest or abdomen is the most useful localizing sign in thoracic cord injury. The abdominal reflexes may help in localization since their innervation originates from segments T8 to T12.

The tapered lower end of the spinal cord, known as the conus medullaris, lies opposite to the first lumbar vertebra (Fig.

8–39). Trauma of the lumbosacral spine may damage the conus or the cauda equina, but the spinal cord above the conus will escape injury. The lumbar and sacral nerve roots of the cauda equina are loosely arranged in the spinal canal. Injury to the roots is, therefore, often irregular, giving rise to patchy and asymmetrical motor and sensory loss in the lower limbs. By comparison, injuries of the lower spinal cord may be identified by a more complete and symmetrical distribution of neurological signs. If it is present, a Babinski response confirms cord involvement but does not exclude nerve root injury.

In patients unconscious from head trauma, spinal cord injury is suggested by absence of reflexes below the level of cord injury, or by the finding of a sweat-level on the trunk. In semicomatose patients, a sensory level to pinprick may be identified by the absence of a withdrawal response below a given dermatomal level.

Radiographic Evaluation (Plain Films)

When the vital signs are stable, anteroposterior and lateral radiographs are taken of the affected region of the spine. To avoid unnecessary movement, the patient remains on the stretcher, or he may be safely transferred to the x-ray table on a radiolucent lifter. If the patient must be lifted from the stretcher without the benefit of a supporting solid lifter, manual or halter traction is maintained in cases of cervical injury.[15] The study is supervised directly by a physician.

In cervical injuries, initial radiographs are taken in the anterior and lateral projections. An open-mouth view of the atlantoaxial articulation is obtained to visualize the odontoid process, fractures of which may be missed on routine projections. Visualization of the lower cervical spine on lateral projections is often obscured by the shoulders. This can be avoided by depressing the shoulders or employing the "swimmer's position," which consists of placing one arm of the patient over his head and depressing the other shoulder. Radiographic examination of the neck is considered adequate only after the entire cervical spine — including the upper and lower portions — has been visualized. If adequate radiographic visualization can-

not be accomplished in the emergency setting, the patient is generally best managed, at least tentatively, as having a potentially serious cervical injury until the situation can be clarified.

If the routine anterior and lateral views are normal, as in cases of cervical sprain from whiplash injury, right and left oblique views are made to visualize the neural foramina. In addition, lateral views in flexion and extension help to exclude subluxation. Skull films are also obtained in patients with neck injury in whom there is any suspicion of cranial trauma. The converse is also true: that patients presenting primarily with head trauma (with or without impaired consciousness) should generally have cervical spine films (in addition to skull films); cervical injury may be present even in the absence of the usual clinical features of spinal injury.[4, 12]

In correlating the films with the clinical findings, it should be remembered that, except in the lumbar region, a particular cord segment lies approximately two spinous processes higher than its correspondingly designated vertebra. The films may not reveal the full extent of the damage; dislocation may be transient and may have reduced spontaneously, so that subsequent roentgenographic evidence is lacking. Furthermore, the films do not reveal radiolucent soft tissue, such as a herniated intervertebral disc or torn ligaments. Myelography, discussed later in this chapter, is of great value for visualization of cord or nerve root compression by disc herniations or other radiolucent tissues.

Traction for Cervical Injuries

All patients with cervical fracture and/or dislocation are best treated with some form of traction, regardless of the extent of neural involvement and regardless of whether surgery will also be performed (Figs. 8–45, 8–46 and 8–48). Exceptions to this statement are fractures of the transverse or spinous processes that require only stabilization with cervical (Thomas) collar or two-poster neck brace and symptomatic care. Patients with cervical cord neurological deficit, but *without* fracture or dislocation, are also best placed in traction, at least intially, until the situation is clarified. The stabilization can do no harm and may prevent an unrecognized subluxation or reduce further injury from a herniated disc or thickened ligamenta flava. Young children can often be managed with a head halter, but adults better tolerate skeletal traction employing Gardner-Wells skull tongs or one of the older varieties such as those designed by Crutchfield, Cone or Vinke. The primary purpose of traction is immobilization; in cases of dislocation with or without fracture, traction is also usually capable of realigning the displaced spine. Apart from decompressing the neural elements, traction may correct impingement of the vertebral arteries which supply the spinal cord and brainstem.

Application of Tongs. Gardner-Wells traction tongs are the simplest of the various types currently available and are the easiest to apply (Fig. 8–48). The tongs may be applied in the emergency department. Aseptic technique should be observed since local infection, including osteomyelitis and epidural abscess, is a potentially serious complication. Although not essential, a small patch of hair may be shaved over both parietal eminences, in line with the mastoid processes, which correspond to the plane of the cervical articulations. The two sites at which the tong points are to be inserted in the scalp are deeply infiltrated with local anesthetic. Without need for a stab incision, the tong points are screwed through the scalp and into the outer table of the skull. One of the two adjustable points is spring-loaded with an indicator that shows when the proper pressure is being exerted. Antibiotic ointment may be applied around each point, and the area should be checked daily for signs of infection.

Amount of Traction. For purposes of stabilization in nondisplaced injuries, only 5 to 10 lbs. traction are needed. If reduction of a dislocation is necessary, 10 to 15 lbs. are initially applied. The head-end of the Stryker turning frame or bed is elevated on blocks about six inches to allow countertraction by the weight of the patient. Serial radiographs are made every 30 to 60 minutes and additional traction up to a maximum of 40 to 45 lbs. for muscular individuals is applied with careful monitoring of the patient's neurological status.

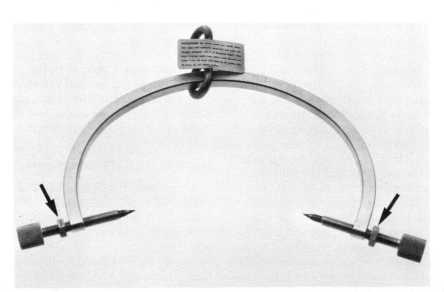

Figure 8–48. *Gardner-Wells tongs for cervical traction. One of the two adjustable points is spring-loaded with an indicator (located on outer flat side of one of the knurled knobs, not seen in this photograph), which shows when the proper pressure is being exerted on the skull. The spring-loading device provides a sharply localized pressure that results in atrophy of the outer table. This atrophy allows the points to advance slightly after the initial setting and to further adjust themselves. Stability is generally reached within 24 hours, after which no further tightening of the points is usually necessary. The pressure-indicator should be checked daily, however, to insure that the proper pressure is being maintained. Note on each side the hexagonal nut (arrow), the purpose of which is to lock the pointed screw to the C-shaped arch; this nut should also be checked daily to insure that the screw does not gradually become loose and slip out of the skull. (Courtesy of Codman and Shurtleff, Inc., Randolph, MA 02368.)*

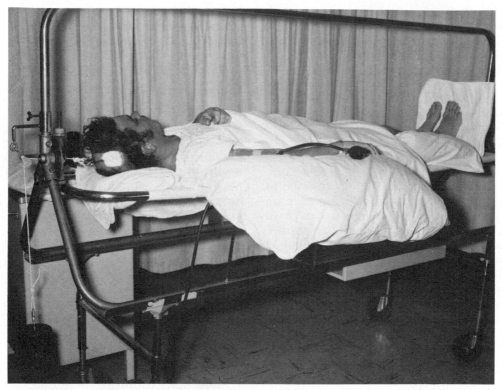

Figure 8–49. *Patient with cervical fracture-dislocation injury on Stryker frame. Crutchfield traction tongs were used in this case. For turning to prone position, a second frame is placed on patient and is secured with bolts at the head and foot ends. Note the vertical prop for the ankles to prevent foot-drop deformity.*

(Byrnes and Ducker[4] use up to 100 lbs. if necessary.)

Because of greater muscular resistance in the lower cervical spine, more traction is generally required for dislocations here than in the upper cervical region. Muscle relaxants can facilitate reduction, especially in the presence of muscle spasm. Gradual addition of weights, with check x-rays, helps to avoid excessive traction which can cause distraction of the vertebrae, spinal cord or vertebral arteries. When reduction is achieved, traction is decreased to a maintenance level of approximately one third the weight that was required to achieve reduction. Repeat x-rays for bony alignment are then obtained every 4–6 hours during the next day; thereafter check films are made every day or every other day during the first week. The weights are checked frequently to assure that they hang freely. A responsible observer should stay with the patient at all times during the initial period until reduction is achieved; the amount of traction is reduced immediately to a maintenance

level at the first sign of any neurological deterioration.

Traction Precautions. When Gardner-Wells tongs are used, the pressure-indicator is checked daily to assure that proper pressure is being exerted on the skull; tightness of the hexagonal nuts is also checked daily to prevent the tong points from gradually slipping out of the skull (Fig. 8–48). Tongs of the Crutchfield type are tightened daily (about one tenth turn) to prevent the points from slipping out. Skull films are obtained every 7–10 days to detect possible penetration of the points through the inner table. Regardless of the type of tongs used, a canvas band or padded face mask should be fitted across the Stryker frame at all times to support the patient's head, when in the supine and prone positions, to prevent further injury to the cord if the tongs should accidentally slip out (Fig. 8–49). When the patient is turned to the prone or supine position, it is necessary to secure the patient between the top and bottom frames with a sufficient number of straps to prevent the patient from a potentially catastrophic fall through the side-opening during the turning. Once the turn is completed, the locking bolts are checked to insure that the frame on which the patient is lying will not accidentally tilt.

Failure of Reduction. If reduction fails to occur within 12–18 hours after instituting traction, this is probably due to locking (overriding) of dislocated facets of the lateral intervertebral joints. In such cases, closed reduction can sometimes be accomplished by altering the angle of traction to slight flexion or extension, depending on the angulation of the locked facets. With the patient supine, a folded sheet under the head causes slight flexion of the neck; a sheet under the shoulders results in slight extension.

Traction beyond 24 hours in an effort to reduce locked facets is not likely to be successful. Consideration is then given to *open* reduction. *With the cervical traction maintained during the operative procedure*, the site of dislocation is explored and the facets unlocked by gently prying with bone instruments under direct vision. Open reduction is far safer than *closed* manual manipulation, which should never be done.

Alternative Traction Methods. Other methods may be employed if tongs are not available or if their use is precluded by a thin skull (as in young children), extensive skull fractures or contaminated scalp lacerations. For example, two burr holes may be placed about 2 cm. from the midline on each side of the skull. On each side, a wire is passed epidurally between the anterior and posterior trephines which are 4–5 cm. apart. The two wires are attached to a weight as in the use of tongs. Alternatively, traction may be applied via a large fish hook (with the barb removed) inserted percutaneously beneath the anterior third of the zygomatic arch bilaterally.

A novel approach to emergency traction has been recommended by Byrnes and Ducker.[4] In anticipation of the possible subsequent need to apply a halo apparatus (Fig. 8–50) for long-term immobilization, they apply the halo portion of the apparatus during the emergency phase. Instead of the usual tongs, the halo is fixed to the skull and attached to weights by a pulley for traction. When traction is no longer necessary, the halo may be attached to a light-weight padded plastic vest for external mobilization, and the patient may then be permitted to assume the upright position.

Thoracic and Lumbar Fractures: Nonoperative Management

The patient may be nursed on a regular bed with a firm mattress or on a Stryker-type turning frame. Cervical traction is *not* used for spinal injuries from T2–S1 since neck traction would not be transmitted below the level of the cervical spine. Pelvic traction, however, may be helpful for fractures situated at T12–L1.

Postural reduction of dislocations in the thoracic or lumbar region may be achieved by positioning the patient and monitoring progress with serial radiographs. In the event of neurological deterioration during postural reduction or pelvic traction, the patient's position is immediately restored or the amount of traction reduced.

Myelography (Contrast Radiography) of Spine

Until recently, this technique was not commonly employed in the evaluation of spinal cord injury because of the risks of spinal motion in performing the procedure. In the past few years, it has become increasingly clear that myelography need not add appreciable risk, and can provide invaluable diagnostic information that may influence the decision regarding surgically remediable compression of the cord or nerve roots (Fig. 8–42). Myelography is undertaken only after the cardiovascular and respiratory status are stable, and after the best possible bony alignment is achieved (by traction for neck injuries and postural reduction for injuries of the thoracic or lumbar spine). In thoracic or lumbar injuries, an oily radiopaque solution (Pantopaque) or air is injected into the lumbar subarachnoid space via a spinal puncture needle. Defects or obstruction in the flow of the "dye" column are observed fluoroscopically. A marker is attached to the skin to aid the surgeon in placing the incision if the patient is to be subsequently explored.

Because of the greater hazard of instability in the cervical than in the thoracic or lumbar region, Byrnes and Ducker[4] recom-

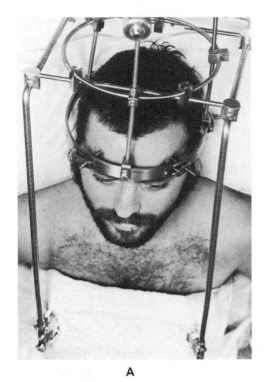
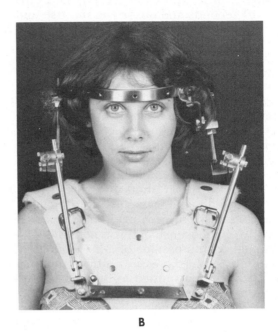

A **B**

Figure 8–50. *For neck injuries, the halo fixation apparatus provides secure external immobilization of the cervical spine and has the major advantage of permitting sitting and ambulation. The halo portion, fixed to the skull by four pins, may be used (instead of tongs) in the acute stage, or the halo may be applied at a later date after bony alignment has been achieved. The halo is fastened by rods to a plaster body jacket (A) or to a lightweight plastic vest (B).*

The halo apparatus may be employed for patients who would otherwise be immobilized for many weeks by skull tong traction alone. In patients requiring surgical decompression and/or internal fixation by fusion, the halo apparatus serves to immobilize the neck during the operative procedure and subsequently during the postoperative period until bony and ligamentous healing has occurred.

mend a "modified" cervical myelogram. This consists of turning the patient face down in traction on the Stryker frame and the injection of approximately 4 to 5 ml. of Pantopaque into the cervical subarachnoid space via a lateral needle puncture at C1–2. Portable radiographs may be made without necessarily moving the patient from the area of resuscitation, which is of particular advantage in patients with multiple injuries. The pooled dye enables visualization of the posterior aspect of the vertebral bodies, in search of cord or nerve root compression by bony fragments or by acutely herniated intervertebral discs not visualized on the plain films. The technique requires no manipulation of the patient other than turning in the prone position. Generally, the patient need not be tipped head up or down, although this may be cautiously attempted, provided neck traction is maintained.

Lumbar Puncture and the Queckenstedt Test in Closed Injuries

Until recently, lumbar puncture was regarded as being a routine test in the evaluation of patients with spinal cord injury. The primary purpose for lumbar puncture in spinal injury was the detection of a spinal fluid block that, when present, would suggest cord compression. In the past few years, however, the value of routine lumbar puncture and the Queckenstedt test has been questioned, since significant cord or root compression may be present even though the spinal fluid dynamics may be recorded as being normal. Another reason for the declining usefulness of the procedure is the increasing acceptance of myelography, which is replacing the Queckenstedt test as the definitive indicator of cord or root compression.

The Queckenstedt test (named for the physician who described the maneuver) consists of compressing the jugular veins for 10 seconds and observing the rise and fall of the cerebrospinal fluid in the manometer attached to a lumbar puncture needle. By impeding venous return from the brain, jugular compression normally produces a transient increase in intracranial pressure, which is transmitted to the cerebrospinal fluid. The fluid in the manometer promptly rises when the jugular compression is applied and falls with release of compression. In the event of a mechanical obstruction in the spinal canal, the cerebrospinal fluid pressure is not transmitted to the manometer during jugular compression, or it may be delayed. A positive Queckenstedt test is confirmed by manual compression of the abdomen, whereby the increased intra-abdominal pressure is transmitted to the spinal fluid via the epidural veins. If the lumbar puncture needle communicates with the subarachnoid space, the increased abdominal pressure produces a rise in the fluid in the manometer, even in the presence of a spinal block. A manometric block is thus confirmed by a differential response between jugular and abdominal compression. A drawback in interpretation lies in the fact that *partial* obstruction of the spinal subarachnoid space by a compressive lesion (such as a bone spicule or herniated disc) may permit enough spinal fluid to bypass the lesion and thereby result in a *misleading* negative Queckenstedt test. For this reason, and the increasing acceptance of myelography, the Queckenstedt test is no longer recommended as a routine procedure in the evaluation of spinal cord injury.

Lumbar Puncture in Penetrating Injuries

In addition to the declining value of the Queckenstedt test, lumbar puncture simply to examine the cerebrospinal fluid does not contribute any useful information in closed spinal injury. In penetrating injuries (stab or gunshot), however, lumbar puncture is of value to rule out meningitis. The examination includes cell count, glucose determination and culture (including both aerobic and anaerobic media); a Gram stain with a drop of the spinal fluid is also performed as this may provide a clue to the immediate selection of appropriate antibiotics without a wait for the culture report. Bloody spinal fluid indicates subarachnoid bleeding, which may occur in both mild and severe injuries of the closed or penetrating variety. Xanthochromia appears as the red blood cells disintegrate.

OPERATIVE TREATMENT

Operation is undertaken only after the patient's general condition is satisfactory; the mortality is unduly high in the presence of surgical shock or respiratory distress. Surgery is carried out for one or any combination of the following three purposes: decompression, fusion (internal stabilization) or debridement for penetrating injuries.

Maintenance of External Fixation

For cervical injuries, *skeletal traction is maintained during and following operation,* which is performed with the patient on the Stryker turning frame. An important trend contributing to the safety of surgery for cervical trauma involves the use of the halo-vest apparatus (Fig. 8–50). The halo portion of the apparatus may be applied in the acute stage for the purpose of skeletal traction, or the halo with vest may be applied days or weeks later to replace standard traction tongs, after satisfactory bony alignment has been achieved. If operation is undertaken for decompression and/or fusion, the procedure is carried out with the patient's neck externally immobilized in the halo-vest apparatus; adjustments in neck angulation may be made by manipulation of the metal rods. Postoperatively, the patient may be mobilized (sitting or standing) with the assurance that the halo-vest apparatus will maintain stability of the neck until bony and ligamentous healing occurs.

Anesthesia and Monitoring of Neurological Function

Endotracheal intubation in cervical trauma is performed cautiously to avoid neck manipulation. Local anesthesia may be considered for patients unable to tolerate general anesthesia. Local anesthesia also has the advantage of enabling monitoring of neurological status during the operation. The technique of cortical evoked responses for monitoring spinal cord function during surgery is a useful new development; this technique was discussed previously in this chapter in relation to Prognosis. The skin overlying a peripheral nerve in the leg is stimulated electrically and scalp EEG responses are monitored by means of a portable signal averaging computer.

Decompression

The principal indication for surgical intervention is mechanical compression of the spinal cord or nerve roots that cannot be relieved by traction (for neck injuries), or by postural reduction (for thoracic or lumbar fractures). Any of the following circumstances warrant a decompressive procedure.

1. Failure of reduction after 12–18 hours if there is evidence or strong suspicion of neural compression.

2. Progression of the neurological deficit. This may be due to cord swelling (edema) or vascular insufficiency of the cord, but it may be difficult to rule out extrinsic compression by bone or soft tissues; a myelogram may be helpful for clarification.

3. Partial or complete myelographic block by a lesion such as bone fragments, herniated disc or extradural hematoma. After satisfactory bone alignment has been achieved by traction or postural reduction, the large majority of patients show no evidence of myelographic block, but it is nonetheless important to identify that small group of patients for whom early decompression may help restore neurological function.

4. Radiographic evidence (on plain films or tomograms) showing bone fragment projecting into the spinal canal.

5. Injuries of the conus medullaris or cauda equina. Exploration in this area is often advisable in cases with neurological deficit, even in the absence of neural compression. The purpose of exploration is debridement of lacerated neural tissues and the evacuation of blood clots; it may be possible in some cases to suture severed motor nerve roots (see also discussion of Regeneration).

Several methods of decompression are available. An anterior approach for discectomy or corpectomy is employed when the neurological or radiographic findings suggest *anterior* cord compression; fusion is carried out during the same procedure by replacing the surgical defect with a bone graft (Fig. 8–51). Figure 8–42 illustrates a lumbar fracture for which an anterolateral approach was employed for decompression and fusion. *Posterior* compression of the cord is relieved by laminectomy; the dorsal bony arch is resected, leaving the articulations intact to prevent spinal instability (Fig. 8–52). If there is associated instability, a fusion is also carried out if the patient's general condition permits, or fusion may be postponed until a second operation weeks later.

For persistent locked facets, a laminectomy is performed, after which the dislocated facets are reduced under direct vision by prying the facets into alignment. Monitoring cord function during this maneuver with cortically evoked responses adds a measure of safety.

In general, surgical decompression by the anterior route is carried out for patients with ventral cord compression involving the spine from C1–T1. Ventral compression from T2–T9 is carried out by an anterolateral costotransversectomy or by a lateral transthoracic approach. Although ventral decompression is technically feasible (though difficult) in the lumbar and lower thoracic spine, experience suggests that ventral compression involving the spine from T10–S1 is usually best managed by a posterior decompression (laminectomy). Thus it is suggested that decompression of the lower spine (T10–S1) be approached by laminectomy whether or not the compression on the neural elements is ventral or posterior. On the other hand, for injuries involving the cervical or thoracic spine down to the level of T9, the surgical approach (anterior or posterior) is generally dictated by the question of whether the main mechanical compression on the cord is anterior or posterior.

A few neurosurgeons advocate exploration in patients with complete neurological loss even in the absence of evidence of cord compression.[10] Incision of the cord to aspirate a hematoma is also performed by some surgeons; the current consensus, however, suggests that the hazard of add-

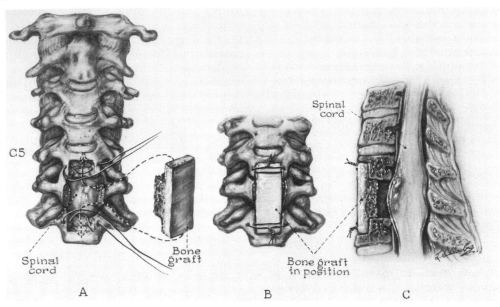

Figure 8–51. *Anterior approach to the spine for relief of anterior cord compression and fusion. This sketch illustrates technique of vertebral corpectomy and interbody strut fusion in the cervical region. (Although wire is shown in this sketch to hold the bone graft, a soft suture material for anterior cervical fusions is preferable, to avoid injury to the adjacent esophagus). (From Schmeisser, G.: Orthopedic aspects of spinal cord injuries. Md. State Med. J. 19:95–99, 1970.)*

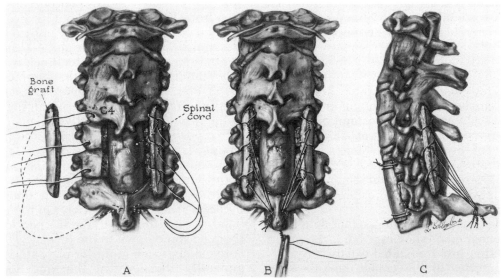

Figure 8–52. *Posterior approach to the spine for decompression or fusion. A laminectomy decompression is carried out when there is posterior impingement on the spinal cord. If there is associated spinal instability, a bilateral strut fusion with wire check reins, is also performed; in the absence of the spinous processes and laminae, the bone struts are wired to the articular facets. In cases with instability but not requiring decompression, fusion may be achieved by fastening the spinous processes together with wire and bone grafts. Lateral view, C, shows combined anterior and posterior fusions performed in cases with severe instability. (From Schmeisser, G.: Orthopedic aspects of spinal cord injuries. Md. State Med. J. 19:95–99, 1970.)*

ing cord damage is too great to justify aspiration, since some patients show partial spontaneous recovery.

Fusion

Bed rest and immobilization in a body cast are often adequate as definitive treatment for thoracolumbar injuries. Similarly in the cervical region, external stabilization with skeletal traction alone often results in *spontaneous* fusion over a 6–8 week period, obviating the need for *internal* (operative) stabilization. Operative fusion is performed when there is a risk of later dislocation resulting from spinal instability when the traction is discontinued. Among the types of lesions for which fusion is indicated are comminuted or teardrop fractures of a cervical vertebral body; such fractures tend to heal by fibrous union, posing a risk of instability and cord compression months or years later.[23] In evaluating other types of lesions, a useful guide in determining the need for operation is the ease or difficulty with which a dislocation is reduced by skeletal traction or postural reduction. Rapid reduction often signifies considerable ligamentous disruption, making fusion advisable.[21] An *anterior* or *posterior* approach is used, depending on the site of instability, and the operation may or may not be combined with a decompressive procedure (Figs. 8–51 and 8–52). Extensive spinal disruption may require both anterior and posterior fusions, as illustrated by the case shown in Figure 8–41. In the thoracic region, internal stabilization may be achieved with Harrington rods.

Operative fusion offers the physical and psychological advantage of early mobilization of the patient and permits an earlier start of intensive rehabilitation. Some form of *external* stabilization, however, must be continued during the 6- to 8-week postoperative period until the fusion is solidly healed. External stabilization of the cervical spine can be accomplished by the *halo* fixation apparatus which permits sitting or ambulation (Fig. 8–51). The halo may also be employed for patients who would otherwise be immobilized by skull tong traction alone, without internal fixation. The halo ring is attached via metal rods to a plaster body cast or to a light-weight plastic vest.

Debridement for Penetrating Injuries

Penetrating wounds with retained foreign bodies in the spinal canal should be explored by laminectomy (Fig. 8–43).[18] Early debridement offsets the development of scarring which may produce pain as well as increase the neural damage.

Surgical indications are less clear-cut in patients *without* radiopaque foreign bodies. For example, in stab wound cases with stable or improving neurological deficit, exploration is probably not necessary, except perhaps in an attempt to reapproximate severed motor nerve roots. On the other hand, a bullet passing through the spinal canal may carry fragments of clothing and generally causes considerable tissue disruption for which debridement is desirable. Leakage of spinal fluid after penetrating injuries is another relative indication for exploration and surgical closure of the dural tear. Wound exploration should also be carried out, with the patient covered by antibiotics, if there is evidence of meningitis, suggesting the possibility of retained debris or a fistulous tract. As was discussed previously in this chapter, lumbar puncture is advisable in penetrating injuries to rule out meningeal infection.

Penetrating injuries of the chest or abdomen, which may be more immediately life-threatening, take precedence over the spinal injury. Although early spinal exploration is desirable, it can be safely delayed several days. Exploration becomes more urgent, however, if there is suspicion that the penetrating spinal injury is associated with cord compression.

SUPPORTIVE CARE FOR MAJOR INJURIES

Respiratory Function

Administration of oxygen in the early stages may help to reduce hypoxic damage to the injured cord. Blood gases are determined initially and are repeated at intervals if there is a question of adequacy of ventilation. Mental confusion is difficult to evaluate; it may be related to associated head injury, to cerebral hypoxia due to impaired ventilation, or to vertebrobasilar arterial insufficiency.

Patients with spinal cord injury are prone to *pneumonia* owing to reduced ventilatory effort, immobilization and failure to clear secretions from the upper respiratory tract. A respirator may be necessary in cases of serious respiratory embarrassment. If respiration is intact, a simple incentive spirometer will help maintain lung expansion. Frequent turning of the patient reduces hypostasis. These patients are also subject to *pulmonary embolus;* this risk may be reduced by the use of elastic stockings and elevation of the legs on pillows to prevent venous stasis in the lower extremities.

Nutrition

Protein depletion with loss of body weight is one of the serious systemic effects of paraplegia. Examination of the serum protein level may reveal the negative nitrogen balance only in the later stages. Anemia resulting from protein loss appears as early as one week after trauma. Protein deficit plays a major role in susceptibility of paraplegics to urinary tract infection and to the development of decubitus ulcers. Vigorous feeding encouragement is given these patients in whom apathy is commonly encountered. Tube feedings may be necessary. A reasonable daily intake for an adult paraplegic is 3500 calories, which should include a minimum of 125 gm. of protein and added vitamins. The fluid intake is aimed at 4000 cc. to promote "irrigation" of the urinary tract.

Skin

Local care of the skin, in addition to dietary measures, makes ulceration an avoidable complication. Skin maceration is minimized by keeping the linens clean and dry. Turning of patients with cervical injuries on the Stryker frame is carried out every two hours day and night in order to

avoid prolonged pressure on bony prominences. Patients with stable compression fractures of thoracic or lumbar spine may be nursed on a regular hospital bed and rolled "as a log" for turning. A pneumatic mattress or a waterbed is useful in protecting the skin, but these devices are not a substitute for frequent turning.

Bladder

Loss of detrusor muscle tone is one of the manifestations of the acute phase following cord trauma. Early in the acute stage, an indwelling urethral catheter prevents excessive stretching of the bladder wall. A cystometrogram is obtained as early as feasible as a baseline for subsequent evaluation of bladder function. *Intermittent* catheterization is started after the first 4 to 6 hours and is generally regarded as the most effective regimen for the prevention of bladder complications and the promotion of bladder training.[3] The patient may be taught to self-catheterize if the upper limbs are not paralyzed. In hospital settings where personnel are not available for intermittent catheterization, continuous catheter drainage is acceptable. Tidal drainage is not recommended. Regardless of the method of drainage, the bladder is irrigated twice daily with 0.25 per cent acetic acid. The patient is given a urinary antibacterial agent, methenamine mandelate (Mandelamine), and ascorbic acid (to acidify the urine).

As spinal shock recedes over a period of days or weeks, *automatic* or *reflex* micturition gradually appears if the bladder has not been damaged by overdistention or infection. This phase is characterized by vigorous involuntary voiding at intervals of one to three hours; catheterization may then be discontinued, if the residual volume of urine in the bladder is minimal. In complete cord lesions, automatic micturition will be permanent, but return of voluntary control is possible in less serious injuries. When sacral segments or nerve roots S2 to S4 are destroyed, the bladder remains permanently *atonic;* evacuation in these cases is achieved by manual compression (Credé maneuver).

Gastrointestinal Function

Oral feeding is withheld immediately following injury until it is clear that paralytic ileus will not pose a problem. If ileus occurs, nasogastric suction, rectal tube insertion and enemas are employed to decompress the bowel. Injections of neostigmine may help to restore intestinal tone. When the acute stage has passed, enemas are given regularly to avoid fecal impaction.

Stress Ulcers. Spinal cord injury, like any severe stress, may trigger an as yet poorly defined neurohumoral mechanism which results in gastric ulceration, followed by hemorrhage or perforation.[5] Stress ulcers occur more frequently during the first week after injury and affect all age groups. Hemorrhage or perforation occurs silently, without pain or distress; there may be sudden deterioration in the patient's condition, such as shock. *Prevention* of stress ulceration consists of a prophylactic ulcer regimen, including antacids, and Cimetidine. Monitoring of vital signs and stool guaiacs are helpful for early detection. Patients given corticosteroids for management of the cord injury should be watched particularly closely for signs of gastrointestinal bleeding. Because sepsis from any source increases the incidence and morbidity of stress ulceration, infection should be treated vigorously.

Rehabilitation

Physical and occupational therapy are begun soon after the patient's general condition has stabilized, usually within a few days after injury. To prevent contractures, all limb joints are ranged daily. When at rest, paralyzed hands are splinted in a functional position with the thumb-web stretched, and the shoulder is placed in abduction and moderate external rotation. A vertical foot board is used to prevent foot-drop deformity. The patient is placed in the sitting position as soon as spinal stabilization is secure.

An optimistic yet realistic approach is adopted in planning the patient's future. The participation of a skilled medical social worker can be invaluable in helping the patient and his family adjust to the new demands imposed by the disability.

New Therapeutic Possibilities

A number of potential treatments for spinal cord injury are currently under investigation. *Local hypothermia* by application of cold saline to the injured cord in animals appears promising, but the results of limited trials in humans thus far have been inconsistent. Additional possibilities under investigation, but not yet studied in man, include (1) *osmotic diuretics,* such as urea[13] and mannitol; (2) agents to *block synthesis of norepinephrine,* local accumulation of which is thought to produce hemorrhagic necrosis at the site of spinal cord injury[20] and (3) *hyperbaric oxygenation.*[14]

MANAGEMENT OF MINOR SPINAL INJURIES

Acceleration (Whiplash) Injuries of the Neck

For cervical sprains (neck pain and muscle spasm) without neurological or radiographic abnormality, several days of bed rest at home are prescribed, followed by gradual ambulation. Analgesics, muscle relaxants and mild heat to the neck are helpful. A light cervical collar (a folded towel may suffice) affords mild immobilization, but its use should be tapered off after 1–2 weeks to avoid loss of muscle tone. Not uncommonly, the symptoms first appear or are aggravated several hours or days after the injury. The large majority of patients with simple cervical sprains recover over a period of 3–6 weeks without residual difficulties. A psychoneurotic response to the injury, with prolongation of symptoms, may be avoided by the physician's careful explanation of the condition, the plan of treatment and the expected course of recovery.[9, 11] Patients whose convalescence is prolonged require neurosurgical or orthopedic evaluation in search of complicating factors, such as disc injury.

Acute Lumbosacral Sprain

Musculoligamentous sprains sustained in falls, heavy lifting or bending represent the commonest cause of acute low back pain. The possibility of referred pain from pelvic or abdominal lesions is considered in eliciting the history. Radiographs of the lumbosacral spine are obtained to visualize the vertebral bodies, intervertebral disc spaces and the apophyseal joints. The radiographs also help to exclude unexpected lesions such as pathological fracture, osteolytic defects or abnormal psoas shadows. On physical examination, sciatica, with limitation of straight-leg raising, suggests nerve root irritation, making disc herniation (protrusion) a possibility. In most cases, symptoms of either back sprain or disc herniation resolve spontaneously on bed rest (with board under mattress) for a few days to several weeks. Analgesics, muscle relaxants and local heat are added. Bladder dysfunction (frequency or retention) or rapidly progressing loss of strength (such as foot drop) signify serious nerve root compression for which neurosurgical intervention may be urgently required. If bladder function is in doubt (question of urinary retention or overflow incontinence), a cystometrogram, or simple measurement of post-voiding residual urine, may clarify the situation.

SUMMARY

When a patient presents in the emergency department with major trauma, priority decisions must be made rapidly in determining the steps of appropriate action. When spinal injury is suspected, the following sequence of attention to presenting problems is suggested:

1. Vital signs, resuscitation.
2. Rapid evaluation of problem, including search for associated injuries.
3. Head-halter traction for evident or suspected cervical injuries; firm mattress for thoracic or lumbar injuries.
4. If spinal cord injury is likely, start corticosteroids, first dose IV, with subsequent maintenance by IM route for 1–2 weeks. Give antacids and possibly an anticholinergic agent to protect gastric mucosa against stress ulceration.
5. Request for specialty consultations as indicated.
6. Indwelling urethral catheter initially, then intermittent catheterization.
7. Detailed clinical evaluation.
8. Radiographic evaluation.
9. Skeletal (e.g., Gardner-Wells) traction for cervical injuries.
10. Decision regarding further manage-

ment (e.g., myelography, lumbar puncture to rule out infection in penetrating injuries, spinal decompression and/or fusion).

11. Supportive care — respiratory function, nutrition, skin, bladder, gastrointestinal function, rehabilitation.

REFERENCES

1. American National Red Cross: Lifesaving: Rescue and Water Safety. Garden City, N.Y., Doubleday and Co., Inc., 1974, pp. 209–214.
2. Black, P., and Markowitz, R. S.: Experimental spinal cord injury in monkeys: Comparison of steroids and local hypothermia. Surg. Forum 22:409–411, 1971.
3. Boyarsky, S.: Management of the neurogenic bladder: Current status and recent developments. Clin. Neurosurg. 20, 1973.
4. Byrnes, D. P., and Ducker, T. B.: Maryland Institute for Emergency Medicine, University of Maryland, Baltimore. Personal communication, 1978.
5. Clark, W. K.: Stress ulceration. Clin. Neurosurg. 18:426–440, 1971.
6. Crosby, E. C., Humphrey, T., and Lauer, E. W.: Correlative Anatomy of the Nervous System. New York, Macmillan, 1962, p. 61.
7. Davis, D., Bohlman, H., Walker, A. E., Fisher, R., and Robinson, R.: The pathological findings in fatal craniospinal injuries. J. Neurosurg. 34:603–613, 1971.
8. Folson, F.: Extrication and Casualty Handling Techniques. Philadelphia, J. B. Lippincott Co., 1975.
9. Frankel, C. J.: Medical-legal aspects of injuries to the neck. J.A.M.A. 169:216–223, 1959.
10. Freeman, L. W.: Injuries of the spinal cord. Surg. Clin. N. Am., 34:1131, 1954.
11. Gay, J. R., and Abbott, K. H.: Common whiplash injuries of the neck. J.A.M.A. 152:1698–1704, 1953.
12. Jackson, F. E.: The Achilles' neck and other vulnerable vertebrae. Emergency Medicine 9:22–41, 1977.
13. Joyner, J., and Freeman, L. W.: Urea and spinal cord trauma. Neurology 13:69–72, 1963.
14. Kelly, D. L., Lassiter, K. R. L., Vongsvivut, A., and Smith, J. M.: Effects of hyperbaric oxygenation and tissue oxygen studies in experimental paraplegia. J. Neurosurg. 36:425–429, 1972.
15. Lewin, P.: Head sling traction technic in cervical spine roentgenography. Am. J. Surg. 8:434, 1930.
16. Locke, G. E., Yashon, D., Feldman, R. A., and Hunt, W. E.: Ischemia in primate spinal cord injury. J. Neurosurg. 34:614–617, 1971.
17. Macnab, I.: Acceleration injuries of the cervical spine. J. Bone Joint Surg. 46A:1797–1799, 1964.
18. Meirowsky, A. M.: Neurosurgical management. In Coates, J. B., and Meirowsky, A. M., eds.: Neurological Surgery of Trauma. Washing-

ton, D.C., Office of the Surgeon General, Dept. of the Army, pp. 307–325, 1965.

19. Ommaya, A. K., Faas, F., and Yarnell, P.: Whiplash injury and brain damage. J.A.M.A. *204*:285–289, 1968.
20. Osterholm, J. L., and Mathews, G. J.: Altered norepinephrine metabolism following experimental spinal cord injury. Part 2. Protection against traumatic spinal cord hemorrhagic necrosis by norepinephrine synthesis blockade with alpha methyl tyrosine. J. Neurosurg. *36*:395–401, 1972.
21. Robinson, R. A.: Anterior and posterior cervical spine fusions. Clin. Orthopaed. *35*:34, 1964.
22. Russo, G. L., Bellegarrique, R., Lucas, J., and Ducker, T. B.: Complete sensory-motor paralysis after cord injury in 273 cases: Recovery and mortality and therapeutic implications. Presented at 26th Annual Meeting of Congress of Neurological Surgeons, New Orleans, Louisiana, Oct. 1976.
23. Schneider, R. C.: Surgical indications and contraindications in spine and spinal cord trauma. Clin. Neurosurg, 8:157, 1962.
24. Schneider, R. C., Gosch, H. H., Norrell, H.,

Jerva, M., Combs, L. W., and Smith, R. A.: Vascular insufficiency and differential distortion of brain and cord caused by cervicomedullary football injuries. J. Neurosurg. *33*:363–375, 1970.
25. Schneider, R. C., and Schemm, G. W.: Vertebral artery insufficiency in acute chronic spinal trauma. J. Neurosurg. *18*:348–360, 1961.
26. Suwanwela, C., Alexander, E., Jr., and Davis, C. H., Jr.: Prognosis in spinal cord injury with special reference to patients with motor paralysis and sensory preservation. J. Neurosurg. *19*:220, 1962.
27. Tarlov, I. M.: Spinal Cord Compression. Mechanisms of Paralysis and Treatment. Springfield, Ill., Charles C Thomas, 1957.
28. Vlahovitch, B., Fuentes, J. M., Choucair, Y., and Verger, A. C.: Valeur prognostique indissociable des fonctions spinothalamique et corticospinale dans les traumatismes médullaires graves. *Neuro-Chirurgie* (Paris) *23*(1): 55–72, 1977.
29. World Wide Medical Press: The $10 unilitter: It supports patients at scene, during diagnosis, therapy. Radiology News 2:4–5, 1977.

CHAPTER 9

INJURIES OF THE EYE, THE LIDS AND THE ORBIT

David Paton, M.D., F.A.C.S.,
Morton F. Goldberg, M.D., F.A.C.S.,
and Jared M. Emery, M.D., F.A.C.S.

The eye and its surrounding structures are subject to serious injury from many forms of head trauma. Treatment of such injuries is the proper concern of an opthalmologist, but most trauma cases are seen first by the emergency treatment room surgeon or other attending physician. For that doctor, the importance of routine examination of the eye, the lids and the orbit can scarcely be overstressed. Whether or not he must accept the responsibility of treating the injuries himself, he must not fail to suspect or discover their presence. Emphasis here is given to the variety of injuries that the examiner should seek and the primary treatment that the more common ones require.

Chemical burns of the eye are probably the only true ocular emergency. Other lesions of prime concern are lacerations of the globe, intraocular foreign bodies, severe lid lacerations and hyphemas. Prompt attention, however, is a matter of hours, not minutes. There is time for adequate examination and time for an unhurried decision regarding optimal management. Too frequently, lacerations of the globe are undetected because tightly swollen lids are not separated by lid retractors for an adequate view of the eye itself. Surgical correction of facial fractures is sometimes

completed without recognition of a "blowout" fracture of the orbital floor because it was not visible on routine skull films. Intraocular bleeding is occasionally unidentified if persons with "black eyes" are simply dispatched with cold compresses, and minor lid lacerations are at times repaired without detection of an unsuspected intraorbital foreign body. It is to the credit of emergency room staffs that these oversights do not happen more often.

Further reason for careful evaluation of the eyes in accident cases is the assistance this may give in general appraisal of the patient's illness and in decisions for his referral to consultants. The pupils can give useful clues to the state of consciousness and to specific intracranial disorders, but these clues can be interpreted only after consideration of the many reasons for abnormal pupillary size and reactions (Table 9–1). Following accidents, double vision is a frequent complaint, with multiple possibilities to be considered in the differential diagnosis (Table 9–2). Loss of vision following an injury should be diagnosed by thorough evaluation (Table 9–3). The position of the eyes, testing of the corneal reflexes and the presence of nystagmus are well-known observations of

TABLE 9–1. Causes of Asymmetry of the Pupils

1. Antecedent causes of unequal pupils.
2. Traumatic mydriasis or miosis from direct blow to eye.
3. Unilateral blindness.
4. Iridodialysis or rupture of iris sphincter.
5. Unilateral use of topical drugs.
6. Intraorbital trauma to ciliary nerves or ganglion.
7. Horner's syndrome from injury to brainstem or cervical sympathetic pathways.
8. Intracranial third nerve palsy.

TABLE 9–2. The Differential Diagnosis of Double Vision Following Head Trauma

1. Orbital fracture (particularly blowout fracture of the floor) causing restricted function of inferior rectus and inferior oblique muscles.
2. Hematoma in orbit and/or ocular muscles.
3. Third, fourth or sixth cranial nerve palsies (orbital or intracranial).
4. Avulsion, contusion or transection of extraocular muscles.
5. Avulsion of pulley of superior oblique.
6. Subluxation of the lens (unilateral diplopia).
7. Edema or detachment of the macula (unilateral diplopia).
8. Decompensation of pre-existing ocular phoria, becoming tropia.
9. "Whiplash" injury, and other diplopias of obscure origin.

TABLE 9–3. The Differential Diagnosis of Post-Traumatic Loss of Vision

1. Lid swelling; blood or foreign material covering cornea; corneal damage.
2. Hyphema; vitreous hemorrhage.
3. Traumatic cataract; luxation of the lens.
4. Central retinal artery or vein occlusion (from markedly increased orbital pressure or embolus).
5. Traumatic retinal edema and hemorrhage of retina from direct or contrecoup blows.
6. Avulsion of optic nerve by lateral orbital wall trauma or contrecoup blow to head.
7. Retinal detachment.
8. Cortical blindness from hematoma, ischemia or anoxia (patient may be unaware of blindness).
9. Intracranial interruption of visual pathways (hemorrhage, foreign body).
10. Acute congestive (angle closure) glaucoma precipitated by emotional trauma of recent accident or from intumescent lens, etc.
11. Hysteria.
12. Malingering.

TABLE 9–4. The Differential Diagnosis of "Blurred" Optic-Nerveheads

CONDITION	VISION	VISUAL FIELDS	RETINAL VEINS	NERVE-HEAD COLOR	RETINAL HEMORRHAGES	PERIPAPILLARY RETINAL EDEMA	VITREOUS CELLS	SYMMETRY OF NERVEHEADS	COMMENTS
Early papilledema	Normal	Normal (except blind spot enlargement)	Slightly distended; early loss of spontaneous pulsations	Pink	±	±	–	Often asymmetrical	Rarely: extension of subarachnoid hemorrhages into the eye; headaches
Advanced papilledema	Normal or, at times, somewhat reduced	Normal (except blind spot enlargement)	Distended without spontaneous pulsations	Very pink to pale	+	+	–	Often symmetrical	Sixth nerve palsies additional clue
Hyperopia and physiological variants	Normal	Normal	Normal	Normal	–	–	–	Often symmetrical	Fundus seen with +lens; central disc-cupping usually present
Optic neuritis	Impaired	Central scotoma, ± peripheral loss	Distended ± spontaneous pulsations	Pink	±	±	±	Unilateral usually	Precipitous onset; may have pain with ocular motility
Optic nerve avulsion	Blind eye	Absent	Sludged	Pale	±	–	±	Contralateral eye normal	Contrecoup or direct trauma
Hyalin bodies of nervehead	Normal	Normal (rarely binasal field cuts)	Normal	Normal	–	–	–	Often symmetrical; hyalin bodies sometimes seen at disc margins in one eye only	Often familial (examine parents and siblings)
Hypotony of eye (after trauma)	Slightly impaired	Usually normal	Distended	Pink	±	Peripheral edema	–	Unilateral	Soft eye; commotio retinae

**TABLE 9–5.   Emergency Room Evaluation of Trauma Affecting
the Orbit, Lids or Eye**

1. Obtain history of previous eye disorders, type of chemical burn or nature of injuring object, and tetanus immunization.
2. Determine visual acuity and screen visual fields by confrontation with test object.
3. Differentiate partially penetrating and completely penetrating (perforating) injuries of cornea and sclera. Use lid retractors. Note uveal prolapse.
4. Note hemorrhages and infections of orbit, lids and conjunctiva. Account for chemosis.
5. Investigate depth of all lid lacerations, noting fat in wound. Seek foreign bodies under lid: evert lid and sweep fornix with cotton swab after use of topical anesthetic.
6. Palpate orbital rim; feel for crepitus through lids; test facial and corneal sensation; auscultate for orbitocranial bruit.
7. Appraise real or apparent anterior, posterior or vertical displacement of globe.
8. Characterize diplopia by analysis of ocular ductions and versions; attempt forced-duction test using forceps and topical anesthetic.
9. Record pupil shapes, sizes and reactions, accounting for asymmetry.
10. Inspect for hyphema, iridodonesis and iridodialysis.
11. Examine cornea for opacities, ulcers, foreign bodies, rust rings and abrasions (use fluorescein paper). Avoid steroid-containing medications.
12. Use loupe or slit lamp to detect foreign body paths in cornea, iris and lens.
13. Estimate comparative depth of anterior chambers for evaluation of intumescent cataract, displaced lens and recessed chamber angle.
14. If traumatized globe is intact and cornea undamaged, measure intraocular pressure with tonometer.
15. Ophthalmoscope: Differentiate various types of intra-ocular hemorrhages. Record appearance of nerveheads, maculae and retinal circulation. Visualize foreign bodies if possible.
16. Get x-rays in all cases of possible retained foreign body in globe or orbit, and whenever orbital fracture is conceivable.
17. Consider value of photographing all injuries.

neurological importance. Evaluation of carotid artery function is often assisted by determination of the relative central retinal artery pressures through ophthalmodynamometry.[21] Papilledema is of concern in all cases of head trauma, but there are several causes of "blurred" optic nerveheads that must be remembered in appraisal of the fundus appearance (Table 9–4).

It is unreasonable to expect a general surgeon to deal comprehensively with traumatic injuries of the eye, but it is important that the surgeon develop a keen awareness of ocular injuries and a practical knowledge of their management. Table 9–5 summarizes the considerations that should be kept in mind for "work-up" examination of various types of injuries of the eye and its adnexa. Figure 9–1 shows a minimal set of equipment essential for emergency room evaluation of ocular trauma.

INJURIES OF THE LIDS

The first step in caring for an injury of the lid is to determine the extent of the injury, paying particular attention to the underlying globe. Small lacerations should be gently probed and at times explored; larger ones can simply be laid open. Prophylactic antibiotics, tetanus immunization and hemostasis are so routine in general surgery that further comment is unnecessary. The same is true of most burns. but these are discussed in more detail later.

For lacerations of the lid, the surgeon should perform a meticulous primary repair, employing instruments and sutures suitable to the delicacy of the task. Many months should then elapse before plastic revision for cosmetic correction of any residual deformities is undertaken; it is remarkable how often a primary repair produces an excellent final result after a year or more of gradual improvement. Permanent deformity of the eyelids is not only of major functional significance to the eye, but it may also cause great damage to the psyche of the patient. Vanity in these matters is a characteristic of far more people than those reputed to be preoccupied with appearance. Surely few other areas of the body require more attention to careful reapproximation of tissue planes and precise reconstruction of defects to assure satisfactory results. However, rarely is scrupulously performed surgery so well rewarded — the rich blood supply of the eyelids, the thinness and laxity of the lid skin and the infrequency of infection all provide an ideal tissue for plastic refurbishing.

Surgical Anatomy of the Eyelids. A

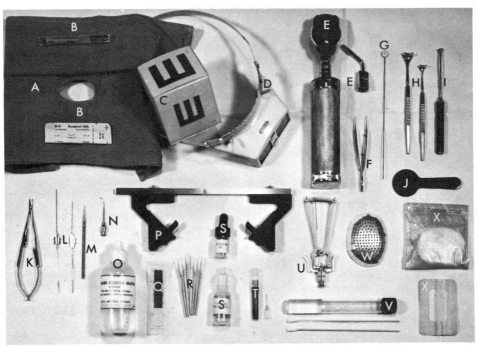

Figure 9–1. *Equipment essential for emergency room evaluation of ocular trauma. A, Drape for minor lid laceration repairs; B, ophthalmic 6-0 catgut and silk sutures; C, "E box" for visual acuity testing; D, loupe; E, hand ophthalmoscope and transilluminator; F, fine, toothed forceps; G, test object for visual field examination; H, lid retractors; I, ophthalmodynamometer; J, pin hole disc for acuity measurement; K, needle holder for ophthalmic sutures; L, lacrimal probes; M, punctum dilator; N, curved, blunt lacrimal irrigation needle; O, squeeze bottle for sterile saline irrigation; P, exophthalmometer; Q, fluorescein paper strips in sterile envelope; R, cotton applicators; S, topical anesthetics; T, disposable No. 25 needles; U, tonometer; V, culture tube; W, protective metal shield; X, eye patches.*

comprehensive review of lid anatomy cannot be included here, but selected features of particular importance in surgical repairs will be mentioned. *The lids should be regarded as double-layered structures: the anterior layer is composed of the skin and orbicularis muscle, and the posterior layer of tarsus and palpebral conjunctiva* (Fig. 9–2). Examination of the lid margins reveals a faint linear demarcation between these two layers: the "gray line," or mucocutaneous junction. Each of the two surgical layers of the lids should be separately closed in all lid lacerations that transect the tarsus. Another important aspect of the two surgical layers of the lids is the inherent convenience of splitting the lids along the gray line so that a sliding flap of skin-muscle can be used to fill a post-traumatic lid defect. Undermining the anterior surgical layer is readily performed; and because of the abundance of skin in the vicinity of the lids, large defects can usually be closed by such flaps, which are

brought over the relatively fixed posterior layer. Defects in the posterior layer of tarsus and palpebral conjunctiva can be filled by bringing across the lid-fissure portions of the same layer from the opposing lid — deficiency of which, if not total, will make little difference to the uninjured tissue from which it is removed.

The conjunctiva is a mucous membrane lining for the entire posterior surface of the lids, reaching from canthus to canthus and fornix to fornix, forming a sac that is open anteriorly at the lid fissure and closed at the limbus. (Fig. 9–2C). The conjunctiva is a distinct tissue layer except where it is firmly adherent to the tarsus of the lids; it has generous recesses (the upper and lower fornix) whose loose folds permit marked lid and eye mobility. Like the skin of the lids, its natural laxity permits extensive mobilization for surgical repairs. Like other mucous membranes, its mucocutaneous junctions are abrupt, smooth boundaries that cannot be emulated by surgical apposition of conjunctiva to skin. Consequently, it is important to salvage as much natural lid margin as possible in lid reconstructions. Mucous membrane grafts *within* the conjunctival sac do exceptionally well. Customarily, they are taken from the contralateral eye or the buccal cavity.

The tarsal "plates" provide the strength and curvature of the lids. The tarsus is composed of dense fibrous tissue containing the meibomian glands whose orifices are posterior to the gray line. There is no cartilage in the lids. Peripheral to the tarsi is the orbital septum, of which the upper and lower tarsi are merely thickened portions in the same fascial plane. The orbital septum attaches to the periosteum at the orbital rim throughout its circumference and forms the anterior barrier between orbital contents and the skin-muscle layer. *If a lid laceration contains fat, the examiner knows that the orbital septum has been perforated.* Superiorly, the septum is pierced by the tendon of the levator palpebrae muscle, which courses from the orbital apex to the skin of the upper lid, inserting near the upper margin of the tarsus and producing the upper lid fold. Traumatic damage to the levator muscle may there-

fore be signaled by the absence of lid fold as well as by ptosis of the lid. Lacerations involving the superior portions of the orbit, particularly in its medial third, sometimes involve the aponeurosis of the levator tendon; this must be recognized and repaired.

The lacrimal gland is located at the lateral aspect of the superior orbital margin. During orbital explorations from lateral or superior approaches, the surgeon must avoid damage to both the gland and its ducts, which enter the conjunctival fornix superotemporally. The eyelids contain the canaliculi of the lacrimal drainage apparatus (Figs. 9–2, 9–11 and 9–12). In repair of lid lacerations, attention should be directed to the functional role of the lids — not only to the fact that the lid must be able to close fully to protect the eyeball but also to the part the lids play in distribution and drainage of tears.[15] Blinking does more than moisten the cornea with tear film. The gentle squeeze of eyelid closure brings the lacrimal puncta of the lids into close contact with the pooled tear fluid of the eye; the contraction of the orbicularis fibers assists in the propulsion of tears into the canaliculi and compresses the lacrimal

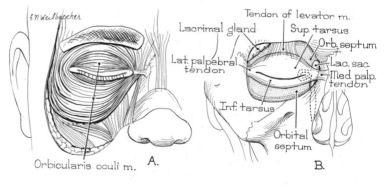

Figure 9–2. *Anatomy of the lids and orbit. (From Paton, D. L., and Goldberg, M. F.: Management of Ocular Injuries. Philadelphia, W. B. Saunders Co., 1976.)*

sac itself, causing the tear flow to proceed into the nose via the nasolacrimal duct. The orbicularis fibers of the lower lid, in particular, should be given great respect at the time of injury repair; surgical skin-muscle flaps or superficial tissue deformity from primary trauma itself can cause irreversible loss of function of the lacrimal drainage passageways, even though the drainage structures themselves were spared from the original trauma.

Finally, it is useful to recall that the orbit has no lymphatics, whereas the lymphatic drainage of the eyelids is divided into two main pathways. The medial two thirds of the lids drain to the submaxillary glands and the lateral one third to the preauricular glands. Inflammation of the eyelids is often associated with palpable enlargement of these glands.

Ecchymoses of the Lids. Direct blows to the eyelids may cause ecchymoses from the plentiful blood supply of the lids themselves. Often there is an associated orbital hemorrhage with proptosis of the eye and hemorrhage under the conjunctiva. What is a unilateral "black eye" one day may spread to the other side in ensuing days, as the blood within the lids seeps subcutaneously across the nasal bridge.

Hemorrhage within the lids is of no consequence per se, but it can signal other more serious injuries to orbital contents. For example, fracture of the roof of the orbit is not infrequently followed by dissection of hemorrhage along the levator muscle, producing subconjunctival hemorrhage superiorly and also ecchymosis of the upper lid. Orbial floor fractures may be associated with hemorrhage in the lower lid and inferior portion of the orbit. As will be described more fully later, there are also various contusion injuries within the eye that can accompany hematomas of the lids.

Treatment of lid ecchymoses themselves is usually limited to initial cold compresses, subsequent hot compresses and the use of sunglasses for a fortnight.

Traumatic Ptosis. It is important to identify the levator muscle during repair of upper lid injuries so that the tendon can be sutured to the upper margin of the tarsus and the muscle function can be restored (Fig. 9–9C).

Any upper lid swelling is associated to some degree with a drooping of the upper lid or narrowing of the lid fissure. Most often that type of ptosis resolves as the edema subsides, and lid function returns to normal. Any persistent soreness or photophobia of the eye will produce a partial "protective" ptosis that will persist as long as the irritation remains. There are times, nevertheless, when a blow to the eye is followed by a prolonged ptosis of the upper lid without evident damage to the third cranial nerve, without evident avulsion of the levator palpebrae muscle and without abnormality of the eye itself. Once the examiner is satisfied that there is no clinical evidence of mechanical interruption of the levator muscle, the only recourse is to wait an extended period of time before surgical repair is considered. Spontaneous correction of traumatic ptosis may require a year or more; thus, ptosis operations must not be considered for many months following such injury.

Anesthesia for Repair of Lid Injuries. The majority of lid lacerations can be repaired under local anesthesia if the patient is cooperative. Figure 9–3 shows the customary sites of injection for those branches of the fifth and seventh cranial nerves that serve the periocular tissues. It is preferable to given retrobulbar anesthesia when lacerations involve the conjunctiva and when orbital hemorrhage or lacer-

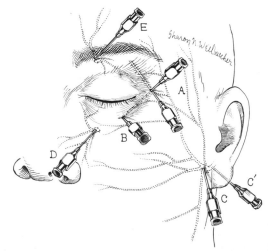

Figure 9–3. Injection points for facial and orbital anesthesia and akinesia. A Van Lint technique of orbicularis infiltration, B retrobulbar injection site, C O'Brien facial nerve block, C' alternative facial nerve block by tympanomastoid fissure injection, D infraorbital sensory block, E supraorbital sensory block. (From Paton, D. L., and Goldberg, M. G.: Management of Ocular Injuries. Philadelphia, W. B. Saunders Co., 1976.)

ations of the globe do not contraindicate increased intraorbital pressure by addition of the anesthetic solution. Topical instillation anesthetics are useful adjuncts, particularly when the effect of the infiltration anesthesia is waning.

Lidocaine (Xylocaine) in 2 per cent solution is currently a favored agent for infiltration anesthesia; longer effect and reduced bleeding are achieved by the addition of 2 drops of 1:1000 epinephrine per 10 ml. of the anesthetic. The amount of lidocaine injection may not exceed 500 mg. if used with epinephrine, or 300 mg. if used without epinephrine. This dosage must be reduced for children and for elderly or debilitated patients. Topical anesthetics that can be dropped onto the eye and the conjunctivae include cocaine 4 per cent, proparacaine hydrochloride (Ophthaine) 0.5 per cent, and others. Cocaine is probably the most effective but has the occasionally undesirable side effect of temporarily reducing corneal transparency.

TECHNIQUES. Paralysis of the orbicularis muscle can be obtained by the O'Brien technique. The zygomatic arch is located and followed back to a point just above the tragus of the ear; the condyloid process of the mandible is felt to slip forward under the finger as the patient opens his mouth. The patient is directed to close his mouth and the injection is made just anterior to the condyloid process, not in the joint itself. At this site, only 2 or 3 ml. of 2 per cent lidocaine is required for good lid akinesia (Fig. 9–3C). This injection does not provide anesthesia of the lids or globe; but, when used in combination with a retrobulbar injection, it helps in avoiding excessive lid swelling when reapproximation of tissues can be facilitated by minimizing edema. Supplementary injections at the supraorbital notch and infraorbital foramen augment anesthesia of the lids (Fig. 9–3D and E).

The Van Lint technique of akinesia and anesthesia of the eyelids employs local injection of the anesthetic into the deep subcutaneous tissues of the orbital margins (Fig. 9–3A). As much as 10 ml. of lidocaine with hyaluronidase and epinephrine can be used in this manner. Hemorrhage from the injection can occur but rarely complicates surgical repairs.

Retrobulbar injection of local anesthetic is a useful and sometimes essential adjunct to repair of lid lacerations, particularly when the bulbar conjunctiva requires surgical manipulation or when ocular motility is undesirable. The technique is simple, but the injection should be made by someone familiar with orbital anatomy (preferably an opthalmologist) because hemorrhage, damage to the globe and inadequate akinesia can result from improper placement of the needle. A 23 gauge by 35 mm. Atkinson retrobulbar needle with a special sharp but rounded point reduces the possibility of orbital hemorrhages. After the skin has been cleansed and a wheal of anesthetic has been produced at the injection site, the patient is directed to look upward and toward his nose. The needle is introduced through the skin just above the junction of the middle and lateral third of the inferior orbital margin (Fig. 9–3B). The needle is passed through the orbital septum and then directed obliquely upward and slightly inward toward the apex of the orbit. The plunger is retracted to determine whether a vessel has been penetrated; if not, 1 to 3 ml. of anesthetic is injected. It is important not to wag the needle tip, as this is the chief cause of retrobulbar hemorrhage. Some surgeons prefer to inject into the muscle cone just posterior to the globe, whereas others insert the needle farther into the apex of the orbit.

A surgeon unaccustomed to lid surgery will too often forget that abrasions of corneal epithelium may occur from contact with instruments, sutures or sponges. Undetected and unattended corneal abrasions can proceed to corneal ulcerations and will create severe discomfort for the patient when the anesthetic has worn off.

Preoperative Preparation for Repair of Lid Wounds. EYELASHES AND BROW. Eyelashes may be trimmed if desired; they regrow promptly, regaining their normal length in 4 to 6 weeks.

In contrast, the brow hair should not be shaved, for in rare cases this hair does not regrow and at times the pattern of new brow hair is irregular. Unusual though these misfortunes may be, the advantages of shaving the brow are slight and do not warrant the possible complications.

CLEANSING THE SKIN AND CONJUNCTIVA. Many techniques for cleaning the skin are acceptable preoperative routines. Preliminary use of liquid green soap is time-honored. The soap (and all other antiseptic agents) should not be used within the conjunctival sac but should be applied only to the skin and the surrounding surgical field. Detergents containing iodine compounds are also used in this manner and are probably superior to soap. Irrigation is the key to adequate wound cleansing. An intravenous set with a suspended 500 ml. bottle of sterile saline is a convenient way to "hose down" the injured region, combining lavage with tissue separation to wash away particulate foreign material. The conjunctival sac is also thoroughly irrigated with saline, and cotton swabs are used to assure absence of foreign bodies in the fornices of the conjunctiva. Alcohol is then used on the skin following completion of the irrigation.

DRAPING, LIGHTING AND MUTUAL COMFORT. Draping of the wound for sterile repair will depend upon the site of the lesion. In all cases, a head towel should be used, and it is considerate to recall that the ear is not a comfortable repository for drainage of blood, saline or tears. It is customary to employ an "eye sheet" with a central 3- to 4-inch round opening when only a small area of exposure is required.

The necessity for a strong, well-directed operating light is obvious. The general surgeon is reminded of the advantages of wound repair from a sitting position. Arm's-length surgery is less conducive to precise manipulations.

Simple Lacerations of the Lids. After debridement, search for foreign bodies and control of bleeding, the actual repair of lid lacerations is similar to wound repair elsewhere *except for the particular importance of separate layer closure and the need for fine suture material.* Prevention of contracture deformity of the lid contours is of vital concern. Poor wound closure can result in abnormally thin or thick scars and resultant impairment of lid function. Ragged wound margins should be trimmed, but as much tissue as possible should be preserved. Healing is surprisingly excellent despite a patchwork of suture lines at the time of primary closure. Hawsers of 4–0 black silk have no place in repair of the lids; 6–0 or 7–0 gut, and 7–0 or 8–0 silk are the mainstays of lid surgery. It is unnecessary to discuss the advantages of interrupted sutures, a symmetrical placement of the suture needle in the skin edges and the

eccentric placement of suture knots so that these do not override the wound itself.

Basic to repair of lid lacerations is the technique of incision along the gray line to obtain mobilization of the skin-muscle layer when a sliding flap is needed. The lid is grasped firmly with forceps and a knife blade tip begins the gray line incision, extending only to a depth of about 3 mm. Separation of the skin-muscle layer from the tarsoconjunctival layer is then completed to the full depth desired by the use of fine blunt scissors, which are used by spreading the blades and obtaining the plane of dissection without injury to the tarsus or the vascular orbicularis muscle (Fig. 9–4). Wounds are rarely as sharp and simple as diagrammed in textbooks. Not infrequently, the tarsus is raggedly torn and needs restoration of neat contours prior to closure. Yet, excision of any portion of the tarsus causes much greater wound stress than does comparable excision of the loose skin-muscle layer, which can be undermined and mobilized readily. Thus, to avoid postoperative notching of the lid margin, the surgeon can trim the ragged margins of the transected tarsus in a slightly curved fashion so that when these curved margins are brought together vertically the straight line of closure will afford slightly greater tarsal width than before the injury (Fig. 9–5). This slight overcorrection (pouting of the lid margin at the site of repair) can produce a smooth-contoured lid when scarring ensues.

For lacerations involving the lid margin, Fox's modification[7] of Minsky's[18] figure-8 splinting suture is a useful means of assur-

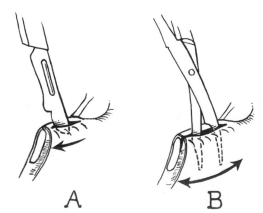

Figure 9–4. *Technique of lid splitting along the gray line.*

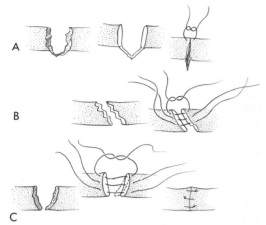

Figure 9–5.   *Techniques of repairing injured tarsus. (From Paton, D. L. and Goldberg, M. F.: Management of Ocular Injuries, Philadelphia, W. B. Saunders Co., 1976.)*

ing good closure of the marginal wound and prevention of lid notching. An intermarginal suture of 4-0 silk is passed into the tarsus within the wound to emerge in the gray line on either side (Fig. 9–6A). The tarsoconjunctiva is closed with interrupted 5–0 or 6–0 chromic gut sutures tied so that the knots lie on the anterior tarsal

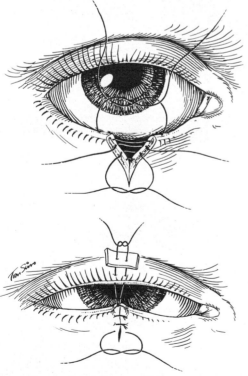

Figure 9–6.   *Fox's modification of Minsky's figure-8 splinting suture for lid laceration repair.*

surface and will be buried within the wound (Fig. 9–6A). The intermarginal suture is then tied and passed through the gray line of the opposite lid margin to emerge in the skin, where it is tied over a peg (Fig. 9–6B). The skin at the laceration site is closed with 6–0 or 7–0 interrupted silk sutures (Fig. 9–6B). The skin sutures are removed after 5 days and the intermarginal suture after 10 days.

Avulsions of the Lid.   Glancing blows can avulse a lid, which then dangles free like a pedicle flap, having little or no loss of its substance (Fig. 9–7). The most important factor in repair of such injuries is identification of the stump of the canthal ligament* from which the lid has been torn so that lid and ligament can be reapproximated, either with synthetic nonabsorbable suture material or fine wire (Fig. 9–8). Because these tissues are edematous at the time of this injury repair, the essential role of the canthal ligaments is not readily appreciated, and it may be weeks before the effect of failure to repair an avulsed ligament is noticeable. Fractures of the orbital walls, particularly the lateral one, can tear the canthal ligament from its bony insertion; this, too, must not be overlooked when the bones themselves are realigned. Clues to the injury are a droopy appearance of the lateral canthus and undue laxity of the lid. At the medial canthus, lid avulsion necessarily involves damage to the lacrimal canaliculi; repair of these injuries will be discussed later.

Extensive Lid Lacerations with Loss of Tissue.   The majority of lid lacerations associated with loss of tissue can be repaired by judicious construction of flaps and free use of lid-splitting along the gray line. Only rarely are free grafts required. The two-layered closure of lid wounds is the basic principle of the surgical approach.

At first glance in an emergency treatment room, lid trauma can produce a startling disfigurement (Figs. 9–7, 9–9A): a scrambled mass of tissue with areas of unnaturally exposed eyeball, twisted lid fragments containing eyelashes displaced toward the brow, sections of exposed and everted tarsus, particles of foreign material throughout the wound and profuse bleed-

*Since the canthal "ligament" unites muscle to bone, it should be referred to as a *tendon*, but the conventional nomenclature is used here.

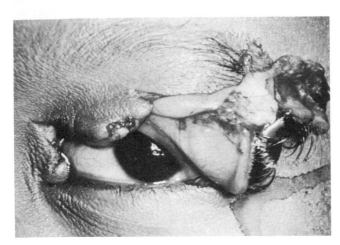

Figure 9–7. Dog bite to upper lid with avulsion of medial canthal ligament.

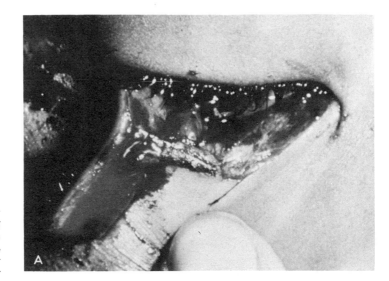

Figure 9–8. A, Traumatic avulsion of the medial canthal tendon; B, demonstration of its repair. (From Paton, D. L., and Goldberg, M. F.: Management of Ocular Injuries, Philadelphia, W. B. Saunders Co., 1976)

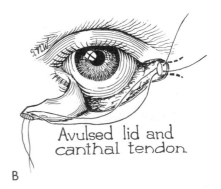

Avulsed lid and canthal tendon

B

ing. Once the injured area has been cleansed and bleeding controlled, the pieces can usually be replaced with surprising completeness, but a logical plan of repair must be formulated. Assuming that the eye has not been injured and that x-rays have failed to disclose a retained foreign body, the surgeon should give attention to the integrity of the lacrimal drainage apparatus, the levator palpebrae tendon and the orbital septum. Repair of lacrimal canaliculi is discussed in a subsequent section.

Reference has already been made to the importance of suturing a severed levator tendon to the upper margin of the tarsus. The fascial layer of septum, tarsus and canthal ligament must be organized and realigned first. Attention is then turned to the lid margins at the angles of the lid fissure. Despite extensive damage to the lateral or medial canthus, there is usually a remnant of the lid angle attached to the canthal ligament, and this is a vital landmark upon which to build the reconstruction. Usually, most of the tissue fragments can be drawn back into their natural position, and denuded strips of tarsus can be salvaged; thus, the tarsoconjunctival layer can be reformed piecemeal by laborious tissue identification and suturing.

A lid needs continuous tarsus at its margin for stability of its contour. This is the most important principle of surgical repair of the tarsus. All but a 2 mm. strip of lid-margin tarsus can be excised (as is commonly done in many parts of the world for trachomatous scarring) without significant residual deformity of the lid contour; however, a continuous strip of tarsus must be retained at the lid margin if deformity is to be prevented. If there is absence of tarsus, a wedge or tongue of the tarsoconjunctival layer can be slid into the defect from the opposing lid (Fig. 9–9B and C), constituting a tarsorrhaphy at this site (which is advantageous in most cases of extensive lid trauma). When, after several months, the lids are separated, the defect in tarsus in the uninjured lid will cause no cosmetic deformity. Damage to the meibomian glands is of no practical consequence.

Once the posterior surgical layer has been reconstructed by securing an avulsed canthal ligament, suturing orbital septal defects and repairing the tarsus, the skin-muscle layer is separately closed. There is marked variation in the laxity of this layer, with slackness more pronounced in the elderly. Simple undermining of the skin-

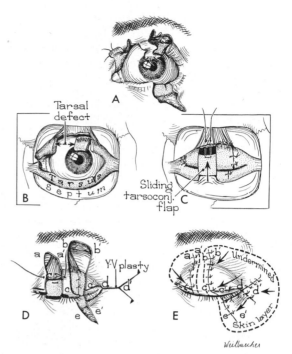

Figure 9–9. The steps necessary for repair of extensive lid lacerations. A, Appearance of the original injury. B and C, In order to demonstrate repair of the tarsoconjunctival layer, the skin and muscle layers have not been shown. D, Heavy lines at the lid margins indicate where gray-line splitting has been used to assist in mobilization of tarsal flaps; the skin incisions for sliding skin flaps to fill the traumatic defects are also illustrated. E, As in most cases of lid lacerations, the skin can be closed without use of skin grafting, if sufficient mobilization of this anterior layer is accomplished. (From Paton, D. L., and Goldberg, M. F.: Management of Ocular Injuries, Philadelphia, W. B. Saunders Co., 1976.)

muscle layer is generally sufficient for mobilization and closure of tissue defects that do not include the lid margin. When skin-muscle defects *do* include the lid margin, wide incision along the gray line is often necessary to obtain a sliding flap. Extensive gray line incision has no disadvantages if the surgeon is careful to find a proper plane and does not split the tarsus itself or damage the muscle by excessive use of the knife blade.

Sliding flaps of skin-muscle are best mobilized from the lateral regions of the lids and the tissue overlying the temporal fossa. Gray line incision and two-layered separation can be extended all the way to the lateral canthus, followed by a partial cantholysis to free the orbicularis insertion from the canthal ligament. A flap of undermined skin and muscle can be brought medially, with or without auxiliary incisions, to prevent lateral skin traction tending to withdraw the flap (Fig. 9–9D and E). The use of

Z- and Y-plasties is often of great convenience in repair of extensive lid lacerations; since these represent well-known surgical maneuvers, they need not be discussed in detail here. It is important, however, to avoid tension on a flap. The sutures should do little more than hold the tissue margins together. When the superficial tissue defect to be filled does not include the lid margin, the sliding flap of skin-muscle need not involve the lid margin; therefore, incision along the gray line is unnecessary.

Unless there is extensive loss of lid tissue and a large field of surrounding trauma, plastic pedicle flaps are rarely needed at the time of primary repair. Efforts to simulate a natural lid margin by a pedicle flap containing brow hair are rarely successful and should not be done at the time of accident room surgery, if at all.

It is seldom necessary to perform free skin grafts for treatment of lid injury, but extensive loss of lid substance occasionally requires them. If the tissues are clean, the results can be excellent. The best site of full-thickness donor skin for lid grafting is the lax skin fold of the contralateral upper lid. No other skin of the body provides so good a color match or is so thin. Possibly another excellent donor site would be the skin of the prepuce or penis, but the usual donor is not enthusiastic about the use of this site. Thus, the next best donor sites are the cephaloauricular angle, and the supraclavicular fossa (if it is not hair-bearing). When defects between the medial canthus and the bridge of the nose are grafted, the surgeon should be especially careful to get good apposition of the graft to the deep underlying tissues; this is facilitated by stab incisions in the graft and by a tightly applied postoperative dressing. Split-thickness skin grafting is an occasionally useful and at times necessary adjunct to the treatment of severe lid burns or denuded skin areas where granulation tissue has already formed. The principles and techniques of skin grafting are not specific for eyelid injuries.

Traumatic Loss of the Lids. In the event of almost complete loss of the eyelids, first attention must be given to protection of the globe, which may be completely spared from the devastation that has destroyed the eyelids. Effective protection of an exposed but uninjured globe, prior to

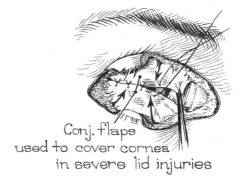

Conj. flaps used to cover cornea in severe lid injuries

Figure 9–10. *A simple method of providing temporary protection to an exposed globe by double thickness flaps of undissected conjunctiva.*

the extensive plastic surgery necessary for rebuilding the eyelids, can be obtained in several ways. The ophthalmologist will usually incise the bulbar conjunctiva around the limbus of the eye and undermine this tissue peripherally so that it can be brought over the cornea either as an apron or as a bridge flap. Surgeons without training in ophthalmology would not want to undertake this dissection of tissue on the globe itself. An alternative method utilizes the laxity of the conjunctiva of the upper and lower fornix.[10] *Without any dissection,* the conjunctiva can be grasped at the upper fornix with forceps and a suture passed through it and then brought through a similar fold from the lower fornix, in the same vertical line. Thus, by using multiple interrupted sutures, a double thickness of conjunctiva can be brought over the globe, and a horizontal straight line closure of conjunctiva across the cornea can be obtained (Fig. 9–10). These sutures will not hold for more than a few days, but this is more than enough time for accomplishing plastic revision of the lids. Rebuilding a lid often requires large pedicle flaps, sliding flaps and mucous membrane grafts — the details of which are not appropriate here, since these are clearly the responsibility of specialists.

Injuries of the Lacrimal Apparatus. The anatomy of the lacrimal drainage apparatus is illustrated in Figure 9–2*B*. Lacerations within the medial fourth of the lids may impair tear drainage to the nose by direct injury to the puncta, the canaliculi, the lacrimal sac or the nasolacrimal duct. Lid injuries may also disrupt lacrimal drainage indirectly if lid deformity causes poor pumping by the orbicularis muscle or poor apposition of the punctum against the eyeball. Thus, in repair of such lid lacerations, attention must be directed to the normal conformity of the lid as well as to the severed canaliculus.

Repair of a canaliculus is not always successful, but it is well worth undertaking. If only the upper canaliculus is injured, there is little likelihood that epiphora (spillage of tears over the lid margin) will result. Some persons whose lower canaliculus has been irreversibly damaged get along well with the upper canaliculus alone, but this is unusual.

For surgical repair, the following procedures are employed. After instillation and injection of local anesthetic, a punctum dilator is used to widen (but not split) the aperture to the canaliculus, permitting passage of probes. The Worst pigtail probe[22] is passed through the upper lacrimal canaliculus around to the lower canalicus where it appears within the wound (Fig. 9–11A). A silk suture is then attached to the probe, which is reversed (arrow, Fig. 9–11A), drawing the suture through the canaliculus (Fig. 9–11B). The pigtail probe is then passed through the lower punctum, and the suture is drawn through the remainder of

the lower canaliculus (Fig. 9–11B and C). The suture is then used to draw a small silicone tube through the canalicular system, as illustrated in Figure 9–11C. The ends of the lacerated canaliculus are sutured together with 10–0 nylon or 8–0 virgin silk sutures (Fig. 9–11D), with the aid of the operating microscope. The lid margin, deeper tissues and skin are also sutured (Fig. 9–11E). The silicone tube is left in place for several weeks.

Occasionally, it is not possible to pass the pigtail probe through the canalicular system, in which case the proximal portion of the canaliculus may be identified by injection of sterile milk through the upper canaliculus while applying pressure over the lower part of the lacrimal sac with a cotton-topped applicator (Fig. 9–12A). An alternative method is to pool sterile saline in the wound and then watch for bubbles while injecting air into the upper canaliculus. Once the proximal opening of the severed canaliculus is identified, canalicular anastomosis remains the greatest challenge; many methods of repair have been advocated.[6] Perhaps the simplest means is to thread a fine silicone tube over a lacrimal probe and pass these two through the punc-

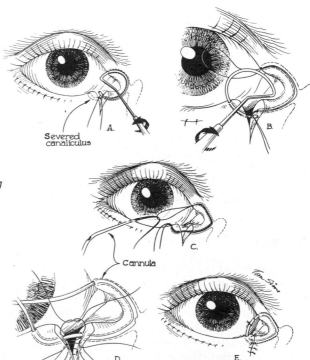

Figure 9–11. *Worst's method of identifying and repairing a severed canaliculus.*

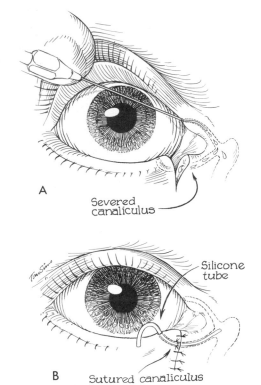

A   Severed
canaliculus

Silicone
tube

B   Sutured canaliculus

Figure 9–12. *A method of identifying and repairing
a severed canaliculus. (From Paton, D. L., and
Goldberg, M. F.: Management of Ocular Injuries,
Philadelphia, W. B. Saunders, 1976.)*

tum, through the distal portion of the canaliculus, and then through the proximal
portion of the canaliculus (Fig. 9–12*B*) — a
final step that is more easily described than
performed. If the lacrimal sac has been
lacerated or exposed in the dissection, it is
sometimes easier to make an incision in the
sac and introduce the silicone tube (or
whatever stent is used) from a retrograde
direction and thereafter maneuver it to the
distal portion of the canaliculus. Once the
tube or similar stent is in position, the two
portions of the canaliculus are sutured to
each other as described above.

INJURIES OF THE ORBIT

Fractures of the Orbit. Facial fractures
frequently include damage to the walls of
the orbit and resultant injury to intraorbital
contents; consequently, they are of importance to the ophthalmologist. In particular,
blowout fractures of the orbital floor are of
prime concern to the eye specialist because
of the frequent impairment of ocular mo-

tility that results when orbital tissue is extruded into the maxillary antrum.

Orbital trauma is typically signaled by
ecchymosis and swelling of the lids, and by
mild to severe proptosis and ophthalmoplegia from hemorrhage within the orbit. In
addition, there may be subcutaneous emphysema (crepitus, palpable through the
lids) from fractures of sinuses, and localized anesthesia of the skin in areas innervated by the supraorbital and infraorbital
branches of the trigeminal nerve along the
roof and floor of the orbit, respectively.
Defects in the orbital rim can sometimes be
detected clinically.

Fractures that cannot be diagnosed until
special x-ray views are obtained can be
suspected from a variety of clinical signs.
For example, fractures of the roof of the
orbit are often followed by hemorrhage into
the upper lid and subconjunctival hemorrhage on the lateral aspect of the globe.
Lateral wall fractures are the ones more apt
to be associated with avulsion of the optic
nerve and profound loss of vision. Medial
wall fractures usually produce orbital emphysema which, even if not palpable, is
frequently visible in x-rays. Systemic antibiotics are indicated, but surgical repair is
not necessarily undertaken if there is no
damage to the orbital contents. The patient
must avoid nose-blowing or muscular
straining if an orbital fracture into one of
the sinuses is suspected.

The percentage of accurate diagnoses is
greatly increased by well-planned, technically excellent x-rays (Table 9–6). Tomography and the use of intraorbital radiopaque contrast material are sometimes
valuable adjuncts to x-ray studies. References to pertinent literature on this subject
have been given in the table.

**Blowout Fractures of the Orbital
Floor.** The alert surgeon will usually diagnose the majority of orbital fractures at
the time of his initial evaluation of an injury. The one fracture that he is most likely
to overlook is the blowout fracture of the
orbital floor, which is often unassociated
with fractures of the orbital rim or other
facial bones.

When the force of a blunt object (such as a
fist or baseball) is exerted upon the orbit,
there is compression of orbital tissues; the
markedly increased hydraulic pressure
within the orbit may result in a blowout at
the site of the weakest portion of the orbit,

TABLE 9–6.   Suggestions Concerning Radiographic Projections for Orbital Injuries*

ANATOMICAL SITE	OPTIMAL RADIOGRAPHIC PROJECTION	ADDITIONAL STUDIES
Orbital roof Superior orbital rim	Caldwell (15° PA)	Tomography: particularly suitable to show isolated fractures of the orbital plate or damage of cribriform plate (preferably pluridirectional)

Medial wall
  upper half
  lower half
	Caldwell
	Special View I (Fueger)†
		Hypocloidal Polytomography

Orbital floor
  "en face"
  profile
	Waters
	Special View I (Fueger)†
	Special View II (Fueger)‡
		Hypocloidal Polytomography

Lateral wall	Caldwell Rheese Special View II (Fueger)‡	Usually not necessary
Infraorbital rim	Waters	Usually not helpful
Optic foramina	Rheese	Tomography (preferably pluridirectional)

*A facial bone survey should always be obtained to determine the extent of facial trauma. A lateral projection should be included to show the facial bones in a second plane. Special projections with narrow collimation should follow the facial bone survey. Technical excellence is necessary. There must be no motion. The density range should be long.

†Fueger I. Forehead-film-position, C/R 30 degrees caudad, to exit one to one and a quarter inches below nasion.

‡Fueger II. Oblique position, sagittal plane rotated 20 degrees, C/R 35 degrees caudad; through affected orbit, to exit one inch below infraorbital rim.

For further information see references 17, 19 and 21.

the floor. Orbital fat may prolapse into the maxillary antrum, and the inferior rectus and inferior oblique muscles are often included with the incarcerated tissues (Fig. 9–13). When these two ocular muscles are caught in the incarceration, not only is their function restricted but they also serve as limiting bands that prevent full range of contraction of other ocular muscles not involved in the fracture. As a result, downward gaze may be reduced because of a pinched inferior rectus, but *upward gaze is often more impaired.* This occurs not only from incarceration of the inferior oblique muscle but also because the superior rectus cannot elevate the globe against the short rein of the trapped muscles beneath the globe.

It is not necessary to obtain a definitive diagnosis of orbital floor fracture at the time of emergency room examination; other injuries may take precedence, and the surgeon often must wait several days until orbital swelling has subsided before adequate clinical examination can be performed. A blowout fracture is never an emergency, whereas simultaneously incurred globe injuries frequently are.

Clinical suspicion of a blowout fracture is based on one or more of the following findings: anesthesia of the ipsilateral side of the nose and skin of the lower lid; diplopia, from limitation of the inferior rectus and inferior oblique (Figs. 9–14 and 9–15); posi-

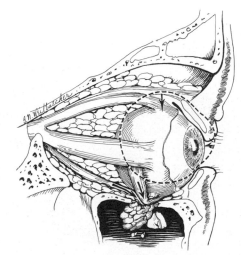

Figure 9–13. Blowout fracture of the floor of the orbit. The dotted line indicates normal position of the globe. The inferior oblique and inferior rectus muscles are restrained by the incarcerated orbital tissues.

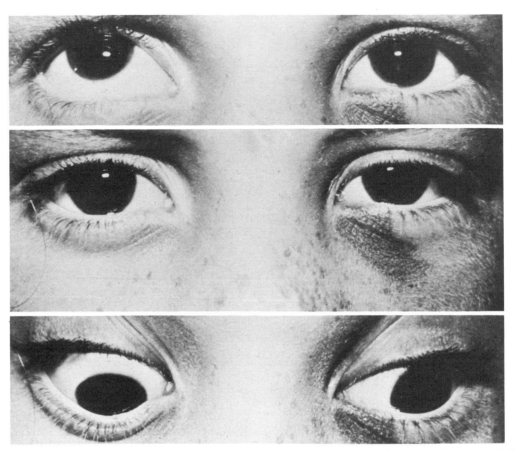

Figure 9–14. *Fresh blowout fracture of left orbit with limitation of upward and downward movement of left eye.*

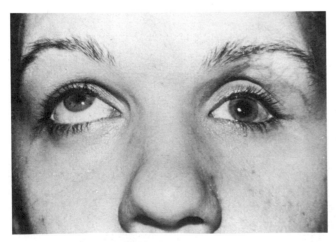

Figure 9–15. *Old blowout fracture of left orbit with enophthalmos and limited upward gaze of left eye.*

tive forced-duction test of the inferior rectus (see later); or, several weeks after injury when orbital swelling has resolved, downward and inward displacement of the globe with increase in the supratarsal sulcus (Fig. 9–15). Confirmation can be obtained by x-ray studies in more than 90 per cent of cases if the proper special views and techniques are employed.[4]

When upward gaze is impaired following trauma, it is helpful to determine the site of injury by the forced-duction test. After topical anesthesia, a forceps is used to grasp the eye at the insertion of the inferior rectus muscle, about 7 mm. above the limbus. The patient is requested to look up and the eye is rotated upward by the examiner; if it then shows full range of motility, the superior rectus or inferior oblique may be paretic. If it does not elevate even with manual force, the eye is being restrained by something — usually the incarceration of tissue in an orbital floor fracture. Of course, the forced-duction test can be used to test the motility of the other rectus muscles as well. When using forced duction, the inexperienced examiner should not mistake posterior displacement of the eyeball for improved ocular motility. Because of lid swelling and the discomfort of forced motility, this test is not always useful for preoperative diagnosis.

Surgical Technique for Repair of Blowout Fractures. Floor fractures should be repaired when incarcerated orbital tissues cause restriction of movement of the globe with significant diplopia or when extensive bony defects are present on x-ray. Small fractures without incarcerated muscles do well without surgery. It is preferable to operate between 5 and 15 days after injury, when orbital edema has subsided, and significant fibrosis of the fracture site has not yet occurred.

The usual surgical approach is accomplished by a lower eyelid incision through skin and orbicularis, followed by incision of the periosteum below and parallel to the inferior orbital rim. The periosteum is then elevated, the orbital floor exposed, and the extent of the fracture is determined. Any incarcerated orbital tissues are carefully removed from the fracture site. *It is important to demonstrate full range of all ocular ductions at the time of surgical repair.* Bony fragments or hinged flaps are restored to their original positions whenever possible. If the restored floor is of inadequate strength or if a defect remains, the floor is reinforced by a sheet of alloplastic material such as Supramid or Teflon. Periosteum and then skin are closed.

In some cases incarcerated orbital tissues cannot readily be freed by the trans-eyelid approach just described. On those infrequent occasions, further exposure must be gained by utilizing the Caldwell-Luc approach in combination with the transeyelid approach. The upper lid is retracted, and an incision is placed in the gingivolabial fold between the second molar and the canine teeth. The maxilla is then exposed in the region of the anterior wall of the maxillary antrum. A bony opening large enough to admit a finger into the maxillary antrum is then chiseled out. This permits exposure of both the superior and inferior aspects of the orbital floor, and simultaneous manipulation of fracture fragments and incarcerated tissues from above and below allows release of the entrapped tissues with the least possible trauma. The Caldwell-Luc approach is best performed by an otolaryngologist. Pre- and postoperative management and orbital surgery are best performed by an ophthalmologist.

Orbital Hemorrhage. Blunt trauma to the orbital region may result in extensive hemorrhage with proptosis and limitation of ocular motility. Occasionally, blood may dissect forward beneath the conjunctiva to produce a firm red mass that interferes with lid closure (Fig. 9–16). In extreme cases, the orbital swelling may cause a serious rise in intraocular pressure, requiring lateral canthotomy and possibly intraorbital injection of hyaluronidase (150 units in 1 ml.). An ophthalmologist should examine such an eye as soon as possible.

INTRAOCULAR AND INTRAORBITAL FOREIGN BODIES

With any puncture wound of the lids or ocular tissues the surgeon should make every effort to exclude the possibility of a retained intraorbital or intraocular foreign body. He should obtain x-rays if the presence of a foreign body is even remotely suspected. However, glass, plastics and a host of other materials are often not visible on the films. Intracranial injuries from

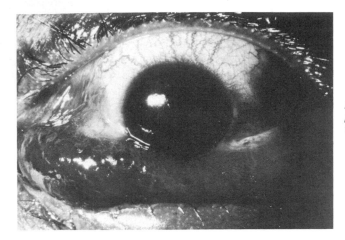

Figure 9–16. Orbital hemorrhage with proptosis and large subconjunctival hematoma preventing lid closure.

transorbital foreign bodies are infrequent but are potentially quite hazardous (Fig. 9–17A and B).

Common sites for lodgment of foreign bodies within the eye and beneath the lids are shown in Figure 9–18. Eversion of the upper lid is extremely important in routine search for small missiles that have struck the eye. To get optimal x-ray views of the anterior segment of the eye, a dental film can be placed deeply near the bridge of the nose, and an oblique x-ray of the anterior

ocular segment can be obtained that is free of bony markings. Several exposures should be made so that artefacts on one film are not misinterpreted as small foreign bodies.

The majority of metallic chips that enter the eye are from a metal-on-metal blow or from a grinding-wheel injury. The generated heat of the struck metal particle probably accounts for sterility, for endophthalmitis is the least likely complication. Iron-containing foreign bodies eventually

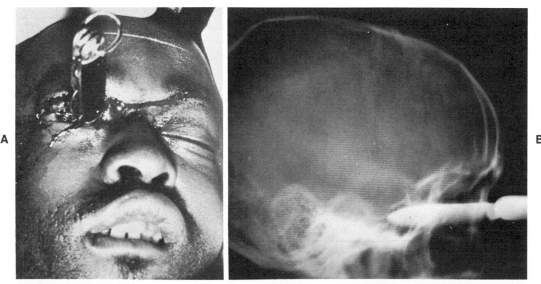

Figure 9–17. A, A 35-year-old male with pen knife embedded to the hilt in the right orbit. There was no light perception of the right eye and total ophthalmoplegia. The globe itself was intact. B, X-ray showing the tip of the blade next to the sphenoid sinus. The knife was removed by simultaneous right frontal craniotomy and orbital exploration. The knife had not entered the dura, but severed the optic nerve and the medial rectus muscle. Except for ophthalmoplegia and loss of vision, the patient's recovery was uneventful. (Case reported previously and photographs published with permission of Dr. David Paton and the authors: Bard, L. A., and Jarrett, W. H.: Arch. Ophthalmol 71:322, 1964.)

Figure 9–18. *Common sites of foreign bodies.*
A, BB pellets and even contact lenses may be
retained in the conjunctival fornix of the upper lid.
B, Corneal foreign bodies are usually found within
the lid fissure. C, Small sharp fragments such as
glass may pass through the cornea and sink into
the angle of the anterior chamber interiorly. D,
Metallic missiles may pass through the cornea,
iris and lens and lodge in the posterior wall of the
eye or remain within the vitreous cavity. Less fre-
quently, they pass entirely through the eye and re-
main within the orbit.

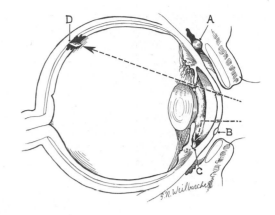

A   B

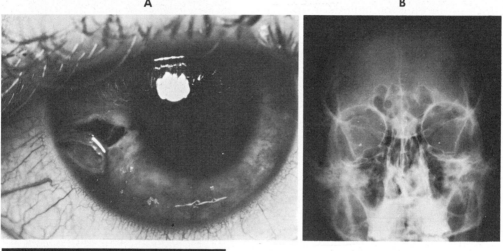

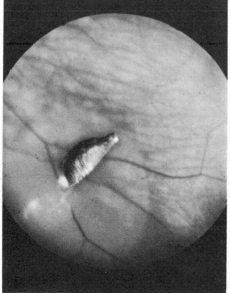

Figure 9–19. *A metal fragment has passed through*
the cornea and iris with little gross evidence of
ocular damage (A). The foreign body is seen by skull
x-ray (B) and, in this case, can also be visualized
with the ophthalmoscope on the surface of the
retina (C).

C

cause siderosis within the eye, and copper-containing metals produce chalcosis. All foreign bodies within the eye create the strong possibility of functional loss of the eye from mechanical damage or secondary inflammation. A safe generalization is that intraocular and intraorbital foreign bodies should be removed as soon after the injury as possible, before they cause damage by disintegration products or become encapsulated by fibrous tissue.

When scout films of the orbit demonstrate a radiopaque foreign body (Fig. 9–19*B*), there are several techniques for determining whether it it located within the globe and, if so, at precisely what location. The Sweet's localization procedure is a classic example;[12] other methods employ a contact lens with radiopaque markers, ultrasound[2] or an electromagnetic sounding device such as the Berman locator (which is primarily of use at the time of operation). The problems and methods of removing these retained foreign bodies are so clearly the responsibility of the ophthalmologist that they will not be discussed here.

BURNS OF THE EYE AND ADNEXA

Chemical Burns of the Eye. Burns of the eye by alkali or acid are the most urgent of all ocular emergencies. The extent of permanent injury is related not only to the nature and concentration of the chemical but also to the time lapse before decontamination.[16] Strong alkalis such as lye and lime cause ischemia and necrosis of conjunctiva and sclera and rapid opacification of the cornea (Fig. 9–20). Unless irrigated within moments, the eye may eventually be lost.

With the rare exceptions of chemicals that react violently with water, the immediate treatment of chemical burns must be copious irrigation of the eyes, using the nearest source of water. The victim's face should be placed under a forceful stream of water from a shower, drinking fountain, hose or bathtub faucet. The lids must be held apart, for severe orbicularis spasm might otherwise prevent the beneficial effect of the irrigation. Particulate matter of the chemical should be promptly removed with cotton swabs: the lids should be evert-

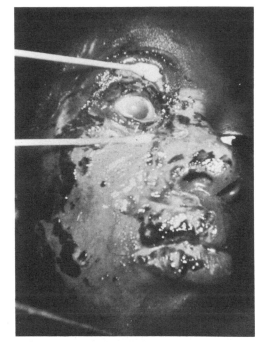

Figure 9–20. *Alkali burn to right eye and skin of face.*

ed and cotton applicators used to sweep the fornices of the conjunctival sac.

After initial lavage, early use of topical anesthetic will greatly facilitate the emergency measures by easing the patient's discomfort. Systemic analgesics are also valuable. As soon as possible, irrigation should be continued with a reservoir of isotonic saline connected to an intravenous tubing set; this should be continued for a minimum of 20 minutes.

Neutralizing solutions have not been found effective in the treatment of chemical burns. There are only a few specific antidotes of proved value in burns with common chemicals. For example, mortar and plaster (which contain calcium hydroxide) are removed with greater ease by the use of 0.01M solution of neutral sodium edathamil (EDTA).[9]

After lavage, mydriatics are instilled to reduce iris adhesions to the lens (atropine is favored because of its prolonged action); it is customary to start treatment with topical steroids to reduce iritis. Cysteine or other collagenase inhibitors may be useful in preventing loss of corneal stroma by the action of collagenase liberated by injured corneal epithelium. In rare cases, severe chemical burns are treated by emergency corneal grafts to preserve the eye when corneal destruction is so extensive that its eventual slough can be predicted. The prognosis for such grafts is poor; therefore, surgery is usually deferred until perforation of the cornea is imminent. Both moderate and severe chemical burns by alkali or acid may lead to scarring of the conjunctiva, with resultant adhesions between the lids and the globe (symblepharon). The use of steroid ointment and a plastic contact lens or other conformer fitted into the fornices within the lids is a means of reducing this scarring, which can be a late complication of great severity.

Thermal Burns. Thermal burns of the lids are treated in much the same way as elsewhere on the body. Marked edema and tissue necrosis are usually present, making examination of the globe dependent upon the use of lid retractors. Tarsorrhaphy is often impossible because of friable lid tissue; exposure of the globe must be prevented in succeeding days, and treatment with artificial tear solution or an ophthalmic ointment is then essential. Thin split-thickness skin grafts (of 0.005-inch thickness) are sometimes required. A convenient donor site is the medial surface of the upper arm. A common late complication of lid burns is cicatricial ectropion, eversion of the lids by scar tissue.

Radiation Burns of the Eye. Ultraviolet radiation is the most common form of radiation is the most common form of radiant energy producing ocular injury; the chief sources are welding arcs, "sun-tan" lamps and carbon arcs. There is an interval of 6 to 10 hours after exposure before symptoms begin; the patient first notes an irritated sensation of the eyes that progresses to severe photophobia, pain and blepharospasm. Examination shows mild chemosis; topically applied fluorescein produces a punctate staining of the cornea. Treatment consists of mydriatic drops, topical ophthalmic ointment and a semipressure eye dressing that restricts lid blinking. Sedatives and analgesics are often required. The eye patches remain in place for at least 24 hours; usually by then, the corneal epithelium is restored and the symptoms gone.

Infrared flash burns are usually of little consequence; the lids develop an immediate temporary erythema, but the eye itself is unharmed. However, prolonged exposure to the shorter wavelengths of infrared rays is responsible for the development of heat cataracts. In the past, glassblowers and metal-furnace stokers who were improperly protected from the radiation developed cataracts after many years of such employment.

Cataract is a late result of ionizing radiation of various types; high-speed neutrons from cyclotron exposure or from atomic blasts are the most typical sources. Beta radiation will also cause cataracts if the eye is exposed to excessive doses; the latent period for development of such lens changes is usually 2½ years.[19]

Changes in the posterior portion of the globe from radiation exposure are rare. Viewing of a solar eclipse is the most notable exception; irreversible damage to the macula can result from failure to protect the eye from the excessive brightness. Since there is no emergency treatment for radiation burns of this nature, further discussion will not be included.

INJURIES OF THE CONJUNCTIVA

Conjunctival Hemorrhage. Conjunctival hemorrhage is the most common accompaniment of ocular trauma but is, in itself, of no consequence. Spontaneous hemorrhages of the conjunctiva occur in adults of advancing age and in others without apparent reason. No known medication will effectively speed resorption of the hemorrhage, but all traces of it should be gone in a week or two. Subconjunctival hemorrhage from orbital bleeding is sometimes so severe that the conjunctiva balloons out between the lids and must be kept lubricated with ointment until the swelling subsides and the conjunctiva returns within the lid fissure. Use of a rubber glove filled with crushed ice is a good way to hasten regression of the swelling.

Chemosis. With or without hemorrhage of the conjunctiva, chemosis is often a serious portent (Fig. 9–21). Benign causes of conjunctival edema are ultraviolet exposure and various forms of allergic conjunctivitis. Chemosis is often characteristic of endocrine exophthalmos, pseudotumor of the orbit and trichinosis. *Following injury, acute chemosis with hemorrhage of pro-*

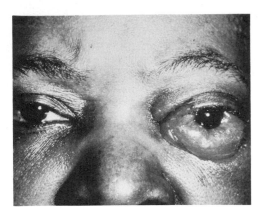

Figure 9–21. *Chemosis in this case was due to traumatic carotid-cavernous fistula. There was an orbital bruit and proptosis of the left eye.*

nounced or minimal amount may be caused by a retained intraorbital foreign body, fracture of the orbit, scleral rupture, carotid cavernous fistula or traumatic asphyxia.

Lacerations of the Bulbar Conjunctiva. Every conjunctival laceration should be carefully explored after use of topical or retrobulbar anesthetic. Again, the possibility of the presence of occult foreign bodies must be considered. Repair of a conjunctival laceration is not necessary unless it is more than a centimeter in length. Interrupted 7–0 or 8–0 gut sutures are sufficient; the only precaution necessary is care that conjunctival edges are properly recognized and that Tenon's capsule (the fascia beneath the bulbar conjunctiva) is not confused with the thinner and more superficial layer.

INJURIES OF THE EXTRAOCULAR MUSCLES

Hematoma of the extraocular muscles is not uncommon following contusion injuries to the orbit or lacerations by a foreign body. These hemorrhages are visible only at exploratory operation, except when they extend along the muscle sheath to the insertion of its tendon on the globe. The only significant consequence of such hemorrhages is the transitory limitation of the muscle's action and the problems in differential diagnosis raised thereby.

The ocular muscles are not often avulsed, but foreign bodies entering the orbit can sever the muscles and render them func-

tionless (Fig. 9–17). See also the earlier section on fractures of the orbit.

INJURIES TO THE GLOBE

Techniques of Examination. Corneal abrasions are often due to a foreign body caught under the upper lid. Every physician should know how to evert the lid, for he will be called on to remove "cinders" or "trash" from the inner aspects of the lids throughout his professional life. The patient should be conveniently seated and directed to look down; the upper lid is grasped by its central lashes and pulled downward and slightly outward; the examiner then presses with a finger or cotton applicator at the upper margin of the tarsus and maintains this gentle pressure while the lid is flipped into the everted position. Key assistance in this maneuver is gained by a cooperative patient who maintains downward gaze and does not squeeze the eyelids. A drop of topical anesthetic should be used beforehand if the eye is painful.

When the eye has been lacerated, pressure on the globe must be avoided. Upper lids can be retracted with the examiner's thumb on the superior orbital rim. If the view is still inadequate, a topical anesthetic is instilled and lid retractors are employed.

Corneal Abrasions and Foreign Bodies. There are many people who know the anguish of a corneal abrasion. There is sudden onset of pain, lacrimation and blepharospasm; blinking and motions of the eyeball serve to aggravate the pain. Eyes so injured are not easily examined until the patient is afforded relief by a topical anesthetic such as proparacaine hydrochloride 0.5 per cent. The cornea should be inspected with a bright hand light, using oblique illumination. If no foreign body is seen, the upper lid should be everted (as described previously). The foreign body is often a tiny piece of grit lodged on the palpebral conjunctiva (Fig. 9–22); this can be removed by a light touch with a moistened cotton applicator.

If no foreign body is found and no corneal abrasion is seen with the hand light, fluorescein dye is an infallible means of demonstrating epithelial injury or denudation. The sterility of aqueous solutions of fluorescein is not readily maintained, and they

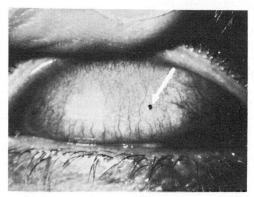

Figure 9–22. *A common lodging site for air-borne dust particles is the tarsal conjunctiva (arrow). Vertical "scratch marks" on the cornea are brought out with fluorescein staining; they suggest the location of the foreign body and account for the marked discomfort that it produces.*

afford an excellent culture medium for *Pseudomonas*; sterile strips impregnated with fluorescein are now in widespread use. A drop of sterile saline is placed on the paper and its tip is touched to the palpebral conjunctiva. Blinking spreads the dye over the cornea; the eye is then irrigated with sterile saline from a plastic squeeze bottle. Green dye remains wherever corneal epithelial cells have been damaged or lost by abrasion.

Once the "cinder" has been removed and the abrasion identified, treatment is primarily that of putting the eye at rest until the corneal epithelium covers the defect. The corneal epithelium, composed of stratified squamous cells, is separated from the corneal stroma by Bowman's membrane. If a foreign body has not entered the stroma, no corneal scarring will result. A short-acting "pupillary dilator" such as homatropine 5 per cent will make the eye more comfortable and reduce the effects of secondary iridocyclitis. A broad-spectrum antibiotic ointment is customarily used to prevent infection, and a semipressure patch is applied for 8 to 48 hours, depending on the severity of the injury (Fig. 9–30). The patient should *never* be maintained on topical anesthetic; it can retard healing, aggravate the keratitis and cause addiction.

Metallic foreign bodies (from grinding wheels, hammering metal on metal, etc.) sometimes lodge in the cornea; if allowed to remain, iron-containing particles will become surrounded by a rust ring within 2 days of the injury. After use of topical anes-

thetics, the metal fragment can often be removed by a small jet of ophthalmic irrigating solution applied with a plastic squeeze bottle, or by a gentle rub with a moistened cotton applicator. If this is unsuccessful, the foreign body should be removed by an opthalmologist as follows:

The patient's head is placed in a comfortable position (with the patient either supine or sitting at a slit lamp) and a foreign body is removed with a dental burr or similar instrument. Deeply lodged foreign bodies must be removed in the operating room by the use of shelved corneal incisions and with proper precautions to avoid collapse of the anterior chamber or loss of the foreign body within the anterior chamber. Rust rings should also be removed, either at the time of the first examination or several days thereafter when they can be more easily curetted with a dental burr.

Fragments of glass, thorns, caterpillar hairs and similar splinter-shaped objects are often difficult to detect without the modification of a slit lamp. For this reason, the patient who feels that he has a foreign body in his eye should not be treated casually if gross examination is negative. Herpetic corneal ulcers sometimes begin with a scratchy sensation in the eye and can be detected only by a fluorescein stain, which displays a characteristic dendritic pattern. Not only can the discomfort of herpetic keratitis simulate a foreign body in the conjunctival sac, but this viral infection may follow a corneal abrasion. Presumably, the herpes simplex virus gains entrance to the cornea at the site of epithelial damage. It is well known that steroids are contraindicated for superficial herpetic infections of the cornea; therefore, *no medication containing a steroid should ever be used in eyes with a corneal abrasion.*

Corneal and Scleral Lacerations. In all cases of post-traumatic lid swelling, deep laceration or damaged periocular tissues, the globe itself should be carefully examined with a determination inversely proportional to the ease of the examination. The only way to see the globe in the presence of severely swollen lids is to separate the lids forcefully with lid retractors.

The appearance of a corneal or scleral laceration needs little description. Occasionally, the signs of trauma are mild (Fig. 9–19A), but usually injury to the globe is readily apparent (Fig. 9–23). The anterior chamber is often flat, and the iris or the ciliary body may be incarcerated in the wound or prolapsed through it. Frequently there is external bleeding from the injured sclera and internal hemorrhage within the anterior chamber (hyphema, described later). It is not always easy to determine whether the lens has been damaged: hemorrhage may obscure an adequate view, and *rapid accumulation of fibrin in the pupillary space is sometimes indistinguishable from flocculent lens cortex*. The entire lens, along with some of the vitreous, can be extruded through the wound; it may be wiped away when the injury is first inspected. If this is the case, such information must be recorded on the patient's record, as it may be of assistance to the ophthalmologist in deciding future management of the injured eye.

Until the time of surgical repair, a lacerated eyeball should be protected from further damage by relief of blepharospasm with analgesics (or facial nerve block if necessary), topical antibiotic *drops* (not ointment) and a protective shield taped over an eyepad. The patient should be prepared for general anesthesia; he should receive nothing by mouth, be sedated, have x-rays of the orbit for possible foreign body and receive tetanus immunization. Broad-spectrum systemic antibiotics should be started promptly, even if surgery must be delayed until other injuries have been investigated.

Cataract from Perforating Injury of the Globe. Hatpins, darts, needles and other sharp objects can cause puncture wounds of the eye with scarcely any residual evidence of the site of entrance other than rapid development of a cataract. Any injury to the lens capsule has a strong likelihood of producing a cataract, which may develop within minutes or within months. Swelling of the lens may ensue, causing shallowness of the anterior chamber and, at times, glaucoma as a result of closure of the chamber angle from the anteriorly bulging cataract; early surgery for lens removal is then indicated. It is true that some small foreign bodies can remain within the lens or pass entirely through it and cause only localized opacity of the lens fibers, but such cases are exceptional. Usually, once there is partial opacity, the entire lens becomes cataractous. A discussion of the management of cataracts is not apropos here, but it is important to recognize injury of the lens. Markedly "swollen" (intumescent) cataracts require early surgery. The degree of intumescence can be estimated by appraisal of the anterior chamber depth.

General Information About Repair of Wounds to the Globe. Many of the problems of surgical repair of a lacerated glove are of concern only to the eye specialist. However, there is one standard practice of ophthalmologists that is pertinent here, since it represents a general philosophy about the necessity for wound repair in seemingly hopeless cases. Unless there is no light perception and almost total destruction of the eyeball, an ophthalmologist will usually make every effort to repair the eye as carefully and completely as possible. Of prime importance is the fact that occasionally some vision can be salvaged. Second, the patient himself will know that every effort was made to save his eye; and if it must be removed in later days, he is more prepared to accept this decision. Finally, there are many times when the injured person is either disoriented, inebriated or irrational; this is a difficult time to request consent for enucleation of the damaged eye. It is better to attempt salvage of every eye, except those with extensive extrusion of intraocular contents and a degree of laceration that defies repair.

Any perforating injury of the eye (especially with prolapse of iris or ciliary body) has a slight but significant chance of inducing sympathetic ophthalmia. This is a bilateral, granulomatous uveitis originating from unilateral injury and probably resulting from injury-induced autosensitivity to uveal pigment. In trauma cases in which iris or ciliary body prolapse has not been

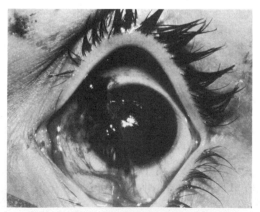

Figure 9–23. *Corneoscleral laceration.*

treated (or the eye enucleated) within several weeks of the injury, the incidence of sympathetic ophthalmia may be as high as 3 to 5 per cent of cases.[13] The frequency of this dreaded disorder has diminished greatly in recent years because of prompt treatment of injuries, early enucleation when necessary, and possibly also from the use of systemic steroids. But sympathetic ophthalmia remains a threat to be considered with every eye injury.

Sympathetic ophthalmia may occur from 10 days to many years following the initial injury. Its usual onset is within the first 2 months after injury to uveal tissue. It is important to decide within the first 10 days whether the patient's repaired eye has a fair chance of providing useful vision; if it does not, enucleation is advisable. Inflammation in the second (uninjured) eye does not occur if the injured eye has been removed prior to the earliest evidence of inflammation in the uninjured eye. Once the second eye is involved, it is doubtful whether enucleation of the injured eye is beneficial. Frequently the sympathetic ophthalmia is so severe that the eye originally injured is eventually the patient's better eye.

Phacoanaphylaxis is probably similar to the pathogenesis of sympathetic ophthalmia. Subsequent to injury to the lens, an eye will sometimes develop a delayed inflammatory reaction and granulomatous uveitis alike in many respects to sympathetic ophthalmia. In rare cases, the uninjured eye may also develop uveitis from sensitivity to lens protein. Sympathetic ophthalmia and phacoanaphylaxis sometimes occur in the same eye.

The use of systemic steroids has been a great boon in the treatment of these two postinjury disorders. Sympathetic ophthalmia can be suppressed by steroid therapy, but if its incidence is decreased by the use of steroids its occurrence is not entirely prevented. Steroid therapy has undoubtedly saved many eyes from complete loss; but it usually must be continued for many years, and the inflammation may become low grade and indolent despite its use.

INTRAOCULAR CONTUSION INJURIES

A clenched fist and a multitude of other missles can strike the eye and cause havoc with its contents. The examiner should take careful stock of the damages (Fig. 9–24).

Hyphema. Hyphema refers to hemorrhage within the anterior chamber. BB shotgun pellets, stones and fists are notorious causes of hyphema. Some hyphemas fill the entire anterior chamber, but most are less in amount and settle inferiorly where they can usually be seen with a hand light (Figs. 9–24C and D and 9–25). An *iridodialysis* is sometimes associated with contusion hyphemas; this is a traumatic disinsertion of the iris from the ciliary body (Fig. 9–26) and indicates the site of bleeding. Hyphema without iridodialysis is commonly caused by rupture of the arterial circle of the ciliary body located near the angle of the anterior chamber.

It is not commonly realized that the presence of blood in the anterior chamber can cause marked somnolence through reflex mechanisms that are poorly understood. Particularly in children, hyphemas can produce such drowsiness that, when coupled with the history of trauma, they will often lead a surgeon to put these patients on a head chart. It is significant that the hyphema alone may account for the lack of alertness, although possible head injury must still be considered.

The management of hyphemas should be conservative. *Patients should be hospitalized and put to bed; both eyes should be covered until the hemorrhage has resorbed.* No miotic or dilating drops should be used in the eye; the only indicated systemic medication is a sedative if this becomes necessary. Unless a hyphema entirely fills the chamber it is not a danger to the eye. However, within the first five days following injury, spontaneous rebleeding is common.

Rebleeding frequently fills the entire chamber and may cause secondary glaucoma. If the hemorrhage does not resorb promptly, blood pigment enters the cornea where it causes prolonged brownish "blood staining."

After a few days, a total hyphema changes from red to black in color (an "eight ball" hyphema); the intraocular pressure is invariably elevated and the prognosis is guarded. Oral carbonic anhydrase inhibitors such as acetazolamide (Diamox) are used to reduce the intraocular pressure; if the hemorrhage does not promptly resorb, surgical intervention is indicated. The anterior chamber is open via a cataract-type incision at the limbus, and the clotted hy-

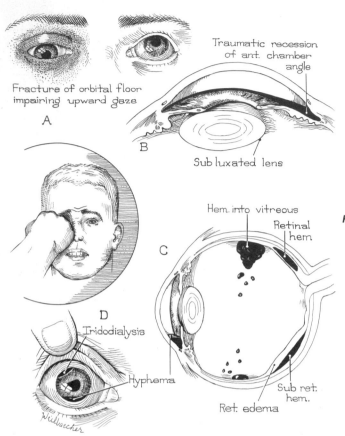

Figure 9–24.   *Common contusion injuries.*

phema is removed as extensively as possible without trauma to the ocular structures. Generally, surgery is avoided in cases of hyphema unless total hyphema with secondary glaucoma is not self-limited within a few days. One indication for surgery is the onset of corneal blood staining, detected by slit-lamp examination.

Traumatic Mydriasis and Miosis. Almost any trauma to the eye may be followed by a mild inflammation of the iris and ciliary body; the intraocular pressure is lower

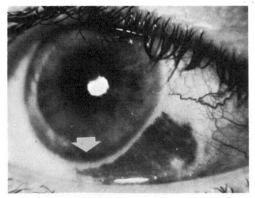

Figure 9–25.   *The photograph shows a conjunctival hemorrhage that is of no consequence per se; the arrow indicates a small hyphema that could easily escape cursory examination but may have serious prognostic significance.*

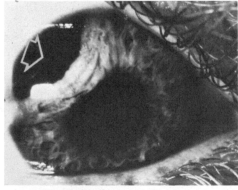

Figure 9–26.   *Following blunt trauma, there is not only a hyphema but flattening of the pupillary contour owing to a large iridodialysis (arrow). The cornea is intact and the damage to the iris will not be discovered unless the upper lid is properly elevated.*

than normal in the early post-traumatic period, and the aqueous humor contains cells and fibrin. More severe blows will, in addition, be accompanied by dilation or constriction of the pupil, a traumatic mydriasis or miosis that may persist for several days. The pupil reacts minimally and is often slightly irregular. Hard blows to the eye can produce a rupture of the iris sphincter and cause permanent deformity of the pupil. The causes of pupillary asymmetry following trauma are listed in Table 9–1.

Traumatic Recession of the Anterior Chamber Angle. It is well recognized that blunt trauma to the eye is a frequent cause of a unilateral glaucoma that may develop months or years following the injury. The blow causes a cleft in the tissues at the anterior chamber angle, the most important site of aqueous drainage from the eye (Fig. 9–24B). Follow-up studies on eyes with traumatic hyphema indicate an incidence of glaucoma of about 7 per cent. Thus, all patients with hyphema should be referred to an ophthalmologist, who should perform studies of the intraocular dynamics, examine the angle of the anterior chamber with a gonioscope and provide long-term follow-up observations.[1, 14]

Contusion Cataract. Even when there is no detectable damage to the lens capsule, contusion injuries can lead to secondary cataract. (Cataracts secondary to perforating injuries have been discussed previously.)

Subluxation and Luxation of the Lens. Blunt trauma to the globe can break the zonular fibers that encircle the lens radially and anchor it to the ciliary body. When 25 per cent or more of these fibers are broken, the lens is loosened and is no longer held as firmly against the posterior surface of the iris (Fig. 9–24B). Thus, with subluxation of the lens, the anterior chamber deepens; there is also a shimmering of the iris (iridodonesis); both of these signs can be detected by hand-light examination of the patient. Certain diseases predispose to zonular fiber disintegration, which can be further increased by relatively minor trauma; Marfan's syndrome and syphilis are the most common examples. Therefore, routine examination of the traumatized eye should include appraisal of the depth of the anterior chamber and a search

for iridodonesis. The lens may be loose in situ or entirely luxated, either into the vitreous cavity or into the anterior chamber; only in the latter instance is emergency surgery required. Removal of a subluxated or luxated lens should not be undertaken without careful evaluation of the risks involved; this is beyond the scope of this chapter.

Scleral Rupture. Blows to the eye sometimes produce rupture of the globe. The most common sites are: in an arc circumferential to the corneal limbus, opposite to the blow impact site; at the insertion of the rectus muscles on the globe; or at the equator of the eyeball. Thus, a scleral rupture can be present without being visible to the examiner. Suspicion of rupture is aroused when the anterior chamber is filled with blood, the eye is soft (as determined with a tonometer) and there is marked hemorrhagic chemosis of the conjunctiva disproportionate to other evidences of injury. A ruptured globe is rarely salvaged by surgery, but the attempt to repair it is almost always justified, particularly if it is the patient's better eye.

Contusion and Concussion Injuries to the Posterior Segment of the Eye. VITREOUS HEMORRHAGE. Vitreous hemorrhage from trauma is usually caused by damage to a retinal vessel. Loss of vision may be sudden and profound, and the site of retinal pathology may be obscured from the examiner's view. The examiner will note a loss of the usual "red reflex" when using the hand light. Often no fundus view is possible with an ophthalmoscope. Patients with eyes with a predisposition to hemorrhage are particularly vulnerable; persons with hypertension, arteriosclerosis, diabetes and sickle cell diseases are examples. The treatment of vitreous hemorrhage is expectant; most vitreous hemorrhages eventually resorb, and the underlying pathology can then be detected and sometimes treated. In some instances recently developed vitrectomy instrumentation allows removal of extensive vitreous hemorrhage via a pars plana incision.

TRAUMATIC RETINAL DETACHMENT. Retinal detachments resulting from ocular trauma are usually late sequelae of the original injury. When the retina detaches soon after contusion of the eye, the detachment is generally due to antecedent vitreoretinal pathology which, after blunt trauma, leads to tears in the retina and the detachment.

A retinal detachment is suspected when there is a history of floating black specks, "light flashes" and a curtain-like defect in the peripheral field of vision. Examination with an ophthalmoscope often reveals a billow of whitish retina which shifts with change in the patient's position. Typical traumatic retinal detachments are usually the result of far peripheral retinal tears which cannot be seen with a hand ophthalmoscope.

Since vitreous hemorrhage damages the vitreous structure and can lead to vitreous bands pulling on the retina, it is easy to understand why retinal detachment can be a late sequela of traumatic vitreous hemorrhage. But contusion injury alone, without hemorrhage into the vitreous, can also cause microdestruction of the vitreous structure and facilitate the late occurrence of retinal detachment. These factors are very difficult to appraise but have medicolegal implications of such importance that they constitute another reason for referral of patients with eye trauma to an ophthalmologist.

RETINAL HEMORRHAGES AND EDEMA. Either direct blows to the eye or contrecoup trauma from blows to the back of the head can produce retinal edema,

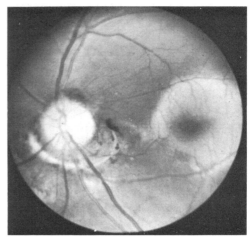

Figure 9–28. Edema and hemorrhages surround the optic nerve head, and there is edema of the macula in this eye, which has sustained blunt trauma.

with or without reduction in vision, depending upon the location. If the examiner is uncertain whether there is retinal edema, comparison with the other eye is helpful.

A short time after concussion injury to the eye, large subretinal hemorrhages may be found (Fig. 9–27); these are often accompanied by intraretinal and superficial retinal hemorrhages, which appear a brighter red than the grayish blue of deep hemorrhages. Macular vision is not necessarily affected unless macular hemorrhage or edema occurs (Fig. 9–28) or unless in the ensuing days hard retinal exudates form in a star configuration at the macula (when the prognosis for macular function is poor). Traumatic edema and hemorrhages of the retina are usually referred to loosely as commotio retinae. The chance of recovering vision is generally good, but coincident contusion injuries of the anterior segment of the eye may account for late onset of glaucoma that eventually affects retinal function if the intraocular pressure is not adequately controlled.

RUPTURE OF THE CHOROID. Severe concussion injury to the globe can produce a rupture of the choroid that, at the time of the emergency room examination, appears as a large retinal hemorrhage at the posterior pole of the eye, often breaking through into the vitreous. Late clearing of this hemorrhage then permits a view of a vertical yellow-white scar, which often transects the macula and causes permanent impairment of vision (Fig. 9–29).

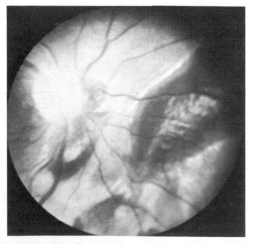

Figure 9–27. Traumatic retinal and subretinal hemorrhages characterize "commotio retinae." In this case, traumatic recession of the chamber angle led to eventual loss of all vision owing to failure of the patient to take medications prescribed for secondary glaucoma.

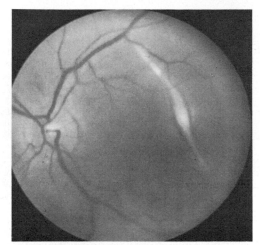

Figure 9–29. Six months following a blow to the eye, vitreous and retinal hemorrhage has cleared. A spindle-shaped scar of choroidal rupture is seen at the posterior pole, damaging macular vision.

CENTRAL RETINAL ARTERY OCCLUSION. Prolonged compression of the eye from external pressure or from severe intraorbital swelling sometimes occludes the central retinal artery. Operating on a patient in the face-down position is one way that this intraocular tragedy can occur; the surgeon must, therefore, be careful to see that the eye is not being pressed upon. The optic nervehead appears pale; the arteries are narrow; and vision is either absent or extremely slight. Edema of the retina ensues, leaving a "cherry-red spot" at the macula where retinal thinness and absence of edema permit transmission of normal fundus coloration from the choroid. Central retinal artery occlusion from trauma is fortunately rare, for treatment is not particularly effective. The patient is directed to breathe from and exhale into a paper bag to attain vasodilation by increase in the carbon dioxide content of the inhaled air; intravenous and oral carbonic anhydrase inhibitors such as acetazolamide are given; and retrobulbar vasodilators such as aminophyllin or tolazoline hydrochloride (Priscoline) are sometimes used. An effort must be made to relieve intraorbital pressure if it exists; a canthotomy may be helpful, and retrobulbar injection of hyaluronidase may be tried. Paracentesis of the anterior chamber is another effective method of managing these patients, and this should be done by an ophthalmologist.

Long-bone fractures can be followed by fat emboli that may pass through the pulmonary circulation and appear as small yellowish spots within the retinal artery branches. Large emboli are potential causes of occlusion of the artery itself.

SWELLING OF THE OPTIC NERVEHEADS. Any patient with a history of head trauma, loss of consciousness or suspected intracranial hemorrhage should have an examination of the optic nerveheads, and a

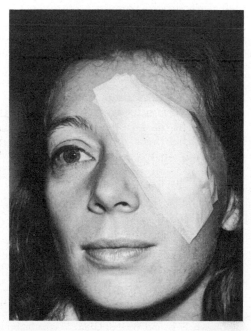

Figure 9–30. A semipressure eye dressing affords comfort and protection when properly applied. The lids are closed under the patch. The tape is placed to avoid impairment of the contralateral side of the face and should be lateral to the nasolabial fold to prevent inconvenience when patient is eating and talking.

description of the findings should become part of the hospital record. It is sometimes very helpful to know the initial appearance of the nerveheads soon after an accident, to detect later the presence of early papilledema. *Papilledema does not occur rapidly.* When "swollen" optic nerveheads are seen immediately after trauma, antecedent causes should be suspected. Factors in differential diagnosis have been listed in Table 9–4.

TYPES OF EYE DRESSINGS

All surgeons know how to apply a simple gauze eye patch or a pressure head dressing, but the common *semipressure dressing* does deserve mention. When eyelid blinking is to be avoided and the injured eye protected from contamination, a firm dressing is highly desirable and should be routinely employed. Two oval eye patches are removed from their sterile envelopes and placed over the closed lids. Strips of paper tape, which hold securely but leave virtually no residue in contrast to regular adhesive tape, are then placed over the soft gauze patches in a diagonal and slightly arcuate line, so that their ends overlap on the central forehead and lower portion of the cheek, respectively (Fig. 9–30). Increased firmness of the dressing is obtained by applying the tape first to the forehead and then *pulling* it firmly toward the cheek before applying the remaining tape end. Generous use of diagonal tape strips affords a good protective dressing that will not come off; horizontal and vertical tapes are unnecessary and uncomfortable. When added protection against trauma to the eye must be guaranteed, a metal eye shield can be used over a single eye patch (Fig. 9–1W). The shield is taped so that its margin touches the brow and cheek. Remember that when an eye dressing is removed it should be done with great gentleness and care.

REFERENCES

1. Blanton, F. M.: Anterior chamber angle recession and secondary glaucoma, a study of the after-effects of traumatic hyphemas. Arch. Ophthalmol. 72:39, 1964.
2. Bronson, N. R., II: Non-magnetic foreign body localization and extraction. Am. J. Ophthalmol. 58:133, 1964.
3. Brown, S. I., and Weller, C. A.: The pathogenesis and treatment of collagenase induced diseases of the cornea. Trans. Am. Acad. Ophthalmol. Otolaryngol., 74:375–383, 1970.
4. Emery, J. M., von Noorden, G. K., and Schlernitzauer, D. A.: Orbital floor fractures: Long-term follow-up of cases with and without surgical repair. Trans. Am. Acad. Ophthalmol. Otolaryngol. 75:802–812, 1971.
5. Emery, J. M., von Noorden, G. K., and Schlernitzauer, D. A.: Management of orbital floor fractures. Am. J. Ophthalmol. 74:299–306, 1972.
6. Fasanella, R. M.: Pitfalls and complications in surgery and trauma of the lacrimal apparatus. In Fasanella, R. M. (ed.): Management of Complications in Eye Surgery. (2nd Ed.) Philadelphia, W. B. Saunders Company, 1965, pp. 110–148.
7. Fox, S. A.: Lid Surgery: Current Concepts. New York, Grune & Stratton, 1972, pp. 18–21.
8. Fueger, G. F., Milauskas, A. T., and Britton, W.: The roentgenological evaluation of orbital blowout injuries. Am. J. Roentgenol. 97:614, 1966.
9. Grant. W. M.: Toxicology of the Eye. Springfield, Ill., Charles C Thomas Co., 1962.
10. Haik, G. M.: A fornix conjunctival flap as a substitute for the dissected conjunctival flap, a clinical and experimental study. Trans. Am. Ophthalmol. Soc. 52:497, 1954.
11. Hanafee, W. N. (ed.): Symposium on Radiology of the Orbit. Radiol. Clin. N. Am. 10:1–182, 1972.
12. Hartmann, E., and Gilles, E.: Roentgenologic Diagnosis in Ophthalmology. (G. Z. Carter, trans.; C. Berens, ed.) Philadelphia, J. B. Lippincott Co., 1959.
13. Hogan, M. J., and Zimmerman, L. E. (eds.): Ophthalmic Pathology. (2nd Ed.) Philadelphia, W. B. Saunders Company, 1962.
14. Howard, G. M., Hutchinson, B. T., and Frederick, A. R., Jr.: Hyphema resulting from blunt trauma. Trans. Am. Ophthalmol. Otolaryngol. 69:294, 1965.
15. Jones, L. T.: An anatomical approach to problems of the eyelids and lacrimal apparatus. Arch. Ophthalmol. 66:111, 1961.
16. Leopold, I. H., and Lieberman, T. W.: Chemical injuries of the cornea. Fed. Proc. 30:92–95, 1971.
17. Merrill, V.: Atlas of Roentgenographic Positions. St. Louis, The C. V. Mosby Co., 1949.
18. Minsky, H.: Surgical repair of recent lid lacerations: Intermarginal splinting suture. Surg. Gynec. Obstet. 75:449, 1942.
19. Newell, F. W.: Radiant energy and the eye. In Industrial and Traumatic Ophthalmology; Symposium of The New Orleans Academy of Ophthalmology. St. Louis, The C. V. Mosby Co., 1964, pp. 158–187.
20. Paton, D., and Goldberg, M. F.: Management of Ocular Injuries. Philadelphia, W. B. Saunders Company, 1976.
21. Weigelin, E., and Lobstein, A.: Ophthalmodynamometry. (Daily, R. K., and Daily, L., trans.) New York, Hafner Publishing Co., 1963.
22. Worst, J. G.: Method for reconstructing torn lacrimal canaliculus. Am. J. Ophthalmol. 53:520, 1962.

CHAPTER 10

EMERGENCY CARE OF MAXILLOFACIAL INJURIES

Milton T. Edgerton, Jr., M.D.

The modern background to treatment of facial fractures may be traced to World War I, when a high incidence of facial injuries required the development of basic principles of surgical management. Kazanjian, Blair, Davis and Gillies were pioneers during that era. Further experiences with large numbers of facial injuries from automobile accidents and later from World War II led American plastic surgeons such as Barrett Brown, Cannon and McIndoe, and Gillies' teams in England, to replace the use of complex external apparatus with direct open reduction and wire fixation of fractured bone. Modern plastic surgery techniques of soft tissue wound management, antibiotics, improved anesthesia, better provision of a nonobstructed airway and appropriate use of blood transfusions have greatly improved the care of these injuries.

The human face is the center for the vital functions of speech, eating, smell, taste, vision and hearing; it is also the most conspicuous part of the exposed anatomy. Facial expressions give man a vast international nonverbal language that conveys both ideas and emotions. Indeed, the appearance of the face is the largest single element in an individual's sense of identification or body image. It is the face that allows us to recognize one another, and we often attempt to judge another's intentions or character by looking at the face. Con-

sequently, deforming injury in this area creates complex and severe stresses in the patient's life.

Surveys of automobile accidents indicate that the head is injured in over 72 per cent of all accidents in which reports of personal injury are filed. The neck and cervical spine are injured in an additional 8.7 per cent, indicating the high frequency of head and neck injuries among victims of highway crashes. Recent federal legislation is aimed at improving the mechanical safety of automobiles. Although this is desirable, new safety features on cars will not alter the fact that emotional turmoil of the driver just prior to an accident plays a big role in many of the high-speed crashes on our expressways. Alcohol is an additional causative factor in over 50 per cent of these casualties. The physician must always consider the possibility of intoxication in any patient with facial injury. Facial fractures involve males 3½ times as often as females; such injuries are relatively uncommon in older people and young children.

INCIDENCE, ETIOLOGY AND SIGNIFICANCE OF FACIAL INJURIES

Incidence. Maxillofacial and cervical injuries are more common with high-speed travel, fast-moving machine parts in industry and high-velocity missiles in warfare. As people all over the world have taken to the highways, facial impacts against windshields and dashboards have multiplied the number of injuries alarmingly.

Other major causes of facial injuries are fist fights, motorcycle and bicycle accidents, falls, epileptic seizures and a variety of athletic and recreational activities.

The recent popularity of the snowmobile in the northern states and Canada has created a new cause of facial injury, as riders are being struck by low branches, wire fences and other unexpected obstacles. Fragments of goggles are not infrequently driven into the soft tissues of the face at the time of impact. Neck injuries have also been common in such cases.

INDIVIDUAL FACIAL FRACTURES. Approximately two thirds of facial fractures involve the mandible alone, one fourth involve the maxillae and associated bones, and one tenth involve both the mandible and the maxillary complex (thus, the mandible is involved in three fourths of all facial fractures). The middle third of the face is involved in one third, and the nasal bones are fractured in one fourth of facial injuries. These figures will vary significantly, depending upon the occupations, ages and living conditions of the populations served by a given hospital and the climate of its area.

Etiology. Seventy-five per cent of all deaths and injuries following crash decelerations are a result of maxillofacial and head impact with a nonyielding object. The Federal Aviation Agency carried out experimental studies in 1965 and again in 1976 to determine the tolerances of the human face to crash impact.[20] In most automobile and aircraft crashes, the head is usually thrown against an object that has some degree of "deformation yield." Such yielding increases deceleration time and allows a larger area of the face or head to receive the shock of the blow. The force that individual facial bones can sustain without fracture of the skull is obviously important.

When man is traveling at a high speed, he is usually surrounded by nonyielding rigid knobs, door posts, rigid tubes and other instruments designed to create a small area of impact when struck by the moving head or face. If this surface could be constructed of medium-weight deformable metal and padded with two inches of "slow return" material, the impact load would be distributed over the available area of the face. Such changes would reduce or almost eliminate maxillofacial fractures in crash impacts. If the deceleration force is measured in "g's," the following impact forces will produce fractures of the human face:

Nasal bones - - - - - - - - - - 35–80g's
Zygoma - - - - - - - - - - - - - 50–80g's
Mandibular condyles - - - - - 70–110g's
  (applied on the chin)
Central maxilla - - - - - - - - - 120–180g's
Frontal bone - - - - - - - - - - 150–200g's

Studies also show that blows to the face in excess of 30 g's will produce unconsciousness lasting from 15 minutes to 2 hours, with or without associated fractures. If design engineers will produce vehicles with dashboards that would deform with head impacts of 40 feet per second, significant reduction in the number of maxillofacial injuries would occur. Since 1976 federal laws have been passed requiring automobile manufacturers to meet minimum "safety design specifications" in production of new car models.

Significance. The physician treating maxillofacial injury has responsibilty to:

1. Save life.
2. Restore function.
3. Prevent and correct resultant deformity.

Injuries to the neck and cervical spine are particularly important, as over 15 per cent of them are fatal and over 8 per cent are "dangerous" (Cornell University Study, 1961). The combination of craniocerebral injury and injury to the long bones has been reported as the most frequent type of major automobile crash injury. All doctors are called upon at times to render emergency care to crash victims at the roadside or in a hospital emergency room. *In few injuries is the final outcome so directly dependent upon early proper care* as with a severe maxillofacial injury.

Facial injuries disturb the functions of chewing, eating, talking, breathing and seeing. In addition, the more subtle problems of appearance, identity, emotional expression — indeed, basic physiognomy — may be altered by deformity. It is in the appearance of the face that the individual has his greatest source of self-identification. It is small wonder that the management of these injuries demands meticulous *attention to detail*. The failure to handle such patients with skill and competence will produce serious medicolegal problems for physicians and hospitals.

The peculiarities of facial anatomy indicate the use of treatments and techniques that, at first glance, seem quite different from methods used to care for injuries to other parts of the body. However, all these techniques are firmly based on sound principles of general surgery. The complex array of headcaps and dental splints that once were widely advocated caused many to lose sight of the elementary principles involved.

Surgeons dealing with facial injuries must be ever alert to the possibilty of occult life-threatening injury elsewhere that must be diagnosed and treated before attention is focused upon less urgent aspects of the facial injury. The proper management of the maxillofacial injury itself will depend upon: (1) an exact understanding of the method of injury, (2) detailed knowledge of the anatomy and physiology of the injured area, and (3) a completely accurate assessment of the injury. This is often obtainable only in the operating room, as the overlapping of bone fragments in radiographs and the rapid development of soft tissue edema and hematoma make x-ray films and physical examinations imprecise.

INITIAL CARE AND TRANSPORTATION OF THE PATIENT WITH FACIAL INJURY

Bleeding from wounds in the head or neck should be arrested by elevation of the head and simple finger or hand pressure exerted on the bleeding point with the aid of a clean handkerchief or dressing. The airway should be cleared by removing blood clots, dentures and foreign bodies from the mouth. If the patient is unconscious the face and mouth should be placed in a dependent position and the tongue pulled forward to allow blood and saliva to escape from the oropharynx by gravity (Fig. 10–1). A dressing should be used around the head only if needed to stop serious bleeding or to splint loose

parts that are painful on movement. If the patient is conscious, he should be allowed to sit up to control airway and oral mucous secretions. Be particularly careful about moving the head if there is pain or spasm in the neck region or any suggestion of anesthesia or paralysis in the extremities. In such circumstances sandbags may be used to prevent unexpected head movements. If the patient must be moved to a stretcher or ambulance, one person should gently exert traction on the neck during the transfer. This is most easily accomplished by placing one hand under the patient's chin and another at the back of the head while others lift the body and limbs.

In dealing with any medical emergency, it is important that the physician have a previously prepared plan of action, including a definite order of priority in the management of the injuries. There are three phases in the management of a patient with severe maxillofacial injury:

1. An urgent period of diagnosis of life-threatening problems, combined with immediate treatment to correct these (e.g., cardiac arrest, obstruction of the upper airway or persistent bleeding).

2. A more leisurely period of determining the exact extent and nature of the problem.

3. A period of definitive treatment, which may be carried out by a team of surgical specialists working under the supervision of a single responsible surgeon.

(Phases 2 and 3 are usually carried out in a hospital emergency department or operating theater.)

URGENT SURGICAL MANAGEMENT

Establishment of Adequate Airway. *The principal cause of death from facial injuries is obstruction to the upper airway.* The number of minutes that a patient may live with a partially obstructed upper respiratory tract varies inversely with the percentage of the lumen that is obstructed and directly with his myocardial reserve. Attention should be given to the establishment of an airway *even before the arrest of hemorrhage* (except, of course, when there is division of a major arterial trunk and active spurting into the wound).

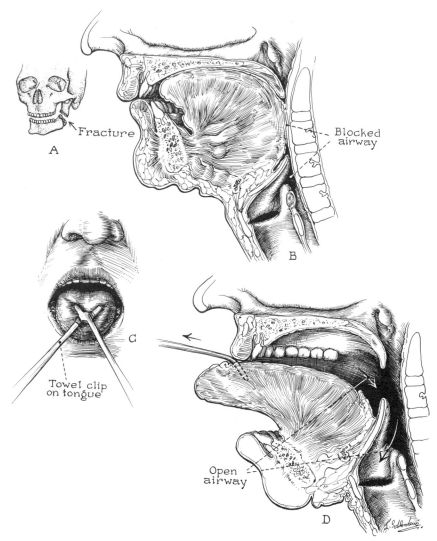

Figure 10–1. *When the bony arch of the mandible is fractured in one or more places as shown in the inset A, the chin is allowed to drift backward carrying with it the geniohyoid, genioglossus and mylohyoid muscles. The base of the tongue is allowed to settle posteriorly as shown in B and obstruct the entrance to the glottis. The patient may be unable to breathe unless the chin is brought forward. It may be necessary to support both the chin and the tongue in a forward position by means of a towel clip inserted near the anterior tongue (C and D). This produces very little discomfort and may be life-saving. Rubber shod clamps of various types are generally ineffective in holding the tongue of struggling airway-obstructed patients. This type of respiratory obstruction is particularly common with bilateral fractures involving the body of the mandible.*

DIAGNOSIS OF RESPIRATORY OBSTRUC-
TION. If the patient is conscious, it is important to ask him if he is "having any difficulty getting his breath." Even if he is unable to speak as a result of injury, he may be able to affirm or deny this by a nod of the head. If the patient is unconscious, the airway should be checked carefully. Do not wait for evident cyanosis; this is too late! It is a sign of impending death — not of respiratory obstruction.

Noisy breathing is an important sign. *All noisy breathing is obstructed breathing.* However, if the obstruction is complete, there will be no noise. Then one must look for intercostal retractions and paradoxical movements of the lower neck and chest with attempted respiratory movements by the patient. If there is any doubt, the examiner should place his ear, the back of his hand or his opened eye near the patient's mouth and nose to gauge the movement of air with breathing. If these maneuvers indicate inadequate exchange and if the patient is still attempting respiratory movements but has poor color, a quick check should be made for compression of the trachea or larynx, a sucking chest wound, flail chest or a tension pneumothorax, as described in the chapter on chest injuries. If these are not present, and instead the chest is moving vigorously and symmetrically, the patient has airway obstruction and the chin should be lifted forward; this will automatically also bring forward the base of the tongue. In the unconscious patient it may be necessary to insert a bite block between the molar teeth in order to open the jaws. The examiner's fingers can then be swept quickly back into the pharynx to locate and remove any clots or foreign bodies. At times, all or part of the patient's missing denture will be found to be driven back into the throat. If the mandibular arch has been fractured, it may collapse and allow the base of the tongue to obstruct the entrance to the larynx. In this event a large towel clip or safety pin may be passed through the anterior tongue, and traction may be used to bring both tongue and mandibular arch forward (Fig. 10–1). If this does not produce an immediately gratifying inrush of air, the examiner should check the position of the maxilla and soft palate. These structures may be impacted downward and backward in severe "midfacial mashes" so as to obstruct the entire oropharynx. If this is the case, the fingers should be passed up behind the free edge of the displaced soft palate to attempt forceful forward elevation of the fractured obstructing bone and soft tissue. An immediate inrush of air may follow this elevation of bone and soft tissues.

Should these measure not *immediately* relieve the obstruction, the tip of a laryngoscope should be inserted behind the tongue base, the vocal cords inspected for damage and an attempt made to pass an endotracheal tube. If the surgeon or anesthesiologist is unable to insert the endotracheal tube promptly, the attempt should be abandoned and a *coniotomy* performed whenever the obstruction is so severe that time does not permit an ordinary tracheostomy.

With *cricotomy* the cricoid cartilage is divided, and in *cricothyrotomy*, *both* the cricoid and thyroid cartilages are split.

Both methods will open the airway in an emergency, but bleeding and late scarring may be significant, and scar deformation of the divided cartilages may later require reconstructive procedures. In doing a *coniotomy* only the skin, fat and avascular membrane *between* the cricoid and thyroid cartilages are divided, thus causing few immediate or late complications. Coniotomy has proved to be of great value in the rapidly worsening patient with glottic or supraglottic airway obstruction who requires emergency establishment of an airway below the level of the larynx. It may be performed with only a pocketknife and without a special tracheal cannula to keep the opening patent. Danger from bleeding or pneumothorax is minimal. This very useful procedure was first described by the French surgeon Vicq d'Azyr in 1805. It consists of a transverse division of the cricothyroid (conic) ligament, which runs from the thyroid cartilages inferiorly to insert on the cricoid cartilage. The ligament is near the skin just below the prominence of the larynx and may be quickly opened with little bleeding using no equipment but a knife. A single suture placed in the skin edge on each side of this incision will keep the soft tissue open. Once divided, any wedge or hollow tubular structure (such as a pipestem or shell of a ballpoint pen) will maintain the opening in the membrane (Fig. 10–2). If available, one or more large (13 gauge) needles may be inserted through this ligament preliminary to the coniotomy to give some immediate relief so that the actual coniotomy may be performed in a more leisurely manner. It is usually wise not to use the coniotomy as a long-term airway. Once the acute air shortage is relieved, the surgeon should perform an elective tracheostomy through the third or fourth tracheal ring, using a transverse skin incision and local anesthesia.

When the airway obstruction is only partial, it is often possible to carry out a tracheostomy as the primary procedure. In such patients it is usually desirable to first insert an endotracheal airway, as it will facilitate the tracheostomy and make it a truly elective procedure. Patients who have major burns about the face and neck or who have had blunt injuries to the anterior larynx may be especially susceptible to the sudden closing off of the upper airway at a period several hours after injury.

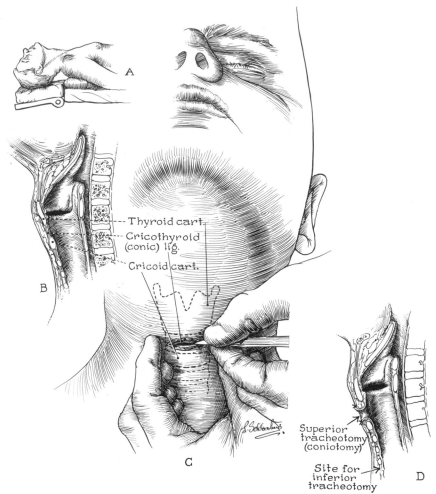

Thyroid cart.
Cricothyroid (conic) lig.
Cricoid cart.

Superior tracheotomy (coniotomy)

Site for inferior tracheotomy

Figure 10–2. *Emergency coniotomy. When there is critical blockage of the upper airway, the patient's head may be quickly extended and a short transverse incision made just above the cricoid cartilage. The index finger and thumb of the left hand are used to press the skin laterally and to fix the trachea in the midline. The knife is held with only a small part of the blade showing so as to avoid injury to the posterior wall of the trachea in a struggling patient. One or two stitches will hold the edges of the skin back from the wound until an elective tracheostomy can be performed.*

(See Chapter 1.) Furthermore, not only may clots from an oropharyngeal source of bleeding obstruct the airway but also the control of such bleeding may not be possible without performing a tracheostomy. One should remember that in children the apex of each pleural cavity extends well up into the base of the neck and lies close to the trachea on either side. If the pleura is inadvertently opened in an already "air hungry" patient while a tracheostomy is being done, a pneumothorax may not be recognized and may produce disaster. In addition, the innominate and thyroidea ima vessels extend high into the base of the

neck in children and must be avoided carefully in performing a tracheostomy.

No patient with questionable airway obstruction should be given any respiratory depressant drugs for the relief of pain. The primary sign of respiratory obstruction is *restlessness.* Any patient with facial injury who thrashes his extremities or struggles to raise his head from the stretcher or bed should be immediately checked for increasing airway obstruction or other cause of hypoxia.

If there is no sign of attempts at respiratory movements of the chest wall, mere provision of a proper airway will obviously do little good. In such patients assisted ventilation should be instituted immediately upon the establishment of an airway. This may be achieved by mouth-to-mouth (or mouth-to-tracheal cannula) assistance until an endotracheal tube and positive pressure equipment may be obtained. Any patient lacking a pulse or cardiac sounds on auscultation requires simultaneous external cardiac massage in addition to provision of an unobstructed airway and artificial ventilation if there is to be hope of resuscitation. (This is discussed in detail in Chapter 2.)

Control of Bleeding. Next to obstructed airway, bleeding is the most common cause of death from facial and cervical injury. Except for instances of division of a carotid artery, cervicofacial hemorrhage is usually readily controlled by simple compression applied over sterile gauze (or even a clean handkerchief) directly against the bleeding point. *It is both unnecessary and dangerous to attempt instrument clamping of vessels deep within a cervicofacial wound.* If the patient is unconscious, elevation of the head and shoulders to a 45-degree angle will help reduce bleeding. If excessive bleeding issues from the nasal or oral cavities, some form of gauze packing against the torn mucosa may be required. With stubborn nasal hemorrhage, rubber catheters may be passed through the nasal cavity into the pharynx and then brought out of the mouth. Sutures are attached to the catheter tips and used to draw a tamponading pack up behind the palate so that the gauze presses against the posterior choanae. Often bleeding will cease after the careful removal of clots overlying the bleeding points within the nasal cavity. On rare occasions the patient must be taken to the operating room and the internal maxillary artery must be ligated to control nasopharyngeal bleeding. This is readily accomplished by a transantral approach with removal of the thin posterior wall of the antrum to expose this artery.

Whenever the surgeon realizes that serious blood loss has occurred from the facial injury, he should immediately start an intravenous infusion with a large-bore catheter, and blood should be obtained for baseline and hematocrit determination, typing and cross-matching and measurement of blood gases. A central venous pressure monitoring system and an indwelling catheter in the bladder to measure the rate of urine output may be established to constantly monitor the effectiveness of intravenous fluid therapy (see Chapter 4).

Arterial bleeding from maxillofacial injury rarely requires ligation of either external carotid artery. Indeed, this often has little effect on facial bleeding. If the patient shows clinical signs of shock without sufficient facial bleeding to produce it, the physician should increase his efforts to locate another source of the bleeding.

Ambulance attendants, family and friends should be questioned as to the *amount of blood* lost at the scene of the accident and en route to the hospital. Major bleeding may have ceased *only* when blood pressure fell to low levels during early exsanguination. An attempt should be made to determine if the patient has a history of hypertension. Systolic readings of 120 mm. of mercury may actually represent significant shock in a usually hypertensive patient.

Early Check and Recording of Vision. Any patient with evidence of a major blow to the head or face should have each eye carefully checked for both central and peripheral vision. Any loss of visual ability *should* be carefully recorded so that subsequent surgical manipulations will not be blamed for unnoticed or unrecorded early blindness. Even a conscious patient may not realize that his injury has already produced a major loss of vision in one eye. An attempt should be made to detect diplopia in the four major quadrants of vision in all conscious patients with facial injury. The fundus should be checked for hemorrhage into the vitreous or dislocation of the lens. Any penetration of the sclera demands prompt attention. If these examinations reveal loss of vision or suspected injury to the globe, the ophthalmologist should be called (see Chapter 9 on eye injuries).

Because maxillofacial injuries are associated with an approximately 13 per cent incidence of concussion, 10 per cent of skull fractures, 8 per cent of rhinorrhea, 5 per cent of neck injuries and 20 per cent of fractures of other bones, as well as a significant incidence of thoracic and abdominal injuries, a search for such injuries should be made as soon as major bleeding and airway obstruction have been attended to and intravenous therapy has been initiated, before progressing to the second phase of management of the obvious maxillofacial injuries.

DIAGNOSTIC STUDIES OF MAXILLOFACIAL INJURIES

Complete Details of History — Initial Photography

An attempt should be made to clarify the exact history of the injury to determine the nature of the force producing the deformity and the direction from which it originated. The patient's previous medical history should be carefully assessed for other disease processes. Pre-existing renal, cardiac, vascular or respiratory disorders should be known before starting definitive treatment. Diabetics with hypoglycemia, epileptics and elderly patients with episodes of cerebrovascular insufficiency often suffer facial injuries when they lose consciousness suddenly and fall. If there is any odor of alcohol, the patient's breath or blood should be tested for alcoholic content. Severe depression of the central nervous system may be partly due to drug or alcohol ingestion and partly to head injury. This combination of causes is seen often in suicide attempts and may confuse the diagnosis. The use of a pressure screw in the subarachnoid space may quickly clarify the diagnosis.

Careful photographs should be taken of any significant external deformity before corrective treatment. These should be taken only *after* the clothing has been removed and blood cleansed from around the wounds. Such records have important medicolegal value and are vastly more accurate than verbal descriptions. Patients are frequently too ill or upset to realize the extent of their original disfigurement. Every modern emergency department should be equipped with simple, readily available photographic equipment, and personnel should be trained to use it.

Key Points in Physical Examination

OCCLUSION OF THE TEETH. Malocclusion is one of the most accurate diagnostic signs of mandibular or maxillary fracture. The examiner must have a working knowledge of normal dental relationships (Fig. 10–9). In the unconscious patient the jaws may be brought together and the meshing of the cusps of upper and lower teeth may be checked. Even small displacements of tooth positions that result from jaw fractures are readily reflected in these dental relationships. If the patient is conscious he will usually volunteer that his teeth "don't fit right." If dentures are normally worn and have been removed, they may be replaced to check the occlusion. If dentures are broken, the segments may be first wired or glued together with epoxy and then reinserted to aid in checking for bony displacement.

POINT TENDERNESS AND MOBILITY OF FACIAL BONES AT LINES OF FRACTURES. Fractured facial bones usually show well-localized tenderness when palpated. In addition, abnormal mobility or even slight asymmetry may yield a clue to the diagnosis of fracture. To determine bony symmetry, the examining fingers of both hands may be simultaneously used to palpate both sides of the face. Key points of the infraorbital rim, the zygomatic arch, the anterior wall of the antrum (with fingers beneath the upper lip), the angles of the jaw and the lower border of the body of the mandible are compared with corresponding points on the opposite side of the face. If this is carried out with the operator standing directly in front of the patient, even small displacements of the facial skeleton may be detected. The upper teeth and the hard palate should be grasped by the operator's fingers and an attempt made to move the upper jaw both up and down and from side to side (Fig. 10–3). Mid-facial fractures of the maxilla may often be detected in this way. If the examiner's little fingers are simultaneously placed in both of the patient's external auditory canals while the latter opens and closes his mouth, movements and symmetry of the mandibular condyles may be easily checked.

Patients seen within the first 2 hours of injury may usually be examined accurately, but some patients are highly susceptible to the rapid development of massive interstitial edema after even modest trauma. Others develop edema slowly but may not be first seen until many hours after a facial fracture. A third group of patients may show minimal formation of edema but will be difficult to examine because of a major localized hematoma, or they may be uncooperative because of alcoholic

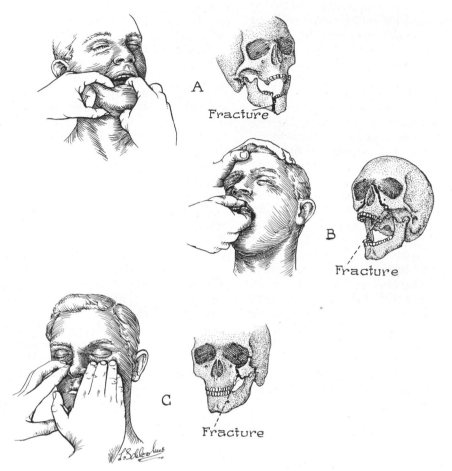

Figure 10–3. *Manual examination for diagnosis of fractured bones of the face and jaws; careful examination with bimanual palpation will reveal the vast majority of facial fractures. In A, a gentle rocking motion of the fingers will reveal movement or pain at the site of fractures of the mandibular body or symphysis. In B, the top of the head is fixed and an attempt is made to move the hard palate by grasping the upper central incisor teeth. Mid-face fractures will often reveal slight movement or pain. In C, the examiner feels for symmetry of the infraorbital rim, or for a step or "notch" along the normal smooth lateral rim of the orbit.*

intoxication. When these conditions are present, it may be wise to admit the patient to the hospital, apply ice packs to the face and defer x-rays and precise examinations until conditions improve.

PALSIES OF THIRD, FOURTH, FIFTH, SIXTH AND SEVENTH NERVES. Careful testing for cranial nerve palsy is important in assessing facial injuries. In particular, anesthesia of the upper lip and central upper teeth suggest fracture of the maxilla near the infraorbital foramen. Palsy of the facial nerve may be revealed by difficulty in closing the eye, elevating the brow or retracting the corner of the mouth. Diplopia or strabismus *may* indicate palsy of extraocular muscles, but the diplopia accompanying facial fractures is much more commonly due to bony deformities of the orbit that displace the positions and tensions of the extraocular muscles or trap them in fracture lines. It is common to find double vision upon re-examination several days after injury when it had not been detectable at the initial examination shortly after injury. This may result from increasing displacement of the globe by hematoma, resolution of early orbital edema or progressive herniation of orbital fat through fracture lines down into the antrum to produce increasing enophthalmus.

ADEQUACY OF NASAL AIRWAY. (See also section on nasal fractures.) A nasal speculum should be used to permit suction of clots and crusts from the nasal cavity and to check the mucosa for lacerations or displaced bone fragments. The position of the nasal septum and the mobility of the nasal bridge should be determined. The patient should be asked to close his lips, and the airway through each side of the nasal cavity may be checked by alternately blocking one nares and then the other with a fingertip as the patient is instructed to inhale forcefully. In the conscious patient, the use of vasoconstrictors (topical vasopressin solution) and topical anesthetics will make the examination much more comfortable for the patient.

PRESENCE OF BLOOD, RUPTURED TYMPANIC MEMBRANE OR BONY INFRACTURE OF THE EXTERNAL AUDITORY CANALS. The external auditory canal should be checked with an otoscope for blood clots or ruptures of the tympanic membrane. Severe blows on the chin will often drive the heads of the mandibular condyles backward with sufficient force to break the bony walls of the external auditory canals. A completely blocked canal with or without bleeding from the ear may then be encountered on otoscopic examination. Middle ear injuries may also be present and require special radiographs and otologic consultation.

MOBILITY AND CREPITUS AT THE TEMPOROMANDIBULAR JOINT. A finger placed in each external auditory canal will allow the operator to determine the position, shape and movement of the head of the mandibular condyles when the jaw is opened and closed. If one condyle does not move or if it is displaced, tomograms of the temporomandibular joints should be obtained.

CEREBROSPINAL FLUID RHINORRHEA. If the patient is placed face down for a short while, any significant leak of cerebrospinal fluid would be detected by the appearance at the nose of a watery nonmucoid liquid. If there is doubt about the nature of this fluid, let some of it dry on a handkerchief. Nasal mucus will stiffen the handkerchief, but cerebrospinal fluid will dry without stiffening. Cerebrospinal fluid will also show glucose on testing.

RE-EXAMINATION FOR OTHER INJURIES. Even those patients who appear to have only maxillofacial injuries at the time of initial examination may develop other problems with the passage of time. The maxillofacial surgeon must keep this possibility in mind and continually check the general condition of his patient as well

as checking for head, neck, thoracic, abdominal and extremity injuries.

PERTINENT RADIOGRAPHS AND LABORATORY STUDIES. Laboratory tests should be kept to a minimum; only those leading to more accurate therapeutic management should be ordered. The cost of medical care today makes it incumbent upon physicians to use laboratory facilities with discretion.

A single stereo-Water's (submentooccipital plane) roentgenogram will give almost all the diagnostic information needed in the emergency care of fractures of the facial bones. If there is also clinical evidence of mandibular fracture, posteroanterior and lateral oblique roentgenograms of the bodies of the mandible and, occasionally, tomograms of the temporomandibular joints may be indicated. Nasal bone roentgenograms are virtually useless since they so seldom affect treatment. A nasal fracture seen only in roentgenogram and without accompanying clinical displacement of the external nose or obstruction to the airway does not require surgical reduction. Conversely, nasal fractures with obvious clinical displacement may not show effectively on x-ray but may require surgical reduction. If there is evidence of injury to the cervical muscles or vertebrae, such as neck pain and spasm or tenderness of the cervical spinous processes, roentgenograms should be taken only with the neck in positions of extension and flexion after a scout film of the cervical vertebrae has revealed absence of any major bony dislocations or fractures. A chest x-ray is valuable even in the absence of thoracic trauma, not only as a preanesthetic screening test for occult cardiopulmonary disease but also to detect unobserved aspiration or developing atelectasis. Similarly, an electrocardiogram may reveal not only pre-existing cardiac disease but also may detect in automobile accident victims an occult myocardial contusion that might produce an arrhythmia or adverse response to anesthetic agents that tend to depress myocardial function.

Central venous pressure determinations, obtained via a subclavian or jugular vein catheter and a catheter in the bladder to determine hourly urinary output, will gauge the effectiveness of intravenous therapy. A baseline hematocrit and urinalysis should be performed. In older patients, particularly those with known intercurrent disease, more comprehensive blood tests are indicated, including a standard screening battery such as the SMA–12.

SPECIALTY CONSULTANTS. Diagnostic consultations may be needed. In many large medical centers it is practical to establish a regular maxillofacial team under central supervision. In other hospital emergency departments, both a general surgeon and a plastic surgeon will usually be called when any patient with a severe maxillofacial injury arrives. Both will normally participate in the diagnostic evaluation and emergency care. It may become apparent that consultations are also desirable in otolaryngology, dentistry, ophthalmology and neurosurgery. Each of these specialists may contribute valuable aid in the management of special problems with the facially injured patient. They should be called as early as it is evident that their services are needed.

Once life-endangering injury has been controlled and an analysis made of the extent of damage to the face, the question of definitive treatment arises. When there are major abdominal injuries such as a suspected rupture of a hollow viscus or organ, it is usually wise to admit the patient for care and observation on the general surgical service, since a sudden change in the abdominal condition might require immediate surgical intervention. Similarly, if there appear to be no abdominal injuries but severe intracranial damage is evident, with loss of consciousness and indications of increasing intracranial pressure, the patient should be admitted on the neurosurgical service for observation and care until the intracranial condition is stabilized. If neither of these conditions exists, it is usually desirable to admit patients with major maxillofacial injuries under the care of a plastic surgeon who has had liberal general surgical training. Attention must be paid not only to the patient's maxillofacial problems but also to the possibilities of delayed appearance of shock or abdominal, thoracic or pelvic problems.

If the injury is less severe and is confined to localized areas, such patients may be best treated by admission to a specialty service such as ophthalmology, dentistry or otolaryngology. It is important in all cases that the responsibility for coordinating the multiple treatment for facial injury be vested in a single responsible physician. In the

case of extensive injuries, this physician should be a surgeon with broad training in the field of general surgery and trauma.

DEFINITIVE EMERGENCY SURGICAL TREATMENT

Proper Time and Location of Surgery. GENERAL EMERGENCY OPERATING PROCEDURES. Maxillofacial injuries should not be treated in the emergency department unless they are of a very simple nature. Soft tissue lacerations of the face not involving nerves, ducts or cartilages and lesser fractures of the mandible with minimal fragment displacement that do not require open surgical reduction may be readily managed without the use of the operating room. In all such instances, local anesthesia should be employed, and careful attention should be given to the principles of wound care.

All patients with major injuries requiring complex operative manipulation, additional incisions for bone fixation or general anesthesia should be transferred to the operating room where adequate assistance, aseptic conditions, proper tools and lighting and complete anesthetic equipment are available. Many times two or even three surgical specialties may be represented as a team in such a definitive emergency reconstruction. The head of such a team must be able and willing to integrate the knowledge and talents of his colleagues in their contributions to the relief of deformity and dysfunction.

IMMEDIATE OR DELAYED REDUCTION OF FACIAL FRACTURES. Several factors should be considered in deciding on the time of fracture reduction.

1. Are there significant advantages for the patient or for the injured part in undertaking immediate treatment?
2. Is facial edema already so marked that it would make manipulation of the tissues difficult and disguise landmarks for proper reduction of fractures?
3. What is the general condition of the patient? Is there any evidence of hemorrhagic shock? Is there a history of recent alcohol intake? Does the injury represent a possible attempt at suicide? What is known of the patient's cardiac status?
4. Is the patient conscious? It is almost never wise to undertake major facial bone reductions in an unconscious patient.

5. Is a significant cerebrospinal fluid leak present, indicating a basal skull fracture? Would early reduction of fractures increase or decrease such leakage?

6. Do you have proper operative permission and adequate relationship with the patient and relatives? Is the patient a minor? Does the family wish other consultants called before definitive treatment is started?

Most severe maxillofacial injuries are best managed in two steps. The definitive phase of urgent care (described previously) is carried out in the emergency department and is followed by a waiting period of several days, during which time ice compresses on the facial area are used to reduce edema. During this period the patient's general condition is evaluated, any additional roentgenograms needed for definitive treatment are obtained, antibiotic therapy is started and further consultations are completed.

Preferably, the patient with facial fractures should be scheduled for well-conceived elective surgery several days after injury, when the facial edema is subsiding. This gives results that are superior to those from middle-of-the-night endeavors undertaken on a massively edematous face.

General Principles of Repair of Soft Tissue Injuries

Blood Supply. Major facial lacerations or avulsions are found in over 40 per cent of patients with facial fractures. Differences exist between the management of soft tissue injury to the face and to other parts of the body that relate primarily to the tremendously rich blood and lymphatic supply to the face. This permits more refined immediate reconstruction and delayed primary repairs. Secondly, the attachment of delicate mimetic muscles of the face directly into the facial skin, which produces those normal and subtle facial expressions, creates special problems in surface healing. The repair of skin and subcutaneous tissue without careful repositioning and reattachment of the face may result in a kinetic deformity that could have been prevented but that is almost impossible to correct later.

Although lacerations in other parts of the body are frequently not closed if they are seen over 6 hours after injury, such treatment is not desirable in the face. Indeed, *clean lacerations of the face may be closed as long as 24 hours after injury with considerable profit to the patient.* Such primary closure is beneficial in minimizing deep cicatrix and distortion of immediately subjacent facial muscles.

Animal Bites. Even in the case of animal bites of the nose, lips and cheeks, the rich blood supply of facial skin will allow the surgeon to do a primary closure. In such instances irrigation should be copious, and any crushed tissue should be carefully debrided. Antibiotic solution (bacitracin and/or neomycin) should be used to irrigate the wound before closing. The use of systemic antibiotics is also prudent with bite injuries, and it is important that they be used as quickly as possible (that is, before the suturing of the wound has been completed).

Extensive facial injuries require protection from tetanus, usually by a booster dose of toxoid; gas gangrene following facial trauma is an extremely rare occurrence. Experimentally, doses of *Staphylococcus aureus* in the magnitude of 10^7 organisms are usually required to produce abscess formation if inoculated into the skin of a healthy human. Lesser doses result only in temporary localized cellulitis, and recovery takes place without tissue necrosis. If the tissue is first traumatized by crushing, or if a bit of sterile suture or blood clot is experimentally placed beneath the skin, the dosage of bacteria required to produce abscess is reduced *approximately ten thousandfold* (10^3 bacteria). Conversely, if the blood and lymphatic circulation to and from a given area of skin is rich (as in the face), many times more bacteria may be managed by the local cellular and humoral defense mechanisms without resultant tissue necrosis than in the case of skin with less capillary flow (such as the skin of the foot or ankle). This wide variance of bacterial defense in different parts of the body explains both the need for meticulous debridement of all crushed or necrotic tissue and the ability to carry out many delayed or primary reconstructive maneuvers on the injured face.

Cleansing of Skin and Wound Irrigations. The preparation of a facial wound before suturing involves preliminary washing of the surrounding skin with soap and water and an antiseptic with lipolytic qualities. Solutions and soaps containing 3 per cent hexachlorophene (G11) have proved quite effective in reducing bacterial flora of skin.

Eyebrows should *never* be shaved, as those of some patients fail to regrow. Local anesthesia may be painlessly injected directly through the cut margins of the open wound and will reduce the discomfort of cleansing and irrigation. This is significantly less painful than injection of the anesthetic through the intact adjacent skin. Lidocaine hydrochloride (Xylocaine) is longer lasting, but procaine hydrochloride (Novocain) is less painful on initial contact with the tissues, and its effect is of adequate duraction for almost any repair.

Gentle soapsuds washing of the wound and surrounding area should be followed by copious irrigation with isotonic saline. When irrigation with large amounts of saline (1 to 3 liters used to *forcefully* flush out the wound in all its recesses) was instituted in The Johns Hopkins Hospital emergency department as standard treatment for all fresh cutaneous wounds, the infection rate dropped to *one third* of the previous level. Prior attempts to reduce these infections by the use of prophylactic antibiotics, stronger germicides on the surrounding skin or topical antibiotics to the wound had all been unsuccessful. After washing of the wound, the surrounding skin (*but not the wound*) may be prepared with benzalkonium chloride 1:1000 (Zephiran) or povidone-iodine solution (Betadine) to reduce concentration of skin bacteria. Recent evidence has shown the effectiveness of some of the newer *topical* antibiotics in reducing the incidence of clinical infections in experimental wounds deliberately inoculated with measured doses of pathogenic bacteria. Bacitracin solution (500 units per liter of physiologic saline) is particularly effective and appears to cause no clinical evidence of inflammation or delay in wound healing. Bacitracin irrigation may thus be indicated in patients with heavily contaminated wounds.

Anesthesia. General anesthesia is occasionally necessary for emergency treatment of extensive compound facial injuries, but its use is generally reserved for reduction of displaced fractures after the facial edema has begun to subside and the general condition of the patient has stabilized and been assessed. Endotracheal anesthesia is invaluable in controlling the airway and in permitting the anesthetic equipment to be placed at some distance from the facial wounds. Ethrane and other new anesthetic agents are valuable in that they permit the use of electrocautery without danger of explosion and reduce greatly the incidence of postoperative nausea and vomiting in comparison with many of the earlier agents. When general anesthesia is used on patients whose jaws must be wired together, it is wise to leave the nasotracheal tube in position until the patient is fully reactive to avoid the dangers of aspiration.

Anesthesia may be infiltrated locally or by nerve block, using 1 per cent lidocaine hydrochloride (Xylocaine) containing 1:100,000 parts of epinephrine or 1 per cent procaine (Novocain). With major soft tissue lacerations, it is desirable to do nerve blocks at either the infraorbital foramen or the mental foramen or, at times, to block the second and third divisions of the fifth cranial nerve where they emerge from the base of the skull at the foramina ovale and rotundum.

Debridement. It is particularly important to carry out *minimal* debridement of facial skin. As described earlier, the rich blood supply to the facial skin provides greater host resistance to bacterial contamination than skin of any other part of the body. Every square millimeter of tissue may be of value to the plastic surgeon in ultimate reconstruction. Even though bits of skin or vermilion may be totally detached and driven into another area, as by high explosive missiles, these valuable fragments should be left and may be made to survive as "grafts" in the new location. They may later be returned, by plastic techniques, to their normal location. Obviously crushed or charred tissue should be trimmed away, and frayed wound margins may be trimmed for better healing, but major debridement is rarely indicated in facial injuries except in the case of very high-velocity missiles, as in modern warfare. It is better to err on the side of attempting to save tissue that may ultimately necrose than to sacrifice any skin, cartilage or mucous membrane that is viable. The surgeon should remember that, except for the lips, there is no vermilion on the body that can be grafted to replace a missing lip segment. Mucous membrane is the best, but it

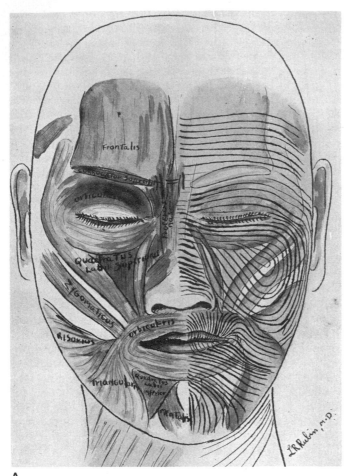

Figure 10–4. A, *This drawing from Rubin[18] shows on the left the position of the major superficial facial muscle groups and on the right the primary lines of skin relaxation produced by the combined effect of these muscles and the elasticity of the skin. Notice that although many of the lines of relaxation are at right angles to the long axis of the underlying muscle, some of the lines are at variance with this principle. In general, any laceration lying directly parallel to one of these underlying lines of relaxation will heal with minimal hypertrophy and thickening, whereas any laceration lying at right angles to one of these functional lines will heal with marked thickening. These lines do not coincide in many instances with the original "lines of Langer."*

A

is an imperfect substitute (Fig. 10–31A and B). When resurfacing of the face is necessary, any skin grafts taken from donor areas inferior to the clavicles will permanently lack the pink "blush" quality of facial skin. At times, facial tissue that is completely avulsed may be replaced as a free graft after careful removal of every vestige of fat clinging to its undersurface. The texture and color of this will be superior to skin grafted from *any other part of the body* at a later date. The inherent vascular pattern gives a ruddy color to the "blush area" which cannot be duplicated by any other tissue.

If an explosion has produced traumatic tattooing or brush abrasions have discolored the underlying dermis with grit or carbon particles, it is important to carry out *immediate* surgical abrasion treatment. The accepted method employs a high-speed engine and a diamond wheel or wire brush. It may be important to spend hours,

if necessary, to remove coal dust, hair or any insoluble pigmented particles. If these are allowed to remain in the skin during healing, hundreds of separate incisions (one over each particle) will be required to remove them later. In 1976 Marsh and Edgerton[15] introduced the technique of "razabrasion" for the removal of multiple foreign bodies from freshly traumatized skin. An ordinary double-edged safety razor blade is bent by the surgeon's fingers and used to remove thin split-thickness skin grafts from the area until the foreign bodies are uncovered and washed away. This is a gentler and more controllable method than use of the wire brush. The technique may also be used on healed wounds.

Suturing Facial Wounds. Incisions in the face that lie parallel to the lines of skin relaxation may be expected to heal in a very kindly fashion, even with minimal skin closure.[18] These lines should not be confused

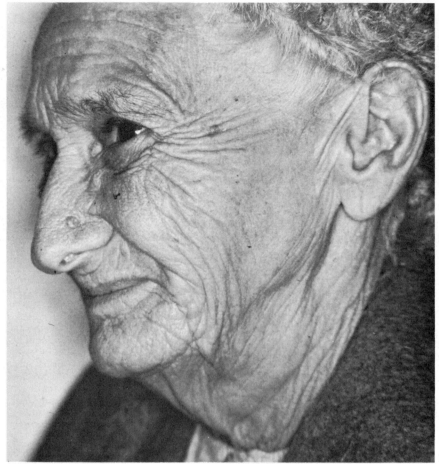

B

Figure 10–4. Continued.   B, *The elderly patient often presents a living example of the normal lines of skin relaxation. Notice that most of the creases in this patient's face coincide with the lines of relaxation in* A. *If primary lacerations cross directly over the more important functional creases, the surgeon may rearrange the laceration by proper use of local flaps even at the time of primary injury. Any additional incisions used to reduce underlying bony fractures should, of course, be placed directly in a functional "line of skin relaxation." (Courtesy of the Journal of Plastic and Reconstructive Surgery* [3:147, 1948].)

with the lines of skin elasticity described by Langer[12] (Fig. 10–4A and B). Patients should be warned of possible unsightly scars when lacerations cut across these lines at right angles. At times immediate Z-flaps or W-plasties may be cut and shifted to prevent later contractures. In some patients the trauma to the skin may make it wiser to plan a later plastic repair.

When lacerations result in beveled or angled cutting of the skin layers, surgical authors formerly recommended debriding these skin margins back to right-angled wound edges. That practice probably should be avoided unless the margins debrided are nonviable because of crush injury. Recent experiments indicate that the oblique slice through the dermis may even

provide superior healing if care is taken to gain *meticulous* apposition of the margins.

Very few subcuticular sutures should be used in the face in the absence of division of underlying muscle bundles. The decision to use subcuticular sutures in the closure of any given facial wound calls for a precise judgment. If the closure will necessitate considerable tension on the skin sutures, it is wise to place subcuticular sutures that may be counted on to secure the wound when the skin sutures are removed. The subcuticular sutures should be placed as deeply as possible within the dermis and with the knots lying in the subcutaneous fat. Skin sutures should be tied loosely and removed in 3 days to prevent permanent "cross-hatch" suture scars. We have seen this hatching persist, in some instances, when tight sutures were removed after only 4 days. During the first 3 to 4 days after closure, the facial wound shows rapid proliferation of, and invasion by, capillaries, but there is little development of tensile strength. Consequently, the skin margins *must* be supported for several days after the early removal of skin sutures in order to prevent disruption or early spreading of the soft scar. This support can be provided by placing collodion gauze strips or adhesive "Steristrips" over the incision for 4 or 5 days after removal of the sutures. Hydroxyproline concentrations of the healing scar and tensile strength determinations show that the facial wounds are reasonably secure after 10 days.

Meticulous hemostasis should be carried out in repairing facial lacerations. This helps to avoid the collection of even small blood clots in the deep recesses of these wounds. Such clots lead to fibrosis and palpable thickening in the postoperative period. If any buried sutures are used, the knots should be tied at the deepest part of the loop, and they should be placed in stout fascia well beneath the surface so as not to encroach on oil glands or hair follicles within the dermis. The choice of the type of suture material is not nearly so important as the method and depth of suture placement. The operator should develop the technique of using skin hooks in place of toothed forceps to handle the wound margins when suturing the face. This will avoid the damaging effects of tissue crushing that are seen even with careful use of fine spring forceps. There should be no need to use cuticular sutures heavier than 6-0 on the face, and the sutures should be placed within 2 to 4 mm. of the wound margin to avoid inversion of edges. They should usually be removed within 3 days. In addition to silk, nylon, mersilene, Polydek and stainless steel sutures are all well tolerated as facial sutures, but most alloys of stainless steel wire lack the flexibility for perfect coaptation of wound edges.

In small children with modest lacerations of the face, it is usually wise to close these wounds, after proper cleansing, by using only adhesive strips, "butterflies," or some type of synthetic strip with skin adhesive (Fig. 10–5). In many instances, the final result will be superior to suturing. The

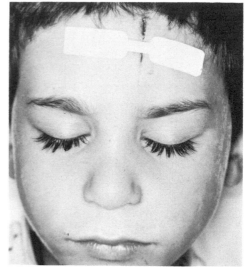

Figure 10–5. *This type of simple butterfly dressing may be used to draw together and approximate wound edges of most fresh facial lacerations. The wounds are first cleaned and irrigated, but no local anesthetic injections are necessary. Usually two or three "butterflies" or other type of adhesive skin strip will suffice to hold the wound without dressing change for a 4- or 5-day period. Many favorably placed lacerations will require no later treatment. Others, such as this vertical laceration of the forehead, may require a later Z-plasty that is best performed on a healed wound. Eyebrows should never be shaved in suturing facial lacerations.*

child also will be spared an unpleasant experience involving injection of anesthetic and placing of sutures. Should further surgical improvement of the scar be necessary, it may be carried out later in an aseptic field with a relaxed and sedated child, with more likelihood of an optimum result. There is little to defend the practice of holding down a crying, frightened, small child while four or five sutures are awkwardly placed.

When soft tissue lacerations lie at right angles to the lines of skin relaxation, muscle pull and movement on these scars will usually produce later hypertrophy and unsightly deformity (Fig. 10–6 A and B). A knowledge of wound dynamics makes it possible for the surgeon to predict accurately most of these complications of healing, and the patient should be warned of these problems at the time of original treatment. Indeed, in many instances, plastic surgeons will resort to primary Z-plasty and local flap shifts in order to prevent the almost certain development of these scar hy-

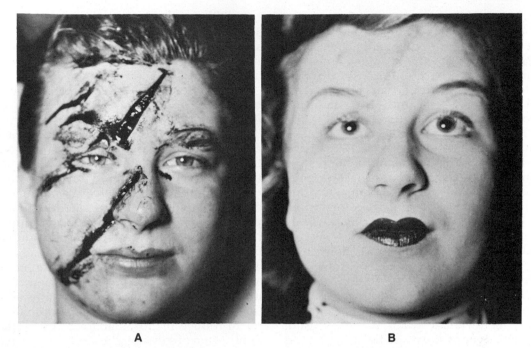

A   B

Figure 10–6. A and B, These lacerations were sustained when the patient's head was thrown against a broken windshield. Many of the lacerations fall along "lines of skin relaxation." The laceration of the central forehead is unfavorably placed and tends to gape more than the others. Part of the levator muscle to the right upper eyelid was also divided. Only a few subcuticular sutures of 5-0 silk were used in the vertical forehead laceration. All other lacerations were closed with fine skin sutures to produce the result shown (B) when the patient returned for minor revision of scars 3 months later. The levator muscle of the right upper eyelid was shortened at the same time. A primary Z-plasty in the forehead scar might also have been used as an alternative method of treatment.

pertrophies. Such "primary flaps" require a knowledge of facial skin circulation and should not be undertaken if the skin has been crushed. When the patient is an Oriental or a dark-skinned black, such immediate flaps are more likely to produce true keloids, and a careful history of skin healing of prior wounds will be a valuable guide in choosing the most appropriate treatment.

Dressing Techniques. Pressure dressings are rarely necessary with soft tissue lacerations of the face and are likely to interfere with eating or breathing and be uncomfortable in the postoperative period. Usually, sutured incisions may be left open for frequent cleansing with weak concentrations of hydrogen peroxide or they may be covered with a light greasy protective ointment to avoid dry crust formation that may block wound secretions. Adhesive or synthetic strips may be placed across the sutured incisions to splint the cheek, lip or forehead and to reduce tension on suture lines. It is important to prevent the accumulation of dry crusts on the sutures if perma-

nent pits and irregularities in the surface healing are to be avoided. After each cleansing of the sutures, a coating of sterile white (mineral) oil will minimize further accumulations. Antibiotics are rarely indicated with lacerating injuries of the face that involve only soft tissues, but are desirable when compound fractures and crushed tissue are also present.

When the eyelid and orbital regions have received an extensive blow, a pressure dressing will be of great value in preventing the development of severe lid and conjunctival edema. If such massive swelling is allowed to occur, some patients will develop exposure and drying of the cornea or permanent skin striae from the irreversible stretching and scarring of lid skin. Care should be taken to avoid the use of "Ace" or *elastic outer bandages* around the injured eye. This may produce excessive pressure over a prolonged time, causing compression of the retinal artery and even blindness. In the cervical region, large flaps that have been elevated may be dressed with the aid of continuous suction catheters beneath them. This utilizes normal atmospheric pressure in keeping the flaps in contact with the underlying bed.

Proteolytic Enzymes. Many pharmaceutical houses have enthusiastically promoted proteolytic enzymes for systemic and localized use in increasing fluid absorption from traumatized areas. Controlled studies to date have *not* established that patients receiving these expensive medications ultimately obtain better results than those in control groups. Resolution of experimental hematomas in human volunteers was not significantly accelerated by use of several commercial enzymes widely used by surgeons. Enzyme therapy such as hyaluronidase (Wydase) breaks down hyaluronic acid in the connective tissue and produces some initial resolution of traumatic edema, but "rebound edema" is common, and ultimate results are not impressively better than when it is not used. Plastic surgeons *have not* been impressed with the value of these expensive drugs.

In contrast to the general ineffectiveness of enzymes in controlling traumatic edema and promoting healing, it is becoming apparent that some of the newer proteolytic enzymes can be of significant value as *debriding agents*. When applied properly and kept moist, some of these agents have shortened the removal of slough on the face from 22 days to 5 days, thus greatly facilitating treatment.

Mandibular Fractures

The large, strong mandibular arch is balanced in position by many strong muscles of mastication. When the jaw is fractured, the mandibular fragments are readily displaced by these same powerful muscles. Thus, strong methods of bone fixation and longer splinting periods are required when the mandible is fractured than in the case of other facial bones. In contrast, the remaining facial bones (the "membranous bones") surrounding the orbit, nose and paranasal sinuses are light in weight and easily comminuted. When fractures of these bones are surgically reduced, the lack of strong muscle pull makes it easier to hold them in the correct positions than to hold mandibular fragments. Membranous bones of the face also tend to unite quite rapidly.

It is of some interest that the central facial bones are highly efficient energy decelerators. This ability of nasal and paranasal sinus bones to absorb great force prevents serious injury to the brain and spinal cord in many individuals when the face meets any solid object with great speed.

Most simple mandibular fractures may be best treated by the method known as *intermaxillary wiring.*

Intermaxillary Wiring or Elastic Band Fixation. It is a happy anatomical fact that the mandible contains hard white structures that are firmly fixed to it and that emerge through the mucous membrane covering its surface. These mandibular appendages, the teeth, serve as convenient handles to manipulate and control mandibular bone fragments following fracture. Teeth are very helpful both in diagnosis and in fixation of jaw fractures. When each major fractured jaw fragment contains adequate dentition, it is usually a simple matter to reduce mandibular fractures by the application of soft metallic arch bars to each of these fragments. These bars contain small metal pegs and are held in place by passing metal ligatures of stainless steel about the neck of each tooth to encompass the bar. Elastic bands are then applied to these bars in such directions that the teeth (and attached jaw fragments) will be drawn into their normal occlusal relationships. By using *elastic* rather than *rigid* bands, the reduction will continue over a period of several days and successfully overcome muscle spasm that might be present at the initial reduction. This technique is called intermaxillary wiring or, more accurately, intermaxillary elastic band fixation (Fig. 10–7). A mandibular fracture may thus be brought back into normal alignment with an intact upper alveolar arch or, conversely, a fractured maxilla by similar elastic traction may be drawn back into alignment with an intact mandibular arch. These arch bars and elastic bands need to be left in place approximately 6 weeks for proper healing. When the bands are removed, bony union must be tested by palpation as x-ray changes will not demonstrate callus formation for several additional weeks. When fractures of the mandible result in unfavorable position of the bone fragments, or when both arches are fractured and badly displaced, a more complex method of treatment is required.

Open Reduction and Wiring (Transosseous). There are certain circumstances

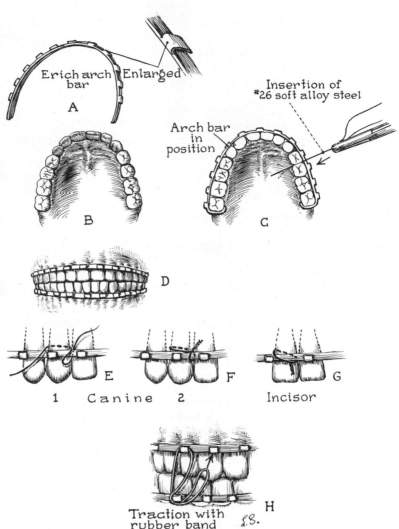

Figure 10–7. Method of applying soft metallic arch bars to upper or lower jaw in preparation for use of intermaxillary elastic band fixation of a fractured maxilla or mandible: The soft metal Erich bar is bent to fit against the dental arch and allowed to curve about the most posterior tooth. Soft steel wires are then passed about the necks of the molar teeth and about the bar to make the latter secure. E, F and G illustrate the variations in applying the wire when it is necessary to use a canine tooth as one point of fixation. This method prevents the tendency of such forces to slowly extract the anchored tooth. Once the arch bars are properly attached, elastic bands may be applied to the metal hooks, as shown in H, to bring the jaw fragments and teeth into satisfactory occlusion.

under which intermaxillary elastic band fixation does not offer sufficient fixation for mandibular fractures. These include:

1. Patients with an edentulous mandible or maxilla.
2. Displaced fractures of the mandible in which one or more fragments do not contain healthy erupted teeth.
3. Displaced mandibular fractures in small children with only deciduous dentition.
4. Patients with traumatic disruption of both arches who will need another point of fixation for realignment.

The first known report on the use of interosseous wiring of the mandible is by the surgeon Gurdon Buck.[5] In 1846 he reported an open reduction of the mandible using malleable iron wire for fixation of the fragments. The fracture involved the lower jaw between the first and second incisor teeth on the left side and occurred when a seaman was struck in the face by a block. To accomplish reduction of the fracture Dr. Buck proceeded as follows:

The lower lip was divided along the median line to the chin, and the flaps dissected up to expose the ends of the bones. The remaining adhesions were divided and a narrow chisel insinuated behind the fragment to be excised in order to protect the soft parts, while with a metacarpal saw, a perpendicular section was effected. The left middle incisor tooth, being loose in the right fragment, . . . was removed. The ends of the bone now admitted of accurate adjustment, so as to bring the teeth of both sides on the proper level. To maintain them in this position, a hole was drilled near the lower angle in each bone, and a piece of malleable iron wire passed through, with the ends drawn forward and twisted, so as to secure the desired object.

Six weeks later Dr. Buck reported: "the opening through which the wire passed was healed up. Union solid. Discharged cured."

In recent years all plastic surgeons have moved steadily toward an *increased* use of open reduction and direct interosseous wiring of mandibular fractures.[7] There are numerous advantages to open reduction:

1. It produces immediate and simple reduction.
2. It provides more precise correction of bony displacement.
3. It relieves pain and provides more comfort than other types of appliances.
4. It avoids the need for constant adjustment of oral or external appliances or the danger of displacement of the bony fragments by muscle pull.
5. It reduces the period of total jaw immobilization.
6. It does not interfere with prompt reduction and positive fixation of fractures in other parts of the body.

The only significant disadvantages to open reduction and direct transosseous wiring are the necessity for the surgeon to be thoroughly familiar with the location of the branches of the facial nerve (so as to avoid injury to them during the operation) and the occasional necessity to remove a steel wire from the bone because of late tenderness or drainage. When drainage is present, there is usually a low-grade localized osteitis of the bone immediately about the wire. It usually clears promptly after the wire is removed. Tenderness, in the absence of drainage and inflammation, may also result from pressure of the twisted wire against the overlying cutaneous nerves. When incisions are properly placed in the lines of skin relaxation (Fig. 10–8), the external scars of open reduction are almost invisible when healed.

Before the reduction of mandibular fractures, the oral cavity should be carefully inspected. Any loose teeth should usually be removed as well as certain teeth lying in the fracture line of the mandible. This is especially true if that tooth root shows evidence of root abscess or fracture and might serve as an inciting cause to the development of osteomyelitis. Many times healthy teeth lying in undisplaced fracture lines may be saved, and they will often contrib-

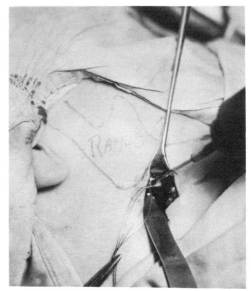

Figure 10–8. *This simple type of exposure is ideal for transosseous wiring with open reduction of fractures of the angle of the mandible body or ramus. The incision is made with a knife only through the skin and fat. The remainder of the exposure is then obtained with gentle blunt dissection, going between parallel branches of the facial nerve. The periosteum of the mandible is elevated at the inferior border to reveal the fracture site. Drill holes are placed as shown in this illustration on either side of the fracture line, and doubled strands of No. 26 steel wire may be used to achieve a hair line reduction. The outline of the mandible is drawn on the skin here only for orientation.*

ute greatly to jaw fixation and mastication after healing. The mouth should be swabbed and the teeth scrubbed with a small toothbrush, using a mild detergent mouthwash.

Many mandibular fractures are compounded into the oral cavity, and it is important that the tears in the mucous membrane be loosely reapproximated with fine sutures. Such closure will avoid continuing massive contamination of the fracture line by gravitational collections of saliva and oral cavity bacteria in the depths of open mouth wounds. If these "saliva pools" are allowed to lie in direct contact with the fracture line, non-union and osteomyelitis will commonly result. It is important that surgeons understand the basic principles of dental occlusion (Fig. 10–9). Recognition of the preinjury occlusion of the teeth is necessary in order to re-establish this original occlusion by the reduction of any jaw fractures. Most patients with jaw injuries readily detect even very minor variations in their normal bite relationships and so advise the surgeon. It is usually desirable to check this with some standard reference for normal occlusion.

Angle's[2] classification of dental occlusion is based on the relationship of the mesiobuccal cusp of the maxillary first molar tooth to the mandibular teeth below (Fig. 10–9). In patients with normal bite relationships, this cusp interdigitates in the mesiobuccal groove of the mandibular first molar tooth. With distoclusion (retroclusion or Class II malocclusion), the mesiobuccal cusp of the maxillary first molar is anterior to the mesiobuccal groove of the mandibular first molar. The reversed displacement is known as mesiocclusion (prognathic occlusion or Class III malocclusion). In this instance, the mesiobuccal cusp of the maxillary first molar is in the space between the first and second mandibular molars. Lateral blows to the upper or lower jaw may produce either a unilateral or bilateral cross-bite as a result of a horizontal fracture and segmental medial displacement of one or both alveolar processes with their contained teeth. In such instances the full vertical height of the mandible or maxilla may or may not also be fractured.

Fractures of the mandible may be divided for simple classification into four groups:

1. *Fractures of the condylar neck.* This is the weakest portion of the mandible and accounts for 35 per cent of the fractures.
2. *Fractures of the mandibular angle, ramus and coronoid.* This portion of the bone lies beneath the masseter and temporalis muscles and accounts for 30 per cent of the fractures of the mandible.
3. *The body of the mandible and/or the alveolar ridge with its contained tooth roots.* This accounts for 25 per cent of mandibular fractures.
4. *Anterior mandibular fractures.* These fractures involve the symphysis and mandible from midline back to the mental foramen on either side. They account for 10 per cent of mandible fractures (Fig. 10–10).

Treatment of these fractures depends on an understanding of the action and force of strong muscle groups acting on each of these major segments of the lower jaw. A fractured anterior mandibular segment will be pulled downward and posteriorly by the depressor-retractor group of muscles (the geniohyoid and digastric muscles). A fracture through the body of the mandible will usually show an upward and medial displacement of the posterior fragment due to the powerful force of the elevator muscles (masseter, medial pterygoid and temporalis muscles). Such a displacement may fail to occur if the fracture has a "favorable" direction (i.e., if the line of the fracture runs posteriorly to anteriorly through the man-

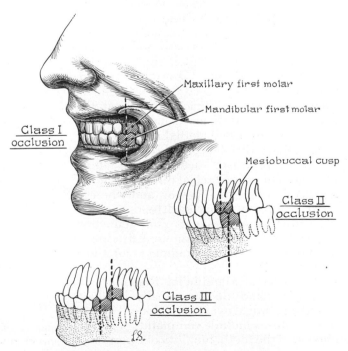

Figure 10–9. *Elementary types of dental occlusion as originally described by Angle. The relationship of the mesiobuccal cusp of the maxillary first molar tooth to the mandibular first molar tooth is used as a guide for normal types of occlusion. Class II occlusion is commonly seen in patients with mandibular retrusion; Class III occlusion is the type seen with prognathism. In fractures of the mandible or maxilla, the surgeon attempts to re-establish the occlusion present prior to the injury.*

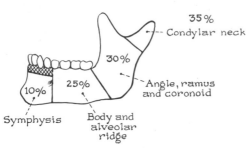

Figure 10–10. *A simple classification of mandibular fractures with approximate incidence is shown in this diagram. Note that the masseter and temporalis muscles tend to pull any attached posterior bone fragments strongly upward. The internal pterygoid muscle tends to pull the neck of the condyle medialward and forward when the latter is fractured. The cross-hatched area of the alveolus shown anteriorly merely indicates that this region of bone is involved not only with fractures through the symphysis but also occasionally with fractures of the body of the mandible, including horizontal fractures of the alveolus itself. Slightly differing methods of fixation are required for each of these four major types of mandibular fracture.*

dibular body as it descends from the alveolar margin to the inferior border of the mandible [Fig. 10–11A]). With such a "favorable" fracture line, the muscle forces tend to impact the mandibular fragments against each other. A fracture line that lies at right angles to this favorable direction will allow the muscles to distract the fragments (Fig. 10–11B).

Fractures through the angle and ramus of the mandible may show minimal displacement, or the posterior fragment may be displaced markedly forward and upward. This often depends upon the fracturing force since the bone of the ramus is thin, making medial or lateral displacements of fragments common. Fractures through the neck of the condyle are usually accompanied by anterior and medial rotation of the proximal mandibular condyle and neck as a result of "protrusor" action of the lateral pterygoid muscle. Each of these muscles of mastication has great power, and when in spasm following injury, each tends to redisplace the bone fragments after reduction unless strong, well-engineered fixation is used to secure the jaw fragments for 4 to 8 weeks.

Diagnosis of Mandibular Fractures. A fractured mandible can usually be diagnosed on clinical evaluation alone. The cardinal features include complaints of malocclusion of the teeth, mobility of a portion of the mandible on bimanual manipulation (Fig. 10–3), frequent compounding of the fracture into the oral cavity (especially if the body of the mandible and alveolus are involved), pain localized at the fracture site on movement or palpation, inability to chew properly, some degree of trismus and edema or hematoma at the site of fracture. If the inferior alveolar artery was torn by the separation of the fracture line, there is usually discoloration of the overlying skin by ecchymosis.

If the mouth was closed at the time of injury, there may be associated avulsion of one or more of the cusps of premolar or molar teeth. Strong lateral forces not only shear off high points on the teeth, but may also cause exposure of dental pulp. Reimplantation of avulsed teeth may be successful, particularly in young children, whose teeth have open root canals, but such decisions should be left to an exodontist.

Roentgenographic examinations are of greatest value in determining (1) the position of bone fragments before reduction, (2) the presence of caries, abscesses or broken roots of teeth in the fractured area, and (3) the position of the bone following surgical reduction.

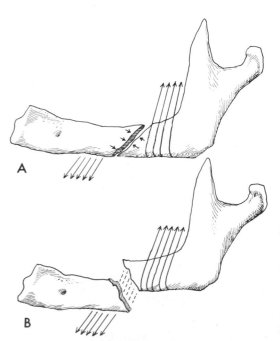

Figure 10–11. *A, Favorable direction of fracture line of mandible. B, Unfavorable direction of fracture line (angle of fracture allows masseter and mylohyoid muscles to pull fragments apart).*

General Principles in Treatment of Mandibular Fractures. Once the diagnosis of mandibular fracture is clearly determined, treatment may be carried out by wiring a section of soft metal arch bar (containing small metal projecting hooks) to the teeth in the upper jaw and to each fractured segment in the lower jaw (Fig. 10–7).

The teeth serve as convenient pegs to which may be wired a separate section of arch bar for each displaced bone and tooth unit. An arch bar is also fixed to the maxillary arch and the mandibular fragments may be drawn into proper position by using small rubber bands (easily made by cutting slices off ordinary soft rubber tubing) to connect the arch bar hooks at corresponding points in upper and lower arches (Fig. 10–7H). This method of "intermaxillary elastic traction" may not produce "instant normal occlusion" when first applied, but over a period of several days the gentle gradual pull of the elastic bands overcomes the spasm of opposing muscles, the high points of tooth cusps tend to slide into the proper "valleys" or grooves between the cusps of opposing teeth and the jaws settle into the desired relationships for healing. When all fracture fragments contain teeth, or when there is minimal displacement of bone, such intermaxillary elastic splinting may be the simplest and best surgical treatment for a mandibular fracture. When there are large bony fragments bearing no teeth, or when tooth-bearing fragments have been markedly displaced and are unstable, other surgical measures are often of value.

Plastic surgeons stress both the simplicity and the effectiveness of direct transosseous wiring of the mandibular fragments (see p. 302). Such wires may be inserted through small (1.5 cm.) incisions, may be left in the tissues permanently and allow the patient to use his jaws at a much earlier postinjury period than in the case of patients treated only by the use of intermaxillary elastic fixation. Open reduction is of special value with displaced fractures of the ramus and with double fracture lines in the region of the symphysis. When direct interosseous wiring is undertaken, the skin incisions should be placed parallel to the lines of skin relaxation (Fig. 10–8); the facial nerve branches may be located just deep to the platysma muscle as the fibers of the latter are bluntly separated. The drill

holes should be placed in the bone on either side of the fracture line at a proper oblique angle to anticipate the direction of muscle pull on the bone.

Direct interosseous wiring may be combined with intermaxillary elastic traction or, in the edentulous patient, with circumferential wiring. Such circumferential wires may be passed so as to encircle the overlapping ends of the fractured edentulous mandible or, when the patient's denture is not broken by the injury, it may be positioned against the oral surface of the fractured mandible and the encircling wires allowed to include both denture and mandible.

A French surgeon, Jean-Baptiste Baudens, appears to have been the first to describe the concept of circumferential wiring for mandibular fractures.[3] In 1840 he outlined his treatment of a soldier with an oblique fracture through the region of the angle of the mandible and severe displacement of the proximal fragment. He was "able to hold the fracture securely with one circumferential wire passed around the mandible with a needle. The two ends of the ligature were fixed over a posterior tooth." Baudens was criticized by Professor Roux, who suggested that the pressure of the metal ligature upon the bony tissue might alter the structure of the bone. Baudens pointed out that the wire had "remained in place for twenty-three days and left the bone in a condition of good health."

In 1852 Cesar Robert modified this treatment by passing the circumferential wire over a small lead plate.[15] In modern times a denture or small acrylic shell is used in place of the lead plate to prevent the wire from cutting into the alveolar ridge.

Most mandibular fractures may thus be managed by a combination of intermaxillary elastic band traction, direct transosseous wiring with open reduction, or circumferential wiring with or without use of the patient's dentures or a dental splint. On occasion an extra plane of fixation is required, particularly in the edentulous mandible or when much destruction of the maxilla has also occurred. Such stability may be gained by drilling a straight steel Kirschner wire through the lower borders of the mandible from side to side after reduction and manual fixation of the arch (Fig. 10–24). A *threaded* K-wire should not be used because the threads may catch and wind their way up the alveolar nerve if it passes too near.

One must remember that the mandible does not produce a dense callus for many months following clinical healing of a fracture line; thus, it is both unnecessary and unwise to wait for radiologic evidence of bony union before stabilizing the jaws in the postoperative period. Clinical bony union is a much more reliable guide as to the time at which jaw function should be resumed. Indeed, mild stress applied to the fracture line in later stages of healing appears to actually accelerate the rate of bony union in some fractures.

Fractures and Dislocations of the Mandibular Condyle. In general, undisplaced or slightly displaced fractures of the condylar neck should be treated conservatively by simply restoring occlusion with intermaxillary wiring for a 3-week period. However, when there has been severe displacement of the head of the condyle, particularly in young children in whom growth arrest would create serious deformity, a very gently performed open reduction, carried out as a primary or delayed procedure,

may be of great value. Exposure of the condyle may be obtained with least danger to the facial nerve by an incision *behind* the external ear. This postauricular approach divides the postauricular muscle fibers and fascia and the full circumference of the cartilaginous external auditory canal. The operator may then reflect the ear, parotid gland and facial nerve forward and downward to reveal the entire lateral and posterior surfaces of the temporomandibular joint. The dissection should be gentle and carried out so as to preserve as much soft tissue attachment (blood supply) to the fractured condyle as possible. If the bone is exposed too widely, aseptic necrosis may develop postoperatively. If both condyles are fractured and displaced, and if the symphysis and body of the mandible are also comminuted, it may be difficult to maintain an adequately forward position of the lower jaw during healing. In such circumstances open reduction and direct wiring of the symphysis and body fractures may be combined with application of a simple plaster headcap or metal halo-type head splint with metal pin fixation to the cranial bones. Whichever device is used, it should contain

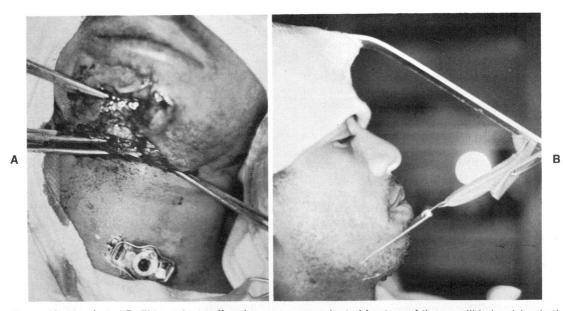

A B

Figure 10–12. A and B, *This patient suffered a severe comminuted fracture of the mandible involving both condyles and both rami, and a triple fracture of the symphysis following a head-on collision in a speeding automobile. Emergency tracheotomy was lifesaving, but transosseous wiring of the mandibular fractures and intermaxillary elastic fixation would not succeed in holding the lower mandibular arch forward in satisfactory position. To restore the arch, a steel pin was passed through the lower border of the body of the mandible and held forward by moderately strong elastic traction supplied by means of a metal rod and plaster head cap as shown in B. The dislocated condyles were gently maneuvered back into position when the severe facial edema had subsided. Good mandibular function resulted.*

a projecting metal arm. This arm may be used to permit elastic forward traction on the condylar fracture lines (Fig. 10–12A and B) by attaching it to the symphysis of the mandible with a Kirschner wire or arch bar.

With all compound mandibular fractures, attempts should be made to suture loosely any lacerated mucosa in the area of the fracture. This accelerates wound healing and reduces the incidence of bone infection. With major avulsions and loss of mucosa, drainage should be carried out in a dependent direction through a small submandibular "stab" incision rather than by "uphill" drainage into the oral cavity.

In the case of explosive wounds resulting in loss of large segments of the mandible, it may be necessary to fix the remaining portions in normal position by means of external skeletal pin fixation (Fig. 10–13). This fixation will retain alignment of fragments until soft tissue healing is complete and may be followed by bone grafting and further plastic repair. At times a small buried bone plate may be used to maintain the space caused by the missing segment of bone. Use of this method is wise only when sufficient skin and mucous membrane is

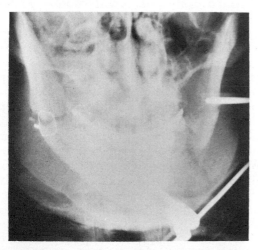

Figure 10–13. *This x-ray shows a necessary combination of three methods of fixation for a compound fracture of the mandible. The injury resulted from a shotgun blast with destruction of approximately 2 inches of the body of the right mandible. Intermaxillary elastic traction has been applied by arch bars to the upper and lower jaw. The fracture of the left angle of the mandible has been reduced by direct transosseous wiring, and external skeletal fixation has been applied across the defect in the right mandible. This large defect in the bone was filled later with an iliac bone graft to retain the lower arch.*

present to allow easy wound closure around the plate.

Dislocation of the Temporomandibular Joint

Spontaneous dislocation of the lower jaw may occur as the result of a sudden interruption in the normal jaw-closing action of the muscles of mastication. It may also result from trauma which suddenly forces the condyle out of the fossa. In the absence of fracture, the dislocation always displaces the head of the condyle in an anterior direction. The chin shifts to the opposite side, and the teeth on the side of the dislocation become locked in an open bite position with considerable pain and muscle spasm.

A writer in the Smith Papyrus (written 25 centuries before the time of Christ) gives advice for treatment for dislocation of the mandible: "If thou examinest a man having a dislocation in his mandible, shouldst thou find his mouth open and his mouth cannot close for him, thou shouldst put thy thumbs upon the ends of the two rami of the mandible on the inside of his mouth, (and) thy two claws (meaning two groups of fingers) under his chin, (and) thou shouldst cause them to fall back so that they rest in their places."[19]

W. B. Johnson[10] first reported that local anesthetic (1 per cent lidocaine hydrochloride) injected unilaterally into the connective tissue of the torn temporomandibular joint capsule brought about consistent spontaneous reduction of the dislocation. When this excellent method is not successful, manipulation may be undertaken. The operator should face the patient with the thumbs placed inside the mouth and the lower borders of the mandible grasped on both sides with the fingers. The posterior mandible is depressed, and the symphysis is elevated. This position is held gently but firmly until the condyle slips backward over the articular eminence. At times muscle relaxing drugs and general anesthesia may be required to effect reduction. Occasional patients habitually reappear in emergency departments with a long history of recurrent dislocation of the temporomandibular joint. Such patients may be effectively cured by a simple reconstructive operation that involves the use of a tendon graft to rebuild the torn anterior joint capsule. Many sufferers of chronic dislocation of the jaw are unaware that such relief is available.

Fractures of Membrane Bones of the Face

Central facial bone fractures involve membrane bones that comminute more easily than the mandible when struck, but they are not so difficult to hold in place after reduction because the muscles attaching to them are not of the strength and leverage of those that insert on the mandible. Consequently, reduction usually does not require strong or prolonged fixation. The thinness of membrane bone and the lack of support provided by adjacent paranasal sinuses cause it to respond to a sharp blow by breaking like an eggshell into many tiny fragments that are often difficult to replace. Such fractures occur in well-defined patterns at weak points in membrane bone. They may be considered under the headings of nasal fractures, zygomatic arch fractures, malar compound and orbital bone fractures, and complex transverse middle-face fractures (mid-face mash).

Nasal Fractures. Diagnosis of a nasal fracture is readily made by finding bleeding from the nose, external displacement of the nose, localized bony tenderness, difficulty in breathing or evidence of septal edema and deformity on intranasal speculum examination. Roentgenograms of the nasal bones are of interest but of little value in treatment; they should not be required to determine whether operative reduction of the nose is required. Their importance has been overemphasized since noses that are clinically straight and without septal deformity need no surgical reduction, even if roentgenograms show minor fracture lines. In the presence of massive nasal and paranasal edema, treatment should be postponed for 7 to 10 days. This will permit the swelling to subside and will improve manual palpation of the position of the bones at the time of fracture reduction.

The prominent location of the nose and its relative structural weakness may be responsible for the fact that nasal fractures are more common than any fracture other than fractures of the wrist. Early treatment is quite important since neglect of a nasal bone fracture may result in a deformity that increases slowly over a period of months or years. Such deformities are extremely difficult to correct by later manipulation and often require formal rhinoplasty.

Most nasal fractures should be treated by simple reduction, using only local anesthesia and a lightly padded elevator placed within the nose that will "snap" the bones back into good position. Although nasal fractures are only rarely compounded through the external nasal skin, the vast majority are compounded through the more delicate nasal mucous membranes. This, in fact, is the usual cause of nosebleed with nasal fracture. After reduction of the bones it is both unnecessary and undesirable to attempt suture of the torn mucosa. Some fractures are complicated by extensive compound soft tissue wounds or by crushing forces that also destroy the central maxillary bone foundation on which the nose normally rests. Such injuries create difficult therapeutic problems.

Nasal fractures in children are of particular importance because of the danger of growth arrest or delayed nasal deformity that may follow improper treatment. The small external nares and air passages in children make it difficult to visualize and evaluate septal fractures. In general, *one should assume that a nasal fracture is present in any child bleeding from the nose after injury.* If there is doubt, children with suspected nasal fracture should be given a general anesthesia and a topical vasoconstrictor should be applied to the nasal septal mucosa to permit determination of a possible fracture. If a badly displaced septal fracture is not properly reduced in a child, later growth problems and airway obstruction may be expected. With the aid of a small exploratory septal incision, any displaced section of septal cartilage may be discovered, gently elevated back into place and held in the midline by light nasal packs.

Diagnosis cannot be adequately made of the extent of damage in the fractured nose without shrinking the edematous nasal mucosa with a vasoconstrictor drug. We prefer to use a 10 per cent cocaine hydrochloride solution applied very *sparingly* (8 ml. will moisten four long cotton applicators) as both topical anesthetic and vasoconstrictor. The patient's history should first be carefully checked for drug sensitivity, and intravenous fluids should be started. Proper supportive anesthetic equipment (oxygen, gas machine, intubation tubes and laryngoscope) should be available in the event of a drug reaction. The development of occipital headache or numbness and tingling in the fingers is indication of toxicity and should be followed by discontinuing the use of the local anesthetic and proper supportive measures.

Treatment of nasal fractures is most easily carried out in the first hours after injury. After the mucous membranes have been shrunk and the extent of damage determined, a blunt elevator covered with a protective thin rubber tubing may be used to raise the depressed or deviated fragments. The thumb may then be used to mold the elevated bones into symmetrical positions. Local block and topical anesthesia is always preferred to general anesthesia except in very young children or for complicated injuries. Simple nasal fractures may often be literally "snapped" back into position and then require no splinting or packing. At times the dislocation of the nasal septal cartilage will be automatically reduced when the external nasal pyramid is lifted into proper position. In addition to a simple elevator, the surgeon usually needs only a pair of Asch forceps, a long-bladed

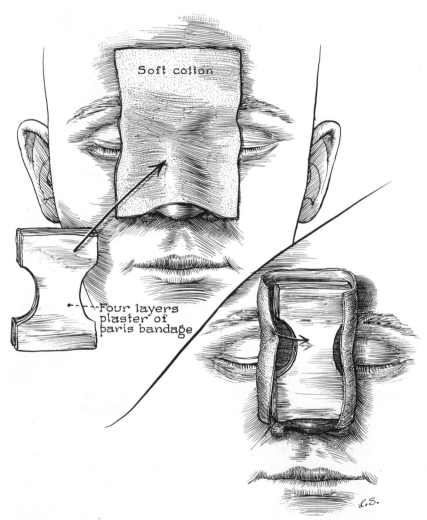

Figure 10–14. *Every surgeon should know how to splint the external nose after reduction of a nasal fracture. Simple materials will provide an excellent splint. One or two thicknesses of soft cotton roll are first placed over the nose after reduction of fracture. Four thicknesses of fast-setting ordinary plaster of Paris may then be cut to relieve pressure over the inner canthus of each eye. The wet plaster is then molded gently to the shape of the underlying glabella and nasal bones. The edges of the cotton are turned upward to protect the skin from the edges of the plaster.*

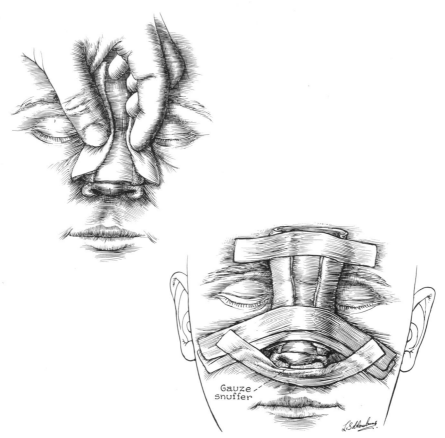

Figure 10–15. *If needed, the surgeon may place two more small strips of plaster along each side of the nose for additional strength in the splint. The fingers are then used to support the plaster in proper position against the bridge until the splint becomes firm. Strips of adhesive are used to secure the splint to the cheeks and the forehead, and a removable gauze snuffer is lightly taped across the end of the nose to control any secretions from the nasal packing. This splint is usually left in place 5 days.*

nasal speculum and a narrow suction tip. Unless nasal fractures are reduced within the first several days following injury, bony fixation may become quite solid, necessitating a formal rhinoplasty for correction. Fixation of most nasal fractures may be provided by combination of light anterior nasal packing and the application of a thin external splint of plaster of Paris (Figs. 10–14 and 10–15), a dental compound or sheet aluminum covered with adhesive.

It is wise to leave the nose packed with gauze only as long as may be required for fixation of the bony parts. Even gauze impregnated with bland ointment creates secondary irritation and edema in the nasal mucous membranes. If such internal splinting is required for more than 4 to 5 days, it is desirable that the gauze be impregnated with an antibiotic in order to minimize the development of infection.

Wide Bridge and Epicanthal Deformities of the Nasal and Infraorbital Region

With many severe blows to the region of the bridge of the nose, the nasal bridge is comminuted, and the thin ethmoid bone of each medial orbital wall is badly crushed and carried posteriorly.

These injuries are often seen in automobile accidents when the face strikes the dashboard or the steering wheel. If the force of the impact is in the region of the glabella above the nasofrontal suture line, the anterior wall of the frontal sinus is often fractured inward. If the impact is somewhat lower, over the nasal bridge, the major displacement is in the interorbital structures. The frontal processes and nasal bones may then be driven backward as a unit between the eyes. The orbital rims are fractured and there is telescoping of the ethmoidal plates and frequently a fracture of the skull base. Cerebrospinal rhinorrhea is common in these injuries. The medial orbital walls are pressed laterally by the force and impinge on the medial rectus muscles. The surgeon's problem is to find a method of reconstructing the bony anterior ethmoidal labyrinth.

In many of these patients the nasofrontal ducts will be obliterated, blocking the frontal sinus. The anterior ethmoidal artery may be lacerated and produce extensive hemorrhage. The trochlea of the superior oblique muscle may be displaced or fractured, producing diplopia, and a high percentage of such patients are left with a deforming traumatic hypertelorism. This type of fracture is one of the most difficult of maxillofacial injuries to correct; and, on many occasions, the plastic surgeon may wish the help of a neurosurgeon to effect correction. In such instances a combined intracranial and extracranial surgical approach may offer many advantages.

If the lacrimal apparatus has been damaged, the discharge of watery tears into the wound may be confused with cerebrospinal fluid, as both will give a test for reducing substances. Clarification may be obtained by placing fluorescein dye in the lumbar subarachnoid space and inserting cotton pledgets within the nose in the sphenoid-ethmoidal recess. If these pledgets are examined with a Wood's light, after 30 minutes the presence of spinal fluid leakage and its location may be established. With such "bridge bashes" it is extremely difficult, by ordinary traction devices or even by lashing lead plate splints against the lateral walls of the nose, to re-elevate the nasal bridge to a normal position and regain a normal shape to the inner canthal regions. In such patients it is of significant help to make small longitudinal incisions anterior to the canthal ligament on either side of the nasion (Fig. 10–25). Through these incisions, the periosteum may be elevated along the medial bony wall of each orbit to expose the fractured ethmoid cells. It may then be possible to gently insert an opened, large, smooth, long-bladed forceps, such as the Asche or Walsham forceps, and gently compress the widened ethmoid bones back to the midline. The two blades of the clamp may be placed superior to the attachment of both internal canthal ligaments and firm pres-

sure can then be exerted in closing the jaws of the clamp. The maneuver is repeated with the blades of the clamp passed inferior to the canthal ligaments.

The forward reduction of the nasal bridge may be further aided if strong anterior traction is applied to a thin padded elevator placed within the nasal cavity alongside the upper nasal septum. If the inner canthal ligaments have been split away from the bony nose, they may be wired to one another across the midline by use of a small drill hole placed through the nasal bridge. This operative reduction of the "bridge bash" seems to be effective only if applied to the face within one week after injury. Within that period it can be very helpful in preventing epicanthus deformity and pseudohypertelorism.

Severe frontal forces applied to the nose may flatten the nasal bones and drive the lacrimal bones and internal palpebral ligaments out of position (the "canthal crush" deformity). Obstruction to the nasolacrimal ducts and to the ostia of the ethmoidal sinuses may result. The cribriform plate and the frontal bone may be damaged. Epiphora and dacryocystitis may result. Permanent pseudohypertelorism may remain and cause a great sense of deformity. Fracture of the quadrilateral cartilage of the nasal septum at its junction with the perpendicular plate of the ethmoid may result in a backward displacement and shortening of the nose, with retraction of the columella and flattening of the upper lip. Subcutaneous emphysema may be present and progressive because of the patient's repeated efforts to use his nasal airway, thus spreading air through the subcutaneous tissues.

At times the severe comminution of the bridge of the nose requires that perforated acrylic or lead plates be applied to the lateral walls of the nose and attached to one another by wires passed across the nasal cavity and out through the holes in the plates. When these wires are tightened the plates draw the bits of nasal and maxillary bone forward and back to the midline, thus narrowing the width of nose and canthus and preventing collapse of the nasal bridge. Rarely, an additional external plaster headcap or skeletal fixation to the cranium is required to provide a stable point anterior to the nose that will allow additional traction to this type of crushed-in nose. When lead plate splinting is used, it should be left on for 10 to 14 days, depending on the amount of comminution with the injury.

Cerebrospinal rhinorrhea may accompany severe nasal fractures. In such circumstances neurosurgical consultation is desirable, but this complication is *not* a contraindication to reduction of nasal or other facial fractures. If the surgeon waits for many days in hopes that this leakage will stop, ultimate reduction of the nasal fracture may be difficult and permanently unsatisfactory. Broad spectrum antibiotics should be given as long as spinal fluid leak continues in order to reduce the danger of meningitis.

Hematomas should not be allowed to remain within the tissues of the nasal septum since they may be followed by narrowing of the airway and progressive deformity of the nose.

The removal of the hematoma requires the shrinking of the edematous mucous membranes. After this shrinkage, a short vertical incision is made through the septal mucosa at the anterior margin of the clot. The latter is then lifted out with a suction tip and all blood is removed from the pocket by irrigation. A careful search is made for any bleeding points. Electrocautery is used to coagulate any open vessels. Care is taken to leave the septal cartilage intact. If it is fractured and displaced it should be repositioned. The incision is loosely sutured and a nasal pack is placed to hold the membranes snugly against the cartilage. Septal work of this type is greatly aided by the use of a headlight. A failure to discover and remove one of these clots may also result in infection, abscess and even septal perforation. There is a tendency for septal hematomas to recur, and the nose should be inspected at reasonable intervals following evacuation of such a clot.

Zygomatic Arch Fractures. Zygomatic arch fractures usually result from direct localized blows just anterior to the ear. When the major part of the malar compound is not fractured, a segment of the arch may be carried inward, producing pain on opening of the jaws and some degree of trismus (Fig. 10–16A). Such fractures may be diagnosed on palpation unless there is extensive associated hematoma or edema. There is point ten-

derness over the arch, and the patient has reduced lateral movements of the lower jaw. The roentgenogram most useful to demonstrate this fracture is a submental-vertical projection of the zygomatic arches. The tube is placed beneath the patient's chin, and the emulsion plate is put behind the occiput and held parallel to the zygomatic arches. The film should be deliberately underexposed to obtain the best detail.

The most popular treatment for zygomatic arch fractures is the approach of Gillies, Kilner and Stone.[9] Some of the hair is shaved in the temple region. A one-inch incision is made, down to and including all of the temporal fascia, to expose temporal muscle fibers. A heavy, long elevator is then passed downward along these muscle fibers until its tip is felt suddenly to dip medially beneath the fractured zygomatic arch. By using a roll of gauze against the side of the head as a fulcrum, the operator elevates laterally the depressed bony fragment; usually he can feel it "click" into place. If a fracture is unstable, it may be retained in a good lateral position by passing a single circumferential wire around the arch and attaching it to an arched and rigid suspension bridge that rests on the temporal bone superiorly and the angle of the mandible inferiorly (Fig. 10–16 B and D). Such support should be maintained for approximately 10 days to establish union. During this period the patient may be allowed to chew soft food.

Fractures of the Malar Compound and Orbital Bones. MALAR COMPOUND. The zygoma or malar compound is a dense bone forming the prominence of the cheek. It has four major "arms" or processes. These articulate with the frontal, maxillary and temporal bones and with the greater wing of the sphenoid bone. The junctions with the sphenoid and zygomatic process of the temporal bone are weak and easily fractured. The medial surface of the zygoma helps to form the greater portion of the lateral floor of the orbit and contributes to the lateral superior wall of the maxillary sinus. Fractures of the malar bone are present in two thirds of all middle-face fractures. The malar bone is usually fractured along with any adjacent articulating bone. When the zygoma is displaced, it usually produces fractures of the orbit, the anterior and lateral walls of the maxillary

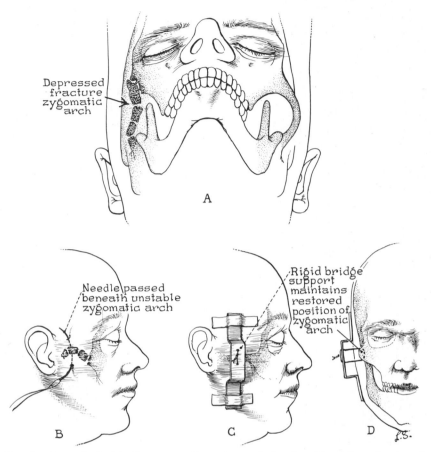

Figure 10–16. *Fractures limited to the zygomatic arch usually involve at least three fracture lines. The swelling and displacement may impinge on the underlying coronoid process of the mandible, causing pain when the jaw is opened. Most of these fractures can be reduced simply by the classic approach of Gillies. This involves passing an elevator beneath the fracture by means of a small incision within the hairline. At times the arch fragments will not remain stable in the reduced position, and this simple device using a bridge splint will maintain the position without undue discomfort to the patient. The wire and splint are usually removed after a 10-day period.*

antrum, the zygomatic process of the temporal bone, and separations of the zygomaticofrontal and zygomaticosphenoid suture lines.

Knight and North[11] have made a most useful classification of zygoma fractures. Based on their studies, there are six common types of malar bone fractures:

1. One in 20 fractures of the malar compound shows no significant displacement, and treatment is not required.
2. One in 10 involves only the zygomatic arch (Fig. 10–17). In this fracture pattern there are typically three fracture lines of the arch, with a "buckling-in" of the fragments.
3. One third of malar compound fractures produce unrotated fractures of the body of the zygoma (Fig. 10–17*B*), with displacement di-

rectly into the antrum (backward, inward and slightly downward).

4. One in 10 fractures of the malar compound is *medially* rotated (Fig. 10–17*C*). The left malar compound in such injuries is thus rotated counterclockwise (or clockwise in the case of a fracture of the right malar compound) when viewed from the front. Examination of the Water's view roentgenogram shows apparent downward displacement at the infraorbital margin.

5. One fifth of the malar compound fractures are *laterally* rotated and apparently caused by blows below the horizontal axis of the bone (Fig. 10–17*D*). When such fractures involve the left malar compound it appears to be rotated clockwise when viewed from the front (i.e., away from the midline). On roentgenogram with the Water's view, these fractures often ap-

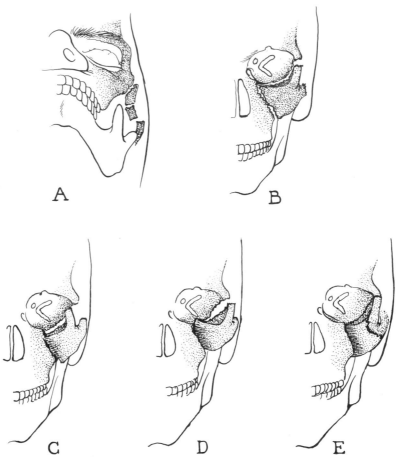

Figure 10–17. *Simple classification of displaced fractures of the zygomatic compound: One tenth involve the arch only (A), one third show inward or downward displacement without rotation (B), one tenth show medial rotation of the upper part of the zygoma toward the midline (C), one fifth are rotated laterally (D), and one fifth are complicated by additional fractures of the central heavy portion of the malar bone (E). These various types of fracture may be readily determined on examination and x-ray, and their recognition is of considerable help in planning operative reductions.*

pear to be displaced upward at the infraorbital margin.

6. Finally, about one fifth of the malar compound fractures are complicated by additional fracture lines through the dense bone of the main fragment (Fig. 10–17E).

Most fractures of the zygomatic compound tear the lining of the maxillary sinus and cause hematoma within the sinus cavity. Ecchymosis and subconjunctival hemorrhage are almost pathognomonic of facial bone fracture. The lateral palpebral ligament is attached to the zygomatic portion of the orbital rim. It may be significantly displaced with zygoma fractures and, if the bone is not replaced, a downward and lateral deformity of the external canthus of the eye is produced.[8] Similarly, the orbital

septum is drawn inferiorly by any downward displacement of the malar compound and infraorbital rim. This will produce a permanent widening of the eyelids with epiphora and lower lid deformity.

Diagnostic features of fractures of the zygoma include flattening of the cheekbone, depression in level of the globe, diplopia, downward displacement of the lateral palpebral ligament, downward retraction of the lower eyelid, subconjunctival hematoma or unilateral epistaxis. Numbness of one half of the upper lip and palpable irregularity, displacement or tenderness of the orbital rim (Fig. 10–3C) will often be present. If the index finger is passed behind the upper lip and used to palpate the anterior wall of the antrum, bony irregularities may be detected with many zygomatic fractures. A stereo-Water's roentgenogram of the face will usually provide all the needed radiographic information for surgical management of this fracture. Occasionally, tomograms taken through portions of the bony orbital walls will be of help in determining fracture lines or herniations into the ethmoids or antrum. Clouding of the antrum is commonly seen and usually represents collected hematoma. Such clots will usually liquefy and spontaneously drain out into the nasal cavity if the antral drainage is not blocked at the ostium by bone impaction. Anesthesia of the infraorbital nerve with numbness of the upper lip is commonly a diagnostic feature with malar compound fractures. Delay in relieving the pressure of fractured bone on the nerve (often at its emergence from the infraorbital foramen) may result in permanent anesthesia or even severe facial neuralgia.

ORBITAL BONES. Diplopia and orbital floor fractures accompany middle-face fractures in over 25 per cent of the cases. "Double-vision" will prove to be transient in about one third, with eye symptoms disappearing within one week along with the absorption of intraorbital hemorrhage and edema; in about one third the difficulty will persist; and in about one third the problem will appear late and will persist. Diplopia may result from several mechanisms:

1. Loss of bony support of the floor of the orbit with downward displacement of the origin of the inferior oblique muscle and the globe.
2. Increase in total volume or capacity of the bony orbit, producing relative enophthalmus and ineffective extraocular muscle control.
3. Anchoring of the inferior rectus muscle in a fracture line of the orbital floor, thus limiting eye movement (especially in upward rotation of the eye). This may be diagnosed by the "forced duction test." The conjunctiva is first anesthetized. The insertion of the inferior rectus muscle is then grasped through the conjunctiva with toothed forceps and an attempt is made to roll the eyeball upward. If the muscle is entrapped in the fracture, this movement will be prevented.
4. Herniation of orbital fat into the antrum through a fracture line in the orbital floor. This herniation of tissue may increase progressively over a period of days or weeks following injury. The movements of the eye seem to massage

orbital fat down through the fracture line. Edema or hematoma within the orbital box may raise orbital pressure and help to extrude additional material into the antrum. Serial tomograms of the antrum will show this increasing displacement in some untreated patients.
5. Partial or complete paralysis of cranial motor nerves that supply the extraocular muscles may result, on *rare* occasions, from direct injury of the original trauma.
6. An increase in volume of orbital contents may appear if hematoma and fibrosis develop within the lateral and inferior bony walls of the orbit. This may produce proptosis and marked limitation of eye muscle movement. Such hematomas have also been associated with nerve palsies of the extraocular muscles that recover only after the clot is removed.
7. Dislocation of the lens of the eye and tears of the iris may produce a form of "monocular" diplopia.

All these mechanisms of producing diplopia create some form of muscle imbalance. Merely dropping the level of the globe produces diplopia by causing an associated abnormal stretch, tear, palsy or ankylosis of one or more extraocular muscles. In many instances diplopia associated with orbital floor fractures will not appear until several days, or even weeks, after injury. The initial support of the globe by traumatic edema may mask incipient double vision for as long as 6 to 8 weeks. At this late date, replacement of the fractured fragments is impossible and the eye function and facial deformity may be corrected only by major complex plastic operations involving bone grafting or synthetic implants (Fig. 10–20 A to C). There is thus good reason to attempt to detect *all* orbit floor fractures during the first few days after injury.

There are two basic types of orbital bone fractures: pure blowout fractures and complex orbital fractures associated with middle face fractures.

The simple blowout is thought to occur from a sudden blow directly on the closed eye, suddenly forcing the globe inward and splintering the thin floor of the orbit by the sudden increase in intraorbital pressure without causing other facial fractures. Often this injury will also cause outfractures of the lateral wall of the orbit and drive the anterior ethmoid bones toward the midline. All of these changes tend to enlarge the total volume of the bony orbit and lead to enophthalmus. Although not

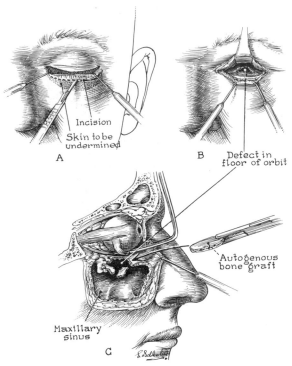

Incision

Skin to be undermined

A

B *Defect in floor of orbit*

Autogenous bone graft

Maxillary sinus

C

Figure 10–18. This simple method of exploration of the floor of the orbit should be utilized in all cases with clinical signs suggestive of a possible fracture to the bony floor of the orbit. The incision should be placed only 2 to 3 mm. below the lash border rather than at a lower level in the eyelid. The orbicularis oculi muscle fibers are gently separated, and the periosteum elevated from the floor of the orbit. An effort should be made not to enter the mucous membrane of the antral cavity. If a defect is encountered in the orbital floor, any completely loose bone fragments in the antrum (C) should be removed and the defect repaired by rotating long orbital floor bone fragments to bridge the opening or by replacement with an autogenous iliac bone graft or a synthetic material such as silicone. Such a procedure will often prevent the late development of diplopia several weeks after the injury. If the defect is left unrepaired, movements of the globe tend to cause the migration of fat and other soft tissue into the antrum with resulting enophthalmus.

rare, *this type of fracture is much less common than the orbital fracture associated with other facial fractures.*

There are five cardinal signs that should lead one to suspect an orbital bone fracture:

1. Bony deformity and tenderness of infraorbital, or canthal, regions on palpation.
2. Subconjunctival hemorrhage and discoloration of the eyelids.
3. Infraorbital nerve anesthesia of over 24 hours' duration.
4. A measurably lowered position of the center of the pupil of one eye in comparison with the other.
5. Early diplopia (this may disappear after a few hours only to return later). In some patients it may be detected only when the eyes are placed in a single position of gaze.

A surgical exploration of the orbital floor is indicated by the appearance of *any* of these signs (Fig. 10–18).

Nicholson and Guzak[16] in 1971 suggested that suspected blowout fractures of the orbit need not be explored and that function would be good on conservative management. This approach is refuted by the significant numbers of patients who seek help each year after conservative manage-

ment of these fractures. Diplopia and enophthalmus are the commonest symptoms and plastic surgeons find the *late* correction of these problems to be much more difficult than at the time of initial injury. There are additional diagnostic studies of value:

1. Tomograms of the orbit may show disruptions of the orbital floor or medial wall.
2. Orbitograms may be made by injecting a few milliliters of radiopaque material along the orbital floor and trying to determine if this material leaks through a fracture line. Although of considerable interest, this technique produces both false positive and false negative results. Since orbital floor exploration has proved to be a safe, simple procedure that may be carried out under local anesthesia and with no residual deformity, it remains the most dependable method of establishing the diagnosis of many orbital bone fractures. Certainly the most serious present-day problems associated with zygoma fractures are *associated with the failure to suspect and discover orbital fractures at an early postinjury date.* Routine orbital exploration is advisable in all suspected cases and will uncover many correctable problems. We have twice encountered a sharp bone spicule displaced from the floor of the orbit, standing vertically, and pressing its sharp edge deeply into the sclera. Later perforation of the globe might

well have occurred in either or both of these cases had routine exploration not been carried out.

Because of the frequency of missed diagnosis of orbital fractures on clinical and roentgenographic studies, it is now our practice to *expose the orbital floor in all cases of suspected orbital bone fracture.* (See section on treatment.)

TREATMENT OF FRACTURES OF THE ZYGOMATIC COMPOUND AND ORBITAL BONES. Treatment of these fractures varies greatly and depends on the stability or instability of the bone fragments following reduction. Unrotated fractures of the malar compound, like fractures of the zygomatic arch, tend to be relatively stable on reduction. Many will remain in good position as a result of the support offered by normal muscular attachments to the bone and by impaction of the fragments at the time of reduction. Certain types of fractures consistently require supplementary fixation after reduction. These include laterally rotated fractures of the body of the malar compound, fractures involving the dense central eminence of the malar compound, and unrotated fractures with gross medial displacement and extensive impaction and comminution of bone.

Until recent years, support and fixation of zygoma and antral fractures was obtained commonly by the use of folded gauze packing placed within the antrum by means of the traditional Caldwell-Luc exposure. This approach involves an incision behind the upper lip in the canine fossa and the removal of a bony window from the anterior antral wall. Although this method of antral packing gives adequate bony support, the reductions are inexact and morbidity is greater than with newer methods. Late complications that have been reported after antral packing include diplopia, malunion, residual facial deformity on subsidence of edema, and even blindness from pressure of the pack against the optic nerve. Antral secretions tend to be blocked from egress; temperature elevations and persistent facial edema may be related to packing; thin bony fragments of the antral wall or orbital floor are sometimes distracted from one another by overpacking or they may later be pulled out of position by catching on the pack at the time of its removal. Thickening of the antral mucosa is a common sequel of this method of management. Such complications may be largely eliminated by newer methods of direct wire fixation of bony fragments.

Antral packs are of historical interest, but our experience has been similar to that reported in 1964 by Dingman and Natvig.[6] We have also encountered many instances of zygomatic fractures in which antral packing and methods of closed reduction have failed to secure ideal replacement of bony parts. When such fractures are treated by open reduction, it becomes apparent that roentgenographic and clinical examinations frequently fail to reveal the degree of displacement. Open reduction and direct wiring of displacements of the zygoma may be carried out through the associated facial lacerations or small esthetic incisions.[4, 17] *This "jigsaw puzzle concept" of replacing facial fractures and attaching each piece of bone to its neighbor with fine wire probably constitutes one of the greatest twentieth century advances in the treatment of maxillofacial injuries.* The wiring should be based on some remaining portion of the skull that is stable and unfractured, and the surgeon should then wire the more mobile fragments.

To expose fractures of the orbital floor, a single incision is made about 3 mm. below the lash border of the lower eyelid (Fig. 10–18A). Since 1971 a number of plastic surgeons have advocated exploring the orbit by means of an incision made through the *conjunctival* surface of the lower lid. This incision is approximately 10 mm. below the border of the lower lid and extends across its entire width. A quite adequate exposure of the bony floor of the orbit is obtained in this manner, and it avoids the need for external lid scars and separation of the fibers of the orbicularis muscle within the lid. The incision is closed with three 6–0 plain catgut sutures, and the subciliary skin incision shown in Figure 10–18 may be avoided. The conjunctival incision does not give quite the wide exposure offered by the subciliary approach and the orbital fat may be troublesome. For these reasons, many surgeons still prefer to approach the orbit through a skin incision at the subciliary level — or even at the lower margin of the eyelid at the level of the infraorbital rim. The healing of these skin incisions is excellent as long as they remain within the thin skin of the true eyelid. If actual wiring of fractures along the orbital rim is required, the skin incision in the lid is preferable to one through the conjunctiva. It is a matter of only a few minutes' dissection to separate the orbicularis muscle fibers, incise the orbital septum and elevate the periosteum of the orbital floor (Fig. 10–18B). The surgeon may then detect displacements in this region far more accurately than is possible by tomograms, planograms or orbitograms. Such explorations are benign surgical procedures with the fine line scar hidden in a normal eyelid crease.

When large sections of the orbital floor are missing or badly crushed, some support must be provided to prevent ptosis of the globe into the antrum. The use of a thin sliver of autogenous bone from the patient's iliac crest is highly satisfactory (Fig. 10–18C). When the patient's nose is undamaged, the quadrilateral cartilage of the nose or even autogenous conchal cartilage from the ear may be used to repair the orbital floor. Recently thin sheets of Teflon, silicone or synthetic collagen have been substituted for the bone. These synthetic materials give adequate support but they have a tendency to migrate or extrude because of their nonadherent surfaces. If used, they should never exceed 30 mm. in AP depth and they should always be perforated and anchored in position to the orbital bone with nonabsorbable sutures. Synthetic implants are best avoided when there are large losses of the mucous membrane lining to the roof of the antral cavity. When they are inserted without adequate soft tissue cover, draining sinus tracts will form, leading into the antrum or orbit or out through the eyelid skin.

With acute simple inward and downward displacements of the malar compound, it is sometimes possible to reduce the fracture by passing a curved metal blunt urethral No. 18 sound through the thin medial bony wall of the antrum in the area just beneath the inferior nasal turbinate (Fig. 10–19A). The tip of this sound may then be used to elevate the dense central portion of the malar compound, forcing it outward to match the bony contour of the opposite cheek. This will produce effective reduction, especially in the case of an unrotated fracture of the zygomatic compound (Fig. 10–19 B and C). In most instances, this form of reduction should be combined with small skin incisions placed beneath the lower eyelid and at the frontal suture. These incisions permit direct interosseous wiring and secure the fragments in a reduced position.

If reduction is not effected within a few hours, severe facial edema or the condition of the patient may complicate immediate reduction and make it advisable to utilize local hypothermia (ice packs) and defer operation for several days. It is unwise to let the patient go without fracture reduction for more than 2 weeks following injury, lest the zygoma become firmly fixed in a position of malunion. McCoy et al.[14] have wisely pointed out the dangers and disadvantages of using the traditional Caldwell-Luc incision (made through the mucosa of the canine fossa behind the upper lip) and of placing gauze packing into the antrum postoperatively. Most plastic surgeons avoid using this approach whenever possible. Eyebrows should not be shaved nor eyelashes trimmed in carrying out reductions of facial fractures. Occasional patients have considerable difficulty in regrowing these specialized types of hair.

It is frequently possible to reduce bleeding during the reduction of facial fractures by injecting the fracture sites with small amounts of local anesthetic containing epinephrine solution 1:120,000. Once the bone fragments are loosened, fixation of the zygoma should begin with its reattachment to the firm zygomatic process of the frontal bone by a single steel wire placed through holes drilled on either side of this suture line. Attention is then turned to the fracture lines located along the infraorbital rim. Again, small drill holes are made with a power drill on either side of the fracture line and a steel wire loop is placed to fix the medial end of the fragment. The zygomaticofrontal incision may next be used to insert a long elevator behind the zygomaticotemporal process to elevate and further rotate this process outward and upward. If the arch of the zygoma is also fractured with these injuries, it may be reduced with fine wire sutures by means of a small direct transverse incision over the fracture line or by the method shown in Figure 10–16. Fractures of the floor of the orbit are always present when the zygoma is fractured.

At times the collection of blood and

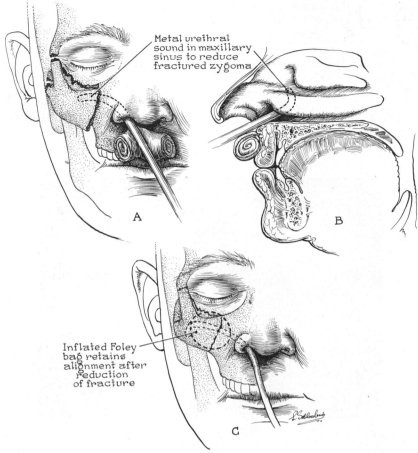

Figure 10–19. *Early nonrotated fractures of the zygoma may at times be effectively reduced by the simple insertion of a metal urethral sound through the thin medial wall of the antrum by means of the nasal cavity. The tip of the sound may then be directed up beneath the solid central portion of the malar bone and a leverage action brought to bear against the bone from within. The roll of gauze acts as a fulcrum to protect the upper lip, and strong outward force can then be brought to bear on the zygoma. At times the bone will actually be heard to "click" back into place. If the zygoma does not remain stable in the reduced position, a Foley bag catheter can be inserted by the same route and the bag inflated until the bone receives adequate support.*

bone fragments within the antrum makes it necessary to explore and debride this cavity. In such instances the Caldwell-Luc exposure through the canine fossa is satisfactory. In opening the antrum, an attempt should be made to retain soft tissue attachments to as much as possible of the bone of the anterior antral wall. Careful irrigation of the cavity and removal of clots will often reveal that much of the antral mucous membrane may be preserved.

In former years many complex headcaps were devised for stabilizing zygomatic and nasal fractures. These have proved to be rarely desirable or necessary in reducing fractures of the zygomatic compound. It is the exceptional patient who benefits from this type of fixation today. In the case of zygomatic compound fractures that remain unstable after direct interosseous wiring

and reduction, the suspension wire technique originally described by Adams[1] is of great value (Fig. 10–23). When the zygomatic compound is not repositioned within the first 2 weeks after injury, it is sometimes very difficult to loosen the bone fragments at the time of the delayed operation. In such cases, very complex late reconstructive procedures, including contour bone grafting and multiple osteotomies, may be required. Even then the result is likely to be only partly satisfactory.

In recent years it has been possible to correct double vision in approximately 80 per cent of patients with persistent traumatic diplopia that resulted from improperly reduced zygomatic compound and orbital floor fractures. This has been achieved at The Johns Hopkins Hospital and at the University of Virginia by means of surgical restoration of lost orbital contents and globe support through use of wedges of the iliac bone or silicone rubber to lift and position the eye (Fig. 10–20 A to D). Although bone is well tolerated, it will sometimes show slow absorption over a period of years and allow some recurrence of deformity. Silicone will not absorb and better methods of fixation have made this

material increasingly successful in correcting diplopia. A careful ophthalmologic consultation is desirable to rule out associated paralysis of extraocular muscles before undertaking the correction of "displacement diplopia" resulting from skeletal malposition with "dropped globe" or from fixation of the inferior rectus muscle in the orbital floor fracture line.

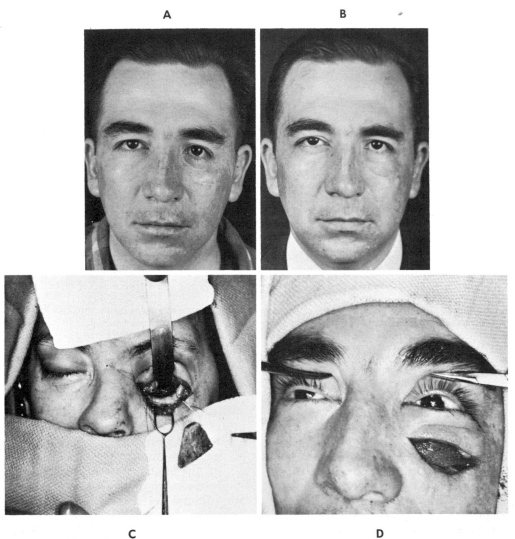

A

B

C

D

Figure 10–20. *This patient had had a fracture of the zygomatic compound with incomplete early reduction, which resulted in the drooping of left lower eyelid and dropping of the globe shown in A. He had troublesome double vision that prevented him from carrying out his occupation as an airplane pilot. Elevation of the left globe and complete relief of the diplopia was achieved 2½ years after the injury by means of bony reconstruction of the left orbit. C shows the badly displaced infraorbital rim at exploration. The periosteum was elevated, and approximately 8 cc. of iliac bone was fitted in along the inferior and lateral walls of the orbit in order to provide additional volume of orbital content. This tended to correct the existing enophthalmus and to stretch forward the cone of extraocular muscles once again. It was firmly wired into position with two steel wires. D indicates the usual amount of over-correction allowed in obtaining the level of the globe. Many complex late plastic repairs could be avoided by a more aggressive approach to reconstruction of the bony orbit at the time of the primary injury. The final result is shown in B. The diplopia was corrected, and the patient is now active as a pilot.*

Fractures of the Maxillae (Middle-Face Fractures)

Incidence. The upper jaw is formed by the two maxillae and the paired palatine bone. At The Johns Hopkins Hospital, fractures of the upper jaw occur about one third as commonly as fractures of the mandible. These fractures are known in Canada by the colorful term "mid-face mash."[8] The ability of the maxillae to absorb great energy in the process of fracturing offers considerable protection to the cranium and its contents. It is a particularly common injury following crashes in automobiles or planes where the passengers must sit facing forward. There has been a strange reluctance of designers of commercial airplanes to face seats rearward despite increasing evidence that this position will greatly reduce injuries on crash. As with the membrane bones of the face, secondary muscle contraction and spasm play only a very small role in the displacement of maxillary fractures; the original impact produces the entire deformity.

Classification. In 1900 René LeFort[13] carried out classic experiments to determine the portions of greatest weakness within the maxilla. His work has resulted in a classification of fractures of the maxilla that is now widely used.

LeFort carried out over 40 experiments, mostly upon cadavers, inflicting trauma to the face and studying the resulting nature of fractures. He concluded:

Fractures of the face, although they are not frequent, nevertheless are much less rare than we have thought and most of them are not discovered by the physician. And . . . quite rarely, nevertheless, the base of the cranium is involved in these fractures. This hardly ever occurs except by bilateral compression of the head, that is, by pressure applied not only to the cranium but also to the face. In such cases, the cranium may be fractured. One almost always notices the independence of the cranium from the face at the pterygoid apophyses and at the lateral plates of the ethmoid which, anatomically, being rather to the face than to the cranium, and which adhere to the maxilla. . . . The most frequent fracture which we have obtained in our experiments corresponds to the great transverse fracture of Guérin. It includes the roof of the palate, the alveolar ridge, and the pterygoid apophyses.

Surgeons and dentists alike have tried to treat fractures of the maxilla with a multi-plicity of external appliances to hold these bones in position. Only in recent years, with the advent of the surgical publications by Milton Adams,[1] Reed Dingman,[6] Frederick McCoy[14] and others, has direct surgical reduction replaced the external appliance methods. The most widely used classification is based on LeFort's early studies.

LEFORT I FRACTURES (transverse maxillary fractures of Guérin). This is a transverse fracture in which the fractured segment contains the upper teeth, the palate, lower portions of the pterygoid processes, and a portion of the wall of the maxillary sinus (Fig. 10–21).

LEFORT II FRACTURES (pyramidal fractures). In these fractures the fractured fragment also contains the nasal bones and the frontal processes of the maxilla (Fig. 10–22). The fracture lines usually run through the lacrimal bones and inferior rim of the orbit, continuing downward near the zygomaticomaxillary suture. The fracture line then extends beneath the malar bone toward the pterygomaxillary fossa. This often produces significant widening of the inner canthus of the eyes, epicanthal deformity of the bridge of the nose and destruction of the ethmoidal sinus cells.

LEFORT III FRACTURES (craniofacial

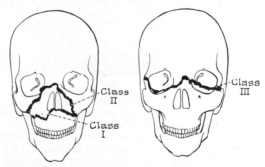

Figure 10–21. *The three major patterns of fracture line seen in middle face fractures were first described by LeFort in 1900 and often assume one of the three classifications shown here. The class I fracture is also known as a transverse maxillary fracture or a Guérin fracture. The class II fracture usually includes the nose in the mobile central fragment and is known often as a pyramidal fracture. The class III fracture includes also both zygomatic compounds in the mobile fragment and is referred to frequently as a craniofacial disjunction. At times, there may be two or three of these classic patterns in a single patient. They represent the lines of least strength in the facial bone skeleton.*

A

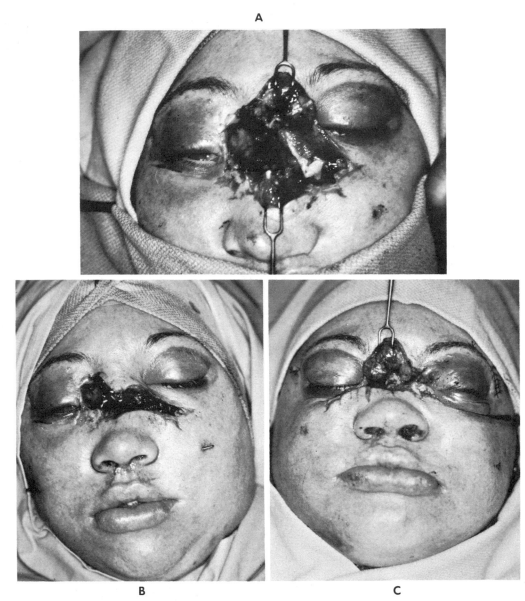

B   C

Figure 8–22. *This young woman was thrown into the steering post of her car in a head-on collision and suffered a severe midface mash, with pyramidal fractures involving the bridge of the nose and left side of the right eye and the marked loss of bone in the region of the nasal bridge and ethmoids. Initial hemorrhage was difficult to control even with packing. In B arch bars have been applied, and the teeth are in good occlusion. The multiple maxillary and antral fractures have been further stabilized by a transverse Kirschner wire pin as advocated by Brown. The eye is still unsupported, and the central face is still elongated. In C a craniomaxillary suspension wire has been applied on the right side (see Fig. 10–23), and the mobile central face has been lifted upward to restore the normal relationship between eyes and mouth. The soft tissue wounds were then repaired primarily, and a later bone graft to the bridge of the nose restored facial balance.*

disjunction). In this fracture, the maxilla, nasal bones and zygomatic compound are all separated as a unit from the cranial attachments (Fig. 10–21). Such injuries usually involve multiple additional fractures within this large mobile segment and, on healing, the patient will be troubled by severe elongation deformity of the central face unless vigorous measures are taken to combat this during early treatment (Fig. 10–23).

In addition to the three major types of LeFort fractures, one may see vertical or segmental fractures through the maxilla that may separate portions of the central face near the midline. Fractures may also occur horizontally through portions of the upper alveolar ridge, or the entire maxilla may be driven upward and backward into the interorbital space.

Diagnosis. Middle-face fractures often produce dish-face deformities in which the patient develops an elongation of the vertical distance between the lips and the eyes. If the surgeon has not seen the patient prior to the injury he may fail to recognize this facial elongation, especially in the presence of severe facial edema.

Malocclusion, involving open-bite de-formity and considerable conjunctival and labial edema, may be seen. Mobility of the maxilla is a cardinal feature of such fractures and may be detected by the examiner's ability to move the anterior hard palate and alveolus manually (Fig. 10–3). Severely impacted fractures may lack this mobility. Malocclusion is not always present, even in the presence of complete craniofacial disjunction, and the surgeon should not be falsely reassured by finding good dental occlusion. The appearance of a watery fluid issuing from the nostrils and having a salty

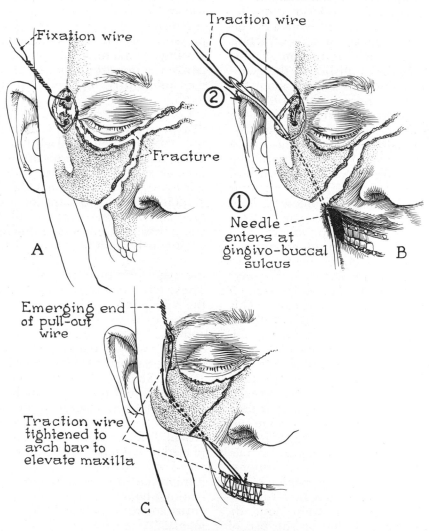

Figure 10–23. *For a unilateral or bilateral LeFort III fracture, a method is needed to secure the central face firmly against the base of the skull to avoid facial elongation. This method of craniofacial suspension is of great value. The zygomaticofrontal suture line is first reunited with steel wire and drill holes, fixing the zygoma firmly to the nonfractured frontal bone. A double loop of steel wire is then passed through the drill hole in the frontal bone and drawn subcutaneously behind the zygoma to emerge in the buccogingival sulcus as shown in B. An arch bar may then be applied to the upper arch, and the two ends of the suspension wire are passed about this arch bar at an appropriate location to provide strong upward and lateral traction to the central bony fragments of the face. After 3 weeks the ends of the wire are cut free of the arch bar behind the upper lip, and the pull-out wire in the region of the brow is used to withdraw the entire suspension wire loop.*

taste to the patient should suggest damage to the cribriform plate. Steroscopic roentgenograms in the Water's position provide an excellent x-ray view for visualizing these fractures. Planograms, using an eccentrically moving source of roentgen rays, may give beautiful bone detail. One should look for disruptions of the frontomaxillary sutures, step irregularities in the infraorbital regions or breaks in the continuity of the lateral wall of the sinus.

Treatment. A severe mid-face mash may produce severe upper respiratory obstruction by impaction of palatal and maxillary bone posteriorly and inferiorly into the oropharynx; as concomitant edema develops in the supraglottic area, obstruction increases. Emergency reduction of this fracture may be accomplished by the examiner if he will hook his fingers about the displaced posterior border of the soft palate and pull forward the fractured bones of the central face. This maneuver may simultaneously establish both the diagnosis and the patient's airway. Hemorrhage can be severe with maxillary fracture because of rupture of the internal maxillary or greater palatine arteries. Massive bleeding from the nose in these patients is usually from multiple tears in the highly vascular mucous membranes of the septum or nasal turbinates. This bleeding may be controlled by inserting a one-inch diameter gauze behind the soft palate and drawing it forward against the posterior choanae. This pack is placed in the nasopharynx with the aid of two rubber catheters passed through the nasal cavity along each side of the septum to emerge in the oropharynx. The pharyngeal tips of the catheters are then grasped by a clamp and are drawn forward through the lips. Each catheter tip is then secured with a heavy silk suture to one end of a wide postnasal pack. The latter is then pulled into the posterior choanae by traction on the nasal catheters. Additional packing of the nose or even ligation of the external carotid arteries may be required.

Middle-face fractures were formerly managed in many clinics by the use of plaster headcaps, external pin fixation and elaborate dental splints. Greater experience has shown these to be unnecessarily complicated, unsatisfactory in securing reduction and unpleasant to the patient. In recent years, the concept of open surgical exposure and direct fitting together of the

pieces of the bony puzzle has gained widespread acceptance. The combined use of interosseous wiring and suspension sling support has markedly improved the results in the treatment of these complex facial fractures. When the mandibular arch is intact, LeFort I (transverse maxillary) fractures may be reduced, and occlusion may be restored, by applying arch bars to upper and lower jaws (Fig. 10–7). To avoid elongation of the middle-face, two wires are then placed through drill holes in each infraorbital rim. The wires are next passed downward through the subcutaneous tissue of the cheeks to emerge in the buccogingival sulcus. The maxilla is firmly pressed superiorly into normal position, closing the fracture lines, and the two suspension wires are tightened about an arch bar previously applied to the upper teeth.

LeFort II fractures (Fig. 10–21) are often displaced posteriorly and require a loosening of the fragments and a bringing forward of the maxillae if the teeth are to regain normal occlusion. Again, intermaxillary wiring and arch bars may be applied if sufficient teeth remain for fixation. In most LeFort II fractures, maxillary suspension wires may be passed downward subcutaneously from anchoring drill holes or wire loops that have been placed through the zygomatic process of the frontal bone. These wires emerge through the mucosa in the sulcus behind the upper lip, and there they may be twisted securely to the upper arch bar. As the wires are tightened, the dental line will rise and the central face will again shorten to its normal length (Fig. 10–23). Small pullout wire loops can be passed around the upper anchor points of these suspension wires to aid in their removal after approximately 3 weeks. Individual transosseous wire loops may be placed through tiny drill holes at any other major fracture lines (especially along the infraorbital rims or at fracture lines of the lacrimal bones). These provide further security and reduction of the lesser bone fragments.

LeFort III (craniofacial disjunction) fractures require combination methods of fixation because of the multiple fracture lines that involve the nasal bones, the zygoma, the maxillae and, often, the palatine bones. Such combinations make use of the usually intact frontal bone for application of craniofacial suspension wires (Fig. 10–23). If intact, the mandibular arch (or one restored by open reduction and wiring) is used as a guide to positioning of the maxillary fragments for proper occlusion. The surgeon must remember that simple wiring of the teeth in the fractured upper jaw to the teeth in an intact mandible may restore perfect dental occlusion, but *leave uncorrected an associated elongation of the central face.* Edema may obscure this deformity initially, but if it is not recognized and treated early, the patient will have a distressing "dish-face" deformity. *The late correction of this deformity is both complex and unsatisfactory in contrast to the excellent results that may be obtained with good emergency management* (Fig. 10–24).

In the event that the mandibular arch is also fractured, it should be realigned by open reduction and direct interosseous wiring in order to provide a proper lower arch as a guidline for the establishment of occlusion in positioning the upper arch bone fragments. Thus, if the surgeon will

follow an orderly plan in facial reductions, working from nonfractured stable bony points to unstable areas, he may be able to replace the pieces of the puzzle quite satisfactorily. In the absence of dentition, if the patient possesses an intact denture, the surgeon may fasten this to the upper or lower jaw by circumferential or direct osseous wiring. The denture may then be drilled to permit the attachment of an ordinary arch bar and utilized much like the patient's remaining natural teeth in securing a normal bite relationship.

Fractures of Frontal Bone and Sinus

In cases of frontal sinus fracture, surgeons formerly recommended that all sinus membrane be removed and that the bony cavity be collapsed inward. This technique of "obliteration of the sinus" is almost always unnecessary and is quite deforming.

When the anterior wall of the frontal sinus has been fractured, care should be

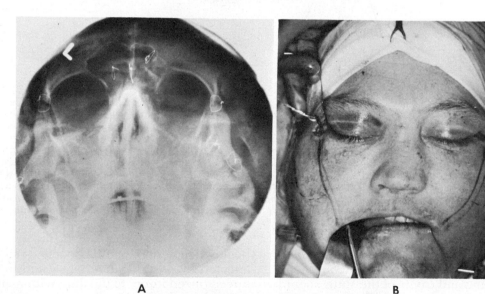

A **B**

Figure 10–24. *Complete craniofacial disjunction occurred in this patient when he was forced to make a crash landing in his private plane and was thrown forcefully against a padded panel. The x-ray shows multiple fracture lines involving bilateral class I, II and III LeFort fractures. The nose was also badly fractured. The mandibular arch was broken in three places, but no major facial lacerations occurred! Reduction was secured by the application of arch bars and intermaxillary elastic traction, by multiple transosseous wiring of the frontal and zygomatic bones, and by bilateral craniomaxillary suspension wires attached to the upper arch bar as shown in B. Note that additional fixation of the mandibular arch was achieved by a transverse Kirschner wire passed through the lower border of the mandible behind an unstable fracture in the region of the right mental foramen. It was not necessary or desirable to pack this man's antral cavities with gauze through a Caldwell-Luc exposure. In B the left craniomaxillary suspension wire has already been placed and may be seen emerging from the left corner of the patient's mouth. A Saunder's fascial needle has been passed behind the right zygoma and is about to be used to draw the right suspension wire along the course marked by ink on the cheek and out of the buccogingival sulcus.*

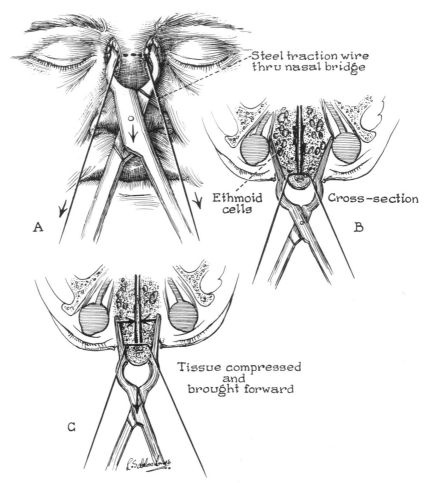

Steel traction wire
thru nasal bridge

A

Ethmoid
cells

Cross-section

B

Tissue compressed
and
brought forward

C

Figure 10–25. *When a head-on blow crushes the nasal bridge back into the ethmoid region, aggressive methods of early reduction are necessary to prevent permanent severe deformity about the nose and inner canthi. Bone of the nasal bridge is often forced toward the corner of the eye on either side, and reduction of the nasal fractures may not correct this deformity. Two longitudinal incisions may be made as shown in (A), and a heavy traction wire may be passed through the dense bone of the nasion. The periosteum along the medial wall of each orbit may then be carefully elevated for a distance of approximately 3 cm. An assistant is then asked to exert strong forward traction on the steel wire through the nasal bridge while the operator uses a wide-jawed and flat-bladed clamp to gently manipulate the ethmoid bone back toward the midline. In this way, a molding and bringing forward of the bridge of the nose may be accomplished during the first few days after such fractures. It is almost impossible to accomplish this reduction once the bones have healed firmly into position.*

taken to reduce it and wire it accurately in place. At the same time, the mucous membrane lining and cavity of the sinus should be explored and irrigated. The nasofrontal duct should be gently probed to be sure that it has not been obliterated by the fracture. The insertion of a metal dilator will often reopen a collapsed nasofrontal duct and, if necessary, a catheter can be placed within this channel as a stent so that one end extends into the nasal cavity. If the posterior wall of the frontal sinus has been fractured, the sinus may still be preserved, provided that the patient is protected from

the development of pneumatocele (readily detected by postoperative x-ray) and from unrecognized injury to the dura with resultant spinal fluid leak. Over the past 15 years, the author has found it unnecessary to surgically obliterate a single frontal sinus following injury!

In the absence of displacement of the frontal bone, the appearance of an air-fluid level on sinus x-ray several days after surgery is highly suggestive of damage to the nasofrontal duct and suggests further study. If unrecognized, such complications can lead to mucoceles or mucopyoceles.

Fractures of the Facial Bones in Children

Every emergency department team is asked to care for children whose faces were injured in automobile accidents. Usually they have been sitting, without protection of seatbelt, between parents on the front seat of the family car. The child is usually frightened and uncooperative, and the face is often badly swollen. The mother is sometimes hysterical. Clinical examination of the damaged facial bones of such a child will be difficult. The nasal cavity is so small that it is difficult to insert a speculum or light. X-rays are badly obscured by the multiple unerupted tooth buds present through the upper and lower jaws of all small children. Paranasal sinuses may not yet be pneumatized. A number of deciduous teeth may be missing, and the child may be totally unable to indicate whether his dental occlusion is satisfactory. In the absence of grossly displaced fractures or other injuries, there is a strong temptation for the surgeon to send the child home and to recommend the application of ice compresses to the face and ask the parents to bring the child back to the clinic 2 weeks later, "when the swelling has subsided." This temptation should be avoided.

Facial bone fractures are relatively uncommon in children, comprising only about 4 per cent of the total number of facial fractures. Fortunately, children have very resilient bone that stands considerable trauma without fracture or, in many instances, with only a greenstick deformity. Young bone is highly vascular and heals very rapidly. It is also more resistant to infection than is adult bone. The paranasal sinuses are small and cause little problem in fractures of the facial bones of children. Several precautions should be stressed in the management of childhood facial fractures; several problems of treatment that are not seen in adults arise with children.

Injury to immature facial bones will sometimes result in the arrest of growth, which may not manifest itself until some years later. This is most likely when the growing suture lines near the base of the skull are displaced. Some surgeons have also reported overgrowth of injured facial bones in children. It is our impression that this is *not* true overgrowth, but rather is the result of early malunion and an increase in asymmetry of the deformity associated with continued growth on the normal side of the face. This is a particularly common problem when a fracture involves the neck of the mandibular condyle. Such a fracture in a small child may be followed by severe progressive asymmetry of the face and by shifting of the chin both backward and toward the side of the injury as the child gets older.

Teeth are small and easily dislodged in children. The roots of deciduous teeth may be partially resorbed at the time of injury. Such teeth may be readily aspirated when dislodged and may produce pulmonary abscesses if they are not discovered and removed. When deciduous teeth are lost prematurely, one may later find abnormal underdevelopment of the alveolar bone and adjacent mandible or maxilla. Between the ages of 6 and 12 children have a period of "mixed" dentition in which the deciduous teeth have such small roots that they will not adequately permit secure attachment of arch bars, and the permanent teeth are likely to be insufficiently erupted to be of value. Tooth buds almost always lie in the fracture line of mandibular or maxillary fractures in small children. If these buds are injured by the fracture or the reduction, dental eruption may be delayed.

Fracture dislocations of the mandibular condyle are so commonly followed in children by severe growth asymmetry that it is usually wise to attempt gentle open reduction and repositioning of the mandibular condyle. This may best be carried out by a retroauricular incision that divides the full circumference of the external canal and permits the surgeon to reflect the ear, parotid gland and facial nerve forward in a single unit in order to expose the fractured condyle. If it is evident that some portion of the face is not developing properly following injury, it may be wise to build up that portion of the anatomy with pedicle flaps and bone or even with various synthetic implants. This will serve to minimize psychologic damage to the child and to keep the soft tissues under sufficient stretch stimulus to provide an adequate pocket for later bone grafting. At adolescence an adult-sized bone graft can be inserted at the time of removal of the synthetic implant.

If these considerations are kept in mind, facial bone fractures in children will respond well to the methods utilized in the treatment of those in adults.

Because of the high vascularity of immature bone, there is rapid healing (but also rapid malunion) of facial fractures in children. If these fractures are not reduced within the first few days after injury, it becomes almost impossible to reposition them later. (Delayed reductions may be practical in adults for 2 to 3 weeks after injury.) Small anatomical parts, susceptibility to edema and the difficulty in obtaining x-rays add to the problems of diagnosis of facial fractures in children; a significant number of nasal fractures are thus unrecognized and untreated. Unreduced nasal fractures may produce progressive deformity with growth. At times the child may have severe nasal obstruction requiring rhinoplastic or septal surgery during adolescence. Children are also susceptible to ankylosis of the temporomandibular joint following trauma to the chin. This is quite common following fractures of the condyle neck. After extensive facial trauma, with craniofacial dysfunction, we have found that some children may have a continuing cerebrospinal fluid leak. This may lead to recurrent bouts of meningitis over a period of months, or even years, until the dural tear is repaired.

Finally, it must be recognized that small children look upon medical treatment with considerable apprehension, and their lack of cooperation in combination with parental anxiety may further complicate the surgeon's task.

What are the therapeutic methods that aid the surgeon in the management of problems encountered with fractures in the faces of children? Both child and parents obviously require gentleness and patience in the examination and the therapeutic manipulations that follow. Local anesthesia may prove quite unsatisfactory even for simple fractures in children, and general anesthesia is often more desirable. Even in the removal of arch bars or pull-out wires, it is wise to utilize heavy sedation and local lidocaine (Xylocaine) in mucous membranes in order to gain cooperation and minimize discomfort and anxiety. Children have a tendency to manipulate "tricky" or removable appliances that may be used for fixation. For this reason as well as because of dental immaturity, open reduction is more often indicated in children than in adults. Further support for the use of open reduction of fractures in children comes from the realization that the late adverse consequences of inadequate closed reduction are much more severe in the case of children than of adults.

Because of the difficulties in obtaining exact diagnosis of facial fractures in children, it is often wise to carry out a diagnostic surgical procedure. At times this may require a general anesthetic. An exploratory incision may be made in the septal mucosa to identify a suspected fracture or dislocation of the cartilaginous nasal septum or an exploration on the floor of the orbit may be indicated for a possible blowout fracture or a fracture of the zygomatic compound. It is important that reductions of these fractures in children be carried out early to avoid rapid bony malunion.

Loose teeth should be repositioned promptly and carefully splinted for at least 3 weeks. Many of them will again become secure. In children, this possibility is increased by the presence of open root canals. If teeth appear to be missing and are not found at the scene of the injury, a chest x-ray will rule out the possibility of the patient's having aspirated the missing teeth. When it is difficult to apply arch bars because of mixed dentition in a child, circumferential wires may be applied so as to include the arch bar and the body of the mandible. These wires will secure an arch bar in good position without the danger of extracting teeth. In the upper jaw, an incision can be made in the sulcus behind the upper lip to expose the bony rim of the nasal pyriform opening. Drill holes may be placed in this bony margin and used to attach steel wires. The ends of the wires may be brought out through the incision and attached to the upper dental arch bar.

Careful consideration must be given to possible consequences of injuries to the facial bones in children. The family should be warned of the possible growth asymmetry that may develop. A failure to do so may be followed by great loss of confidence in the surgeon when such deformity appears at a later date.

If the entire external ear, or some major portion of it, is amputated, one cannot hope for resuturing to be successful. In such instances, the posterior skin and subcutaneous tissue may be removed from the cartilage and the latter preserved by grafting the lateral ear skin and cartilage onto the mastoid region as a composite graft. Several large windows are made in the ear cartilage to allow circulation to reach the skin. Six weeks later the ear skin and cartilage are dissected away from the mastoid bone and a skin graft is placed in the elevated angle. In this way, the valuable auricular fibrocartilaginous framework and thin specialized ear skin may be preserved.

Injuries to Specialized Facial Features

Eyelids and Orbit. Eyelid skin is the thinnest skin on the surface of the body. As a result, it is difficult to replace it exactly with skin grafting, and the lid is susceptible to massive edema that may produce stretching and rupture of elastic fibers and permanent lid striae (Fig. 10–26). Eyelid skin withstands thermal injury poorly because of its thinness. Slight displacements of the mobile skin during healing may produce secondary deformities of the lash border, which are very troublesome to the patient from the standpoint of both appearance and function.

Severe injuries to the lids and orbit call for protection of the cornea by early closure of the eyelids with or without suturing and by the application of a firm compression dressing to control traumatic edema. If this is not done, proptosis and severe conjunctival edema may follow, producing disability and deformity similar to that shown in Figure 10–26A. Even then, it may be possible to protect the cornea by performing a tarsorrhaphy between the upper and lower eyelids until the traumatic edema subsides (Fig. 10–26B). The closed eyelid is also the best possible treatment for corneal abrasions that may have occurred with the original injury. (See Chapter 9.) Pressure dressings do not threaten the eye unless they are applied with elastic (Ace-type) outer layers. That type of compression can produce retinal artery occlusion and should be avoided. Elevation of the head and use of ice compresses will serve with many patients, and should be used especially when that particular patient shows disorientation when the eyes are bandaged (approximately 20 per cent of the adult population). At times, lacerations involving the region of the inner canthus of the eyelids may divide one of the canaliculi on its route from the eyelid to the nose. The loss of the lower canaliculus is more important than loss of

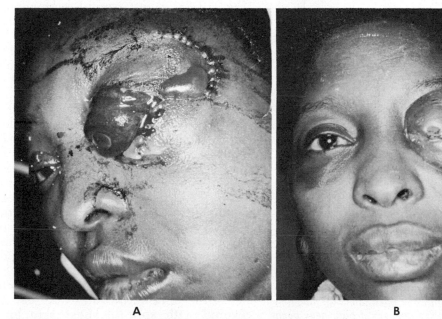

| A | B |

Figure 10–26. A and B, This patient suffered class III fractures of the frontal bone, orbit and zygoma. Rapidly developing hemorrhage and ocular edema produced the severe proptosis and chemosis of the left eye. A protective double tarsorrhaphy performed earlier would have prevented much of this complication. In order to protect the cornea from drying and ulceration, a full lid closure was carried out as shown in B, and a compression dressing was used to bring about further resolution of the severe edema. Loss of a major portion of an eyelid requires urgent reconstruction to protect the cornea from secondary perforation.

the upper and is likely to result in troublesome epiphora if not corrected. It is usually possible to find the two ends of a freshly divided canaliculus and repair them by the method illustrated in Figure 10–27. In the past few years the use of microsurgical techniques has greatly improved the reliability of reconstructive methods on small structures such as canaliculi, facial nerves, the parotid duct and small but important blood vessels.

Full-Thickness Losses of Portions of the External Nose. Certain injuries to the nose involve full-thickness losses of the tip or nasal alae. Many times these can be repaired primarily with a proper appreciation of plastic techniques. A nasal rim that has been sliced off may be replaced if the missing segment is located and brought to the emergency room with the patient. In its

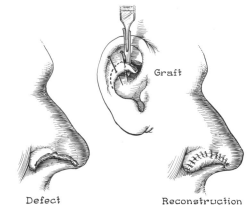

Figure 10–28. *Moderate full thickness losses of the nasal rim or tip may in some instances be repaired either by resuturing of the amputated skin and cartilage or, when the missing segment is crushed or cannot be located, a primary composite graft can be removed from the antihelix of the ipsilateral ear including the necessary supporting cartilage. Such primary reconstruction should not be undertaken in cases of nasal losses from dog bites or human bites or when the wound is badly contaminated. The composite graft may be more easily handled if the several layers are first transfixed with sterile pins through all layers and the cartilage.*

absence, a composite graft, consisting of two thicknesses of ear skin and the contained cartilage, may be transferred into the defect to replace the amputated segment (Fig. 10–28). Very careful postoperative splinting is necessary for successful "take" of these thick grafts.

Full-Thickness Losses of All or Part of the External Ear. Completely amputated portions of the ear helix or lobule that are less than 1 cm. in thickness or width can often be returned as a composite graft by resuturing the amputated part. The blood supply of the ear is excellent, and very small remaining pedicles of soft tissue will often support long and badly lacerated pedicles of ear skin and cartilage. With larger losses of soft tissue that expose significant amounts of underlying ear cartilage, local pedicle flaps may be designed from the area of the mastoid region or the nonhair-bearing preauricular skin (Fig. 10–29A and B). Island arterial flaps may even be removed from the fascia and subcuticular tissue of the temple, moved to the ear and covered with split-thickness skin grafts taken from the lateral neck.

Lips and Cheeks. The lips are commonly perforated by the patient's own teeth, producing a dirty wound that should be closed very loosely by sutures, if at all.

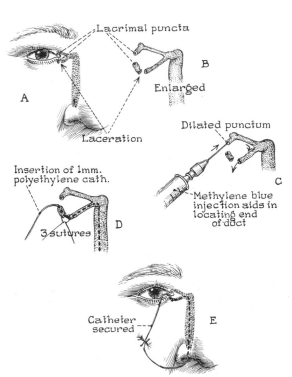

Figure 10–27. *Technique of identification and repair of divided canaliculus: The proximal end is located by dilating the punctum with a lacrimal probe and passing it to the point of division. The distal end may be found by injecting a small amount of methylene blue through the noninjured punctum or directly into the lacrimal sac if both have been divided. A tiny polyethylene catheter is then passed through the divided duct into the sac to emerge in the nasal cavity. After closure of the duct with fine sutures, the two ends of the catheter may be sutured together to complete the circle until healing has occurred.*

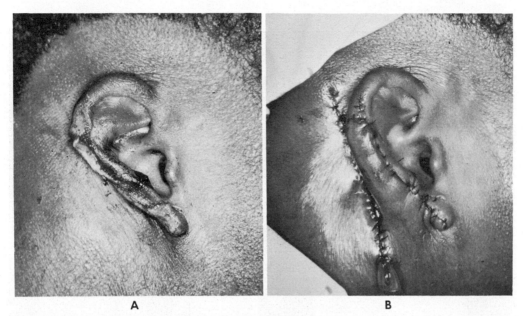

A   **B**

Figure 10–29.   *A, A knife wound resulted in the loss of approximately 30 per cent of this man's external ear, with marked exposure of the remaining ear cartilage. To facilitate healing, prevent a spreading chondritis and reconstruct the helix of the lower ear, an immediate mastoid flap (B) was elevated on an inferior pedicle and brought forward to cover the exposed cartilage. The lower pedicle of this flap was divided later and shaped into an ear lobule. The mastoid donor defect has been closed by undermining and advancement.*

When areas of the vermilion have been lost, they may require later substitution in the form of mucous membrane flaps taken from the inner surface of the lip or from the lateral side of the tongue.

Children commonly suffer severe electrical burns of the lips and tongue when they find an extension cord on the floor that is still connected to the house current but not to a lamp. These extension cord heads are often a chocolate color and invite the child to place them in his mouth. The result is a painful third-degree burn involving the commissure of the mouth and tongue, generally requiring delayed and complex plastic surgery to open and shape the mouth properly. Although some surgeons have advocated early resection of the necrotic muscle of the lip in these injuries, most plastic surgeons think that a better result can be obtained with delayed repair. Secondary hemorrhage may develop in these wounds after 10 to 12 days and may cause profound hemorrhagic shock if it occurs during sleep.

When considerable cheek substance has been lost from electrical or traumatic injury (Fig. 10–30A), repair must be designed not only to provide skin replacement to the cheek but also to replace the missing mucous membrane lining and necessary bulk within the cheek. To avoid unsightly contour depression, it is often necessary to elevate a pedicle flap from the neck or chest and to transfer one end to the defect after lining its undersurface with a skin graft (Fig. 10–30B). Three weeks later the lined flap may be divided and the pedicle returned to the neck. Removal of the excess fat will produce, in such instances, an adequate reconstruction of the cheek and corner of the mouth (Fig. 10–30C).

Parotid Duct.   Compound wounds of the face often involve transection of the parotid duct just prior to its entrance into the oral cavity. The surgeon should bear in mind carefully the normal location of the parotid duct. It is usually on a line between the base of the nostril and the lobe of the ear. It emerges from the parotid substance to run across the lateral surface of the masseter muscle and then to dip medially at the anterior border of the masseter to pass between some of the upper fibers of the buccinator muscle. A branch of the facial nerve usually travels with this duct over the proximal half of its course. Thus, injury to the nerve should be suspected whenever the duct is divided. The availability of operating microscopes in most modern operating rooms greatly improves the accuracy of reconstruction of these structures. If the two

A

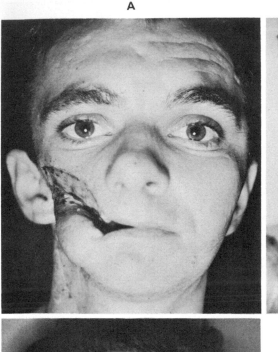

B

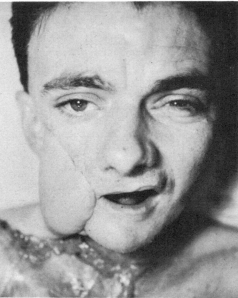

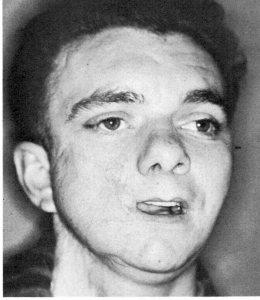

Figure 10–30. A, *This young man suffered a traumatic avulsion of the full thickness of the right cheek. A split graft has been applied to the defect above and over the mandible to provide the initial healing. Reconstruction requires the transfer of a lined pedicle flap to provide skin mucosal replacement of the cheek and sufficient bulk for contour. In B a cervicothoracic flap has been elevated with its base on the right shoulder and with a split thickness graft lining its undersurface. In C the flap has been fitted into the cheek, the extra bulk has been removed, and the pedicle has been returned to the shoulder. A free skin graft on the neck replaces the donor flap.*

C

ends of the duct can be located and a small polyethylene cannula threaded along the lumen, it is possible to carry out careful end-to-end suture of the duct over this indwelling catheter. For the best results care should be taken not to let the sutures enter the lumen of the duct. The catheter tip should be allowed to project into the oral cavity and should be sutured into position for several weeks (Figs. 10–31 and 10–32).

Facial Nerve Injuries. Major lacerations involving the cheek that cross the

course of the facial nerve may divide important branches.

In 1972 evidence was presented from several sources to indicate superior results with facial nerve injury if immediate repair is carried out. This is in part due to the ease of finding the divided nerve ends before nerve degeneration has occurred. Muscle contraction on stimulation of the distal nerve fragment is usually lost after one week. Facial nerve repair should probably not be undertaken by any surgeon who is without experience in the use of the operat-

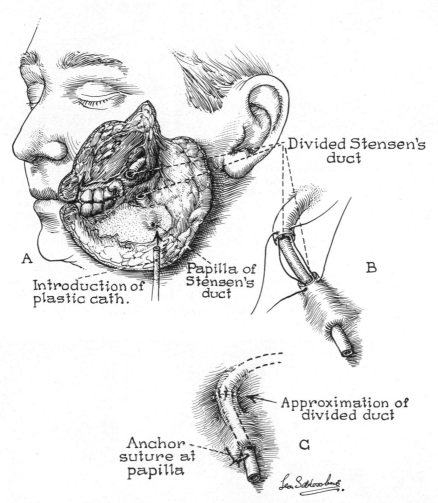

Figure 10–31. *Explosion injury to the cheek resulted in multiple fractures with division of the parotid duct approximately 1½ inches before its entrance into the oral cavity. The proximal end of the duct was found at operation and identified by the slow discharge of serous parotid secretion. The distal cut end was found by a retrograde threading of a polyethylene catheter from the duct papilla on the oral mucosa. Six-zero silk sutures were then placed in the submucosa of the duct to carry out fine closure of the divided duct with interrupted sutures. The catheter was anchored to the oral mucosa to prevent its slipping out in the postoperative period and was removed 2 weeks later.*

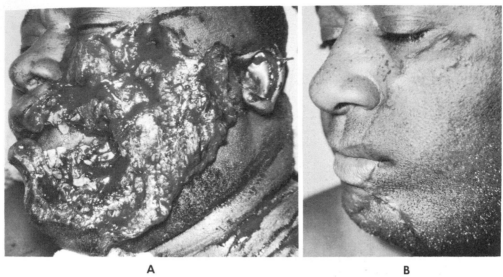

A   B

Figure 10–32. A and B, *This patient received an explosive wound of the face with compound fractures of the upper and lower jaw, loss of several teeth, extensive lacerations of the left cheek involving transection of the parotid duct, and loss of vermilion at the left commissure of the mouth. After thorough irrigation and clean-up, arch bars were applied to the upper and lower jaw for intermaxillary elastic traction; and a repair of the parotid duct was carried out as illustrated by the technique in Figure 10–31. B shows early result, including a patent left Stensen's duct. The loss of vermilion in the left corner of the mouth is evident and requires a mucous membrane flap from behind the upper lip. The arch bars were left in position for 6 weeks.*

ing microscope. (Microsurgery teams are available in most major medical centers as a standard technique where plastic surgery teams are available for emergency calls.)

Sutures of 10–0 nylon plus a fibrin "fixation" technique will provide a highly reliable degree of nerve recovery. The nerve ends may be located by careful use of a

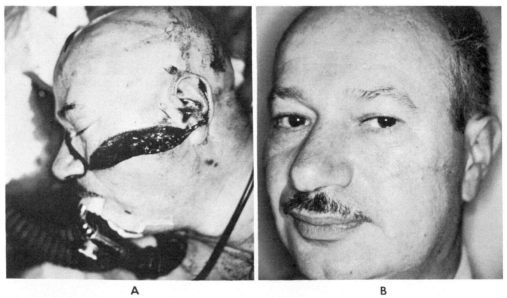

A   B

Figure 10–23. A shows a deep hatchet wound of the cheek sustained when this grocery store owner was attacked by a hold-up man. Both his parotid duct and three large branches of the facial nerve were divided. Other injuries of the extremities made the use of general anesthesia desirable. Careful repair of the parotid duct and resuture of the three branches of the facial nerve were carried out at primary operation. Four months later, the result shown in B indicates a definite return of tone in the facial nerve branches supplying the upper and lower lip. The nerve branches to the forehead and right eyebrow have largely recovered, and very little brow ptosis is present.

nerve stimulator to detect the distal branches and by careful anatomical dissection to locate the proximal branches. Whenever possible, these tiny nerves should be brought together and sutured with one or two very fine sutures of nonabsorbable (7–0) material. Surprisingly good function can be achieved by the resuture of the facial nerve. Indeed, the facial nerve and the digital nerves in the hand seem to be those nerves most likely to have good function restored if they are carefully repaired by suture or nerve grafting following trauma (Fig. 10–33A and B).

At times a portion of the facial nerve may be avulsed by a primary injury or a section may be removed because of tumor. In such instances, primary neurorrhaphy may not be possible. Autogenous facial nerve grafting may produce excellent results. We have preferred to use the sensory branches of the great auricular nerve as the most suitable

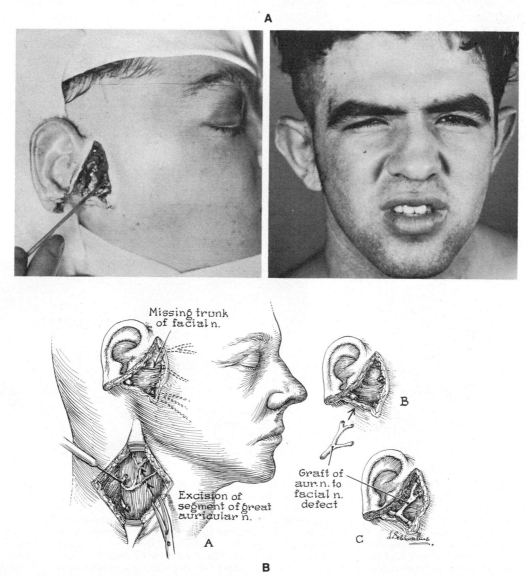

Figure 10–34. A *shows a rotary blade avulsion injury of the cheek and ear with a mission section of the lower ear and a gap of approximately ½ inch in the facial nerve. The distal ends of the nerve were located with a small electrical stimulator, and the proximal trunk was picked up just beneath the external auditory canal. A donor nerve graft of appropriate length was then removed from the great auricular nerve where it crosses the posterior border of the sternomastoid muscle. The technique is illustrated in B. The three distal branches of the great auricular nerve graft were each sutured carefully to the three branches of the facial nerve which could be located in the cheek. C shows the tone and balance that have returned to the face approximately 6 months following the primary injury and just prior to a small plastic operation designed to readjust the lateral position of the ear cartilage. If facial nerve repair is not successful by suture or grafting, dynamic muscle transfers will offer the patient considerable relief from the distressing deformity of facial palsy.*

donor nerve. This nerve may be easily exposed through a short transverse incision in the lateral side of the neck, and the number of branches removed can be made to coincide with the number of major distal trunks of the facial nerve to be repaired. It is important for good regeneration that the nerve be placed in the defect without tension and that a bed of rich vascularity be supplied to the graft. When applied to a primary injury, such nerve grafts are likely to be highly successful (Fig. 10–34A through C).

Major Compound Injuries of the Face with Gross Loss of Bone and Soft Tissues. In the case of explosions or high-velocity missile injuries, such as are commonly seen in hunting accidents or in the war-wounded, an entirely different problem in reconstruction may confront the surgeon. Such patients have lost such an ex-

tensive amount of soft tissue that there is little covering material for the damaged bone and a lack of soft tissue substance to rebuild features. Such patients are likely to require a long and complex series of reconstructive steps which, at times, run over the course of 1 or 2 years. The initial management should be aimed at control of hemorrhage and the establishment of a safe airway. The control of infection and the preservation of all possible damaged tissue may be of value for later reconstruction. Unlike the construction of a house in which the foundation is built first, the reconstruction of a major portion of the missing face must be carried out from the outside surface, working inward. Thus, the surgeon must first think of providing sufficient skin and lining to the cheeks, lips and oral cavity into which he may later insert proper bone grafts to provide stability and, perhaps, a

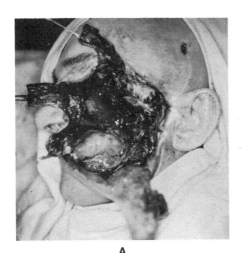

A

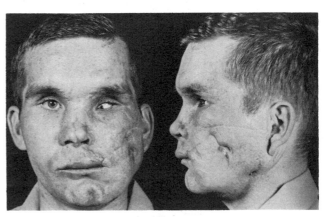

B

Figure 10–35. *A shows a young man who looked into a cylinder of highly explosive gas just as it was ignited by the flame of a match. The left eye, the left maxilla, the left zygoma, and the left mandible with parotid gland and much overlying cheek tissue were all badly destroyed. At the time of primary repair, an effort was made to save all remaining tissue after thorough debridement. A plastic conformer was sutured into the left conjunctival sac and a gold implant was placed inside Tenon's capsule to complete the enucleation of the left eye. Portions of the mandible were rewired, and the soft tissue flaps were closed over the wound. Six weeks later, the patient developed swelling and drainage in the left cheek (B). It was obvious that the lack of soft tissue attachments and blood supply had resulted in infection of some bone fragments. Exploration revealed sequestration and osteomyelitis in eight fragments of mandible. These eight fragments were removed (C). Six months later a rib graft was inserted to reconstruct the mandible (D), and a reasonable repair of the deformity resulted (E). This patient has obtained an artificial left eye and is now married and supporting his family despite the magnitude of his original injury.*

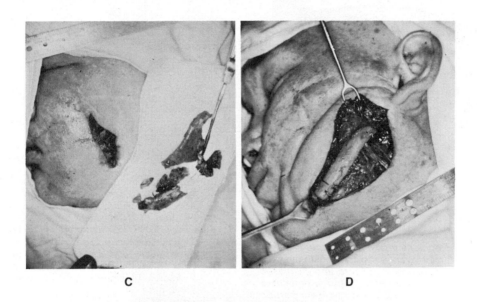

C   D

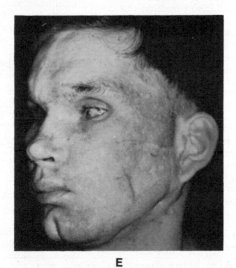

E

Figure 10–35 (Continued)

cessful and creative jobs in the community. The expense of this type of medical care is tremendous and, in the absence of its assumption by some governmental or insuring agency, the private citizen is unlikely to be able to meet the burdensome expenses of this type of care (Figs. 10–35 and 10–36).

REFERENCES

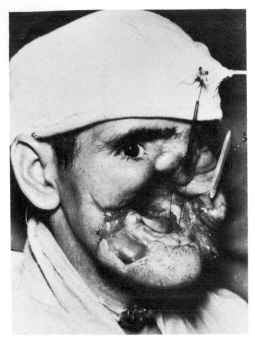

Figure 10–36. *This young man sustained a high-velocity shell fragment injury of the entire middle face during World War II. A tracheostomy tube was inserted as a lifesaving measure, and the plastic splint was wired circumferentially to the remaining mandibular fragments to support the lower portion of the face. Because of bony instability, a plaster head cap was applied, and elastic support traction was provided to the left zygoma and mandibular symphysis. Fortunately, reasonable vision remained in one eye. This young man and many others like him came under the care of the Plastic Surgery Unit at the Valley Forge General Hospital, then under the supervision of Dr. James Barrett Brown and Dr. Bradford Cannon. Under their direction, six or eight different plastic surgeons operated on this patient over a period of approximately 2½ years before he was finally rehabilitated and returned to his home. He is now, thirty years later, married and the proud father of atttractive children. He supports his family and is a useful and effective citizen. The courageous example set by this man and many of his colleagues-at-arms should be an inspiration to all those interested in rehabilitation of the facially injured.*

proper ridge on which a denture may be seated. Following the build-up of cheeks and jaw, it may be necessary to bring distant pedicle flap tissue to the face for the reconstruction of an external nose, the building of eyelids or the reconstruction of external ears. The value of proceeding with this multistaged type of reconstruction has been evidenced in considerable numbers of young men injured in World War II and the conflicts in Korea and Viet Nam. Indeed, many of these young men are now supporting families and carrying out suc-

1. Adams, W. M.: Internal wiring fixation of facial fractures. Surgery *12*:523, 1942.
2. Angle, E. H.: Classification on malocclusion. Dental Cosmos *41*:248, 1899.
3. Baudens, J. B.: Fracture de la machoire inférieure. Bull. Acad. de Méd., Paris 5:341, 1840.
4. Brown, J. B., Fryer, M. P., and McDowell, F.: Internal wire-pin fixation for fractures of upper jaw, orbit, zygoma, and severe facial crushes. Plast. Reconstr. Surg. 9:276, 1952.
5. Buck, G., Jr.: Fracture of the lower jaw, with displacement and interlocking of the fragments. Annalist, New York *1*:245, 1846.
6. Dingman, R. O., and Natvig, P.: Surgery of Facial Fractures. Philadelphia, W. B. Saunders Co., 1964, p. 11.
7. Edgerton, M. T., and Hill, E.: Fractures of the mandible. Surgery *31*:933, 1952.
8. Gerrie, J. W., and Lindsay, W. K.: Fracture of maxillary-zygomatic compound with atypical involvement of orbit. Plast. Reconstr. Surg. *11*:341, 1953.
9. Gillies, H. D., Kilner, T. P., and Stone, D.: Fractures of the malar-zygomatic compound, with a description of new x-ray position. Br. J. Surg. *14*:651, 1827.
10. Johnson, W. B.: New method for reduction of acute dislocation of the temporomandibular articulations. J. Oral Surg. *16*:501, 1958.
11. Knight, J. S., and North, J. F.: Classification of malar fractures: An analysis of displacement as a guide to treatment. Br. J. Plast. Surg. *13*:325, 1961.
12. Langer, C.: Zur Anatomie und Physiologie der Haut. Sitzungst. d. k. Acad. Wissensch. *45*:223, 1861.
13. LeFort, R.: Fractures de la machoire supérieure. Cong. internat. de méd. C. -r., Paris, 1900, Sect. de chir. gen., pp. 275–278.
14. McCoy, F. J., Chandler, R. A., Magnan, C. G., Jr., Moore, J. R., and Siemsen, G.: An analysis of facial fractures and their complications. Plast. Reconst. Surg. 29:381, 1962.
15. Marsh, J. L. and Edgerton, M. T.: Razabrasion: An alternative approach perioral rhytidies. *In* Rogers, B. O. (ed.): Aesthetic Plastic Surgery. New York, Springer-Verlag, 1978.
16. Nicholson, L. T., and Guzak, B. F.: Blindness after blow-out fractures of the orbit. Arch. Ophthalmol. 86:369, 1971.
17. Robert, C. A.: Nouveau procede de traitement des fractures de la portion alveolaire de la ma-

choire inférieure. Bull. Gen. de Therap. Méd. et Chirurg. 42:22, 1852.
18. Rubin, L. R.: Langer's lines and facial scars. Plast. Reconst. Surg. 3:147, 1948.
19. Smith Papyrus: Translations by G. Kasten Tallmadge. *In* Dingman, R. D., and Natvig, P.: Surgery of Facial Fractures. Philadelphia, W. B. Saunders Co., 1964.
20. Swearingen, J. J.: Tolerances of the Human Face to Crash Impact. Report from the Office of Aviation Medicine, Federal Aviation Agency, July, 1965.

CHAPTER 11

THE MANAGEMENT OF NECK INJURIES

Thomas J. Balkany, M.D.
Bruce W. Jafek, M.D.
Robert B. Rutherford, M.D.

INTRODUCTION

Relative to its size, the neck contains a greater concentration and variety of organs and structures than any other part of the body. Unlike the contents of the head, chest and pelvis, those of the neck are not protected by surrounding skeleton, but as in the abdomen, partial protection is provided by the investing musculature and by adjacent structures, e.g., the spine, mandible and shoulders.

Most neck injuries are caused by forces of large mass and low velocity, which cause relatively minor soft tissue damage. The most serious neck injuries result from high-speed vehicular accidents or gunshot wounds, exemplifying the principle that tissue damage is proportional to the square of the velocity of the injuring force. Automobile accidents account for the majority of cervical injuries in civilian populations. In fact, the neck is significantly injured in approximately 10 per cent of automobile accidents, by striking the dashboard, windshield or steering wheel, or by sudden acceleration-deceleration forces.[14]

The majority of serious neck injuries involve the upper respiratory and digestive systems (larynx, trachea, pharynx and esophagus). Less common but more life-threatening are injuries to the major vessels of the neck, the cervical vertebrae and

spinal cord. Serious injuries to the cervical nerves or the glandular structures of the neck are rare.

Anatomical and other differences between adults and children, which are responsible for the different spectrum of injuries encountered in the two groups,[13] should be kept in mind. First, a young child's larynx is located more cephalad than an adult's so that it is better protected by the mandible and hyoid bone and therefore is less frequently injured. It does not descend and assume its final position until early adulthood. Second, because a child's head is proportionately larger than an adult's, the supporting neck structures are much more susceptible to acceleration-deceleration injuries. This susceptibility is partially offset by the greater elasticity of the child's cervical structures, which allows greater displacement without serious injury. Third, the child's weight is less than an adult's so less force is applied to the neck in deceleration injuries. Finally, the types of trauma to which the child is exposed differ signficantly from those of the adult.

The general principles of trauma resuscitation, including the managment of shock and airway problems, have been covered in other chapters (4 and 12 respectively). In addition, the management of certain other cervical injuries, such as those of the cervical spine (Chapter 8), are also discussed elsewhere in this book. Therefore, this chapter will deal primarily with the general principles of managing both blunt and penetrating neck injuries as well as the specific management of the remaining cervical visceral injuries.

BLUNT AS OPPOSED TO PENETRATING INJURIES OF THE NECK

In terms of the injuring agent, penetrating injuries in the neck do not differ greatly from those inflicted on other parts of the body. In contrast, blunt trauma involves a number of injuring mechanisms that are unique to the neck. Because the head and chest project farther anteriorly than the neck, they are more likely than the neck to be involved in direct impact with large objects or surfaces. On the other hand, when either the chest or the head alone is struck, sudden flexion or extension of the neck, associated with significant compression or shearing forces, commonly occurs. This is reflected in both the frequent association of cervical spine injury with serious head trauma[22] and "whiplash" injury with steering wheel injury to the chest.[6] Of course, smaller objects can inflict blunt trauma directly to the neck. Violent examples of this include garrotting, strangling, hanging or "clothes-lining." In recent years the latter type of injury has been seen with increasing frequency in snowmobile accidents, in which the driver fails to see an obstacle such as the upper strand of a wire fence projecting above the surface of the snow. Blunt cervical injuries also differ from penetrating trauma in that, like abdominal injuries, the former are explored only for specific indications, whereas the latter are more often explored routinely, even in the absence of specific signs.

Penetrating wounds of the neck are commonly caused by knife, gunshot or accidental impalement with any sharp object and frequently result in injuries to the vascular, nervous, visceral or skeletal structures of the neck. Injury to a major blood vessel is the most common cause of death following a penetrating neck wound. Penetrating cervical vascular injuries may produce exsanguination, air embolism, traumatic aneurysm, arteriovenous fistula or stroke. Only the latter is likely following blunt trauma.[15] Blunt trauma is more likely than penetrating trauma to be associated with extracervical injuries, particularly maxillofacial, head or chest injuries, but is less likely to be associated with injuries to other structures in the neck that may complicate the local management of a vascular injury, such as contaminating wounds of the airway, pharynx or esophagus.

Management of Penetrating and Nonpenetrating Neck Injuries. Prevailing surgical opinion advocates routine exploration of all penetrating neck wounds.[1, 10] The rationale behind this relates to the following five observations: (1) Most penetrating neck wounds harbor significant injuries.[16] (2) The mortality and morbidity of a negative exploration of the neck is almost negligible and certainly less than that associated with the delayed management of missed injuries.[17] (3) The hospital stay of patients with a negative neck exploration is similar to that of those managed by expectant observation.[27] (4) The selective management of penetrating cervical injuries requires more physician time and effort because of the need for careful repetitive examination. (5) Selective management requires greater experience, judgment and skill in diagnosis as well as the ready availability of special diagnostic studies, e.g., arteriography, endoscopy and contrast studies of the upper aerodigestive tracts.

In spite of these considerations, it must be admitted that there have been several large series of penetrating neck injuries that have been effectively managed by selective surgical exploration.[8, 24] This must be taken into consideration when dealing with patients with other major wounds requiring attention, patients in whom factors are present that increase the anesthetic risk (a full stomach, alcoholic intoxication, serious cardiopulmonary disease) but who have no evidence of serious visceral injury, and patients who have already been "selected out" for observation by delay in presentation. Thus, while the authors support the accepted policy of routine exploration of penetrating cervical wounds, they also recognize that there will be circumstances in which the neck should not be explored in the absence of "mandatory" indications. These are essentially the same indications employed in the management of blunt cervical trauma and include evidence of active bleeding (hemoptysis, epistaxis, expanding hematoma or significant wound bleeding), vascular occlusion (loss of carotid pulse, neurologic deficit) or penetration of the upper airway or digestive tract (bubbling wound, subcutaneous emphysema, tenderness, dysphagia, dysphonia). It is also worth pointing out that exploration of the "negative" neck must be equally thorough if not more so than when there are indications of visceral injury and as such requires at least an equal level of surgical skill.

Finally, the zone of the neck involved in a penetrating wound must be taken into consideration in deciding whether immediate exploration should be undertaken in the absence of "mandatory" indications.[3, 18] Most penetrating wounds involve the middle third of the neck, the structures of which are easily explored and repaired. However, wounds at the base of the skull or root of the neck are considered more difficult to manage. Therefore, in penetrating wounds at the base of the skull or root of the neck that are not accompanied by mandatory indications for exploration, it is advisable first to obtain an arteriogram. If an arterial injury is demonstrated, explora-

tion can then be carried out with knowledge of its nature and location and the exposure and reconstructive procedure that will be required. On the other hand, if the arteriogram is normal, exploration can be safely deferred in favor of continued careful observation. This approach, in algorithm form, is outlined in Table 11–1.

TREATMENT PRIORITIES.   For management purposes, injuries of the neck may be classified according to their severity, in a manner similar to that applied for triage purposes to injuries to other regions of the body:

I. Injuries that are immediately life-threatening.

II. Injuries that are severe but not immediately life-threatening.

III. Injuries that require additional evaluation and definitive treatment.

IV. Minor injuries.

For example, a crushed larynx causing nearly total airway obstruction would receive a priority of I and require immediate treatment, a lacerated esophagus would fall into category II, an enlarging cervical hematoma would represent category III and a superficial laceration would be as-

TABLE 11–1.   Management Plan for Penetrating and Nonpenetrating Neck Injuries

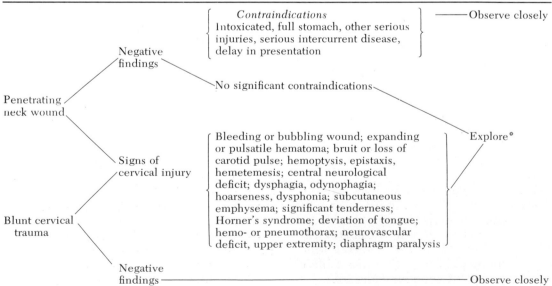

*Preoperative arteriogram if wound in Zones I or III.

signed to category IV. Multiple injuries should be cared for, in order, from highest to lowest priority.

There are three life-threatening or category I types of cervical injuries. The most common are those that cause obstruction of the upper airway with ventilatory impairment. Next in frequency are vascular injuries that may result in exsanguination, stroke or air embolism. The third are injuries to the cervical spine that may cause paraplegia. Therefore, *establishing an adequate airway, controlling hemorrhage and stabilizing the cervical spine are the first orders of business in dealing with cervical injuries.* Only after these problems have been specifically sought and attended to should one proceed with a more orderly examination and initiate diagnostic studies to determine the exact nature of other, less threatening neck injuries. Thus, the management of cervical injuries can be divided into three phases representing the three R's of trauma: *resuscitation, recognition and repair.*

Resuscitation and Initial Management of Serious Neck Injuries. All serious neck injuries should be treated as though there was a cervical spine fracture. The head and neck should be immobilized between sand bags until cervical spine x-rays have been obtained. A cervical collar is undesirable for this purpose because it not only interferes with examination but also with tracheostomy if that suddenly becomes necessary. Further treatment is detailed in Chapter 8.

Establishment of an adequate airway takes priority over attention to all injuries except a spurting laceration of a major artery. The signs of airway obstruction depend on the location of injury, the degree of obstruction and the mental status of the patient. Thus, laryngeal injury generally produces more stridor than tracheal injury and, whereas a conscious patient may describe his symptoms or point to the site of injury, evaluation of the unconscious patient is more difficult and requires rapid, systematic examination.

Stridor (upper airway noise during inspiration or expiration) is the most common sign of laryngeal or tracheal obstruction. By placing the ear above the patient's nose and mouth, one can roughly assess the adequacy of air exchange, since the injured patient tends to hyperventilate. In

severe obstruction, stridor may be absent due to lack of airflow, but secondary signs of upper airway obstruction — supraclavicular, intercostal and suprasternal retractions — are then prominent. In the obstructed patient, examination of the chest reveals vigorous and symmetrical efforts being made, in contrast to the lack of effort observed when poor ventilation is due to central nervous system depression from head injuries, hypoxia or drugs. The initial steps are the same in establishing an airway in either case, but the additional maneuvers to eliminate an obstructing object, the difficulties of these maneuvers in a semiconscious and possibly struggling patient, and the more likely need for tracheostomy make the former situation infinitely more challenging.

Establishment of an airway may be as simple as clearing secretions or foreign bodies from the hypopharynx with the forefinger. Care must be taken, however, not to impact a foreign body deeper into the airway or stir up more bleeding during digital exploration. In fractures of the mandible, grasping the tongue and pulling it anteriorly may be sufficient to establish the airway, as in this instance the obstruction is due to loss of anterior attachments and retrodisplacement of tongue into the airway. Orotracheal or nasotracheal intubation are occasionally life-saving; however, great care must be taken not to reduce a marginally adequate airway into an inadequate one with attempts at blind intubation. Endotracheal intubation may be made difficult or impossible by upper laryngeal edema, hematoma, fracture dislocation or brisk bleeding. A potentially serious problem with endotracheal intubation is the need for extension of the neck in patients in whom cervical spine injury has not been ruled out. Cord transection may occur during attempts to visualize the larynx for intubation. Therefore, all patients with significant neck injuries must be assumed to have cervical spine fracture or dislocation until proven otherwise and if the airway is obstructed, a tracheotomy may be required.

The principal *neck* injuries for which tracheostomy is indicated are (1) laryngeal fracture or destruction, (2) laryngotracheal separation, (3) tracheal separation or destruction, (4) concomitant major maxillofacial injury, especially with edema or hemorrhage into the floor of the mouth or base of tongue. Relative indications, such as provisions of an airway in the obtunded patient or one whose airway is being compromised by an expanding hematoma, can often be at least temporarily handled by intubation. In patients with cervical spine instability, an airway may be established by either nasotracheal or "blind" endotracheal intubation.

Cricothyrotomy, or tracheotomy through the cricothyroid membrane, may be employed as a temporary emergency measure. This membrane underlies a relatively nonvascular area in which the airway is close to the anterior cervical skin. A horizontal stab incision is made directly into the airway and the wound held open with the best available object, e.g., the barrel of a ballpoint pen, a scissors inserted and opened vertically or dining utensils. It is important to recognize that the cricoid cartilage is put at risk during cricothyrotomy. Perichondritis or chondritis of the cricoid may result in eventual narrowing of the airway by cicatrix. Tracheal cartilages are not as prone to this complication owing to the incomplete nature of their rings. For these reasons, cricothyrotomy should be replaced by a formal tracheostomy as soon as feasible (see Chapter 12 for more details).

Failure to appreciate the suddenness with which apparently minor airway obstruction may become life-threatening can be catastrophic, particularly since this obstruction may not occur until several hours following injury. Therefore, unless tracheostomy is performed initially, patients with cervical injuries with stridor or large hematoma should be observed in an intensive care ward with a tracheostomy set at the bedside.

Finally, all cervical wounds that are actively bleeding or bubbling should be controlled by compression using a sterile dressing until the patient has been intubated, anesthetized and is being ventilated using continuous positive pressure and is ready for skin preparation and exploration. Further details of the management of vascular injuries are provided later in this chapter.

DIAGNOSTIC EVALUATION OF PATIENTS WITH CERVICAL INJURY

After attending to the potentially life-threatening cervical injuries just described, one can proceed to the next phase, definitive diagnosis, by performing a thorough physical examination and obtaining the appropriate diagnostic studies to identify specific injuries. It should be emphasized here that in many cases (and in most cases of penetrating injury), surgical exploration may constitute the final, definitive diagnostic procedure. Nevertheless, the more specific information one can obtain prior to exploration the better, as long as the attempts to gain such information do not contribute unduly to the preoperative delay or are not associated with a risk that offsets the potential benefit of the additional information obtained.

If there is a penetrating cervical wound to attact the attention, it is common for the attending physician to proceed directly with examination of the neck. However, there is much to be learned by taking a history from the patient or witnesses to the accident. The wounding agent or the mechanism of injury can be identified and the occurrence of serious hemorrhage, which may have abated by the time of arrival in the emergency department, can be documented. Also the conscious patient can supply important information regarding the presence, severity, character and localization of cervical pain and whether or not he is having difficulty breathing, swallowing, speaking, seeing, hearing or smelling, or in moving or feeling certain body parts. In fact, he should be specifically questioned regarding these functions.

It is axiomatic that the physical examination should include a methodical inspection, palpation and auscultation. More importantly, these maneuvers should be carried out with an acute awareness of the clinical signs that are associated with specific cervical injuries. With this in mind, a list of findings commonly associated with injuries to the vessels of the neck, aerodigestive system, cervical nerves and glands is presented in Table 11–2.

TABLE 11–2. Clinical Findings Associated With Specific Cervical Injuries

1. Vascular injuries°
   a. Vigorously bleeding wound
   b. Progressively expanding or pulsatile hematoma
   c. Bruit
   d. Absent carotid, superficial temporal or ophthalmic artery pulsations
   e. Hemiplegia, hemiparesis, aphasia, monocular blindness or other signs of hemispheric cerebral vascular accident
2. Upper aerodigestive injuries
   a. Decreased ventilatory exchange
   b. Stridor
   c. Bubbling wound or subcutaneous emphysema
   d. Dysphonia
   e. Dysphagia
   f. Hemoptysis, espistaxis or hematemesis
   g. Unexplained wound tenderness
3. Cervical nerve injuries°
   a. Deviation of tongue
   b. Drooping of corner of mouth
   c. Horner's syndrome
   d. Cervical sensory deficits

°With penetrating wounds low in the neck, thorough examination of the upper extremity for neurovascular injury and the chest for pneumothorax or hemothorax or paralysis of the diaphragm is mandatory.

Almost all patients suspected of having sustained a cervical injury should have a chest x-ray and x-rays of the neck. For most penetrating wounds, anterior-posterior and lateral cervical views (the latter with soft tissue technique) are all that is required, but in severe blunt trauma, a complete cervical spine series should be ordered. The indications for more specialized studies, such as arteriography to identify vascular injuries, laryngoscopy, esophagoscopy and esophagograms to identify injuries of the upper aerodigestive system, will be discussed in detail in relation to specific injuries.

DEFINITIVE MANAGEMENT OF SPECIFIC CERVICAL INJURIES

Injuries to the Larynx and Trachea

Anatomy. The supporting structures of the larynx include the hyoid bone, epiglottis, and thyroid, cricoid and arytenoid cartilages. The hyoid bone of the adult is anterior to the base of the tongue and epiglottis. It is suspended below the mandible and, in turn, suspends the rest of the larynx. The thyroid cartilage surrounds the vocal cords anteriorly and laterally. The anterior prominence of the thyroid cartilage (Adam's apple) is an important anatomical structure in the adult male that may be collapsed in laryngeal trauma. The cricoid cartilage can be palpated directly below the thyroid cartilage; the cricothyroid membrane connecting the two is easily recognized and may be used for emergency tracheotomy. The cricoid, like the hyoid, is hyaline cartilage and a transitional structure between larynx and trachea. It is the only completely encircling ring of cartilage in the airway. In females and prepubertal males the thyroid prominence is usually not palpable, making identification of the cricothyroid space more difficult. In these patients, palpation of the superior thyroid notch identifies the thyroid cartilage and leads one to the cricothyroid space immediately inferior to it.

Epidemiology. Upper airway obstruction is the second most common cause of death resulting from head and neck trauma and the commonest cause of upper airway injury is vehicular accidents.[12] In recent years the relative frequency of injuries of the larynx and trachea has significantly increased[23] for two reasons. First, more people are surviving serious automobile accidents owing both to a number of automotive safety devices and to improved transportation and emergency medical care. Second, the use of "lap" seatbelts increases the likelihood of cervical injury.[7] The site of head and neck injury in an automobile accident depends on the configuration of the passenger compartment, the distance from initial passenger position to impact and the use of a seatbelt. When the passenger is close to the object struck, facial injuries predominate. When he is farther away, the changing momentum causes the neck to extend and the chin to rise and expose the larynx and trachea to injury. The two-point ("lap") seatbelt causes the passenger to flex at the hips and increases the frequency of nonfatal head and neck injuries. The three-point seatbelt is more effective in preventing such injuries, as may be the airbag.

The larynx is frequently crushed between the object struck and the cervical vertebrae, typically leading to fracture of the thyroid cartilage, anterior subluxation of the arytenoid cartilages or dislocation of the cricothyroid joint. The most frequent fracture of the thyroid cartilage is a vertical anterior fracture, often extending from the thyroid notch to the cricothyroid membrane. With this fracture, the anterior vocal cord attachments may be avulsed or involved in hematoma.

Fractures of the hyoid bone are uncommon due to its protection by the mandible. They are painful but usually not dangerous. The body of the hyoid is most commonly fractured, owing to the greater re-

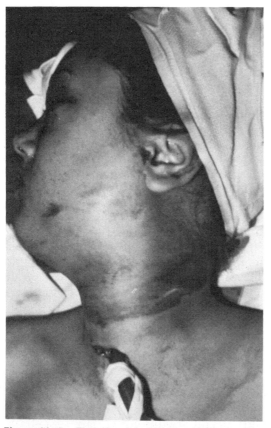

Figure 11–1. *This 19-year-old girl was beaten about the face and anterior neck with a 2 × 4 board, sustaining mandible and maxillary fractures as well as a laryngeal fracture. Evidence of the trauma to the anterior neck is apparent with some (subtle) evidence of flattening of the neck. She was hoarse, and examination showed cervical subcutaneous emphysema. These signs comprise the classic triad indicating a laryngeal fracture.*

siliency of the cornua. Fractures of the hyoid are more common in women because of their relatively longer necks with greater exposure of the hyoid beneath the protection of the mandible.

Signs and Symptoms. The most common signs and symptoms of laryngeal fractures are stridor, shortness of breath, change of voice, tenderness and subcutaneous emphysema (Figs. 11–1, 11–2). Air may be forced by fits of coughing into the soft tissues of the neck through tears in the laryngeal mucosa. This subcutaneous emphysema may reach massive proportions and extend from clavicle to scalp or beyond. Dissection along cervical facial planes may reach into the mediastinum and travel down to the pericardium. Occasionally, especially in the young, the air forced into the tissues may compress the upper airway and cause further respiratory embarrasment.

Dysphonia, a change in voice, may be caused by loss of the anteroposterior dimension of the larynx. This can occur with both vertical anterior thyroid cartilage fracture and anterior subluxation of the arytenoid cartilages. Both result in considerable hoarseness, which may be permanent if early diagnosis and reduction are not carried out. Paresis of one or both of the recurrent laryngeal nerves may also result from their being crushed in the cricothyroid articulation. Hematoma is another common cause of dysphonia. Although most common in the supraglottic larynx above the vocal cords, hematoma may occur anywhere in the upper airway. Dysphonia is also occasionally caused by displacement of the anterior vocal tendon, resulting in shortening and laxity of the vocal cords, and occasionally, loss of superior-inferior alignment.

Pain is often associated with neck motion, cough and swallowing. Dysphagia (difficulty in swallowing) and odynophagia (pain with swallowing) are both common in laryngeal fractures. During the second stage of swallowing the larynx is raised superiorly, causing distraction of fractured cartilage and disrupted tissue.

The most threatening signs of laryngotracheal damage are those of airway obstruction and stridor, as discussed previously in regard to the initial management of serious neck injuries. It is important to re-emphasize that upper air-

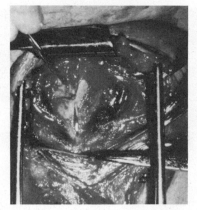
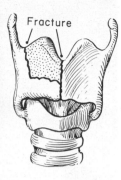

Fracture

Figure 11-2. *Surgical field in patient in Figure 11-1 with diagrammatic representation of the midline laryngeal fracture with horizontal fracture extending to the right. Because the internal mucosa was not disrupted, repair of the larynx was accomplished with fine wire sutures over a finger-cot stent.*

way injuries that appear minimal at first may rapidly progress to complete airway obstruction. The submucosal tissues of the supraglottic larynx permit rapid accumulation of fluid. The resulting edema or hematoma may obstruct the airway and prevent intubation. Too often this occurs while the physician's attentions are directed toward other more obvious injuries so that progression to severe airway obstruction results in hasty, disorderly tracheotomy. Occasionally, attempts at endoscopy in the emergency department may worsen a partial laryngeal obstruction by increasing the edema or hematoma formation. Endoscopy should be part of the definitive management, not the initial examination.

The loss of cartilaginous landmarks is common in laryngotracheal injury. The profile of the anterior neck is flattened and the thyroid prominence may not be palpable.

When mucosal tears allow escape of air into the tissue spaces (subcutaneous emphysema) it must be assumed that upper respiratory secretions and saliva have also reached the deep tissues of the neck. This contamination may spread via fascial planes into the mediastinum. Thus, pneumomediastinum following laryngotracheal injuries suggests the need for drainage and antibiotics.

Radiological Evaluation. When it is determined that the patient is in no immediate danger of acute respiratory obstruction, further diagnostic procedures can be initiated. These include chest x-ray, cervical spine x-ray and soft tissue lateral neck x-ray. A force great enough to fracture the larynx, face or mandible is also great enough to fracture or dislocate the cervical

vertebrae. Dislocations of C2, C3 or C4 are the most common associated cervical spine injuries.[21] These may occur in the absence of neurological signs and only be tragically discovered when manipulation of the neck during endoscopy or exploration compresses or transects the spinal cord.

Free air in the neck as seen on a soft tissue lateral view of the neck may be the only sign of disruption of the upper airway. In this circumstance, the chest x-ray should be carefully studied for the presence of air in the mediastinum for it implies that this has been contaminated by upper airway secretions as well as air (Figs. 11-3, 11-4).

Anteroposterior tomography of the larynx may show supra- or subglottic hematoma formation, arytenoid dislocation or avulsion of the vocal cords. However, this study is time-consuming, requires considerable technical expertise and is usually not available on an emergency basis. Contrast laryngograms are anterior-posterior views of the larynx taken while radioopaque material is dripped into the hypopharynx. It shares the limitations of laryngeal tomography so that both are more commonly used in cases involving late complications. Xeroradiography has been used in the diagnosis of laryngotracheal trauma but offers little additional information.

Laryngoscopy. Indirect mirror laryngoscopy, invaluable in the diagnosis of other diseases of the larynx, is less helpful in evaluating severe laryngeal trauma because of the state of anxiety of the patient, the tenderness associated with the injury and the obstruction of vision by edema and

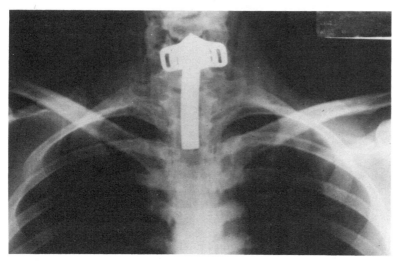

Figure 11–3. *Cervical and upper chest x-ray of a 22-year-old man who drove his open sports car under a chain stretched across a private driveway and was jerked out by the neck. Physical examination showed cervical subcutaneous emphysema with flattening of the anterior neck. The x-ray illustrates cervical, mediastinal and pericardial subcutaneous emphysema with the tracheotomy in place.*

hematoma. Its main use is in minor trauma to rule out significant damage to the endolarynx.

Ninety-degree wide angle fiberoptic laryngoscopes and flexible fiberoptic laryngotracheoscopes are more helpful. However, prolonged attempts at indirect visualization of the larynx may only result in worsening of the airway obstruction and direct laryngoscopy is usually necessary for definitive diagnosis of endolaryngeal damage. Direct laryngoscopy is best performed under general anesthesia. In cases of minor laryngeal trauma, the patient's trachea may be orally intubated and direct

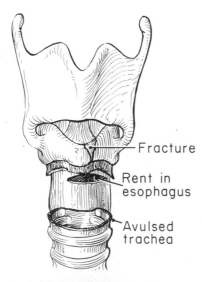

Figure 11–4. *Diagrammatic representation of the cricoid fracture, esophageal laceration and tracheal avulsion found at exploration of the patient shown in Figure 11–3.*

laryngoscopy then performed. However, more commonly in cases of significant laryngeal trauma, tracheotomy is first performed under local anesthesia, after which the patient is given a general anesthetic to allow direct laryngoscopy, following by exploration and repair as necessary.

Treatment. Initial treatment always involves assurance of an adequate airway. Tracheotomy is always indicated in neck injuries for severe or progressive loss of airway (Fig. 11–5). Tracheotomy accomplishes two purposes. First, an airway is provided without the risk of attempting to pass an endotracheal tube through an area of damage in which normal landmarks may be absent. Second, the tracheotomy prevents air, blood and upper respiratory tract secretions from being forced into the soft tissues of the neck by cough. In injuries of the larynx and upper trachea, the tracheotomy should be placed at least one ring below any injury. In injuries of the lower cervical trachea, the tracheotomy may have to be placed through the area of injury.

Early exploration and repair of cartilaginous and soft tissue defects is mandatory. The usual approach is made through a transverse incision at the level of the middle of the thyroid cartilage; this allows good exposure of the most commonly injured structure, the thyroid cartilage. When a vertical incision has been used for the tracheotomy, it may be extended to the level of the superior thyroid cartilage for good exposure or a transverse limb added to the level of the mid-thyroid cartilage. However, extended midline vertical neck

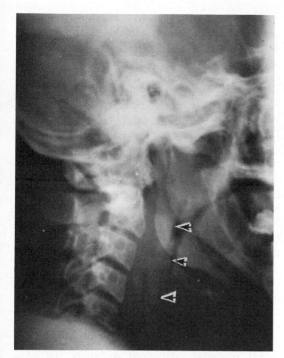

Figure 11–5. Lateral cervical x-ray of a 45-year-old man injured in an automobile accident; he sustained a laryngeal fracture as part of the "padded dash syndrome."[17] Anterior displacement of the posterior cervical-pharyngeal air shadow is seen (arrows) with cervical subcutaneous emphysema (vertical lucencies). Severe compromise of the airway is easily appreciated. The cervical vertebrae are intact and nondisplaced.

incisions often result in "banjo string" contractures and should be avoided. The skin and platysma are elevated superiorly and inferiorly and the strap muscles are separated in the midline to visualize the thyroid and cricoid cartilages. In the common vertical fracture of the thyroid cartilage, the larynx may be gently opened. When this does not occur, a vertical thyrotomy is created in the anterior midline of the thyroid cartilage. It is usually necessary to divide the anterior vocal tendon sagitally and separate the cords to afford good exposure of the interior of the larynx. For additional exposure, the laryngofissure may be extended inferiorly through the cricothyroid membrane and the cricoid itself.

Mucosal tears are repaired with 5–0 interrupted absorbable sutures (Fig. 11–6). Cartilaginous fractures are reduced and wired in place with 26 or 28 gauge monofilament stainless steel sutures. Most hematomas do not require specific treatment; only larger ones need be aspirated. In cases of large hematomas, severe disruption or loss of mucosa or comminution of laryngeal cartilages, an endolaryngeal stent is necessary. Prefabricated silicone rubber stents are manufactured that are formed to the contour of the interior lar-

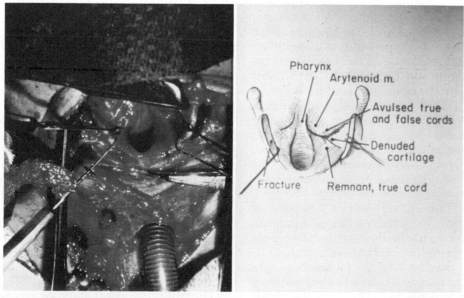

Figure 11–6. Operative field and diagrammatic representation of laryngeal fracture sustained by a 27-year-old woman in an automobile accident. Avulsion of the true and false cords away from the underlying thyroid cartilage on the left side is visible. These were replaced anteriorly with absorbable sutures, and the larynx was closed over a soft stent.

ynx.[19] When such stents are not available, a finger cot filled with sterile sponge rubber may be used. Stents are transfixed with heavy monofilament nylon, which is then tied over external buttons to prevent dislocation and motion during swallowing. Stents usually remain in place for 6 to 8 weeks except in the case of hematomas (2 weeks) and should extend across the vocal cords to below the area of injury.

As mentioned, supraglottic injuries are prone to hematoma formation and extensive edema. When the epiglottis is torn from its anterior attachments to the base of the tongue and larynx, exision may be required. Attempts to reposition a badly torn and displaced epiglottis are attended by a high rate of supraglottic stricture. Rarely, supraglottic laryngectomy is required in such cases along with excision of the epiglottis.

Subglottic injuries require greater exposure and meticulous stenting because they are more likely to lead to stenosis. The most important subglottic structure is the cricoid cartilage. In subglottic injury, the larynx often must be opened from the thyroid notch to the upper tracheal rings. Preformed silastic T-tubes are especially good for subglottic and upper tracheal injuries, with the middle limb of the T being used for the percutaneous portion of the tracheotomy. Lower tracheal injuries may be resected or stented open, depending on the degree of comminution. All injuries in which the mucosa of the upper airway has been opened require external drainage. Because the mucosa of the larynx and trachea is thin and tightly adherent to supporting cartilage, all laryngeal fractures are considered to be compound (contaminated by upper airway secretions). Therefore, prophylactic broad spectrum antibiotics are recommended in all upper airway fractures. Steroids may be combined with antibiotics to decrease inflammation and edema.

Other Laryngeal Injuries. Separation of the larynx from the trachea or separation between two tracheal rings may also occur. In such cases, attempts at endotracheal intubation may be fatal. A tracheotomy tube should be inserted below the separation if possible and the structures reapproximated in layers. Hyoid release may be necessary to relieve tension on the suture lines.

Thermal and chemical burns of the larynx also occur. These are generally treated with nasogastric feeding tubes, steroids and antibiotics. Endolaryngeal stents may be required in the supraglottic area, since that is the usual site of burn damage. This is discussed in detail in Chapter 23. Finally, tracheal injuries that are below the level of T2 must be approached simultaneously through the neck and thorax.

Complications. Subcutaneous emphysema in itself is innocuous unless it produces compression of the airway, heart (pneumopericardium) or great vessels. Mucosal tears, however, allow contamination of the fascial spaces of the neck and may lead to cellulitis and abscess formation. Injury to the perichondrium is associated with subperichondrial hematoma and consequent devascularization and necrosis of cartilage. Chondritis and perichondritis with later stenosis usually result.

All internal laryngeal wounds are contaminated with upper respiratory flora, which results in delayed epithelialization and an exaggerated inflammatory stage of healing. Excessive granulation and cicatrization may result and lead to stenosis after even apparently minor laryngeal trauma. Injuries of the cricoid are especially prone to stenosis because it is the only complete cartilaginous ring in the airway.

Injuries to the Hypopharynx and Esophagus

Anatomy and Physiology. The cervical esophagus is a musculomembranous tube that runs in a posterior-inferior direction between the hypopharynx and thoracic inlet. The upper esophageal sphincter (cricopharyngeus) is 16 cm. from the incisors in the adult and 10 cm. in the child. The esophagus is not fixed in its midline position but freely mobile, restricted only by surrounding structures. It is normally collapsed during its cervical course. These characteristics, plus the protection afforded by the surrounding structures, shelter it from most external injuries. However, the walls of the cervical esophagus are very delicate and easily penetrated.

During the second stage of swallowing, the tongue pushes the bolus into the pharynx, the soft palate seals off the nasopharynx and the larynx rises under the epiglottis. Peristaltic intraluminal pressure rises, forcing the bolus into the hypopharynx and the upper esophageal sphincter opens, allowing passage into the esophagus. This same intraluminal pressure increase may also force secretions and food into the fascial planes of the neck following lacerations of the hypopharynx or esophagus.

Laceration and Rupture. The esophagus may be perforated by internal or external trauma. Most common is internal penetration during endoscopic procedures, or foreign body ingestion in children. Thus, the most common esophageal injury is an internal perforation located in the cervical esophagus. "External" perforation may be caused by either penetrating neck wounds or blunt trauma, but the former are usually accompanied by injuries to more critical adjacent structures whereas the latter are almost invariably located in the distal third of the thorax (see Thoracic Injuries, Chapter 13), where they cause more serious problems.

Violation of the upper digestive passage is one of the most common indications for exploration in large series of neck injuries. The common signs of pharyngeal or cervical esophageal injury include tenderness, dysphagia, drooling and crepitus. Neck infection and mediastinitis are later developments that usually require immediate drainage.

Soft tissue neck films, contrast esophagograms and esophagoscopy are usually diagnostic. Esophagograms should be performed whenever violation of the hypopharynx or cervical esophagus is suspected. If they are positive, esophagoscopy is then performed under anesthesia prior to surgical exploration.

Treatment. Simple mucosal tears of the nasopharynx and oropharynx usually do not require closure. They can be treated with warm saline irrigation, giving nothing by mouth and administering systemic antibiotics. In contrast, hypopharyngeal and esophageal mucosal tears are associated with salivary extravasation, probably because of increased intraluminal pressure during swallowing, and, if not explored, repaired and drained, may lead to serious deep cervical space infections, and often mediastinitis. Thus repair of the esophageal mucosa should be accomplished early. After 12 hours the involved

tissues often become so friable that closure is extremely difficult; adequate drainage, plus the use of a nasogastric tube and systemic antibiotics, becomes the standard treatment. Morbidity and mortality are directly related to the interval between injury and surgical exploration. Injuries to the esophagus down to the level of T2 may be approached through the neck. Those below this level require a thoracic or combined approach. Closure should employ an internal mucosal-submucosal layer of absorbable interrupted sutures and an outer muscular layer of nonabsorbable interrupted sutures; the wound should always be drained.

Vascular Injuries

Background and General Principles of Management. With the possible exception of injuries to the spinal cord, injuries to the major blood vessels carry the highest mortality and morbidity of all those affecting the structures in the neck. The most serious consequences of cervical vascular injuries are exsanguinating hemorrhage, extrinsic airway obstruction, air embolism and stroke.

Injuries to the vessels in the neck differ from those in the extremity in several important ways. First, in the absence of a gross neurological deficit secondary to cerebral ischemia, cervical vascular injuries may be difficult to diagnose. It may be impossible to palpate pulses distal to the injury. In addition, cutaneous signs of circulatory insufficiency are not present as they are with peripheral arterial injuries. Second, in both severe blunt and penetrating neck injuries, it may be difficult to determine whether the patient's neurological abnormalities are due to a vascular injury, hypoxia or direct damage to the nervous system. A third and most important difference is that cervical vascular injuries require immediate treatment. There is no "golden period" following the onset of cerebral ischemia during which repair will restore its integrity. Finally, delayed revascularization in the extremity rarely makes matters worse, whereas restoration of carotid artery flow, once a cerebral infarct has developed, may convert this from an anemic to a hemorrhagic infarct, with devastating consequences.

The vascular structures that may be injured are, of course, the arteries, veins and lymphatics. Lymphatic injuries are ordinarily of little consequence except for penetrating wounds involving the thoracic duct, in which a persistent lymph fistula can result. It should be kept in mind that any time one is exploring a penetrating wound at the confluence of the internal jugular and subclavian veins, injury to the thoracic duct should be specifically sought even if lymphatic leakage is not apparent. If an injured thoracic duct is not identified and ligated, a lymphocele or lymph fistula will commonly result.

Injuries to major cervical veins, even the internal jugular vein, rarely result in serious consequences. They usually present as a large or expanding hematoma. Associated venous thrombosis is ordinarily an occult event, except in the rare circumstance that both internal jugular veins are involved or there is significant propagation of the thrombus. A significant pulmonary embolus from cervical venous thrombosis is almost unheard of.

The most serious complication of penetrating cervical venous injuries is air embolism. This is one of the reasons for prohibiting the exploration of penetrating cervical wounds in the emergency department under local anesthesia. General endotracheal anesthesia with continuous positive pressure applied throughout the respiratory cycle removes this threat.

Cervical arterial injuries, when associated with penetrating wounds, may result in exsanguinating hemorrhage. Over 40 per cent of patients presenting to the Parkland Memorial Hospital with penetrating cervical arterial injuries arrived in shock.[25] Occasionally, hemorrhage from a penetrating arterial wound may produce serious airway obstruction by extrinsic pressure on the larynx and trachea. However, once hemostasis and an adequate airway have been assured, the main determinant of the outcome of cervical arterial injuries is the presence or absence of cerebral ischemia, and more specifically, the severity and duration of any preoperative neurological deficit. In Thal's report of 60 penetrating cervical arterial injuries, only 6 of 41 patients with no preoperative neurological deficit developed deficits postoperatively.[25] Even 5 of 6 patients with mild preoperative neurological deficit recovered without any residual deficits, whereas 4 of

13 patients with a severe deficit died. As will be discussed later, the presence or absence of a preoperative neurological deficit strongly influenced not only the outcome but also the indications for exploration and repair.

In general, injuries to the internal carotid artery commonly present with a neurological deficit and are difficult to repair, injuries to the vertebral artery rarely cause a neurologic deficit but are difficult to repair, and injuries to the common carotid and innominate arteries rarely produce neurological deficits and are easily repaired. Injuries to the subclavian arteries at the base of the neck almost never cause neurological sequelae and are easily repaired once the challenges of exposure and hemostasis have been overcome.

The initial approach to cervical vascular injuries has already been discussed because these injuries and their recognized complications greatly influence the overall approach to neck injuries. Similar to the management of trauma to other systems, there is an initial period when recognition and treatment of life-threatening injuries take precedence. Thus, establishing hemostasis, an adequate airway and ventilatory exchange, restoration of blood volume and stabilization of the cervical spine as well as similar attention to life-threatening injuries elsewhere all precede the formal examination of the neck and the diagnostic studies to be described.

DIAGNOSTIC EVALUATION. In evaluating a patient for the presence of a cervical vascular injury, the examiner should *look for* any asymmetry, swelling or discoloration and consider the relationship of these and any cervical wounds to the known course of the major cervical vascular structures. Bleeding from any cervical wound should only be briefly observed regarding its color, rate, synchrony with heart beat or respirations and association with sucking sounds or bubbling action before firm pressure is applied with a clean or sterile object.

Under *no* circumstances should cervical wounds, however innocuous appearing, be probed in the emergency department, for fear of restarting serious hemorrhage or allowing air to be sucked into lacerated veins. Pressure will control almost any hemorrhage. Clamping in the depths of a bleeding wound usually results in more blood loss and may not only damage adjacent structures but also the vessels themselves, making direct repair more difficult or impossible. The examiner should also *feel* the relationships of these wounds or swelling to specific anatomic landmarks as well as *palpate* for the pulsations of the carotid arteries or their branches (e.g., superficial temporal artery) and the size, firmness and pulsatility of any cervical mass.

Auscultation for bruits should be performed thoroughly and repeatedly following penetrating injuries. With injuries at the base of the neck, examination of the chest for pneumothorax or hemothorax and the upper extremities for signs of nerves or vascular injury is mandatory. Finally, a thorough neurological examination is an essential part of the diagnostic evaluation of all neck injuries. Any neurological findings should be confirmed by a neurologist or neurosurgeon if the attending physician does not frequently perform complete neurological examinations.

Ancillary Studies. NONINVASIVE METHODS. The noninvasive methods developed recently for detecting extracranial and extremity arterial occlusive lesions should prove valuable in evaluating patients with injuries to the brachiocephalic vessels, though no such experience has yet been reported. Even diagnostic methods that are not normally sensitive enough to detect chronic, partially occlusive carotid lesions, such as ophthalmodynamometry and frontal thermography, will accurately detect acute total occlusions. Oculoplethysmography, radionuclide flow studies performed at the time of brain scanning and ultrasonic imaging techniques, although sensitive enough, are of little practical value in evaluating cervical vascular injuries because they are neither portable or readily available for most emergency situations. However, the Doppler ultrasonic velocity detector or "probe," a simple, portable, inexpensive instrument that should be available in every emergency department, can be extremely useful in the evaluation of brachiocephalic vascular injuries.

First, the Doppler probe can be used to "listen" over the course of these vessels to determine the presence and quality of their flow. This relatively simple method should detect most occlusions of the common carotid and subclavian arteries and the internal jugular and subclavian veins. The patency of the vertebral artery can be checked low in the neck just lateral to the internal jugular vein or higher up just below the occiput. Second, by using the Doppler probe as a means of detecting the return of flow as sphygmomanometer cuffs are deflated below systolic pressure, systolic pressures can be segmentally determined in the upper extremities. These provide a more sensitive index of innominate or subclavian artery occlusion than simply feeling the radial pulse or monitoring the brachial blood pressure by the usual method. Finally, using a directional Doppler probe to evaluate the presence and direction of flow through specific branches of the internal and external carotid and its response to compression of collateral vessels, obstruction of flow through the main arteries themselves can be detected with accuracy.

The requisite maneuvers and the interpretation of this periorbital Doppler examination are well described by Barnes.[2] It will usually begin to become positive at 50 per cent stenosis and will detect all *chronic* internal carotid stenoses of 75 per cent diameter or more. Therefore, it should detect essentially all *acute* traumatic occlusions. The examination is based on the fact that flow through the supraorbital and/or frontal arteries, which are branches of the ophthalmic and therefore the *internal* carotid artery, is normally upward or antegrade and collateralizes on the forehead with branches of the superficial temporal artery, the terminal branch of the *external* carotid. If the superficial temporal artery is compressed, there is an ischemic stimulus to the supraorbital artery and its flow should be augmented. Therefore, a normal study would reveal upward supraorbital artery flow that increases with superficial temporal artery compression, whereas downward flow diminished by superficial temporal artery compression would indicate an abnormal test and a significant internal carotid occlusive lesion.

Radiographic Studies. Anterior-posterior and lateral cervical x-rays and, in lower cervical penetrating wounds, an upright 6' AP chest film should always be obtained. The indications for arteriography are less absolute but it is usually desirable whenever an arterial injury is suspected. Both Blaisdell[3] and Monson[18] have related the indications for arteriography to the location of the penetrating wounds. They divide the neck into three zones by two horizontal planes through the top of the head of the clavicles and the angles of the mandible (Fig. 11–2) and recommend that arteriography be obtained for all penetrating wounds in the lower and upper zones (I and III, respectively). The rationale for obtaining an arteriogram for all zone I wounds rather than only those with a wide mediastinum, ipsilateral hemothorax or upper extremity pulse deficit relates to the special problems of obtaining exposure and gaining hemostasis in vascular injuries to this area, especially when the subclavian artery is involved. The value of a preoperative arteriogram for zone III wounds also relates to the difficulties in obtaining exposure and hemostasis with high internal carotid injuries and also to the importance of knowing whether or not there has been thrombotic occlusion of the distal (intracranial) internal carotid, for this will determine the feasibility of a reconstructive procedure as opposed to ligation. Because the choice of incision and the exposure and control of the major vessels in zone II present no particular problem and are regularly performed during the routine exploration of penetrating neck wounds without signs or symptoms, arteriography is not recommended for wounds in the intermediate zone. However, the authors prefer arteriography even in zone II wounds if the signs and symptoms, or the Doppler examination, indicate the likelihood of an arterial injury.

Treatment. The third phase of management, following resuscitation from life-threatening complications and diagnosis, is definitive surgical treatment. The rationale for exploring all penetrating wounds has already been discussed. If one does not follow the policy of routine exploration, the following are indications for exploration, whether or not the inflicting trauma is penetrating: the detection of a bruit; a large, rapidly expanding or pulsatile hematoma; the absence of pulsations or detectible flow in the carotid artery or its major branches; or the presence of a neurological deficit that cannot be explained by direct injury to the nervous system. What is less clear is whether or not to explore a patent carotid artery with mural

or periadventitial hemorrhage encountered during the course of a routine exploration or one dictated by nonvascular indications, and what, if any, procedure should be performed in patients with carotid injuries that have already caused a neurological deficit. These decisions are discussed in the following paragraphs.

PREPARATION OF THE PATIENT AND ANESTHESIA. It is important that blood volume be adequately restored prior to induction of anesthesia and, if necessary, hemostasis should be maintained by manual compression until this has been achieved and additional blood is available for transfusion. The patient should be in the supine position with the head extended and the occiput resting on a rolled gauze "donut." A rolled towel should also be placed under the upper thorax to allow hyperextension; intravenous catheters and blood pressure cuffs are best applied to the arm contralateral to the injury. If an additional IV catheter is required it should be placed through the great saphenous vein at the ankle and the other leg prepped in case a saphenous autograft is needed. However, in most cases the upper cephalic vein can be exposed in the same field and will serve quite satisfactorily. The chin should be turned away from the side of the injury and the entire neck, up to and including the lower chin and mandible, the base of the ear and the posterior cervical and supraclavicular regions, should be prepared and draped into the field. In low cervical injuries, the anterolateral thorax and the proximal upper extremity should be included in the surgical field bilaterally.

A smooth induction is important and pressure should be maintained over any penetrating wound during induction to prevent hemorrhage and/or air embolism. In general, an anesthetic agent that will increase cerebral blood flow in relation to cerebral metabolism, such as halothane or enthrane, should be used. The patient should be kept normotensive and eucarbic during the conduction of the anesthesia and skin preparation should be gentle to avoid embolism from mural thrombi in injured vessels. Allowance should be made for the possible need to perform intraoperative arteriography.

INCISIONS. A long incision along the anterior border of the sternocleidomastoid muscle gives the best exposure for most vascular (and other) injuries, particularly if they are unilateral. This incision can be readily continued downward by splitting the upper sternum in the midline to obtain more proximal exposure of the brachiocephalic vessels, including the subclavian artery. However, with injuries to the subclavian artery due to a penetrating injury low in the neck, the approach recommended by Brawley[4] is preferred. If there is no immediate problem with control of bleeding through the wound or into the pleural space below, an incision can be made along the medial clavicle, resecting its medial third or half. If hemostasis *is* or becomes a problem, an anterolateral third intercostal space incision should be made through which compression can be applied to the apex of the pleural cavity from below to provide immediate hemostasis. Then if further exposure is needed the medial ends of these two incisions can be jointed vertically by a median sternotomy. This allows the entire upper thorax to be hinged outward, giving very ample exposure of the subclavian vessels. The vertebral artery origin can also be exposed in this manner. The more limited exposure used for elective procedures on the proximal vertebral artery will not suffice when this vessel is bleeding. Recently, Brink et al.[5] reviewed a series of vertebral artery injuries and demonstrated how this artery can be exposed at three levels throughout its course.

The techniques for obtaining control of injured vessels and the principles of repair differ from those described for peripheral vessels (Chapter 19) in only a few respects. In dealing with an injured carotid artery, special attention must be given to the possible need for maintaining flow during the repair by means of a temporary indwelling silastic shunt. A shunt does not need to be inserted if the carotid has been occluded for some time and no neurological deficit has developed. It has been reported that as long as the blood pressure has been restored and is maintained, occlusion times from 60 to 110 minutes without shunting are well tolerated.[9] Futhermore, it has been shown that the main cause of a neurological deficit developing during carotid surgery is embolization from an ulcerated plaque rather than interruption of carotid flow. This should be kept in mind

in the dissection of injured carotid arteries that may contain loosely adherent mural thrombus.

Since shunts are required in only about 10 per cent of the patients undergoing elective carotid surgery, it is important to identify that group of patients and avoid the inconvenience and complications of inserting a shunt in the others. The best approach is to measure the retrograde pressure from the distal internal carotid beyond occluding clamps on the common and external carotid arteries.[20] If this "stump" pressure is greater than 40 mm. Hg and the patient has not had a recent cerebral infarct, a shunt is not necessary. Otherwise, it is preferable to insert a Javid or Brenner shunt, secured proximally and distally with Rummel tourniquets, during the exploration and repair.

If one encounters a patent carotid artery with signs of mural periadventitial hemorrhage, that artery should be explored *if* the carotid "stump" pressure is adequate. If the pressure is low, an operative arteriogram should be performed and if it is positive, exploration should be performed using a shunt; the likelihood of the latter circumstance is small.

Another important question is whether to explore an injured artery that is already occluded. If there is no neurological deficit or the deficit is a minor one and arteriography shows that there is no thrombotic or embolic occlusion in the distal tree, the artery should be explored and repaired. If, on the other hand, there is a *major* neurological deficit *or* there is embolic or thrombotic occlusion in the distal tree, the artery should be ligated. This situation is most likely to be encountered with internal carotid injuries.

The other predicament encountered in dealing with *internal* carotid artery injuries is difficulty in gaining exposure and hemostatic control and performing a repair when the injury is high, particulary if it is still bleeding. Occasionally, distal control can be achieved by passing a Fogarty catheter up through a small proximal arteriotomy and inflating the balloon above the injury near the base of the skull.

If there is sufficient arterial destruction to require interposition of a venous autograft, it must remembered that when the neck is brought back to its normal position considerable shortening may occur; if the vein graft is too long, kinking may occur with thrombosis at one of the anastomoses. If a vein graft is necessary, it is usually wise to insert a temporary shunt to maintain flow while the graft is being harvested and prepared for interposition. The vein graft can even be slid over the shunt and the upper and part of the lower anastomosis performed before the shunt is removed. The saphenous, cephalic or even external jugular vein may be used to repair the common or internal carotid arteries. Because the neck has good vascularity and the carotid artery flow is high, the risk of infection or thrombosis of prosthetic grafts is not as high as with peripheral placement. Therefore, while they are not as suitable as an autograft, a Dacron velour or expanded polytetrafluorethylene graft should give satisfactory results in this position. These are relatively contraindicated, however, in the significantly contaminated neck injury.

Finally, because the vertebral arteries supply less than 10 per cent of cerebral blood flow and are difficult to expose and repair, it is unlikely that reconstruction of vertebral artery injuries will be carried out in most circumstances. The likelihood is less than 2 to 3 per cent that developmental anomalies present in the contralateral vertebrae would cause ligation of one vertebral artery to result in infarction.[26]

Delayed Vascular Injuries. Although false aneurysms and arteriovenous fistulas are usually considered delayed forms of arterial injury, they are really the result of delayed recognition and treatment. In general, the same principles apply to their management in the neck as in the extremity; they should be explored as early as possible, preferably when they are still only a poorly organized and/or communicating hematoma, and repair should be performed after proximal and distal control is carefully obtained.

Cervical Nerve Injuries

One must be aware of the possibility of cervical nerve injuries, particularly in penetrating wounds of the neck. Even though it is unlikely that primary repair will be undertaken, the existence of such an injury gives important information about the anatomical course of the penetrating wound.

Thus, deviation of the tongue and difficulty with fricative sounds in speaking would not only indicate a hypoglossal nerve injury but also the possibility of involvement of the carotid artery above its bifurcation. Similarly a high vagus nerve injury, which would also involve the fibers to the recurrent nerve, would cause paralysis of one vocal cord and hoarseness or a weak, husky voice. Thus, one should also specifically look for Horner's syndrome (cervical sympathetics), paralyzed diaphragm (phrenic), drooping of the corner of the mouth (mandibular branch of the facial), and trapezius weakness (accessory). The principles of treatment are similar to those discussed for peripheral nerve injuries, except that, with the exception of the hypoglossal nerve and possibly the mandibular branch of the facial, reanastomosis of injured cervical nerves in the neck is rarely successfully performed. Compensating procedures such as a fascial sling to the corner of the mouth for the latter injury or injection of Teflon into the vocal cord for high vagus or recurrent nerve injuries are often all that can be offered to offset the disability.

Glandular Injuries

The *thyroid gland* has a rich vascular supply and may bleed profusely when lacerated. Such hemorrhage can even lead to respiratory distress.[11] Loss of its endocrine function, however, is extremely uncommon, in part due to its rich vascular supply. In cases where major tissue loss of the anterior neck has occurred, however, hypothyroidism should be considered. A history of tiredness, constipation, brittle hair, thickening of the skin and deepening of the voice should be sought, and thyroid function studies should be performed.

When injury of the thyroid gland is noted during neck exploration, devitalized tissue should be removed and hemostasis obtained. It should be remembered that the recurrent laryngeal nerves are located at the posterior lateral margins of the thyroid gland in close approximation to the inferior thyroid arteries. Extreme care must be taken during clamping of any vascular structures near the tracheoesophageal groove to prevent inadvertent injury to the recurrent nerve. Traumatic loss of the entire thyroid is usually accompanied by carotid artery injury and airway disruption so that survival is unlikely.

Simultaneous injury to all parathyroid glands is most uncommon due to their distribution. When a parathyroid is identified in a devitalized area of the thyroid or found free elsewhere in the wound, it should be carefully dissected free, thinly diced or sliced and reimplanted in muscle. Implantation into the forearm muscle allows the function of the implant to be independently monitored.[28]

Salivary gland injuries, in general, are handled by debridement, hemostasis and drainage. It should be remembered that the tail of the parotid gland commonly extends into the neck. Injuries to this portion of the gland may include the posterior facial vein. However, crucial structures, such as the facial nerve and Stenson's duct, which are commonly injured in facial parotid gland lacterations, are not at risk in the cervical parotid.

The submandibular gland is encapsulated by the superficial layer of the deep cervical fascia and may be removed intact when severely injured. The juxtaposition of the marginal mandibular branch of the facial artery must be kept in mind during surgery in this area. Wharton's duct should be double ligated during excision.

Soft Tissue Injuries of the Neck

Soft tissue injuries of the neck are especially common in children and usually are not life-threatening. Appropriate early care often prevents later complications. The terminology regarding soft tissue injuries is frequently unclear, so a brief review is appropriate. An *abrasion* is a superficial wound produced by friction. It is usually caused by a large mass moving at low velocity and striking the skin tangentially. A *contusion* is a deeper injury with tissue damage (primarily vascular) occurring in the absence of surface disruption. *Laceration* implies skin disruption. A *puncture wound* extends to the deep underlying tissues with minimal disruption of the surface tissues.

Gunshot wounds produce a special type of problem in addition to the entrance laceration and trauma caused by the missile; that is, the cone of injury, caused by the production of secondary missiles of bone

or fragments, by ricochet or by the force of the blast.

In the management of lacerations or abrasions of the neck, the status of tetanus immunization must be determined. In general, active immunization is recommended in the nonimmunized individual. A booster injection (tetanus toxoid 0.5 ml. IM) is recommended for immunized patients who have not received a booster within 5 years. In severe injuries involving extensive contamination or massive tissue devitalization, a tetanus booster should be given along with 250 to 500 units of human tetanus immune globulin (Hyper-tet).

Deep abrasions should be scrubbed under anesthesia to remove all foreign material. Foreign bodies such as wood, asphalt, gravel or glass are meticulously searched for and removed. Greases are more easily removed if a mild detergent is added to the cleansing solution. Acetone and alcohol may be used in superficial wounds; however, these may damage tissue and must be used with care. Organic iodide solution such as Betadine cause minimal tissue injury and are available in soaps. Hydrogen peroxide is irritating to deeper tissues and is not recommended.

Lacerations should be cleaned of clots and foreign materials, scrubbed with aqueous iodine-iodide solution and irrigated carefully. Local anesthesia is recommended, but general anesthesia may be required for more extensive lacerations.

Once the laceration has been cleansed, devitalized tissue should be conservatively debrided. Wound edges should be at right angles and the closure planned to lie in natural skin lines when possible.

Deep structures must be evaluated prior to closure of any laceration. Once injury to vital structures has been ruled out, the deeper tissues should be approximated with absorbable sutures in layers. The subcutaneous tissues are next closed with interrupted subcutaneous sutures, and the skin with nonabsorbable monofilament. Smaller lacerations can often be closed with a running subcuticular suture, which is easily removed in a small child. In either case, the skin edges are accurately reapproximated with slight eversion. Interrupted sutures can be removed from the neck at 4 to 5 days with sterile tape reinforcement for an additional week.

The primary closure of cervical lacerations can be accomplished up to 12 to 18 hours following injury because of the excellent blood supply of the neck. Beyond that time, or in grossly contaminated wounds, closure should be delayed for 72 hours. The laceration can then be sutured loosely or closed with adhesive strips, if clean. Subsequent scar revision will probably be required. Scars of the cervical skin frequently widen in children owing to increased elasticity of their tissues, and parents should be forewarned of this.

REFERENCES

1. Ashworth, C., Williams, L. F., and Byrne, J. J.: Penetrating wounds of the neck. Am. J. Surg. 121:387, 1971.
2. Barnes, R. W., Russel, H. E., Bone, G. E., and Slaymaker, E. E.: Doppler cerebrovascular examination: Improved results with refinements in technique. Stroke 8:468, 471, 1977.
3. Blaisdell, F. W., in discussion of Cohen, A., Brief, D., Mathewson, C.: Carotid artery injuries. Am. J. Surg. 120:210, 1970.
4. Brawley, R. K., et al.: Management of wounds of the innominate, subclavian and axillary blood vessels. Surg. Gynecol. Obstet. 131:1130, 1970.
5. Brink, B. E., Meier, D., and Fry, W. J.: Operative exposure and management of lesions in the vertebral artery. Arch. Surg. In press.
6. Bryce, D. P.: The surgical management of laryngotracheal injury. J. Laryngol. Otol. 86:547, 587, 1972.
7. Butler, R. M., and Moser, F. H.: The padded dash syndrome: Blunt trauma to the larynx and trachea. Laryngoscope 78:1172, 1968.
8. De La Cruz, A. C. Jr.: Management of penetrating wounds of the neck. Surg. Gynecol. Obstet. 137:458, 1973.
9. Fitchell, V. H., Pomerantz, M., Butsch, D. W., Simon, R., and Eiseman, B.: Penetrating wounds of the neck. Arch. Surg. 99:307, 1969.
10. Fogelman, M. J., and Stewart, R. D.: Penetrating wounds of the neck. Am. J. Surg. 91:581, 1956.
11. Grace, R. H., and Shilling, J. S.: Acute haemorrhage into the thyroid gland following trauma and causing respiratory distress. Br. J. Surg. 56:635, 1969.
12. Harris, H. H., and Tobin, H. A.: Acute injuries of the larynx and trachea in 49 patients. Laryngoscope 80:1376, 1970.
13. Jafek, B. W., and Balkany, T. J.: Injuries of the neck (Chapter 77). In Bluestone, C. D., Stool, S. E. (eds.): Pediatric Otolaryngology. Philadelphia, W. B. Saunders Co., (in press).
14. Jafek, B. W., Butler, R., and Ward, P. H.: Blunt laryngotracheal trauma. California Medicine 115:67, 1971.
15. Jernigan, W. R., and Gardner, W. C.: Carotid artery injuries due to closed cervical trauma. J. Trauma 11:429, 1971.
16. McInnis, W. D., Cruz, A. B., and Aust, J. B.: Penetrating injuries to the neck. Am. J. Surg. 130:416, 1975.
17. Markey, J. C. Jr., Hines, J. L., and Nance, F. C.: Penetrating neck wounds: A review of 218 cases. Am. Surg. 41:77, 1975.
18. Monson, D. O., Saletta, J. D., and Freeark, R. J.: Carotid vertebral trauma. J. Trauma 9:987, 1969.
19. Montgomery, W. W.: Surgery of the Upper Respiratory System, Vol. 2. Philadelphia, Lea & Febiger, 1973, p. 543.
20. Moore, W. S., and Hall, A. D.: Carotid artery back pressure. Arch. Surg. 99:702, 1969.
21. Pennington, C. L.: External trauma of the larynx and trachea. Immediate treatment and management. Ann. Otol. Rhinol. Laryngol. 81:546, 1972.
22. Rogers, W. A.: Treatment of fracture-dislocation of the cervical spine. J. Bone Joint Surg. 13:245, 1942.
23. Saletta, J. D., Folk, F. A., and Freeark, R. J.: Trauma to the neck region. Surg. Clin. N. Am. 53:73, 1973.
24. Stein, A., and Kalk, F.: Selective conservatism in the management of penetrating wounds of the neck. S. Afr. J. Surg. 12:31, 1974.
25. Thal, E. R., Snyder, W. H. III, Hays, R. J., and Perry, M. O.: Management of carotid artery injuries. Surgery 76:955, 1974.
26. Thomas, G. I., Anderson, K. N., Hain, R. F., and Merendino, K. A.: The significance of anomalous vertebral-basilar artery communications in operations of the heart and great vessels. Surgery 46:747, 1956.
27. Weaver, A. W., Sankarin, S., Fromm, S. H., Lucas, C. E., and Walt, A. J.: The management of penetrating wounds of the neck. Surg. Gynecol. Obstet. 133:49, 1971.
28. Wells, S. A., Gunnels, J. C., Sheldurne, J. D., et al.: Transplantation of the parathyroid glands in man: Clinical indications and results. Surgery 78:34, 1975.

CHAPTER 12

TRACHEOSTOMY

Margaret M. Fletcher, M.D.

Tracheostomy is a procedure that has been done for more than two thousand years to relieve upper airway obstruction. In the past, it was performed as an unplanned terminal event in diseases such as diphtheria. Because the patients usually died from their primary disease, tracheostomies were seldom done. During the past 30 years, however, the management of the acutely ill patient has changed a great deal. One notes, as well, an attendant change in the indications and complications of tracheostomy.

The initial evaluation and treatment of the injured patient has been discussed in previous chapters. In the severely injured or acutely ill patient, inadequate ventilation and inadequate circulation rapidly lead to central nervous system anoxia. Three to five minutes of central nervous system anoxia lead to irreversible damage and death.

The purpose of this chapter is to provide guidelines on how to manage a patient who requires tracheostomy. These will include:

1. Location of the ventilatory problem.
2. Indications for tracheostomy.
3. The steps involved in performing a tracheostomy.
4. The importance of nursing care following tracheostomy.
5. The management of early and late complications.

LOCATION AND MANAGEMENT OF VENTILATORY PROBLEMS

Head and Spinal Cord Injury

Seventy-one per cent of the victims of automobile accidents sustain injury to the head, midface or upper airway.[16] Sixty-four per cent of these patients die from intracranial and ventilation complications. Several mechanisms are responsible for ventilatory problems. First, cerebral edema seen with head trauma or direct damage to the respiratory center can decrease ventilatory rate and cause anoxia. Second, with unconsciousness, the tongue, pharynx and mandible become posteriorly displaced and obstruct the upper airway. Third, the cough reflex is obliterated. Secretions, blood and foreign bodies can obstruct the airway and cause aspiration pneumonitis. Unconsciousness and/or brainstem involvement often result in copious, uncontrolled secretions of saliva and mucus which, when aspirated, cause severe and often irreversible pneumonitis. It is important to consider this problem early in patients with head trauma. Tracheostomy is done to maintain an airway, to maintain ventilation and to assist in the removal of tracheal secretions and aspirated materials. Once aspiration pneumonitis is established, it is difficult to treat. The mortality rate is approximately 70 per cent.[1, 3]

The diagnosis of head trauma is reviewed in Chapter 8. A brief checklist when considering the airway would indicate the following:

1. Closely observe the patient's mental status and level of consciousness.
2. Lacerations, contusions and palpated fractures of the face or skull may indicate possible central nervous system damage.
3. Cerebral spinal fluid otorrhea and rhinorrhea may indicate meningeal tear and impending brainstem compromise.
4. Cranial nerve impairment may be shown by hoarseness (X), weak shoulder (XI), weak tongue muscle (XII) or cerebel-

lar deficits that indicate brainstem involvement.

5. Respirations may be irregular and deep with coarse inspiratory stridor.

An airway can usually be established by protrusion of the mandible, oral airway and mouth-to-mouth respiration. An endotracheal tube is inserted to maintain the airway, to provide respiratory assistance, if necessary, and to assist in the removal of secretions or blood from the pharynx. If the endotracheal tube must be in place for more than 48 hours, the trachea should be examined daily with a fiberoptic bronchoscope. Some patients may tolerate endotracheal tubes well for several days. If tracheal cartilage is noted, a tracheostomy is indicated.

Pharynx

The pharynx is the most common site of upper airway obstruction; it is also the easiest to manage. Unfortunately, it is often forgotten. If a patient has total airway obstruction, there will be no stridor — only paradoxical chest movements. These movements have often been mistaken for adequate ventilation, but auscultation of the chest and examination of the mouth reveal that no air is being exchanged. Many lives have been saved by pulling the jaw and tongue forward and by scooping gastric contents, blood, dentures, food and secretions out of the hypopharynx with the fingers or with suction, if it is available.

The *diagnosis* of pharyngeal obstruction is made by evaluating the respirations and examination of the pharynx:

Respirations: Before complete obstruction, breath sounds are coarse with palatal and pharyngeal stridor, similar to exaggerated snoring. With complete obstruction, there is no movement of air.

Rate: Tachypneic and labored.

Movements: Suprasternal and intercostal retractions with each attempted inspiration.

Color: Cyanosis is not present unless the patient has 5 gm./100 ml. of reduced hemoglobin circulating. It may not be present if the patient is being administered nasal oxygen or if he is in shock and vasoconstricted.

Other traumatic causes of pharyngeal obstruction include displaced maxillary and mandibular fractures. These can sometimes be disimpacted by a constant pull against the muscles of mastication. If this is not readily accomplished, it is best to insert an oral airway or endotracheal tube or to proceed with a tracheostomy. Thermal burns of the head and trunk may also involve the mucosa of the oral cavity and pharynx. These are diagnosed by redness and edema of the palate and epiglottis, hoarseness, cough, pain and sometimes inspiratory stridor. Chemical burns are usually the result of caustic lye ingestion. Normal mucosa is replaced by a white fibrinous membrane, surrounded by redness and edema. Intubation may cause further damage. Tracheostomy is indicated early.

Hematomas of the retropharyngeal, parapharyngeal and visceral spaces occur as a result of cervical spine, carotid artery, internal jugular vein, thyroid, laryngeal and tracheal injury. Hematomas can cause severe airway obstruction and often extend deep into the mediastinum. Tracheostomy is often of little benefit in these instances; instead, it is important to intubate the patient, evaluate the hematoma and explore the injured sites for control.

Larynx

Vocal Cord Adduction. Incomplete laryngeal obstruction may have a characteristic high-pitched inspiratory crow. This is a result of air passing between two tightly opposed or edematous vocal cords. It is commonly associated with acute inflammation or extubation after anesthesia. Foreign bodies, mucus, blood and thermal burns in the larynx may also cause laryngospasm. Bilateral recurrent nerve paralysis and brainstem injury to the nucleus ambiguus bilaterally are less common causes of vocal cord adduction.

Laryngeal Fracture. Hoarseness, cough, hemoptysis, subcutaneous emphysema and neck contusions, when present with or without head injury, should indicate laryngeal fracture until proven otherwise.

The diagnosis can be confirmed by indirect examination. Complete airway obstruction may develop suddenly. Once a diagnosis of laryngeal fracture is made, tracheostomy is indicated. As soon as the patient's condition has stabilized, the laryngeal fracture should be reduced, mucosal lacerations repaired and an endotracheal stent inserted.

Tracheal, Pulmonary and Chest Wall Injuries

The diagnosis and management of these problems are covered in Chapter 13. Tracheostomy is important in a patient with tracheal laceration, multiple rib fractures or flail chest. It is done to assist ventilation and to remove bronchial secretions. Tracheostomy provides a means for ventilation in patients with lung contusions.

The usual causes of ventilatory problems in an injured patient are an upper airway obstruction, chest injury, or loss of central nervous system control due to head injury. The diagnosis and immediate management of each of these problems have been discussed. In each instance, a tracheostomy may be indicated, but only rarely is it used as the first line of defense of treatment. Instead, patient position, jaw and tongue position, clearing of secretions, foreign material, oral airway and mouth-to-mouth resuscitation are all that are necessary.

If ventilation cannot be maintained with these maneuvers, than an endotracheal tube should be inserted. The technique of intubation is discussed in Chapter 2. Once an airway is established, the emergency situation is under control, and the tracheostomy is then a planned procedure.

Endotracheal intubation causes a certain amount of injury in every patient. When compared with the life-saving aspects of this procedure, the early injury is usually of no consequence and is acceptable. After 30 to 40 hours of intubation, mucosal ulceration occurs on the laryngeal surface of the epiglottis, the arytenoids, glottis and subglottic space. Inflammation increases with time and after 5 days, 80 per cent of intubated patients demonstrate laryngeal cartilage necrosis.[8] Laryngotracheal injury may be seen by direct examination. Subsequent tracheostomy may be indicated if continued ventilatory support or an airway is needed.

INDICATIONS FOR TRACHEOSTOMY

Upper Airway Obstruction. If position change or intubation does not relieve the upper airway obstruction, a tracheostomy is necessary. This may occur in patients with the following problems: (1) Impacted fractures, uncontrollable hemorrhage or congenital deformities of the face or jaw. (2) Epiglottitis, neoplasm, space abscess or a foreign body in the pharynx. (3) Trauma, fracture, laceration, stenosis, bilateral vocal cord paralysis, benign lesions or papillomas of the larynx or trachea.

Prolonged Ventilatory Support. The most common indication for tracheostomy is the need to provide access to the trachea for ventilatory support. Positive pressure to both lungs requires a leak-proof cuffed tracheostomy tube. An endotracheal tube is used when ventilatory support is required for a few days. A tracheostomy is performed when tracheal erosion or injury from the endotracheal tube is noted by fiberoptic examination or if tracheobronchial secretions are inadequately handled by suctioning the endotracheal tube. Abnormal ventilation requiring prolonged ventilatory support is often found in patients with the following conditions: (1) Central neurological disorders causing respiratory depression such as drug overdose, mass lesion, or ischemia (CVA, MI). (2) Neuromuscular disorders causing respiratory depression such as amyotrophic lateral sclerosis, poliomyelitis or Guillain-Barré syndrome. (3) Chest disorders such as flail chest, or chronic obstructive pulmonary disease.

Tracheal Toilet. This removal of tracheobronchial secretions and plugs can be a major problem in some patients following surgical procedures or in those with established pulmonary disease.

Caution: the advantage of clearing heavy secretions via tracheostomy must be weighed against the disadvantages of an unprotected airway and possible aspiration.

TRACHEOSTOMY TECHNIQUE

Once the need for tracheostomy is established, an endotracheal tube or bronchoscope is inserted, after topical lidocaine 4 per cent. The airway can then be suctioned and ventilation begun.

Despite its apparent simplicity and frequency of performance, tracheostomy may be a hazardous procedure and should be performed in the operating room. Before proceeding, one should take a few minutes to check on *four details*. This time will often save hours spent managing complications that otherwise might occur.

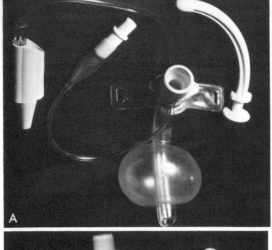
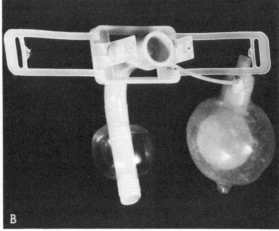
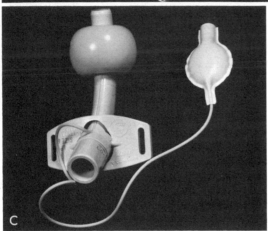

Figure 12–1. A, *National Catheter Pitt Speaking tracheostomy tube. It features a soft "hi-lo" cuff to minimize tracheal damage and a pilot tube in the wall for speaking. The length is adjustable, and it has an obturator and a double swivel adaptor for ventilation equipment.*

B, Lanz Controlled Pressure Cuff tracheostomy tube. The amount of air injected in the cuff is immaterial. When the cuff is inflated, the regulating valve maintains the cuff pressure at 20 mm. Hg. Tube length is adjustable. Includes an obturator and a 15-mm. adaptor for ventilation equipment.

C, Shiley Cuffed tracheostomy tube. It features an inner cannula for cleaning, an obturator and a 15-mm. adaptor.

1. Prepare for possible cardiac arrest and pneumothorax. These problems occur often in injured patients with ventilatory and circulatory compromise.

2. Prepare tracheostomy tube (Fig. 12–1). Determine type and size to be used and check cuff for leaks. The tube should be ready for insertion *before* the incision is made.

3. Prepare a culture tube and suction. When the tracheostomy is performed, the cough reflex produces a large amount of pus. Take a Gram stain and culture, then suction the secretions.

4. Recognize the importance of light and position; one can get into trouble if these simple details are ignored. A patient who is awake with an endotracheal tube in place experiences a great deal of pain when the neck is in a hyperextended position. It is better to have the nurse place a bolster (pillow or rolled sheet) under the patient's shoulder after the surgeon has scrubbed and everything is ready.

SURGICAL TECHNIQUE

Preparation. Scrub the skin from the mandible to below the clavicle. Palpate the midline structures to identify the hyoid bone, thyroid notch, cricoid cartilage and suprasternal notch. Next infiltrate the skin and subcutaneous tissues with 1 per cent lidocaine in a transverse line halfway between the cricoid cartilage and suprasternal notch.

Incision. Make a transverse incision halfway between the cricoid cartilage and the suprasternal notch (Fig. 12–2), extending through the skin and subcutaneous tissue down to the superficial layer of deep cervical fascia. Small dermal vessels will be encountered and bleeding is easily con-

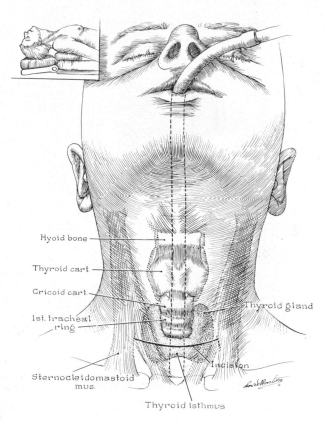

Figure 12-2. *Illustration of position for tracheostomy, midline structures and incision.*

Hyoid bone

Thyroid cart.

Cricoid cart.

1st. tracheal ring

Thyroid gland

Incision

Sternocleidomastoid mus.

Thyroid isthmus

trolled by pressure or clamping. Then identify the midline by palpating the cricoid cartilage and visualize the linea alba seen between the bellies of the sternohyoid muscles. Incise the cervical fascia vertically in the midline from the cricoid to 1 cm. above the sternal notch. The anterior jugular veins are located laterally and the anterior communicating veins are located inferiorly. They should not be in the line of dissection.

Visceral Compartment. If the thyroid isthmus is freely movable, it can be displaced superiorly or inferiorly with a vein retractor. In adults, the thyroid is often more fibrotic and firmly attached to pretracheal fascia. In these instances, it is preferable to clamp, divide the suture, ligate the isthmus (Fig. 12–3) and bluntly dissect it off the trachea. Insert a tracheal hook beneath the first ring and retract the trachea superiorly and anteriorly.

Instruct the anesthesiologist to deflate the endotracheal tube cuff. Then instill 1 ml. of lidocaine into the trachea and make a cruciate incision (Fig. 12–4) between tracheal rings 2 and 3. Do not remove a window of cartilage because this is associated with an increased incidence of tracheal stenosis. Remove the endotracheal tube, obtain a culture and smear and suction the trachea. Insert the tracheostomy tube with its obturator in place (Fig. 12–5). Remove the obturator and the bolster, then flex the head and tie the tracheostomy ribbons with a square knot. Wound sutures predispose to the development of subcutaneous emphysema.

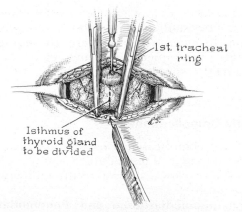

1st. tracheal ring

Isthmus of thyroid gland to be divided

Figure 12-3. *Transection of thyroid isthmus.*

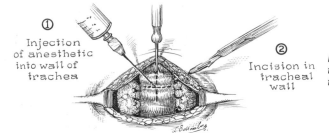

Figure 12-4. Incision between tracheal rings two and three after injecting with local anesthetic.

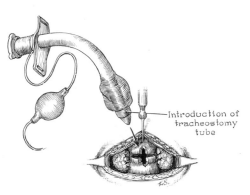

Figure 12-5. Insertion of tracheostomy tube.

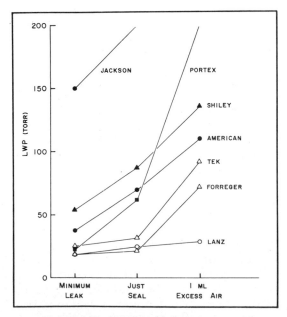

Figure 12-6. Lateral tracheal wall pressure increases sharply after obtaining minimal occlusion. No resistance can be felt during inflation of the new tracheostomy cuffs. One should listen for air passing around the cuff and should stop inflation when seal is first noted. This should occur at 15-20 cm. H₂O. (Courtesy of Dr. H. Turndorf, Critical Care Medicine 1:202, 1973.)

THE TRACHEOSTOMY TUBE

Proper selection and use of the tracheostomy tube is important in reducing complications of tracheostomy. The problem of tracheal stenosis resulting from cuff injury has almost been eliminated because of recent information about cuff pressure. The important conclusion is that the larger tube requires less air and seals at a lower pressure. In addition, the 1 cc. of excess air inserted just after seal results in a very sharp increase in lateral wall pressure (Fig. 12–6).

The cuff should be a high-volume low pressure type with complete protection from aspiration, including no leak ventilation. It should include signalling devices of under- and overinflation, and an automatic device to limit pressure on the trachea. The cuffed diameter should be greater than tracheal diameter and it should gently conform to the trachea without distortion.

POSTOPERATIVE CARE AND COMPLICATIONS

Once the airway has been established by tracheostomy, complications may arise from the operative procedure, the equipment, inadequate nursing care and changed respiratory physiology.

Early Complications

Early complications may be associated with the surgical procedure. Some ways to avoid these are discussed in the following paragraphs.

Pneumomediastinum and Pneumothorax. Secure control of the trachea after making a tracheal incision with the tracheal hook, or stay sutures, in place. Suction the trachea and insert a tracheostomy tube without delay. Do not suture the wound, and do not ventilate the patient with high pressures that rupture alveoli. Lateral dissection in a struggling patient predisposes to cutting lung apices, though this is uncommon. Intubation preoperatively allows a less hurried operation with less struggle.

Air Embolism. This results from transecting anterior jugular veins or subclavian veins without control or recognition.

Hemorrhage. Early hemorrhage is due to improper suture ligation of the thyroid isthmus, poor control of venous drainage, or inadvertent incision of the subclavian vein in the subclavian fossa. For purposes of management, identify source and secure hemostasis with suture or cautery.

Tracheoesophageal Fistula. Tracheoesophageal fistula is usually the result of using too much downward pressure with a large scalpel blade while making tracheostomy. The esophagus may be distended in a struggling patient. Immediate exploration of the neck is done with primary closure of the fistula.

Apnea. After tracheostomy has been performed, the patient is relieved of his airway obstruction and the hemoglobin is oxidized. He has lost his hypoxic drive and becomes apneic. Respirations should be assisted during this period with a respirator or manually with an Ambu bag.

Dislodged Tracheostomy Tube. If tracheostomy ribbons are tied while the neck is hyperextended, they may be too loose when the bolster is removed. This allows the tracheostomy tube to be coughed out during suctioning. For the same reason, bulky dressings should be avoided on the tracheostomy wound. If the tracheostomy tube becomes dislodged within the first 24 hours, one again has an emergent obstructive problem to manage and the steps should follow a logical sequence.

Light, position, suction, tracheostomy tube, hook and retractors are all necessary tools to be used again during reinsertion. If the tube cannot be reinserted with direct visualization, it may be inserted over a fiberoptic bronchoscope. Valuable time is often lost by trying to thread a tracheostomy tube over a suction catheter, ostensibly in the trachea.

Late Complications

Inspissated Mucus. The most common cause of death from tracheostomy is obstruction due to inspissated mucous plugs. This can be avoided by efficient humidification to the tracheostomy by a "tracheal mask" or by the ventilatory apparatus. Suctioning is necessary almost every 30 minutes during the first 24 hours, then every 1 to 2 hours thereafter, more often if necessary. If secretions continue to be dry, one should be aware of the patient's general state of hydration, replacing known deficits. One to three ml. of sterile saline may be instilled within the trachea before suctioning.

Aspiration Pneumonitis and Tracheobronchitis. After 48 hours, almost all tracheostomies have a culture of *Staphylococcus aureus, Pseudomonas aeruginosa, Proteus vulgaris* or *Escherichia coli*. The cause of this is believed to be related to the tracheal foreign body (tube) in an unprotected airway. More importantly, the aspiration of saliva has been documented in at least 70 per cent of patients with tracheostomy. Saliva can destroy respiratory epithelium, predisposing it to local infection, tracheobronchitis, lobar pneumonitis and tracheal erosion. Aspiration may be related to incompetent glottic closure in patients who continue to swallow. Tracheostomy cuff pressure of about 15 mm. Hg is believed to prevent aspiration. If the cuff pressure is well below arteriolar pressure in the trachea, then cuff deflation is not necessary as often as was previously believed.

The pulmonary complication rate from aspiration is high. The best management is prevention since the mortality rate can be as high as 40 to 90 per cent once aspiration has been established. In order to decrease aspiration:

1. Use an endotracheal tube instead of a tracheostomy tube as long as there is no tracheal injury and tracheobronchial secretions can be easily removed.

2. Keep a low pressure cuff at minimal occlusive pressure for longer periods, providing it is well below arteriolar pressure.

3. Suction oral cavity and nasopharynx prior to cuff deflation.

4. Place patient in semi-Fowler's position if possible, teaching him to "bear

down" in order to consciously close glottis with swallowing.

5. Consider nasopharyngeal sump pump in patients with overwhelming pharyngeal secretions (Guillain-Barré syndrome, amyotrophic lateral sclerosis).

Granulation Tissue. Granulation tissue develops after respiratory mucosa becomes ulcerated and the lamina propria is destroyed. This may occur as a result of pressure necrosis from the tracheostomy tube at the stoma, cuff or tip. Foreign body reaction from the tracheostomy tube also stimulates granulation tissue. When the tracheostomy tube is removed, granulation tissue can act like a ball valve obstruction. Hemorrhage is common. Granulation tissue can be excised and cauterized. Removing the tracheostomy tube (foreign body) is most helpful.

Tracheal Stenosis and Tracheomalacia. Further progression of tracheal injury from tracheostomy tubes, especially in patients on respirators, results in chondritis and cartilage necrosis. With loss of cartilage support, the trachea may collapse when the rigid tube is removed. Obstruction may occur after decannulation. The mechanism of tracheal injury is related to the type of tracheostomy tube and its cuff (see p. 366) and abrasive trauma related to movement of the tracheostomy tube with ventilation. Other problems such as excessive removal of tracheal cartilage, infection, aspiration and loss of consciousness increase the problem of tracheal injury. A movable adaptor between the tracheostomy tube and ventilation equipment is helpful along with support and suspension of ventilator tubing.

Delayed Hemorrhage. Bright red blood seen in tracheal secretions 3 to 5 days after tracheostomy indicates ulceration of tracheal mucosa. This might be a superficial ulceration from traumatic suctioning, i.e., the catheter is too large and is used too often. It could also indicate deep erosion of the trachea, esophagus and/or innominate artery. Fifty per cent of cases of massive exsanguination are preceded by a small, bright, bloody ooze. When blood is obtained from the trachea, it should be a cause for alarm. The physician is obligated to identify its source by direct visualization and then to take necessary measures to stop it.

It is important to remove the tracheostomy tube and examine the stoma and trachea with a laryngoscope or fiberoptic nasopharyngoscope. The stoma, cuff site, and tip site should be carefully evaluated for types of secretion and depth of ulceration. AP and lateral chest x-rays are helpful.

Once the diagnosis has been made, one can change suction catheters to size 12 French and re-examine the technique of suctioning. The length of the tracheostomy tube may be changed so that the cuff is at a higher or lower position. Examine the respirator equipment for drag.

Innominate Artery Erosion. This is a hazard that was seen more commonly with long, silver Jackson tubes but it still occurs. In reported cases,[19-21] most of the patients had neurological problems and were on respirators. Cough, retrosternal pain, pulsating tracheostomy tube and a bloody ooze often precede the final event by several hours. Rigid cuffed tubes, unusual pressure, drag of respirator tubes, tip erosion and infection predispose to innominate artery erosion. Inflation of a large cuff produces tamponade and may allow a brief period to administer blood and perform a median sternotomy.

Tracheoesophageal Fistula. Tracheoesophageal fistula occurs after the seventh to tenth day and is a result of high-pressure cuffs. It is more common in patients who are unconscious with nasogastric tubes. This complication is usually lethal. Patients cannot tolerate thoracotomy well in face of severe aspiration pneumonitis.

Tracheocutaneous Fistula. Most tracheostomies heal by secondary intention and are closed after 48 hours. If mucosa is continuous with skin, a fistula can be excised with a local anesthetic and the wound closed in mucosal, subcutaneous and skin layers.

Cosmetic Defects. Vertical midline incisions tend to heal with contractures. This is unappealing and requires a Z-plasty procedure for its correction.

CRICOTHYROTOMY

A recent report by Brantigan showed that cricothyrotomy done in a noninfected trachea for ventilatory support had definite advantages over tracheostomy and that the complications of perichondritis, subglottic stenosis and laryngeal stenosis were rare. The advantages include ease of accessibility and lowered incidence of bleeding. Complications such as pneumothorax, dislodged tracheostomy tube, tracheoesophageal fistula and innominate artery erosion were absent.

Indications are prolonged ventilatory support in a noninfected airway and airway obstruction. When cricothyrotomy is done in patients with infection, consider moving the tracheostomy lower. Contraindications arc conditions in the larynx such as fracture, carcinoma, chemical or smoke inflammation, and infectious diseases such as laryngotracheobronchitis, diphtheria, tuberculosis. Children less than 12 years should not be considered for cricothyrotomy.

Technique

The patient should be intubated if possible, with the neck in slight hyperextension. Palpate the hyoid, thyroid notch, cricothyroid interval and the sternal notch for orientation. Stabilize the thyroid cartilage with the left hand. Make a 2 cm. horizontal incision in the cricothyroid interval. Reverse the scalpel and insert the handle into the incision and rotate to open an airway. Then deflate the endotracheal tube, cuff and remove. Suction and culture the tracheal secretions. Measure the subglottic diameter. Insert a tracheostomy tube one size smaller than with ordinary tracheostomy. Flex neck, tie.

Caution: do not cut or remove cricoid or thyroid cartilage. These cartilages can resist perichondritis if blood supply and perichondrium remain intact.

The postoperative care is similar to that for tracheostomy.

Hazards

1. *Subglottic stenosis* is the most difficult region in the upper airway to reconstruct. Information regarding incidence is not available.

2. *Perichondritis* and granulation tissue on cartilage can be avoided by controlling infection and cartilage injury by the tracheostomy tube or surgical technique.

3. *Laryngeal* stenosis occurs when infection or injury extends superiorly to the glottis.

4. *Vocal cord paralysis, hoarseness* may occur because the recurrent laryngeal nerves are located near the cricothyroid joint, and may be injured by extending the incision. Hoarseness may be noted by cutting the cricothyroid muscles.

Evaluation of the larynx and subglottis should be done frequently with the fiberoptic laryngoscope.

POSTOPERATIVE ORDERS

Patients with tracheostomy should be transferred to an intensive care unit or have special-duty nurses 24 hours each day. Nurses should be specially trained in aseptic technique to care for these patients. It is always the physician's responsibility to know whether or not the patient is getting adequate care. Casual observation by physicians is dangerous to the patient. Instead, he must personally suction the tracheostomy after the nurses, and he must observe the technique of cuff deflation, wound and tube care — not once, but on every shift and with every change of personnel. Postoperative procedures are briefly delineated as follows:

1. Transfer patient to intensive care unit or provide special duty nurses for every shift.

2. a. Suction tracheostomy every 30 minutes for the first 6 hours, then every hour or more often, as needed.

   b. Use No. 12 French catheters for adults.

   c. Instill 1 to 3 ml. normal saline prior to suctioning if secretions are thick or dry.

   d. Suction trachea prior to and after deflation of tracheostomy tube cuff.

   e. Suction trachea prior to and after turning the patient.

   f. Suction trachea after each feeding.

   g. Suction oral cavity and anterior nares each hour — after tracheal suctioning and with number 16 French catheter.

3. Apply cold steam mask to tracheostomy at all times.

4. Provide bell at patient's side to notify nurse.

5. Provide magic slate and marker (or paper and pencil).

6. Be certain that No. 36 (or appropriate

size) tracheostomy tube, obturator, tracheal hook and dilator are at bedside or readily available.

7. Secure overhead light or gooseneck lamp.

8. Deflate cuff for 5 minutes every 2 hours. Reinflate cuff to point where no leak is heard in oral cavity. Measure cuff pressure. Call physician if greater than 20 mm. Hg.

9. Observe for wheezing from tracheostomy tube (plugs), bleeding, unusual tracheal pulsations, subcutaneous emphysema, chest pain, gastric secretions or food in trachea. Notify physician if any of these occur.

10. Auscultate tracheostomy every 4–6 hours, noting absent or unusual breath sounds.

11. Make chest x-ray (portable) on arrival in room. Call physician when it is available.

REFERENCES

1. Awe, W. C., Fletcher, W. S., and Jacob, S. W.: The pathophysiology of aspiration pneumonitis. Surgery 60:232, 1966.
2. Belts, R. H.: Post tracheostomy aspiration. N. Engl. J. Med. 273:155, 1965.
3. Bigler, J. A., Holinger, P. H., and Johnston, K. C.: Tracheostomy in infancy. Pediatrics 13:476, 1954.
4. Brantigan, C. O., and Grow, J. B.: Cricothyrotomy: Elective use in respiratory problems requiring tracheostomy. J. Thorac. Cardiovasc. Surg. 71:72, 1976.
5. Cameron, J. L., Anderson, R. P., and Zuidema, G. D.: Aspiration pneumonia: A clinical and experimental review. J. Surg. Res. 7:44, 1967.
6. Cameron, J. L., Mitchell, W. H., and Zuidema, G. D.: Aspiration pneumonia. Arch. Surg. 106:49, 1973.
7. Cameron, J. L., Reynolds, J., and Zuidema, G. D.: Aspiration in patients with tracheostomies. Surg. Gynecol. Obstet. 136:68, 1973.
8. Carroll, D., and Dutton, R.: The management of respiratory problems in critically ill medical patients including indications for and results of tracheostomy. Johns Hopkins Med. J., 85:(No. 3):163, 1969.
9. Carroll, R. G.: Evaluation of tracheal tube cuff designs. Crit. Care Med. 1:45, 1973.
10. Carroll, R. G., and Grenvik, A.: Proper use of large diameter large residual volume cuffs. Crit. Care Med. 1:153, 1973.
11. Carroll, R. G., Kamen, J. M., and Grenvik, A.: Recommended performance specification for cuffed endotracheal and tracheostomy tubes. Crit. Care Med. 1:155, 1973.
12. Ching, N. P., and Nealon, T. F.: Clinical experience with new low pressure, high volume tracheostomy cuffs. N.Y. State J. Med. 74:2379, 1974.
13. Cooper, J. D., and Grillo, H. C.: The evolution of tracheal injury due to ventilatory assistance through cuffed tubes: A pathologic study. Ann. Surg. 169:334, 1969.
14. Flege, J. B.: Tracheoesophageal fistula caused by cuffed tracheostomy tubes. Ann. Surg. 166:153, 1967.
15. Glas, W. W., and King, O. J.: Complications of tracheostomy. Arch. Surg. 85:72, 1962.
16. Gosch, H. H., and Kindt, G. W.: Head injury — Some current concepts in management. Univ. Michigan Med. J. 37:74, 1971.
17. Haller, J., and Talbert, J. L.: Clinical evaluation of a new silastic tracheostomy tube for respiratory support of infants and young children. Ann. Surg. 171:915, 1970.
18. James, A. E., MacMillan, A. S., et al.: Radiological considerations of granuloma and stenosis at tracheostomy site. Radiology 96:513–520, 1970.
19. Lowbury, E. J., Thom, B. T., et al.: Sources of infection with Pseudomonas aeruginosa in patients with tracheostomy. J. Med. Microbiol. 3:39, 1970.
20. Lu, A. T., and Tamura, Y.: The pathology of laryngotrachial complications. Arch. Otol. 74:323, 1961.
21. Mathog, R. H., and Hudson, W. R.: Delayed massive hemorrhage following tracheostomy. Laryngoscope 79:107, May, 1969.
22. Meade, J. W.: Tracheostomy — Its complications and their management. N. Engl. J. Med. 265:519, 1961.
23. Nealon, T. F., and Ching, N.: Pressures of tracheostomy cuffs in ventilated patients. N.Y. State J. Med. 71:1923, 1971.
24. Neuman, M. M.: Tracheostomy. Surg. Clin. N. Am. 49:6, 1969.
25. Pearson, F. G., Goldberg, M., and Da Silva, A. J.: A prospective study of tracheal injury complicating tracheostomy with a cuffed tube. J. Laryng. Otol. Rhinol. 71:867, 1968.
26. Rabuzzi, D. D., and Reed, G. F.: Intrathoracic complications following tracheostomy in children. J. Laryng. Otol. Rhinol. 85:939, 1971.
27. Seed, R. F.: Traumatic injury to the larynx and trachea. Anesthesia 26:55, 1971.
28. Silen, W., and Spieker, D.: Fatal hemorrhage from innominate artery after tracheostomy. Ann. Surg. 162:1005, 1965.
29. Skaggs, J. A., and Cogbill, C. L.: Tracheostomy: Management, mortality, complications. Am. Surg. 36:393, 1969.
30. Wu, T., Lim, I., Simpson, R. A., and Turndorf, H.: Pressure dynamics of endotracheal and tracheostomy cuffs. Crit. Care Med. 1:197, 1973.

CHAPTER 13

THORACIC INJURIES

Robert B. Rutherford, M.D.

THE PROBLEM

Approximately 25 per cent of all civilian traumatic deaths in this country result primarily from chest injuries, and in another 25–50 per cent they contribute significantly to the lethal outcome; yet the relative contribution of chest injuries to mortality after trauma victims have reached the hospital ward is small. Although a significant number of these people die before reaching a medical facility, and others, in spite of vigorous and well-directed attempts at resuscitation, expire shortly after arrival in the emergency department, the fate of many patients with chest injuries is determined by the responses of the physicians who first attend them.

It has also been shown that thoracotomy is required in less than 10 per cent of cases of major thoracic trauma. Furthermore, most of the resuscitative procedures that suffice in the remainder should fall within the capabilities of the primary physicians who staff emergency departments: thoracentesis, intercostal nerve block, endotracheal intubation, tracheostomy, pericardiocentesis, blood transfusion, tube thoracostomy and nasotracheal suction. This is fortunate, because many of these injuries occur in areas far removed from major medical centers served by thoracic surgeons; furthermore, the resuscitation of the critically injured patient with serious chest injuries usually cannot await his arrival.

This combination of therapeutic potential and necessity emphasizes the importance of the ability of "frontline" physicians to recognize and treat the various types of thoracic trauma. Van Waggoner[69] estimated, from an analysis of over 600 traumatic deaths occuring in patients *after* arrival at the hospital, that one sixth could have been prevented by prompt diagnosis and that an additional one sixth of the patients could have been salvaged by institution of correct treatment. The best results will be obtained by the physician who has a preconceived plan of action and the proper equipment with which to carry it out. Such a plan should be based on a high index of suspicion for specific injuries, an understanding of their pathophysiology and the knowledge of how to correct these physiological abnormalities with the quickest, simplest means available. In more severe cases, the three R's of trauma — recognition, resuscitation and repair — cannot be executed in orderly sequence punctuated by periods of contemplation. Therefore, before discussing in detail each of the different kinds of thoracic trauma, a general approach to the initial evaluation and management of chest injuries is presented, with emphasis on the critically injured. Later, the mechanisms and pathophysiology of the different types of thoracic trauma will be separately discussed.

Much of the basic equipment and the techniques used in the resuscitation of the injured patient are discussed in the chapters on "Initial Evaluation and Resuscitation," "Cardiopulmonary Resuscitation" and "The Treatment of Hemorrhagic Shock" and need not be enumerated here. Materials and methods peculiar to the resuscitation of chest trauma patients are described in conjunction with the condition to which they apply.

Pathophysiology and Pathodynamics of Thoracic Trauma

Chest injuries are classically divided into two categories — penetrating and nonpenetrating. This separation has clinical importance beyond the simple consideration of the mechanisms of injury, because certain injuries fall almost entirely in one or the other group. For example, cardiac tamponade is encountered in an emergency department almost always only after *penetrating* trauma, because myocardial rupture following blunt trauma is almost always immediately fatal and more minor pericardial bleeding usually either goes unnoticed or presents as a delayed pericardial effusion with or without tamponade as the red cells undergo lysis. By the same token, blunt trauma, as typified by a steering wheel injury, may be associated with sternal and rib fractures, flail chest, pulmonary or myocardial contusions, rupture of the thoracic aorta, diaphragm, or a major bronchus and other injuries rarely encountered following penetrating trauma. This type of knowledge contributes to the experienced physician's "index of suspicion."

Currently, blunt trauma causes the majority of serious (patient admitted) chest injuries with traffic accidents (55 per cent) and falls (15 per cent) contributing most heavily. However, in large urban medical centers receiving more patients with stab and gunshot wounds, this relationship may be reversed. The mortality associated with blunt or nonpenetrating thoracic trauma is gerater only to the degree with which it is associated with multisystem injuries. The mortality of isolated chest injuries is in the range of 4–12 per cent, but increases to 13–15 per cent with another system involved and to 30–35 per cent with two or more systems involved.[6] The head, abdomen and extremities are affected in that order of frequency.

Stabbings account for almost three fourths of penetrating chest injuries in most large civilian hospitals, but this is changing with an increasing preference for firearms among the criminal element. The mortality from stab wounds of the chest is lower (2–3 per cent) than from gunshot wounds, which approximates that of nonpenetrating chest trauma with involvement of another system (i.e., 14–20 per cent).[6] Nevertheless, hemothorax and hemopericardium caused by penetrating wounds still constitute the major indications for thoracotomy following chest trauma.

Understanding the effects of a penetrating injury may be as simple as tracing the trajectory of a knife or low-velocity missile through the structures in its path or as complicated as appreciating the degree of "blunt" trauma caused by temporary cavity formation perpendicular to the trajectory of a high-velocity missile.[8] Blunt trauma may be inflicted by a variety of direct and indirect forces, the latter being more important than the striking object. Classically, the extent of injury from a direct impact may be related to magnitude and duration of the applied force, its velocity (rate of onset and decay) and duration and the area to which it is applied. Indirectly, within the thorax, these forces are translated into those of acceleration, torsion, compression and shear. Acceleration and deceleration themselves, over and above direct impact, may be responsible for serious intrathoracic trauma, as may be appreciated from Figure 13–1 A to D. By comparison a force of 20g's may be associated with 40 mph and 60g's by 60 mph impacts.[6] Shearing forces may result from differences in the degree of fixation or mobility of adjacent tissues, as in the site of predilection for disruption of the thoracic aorta near the ligamentum arteriosum, where there is a transition between mobile and fixed segments of the thoracic aorta. Compression and/or decompression may play a major role in producing pulmonary contusions since the work of both Border[10] and Rutherford[61] and their co-workers suggests that a closed airway (glottis or experimentally, an obstructed endotracheal tube) increases the likelihood and severity of pulmonary contusions.

AN APPROACH TO THE PATIENT WITH SERIOUS CHEST INJURY

Diagnosis. Fortunately, the different forms of thoracic trauma capable of causing *severe* cardiorespiratory embarrass-

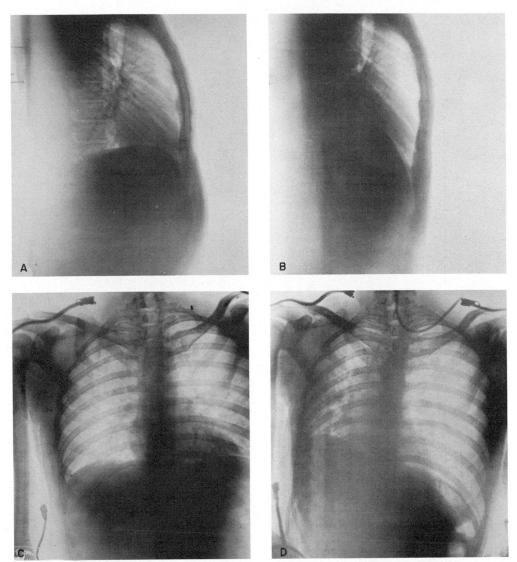

Figure 13–1. Displacement of the intrathoracic contents produced by a 5 G accelerating force in forward (A-B) *and lateral* (C-D) *directions. The distortion of the diaphragm, shift of the heart and mediastinum and change in the density of the pulmonary parenchyma in relation to the direction of acceleration (to the reader's right) can be seen in B and D. (Courtesy of Dr. Edward J. Hershgold: Aerospace Medicine 31:213, 1960.)*

ment *soon* after injury are limited in number and are usually readily recognized if specifically sought. Thus, whenever ventilatory and/or circulatory insufficiency (shock) develop *soon* after chest trauma, initial examination should be quickly directed toward six conditions: open pneumothorax, airway obstruction, flail chest, tension pneumothorax, massive hemothorax and cardiac tamponade. (Myocardial rupture is not included here because it almost invariably causes death before the patient reaches medical attention: airway obstruction is not strictly a "chest injury"

but naturally falls into place here during the evaluation of ventilatory exchange and thoracic motion in the injured patient.)

In addition, there are another half dozen potentially serious (i.e., possibly lethal) conditions that may be causing only modest cardiorespiratory difficulties at the time of admission and that are usually not readily diagnosed on the basis of physical findings. These include rupture or tear of the aorta, diaphragm, esophagus or tracheobronchial tree and pulmonary or myocardial contusion. The first five can often be diagnosed, or at least strongly suspect-

TABLE 13–1. Initial Assessment

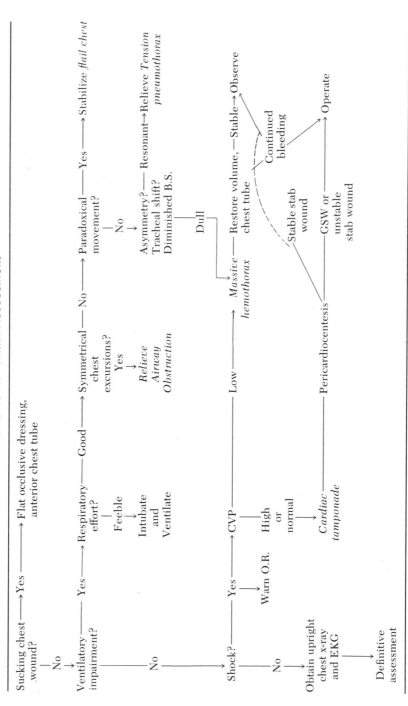

ed, after viewing an upright chest film with these conditions specifically in mind. An EKG may provide the only clue to a myocardial contusion.

Beyond this "dirty dozen," the need for early diagnosis and treatment is less critical, for most of what remains are "routine" problems such as fractured ribs and lesser degrees of hemothorax or pneumothorax. This forms the basis for the following advice: perform a brief examination to determine if there is either ventilatory or circulatory insufficiency and look for any obvious physical findings that point to their cause (e.g., sucking chest wound, stridor and intercostal retractions, paradoxical chest motion, tracheal deviation with unilaterally absent breath sounds, precordial wound bulging neck veins and diminished heart sounds). If these are not found, appropriately positioned chest tubes may be inserted for obvious pneumothorax or hemothorax, but otherwise one should immediately obtain a good upright chest x-ray and examine it with special regard for the telltale signs of rupture of the aorta, diaphragm, esophagus or bronchus or a pulmonary contusion. Finally, in patients with blunt trauma, especially a "steering wheel" injury, an EKG should be obtained to rule out myocardial contusion. This approach is shown in algorithm form in Table 13–1. The remainder of this section will be devoted to elaborating on this initial approach.

The condition responsible for the patient's distress may be suspected immediately if one hears the characteristic sound of a sucking chest wound or the stridor or coarse rhonchi of airway obstruction. Knowledge of the wounding mechanism may suggest one condition above the others and alter the order of examination. For example, cardiac tamponade is considered in patients with precordial wounds; massive hemothorax with any penetrating wound; and flail chest, rupture of the aorta, bronchus, esophagus or diaphragm with steering wheel injuries.

Usually, gross assessment of the degree of ventilatory and circulatory impairment should come first. This may immediately orient the examiner toward certain lesions, since some produce mainly ventilatory insufficiency (e.g., sucking chest wounds, airway obstruction, flail chest, tension pneumothorax) and others mainly circulatory impairment (e.g., massive hemothorax, cardiac tamponade). If one places an ear close to the patient's mouth and nose, watches the movements of the bared chest and palpates the pulse at the wrist, much valuable information can be obtained (Fig. 13–2). With a little experience one can gauge the adequacy of ventilatory exchange by the force, duration and frequency with which the expired air strikes the ear. A strong blast of air would eliminate the possibility of significant interference with the ventilatory mechanism; and if such a patient was in shock, cardiac tamponade or massive hemothorax would be the primary consideration.

On the other hand, if the exchange is

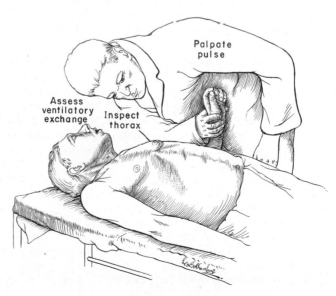

Figure 13–2. *Initial evaluation for chest injuries. Assessment of the adequacy of ventilatory exchange, the integrity and movements of the thoracic cage, and the degree of circulatory impairment provide a quick orientation to the nature of the patient's problem.*

Palpate pulse

Assess ventilatory exchange   Inspect thorax

poor in spite of good effort, inspection of the chest may provide the answer. An open pneumothorax should be obvious, as should any paradoxical movement of the chest wall severe enough to cause respiratory embarrassment, particularly since the flail segment usually involves the anterior or lateral thorax. On the other hand, if the exchange is poor in spite of symmetrical and vigorous respiratory efforts, airway obstruction probably exists. This is not necessarily associated with stridor, crowing or audible, coarse rhonchi. However, if one hemithorax is *prominent* and does not move well with respiration, the problem is probably a large pneumothorax or hemothorax (whereas the involved hemithorax is *diminished* in volume when poor excursions are the result of splinting against painful rib fractures or massive atelectasis). Before proceeding further with examination of the thorax, the neck should be examined to determine the relative position of the trachea, the presence of subcutaneous emphysema and fullness of the neck veins (independent of straining efforts). Both tension pneumothorax and a massive hemothorax may produce a prominent hemithorax with poor excursions, diminished breath sounds and a shift of the trachea to the opposite side. The former is more likely to be associated with subcutaneous emphysema and prominent neck veins, but a hyperresonant percussion note is of greater diagnostic significance. Massive hemothorax, on the other hand, is associated with a dull percussion note *posteriorly* and the neck veins are not full. Since two thirds to three fourths of patients with hemothorax also have some degree of pneumothorax, the percussion note anteriorly and superiorly may be misleading.

Ventilation is not usually interfered with in cardiac tamponade and not until late in massive hemothorax. Therefore, if initial assessment discloses a diminished pulse but fairly adequate air exchange, consideration should first be given to these two conditions or to some extrathoracic cause of shock. The signs of hemothorax have already been mentioned. Cardiac tamponade should be suspected if there is a wound over or near the precordium. The diagnostic triad of low arterial pressure, elevated venous pressure and a small, quiet heart described by Beck[5] is not always present or readily apparent. A low arterial pressure is a common denominator in many traumatic conditions, and the struggling or straining of a patient may produce a misleading bulging of the neck veins. The muffling of heart sounds may be subtle and hard to ascertain in a noisy emergency department. A tension pneumothorax on the left can easily be mistaken for cardiac tamponade. It may give bulging neck veins and, because of mediastinal shift, heart sounds over the normally precordial area may be absent or faint. Another "diagnostic" sign of cardiac tamponade, pulsus paradoxus, represents a fleeting stage in the development of cardiac tamponade and is elicited in only about one third of such cases. The practice of using a central venous catheter in the management of patients in shock has particular value in this situation. If the central venous pressure is low, one can assume that there is low circulating volume and proceed with volume-expanding infusions. If, however, it is high in the face of shock or if it is normal and becomes quickly elevated with infusions, one should suspect cardiac tamponade and proceed with pericardiocentesis.

The approach just outlined is admittedly oversimplified, but it is designed to detect only lesions of sufficient magnitude to cause early cardiac or respiratory embarrassment. Lesser degrees of these and other conditions may be missed while a search is made for the major threat to the patient's life. However, if this primary purpose is achieved, such lesser injuries can be detected when time allows a more painstaking examination and chest x-rays. The main failing of such an approach occurs in patients whose critical condition is the result of many injuries, none sufficient to be obvious on such a cursory examination. This is particularly true when multiple systems are involved. Such an examination, of course, represents only one part of the overall evaluation of the critically injured patient.

Initial Resuscitation. The simplest effective resuscitative measures must be employed initially. Valuable time may be wasted waiting for the means to apply more involved methods, although they may be more effective. Consider again the six conditions just discussed. The simple covering of a sucking chest wound with a sterile towel or a gloved hand will transform it functionally into closed pneumothorax, which is reasonably well tolerated. With the major physiological abnormality corrected, a definitive dressing can be prepared when assistance is available, following which a chest tube can be inserted.

An open airway should be established by the simplest effective means. In the past, tracheostomy was employed too often and too early in combating the various forms of airway obstruction. In the unconscious patient simply clearing the pharynx and inserting an oropharyngeal airway may bring significant relief. If not, insertion of an endotracheal tube should be the next step. Emergency tracheostomy should be reserved for patients with mechanical obstruction or those in whom simpler measures bring only transient relief. Tracheostomy can be a risky and time-consuming procedure when carried out under the suboptimal conditions common in many emergency treatment rooms.

Similarly, placing the hands gently but firmly on a flail chest segment or laying the patient with the injured side down reduces the paradoxical movements that interfere with the thoracic bellows' ability to move air. Later, a tracheostomy may be performed and the patient placed on a positive pressure respirator, which is now considered the definitive treatment of flail chest.

The quickest way to eliminate the lethal potential of a tension pneumothorax is to insert an intravenous needle through the chest wall into the involved pleural space, allowing it to equilibrate with atmospheric pressure. This maneuver converts the situation into that of an open pneumothorax, but with an opening so small that functionally it is little worse than a simple pneumothorax. Oxygen is then administered, by bag and mask if the patient's respiratory efforts are weakened, because severe hypoxia is characteristic of advanced stages of tension pneumothorax. By these maneuvers, the patient's condition should be immediately improved, so that there is ample time to insert a chest tube and apply suction to expand the lung.

In patients with massive hemothorax, restoration of the blood volume holds first priority. Only after this is well under way (usually with *two* large-bore intravenous conduits established) *should the blood be evacuated* from the thorax by a posterolaterally placed chest tube. If large volumes are removed or the patient's response to these measures is inadequate or poorly sustained, immediate operation will usually be necessary.

Pericardiocentesis relieves nearly all patients with cardiac tamponade *initially*, and in a significant but selected number may be the only intervention necessary. Further details of resuscitation and definitive treatment in these and other conditions are provided later in this chapter.

X-ray. As previously mentioned, an upright chest film should be taken as soon as the initial evaluation and resuscitation have been accomplished. This does not mean that the patient should be "sent to x-ray." The attending physician's surveillance of the patient should not be interrupted by this examination. In the same vein, although one should take full advantage of the interpretation of the film by a radiologist if he is in attendance, the treating physician should always bring his own index of suspicion to bear on this x-ray.

A widening of the mediastinal shadow may be the only clue to a temporarily contained rupture of the thoracic aorta. In a patient who has sustained severe blunt trauma to the thorax, such a finding, if unequivocal and associated with shock and a left hemothorax, constitutes a valid indication for immediate thoracotomy. If the widening is equivocal or if there is no associated hemothorax and if the patient's condition is stable, the operating room should be alerted to stand by for emergency thoracotomy while a diagnostic aortogram is performed. This is necessary because there are other causes of mediastinal narrowing and not all aortic tears occur near the ligamentum arteriosus and may be difficult to deal with through the usual posterolateral thoracotomy.

Rupture of the esophagus, though a rare complication of chest trauma, should be considered whenever there is pneumomediastinum or left pneumothorax of traumatic origin, particularly if there are no fractured ribs or penetrating wounds on that side. In approximately two thirds of esophageal ruptures secondary to blunt trauma, an epigastric rather than a thoracic blow is responsible. Mediastinal widening is usually a late finding with this condition, but occasionally the telltale stippling of air may be seen in the left cardiophrenic area. A swallow of contrast material (Hypaque) is a simple and harmless way to confirm this suspicion and may be life-saving, since failure to diagnose this condition is mainly responsible for the reported 80 per cent mortality rate (two thirds of reported cases being discovered at autopsy).[74]

Although a fully developed contusion pneumonitis or "traumatic wet lung" can usually be diagnosed by physical signs, an area of diffuse or fluffy opacification on the initial chest x-ray, signaling pulmonary contusion, may provide an early clue. Whenever marked changes such as this are already evident on a chest x-ray taken soon after injury, a severe degree of contusion pneumonitis can be anticipated. The importance of this early recognition is that the development of this "traumatic wet lung" can be suppressed by early tracheostomy and positive pressure ventilation.

Thoracoabdominal injuries, particularly rupture of the diaphragm, may be fatal unless diagnosed and treated early. Penetrating wounds of the diaphragm may be suspected by reconstructing the trajectory of the wounding agent, considering the victim's position at the time of impact. Operation is frequently dictated by penetration of the subjacent abdominal viscera with attendant bleeding or peritonitis. On the other hand, rupture of the diaphragm from blunt trauma is more likely to present acutely with herniation of abdominal viscera up into the thorax through a large defect. Herniation of air-containing viscera through a tear in the diaphragm may be misinterpreted as a "high stomach bubble." Similarly, an "elevation of the diaphragm" may be more apparent than real and should lead one to suspect diaphragmatic rupture.

Such suspicion can be confirmed by radio-contrast studies of the stomach or colon or by "diagnostic" pneumoperitoneum. An "elevated diaphragm" must also be distinguished from a subpulmonary collection of blood. Subpulmonary hematomas will usually layer out in a lateral decubitus film. Herniation of the liver through the *right* leaf of the diaphragm is rare and harder to diagnose but should be considered whenever the right leaf of the diaphragm is "elevated." Concomitant elevation of the lower border of the liver shadow strongly supports this suspicion.

The initial chest x-ray may also detect less obvious degrees of trauma that may have been missed in the initial examination. Even the lack of radiological evidence of significant intrathoracic injury is valuable information and provides a baseline for later comparison. A preliminary chest x-ray will also facilitate the removal of foreign bodies at the time of thoracotomy indicated for other reasons. Finally, in extensive open wounds of the thorax, an accurate localization of the sites of fracture may be extremely valuable in planning reconstruction.

Reassessment. During the initial period of evaluation and resuscitation, the patient's cardiorespiratory function should be continually reassessed to determine whether his condition has deteriorated further or is responding satisfactorily to treatment.

Changes in the patient's condition with time, particularly his response to resuscitative measures, may be just as important as the type of injury sustained in determining the need for operative intervention. This requires more than merely checking the vital signs. In the past it was common to place almost sole reliance on the blood pressure in assessing the patient's hemodynamic status. However, it is well recognized that a 15 to 25 per cent loss in blood volume may be sustained before there is a significant decline in the blood pressure. During this period tachycardia, tachypnea and complaints of thirst may be the only warning signs of impending collapse but, unfortunately, these are nonspecific. In addition, not all hypotension following chest trauma is due to hypovolemia. Pericardial tamponade, severe acidosis, respiratory insufficiency and impaired venous return from the loss of negative intrathoracic pressure may be important contributing factors.

We have found the *central venous pressure* to be a valuable parameter to monitor in such patients. A large-bore plastic catheter inserted into the superior vena cava through the internal jugular or subclavian vein produces not only a major route for intravenous therapy but a reasonably sensitive index of the functional circulating volume in this trauma setting. While admittedly it is not a reliable means of avoiding overinfusion, it detects hypovolemia with reasonable sensitivity and will be elevated, or in the upper normal range, in essentially all cases of the one normovolemic cause of shock, cardiac tamponade. In addition to this, the rate of urine formation by the kidneys is a valuable guide to adequate tissue perfusion. Serial measurements of arterial and central venous pressures and urinary output are the most practical means of assessing the hemodynamic state of the injured patient.

The adequacy of the respiratory exchange may be grossly estimated by the patient's color, the respiratory excursions of the thorax, and the rate, force and volume of air exchange. However, it must be remembered that although cyanosis is a valuable diagnostic sign when present, its absence should not be reassuring. Recent experience has taught us that significant degrees of respiratory insufficiency may not be appreciated without arterial blood gas analysis (pH, pCO_2 and pO_2). This diagnostic capability is particularly desirable in evaluating the need for or the adequacy of artificial ventilation by a respirator.

If a chest catheter has been inserted, the chest drainage bottles should be carefully inspected since they may provide information about the size of the air leak, the pressure gradients being developed within the pleural space or the rate of bleeding into the chest.

The above guides, supplemented with repeated physical and x-ray examinations, are the keys to the continuing assessment of the patient with severe chest trauma. If the patient's condition continues to deteriorate or if the response to resuscitation has been only temporary, it may be necessary to proceed immediately with exploratory thoracotomy. Cases that demand such bold action almost invariably involve hemorrhage from the heart or great vessels. In most cases, however, the patient's condition will respond to the appropriate resuscitative measures and allow time for more definitive diagnostic study.

Indications for Early Thoracotomy. These must be individualized for each patient and trauma to other systems as well as intercurrent diseases must be taken into account.

The following are *relative* indications for immediate or, at least, early thoracotomy: (1) massive or unrelenting intrapleural hemorrhage; (2) cardiac tamponade from a gunshot wound or from a stab wound if it recurs quickly or is ineffectively relieved by pericardiocentesis; (3) widened mediastinum with a left hemithorax or aortogram confirming aortic disruption; (4) ruptured esophagus; (5) open pneumothorax with major chest wall defect; (6) massive pleural air leak, subcutaneous emphysema, hemoptysis or complete unilateral atelectasis of a degree suggesting ruptured bronchus; (7) gross contamination of the pleural space with foreign bodies; (8) traumatic diaphragmatic hernia (usually requiring laparotomy); (9), valvular or septal cardiac injuries with acute heart failure. These indications will be further qualified, along with less pressing indications, in the discussion of the individual conditions that follows.

THE THORACIC CAGE

Soft Tissue Injuries

The principles that apply to the management of soft tissue injuries in general apply equally to injuries of the musculocutaneous superstructure of the thorax and need not be reviewed at this point.

Subcutaneous Emphysema

Subcutaneous emphysema results when air is forced into the subcutaneous tissues from any source. There are three routes by which air can reach and travel along anatomical pathways of least resistance (Fig. 13–3): (1) through a major disruption of the pleura and intercostal muscles, e.g., a pneumothorax associated with rib fractures; (2) as an outward dissection of mediastinal emphysema, e.g., rupture of bronchus or esophagus, or pneumothorax with a break in the mediastinal pleura; or, rarely, (3) by direct connection with the external wound. Although the air is truly subcutaneous in many areas, the real planes of dissection are the various fascial planes of the neck that connect with those of the mediastinum and the loose areolar tissue plane between the chest wall proper and musculature of the shoulder girdle.

Though it is an important sign following chest trauma, subcutaneous emphysema itself is usually of little significance,

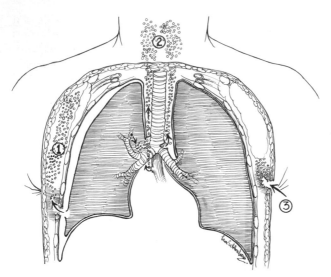

Figure 13-3. *The three major sources of subcutaneous emphysema as described in the text.*

amounting to no more than an annoyance to the patient. Occasionally, air dissecting the deeper fascial planes of the neck may lead to changes in phonation or even mild laryngeal obstruction, but the most annoying problem from the dissection of air in the subcutaneous plane is usually closure of the eyelids. Secondary infection of the involved tissues rarely occurs. The patient rarely complains of the condition once he is assured that it is innocuous.

Whenever the unmistakable crepitus in the skin is encountered, its extent and the area of maximal development should be noted. When associated with a traumatic pneumothorax it is maximal in the area of rib fractures. Occasionally it is detected in the area overlying rib fractures without an apparent pneumothorax. Although this is theoretically possible (that is, if there is underlying pleural symphysis), the more probable explanation is the failure to detect a small degree of pneumothorax that has almost completely evacuated itself along the lines of least resistance through a defect in the pleura and intercostal muscles. As an outward expression of mediastinal emphysema, subcutaneous air first appears in the neck and is maximal in its development there. This carries a more serious connotation. Whenever it is extensive or progressive, disruption of the aerodigestive structures in the neck or chest must be assumed to have occurred. Subcutaneous emphysema associated with an external wound is usually limited in extent and not progressive.

Treatment. Subcutaneous emphysema will progress no further and will be resorbed gradually once its source has been controlled. Therefore, treatment should be directed toward the underlying cause rather than the emphysema itself. In this regard, a halt in the advancing perimeter of the subcutaneous emphysema or its retreat may serve as an important indication of the effectiveness of treatment. Patients with chest injuries not infrequently require tracheostomy. Subcutaneous emphysema may develop secondary to this procedure if the skin is closed too tightly around the tracheostomy. Conversely, subcutaneous emphysema in the neck from other causes may vent itself through an open tracheostomy incision. In addition, both tracheostomy and evacuation of a pneumothorax by tube thoracostomy and suction will arrest the progress of subcutaneous emphysema by eliminating or at least decreasing the pressure differentials that force air into the tissues. The breathing of pure oxygen will also help to speed the reabsorption of subcutaneous air by washing nitrogen out of the blood and improving its diffusion from the sequestered air into the circulation, but this alone is not usually considered sufficient justification for its use. Subcutaneous emphysema will usually yield to such measures. The use of cervical mediastinotomy, venting skin incisions and needle aspiration should be reserved for the uncommon instances in which the subcutaneous emphysema is massive and symptomatic.

Rib Fractures

A simple rib fracture is usually considered a trivial injury by the physician if not the patient, but even a simple rib fracture can lead to serious consequences if treated too lightly. This is particularly true in elderly patients whose more rigid, brittle thoracic skeleton can be fractured by relatively minor trauma. Such a patient, with limited cardiorespiratory reserve, fares poorly if atelectasis or pneumonitis develops secondary to splinting from failure to control pain.

Rib fractures do not occur frequently until adult life and even then, during the third and fourth decades, require a well-directed blow of considerable force. Such a forceful blow may result in other more subtle intrathoracic injuries that may not be apparent on initial evaluation. Nor will their subsequent development be anticipated unless the force of the trauma and the manner in which it was inflicted are considered. The number, position and type of rib fractures incurred can provide such information.

The upper ribs are somewhat protected anteriorly by the clavicle, posteriorly by the scapulae and laterally by the arms, as well as by the heavy musculature of the upper thorax and its appendages. For this reason fractures above the fifth rib imply that there has been considerable trauma, and they are not uncommonly associated with serious intrathoracic injuries. Fractures of at least one of the first three ribs were present in 91 per cent of all patients over the age of 30 with rupture of the tracheobronchial tree.[14] Posterior fractures of the upper ribs, especially the first rib, are not infrequent in deceleration accidents when the arms have been held stiffly in extension to brace against the impact, as in automobile and mortorcycle collisions. The lower ribs are more mobile and are rarely fractured by indirect forces. However, the lower ribs may be fractured posteriorly by a direct blow and, in such cases, associated injury to the spleen or kidneys should be sought.

The middle ribs, the fifth through the ninth, sustain most blunt thoracic trauma and are the site of most rib fractures. Anteroposterior compression of the thorax causes a decrease in the radius of the rib curvature and results in an *outward* breaking in the mid-shaft. This "spring fracture" rarely results in damage to the underlying lung. On the other hand, a direct blow may fracture one or more ribs directly under the point of the impact. The more localized and severe the force, the greater the possibility that fractured rib ends are driven *into* and damage the underlying lung and pleura. A hemothorax or pneumothorax is naturally more common with this latter type of injury. Severe but more *diffusely* applied blows, on the other hand, are more likely to fracture the ribs on either side of the point of impact. Fracture of a series of ribs in more than one plane may so destroy continuity with the rest of the thorax that the involved area may move paradoxically, responding to changes in the intrapleural pressure rather than to the muscles of respiration. This serious consequence, known as "flail chest," will be discussed separately later.

Diagnosis. The conscious patient with rib fractures will usually complain of localized chest pain that is aggravated by coughing, deep breathing or changes in position. Pressure on the area indicated by the patient usually elicits point tenderness, and occasionally bone crepitus is felt. A grating sound may be heard by auscultation of this area as the patient breathes. On the other hand, the patient may not complain of specific discomfort in the period immediately following the trauma. Splinting of respirations on the involved side may be the only clue. Anteroposterior compression of the thorax during the examination will often elicit pain and localize an unsuspected rib fracture and is a useful maneuver in the examination of the injured. This reproduction of the patient's pain by pressure in an area away from the fracture site also helps to differentiate rib fracture from a "strained" or "pulled" intercostal muscle. Pain associated with rib fractures may result in marked splinting and so limit the respiratory excursions and transmission of breath sounds in the involved hemothorax that the presence of fluid or air in the pleural space is suspected.

X-ray examination is important in evaluating such patients. This is not because it is a much surer method of detecting rib fractures. On the contrary, even with special views, overpenetration and the grid technique, it is still difficult to demonstrate some fractures, particularly those located anteriorly and mid-laterally. X-rays are superior to physical examination, however, in detecting rib fractures in the more protected parts of the thorax, especially in heavily muscled or obese patients. More important, x-ray films make it possible to diagnose associated intrathoracic injuries with more certainty, to demonstrate the presence or absence of air or blood in the pleural space and to localize accurately the position and displacement of the rib fractures. Even the x-ray documentation of a simple rib fracture has occasionally proved important in obviating operation for a "pseudotumor" of the rib some time after the original injury had been forgotten.

Treatment. The decision as to how and where to treat the patient with a fractured rib must be individualized. Some of the considerations that govern the decision to admit the patient with rib fractures to the hospital are (1) advanced age, (2) underlying cardiorespiratory disease, (3) significant associated injuries, (4) inability to cooperate because of deficient intelligence or personality, (5) jagged rib fragments with marked inward displacement, (6) bleeding dyscrasia or concurrent anticoagulant therapy, (7) multiple fractures and (8) lack of control of the pain with moderate analgesics. Most simple fractures sustained by young or middle-aged patients who are otherwise healthy can be managed on an outpatient basis with the use of analgesics alone. In such cases one should assess the response to the proposed medication before allowing the patient to leave the hospital, noting particularly the patient's ability to breathe deeply after the analgesic has taken effect. Those not admitted should return within 24 to 48 hours for a follow-up examination and chest x-ray

to rule out late complications (bloody effusion, atelectasis). They should be instructed to take their temperature twice a day and to cough and breath deeply periodically, preferably at the time of maximal analgesic effect.

INTERCOSTAL NERVE BLOCK. One of the best means of managing severer degrees of pain from rib fractures is by intercostal nerve block. In the past, the inability to obtain reliable pain relief beyond 3 to 4 hours made this approach impractical, but with the introduction of newer local anesthetic agents providing relief for 12 hours or more, it is being employed more frequently. Nevertheless since the procedure is associated with a small but definite risk of pneumothorax, it should be reserved for situations in which pain control is difficult or impossible to obtain by simpler measures.

Intercostal block is only feasible if the rib fractures are reasonably discrete, since one or two spaces above and below the level of the rib fracture must be infiltrated. The technique is similar to local infiltration prior to thoracentesis except that the nerves are blocked in the paravertebral plane and the infiltrating needle is walked *under* the rib to reach the nerve rather than over it to avoid intercostal vessels (Fig. 13–4). A wheal is made over each of the interspaces proposed for block about three finger breadths lateral to the vertebral spine. A small amount of local anesthetic (0.5 per cent Marcaine) is infiltrated as the needle is advanced toward the lower edge of the rib. The needle is walked underneath the lower edge of the rib and at this point, after aspiration to make sure a vessel has not been entered, approximately 3 ml. of the agent is infiltrated.

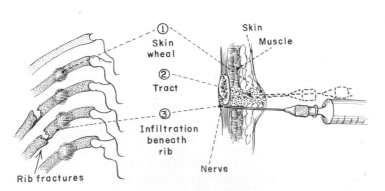

Figure 13–4. *The technique of intercostal nerve block as described in the text. Note that the infiltrating needle is "walked" under the lower rib margin, unlike the technique of thoracentesis.*

If several rib fractures have been sustained, the patient may have difficulty localizing the pain well enough to determine the intercostal levels that need blocking. Here x-ray localization will be helpful. Extensive intercostal blocking has the theoretical disadvantage of producing, by summation of intercostal nerve paralysis, almost as much interference with respiration as do narcotics. This fear has not been justified in our experience. In practice, patients with multiple rib fractures requiring such extensive blocks often have "flail chest" and will be managed by tracheostomy and a respirator, in which case control of respirations allows the liberal use of narcotics.

ADHESIVE STRAPPING OF THE CHEST. Controversy exists over the use of adhesive strapping of the chest to control the pain of rib fractures. Although this measure undoubtedly makes many patients more comfortable and may be employed without penalty in good-risk patients with simple rib fractures, enthusiasm over its use is tempered by the following: (1) it limits the expansion of the thorax and therefore predisposes to atelectasis and secondary pneumonitis; (2) the wide expanse of adhesive tape interferes with examination of the chest; (3) it often leads to a blistering dermatitis, which can be more uncomfortable than the rib fracture itself; (4) it is often no more effective than moderate analgesics, particularly in obese patients and in women with large breasts, which make it difficult to get good splinting with the tape; and (5) it is most effective in controlling pain in patients with lower rib fractures, which constitute a decided minority. Therefore it is rare to see this measure used today in the treatment of painful rib fractures. Instead, in lower rib fractures at least, the use of a circumferential "Velcro" binder or a corset has been found to be of more practical value. Antibiotics are not ordinarily administered, although they may be justified if there is associated cardiorespiratory disease, such as chronic bronchitis and emphysema.

Sternal Fractures

Fracture of the sternum occurs about once in every 20 instances of severe chest trauma, but rarely requires operative reduction. Laustela,[41] in reporting 304 cases

of major chest trauma, noted 17 sternal fractures, only four of which required reduction. The mortality rate associated with sternal fractures, however, is high — ranging from 25 to 45 per cent. This, of course, is not the result of the sternal fracture itself, but of associated injuries. A blow severe enough to cause a sternal fracture will frequently cause serious damage within the thorax. This is attested by the *relatively* frequent association with sternal fractures of disruption of the thoracic aorta, tracheal or bronchial tears, ruptured diaphragm or esophagus, flail chest and contusion of the myocardium or lung. Head injuries are also a frequent accompaniment. It is reported that three fourths of the sternal fractures resulting from steering wheel injury are associated with head trauma.[30] For these reasons, all patients with sternal fractures, even those with minimal displacement and discomfort, should be admitted to the hospital and observed closely.

The diagnosis is usually suspected from the nature of the trauma and the patient's complaint of sternal pain aggravated by deep breathing. Localized tenderness, deformity, crepitus and/or false motion over the sternum at the site of fracture (commonly near the junction of the upper and middle thirds) are the physical signs, but there is usually no cause for vigorous attempts to demonstrate the latter two. Nevertheless, it is common for sternal fractures to be discovered hours or even days after the accident because the patient may have been distracted initially by other discomforts and may not complain of sternal pain. X-ray views of the sternum will usually confirm the diagnosis, although lateral films of excellent quality may be required to demonstrate undisplaced fractures.

Treatment in the form of reduction and fixation is usually required for completely displaced fractures and for partially displaced fractures with false motion. Some completely displaced sternal fractures are not exceedingly painful, but the deformity and restriction of thoracic movements usually warrant reduction. Pain from false motion justifies reducing some incompletely displaced fractures, but there is no indication for interfering with an impacted fracture or a partially displaced fracture that is not causing significant discomfort. The pain from most sternal fractures gradually subsides over the first 2 weeks even though a firm union may not occur for 6 to 8 weeks.

It is neither necessary nor desirable to undertake reduction of the sternal fracture immediately since the threat of associated injuries takes precedence. The most commonly employed procedure is open reduction, with the use of heavy wire sutures to achieve fixation. Although closed reduction may occasionally be achieved by pressure over the more anterior of the two fragments with the patient's thorax at full inspiration and the arms extended over his head, this maneuver is usually too painful to be undertaken without general anesthesia, and once this step is taken it is better to assure both accurate reduction and proper fixation by operative means.

Flail Chest

One of the most serious consequences of blunt thoracic trauma is what has been variously called flail, floating, or crushed chest. With the greater frequency of high-speed automobile accidents this condition has gained an important position in the spectrum of chest trauma. It is relatively more common in older patients because their less resilient rib cages fracture more readily, and because their declining agility makes them more prone to auto-pedestrian accidents and heavy falls.

When several ribs are fractured on both sides of the point of impact, the intervening rib segments may lose their firm continuity with the rest of the thorax so that this region responds to intrapleural pressure changes rather than to the pull of the muscles of respiration. As a result, the involved area moves in an opposite direction to the rest of the thorax during the respiratory cycle (Figs. 13–5A, 13–6A); hence the term "paradoxical" chest movement.

Similar paradoxical movements occur after extensive thoracoplasty. One of the first to appreciate the deleterious effects of

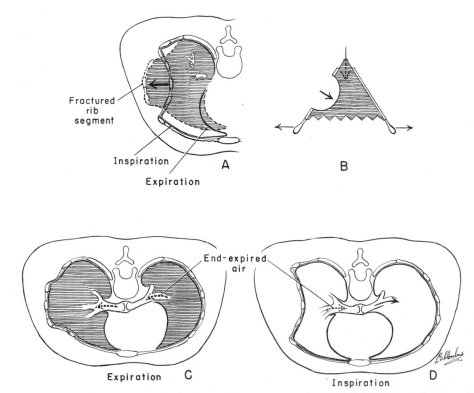

Figure 13–5. *The pathophysiology of flail chest. A, Cross-sectional cut of the involved hemithorax showing (exaggerated) paradoxical motion. B, The mechanical interference with the function of the thoracic cage is likened to that of a bellows in which one of the right sides has been partly replaced by a semielastic membrane. C and D, Cross-sectional views in expiration and inspiration showing the to-and-fro movement of end-expired air across the carina between the two lungs during the respiratory cycle as suggested by the concept of "pendelluft."*

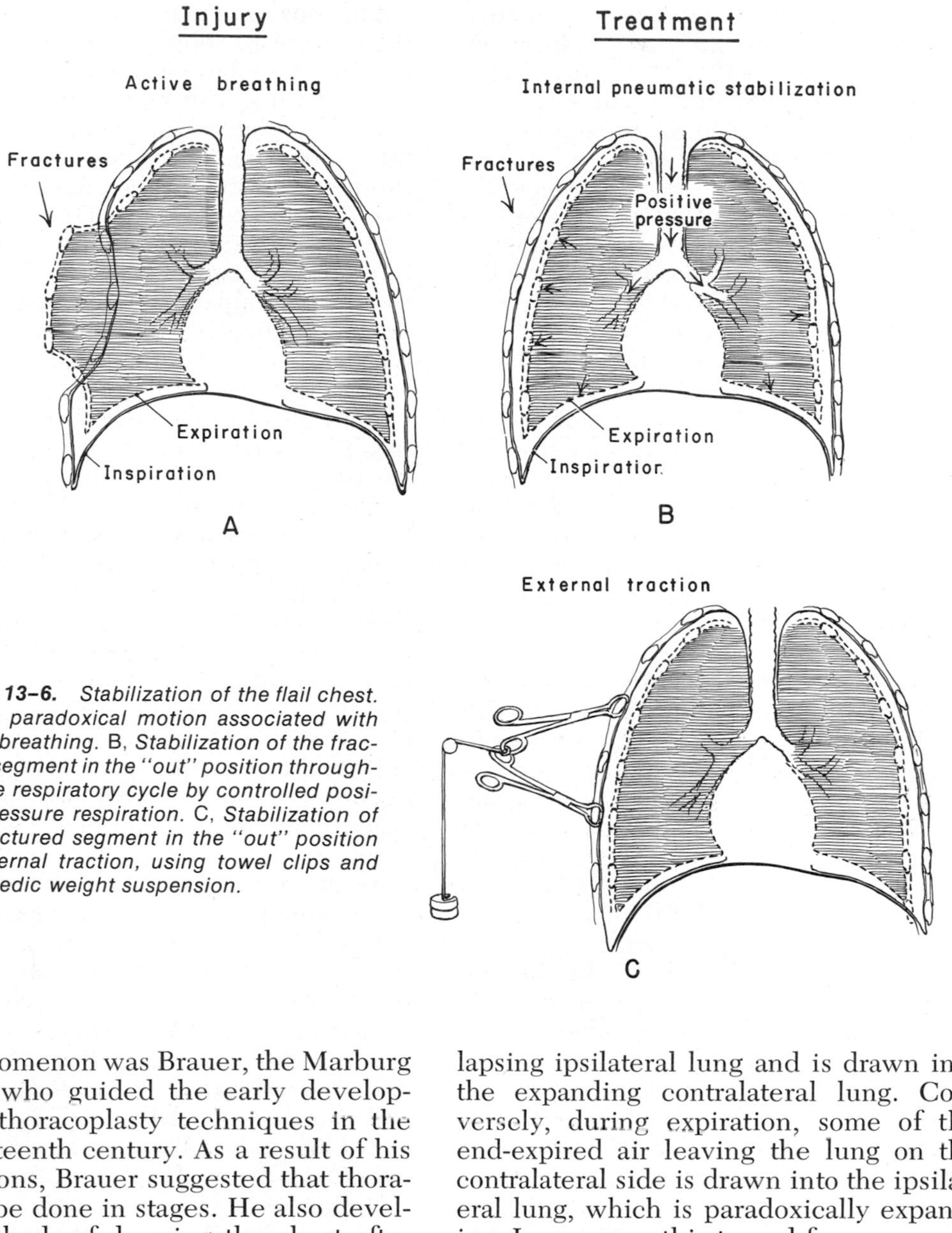

Injury

Active breathing

Treatment

Internal pneumatic stabilization

Figure 13-6. Stabilization of the flail chest. A, The paradoxical motion associated with active breathing. B, Stabilization of the fractured segment in the "out" position throughout the respiratory cycle by controlled positive pressure respiration. C, Stabilization of the fractured segment in the "out" position by external traction, using towel clips and orthopedic weight suspension.

this phenomenon was Brauer, the Marburg internist who guided the early development of thoracoplasty techniques in the late nineteenth century. As a result of his observations, Brauer suggested that thoracoplasty be done in stages. He also developed methods of dressing the chest after thoracoplasty to minimize the paradox, and these were later adopted in the treatment of traumatic flail chest.

Pathophysiology. The mechanisms advanced to explain the respiratory embarrassment associated with this condition are still unsettled. The German concept of *pendelluft*, signifying a to-and-fro movement of useless end-expired air between the two lungs during the respiratory cycle, is still popular in modern texts. Shown diagrammatically in Figure 13–5 *C* and *D*, it suggests that during inspiration end-expired air leaves the paradoxically col-

lapsing ipsilateral lung and is drawn into the expanding contralateral lung. Conversely, during expiration, some of the end-expired air leaving the lung on the contralateral side is drawn into the ipsilateral lung, which is paradoxically expanding. In essence, this to-and-fro movement of end-expired air results in an increase in the respiratory dead space. This may be so great that the patient is unable to compensate for it by hyperventilation, particularly in the presence of painful rib fractures.

Recently doubts regarding the soundness of this theory have been given experimental support. Maloney et al.[47] point out that such an explanation must assume that pressure differentials can exist between the two hemithoraces. They have shown that such differentials do not exist in a dog when flail chest is produced by a large extraperiosteal thoracoplasty. In their experiments the lungs acted as if suspended in a single chambered thorax. Moreover, their work suggests that during inspiration the lung on the side of the flail undergoes net expansion even though the lung subjacent to the flail segment sinks in. Finally, they were unable to detect any to-and-fro movement of end-expired air by continuous CO_2 measurements in each main bronchus. Since this experiment measured the effects of a standard-sized flail segment on an anesthetized animal known for its flimsy mediastinum, it is not possible to say with certainty that some degree of *pendelluft* does not occur in the unanesthetized human with large flail segments and a more rigid mediastinum. In experiments with tension pneumothorax in goats and monkeys, animals that have a more substantial mediastinum, it has been shown that pressure gradients can exist across the mediastinum between the two pleural spaces.[60]

Nevertheless, logic favors the alternative view that the major difficulty in flail chest stems from the fact that pressure gradients developed by the thoracic bellows are dissipated by the paradoxically moving segment of chest wall so that the ability to exchange air against atmospheric pressure is greatly hampered (Fig. 13–5B). Air could be exchanged after the flail segment has completed its displacement, but the extra effort required for this would be limited by the pain of the rib fractures.

The clinical observation offering best support for the theory that it is the bellows function of the thorax that is crippled by the flail segment is: patients who have a central flail segment from rib fractures on either side of the sternum have just as much ventilatory embarrassment as those with unilateral flail chest. Since this segment straddles both hemithoraces, one cannot incriminate a *pendelluft* mechanism.

Even with mild degrees of flail chest, a considerably greater respiratory effort than normal is required to effect adequate ventilation. The pain of multiple rib fractures will discourage this extra effort, and even if such compensation is made initially, fatigue, central nervous system depression or accumulating tracheobronchial secretions eventually tip the scales against the patient.

Diagnosis. Paradoxical movement of the chest wall should be looked for in any patient who has sustained severe blunt chest trauma. The flail segment is usually anterior or lateral since the posterior thorax is not struck as commonly and is more protected by its heavier musculature and the shoulder girdle. The paradoxical movement is often obvious on inspection, but subtler degrees may not be apparent except by palpation, when the abnormal movement may be detected by comparison with the other hand placed on the normally moving side. This technique is particularly useful when the lighting is poor, in obese patients or in women with large breasts.

The visualization of multiple rib fractures on a chest x-ray is supportive evidence but does not identify the pathognomonic paradoxical motion and, even though it is possible to do this fluoroscopically, this is rarely necessary. As the patient's respiratory efforts become more painful and labored, particularly if he characteristically grunts or groans while splinting against the pain of multiple rib fractures, the paradoxical motion becomes accentuated to the point that it is quite obvious.

Treatment. The diagnosis having been made, there are several therapeutic alternatives. The most expedient of these is to stabilize the flail segment by firm but gentle manual pressure. Although this decreases the thoracic volume, it allows the action of the thoracic bellows to be more effective in producing the exchange of air, and can be a useful temporizing maneuver. The same effect can be obtained by using sandbags. However, their weight and the restrictive dressings needed to hold them in place limit their usefulness. Another useful approach at the scene of the accident is to place the patient with the injured side down. Flail chest is said to be the only condition in which this commonly recommended position has been shown physiologically to be beneficial.[64]

However, it is obviously more desirable to stabilize the flail segment in the "out" position, and many ingenious methods have been devised to achieve this. One of the simplest employs large towel clips passed percutaneously around each of several ribs in the flail segment. Traction is then applied to these towel clips by a cord to which are attached weights via an orthopedic suspension, as shown in miniature in Figure 13–6C.

This method has the advantage of being easily applied with equipment that is usually readily available. However, this traction system interferes with attempts to move the patient or to care for him in other ways. Particularly significant, in extreme degrees of flail chest, is the increased work the respiratory muscles must do in moving the thorax against the traction force applied to it. Nevertheless, it is an expedient but effective procedure for treatment of mild to moderate degrees of flail chest. It should be kept in mind in disaster situations in which the demand for respirators may exceed their availability.

Operative fixation of multiple fractures was popular until the introduction of the respirator for managing flail chest in 1955. Now, 2 decades later, it is enjoying renewed interest, particularly in Europe.[50, 52] It is obviously not feasible to perform open reduction and external fixation on *each* of the multiple rib fractures, but the judicious placement of several Kirschner wires, or even intramedullary wires, may stabilize the chest sufficiently that paradoxical motion is negligible and long-term artificial ventilation can be avoided. Rather than multiple incisions over each fracture, formal thoracotomy is carried out, and a hand placed inside the chest both pushes the fractured ribs out and guides the placement of the wires. No studies have been reported that define when if ever its use is better than respirator therapy, but it would seem that it would be preferred any time thoracotomy had to be performed for other injuries and occasionally when the chest was so unstable that respirator therapy would have to be unduly prolonged.

Tracheostomy is beneficial in patients with flail chest[10] although one must use a large cannula (No. 9 or No. 10) placed low in the cervical trachea. In this way, dead space may be decreased and airway resistance lessened so that air can be exchanged with less effort. This also facilitates removal of tracheobronchial secretions that accumulate because of the patient's ineffective cough. In fact, short of continuous positive pressure ventilation,

tracheostomy is probably the simplest and most effective measure in that it both reduces the degree of flail and allows control of secretions.

At the present time, the other methods of stabilization referred to earlier in this discussion have been largely superseded in the management of the patients with significant degrees of flail chest by what has been termed "internal pneumatic stabilization." This approach, first introduced in 1955 by Avery, Mörch and Benson,[3] employs controlled continuous positive pressure ventilation (CPPV), adjusted to just beyond the point of apnea. By this means the flail segment is "floated" out into a reduced position by the positive pressure from within; and since there are no active inspiratory efforts by these apneic patients, the flail segment is never drawn in (Fig. 13–6B). At the point of apnea there is a mild degree of alkalosis. This has a sedative effect and reduces the analgesic requirements, although with respiration controlled such agents may be given without fear of respiratory depression. The respirator not only assures an adequate exchange of air but eliminates the work of breathing. No surgery other than tracheostomy is required, and this is often indicated anyway for removal of blood and secretions from the trachea. The use of positive pressure has the added advantage of minimizing the outpouring of bronchial secretions and pulmonary transudates that are frequently associated in the form of "wet lung" or contusion pneumonitis.[59]

Trinkle[67] has recently reported that 10 patients with this combination who were treated only for the underlying pulmonary contusion did "better" than 19 patients in whom the primary therapy was directed toward the flail chest; that is, they received respirator therapy. The therapy employed for pulmonary contusion included intravenous fluid restriction, furosemide, methyl prednisolone and salt-poor concentrated albumin. Lost blood was replaced with plasma or whole blood but not crystalloid solutions. The patients also received vigorous pulmonary toilet, morphine and intercostal nerve blocks to control pain plus supplemental nasal oxygen, but mechanical ventilation was delivered only briefly when arterial PO_2 could not be maintained above 60 mm. Hg. Unfortunately, the degree to which these measures were applied to the "respirator" group was not detailed; the combination of these two approaches may be better than either alone and should be selectively combined, in this author's opinion, rather than artificially contrasted.

Nevertheless, few would disagree with the statement that CPPV is still the most effective means of treating flail chest. But since no treatment, and certainly not respirator therapy, is without risk, the question remains: Do all patients with multiple rib fractures with some degree of paradoxical motion need it? One must remember that one is usually committing the patient to at least 10–14 days of respirator therapy — the usual time required for sufficient chest wall stabilization to allow CPPV to be discontinued — and that even by this time fixation is not complete, and a certain amount of the reduced or "out" position will be lost to the continuous inward pull of the negative intrapleural pressure. In patients with *lesser* degrees of flail, significant ventilatory impairment initially and a restrictive type of pulmonary functional impairment eventually are *not* important considerations, and the major problems of control of pain and tracheal toilet can be handled by other means.

In general, the following can be considered as indications for respirator (CPPV) treatment of flail chest: (1) significant mechanical interference with ventilatory exchange; (2) significant associated pulmonary contusion; (3) uncooperative patient (e.g., comatose from head injury); (4) the need for general anesthetic and surgical intervention for associated trauma; (5) need for more than 5 to 6 l./min. O_2 to maintain reasonable arterial oxygen tension; (6) a need for voluminous IV fluid therapy for other injuries; (7) significant initial impairment of or deteriorating blood gases; (8) preexisting underlying lung disease; (9) increasing respiratory distress, tachypnea, increased work of breathing and signs of fatigue; and (10) involvement of over five ribs in the flail segment.

Earlier problems with the respirator treatment of flail chest have largely been overcome by the development of more efficient humidification devices and the routine use of prophylactic bilateral chest tube drainage to avoid the constant threat of tension pneumothorax that positive pressure breathing and multiple rib fractures create. A controversy once raged concerning pressure- versus volume-regulated respirators in regard to treatment for this condition. Although most investigators thought that volume-controlled respirators had the advantage of providing adequate ventilation without requiring adjustment for changes in compliance, this argument became academic with the evolution of prototype respirators. These machines have control settings that establish the operating limits for both pressure and volume *simultaneously*.

In summary, a flail chest associated with respiratory embarrassment should be immediately stabilized by the most expedient method, whether external compression or traction with towel clips. Then, as soon as feasible, a low cervical tracheostomy should be performed and a large-diameter cannula inserted. If after this a significant degree of flail persists, or any of the previously mentioned indications are met, one should place the patient on continuous positive pressure ventilation. Occasionally, with lesser degrees of flail, careful tracheostomy care, oxygen inhalation and control of pain by intercostal nerve block may suffice. At other times, particularly when thoracotomy is indicated for other injuries, Kirschner wire fixation of the involved hemothorax may be employed to avoid prolonged artificial ventilation. Serial blood gas analyses are extremely helpful, though not essential, in determining the adequacy of therapy, particularly in regard to the use of a respirator.

Flail chest is associated with a high mortality rate, almost 40 per cent in the recent large series of Conn et al.[18] More universal application of recent advances in treatment should reduce this, but it must be recognized that many of these deaths are at least partly related to serious associated injuries.

Open Pneumothorax and Chest Wall Defects

Open pneumothorax is more likely to be encountered in combat casualties, but occasionally it is seen in civilian practice as a result of shotgun wounds at close range or bizarre accidents in which the patient is impaled or struck by a flying object.

However, this condition was the focal

issue in the early development of the treatment of chest injuries. For six centuries interest in the treatment of chest injuries was kindled by the controversy between the "closed" versus the "open" treatment of the sucking chest wound. This controversy can be traced to 1267 when Theodoric advised closing such wounds so that "the natural heat would not escape or cold air enter the chest." This contradiction of then-accepted practice gained little immediate support. Even 3 centuries later Ambroise Paré, an authority in his time, insisted that although it was permissible to close small sucking chest wounds immediately if they were not associated with internal bleeding, it was best to allow the remainder to drain openly for 2 or 3 days before closure.

In 1767 William Hewson recorded his observations of a patient with marked respiratory distress from such a wound who was promptly relieved when the wound was covered. Forty years later Baron Larrey, Napoleon's surgeon, gave the concept of closed treatment its first authoritative backing after a similar personal observation. He had elected to cover the wound of a soldier near death from an open hemopneumothorax — ostensibly to hide it from the sight of other wounded men with whom the patient was quartered. To his surprise the patient not only responded but survived. Further bolstered by experiences during the Crimean War, this approach was given an extensive trial in the American Civil War, but the favorable initial response was so frequently followed by a fatal empyema that it was again abandoned.

Gradually, by the late nineteenth century, opinions exclusively favoring one or the other approach yielded to the realization that the problem lay between the immediate consequence of respiratory insufficiency from an open pneumothorax and the late complications of an undrained, contaminated hemopneumothorax if the wound were closed. Some selected one or the other approach, the decision depending on the size of the opening or the amount of bleeding and contamination. Others compromised by covering the wound with voluminous dressings in which a drain was incorporated. The eventual development of tube thoracostomy drainage made such compromises unnecessary.

PATHOPHYSIOLOGY. One of the most important outgrowths of this controversy was an aroused interest in the physiology of the open pneumothorax. In 1896 Paget, in the first major work devoted entirely to chest surgery, expressed the opinion that "vibration" of the mediastinum in open pneumothorax destroyed the piston action of the diaphragm. This same year Quénu and Lonquet brought the experimental method to bear on this problem. Their work suggested a method of sustaining expansion of the lung with the chest open by maintaining a positive differential between the intratracheal and intrapleural pressures. Frasier had suggested earlier that the thoracic wound competed with the natural airway; thus, whenever it was of greater diameter than the glottis, it offered less resistance to air flow so that the major portion of the air moved by the thoracic bellows passed through the open wound.

From the German literature came the concept of *pendelluft*, the to-and-fro motion of air, which was used to explain the ventilatory impairment associated not only with open pneumothorax, but with other forms of paradoxical respiration such as flail chest and paralyzed diaphragm. This concept has been described earlier in this chapter in relation to flail chest, and Figure 13–7 shows how it is thought to apply to open pneumothorax. Maloney et al. have cast doubt on its occurrence in flail chest,[47] and carbon dioxide analysis from the trachea and mainstem bronchi in experiments in the author's laboratory suggests that although it may occur to some degree it is not the major cause of ventilatory impairment in open pneumothorax.

A more logical explanation for the ventilatory embarrassment associated with open pneumothorax is that rapid equilibration of atmospheric and pleural pressures occurs through the open defect. This limits the ability of the thoracic bellows to develop the necessary presssure gradient for air exchange (Fig. 13–7). Other factors undoubtedly contribute as well. The loss of intrathoracic negative pressure decreases the efficiency of venous return to the heart. Intermittent torsion of the caval-atrial junction by mediastinal shift or "flutter" may further impede this. Inability to build up pressure against a closed glottis, as required for effective coughing, may eventually lead to retention of bronchial secre-

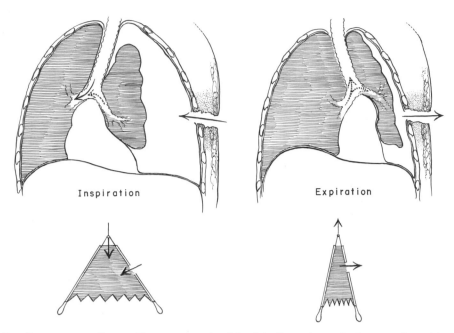

Figure 13-7. *Open pneumothorax. The movements of the intrathoracic contents occurring with open pneumothorax are shown in the inspiratory and expiratory phases. The broken arrows in the upper diagrams denote the transcarinal movement of end-expired air suggested by the "pendelluft" concept. The mechanical interference with function of the thoracic "bellows" is depicted below.*

tions. The relative contributions of the several mechanisms mentioned earlier in the discussion have not been determined.

DIAGNOSIS.   There should be no problem in diagnosing an open pneumothorax. The sucking chest wound is usually obvious on inspection, and it makes a characteristic sound as air moves through it. No further examination should be carried out before covering the wound.

TREATMENT.   Often the wound will already have been covered by the time the patient reaches the hospital, although the dressing used may not be adequate and may have to be replaced. Occasionally, in patients with pneumothorax secondary to a penetrating wound of the chest, the communication may be reopened by unnecessary manipulation of the wound at the time of examination. For this reason it is wise to dress all chest wounds definitively.

It is axiomatic that the sucking chest should be covered immediately. This simple maneuver converts the condition to that of a closed pneumothorax and eliminates the major physiological abnormality. Because time is required to prepare a definitive dressing, one should cover the wound first by the cleanest available means, pref-

erably a sterile towel or sterile gloved hand. This coverage can then be maintained until a definitive dressing can be prepared. Such a dressing should consist of several layers of gauze, the innermost impregnated with petrolatum or some other means of rendering it impervious to air. It should be wide enough to extend 2 inches or more beyond the wound margin in all directions. It should be applied to the chest with several strips of adhesive. "In the field," no attempt should be made to completely seal the dressing to the chest wall with adhesive. In that way the dressing can not only prevent air from entering the chest on inspiration, but allow it to exit during expiration or at least whenever positive pressure builds up within the thorax. This could allow gradual expansion of the collapsed lung, but more importantly, it acts as a safety valve against the development of tension pneumothorax. These considerations are not usually important once the patient has reached the hospital, since a chest tube will be inserted shortly after application of the dressing and immediately connected to water-seal drainage or suction. Thus, in the most common situation — civilian emergency department practice — the dressing can and should be occlusive.

Under no circumstances should such wounds be "packed" with gauze impregnated with such substances as petrolatum because vigorous inspiratory efforts may suck the packing into the pleural cavity, forcing an otherwise unnecessary thoracotomy.

With evacuation of the pleural space and expansion of the lung, the resuscitative phase is completed. If operative debridement and repair of the chest wound are indicated because of the degree of contamination loss or devitalization of the chest wall tissues they can and should be delayed until the patient is thoroughly evaluated and resuscitated from other significant injuries. It is desirable to obtain chest x-rays at this point. In addition to the usual upright chest film, additional views of the ribs and soft tissues in the area of the wound should be made in anticipation of the problems of reconstruction that may become apparent at the time of wound exploration. A lateral chest film should also be taken if there is an intrathoracic foreign body whose removal is planned at the time of surgery.

Repair of Traumatic Defects in the Chest Wall. Not all thoracic wounds require formal exploration and debridement. In civilian practice, the majority can simply be covered with a dressing and allowed to heal by secondary intention. However, any large or grossly contaminated wound should be debrided. This is particularly true of the high-velocity gunshot or close-range shotgun wounds in which considerable tissue damage can be expected. Once debrided, the larger wounds may present reconstructive problems, since more than mere skin coverage may be required. Integrity of the chest wall must be restored so that it not only is airtight but also does not allow significant paradoxical movement. Often this can be satisfactorily achieved by mobilizing a flap of adjacent muscle into the defect.

In the case of larger defects in which much of the overlying muscle has been destroyed or removed by debridement, it may be impossible to accomplish this end by using the available surrounding muscle. Instead, it may be necessary to mobilize a rib from the upper or lower margins of the wound and swing it diagonally across the wound as a strut to stabilize this segment of the thoracic cage. Skin coverage is usually no problem since the surrounding skin can be readily mobilized or, if necessary, a large flap can be swung to fill the defect. Fortunately, the huge chest wall defects that tax the ingenuity of the surgeon dealing with cancer are rarely encountered with trauma. Therefore a discussion of the reconstructive procedures involved is beyond the scope of this chapter.

The techniques that have been developed to repair defects following the en bloc removal of invasive chest wall tumors involve the use of not only rib struts and large pedicle grafts but, occasionally, sheets of prosthetic material such as heavy Marlex mesh or tantalum wire. These techniques may not be applicable to traumatic defects because of damage to adjacent structures that might be used in reconstruction and because of the undesirability of using prosthetic material in the grossly contaminated wound.

With the advent of safer and more sophisticated respirators, we have not hesitated in recent years to maintain patients with the more complicated open chest wounds on a respirator after thorough debridement and simply to dress the wound, exposed lung and all, until fixation occurs and granulation tissue can cover the defect. Skin grafting follows and definitive chest wall reconstruction, if functionally indicated, can be done later when one will be dealing with tissues that have healed and are no longer contaminated.

THE PLEURAL SPACE

Hemothorax

Hemothorax is one of the most common presenting problems following major chest trauma. In the companion studies of Gray et al.[32] and Harrison and associates[35] of penetrating and major nonpenetrating injuries to the chest from all causes, there was a 79 and 70 per cent incidence of hemothorax, respectively. In these reports the mortality associated with hemothorax was 4 per cent with penetrating injuries and 49 per cent with nonpenetrating injuries. The latter mortality rate is misleading because it is mainly a reflection of the severity of associated injuries. In fact, with the exception of traumatic disruption of the arch of the aorta, blunt trauma usually results in less

severe degrees of hemothorax, whereas hemothorax resulting from penetration of the
heart or great vessels provides one of the
major indications for *immediate* thoracotomy.   .

At one extreme, the hemothorax may be
so small that it is not detected initially. (A
hemothorax of less than 300 ml. is often not
demonstrable on an upright chest film.) At
the other extreme, 30 to 40 per cent of the
blood volume may be rapidly lost into one
pleural space, with little resistance offered
by the lung. Such major intrathoracic
bleeding invariably stems from the heart,
great vessels or a major systemic artery
rather than the pulmonary parenchyma,
which is perfused at low pressures, is rich
in thromboplastins and tends to collapse
around the bleeding site.

Diagnosis. A hemothorax of major proportions should rarely be missed. Shock
will be the major feature and will precede
and overshadow the ventilatory embarrassment that results from compression of the
lung and the shift of the mediastinum.

Although only about 25 per cent of hemothoraces are large enough to produce
shock, loss of blood into the pleural space is
still the most common cause of shock following chest trauma. In Andersen and Halkier's large series of chest injuries,[1] shock
developed in 48 patients, hemothorax
being the cause in 31. The associated physical findings are diminished breath sounds
and dullness to percussion posteriorly over
the involved hemothorax, which may appear more prominent but move poorly with
respirations. With major degrees of hemothorax, tracheal shift to the opposite side
may be detected. In lesser degrees of hemothorax, these signs may be difficult to
elicit, particularly when there is an associated pneumothorax. Fortunately, there is
time for a chest x-ray in these cases. The
importance of the *upright* chest film is underscored by the observation that almost a
liter of blood may produce only a slight,
diffuse increase in density over the involved hemothorax on a supine film. A
missed hemothorax may present later as a
pleural effusion and is a more common
cause of delayed post-traumatic pleural effusion than the usual suspect, chylothorax.
Aspiration of blood by thoracentesis establishes the diagnosis. This confirmation
is not academic, for an esophageal rupture

can produce shock and an x-ray picture not
unlike pneumohemothorax.

Treatment. If shock is present, restoration of the blood volume should be the first
therapeutic measure. The general principles of treating hypovolemic shock have
already been discussed and will not be
restated here.

It should be emphasized, however, that a
central venous catheter is invaluable in
treating shock from intrathoracic bleeding,
not only as a major route and sensitive
guide for massive volume replacement but
also because the central venous pressure
will allow detection of the other major
cause of early shock after chest trauma,
cardiac tamponade.

Once efforts at blood volume replacement are under way, a chest tube should be
inserted through the sixth intercostal space
in the mid-axillary line and connected to
constant gentle suction (−20 cm. water).
This is designed to accomplish the following: (1) re-expand the collapsed lung; (2)
remove the blood from the hemothorax,
thus reducing the risk of fibrothorax from
organizing blood clots and the risk of empyema by removing a source of bacterial
nutrition; (3) reduce further bleeding by
negative pressure coaption of the pleural
surfaces; and (4) provide an accurate guide
to the rate of continuing blood loss.

Today few would argue against the use of
chest tube drainage in dealing with a major
hemothorax. However, the choice between
this approach and needle aspiration for evacuating moderate degrees of hemothorax is
another matter. Such a debate is academic
in many instances, since a chest tube will
be indicated for the pneumothorax that will
coexist in at least half of the cases.

During World War I there was debate
over the desirability of evacuating the
blood at all, those opposed arguing that the
accumulating· blood tamponaded the
bleeding. This opposition gradually faded
following the war, and by the time of World
War II it was the method of evacuating the
blood that had become controversial. It was
not until the Korean conflict that advocates
of chest tube drainage gained the upper
hand. However, a review of civilian experiences suggests that this increasingly aggressive attitude may not be without some
penalty. Three consecutive experiences
with penetrating chest trauma reported

from Grady Memorial Hospital for the years 1922 to 1935, 1936 to 1942, and 1948 to 1957[32] showed a drop in mortality from 13 to 6.4 to 3.8 per cent. However, they also document a rise in the incidence of empyema from 1.6 to 2.0 to 3.3. per cent. In their most recent series, four out of five cases of hemothorax were managed by a single aspiration with no instance of empyema. Multiple thoracenteses carried a 2.3 per cent incidence of empyema, and when chest tube drainage was employed, the incidence of empyema was 10 per cent. This is partially explained by the selection of chest tube drainage for the more complicated cases that are associated with a higher incidence of shock and multiple injuries.

In spite of this and other retrospective evidence that a clear majority of cases could be adequately handled by thoracentesis alone, the author still favors the chest tube in managing traumatic hemothorax in the majority of cases because this judgment is difficult to make *prospectively*, particularly soon after the injury, and because tube thoracostomy represents a more decisive and practical approach to the problem in the emergency department setting. Physical examination alone is notoriously inaccurate in gauging changes in the degree of hemothorax; and taking chest x-rays every few hours is not a practical way to ease this uncertainty. To state this in more specific terms, tube thoracotomy is indicated in the management of traumatic hemothorax (1) if it is already of major proportions shortly after injury, e.g., causes shock, covers the dome of the diaphragm on x-ray or exceeds 500 ml. on thoracentesis; (2) if it is associated with pneumothorax; (3) if there are significant associated injuries and particularly if they will require operative treatment; and (4) if a significant hemothorax recurs shortly after initial treatment by thoracentesis. On the other hand, whenever more than an hour or two has passed since the injury, even a moderately large hemothorax can be reasonably managed by thoracentesis alone, if it is essentially an isolated injury. Minor degrees of residual hemothorax may be ignored, since it is difficult to "tap the chest dry" without causing a pneumothorax and even moderate-sized hemothoraces, if they don't become secondarily infected, will usually resorb with surprisingly little residual evidence. This

realization has caused us to be less aggressive with "clotted hemothorax" as an indication for early thoracotomy, preferring to wait at least 6 weeks to see if the degree of restrictive pulmonary dysfunction is significantly greater than that which may result from thoracotomy.

THORACOTOMY FOR MASSIVE HEMOTHORAX. Whenever a patient arrives at the hospital *in shock* from a hemothorax, the operating room should be alerted. Failure to respond satisfactorily to vigorous resuscitative measures or to maintain that response justifies immediate thoracotomy. Although this approach may seem bold, the benefit to those who could be saved only by immediate thoracotomy outweighs the cost to those whose injury *might* have been controlled without such a step.

Even if a patient's response to volume replacement can be maintained, one may still be justified in proceeding with thoracotomy under the following circumstances: (1) bleeding that continues at a significant rate, arbitrarily set at greater than 500 ml. per 8 hours after initial replacement, (2) a rate of bleeding that is steadily increasing rather than decreasing, (3) inability to empty the chest of large amounts of clotted blood, or (4) association of a widened mediastinum with a left hemothorax (i.e., suspected rupture of the thoracic aorta).

A lateral thoracotomy should be employed in the fifth interspace unless otherwise indicated by the trajectory of the penetrating agent, a widened mediastinum or other factors. In critical cases the chest is opened without the usual concern for chest wall hemostasis, the blood clots are evacuated, and the source of bleeding is sought first in the region of the heart and great vessels. If possible, the bleeding should be controlled with pressure, until the blood volume is replaced (usually 1 or 2 units beyond return to normotensive levels). It is foolish to attempt to repair the site of bleeding immediately if it can be controlled by pressure. This interval can be well spent gaining better exposure, controlling bleeding from the wound edges and obtaining proximal and distal control of the site of hemorrhage. Specific details of the operative management of bleeding from the heart and great vessels, which constitute the majority of cases of massive hemothorax, will be dealt with later in this chapter.

Major sources of bleeding from lesser systemic vessels, usually either the intercostal or internal mammary arteries, can be managed by proximal and distal suture ligation while being controlled by finger pressure. Lacerations of the pulmonary parenchyma are rarely a source of major or uncontrolled hemorrhage and can usually be controlled by suture ligatures. Unless the parenchyma has been severely disrupted or the major hilar vessels have been torn, there is little reason to resort to pulmonary resection to control hemorrhage.

Pneumothorax

Traumatic pneumothorax follows both penetrating and nonpenetrating chest injuries. In both instances, there is usually some degree of associated hemothorax. In the case of penetrating wounds, the wounding agent determines the frequency of this association. For example, icepick wounds frequently result in pneumothorax alone, whereas an associated hemothorax most frequently follows gunshot wounds. In nonpenetrating wounds, the pneumothorax will usually be associated with and often caused by rib fractures, which are present in 90 per cent of the adult cases of traumatic pneumothorax secondary to blunt trauma.

Pathophysiology. The respiratory embarrassment caused by a simple pneumothorax depends on the degree of collapse, but even when collapse is complete, the other lung is normally capable of carrying on adequate ventilation. Lesser degrees of pneumothorax are so easily compensated for that patients with *spontaneous* pneumothorax frequently experience little respiratory distress. Pneumonectomy could not be tolerated without this pulmonary reserve. However, this comparison can be carried further. Even patients in whom preoperative pulmonary function studies predict sufficient residual capacity for adequate ventilation after pneumonectomy may have difficulty getting through the immediate postoperative period to fulfill this prediction. The differences between the postoperative and the recovered state following pneumonectomy are not unlike those between the traumatic and spontaneous pneumothorax in that the ability of the remaining functional parenchyma to compensate may be interfered with by the complications of retained secretions and chest pain.

In addition to the simple loss of functioning lung tissue, blood circulating through the collapsed pulmonary parenchyma does not become fully saturated with oxygen. Fortunately, the degree of unsaturation resulting from this pulmonary "arteriovenous" shunting is somewhat reduced by increased resistance to flow through hypoventilated areas.

Diagnosis. The physical signs associated with significant degrees of pneumothorax are diminished breath sounds, hyperresonance to percussion and a prominent but poorly moving hemithorax. Each of these signs implies a comparison with the normal side. Such a comparison may not be entirely reliable in severely traumatized patients, especially if there are painful rib fractures. Tracheal deviation is an important sign when present, but it is not specific for pneumothorax since it occurs in other traumatic conditions such as hemothorax, mediastinal hematoma and pulmonary collapse distal to a totally severed bronchus. The sign that is most diagnostic, of course, is hyperresonance to percussion.

Although major degrees of pneumothorax can be diagnosed by physical examination, a chest x-ray is usually required to rule out a minor pneumothorax. Even this may not consistently demonstrate a pneumothorax of less than 10 per cent. *Expiratory* films of good quality may be required to reveal minor degrees of pneumothorax, and patients with chest pain may not be able to cooperate sufficiently for these. Even greater degrees of pneumothorax may be missed on emergency chest x-rays unless specifically sought. The appearance of a rib fracture or subcutaneous emphysema should alert the examiner to this possibility, and the lung markings should be followed to the periphery along the involved side to detect the separation of the parietal and visceral pleurae.

Treatment. Traumatic pneumothorax should be treated by tube thoracostomy through the use of either water-seal drainage or constant gentle suction. Needle aspiration and/or observation of "minor" degrees of traumatic pneumothorax are even less defensible than in spontaneous pneumothorax. This so-called conservative approach is associated with a much lower success rate than when used for spontaneous pneumothorax. In one series, it was successful in only 53 per cent of *selected* cases, which can be compared to a 97 per cent success rate obtained through use of a chest tube. In addition to being a surer and safer method of evacuating a pneumothorax, tube thoracostomy is less time-consuming in the long run, requires less frequent personal re-evaluation of the patient and results in earlier expansion of the lung.

The tube thoracostomy drainage system also provides important information regarding the persistence and relative magnitude of an air leak. For example, persistent large air leaks, which cause bubbling in the chest bottle during inspiration as well as expiration, may signify a tear in a major radical of the tracheobronchial tree. Small leaks cease fairly promptly, if indeed they still persist by the time the chest tube is inserted. Failure of the chest tube to bubble when the patient coughs is a reliable sign that the air leak has closed, provided that respiratory excursions of the fluid level in the drainage tube assure its patency. Such information allows this condition to be managed with a sureness and decisiveness that is gratifying to all concerned. Statistics do not justify the fear that infection may be introduced by tube thoracostomy (unlike the situation that may exist for hemothorax), nor is there any evidence that the use of *gentle* suction results in persistence of air leaks. An additional benefit from this method of management is shorter hospitalization for the patient.

Tension Pneumothorax

Except for patients in whom underlying disease limits cardiorespiratory reserve, total collapse of one lung, as occurs in simple pneumothorax, is well tolerated. However, in some cases the communication that permits air to enter the pleural space may act as a one-way valve, allowing air to enter during expiration but not exit during inspiration. As a result, there may be progressive accumulation of air under pressure in the pleural space, a situation that may prove fatal if not promptly detected and treated. This condition may develop in a number of ways. An oblique laceration in the pulmonary parenchyma may be so situated that a flap of tissue lies over a bronchial communication. If a rupture of the

main bronchus communicates with the pleural space through a tear in the mediastinal pleura that does not lie directly over the bronchial tear, this pleural flap may similarly act as a one-way valve over the bronchial opening. Obliquely communicating chest wounds rarely may allow movement of air between the pleural space and the outside atmosphere in an inward direction only. Today, with tracheal intubation and artificial ventilation becoming so commonplace during the course of cardiopulmonary resuscitation, a new and *relatively* frequent cause of tension pneumothorax is puncture of the lung by a fractured rib when positive pressure ventilation is being applied. It is the reason why all patients with flail chest treated by positive pressure ventilation should have prophylactic chest tubes inserted and why tension pneumothorax should be considered as the cause of unexplained deterioration in any patient with chest injuries being artificially ventilated.

Pathophysiology. As air builds up under pressure in the pleural space, the mediastinum is pushed to the opposite side, with compression of the lung on that side. Progressive impairment of the venous return and ventilatory exchange occurs. It has been suggested that the venous return eventually becomes obstructed by distortion of the caval-atrial junction, secondary to mediastinal shift. Others think that the obstruction is due to collapse of the intrathoracic venae cavae from positive pressure. Our experiments with goats and monkeys[60] suggest that impairment of venous return is related to the progressive increase in intrathoracic venous pressure in relation to that in the peripheral veins and, in the final stages, resistance to blood flow through the compressed pulmonary parenchyma may further impede the right side of the circulation. Ventilatory impairment results not only from a loss of functioning pulmonary parenchyma but also from the progressive difficulty of the thoracic bellows in achieving sufficient negative pressure gradients for adequate inspiration.

These experiments further suggested that the major lethal factor may be respiratory rather than circulatory since blood pressure and cardiac output were maintained long after respirations ceased. Initially, the goats compensated with increased respiratory effort and rate,

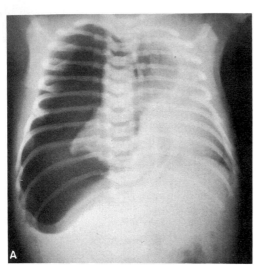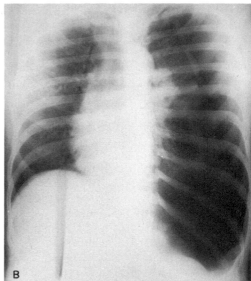

Figure 13–8. *The x-ray appearance of the tension pneumothorax in a child (A) and an adult (B). In both instances there is a characteristic downward depression of the diaphragmatic contour. However, note the marked degree of the shift of the heart and mediastinum and the infringement upon the contralateral lung seen in the child.*

maintaining their minute volume, pCO_2 and pH close to normal. Yet from the outset progressive hypoxia occurred because of a marked degree of shunting through nonventilated portions of the pulmonary capillary bed. Finally, as hypoxia deepened, compensatory efforts gradually weakened until respirations ceased. Although it is likely that the same mechanisms observed in goats are involved in the lethal outcome of tension pneumothorax in humans, their relative contributions may, of course, differ — particularly in children, in whom mediastinal shift is more marked and circulatory impairment appears to assume a more dominant role (Fig. 13–8 A and B).

Diagnosis. Both ventilatory and circulatory impairment may be evident in advanced stages of tension pneumothorax. The involved hemithorax may be prominent, move weakly with respirations and transmit breath sounds poorly. There may be a shift of the trachea to the opposite side, with distention of the neck veins and subcutaneous emphysema. However, the most important sign is hyperresonance to percussion over the involved hemithorax. A tension pneumothorax of this degree of severity should be readily suspected on the basis of physical examination alone and

treatment instituted immediately without further diagnostic measures. Occasionally, however, it will not be realized until a chest x-ray demonstrates a shift of the mediastinum that what was thought to be a simple pneumothorax has already progressed to a tension pneumothorax (Fig. 13–8).

Treatment. The most expedient form of treatment for a tension pneumothorax involves equilibration of the pleural space with atmospheric pressure by percutaneous needle puncture of the involved hemithorax. This maneuver converts the condition into an open pneumothorax but with an opening so small that it is functionally little worse than a simple pneumothorax. If done early enough, the patient's condition will improve dramatically. There is then time to insert a chest tube and to expand the lung with suction. However, if the situation has progressed to a point at which the respiratory drive is failing, and before chest tube insertion, aritificial ventilation with oxygen should be employed in addition to the venting of the pleural space.

The common association of tension pneumothorax with rupture of the bronchus should not be forgotten. Such a possibility should also be considered whenever there is a large and persistent air leak with almost constant bubbling in the chest drainage bottle and difficulty in expanding the lung.

Traumatic Chylothorax

Ordinarily, the problem of chylothorax does not arise early in the management of chest trauma. It rarely becomes clinically manifest until several days after the injury. Because thoracic duct flow is depressed while diet and activity are restricted, it takes time for a significant chylothorax to accumulate. Also, until diet is resumed and the thoracic lymph turns milky, it may be thought that one is dealing with a simple pleural effusion. The true incidence of traumatic chylothorax is probably greater than reports would indicate because many minor degrees of chylothorax go undetected and others "dry up" before the diagnosis is established. Only 90 instances of traumatic chylothorax had appeared in the literature at the time of Goorwitch's review in 1955.[31] However, subsequent reports have almost doubled this total.

Surgery and automobile accidents contribute the majority of the cases of traumatic chylothorax seen today. With the exception of the troublesome cases seen after cavopulmonary shunt, the problems presented by this condition are basically the same regardless of the original injury. Initially, chylothorax presents the problems of systemic loss of protein-rich fluid and the space-occupying effects of fluid accumulating in the pleural space. Eventually, persistent chylothorax may lead to fibrothorax, but secondary infection is rare, possibly because of the bacteriostatic properties of chyle.

Diagnosis. The diagnosis is usually not suspected until milky fluid is aspirated from the chest, and even then empyema is usually the first thought. The differentiation can be readily made because the chylous effusion is sterile on culture, contains predominantly lymphocytes rather than polymorphonuclear cells and will lose its milky color on shaking with ether. Refractile droplets may be seen under the microscope and can be demonstrated to take up lipophilic stains. Ingestion of vegetable dyes that are absorbed from the intestines will color the effusion and confirm the diagnosis in difficult cases.

Treatment. Until Lampson[40] first successfully controlled a case of traumatic chylothorax by thoracic duct ligation in 1948, the treatment had always been nonoperative, with the use of multiple thoracenteses. Lampson's approach was further supported by Goorwitch's review, which pointed to the 10 per cent mortality in patients having duct ligation as compared to 19 per cent in those treated nonoperatively. Transthoracic ligation of the thoracic duct just above the diaphragm was recommended if thoracenteses did not result in spontaneous closure of the fistula in 2 weeks.

It has been pointed out that the difference in mortality between the operative and the nonoperative approach reported by Goorwitch could be attributed to general advances in patient care, since all the cases treated by ligation had occurred in the 6 years prior to 1954, whereas the nonoperated cases dated back to 1695. More recent reports, particularly those of Maloney and Spencer[48] and Williams and Burford,[72] have swung the pendulum back toward a more prolonged attempt at nonoperative management. Williams and Burford pointed out that almost any chylothorax will close in the absence of malignant obstruction or abnormal superior caval pressures.

At present, the following indications for surgical intervention are used: (1) a general deterioration of the patient because of large amounts of protein-rich fluid being lost; (2) inability to maintain expansion of the lung, with the threat of a "trapped" lung from fibrothorax; and (3) prolonged persistence of the chylothorax. One must consider the socioeconomic impact of indefinite hospitalization on the patient. In the majority of cases, spontaneous closure of the chylous fistula will occur in 2 to 4 weeks. Maloney and Spencer noted that the rate of reaccumulation has no prognostic significance since a sudden cessation of the drainage was more common than a gradual diminution. Attempts to accelerate spontaneous activity and diet have experimental backing but have the disadvantage of aggravating the nutritional drain resulting from the loss of protein-rich chyle and of conflicting with the goal of progressive mobilization of the patient.

Recently, it has been proposed[21] that chylothorax is better managed by chest tube drainage using continuous negative pressure. This is thought to help close the fistula by apposition of the pleural surfaces and to reduce the risk of infection and fibrothorax that may attend management by multiple thoracenteses. Although experience with this approach is still limited, it appears to have merit on theoretical grounds at least.

In the minority of patients in whom operative intervention is indicated, ligation of the thoracic duct just above the diaphragm through a right lower thoracotomy will suffice. It is helpful to use dyes to aid in localizing the thoracic duct at surgery. The passage of a long tube into the upper small intestines preoperatively will allow one to instill a blue vegetable dye after the chest has been opened. Earlier instillation of the dye may stain the entire thorax by the time the chest has been opened. Williams suggests a simpler approach in which a small amount of cosmetic blue dye is injected into the wall of the lower esophagus at the time of thoracotomy. Lymphangiogram may occasionally be helpful in localizing the leak preoperatively.

In cases of long-standing chylothorax, concomitant decortication may be necessary. This possibility should be considered preoperatively in a left-sided chylothorax since the usual right-sided approach to the thoracic duct would have to be modified.

Procedures Used in Evacuating the Pleural Spaces

The choice between thoracentesis and tube thoracostomy drainage in the management of pneumothorax or hemothorax has been discussed in preceding sections of this chapter. The site chosen for evacuating the pleural space depends on whether one is dealing with a pneumothorax, a hemothorax or significant degrees of both. Since free air rises to the top of the pleural space, its evacuation is usually carried out through an upper interspace. With the patient in a semiupright position, the highest point in the pleural space is anterosuperior. For this reason, and because it is a reasonably avascular location in a wide interspace, the second intercostal space in the midclavicular line is usually selected for evacuation of air (Fig. 13–13A). However, in less urgent situations, and particularly in women in whom overlying breast tissue and cosmetic

considerations make this location less than desirable, one can insert the chest tube in the axilla below the hairline and just behind the edge of the pectoralis major where the third and fourth intercostal spaces are close to the skin and easily palpable.

On the other hand, if one wishes to evacuate blood or other fluid, a dependent location should be chosen. Because the moving diaphragm constantly changes the size and contour of the lower pleural recesses and is itself subject to injury during these procedures, the sixth interspace is preferred rather than a lower point in the thorax. For tube thoracostomy, insertion in the midaxillary line with tunneling posteriorly is chosen so that the patient will not lie upon and obstruct the chest catheter (Fig. 13–13B).

It has been previously noted that variable degrees of hemothorax and pneumothorax frequently coexist following chest trauma. If there are significant degrees of both, it is not always wise to try to evacuate them through a single chest catheter but rather to apply the method indicated for the treatment of each. Some blood may be evacuated through a superiorly placed chest tube, but this cannot be efficiently accomplished in the face of persistent air leak, because only air, which offers the least resistance to evacuation, will be obtained. Even the choice of a dependent site for tube thoracostomy in this situation may fail to completely evacuate the hemothorax.

If a hemothorax is associated with a small pneumothorax without continuing air leak, one can insert a low, posterolateral chest tube for the hemothorax and initially evacuate the pneumothorax by keeping the patient in the anterolateral supine position for a few minutes before returning him to the semiupright position. If, however, an air leak is still present, a second, high anterior chest tube should be inserted to deal with this. Generally, a pneumothorax should be evacuated through an anterosuperior chest tube and suction applied if an air leak persists. As previously stated, the indications for thoracentesis versus tube thoracostomy for hemothorax are subject to considerable differences of opinion. It is our practice to aspirate even minor hemothoraces initially, to confirm the diagnosis and to rule out chylothorax and particularly, ruptured esophagus. In addition, a minor hemothorax may obscure the radiological signs of ruptured diaphragm. For any major hemothorax, the authors prefer posterolateral tube thoracostomy with suction drainage. Lesser degrees of hemothorax may be aspirated or even watched as long as they produce only a blunting of the costophrenic or cardiophrenic angles. Whenever the fluid spans the width of the hemithorax, tube thoracotomy is justified.

Technique of Thoracentesis (Fig. 13–9). The patient should be seated or semierect. The interspace chosen is identified by counting ribs but in an emergency may have to be approximated. The second interspace anteriorly is broad and is level with the sternal prominence, the angle of Ludwig or Louis. To identify the sixth or seventh interspace posterolaterally it is easier to count backwards from the twelfth rib. One should not rely on the fact that the eighth normally lies at the tip of the scapula since changes with shift in position may be misleading. The area is prepared with an antiseptic solution and draped with sterile towels. An intradermal wheal is raised with 1 per cent Xylocaine using a 25-gauge needle. Then a #20 G needle is advanced with gentle infiltration toward the upper border of the lower rib of the interspace. The needle is passed, or walked, over the upper border of this rib, at which point an additional 2 ml. is infiltrated before the pleural cavity is entered.

After aspiration of air or fluid establishes the proper depth of insertion, the needle is clamped at the skin level to mark the distance required for its entrance and then it is withdrawn. At this point, a change is made to a larger syringe (50 ml.) and needle (#18 G or larger). The new needle is clamped at the same distance from the tip as the needle used to infiltrate, to serve as a constant guide to the correct depth of insertion, and attached to the syringe by a three-way stopcock. It is then introduced along the same tract into the pleural space. The three-way stopcock allows each 50 ml. aspirated to be discharged through a side arm without disconnecting or withdrawing the needle. The volume removed should always be measured. Aspiration is continued until no longer productive, or until over 500 ml. of blood or 1000 ml. of air have been removed, at which time tube thoracostomy usually should be performed.

Closed Tube Thoracostomy. (Fig. 13–

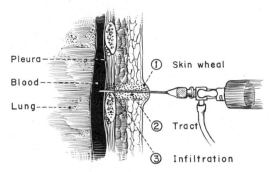

Figure 13-9. *The technique of thoracentesis as described in the text.*

10). Small catheters (16 F) connected to water-seal drainage are used to evacuate modest air leaks. Larger leaks, indicating communication with a sizable bronchial radical, may require even more than one larger (24–28 F) catheter attached to suction. Larger catheters (32–36 F) are also used to evacuate a hemothorax. The initial technique is similar to that described for thoracentesis except that thoracentesis for blood is best performed through the fifth interspace in the mid-scapular line with the patient seated upright, whereas tube thoracotomy for hemothorax is usually performed in the sixth intercostal space in the mid-axillary line with the patient supine and in the lateral decubitus position. (Fig. 13–13C).

The chosen interspace is prepared and draped, and a tract into the interspace is infiltrated with 1 per cent Xylocaine but more widely than for thoracentesis. Specially designed trocars are available for inserting the catheter but are not widely used, because of the potential danger of damaging the underlying lung or diaphragm. However, if there is a sizable pneumothorax or hemothorax, the lung will not be near the chest wall and this risk is minimal. We prefer to make a small incision and develop a tract through the underlying subcutaneous tissue and muscles down to the pleura by advancing a large Kelly clamp in increments and spreading it gently (Fig. 13–13D). The pleura is entered with a short quick thrust of the clamp. (The danger of damaging the underlying lung is minimal with this small instrument because it is separated from the parietal pleura by the accumulated air or fluid and there need be no fear of creating or increasing a pneumothorax since the pleural space

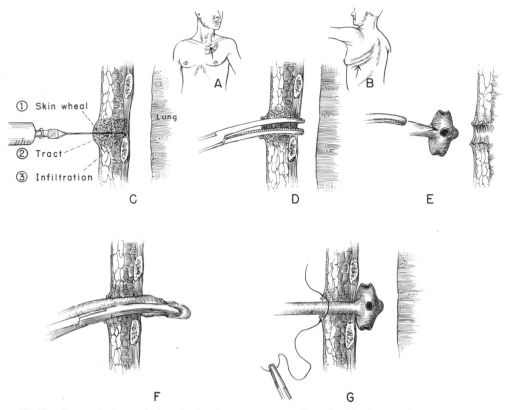

Figure 13–10. *The technique of closed tube thoracostomy as described in the text. The second interspace in the midclavicular line* (A) *is selected for the removal of air and the 6th or 7th intercostal space in the posterior axillary line* (B) *for the removal of fluid.*

will soon be completely evacuated.) Then a catheter of appropriate size, clamped at its distal end, is grasped by its forward tip and introduced into the pleura through this tract (Fig. 13–13*E* and *F*). The skin is snugly closed around the catheter with a heavy silk or wire suture, which is then used to anchor the chest tube (Fig. 13–13*G*). "Mushroom-tip" or Malecot catheters used to be popular since they can be pulled back until the flange abuts the parietal pleura, assuring the position of the tip of the catheter at the proper depth. However, clear plastic "Argyle" catheters with multiple holes near the end and a radiopaque marker to indicate position of the tube and its outermost hole on the chest x-ray are now the most popular type of chest tube. The clear plastic material allows ready visualization of the contents of the tubing and inhibits adherence of blood clots. In fact, few hospitals continue to stock the old latex chest catheters. However, if their features are desirable in a given situation, an inflatable bal-loon-tipped (Foley) catheter can be used. An occlusive dressing may be applied around the tube, but this is usually not necessary if the suture is properly placed. The tube is unclamped after it has been securely connected (with adhesive tape) to the drainage system.

Pleural Drainage Systems. There are basically two types of pleural drainage systems. One employs a one-way water-trap mechanism, the other uses continuous suction. Their relative merits and indications are discussed in relation to the condition for which they are used.

The so-called water-trap or water-seal drainage achieves its purpose of allowing only the egress of pleural contents by the placement of the end of the drainage tube just under water some distance below the level of the patient's chest. The usual drainage bottle used for this purpose is illustrated in Figure 13–11 *left*. Pleural air or fluid will exit through the system whenever intrapleural pressure exceeds atmospheric pressure by more than the distance the drainage outlet is submerged below the water. This usually occurs during expiration, coughing or straining. During inspiration, however, the intrathoracic negative pressure must exceed the distance between the chest and the water level in the drainage bottle in order for fluid to rise up and enter the chest. Since this distance is usually 80 cm. or more, the system progressively evacuates the pleural contents with each expiration. If only fluid is involved, its egress will be further promoted by a siphon effect. Such a system is adequate for evacuating air and fluid accumulating at a modest rate and will prevent tension pneumothorax.

USE OF SUCTION SYSTEMS. The one-way drainage systems just described depend upon changes in intrapleural pressure to evacuate the pleural space. Their efficiency can be enhanced by having the patient cough, strain or breathe deeply, but if the rate of air leak or hemorrhage is rapid, this system will not keep the pleural space evacuated. This can be accomplished by applying negative pressure to the system. A number of devices, from complex pumps to simple faucet attachments, are used as the suction source, but the most important consideration is control of the degree of negative pressure applied. A simple and effective means of achieving this employs a regulating bottle interposed between the suction source and the primary chest drainage bottle, as shown in Figure 13–11 *right*. In it a glass tube open to the atmosphere at one end and submerged below water at the other is used to limit the maximum degree of negative pressure that can be developed in the drainage system. When the negative

pressure in the system begins to exceed the distance its tip is submerged below the water, outside air will be drawn in through the tube and will bring the pressure within the system back to this level again. Thus, by filling the regulator bottle to the desired level above the tip of this tube (usually between 5 and 20 cm.), one can limit the negative pressure applied, regardless of the amount of suction, and, as long as bubbles are emerging from the tip of this tube, this level of negative pressure is assured. The system is usually completed by a third, or trap, bottle interposed between the regular bottle and the suction source to protect the latter against accidental spillover. (In most situations today, in which the source of suction is "piped in" rather than being supplied by a small electric motor, this trap bottle is unnecessary.)

The basic "three-bottle system" or minor modifications of it is the most common pleural suction apparatus used in this country. It has the advantage of being simple and inexpensive. There are more elaborate commercial systems available that are based on the same principles; their chief advantage lies in their capacity to remove larger volumes rapidly at relatively low negative pressures. This is useful for large air leaks, from which air may accumulate more rapidly than the conventional three-bottle system can remove it. It is also claimed that evacuating the pleural space at a lower pressure differential is less likely to delay the closure of air leaks. These features, though desirable, are a significant advantage in only a small minority of cases. In most instances the three-bottle system is quite adequate.

MANAGEMENT OF CHEST DRAINAGE

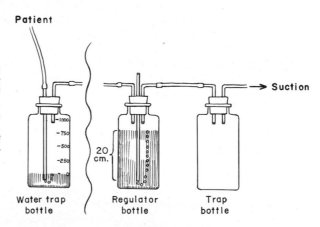

Figure 13–11. *Pleural drainage systems. To the left is shown in the simple water trap bottle that utilizes respiratory excursions in intrapleural pressure to provide egress of the pleural contents. The suction drainage is provided by the addition of the two bottles on the right, the degree of suction being controlled by the depth of the middle tube below the water in the regular bottle. See text for full description.*

Patient

Suction

20 cm.

Water trap bottle

Regulator bottle

Trap bottle

SYSTEMS. Frequent checks should be made to see that all connections are secure and airtight and that the drainage tube has not become inadvertently occluded by the patient's sitting on it, by the inertia of fluid filling a bend in the tubing or by a fibrin or blood clot. These hazards can usually be avoided by seeing that the drainage tube has no excess length and by periodically "milking it down." Much practical information can be gained from careful periodic inspection of the chest bottles and tubing. Oscillations of the air-fluid level in the drainage tube in response to respirations, if greater than 1 to 2 cm., indicate that the system is patent. A persistent air leak is signaled by air intermittently bubbling out from the bottom of the drainage tube. This usually occurs only during expiration.

If bubbling occurs throughout the respiratory cycle in a water-seal drainage system, a large-volume air leak is present and the presence of a ruptured bronchus should be considered. When suction is applied, the rate of air leak will be partly dependent on the degree of negative pressure applied as well as the size of the bronchopleural communication. The hourly rate of bleeding can be documented by marking a vertical strip of adhesive tape on the side of the bottle. The color of the blood may be helpful, but it must be kept in mind that if air is being evacuated through the tube with the blood, the latter can become oxygenated, misleading one as to its possible source.

REMOVAL OF CHEST TUBES. Chest tubes are removed whenever they are no longer functioning or when blood or air has stopped accumulating. A petrolatum-impregnated gauze dressing such as is used to cover an open pneumothorax is prepared, and the anchoring suture is removed. The patient is instructed to hold a forced expiration for the period commanded and, after practice assures that this will be done, the tube is quickly withdrawn during the expiratory phase. The communication is immediately occluded with the dressing, which is then firmly taped in place. Another alternative is to use a twisted wire or heavy suture to anchor the suture initially and to close the tract by tying this down at the time of removal of the chest tube.

THE LUNGS

Intrathoracic Foreign Bodies

The proper management of intrathoracic foreign bodies is a problem associated with penetrating thoracic injuries, particularly those resulting from military action. The problem is rarely urgent. However, after successful completion of the resuscitative phase, a decision should be made regarding the need for removal because if prophylactic removal is indicated, it is best done early. Factors influencing this decision are the nature of the foreign body, its size, shape and position, and the degree of contamination associated with its penetration of the thoracic cavity. Generally, foreign bodies in or near the tracheobronchial tree, the heart or great vessels warrant removal. One should also consider early removal of those that are large, (i.e., over 2.5 cm.), sharply contoured or associated with gross contamination. Objects that do not in themselves constitute an indication for surgical removal should nevertheless be removed when feasible during thoracotomy for other indications.

The removal of foreign bodies in or intimately associated with the heart and great vessels is dealt with later in this chapter. The majority of the remainder involve the lungs or pleura. In general, these are best left alone until they produce symptoms. Laustela[41] followed 502 Finnish casualties of World War II who had this complication and found that only 20 per cent developed complications requiring subsequent removal. Of the 104 presenting with late symptoms, 39 had chronic bronchitis; 31 developed lung abscess; 24 had empyema; 5 had bronchiectasis; and 5, bronchopleural fistula. Thus, the major problem was secondary infection.

The mortality from removal of intrathoracic foreign bodies in Korean War casualties was only 1 per cent when surgery was delayed until symptoms developed.[68] In 60 per cent of the cases the indication for operation was secondary infection. However, 85 per cent of the foreign bodies necessitating subsequent removal were shell fragments. In civilian practice the incidence of late complications would be even less. Indeed, in the Korean War experience, only 10 per cent of bullets lodged in the pulmonary parenchyma caused secondary infection. In spite of a few memorable exceptions, the generalization can be made that complications from foreign bodies develop relatively early, since many of the infections are related to the initial contamination and because it is rare for foreign bodies to migrate after the first few weeks unless they are closely related to hilar structures, are wholly intrapleural or are very sharp.

Direct Pulmonary Parenchymal Trauma

Trauma to the pulmonary parenchyma did not receive much attention in this country until widespread interest was aroused by the World War II experience with "wet lung."[12, 13] Just as there was a higher incidence of serious blast and blunt injuries to the thorax in that war, there has been a progressive increase in serious nonpenetrating thoracic injuries in civilian practice in the subsequent 2 decades. Penetrating injuries of the pulmonary parenchyma, excluding those from high-velocity missiles, are relatively well tolerated. The reparative ability of the pulmonary parenchyma is remarkable. Unless hilar structures are damaged, the leakage of air and blood soon stops, and resections are rarely necessary for peripheral parenchymal damage. In the absence of a foreign body and gross contamination, infection is rare. On the other hand, although blunt trauma to the pulmonary parenchyma usually produces lesser degrees of local injury, it can result in far more serious, even life-threatening consequences by the summation of multiple lesions and secondary reflex changes.

The separation of various types of parenchymal damage is somewhat artificial since they so often occur in combination. In addition, with the exception of blast injuries, parenchymal lesions from nonpenetrating trauma are often associated with other intrathoracic damage.

Localized Pulmonary Contusion. This is a common sequel to thoracic injury. In its simplest form it represents suffusion of blood from disrupted vessels through air spaces into the surrounding parenchyma.

As an isolated lesion it has little importance, although occasionally if there is bleeding into a main order bronchus, consolidation of the entire distal parenchymal segment may result. Nevertheless, when there is no significant disruption of the pulmonary parenchyma, resorption will be prompt.

Parenchymal Laceration. Tearing of the pulmonary parenchyma may disrupt both blood vessels and air passages. Subsequent developments partially depend on whether the laceration connects with the pleura. If there is communication with the pleura, either a hemothorax, a pneumothorax or a pneumohemothorax will be produced. The latter is the most common occurrence with penetrating injuries. On the other hand, parenchymal disruptions resulting from blunt trauma are not infrequently localized in the region of the intermediary bronchus, so that the extravasated blood and air accumulate in the space created by the parenchymal laceration, resulting in either pulmonary hematoma or cystic cavities.

Pulmonary Hematoma. In contrast to the consolidation of pulmonary parenchyma with suffused blood occurring after contusion, pulmonary hematoma implies the accumulation of extravasated blood in a space created by parenchymal disruption. This is a much more common sequel to blunt chest trauma than generally appreciated. In a review of 124 cases of nonpenetrating injury to the thorax, Westermark[71] found radiological parenchymal abnormalities in 94. In 14 of these, slightly over 10 per cent, lesions suggestive of single or multiple pulmonary hematomas were observed.

Errion et al.[26] reviewed 50 cases of pulmonary hematoma resulting from blunt thoracic trauma and made the following observations: When present, pain and hemoptysis were moderate in degree, usually disappearing in less than a week. Low-grade fever and dyspnea were not uncommon, the latter being characteristically greater than expected from the radiological appearance of the parenchymal lesion. Typically, these lesions appear fuzzy in outline on initial films but in a few days, as the surrounding suffusion of blood resorbs, the outline sharpens. This creates a parenchymal lesion that may be indistinguishable from other coin lesions without the benefit of earlier films. The hematomas are ordinarily 2 to 5 cm. in diameter and characteristically are located posteriorly in the lower lobes. In 18 of the 50 cases, a radiolucency developed later in the lesion. Resolution usually took place in 2 to 4 weeks.

Their characteristic location has suggested to some that pulmonary hematomas following blunt trauma result from a contrecoup mechanism in which shearing forces develop in the region of the intermediary bronchi. The main clinical problem created by such pulmonary hematomas results from failure to recognize their traumatic origin. This dilemma usually develops when there is no pretrauma x-ray available for comparison and the early evolution of these lesions is also not observed. Thus, there may be no way to distinguish them from a pre-existing coin lesion. The problem may be resolved by progressive resolution of the lesion, but if this has not occurred in 3 weeks, the lesion should be excised to establish its identity.

Another problem that occasionally arises during exploration for other indications is whether something should be done about coexisting hemorrhagic parenchymal lesions. In view of the remarkable reparative properties of the pulmonary parenchyma, resection is recommended only for extensive parenchymal damage. Otherwise, bleeding and air leaks should be controlled by suture ligation, the laceration left open, and a chest tube placed near this area and connected to suction.

Traumatic Pulmonary Cavity. More rarely, the disruptive forces mentioned previously will tear a small bronchiole without significant vascular damage, resulting in the formation of a pulmonary cavity. These usually resolve spontaneously without secondary infection but occasionally, if associated with disruption of a main order bronchus, they may fail to regress and actually enlarge. These exceptional cases require operative control of the bronchial communication, after which the opened cavity will collapse with catheter drainage and suction.

Contusion Pneumonitis or "Traumatic Wet Lung." Although a clear description of this entity was published many years ago by Morgagni and further elaborated in European — particularly French — literature, it was not until Brewer[11] and Burford[12] and their respective associates reported their experience with this condition during World War II that it became widely appreciated in this country. Brewer felt that "persistence of fluid in the pulmonary tree" resulted from increased production and decreased removal of this fluid — bronchial secretions, serum and blood. Drinker and Warren[23] elucidated some of the factors contributing to increased pulmonary fluid production, emphasizing anoxia, changes in tissue permeability, increased respiratory movements and tracheal obstruction. In addition, it was suggested that the extravasated blood produced a reflex bronchospasm.

Probably one of the most important factors limiting the patient's ability to clear these fluids from the air passages is the inability to cough because of uncontrolled chest pain. Similarly, any interference with effective coughing (e.g., flail chest, elevated diaphragm, central nervous system depression) will aggravate the situation. These factors initiate a vicious cycle that produces progressive ventilatory impairment.

What determines why one patient with blunt chest trauma ends up with only a localized pulmonary contusion and in another this process progresses to the diffuse secondary consolidative changes of "traumatic wet lung" is not clear. The severity of the trauma itself is one obvious factor, and the volume of intravenous fluids administered after the injury may be another. Rutherford and Valenta[62] have succeeded in producing pulmonary contusions in dogs that spontaneously progressed into a lethal "traumatic wet lung" by high-velocity, low-mass blunt trauma inflicted during tracheal obstruction, suggesting the importance of a closed glottis at the moment of impact. Histologically, the secondary areas of consolidation were indistinguishable from those of "shock lung" and other pulmonary parenchymal consolidative lesions of traumatic origin, adding to the conviction that the lung responds in a common manner to all forms of insult and injury. Hypoxia secondary to pulmonary vascular "shunting" through consolidated areas, decreased compliance and hyperventilation with hypocarbia were the main physiologic abnormalities observed.

DIAGNOSIS. After a variable period of delay, the patient usually develops an ineffective cough and progressive hyperpnea and dyspnea. Physical examination reveals scattered bronchial rales. These may be fine or "sticky" and do not completely clear on coughing. Local areas of wheezing are often a prominent finding. The overall picture resembles that of pulmonary edema associated with a degreee of bronchospasm but is more variable in degree and distribution than seen on the initial x-ray.

The x-ray picture is characteristic but may not correspond temporally to the developing clinical picture. A few fluffy opacifications seen on the initial x-ray may quickly progress into a veritable "snowstorm" in which little functional parenchyma would appear to remain. Usually these lesions appear first on the side of impact, and the changes in this area will be more marked, even though scattered lesions may subsequently appear bilaterally. Blood gas analysis will usually show decreases in oxygen and carbon dioxide tension in the arterial blood.

TREATMENT. Treatment depends on the severity of the condition. If the contusion pneumonitis remains relatively localized, it may be weathered without specific therapy. However, one has no assurance, when this localized process is first discovered, that it will not progress into the severe, widespread form. The latent period between the development of symptoms and the rate of progression are only rough guides. Early vigorous therapy should not be delayed until serious symptoms develop. The patient should be placed in a semiupright position in an oxygen-rich, humidified atmosphere. Chest pain must be controlled by analgesics or, if necessary, intercostal block. This alone may allow the patient to maintain a clear airway by coughing. Otherwise, nasotracheal suction should be used. Bronchodilators have proved helpful, particularly the use of small doses of aminophylline.

Although saline infusions have made experimental models of wet lung worse,[20] the inference that patients should be kept dehydrated does not appear justified. This may result in more viscid bronchial secre-

tions that complicate tracheal toilet. However, one should assiduously avoid overhydration whenever intravenous fluids are being administered. If overhydration has taken place during the course of the initial resuscitative efforts before the diagnosis of pulmonary contusion was made, the intravenous administration of a diuretic such as furosemide is indicated. Expectorants and mucolytic agents have been advocated, but their benefit has not been clearly shown. Antibiotics should be administered. In Westermark's series, 26 of the 28 patients who developed clinical bronchitis with purulent sputum after blunt chest trauma had x-ray evidence of contusion pneumonitis on earlier films.

The role of steroids in this situation is still unclear. They have been found to be beneficial in experimental studies of various types of post-traumatic pulmonary consolidative lesions, possibly because of their effect on membrane permeability. More specifically, Franz et al.[28] have shown that methyl prednisolone succinate (30 mg./kg.) reduced the size of a standard pulmonary contusion. Nevertheless, in spite of some suggestive clinical reports,[66] steroids have not been proven, in *controlled clinical* trials, to ameliorate significantly the natural course of pulmonary contusions.

Although a significant proportion of patients will respond satisfactorily to these measures, it has become common practice in recent years to intubate and place the more severely affected patients on positive pressure ventilation, using a respirator. The indication for tracheal intubation here is inability to control secretions in spite of other measures. It has the additional benefit of decreasing airway resistance, respiratory dead space and the work of breathing. The benefit of positive pressure breathing has been implied from the report of Ransdell et al.[59] of a series of patients with traumatic flail chest treated with and without a respirator. Four of 17 treated without a respirator developed the wet lung syndrome, while none of the 16 placed in a respirator developed this complication. This agrees with carlier experience with the use of positive pressure oxygen therapy in the treatment of acute pulmonary edema.

In the previously mentioned experimental study,[62] the author showed that lethal outcome from a severe pulmonary contusion could be reduced from 70 to 10 per cent by only an hour of positive pressure ventilation if it was applied soon after the injury. While the value of prophylactic or, at least early, respirator therapy seems clear, the practical problem of selection remains, since the majority of patients — those with mild, localized pulmonary contusions — will not need this form of treatment. Our experiments showed that pulmonary scans are much more sensitive than chest x-rays in predicting the severity of the parenchymal involvement, but this is not a practical diagnostic approach in most hospitals. Instead, we rely heavily on serial blood determinations. In general, the use of continuous positive pressure ventilation should be considered in the treatment of pulmonary contusions under the following circumstances: (1) multiple large pulmonary contusions are evident on the admission x-ray, (2) the contusions are associated with many (more than five) rib fractures or even minor degrees of flail chest, (3) surgery under general anesthesia will be necessary for associated injuries, (4) arterial blood gases are significantly depressed below normal, (5) voluminous intravenous fluid therapy is anticipated in the treatment of other injuries, (6) underlying dysfunctional lung disease exists (e.g., asthma, emphysema), (7) serial x-rays show progressive opacification, and (8) in the absence of other criteria if rapid labored respirations ensue.

Respirator Therapy of Chest Injuries. In addition to flail chest and contusion pneumonitis, there are a number of other "traumatic" forms of pulmonary parenchymal consolidation that may benefit from use of CPPV (e.g., shock lung, fat embolism, smoke inhalation, aspirative pneumonitis, "pump-oxygenator lung"). Because of their increasing importance, a separate chapter has been assigned to deal with them (Chapter 6). Only the basic principles of respirator therapy as applied to severe contusion pneumonitis will be reiterated here. For a more comprehensive review of respirator therapy the reader should seek other publications.[6, 56]

Serial arterial blood gas analyses and daily chest x-rays still provide the most objective guide for institution and discontinuation of respiratory therapy. Another aspect worth comment concerns the choice of respirator and, more specifically, the controversy over the choice between pressure-cycled versus volume-cycled ventilators. In this particular setting, with changing degrees of parenchymal consolidation, the volume-cycled respirator is definitely superior. Pressure-cycled respirators cannot be relied upon to produce adequate ventilatory exchange in the face of increased and *changing* pulmonary compliance. Furthermore, most of them do not have a very high peak-pressure capacity or good control of inspired oxygen concentrations. Time-cycled devices, such as the original Engstrom respirator, will deliver the required tidal volume with high pressure capacity but have the disadvantages of a fixed inspiratory: expiratory ratio and cannot be patient-cycled. The volume-cycled respirators deliver a metered amount of air at whatever delivery pressure is required. However, some of the newer respirators such as the Ohio 560 and Bennett MA-1 have such a variety of features that these arguments become almost academic. Although they are basically volume-limited ventilators with range-controlled high-pressure capacity in which the inspired oxygen concentration can also be accurately controlled, they have a wide range of flow capacities, a spirometer to monitor each tidal volume, built-in warning devices, a sigh mechanism to protect against atelectasis, an ultrasonic nebulizer and the important capability of applying positive end expired pressure (PEEP) or the inflationary hold (IH).

While tidal volumes of 10 ml./kg. and a rate of 12–14 breaths per minute are sufficient in dealing with most forms of respiratory insufficiency, minute volumes of more than twice this level are commonly required in dealing with traumatic parenchymal problems. The resultant hypocarbia and alkalosis are then combated by adding 1 to 3 feet of dead-space tubing between the trachea and the expiratory valve. In an attempt to keep the inspired oxygen concentration below 40 per cent and avoid superimposing an oxygen toxicity lesion on an already damaged lung, one may have to accept slightly subnormal arterial oxygen tensions and, of course, supranormal levels are inexcusable in a properly functioning respiratory care unit.

Rather than increasing inspired oxygen concentration for any extended period of time, it is worth trying other ancillary measures. One of the most popular of these is PEEP, in which, by a special expiratory valve, 6 to 7 cm. of positive and expiratory pressure can be maintained. This maintains a larger functional residual capacity with which more alveoli may remain open and better ventilation: perfusion ratios may be achieved. Another occasionally useful technique is that of "inspiratory hold" in which peak inspiratory pressure is held for ½ to 1½ seconds to allow additional time for alveolar recruitment and more effective distribution of inspired air throughout the lungs. These maneuvers can interfere with venous return to the heart in normal subjects, but this is less of a problem in the patient with "traumatic wet lung" because the noncompliant lungs dissipate these higher pressures so that they do not result in comparable rises in intrapleural pressure. In fact, when these adverse hemodynamic effects occur in these patients, it is usually because their blood volume is diminished and the appearance of these effects is cause for volume restoration rather than discontinuation of respiratory therapy.

The Tracheobronchial Tree. Although the tracheobronchial tree may be violated by a variety of penetrating objects, most tracheobronchial tears are the result of severe blunt trauma. There were 61 instances of this complication recorded in the medical literature in 100 years prior to 1948 and 94 in the decade that followed.[4] This fifteenfold increase in the reported incidence is attributable in part to increased frequency of severe blunt trauma and in part to the interest generated by successful surgical treatment, first achieved by Griffith in 1948.[33] Since that report, excellent results have been achieved in over 60 per cent of the operated cases reported.[51]

By far the majority of these injuries involve the mainstem bronchi. Only 18 of 98 patients reviewed by Hood and Sloan[37] had tracheal tears, and of the remaining 80, all but six were in the main bronchus. The distribution between right and left side was roughly equal. The mechanism involved has not been established, but shearing forces, compression of the trachea against the vertebral column, airway distention

against a closed glottis and sudden vertical stretch of the tracheobronchial tree all have been suggested.[17] Whichever theory is valid must explain the fact that over 90 per cent of the tears occur within an inch of the carina. The typical tear in the bronchus is circumferential and incomplete. The less frequent tracheal tears are usually vertical along the line of membranous-cartilaginous transition. Complete division of the trachea at this level, however, is extremely uncommon.

DIAGNOSIS. The manner of presentation varies considerably (Fig. 13–12). The lesion may prove rapidly fatal or allow survival without surgical intervention. In more severe cases only prompt recognition and resuscitation will achieve survival. In Burke's series,[14] 52 per cent of the deaths occurred within 1 hour of injury and an additional 44 per cent within 4 days of injury. Fortunately, the majority of patients do not present in critical condition. In the same series, immediate operation was carried out in only 11 per cent, 21 per cent presented with a collapsed lung that resisted attempts at re-expansion and were explored after bronchoscopic confirmation of the injury; and the remaining 68 per cent presented later with bronchial stenosis or other delayed forms of presentation. This is similar to the observation of Hood and Sloan that the diagnosis was made within 24 hours of injury in only one third of the cases.

Depending on the location and size of the tear and the involvement of bronchial vessels or the mediastinal pleura, patients with these injuries may present with one or more of the following: massive hemoptysis, airway obstruction, progressive mediastinal and subcutaneous emphysema, tension pneumothorax, pneumothorax without tension but with persistent air leak, or massive collapse of the lung (Fig. 13–12). Although the patient with a ruptured bronchus is said to present characteristically with dyspnea and cyanosis, subcutaneous and mediastinal emphysema, fractured ribs, pneumothorax and hemoptysis, over two thirds of the patients in Burke's series did not show this combination. In one of seven, the thoracic contents appeared normal on the initial chest x-ray.

Pneumothorax was found in only 55 of the 82 patients reported by Hood and Sloan

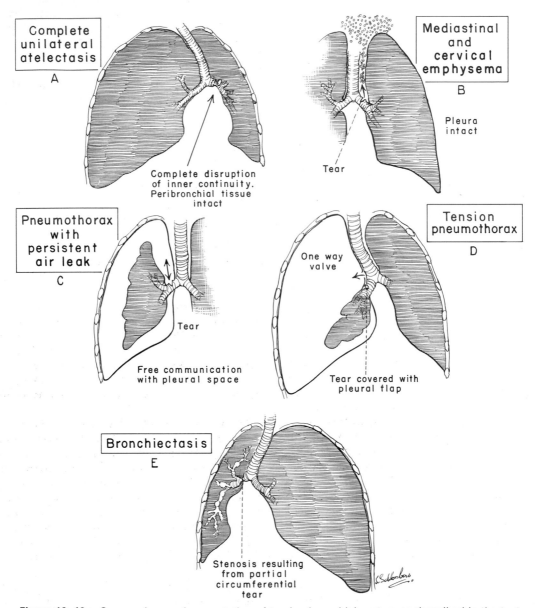

Figure 13–12. Cmmon forms of presentation of tracheobronchial rupture as described in the text.

and tension pneumothorax in only 21. Subcutaneous emphysema was present in just over one half the patients and hemoptysis and thoracic skeletal fractures were demonstrated in only one fourth. Furthermore, one cannot always depend upon other evidence of severe thoracic trauma to alert one's suspicions, for this injury may show remarkable selectivity. In 42 of the 80 bronchial tears reported by Hood and Sloan, this was the only major intrathoracic injury. Although one cannot expect to find all the "characteristic" features in any one patient, any one of them should arouse suspicion. This association of rib fractures is high *if* one considers only the age group in which rib fractures readily occur. Thus, 91 per cent of patients over 30 years of age had fractures involving one of the upper three ribs, and all had a fracture of at least one of the upper five ribs.[4]

Similarly, mediastinal and cervical subcutaneous emphysema should raise the question of such an injury. This is likely to be prominent in tracheal tears or bronchial tears on which the mediastinal pleura remains intact. However, if the pleura is torn, a pneumothorax results. This usually presents either as a tension pneumothorax or a pneumothorax with persistent air leak. A tension pneumothorax often is produced because the tear in the mediastinal pleura occurs some distance from the point of airway rupture so that a valve-like mediastinal flap exists. However, tension pneumothorax is not so common an association as it once was thought to be.

Another common variation is for the edges of a complete bronchial tear to be separated, yet for the surrounding tissues to remain intact so that pneumothorax does not occur. These patients may present early with complete unilateral atelectasis or late with bronchial stenosis. Most bronchial tears bleed, but hemoptysis may be absent because the bleeding may have stopped by the time the patient is seen or the blood may not have been coughed up. Nevertheless, there are instances in which the hemoptysis is massive, presenting a difficult problem in management. Significant hemoptysis following chest trauma is a symptom that should not be ignored and, even in the absence of other symptoms suggesting tracheobronchial rupture, it is an indication for bronchoscopy.

TREATMENT. Patients presenting with massive hemoptysis, airway obstruction or tension pneumothorax need immediate resuscitative measures. Emergency tracheostomy may be necessary to remove accumulating blood. It also helps to minimize the subcutaneous emphysema and to reduce the rate of air leak. The lethal potential of a tension pneumothorax can be eliminated by percutaneous needle puncture of the involved hemithorax. This should be followed by tube thoracostomy and evacuation of pleural air by suction. A large intercostal catheter and an efficient (low pressure and high volume) suction system may be required to evacuate the pleural space if there is a large air leak. In such cases, a point may be reached beyond which the rate or removal of pleural air prevents adequate intake of air into the lungs. Such an impasse, of course, demands immediate thoracotomy. Until this can be accomplished, it is better to settle for a pneumothorax without tension than to persist with more vigorous attempts to expand the lung.

Fortunately, such cases are not common. More commonly, these patients present with mediastinal and subcutaneous emphysema and a pneumothorax without marked tension. The initial treatment has often been tube thoracostomy with simple water-seal drainage. It may be some time before the diagnosis is suggested by the fact that the air leak is unusually large and persistent or that the lung has failed to expand completely even though suction has been applied. Such clues will arouse the suspicion of the alert physician and will lead to bronchoscopic confirmation of the diagnosis. Not only are the bronchoscopic findings diagnostic but they may determine the need for definitive repair. For example, if there is only a fourth to a third circumferential tear, or a tear of less than one inch, tracheostomy alone may be tried since the majority of such tears will heal without stenosis. On the other hand, all large or irregular incomplete tears and all complete tears should be repaired.

Repair. If repair is indicated it should be done as early as feasible. Recent years have witnessed an increasing realization of this goal. Previously, most of the operations for tracheobronchial rupture followed the development of bronchial stenosis. Pulmonary resection was usually carried out, but this is now reserved for irreversible parenchymal damage secondary to infection. It has been shown that in the absence of superimposed infection, significant function may be restored by reanastomosing a lung that has been totally collapsed for years.[45] However, such remarkable instances of late functional restoration are exceptional and, in most cases, one can expect a progressive loss of recoverable function beginning between 2 and 6 months after bronchial occlusion. Fortunately, total bronchial occlusion almost never results in bronchiectasis or serious parenchymal infection. These complications are usually seen as a result of the incomplete obstruction that develops after a partial bronchial tear.

Immediately following injury, primary anastomosis can usually be accomplished after simple debridement of the edges of the tear. The exposure may be difficult on the left side because of the aortic arch. Except for smaller air leaks that can be controlled by intermittent finger pressure, it is preferable to have the anesthetist use a Carlens catheter (a bifid endotracheal tube with separate lumina for each stem bronchus) or advance an endotracheal tube into the opposite bronchus. Cardiopulmonary bypass has also been used to allow reconstruction of extensive tears. Delayed repair is technically more difficult because of inflammatory or scirrhous reaction in the surrounding tissues. These operative difficulties have prompted some to recommend dilatation for late bronchial stenosis, but this is rarely successful except for mild strictures. Resection of the stricture and reanastomosis is preferable to bronchoplastic techniques whenever possible. The latter are more applicable for the long, postinflammatory strictures for which they were originally devised.

Airway Obstruction

Patency of the airway and adequacy of the respiratory exchange should be among the first considerations in the evaluation and management of the injured patient. The stridor of laryngeal obstruction or the noisy rhonchi emanating from a trachea filled with retained secretions or blood demand immediate attention. More commonly, however, the airway obstruction asso-

ciated with chest injuries is subtle in presentation. It may be completely absent on initial examination and vary in degree from moment to moment. The cause is often extrathoracic. Head injuries frequently accompany thoracic trauma, particularly when automobile collisions are involved. Depression of the state of consciousness from this, the effects of alcohol or indiscriminately administered narcotics are three common factors contributing to airway obstruction.

As noted, the adequacy of the ventilatory exchange can be grossly assessed by placing one's ear close to the patient's face and, at the same time, watching the respiratory movements of the thorax. By this maneuver one can evaluate not only the ventilatory exchange but the effort used to produce it. Initially, the patient may be able to compensate for minor degrees of obstruction with extra effort. Later, exhaustion, depression in the state of consciousness or accumulating tracheobronchial secretions may tip the scales against the patient.

Treatment. When the obstruction is positional, secondary to the relaxation of the muscular support of the tongue and mandible, manual repositioning of these structures will relieve the obstruction temporarily. This gain should be consolidated by an oropharyngeal airway or even an endotracheal tube. Because of improvements in design and fabrication, these may be left in for several days, beyond which time tracheostomy is indicated. Ordinarily, however, tracheostomy should wait until other serious injuries have been dealt with and the patient's condition has stabilized.

In the conscious patient, on the other hand, airway obstruction usually develops because of retained secretions and blood. This is particularly true of patients with multiple rib fractures, flail chest or contusion pneumonitis, although it may be seen in any patient with chest trauma in whom pain is not properly controlled. There will often be a variable period of delay before this problem becomes manifest, a period during which its appearance may be prevented by control of pain by intercostal block, restoration of the integrity of the thorax, evacuation of the pleural space or attention to nasotracheal toilet. In severe cases, even these measures may not suffice and one must resort to tracheostomy.

Obviously, the methods used to maintain

the airway free of blood and tracheobronchial secretions must be chosen to fit the individual case. A brief description of some of the techniques recommended earlier in the discussion is included here. Others will be found in Chapters 2, 5 and 12.

NASOTRACHEAL SUCTION. This maneuver, introduced by Haight in 1942, is a valuable means of providing adequate pulmonary toilet after thoracic trauma. The technique can be easily learned. If possible, the patient is seated in an upright position. He is instructed to project the mandible forward and protrude the tongue. The latter is grasped with a gauze sponge and drawn gently forward. A sterile No. 14 to 18 French catheter is introduced into the posterior oropharynx through a nostril so that its tip lies pointed above the glottis. The depth of insertion can be guided initially by watching its passage down from the nasopharynx through the open mouth. Its arrival over the glottis is signaled by a "nearness" of the breath sounds heard through the proximal end of the tube. Once the catheter is in this position, the patient is induced to take a deep breath, at which moment the tube is quickly advanced through the open glottis. Even uncooperative patients will open the glottis after a cough or breath holding.

The successful introduction of the catheter into the trachea will result in vigorous coughing unless the patient has a depressed cough reflex. In such cases, the patient's inability to phonate or the forceful jet of air coming through the end of the nasotracheal catheter with each expiration will serve as a clue. At this point, the catheter is connected to a suction source by a Y-connector and intermittent tracheal aspiration is carried out with *brief* periods of suction, lasting no longer than 10 seconds or the length of time this patient can hold his breath. More prolonged suctioning is contraindicated because much of the inspired air is being removed. Even when passage of the nasotracheal tube is not successful, the paroxysms of cough resulting from the attempts partly achieve the desired goal. This procedure may have to be repeated at 4- to 6-hour intervals. If much more frequent tracheal aspiration is indicated, a tracheostomy is usually warranted.

TRACHEOSTOMY. The technique and care of a tracheostomy are described else-where in this book (Chapter 12). The following comments are directed toward its role in the treatment of thoracic trauma. For more than a century after Trousseau reported its use in 200 diphtheritic children in 1833, tracheostomy was employed only to relieve airway obstruction. In 1943 Galloway suggested its use in aspirating the tracheobronchial tree, and considerable experience with its use for this indication was obtained during poliomyelitis epidemics, particularly in Scandinavia in 1952 and 1953. At about this time, its potential in the treatment of chest injuries, particularly crushed chest, became more fully appreciated following reports of Carter and Giuseffi.[16] The progressive wave of enthusiasm that followed has only recently been tempered. Unfortunately, the procedure has become a "prophylactic" or "routine" measure in the hands of many. It was often said that "the time to do a tracheostomy is when you first think about it." However, the need for following strict indications can be appreciated if one considers the risk this procedure carries in terms of serious complications.[39] Furthermore, this risk is trebled when tracheostomy is performed as an emergency procedure under suboptimal conditions. This is not to deny the value of this important resuscitative procedure but rather to stress the need for indications based on attainable objectives.

Mechanical obstruction to the upper air passage is an unchallenged indication and is one of the few indications for emergency tracheostomy. Fortunately, injuries resulting in true mechanical obstruction to the air passage proximal to the cervical trachea are not frequent. They are discussed in the chapter on neck injuries.[11] More often, it is the associated bleeding from such injuries that prompts tracheostomy.

As previously mentioned, position obstruction secondary to central nervous system depression is common, but this can be initially treated by insertion of an oropharyngeal airway or endotracheal tube, with tracheostomy performed later when the patient's condition has stabilized and the long-term need for tracheal intubation has been established.

Another relative indication for tracheostomy is the accumulation of tracheobronchial secretions. Maloney and MacDonald[46] have cautioned that most of the secretions removed from an established tracheostomy are aspirated saliva since it is known that some degree of laryngeal incompetence frequently follows tracheostomy. However, there remains a definite role for tracheostomy when simpler measures have failed to remove retained tracheobronchial secretions and blood.

It has been suggested that tracheostomy reduces dead space and resistance to air flow and in this way decreases the work of breathing. Indeed, the respiratory dead space can be reduced by tracheostomy although not by so much as once thought. Estimates based on anatomic studies assume that all the respiratory exchange passes through the tracheostomy cannula, an assumption that is valid only if cuffed tubes are used. The reduction in dead space that can be expected is therefore closer to one third than the two thirds formerly predicted. It should also be pointed out that resistance to airflow is reduced only when large-diameter tracheostomy cannulae are used. It has been shown by Garzon et al.[29] that the work of breathing through a No. 7 or 8 cuffed tracheostomy tube is equal to that of mouth breathing. Only when a No. 9 or 10 tube is used can a significant reduction in resistance be expected. Thus, whenever relief of the work of breathing is the major goal, a respirator should usually also be employed.

By the same token, if one wishes to reduce the paradoxical movement of a flail chest by tracheostomy, it is necessary to use a large cannula placed low in the cervical trachea. This allows air to be exchanged at relatively lower pressure differentials and, in some cases, reduces the paradoxical movements of the flail segment enough so that use of a respirator is not necessary. However, need for prolonged artificial ventilatory support is the major indication for tracheostomy in this case.

With these qualifications, tracheostomy remains one of the most valuable resuscitative procedures available to the physician treating chest injuries. The indications for its use are summarized as follows:

1. True mechanical obstruction of the upper air passages.

2. Positional airway obstruction secondary to central nervous system depression, if prolonged for several days.

3. Retention of tracheobronchial secretions and blood that *cannot* be controlled by simpler methods.

4. Use of a respirator.

5. Rarely, massive or progressive cervical subcutaneous emphysema.

6. Minor tears of the tracheobronchial tree (less than 1 cm. or one third of the circumference).

7. Flail chest (use with or without a respirator).

8. Traumatic tracheoesophageal fistulas.

THE ESOPHAGUS

This section will deal with injuries to the thoracic esophagus. Injuries to the cervical esophagus are discussed in Chapter 11, and since caustic burns of and foreign bodies in the esophagus are primarily encountered in children, these are dealt with in Chapter 24. All other significant forms of esophageal injury involve disruption of its wall by one mechanism or another. The esophagus may be perforated from within by instrumentation or a swallowed foreign body, penetrated from without by a bullet or other missile or ruptured by blunt trauma to the abdomen or chest. Except for missile perforation, which may occur anywhere, these different mechanisms have characteristic sites of predilection. Perforation from instruments (esophagoscope, dilator or biopsy forceps) or by ingested foreign bodies almost invariably occurs at the site of esophageal narrowing, either at the three natural points of constriction (the pharyngoesophageal junction, the level of the aortic arch and the cardia) or at the site of an inflammatory or neoplastic stricture. The esophagus usually ruptures from blunt trauma at the same site in the lower third of the esophagus above the cardia at which "spontaneous," or postemetic, ruptures occur. The relative weakness of this area has been clearly demonstrated by MacKenzie[42] and Mackler.[44] Rupture following a blast injury frequently occurs at this point too.

Diagnosis. Although these various mechanisms all result in disruption of the esophageal wall, the clinical picture may be quite variable, depending on the site of rupture and the degree of contamination. At one extreme is the relatively benign course that follows instrumental perforation at the pharyngoesophageal junction when it is immediately recognized and the patient given nothing by mouth. At the other is the fulminant and often fatal condition that results when the gastric contents are ejected up through a tear in the wall of the lower esophagus. In the former, discomfort may be minimal and noticed only with swallowing; with the latter, pain may be so excruciating that a coronary occlusion or some intra-abdominal catastrophe is suspected.

Mediastinitis, of course, is common after perforation of the thoracic esophagus. It characteristically occurs after internal perforations that do not violate the pleura. The dissection of air throughout the mediastinum may be detected on physical examination, if a "mediastinal crunch" is heard on auscultation, or if it reaches the neck so that the subcutaneous emphysema in the suprasternal area is noticed. The diagnosis may be confirmed, or even first suggested, by chest x-ray if stippling of the mediastinum with air is visible. Widening of the mediastinum is a late sign, and its absence should not delay the diagnosis.

Larger perforations, missile injuries and rupture of the thoracic esophagus secondary to blunt or blast injury are usually associated with a pneumothorax. Depending on the degree of contamination of the pleural space, there will be a variable amount of reactive pleural effusion. When gastric contents have been ejected into the esophagus and out through the tear, the pleural space may contain more fluid than air. The fluid losses resulting from such contamination of the mediastinum and pleural space may be massive.[73]

Patients with esophageal rupture secondary to blunt or penetrating trauma may be thought at first to have a simple pneumothorax or hemopneumothorax. However, once a chest tube is inserted the diagnosis should become obvious from the appearance of the drainage. The diagnosis should also be considered whenever there is a pneumothorax with a persistent air leak. Dyspnea, cyanosis and shock are common in severe cases but are late signs. Hematemesis is a helpful but inconstant sign.

It is important to establish the diagnosis as early as possible. If esophageal rupture is even remotely possible, the patient should be made to swallow an absorbable contrast medium (not barium) and x-rays should be taken. This study is desirable even if the diagnosis is obvious, since it is important in planning the operative approach to know the site of the tear and whether it communicates with one or both pleural spaces. However, this examination should not delay or take precedence over vigorous resuscitative efforts.

Treatment. Common to the treatment of all esophageal tears should be vigorous intravenous fluid administration, massive doses of antibiotics and restriction of oral intake. These are the mainstays of nonoperative treatment, an approach that should be limited to *selected* cases of cervical esophageal perforation. In most instances, these measures are intended only as support for definitive surgical intervention. In addition to these measures, the pleural space should be drained as early as possible by closed tube thoracostomy.

The earlier the exploration, the better the result. Operation should not be delayed indefinitely while awaiting optimal response to supportive measures. As soon as a reasonable initial response has been obtained, the patient should be explored with these supportive measures vigorously continued during surgery. The central venous pressure is a valuable means of determining the rate at which intravenous therapy should be administered. The work of Ware and Strieder,[70] showing no improvement in survival of animals given antibiotics and intravenous fluids alone, gave further impetus to the policy of early operative intervention. Also, early exploration allows definitive repair to be carried out before inflammatory changes in the tissues at the site of the tear have occurred. It should be emphasized, therefore, that severe debilitation, shock and moribund appearance are not contraindications to surgery, but indications for more aggressive supportive care before and during operation. Even in delayed cases in which primary closure of the tear cannot be expected to succeed, operative drainage of the site of rupture can be life-savings.

The operative approach will be determined by the site of rupture. Generally, upper third perforations should be explored through the neck; middle third, through the right chest; and lower third, through a left thoracotomy. If possible, repair should be performed in two layers. A drainage tube should be placed with its tip *near but not on* the suture line and the pleura left open to avoid mediastinitis and abscess formation should the repair not hold.

If the tissues will not hold sutures, as may be the case if there has been considerable delay, one may have to rely on this drainage tube alone, accepting the fistula that will develop. If repair is possible, drainage of the suture line should be continued until it has been tested first by esophagogram and then by oral feedings. Concomitant gastrostomy used to be performed routinely to allow management of the patient during this period; the success of intravenous hyperalimentation regimens has made this no longer mandatory. Esophageal stricture not infrequently follows a difficult repair, particularly if a fistula forms. Unless a pseudo-diverticulum develops with luminal distortion, these can usually be managed by dilations.

Results. The outcome of esophageal rupture depends upon the mechanism of injury, the site of perforation, the degree of contamination and the delay in treatment. Instrumental perforations carry the best prognosis and rupture secondary to blunt trauma the worst. The high mortality (80 per cent) in the latter situation is mainly the result of failure to make the diagnosis, which was not suspected until autopsy in two thirds of the recorded cases.[74] That better results can be obtained is reflected by the statistics for post-emetic rupture. Prior to 1951, only 13 of 100 reported patients had survived. However, the prognosis has steadily improved since then and in several recent series this mortality rate has almost reversed. This improvement stems as much from early diagnosis and operative repair as from a more aggressive supportive therapy.

Post-traumatic Tracheoesophageal Fistula

As a consequence of blunt chest trauma, this condition stands somewhere between esophageal and tracheobronchial rupture, both in incidence and development. It most commonly occurs after automobile or auto pedestrian accidents and rarely occurs in association with externally penetrating injuries. Up to 1965, 98 cases had appeared in the literature since Vinson's first report in 1836.[2] Like tracheobronchial rupture it is located near the carina, and the same mech-

anism is thought to be involved in the development of both conditions, with a fistula resulting when the adjacent esophagus is also damaged. Because of the late presentation of the majority of cases, it has been suggested that an abscess develops at the site of tracheal rupture and that this later breaks through the weakened esophageal wall.

Diagnosis. The initial symptoms are similar to those following a small localized bronchial or esophageal tear with localized mediastinitis. Later, the patient develops a paroxysmal cough aggravated by feeding. This pathognomonic feature should suggest the diagnosis, although it may be attributed erroneously to a degree of laryngeal incompetence associated with tracheostomy that has been performed. Confirmation may be obtained by an esophageal swallow using contrast material suitable for bronchography.

Treatment. The timing of the repair will be dictated largely by the patient's condition at the time of diagnosis. Although definitive repair would be preferable, delay in development or diagnosis usually prevents this, and commonly several months intervene between injury and definitive surgery. Once operation has been delayed, it is better to wait for local inflammatory changes to subside. During this period tracheostomy and feeding gastrostomy or intravenous hyperalimentation are used to avoid further complications. The dissection is frequently difficult, particularly in delayed cases. Small fistulas may be ligated and divided. Moderate-sized fistulas should be excised and the ends inverted. Excision of larger fistulas may result in defects of such magnitude that other tissues must be employed to bridge the gap. In such situations, the bronchoplastic techniques developed for postinflammatory strictures and the vascularized pericardial flap may be useful adjuncts.

Results. The mortality associated with post-traumatic tracheoesophageal fistulas is much less than that with esophageal or bronchial rupture alone. Survival rates range between 70 and 85 per cent. This may be because the very nature of a fistula implies that the injury has been confined by surrounding tissues and that it develops relatively late when survival from other injuries has already been achieved.

THE DIAPHRAGM

The integrity of the diaphragm may be violated by either penetrating or nonpenetrating injury. Recent experiences[75] suggest that the incidence of diaphragmatic injuries has steadily increased since World War II, mainly as a result of the increase in automobile accidents. Today the majority of diaphragmatic disruptions are caused by blunt trauma rather than penetrating injuries. Automobile accidents are responsible for over 80 per cent of tears following blunt trauma, with falls from great heights and crushing injuries providing most of the remainder. Penetrating wounds, of course, are usually the result of a stabbing or shooting.

Blunt trauma results in larger diaphragmatic tears, a higher incidence of acute herniation, less external evidence of trauma and, because of the common association with other serious injuries, a higher mortality rate than are seen with penetrating wounds. The latter usually result in small defects that either are discovered early during exploration for other indications or present later with intestinal obstruction from an incarcerated or strangulated diaphragmatic hernia. Occasionally, the condition may be discovered on coincidental chest x-rays or when interval complaints of dyspepsia, discomfort in the left chest or shoulders, flatulence or postprandial fullness are being investigated.

Regardless of the type of injury, there is an overwhelming left-sided predominance in clinically manifest diaphragmatic tears, often as high as 90 per cent. This can be explained by the buttressing of the right diaphragm by the liver, the predominance of right-handed assailants, and the left-sided position of the usual intended target, the heart. Penetrating injuries may involve any area of the diaphragm, although knife wounds are characteristically anterolateral. Blunt trauma most commonly ruptures the diaphragm at the junction between the tendinous and posterior leaves, a weak point related to the fusion of two of the diaphragm's embryonic components. These tears are usually radial. They may extend to, but rarely through, the hiatus or may even involve the pericardium. Occasionally, the diaphragm will tear loose from its peripheral attachments. Distortion of the diaphragm by the changes in gravitational force that accompany decelerating accidents can be appreciated from inspection of Figure 13–1B and D.

Larger tears usually result in acute herniation of the abdominal viscera into the chest. The stomach, spleen, left colon, small bowel and the left lobe of the liver may pass through the defect. Herniation of the liver through the right leaf of the diaphragm is rare but can occur with the large tears associated with blunt trauma. Progressive herniation through the larger defects may be encouraged by the increased pleuroperitoneal pressure differential caused by labored respirations. A progression of events similar to those occurring in patients with congenital diaphragmatic hernia may eventually lead to almost total collapse of one lung and infringement on the other as mediastinal displacement occurs.

Diagnosis. If acute herniation has occurred, the earliest complaints are usually shortness of breath and left chest pain that may be referred to the shoulder. With small hernias the physical examination may reveal nothing abnormal or, at most, a small area of dullness and diminished breath sounds with limited excursion of the diaphragm. In the acutely injured patient, these signs are hard to elicit and even harder to interpret, particularly since the respirations on that side are usually splinted and some degree of hemothorax is commonly associated. One cannot expect the classic combination of diminished breath sounds and audible peristalsis over the lower hemithorax that greets the physician who examines such a patient in the interval following recovery.

With larger degrees of herniation, the examiner may be perplexed by a strange mixture of areas of dullness and tympany on percussing the chest. Peristalsis is usually suppressed initially, so that chances of auscultating bowel sounds over the thorax are slight. A shift of the mediastinal structures to the opposite side may occur with larger hernias, but by this time respiratory distress, cyanosis and even shock may have entered the picture and the finer points of physical diagnosis have to be abandoned.

The diagnosis usually rests on proper interpretation of the chest x-ray. An associated hemothorax not uncommonly obscures both the physical and radiological signs of herniated viscera, a good reason for repeating chest films after evacuating a hemothorax. The diagnosis should be suspected whenever the left diaphragm is high following injury to the chest or abdomen, or when radiolucent areas appear above the usual level of the diaphragm. Common misdiagnoses are "loculated pneumothorax in the lower chest due to pleural adhesions" or "elevation of the diaphragm secondary to acute gastric dilatation." Passage of a nasogastric tube at this time may provide an important clue. If the stomach has herniated into the chest, distortion of the cardia may impede passage of the tube or, if it can be passed, it may be seen to deflect upward into the thorax. Upright films taken after induced pneumoperitoneum may result in the collection of air in the thorax. Finally, contrast studies with barium in the stomach or the colon may be attempted if the patient's condition permits. Before one diagnoses traumatic herniation of the liver into the right chest on the basis of a high diaphragm, one should take lateral decubitus films to rule out the subpulmonary entrapment of a hemothorax. A further clue here is elevation of the x-ray shadow of the inferior border of the liver.

The small diaphragmatic tears resulting from penetrating injuries can result in acute herniation, but they are just as likely to be discovered incidentally during exploration for other indications. One might expect all such injuries to be discovered early because of the common policy of exploring all penetrating wounds entering below the level of the nipple. However, small diaphragmatic wounds may be overlooked during exploration. Furthermore, the possibility of penetration of the diaphragm may not be entertained unless the physician is aware of the height to which the diaphragm may rise in the crouching or straining patient. Thus, the penetrating chest wound may be thought to involve only the thorax, and the associated pneumothorax or hemothorax may be treated simply by chest tube drainage.

Initially, only a piece of omentum may herniate through the small defect. Sometime later, even years later in many cases, a sudden increase in intra-abdominal pressure may push the abdominal viscera through the defect in the diaphragm maintained by the omentum's "toe in the door." This mechanism was responsible for the long-held belief that diaphragmatic wounds do not heal well. Since these diaphragmatic defects are usually small, delayed cases commonly present with obstruction and even strangulation of the herniated viscera. The pain associated with this delayed presentation may be severe enough to suggest coronary occlusion. X-rays at this stage should be diagnostic, but because of a remote history of injury and overlooked small scar, they are frequently misinterpreted. Common misdiagnoses include multiple lung abscesses, cystic disease of the lung, multiloculated empyema or atypical pneumothorax secondary to pleural adhesions.

Treatment. When diagnosis is made in the acute period, operative reduction of the hernia and repair of the diaphragmatic tear should be undertaken as soon as feasible. A brief delay for further evaluation of significant associated injuries is permissible if the hernia is small and is causing little or no cardiorespiratory embarrassment. In any event, an attempt should be made to decompress the stomach by nasogastric tube as soon as possible.

There is some difference of opinion as to whether a thoracic or abdominal approach should be used. Because of the significant incidence of associated injury to abdominal viscera, the abdominal route is preferred for acutely presenting diaphragmatic tears secondary to a penetrating injury. However, because of adhesions that develop between the herniated viscera and intrathoracic structures, hernias with delayed presentation should be initially explored through the chest. This approach may also be selected for hernias secondary to blunt trauma, hernias in which there is a major hemothorax or evidence of other significant intrathoracic injury, or if previous abdominal operations are expected to interfere with the abdominal approach. Regardless of the initial incision, one should not hesitate to combine the abdominal and thoracic approaches in difficult cases, and the patient should be prepared and draped for such an eventuality. The repair should employ two layers of interrupted nonabsorbable suture and the chest should be drained.

THE HEART

Penetrating Injuries of the Heart

The management of penetrating injuries of the heart has challenged the judgment and technical skill of physicians for centuries. Even at the present time, surgeons in the medical centers with the greatest experience with this type of injury are unable to agree on its management.

In most reports of penetrating wounds of the heart, emanating as they do from urban medical centers and reaching back for many years, stab wounds outnumber gunshot wounds by a ratio of 3 or 4 to 1. This not only reflects a preference for the knife or icepick rather than the gun in choice of weapons but also the fact that fewer victims shot in the heart survive to reach the hospital for treatment. Randall and Glass's[58] report in 1960 of 20 cases of cardiac gunshot wounds was the first sizeable experience with this type of injury reported from a civilian hospital.

Penetrating wounds of the heart may present in several different ways. Most commonly, the problem is one of hemopericardium with cardiac tamponade. However, if the pericardial wound communicates freely with the pleural space, exsanguinating intrathoracic hemorrhage may dominate the picture. Only rarely will traumatic hemopericardium lead to recurrent pericardial effusion or constrictive pericarditis. Penetrating wounds of the heart may occasionally result in rather selective injury to certain vulnerable parts of the heart's anatomy so that valvular or septal defects, infarction from injury to a coronary vessel or arrhythmias from damage to the conducting system may be encountered. A final point of consideration in such wounds is the problem of intracardiac foreign bodies.

Nonpenetrating Injuries to the Heart

At one time cardiac injury secondary to blunt thoracic trauma was thought exceedingly rare. This was partly because myocardial rupture, the greatest threat in such injuries, is almost invariably fatal and thus seen by the pathologist rather than the clinician. It was also due in part to the fact that cardiac contusion, the most common clinically presenting problem, was not fully appreciated until recent years when serial electrocardiograms and serum enzyme determinations were used to study chest trauma victims. Although nonpenetrating chest trauma can cause, with the exception of intracardiac foreign bodies, the same forms of injury mentioned in regard to penetrating trauma, these occur so rarely that only cardiac contusion warrants separate discussion.

In the following sections the management of cardiac wounds is discussed according to the type of problems they present clinically.

Cardiac Tamponade

In penetrating wounds of the heart, bleeding is usually significant enough to produce either cardiac tamponade or, if the penetrating agent has also produced a large enough pleuropericardial communication, massive hemothorax. Because many wounds penetrating the pericardium are located anteriorly where it is not in contact with the pleura and because, in many others, the traumatic pleuropericardial defects are not large enough to effectively vent the hemopericardium, the most common form of presentation is cardiac tamponade.

Diagnosis. With each systolic contraction, blood spurts from the myocardial laceration into the pericardial sac; and as it accumulates, it leaves less and less space for the heart to occupy in diastole. Therefore, diastolic filling and stroke volume progressively decline. Initially, cardiac output can be maintained by increasing rate, but eventually this can no longer compensate for impaired venous return and cardiac output falls. At this point there will be an elevation of venous pressure and decline in arterial pressure that, along with the muffling of heart sounds by the hemopericardium, constitute Beck's triad.[5]

Another feature of cardiac tamponade is an accentuation of the *normal* tendency for cardiac output to decrease during inspiration. This was originally observed as a weakening of the pulse during inspiration and still bears the name pulsus paradoxus. A more objective criterion is a greater than 15 mm. Hg decrease in systolic pressure during normal inspiration. The underlying mechanism is still unsettled. One theory is that, although the decreased intrathoracic pressure during inspiration normally enhances venous return and compensates for concomitant expansion of the pulmonary vascular bed, this is prevented because tamponade impedes venous return. Another explanation is that tensing of the pericardium by diaphragmatic descent during inspiration increases the tamponading effect of the hemopericardium.

It might seem that the diagnosis of cardiac tamponade would be a simple matter of finding Beck's triad or pulsus paradoxus in a patient with a penetrating chest injury. However, as previously pointed out, hypotension is common to many forms of injury. The loudness of heart sounds may be difficult to assess in a noisy emergency department. Bulging neck veins may be absent if much blood has been lost, although they may occur, in the absence of tamponade, in a straining patient or in a patient with tension pneumothorax or compression of the superior vena cava by hemorrhage into the mediastinum. A *left* tension pneumothorax may superficially mimic cardiac tamponade by producing hypotension and bulging neck veins and is responsible for the inability to hear heart sounds clearly when listening over the precordium. Finally, Beck's triad is absent in one third to one half of patients with traumatic hemopericardium when they first arrive in the emergency department.

If one considers the problem as that of a patient presenting with shock *without* significant ventilatory impairment after chest trauma, the diagnosis usually rests between exsanguinating hemorrhage and pericardial tamponade. If the differentiation is not readily apparent, a central venous catheter should be advanced into the superior vena cava through the external jugular or subclavian vein. (See Chapter 4.) If the central venous pressure is low, cardiac tamponade is unlikely and one can then use this catheter as a central channel for vigorous blood volume expansion. If it is high or soon becomes elevated in response to intravenous infusion, the diagnosis of cardiac tamponade is virtually assured. The importance of serial determination of the central venous pressure in such a situation has been emphasized by two studies,[55, 76] which showed that one third of patients

developing tamponade after penetrating injury to the heart did not have a significant elevation of the venous pressure on the initial determination, but elevation occurred later when blood volume had been restored.

One of these reports also noted that pulsus paradoxus was detected in only one third of the cases. This is because pulsus paradoxus represents a transient stage early in the development of acute tamponade and has usually disappeared by the time severe shock has developed. However, it is a valuable warning sign of the redevelopment of tamponade after pericardiocentesis.

X-RAY. Several authors have referred to the diagnostic significance of enlargement of the cardiac silhouette on chest x-ray. However, as Doubleday[22] has pointed out, patients can succumb with as little as 200 ml. of blood in the pericardium, yet 300 or more ml. can be present without a detectable increase in the cardiac silhouette. In addition, one rarely has a chest x-ray adequate enough to be sure of increased heart size without previous films for comparison. Some success has been reported using fluoroscopy to detect diminished pulsations of the cardiac silhouette, but this finding may be equivocal and lack of time and facilities limits this approach.

Treatment. There is little disagreement regarding the indication for immediate pericardiocentesis once the diagnosis of cardiac tamponade is made or even, in more desperate situations, strongly suspected. Sudden and dramatic relief may follow the removal of even 30 ml. of blood although as much blood should be aspirated as possible. The technique of pericardiocentesis is described later.

It is important to be sure that the blood obtained by this maneuver has been aspirated from the pericardium and has not been obtained by puncture of the heart through an empty pericardial space. Several considerations will help in making this distinction. First, blood aspirated from the pericardium should not clot in the syringe, having been defibrinated within the pericardial sac by the motion of the heart. Second, the removal of blood should be rewarded by hemodynamic improvement on the part of the patient. On the other hand, if the heart has been entered, pulsations transmitted to the needle and syringe will usually be felt and, since patients in the acute stages of shock become hypercoagulable, the blood obtained should rapidly clot in the syringe, particularly in a glass syringe.

It is at the point at which the immediate threat of pericardial tamponade has been relieved by aspiration that a divergence of opinion concerning management exists. The history of the treatment of cardiac tamponade is interesting in this respect. In 1649 Riolanus first suggested the use of pericardiocentesis in the treatment of cardiac tamponade. The first successful outcome of such treatment was reported in 1829 by Larrey. However, in 1868 Fischer,[27] in a collective review of 425 cases, reported an 84 per cent mortality following use of pericardiocentesis and its popularity waned. It was not fully appreciated, however, that in most cases pericardiocentesis had been used in combination with venesection. Following Del Vecchio's experimental work in 1895, Rehn reported the first successful control of a bleeding heart wound by cardiorrhaphy. There followed a period of popularity for the direct surgical control of penetrating heart wounds. Not until the classic paper of Blalock and Ravitch[8] in 1943 reporting survival in 17 of 18 patients in whom pericardiocentesis was used did this approach become popular again.

In review of the experience at The Johns Hopkins Hospital by Isaacs[38] in 1960, 40 of the 60 patients reported were treated by a pericardiocentesis alone, with only 1 death. In the remaining 20 there was a 50 per cent mortality from surgery regardless of the employment of preliminary pericardiocentesis. This experience has been shared by some institutions[18, 25] but not others[11, 49] so that a divergence of opinion still exists between those recommending immediate operative intervention in *all* such patients and those who believe that the percentage of patients whose condition can be controlled by pericardiocentesis alone is significant enough to justify the attempt. This difference of opinion is in part related to the wounding agent predominating in the experience reported, since stab wounds of the heart are more likely to be manageable by pericardiocentesis than gunshot wounds.

Adopting a position at either extreme seems unwise. Experience indicates that certain patients are not likely to be successfully managed by pericardiocentesis alone. These are patients who are also bleeding into the chest through a pleural-pericardial laceration, patients with cardiac wounds from large knives or large-caliber bullets, and patients with a partially clotted hemopericardium that yields only a small volume on aspiration so that continued bleeding will quickly lead to tamponade again. In such patients, or in any patient whose response to pericardiocentesis is weak or evanescent, immediate surgical intervention is indicated. A practical approach is to take all patients with traumatic hemopericardium to the operating room after the tamponade has been relieved by pericardiocentesis. During transit and preparation for thoracotomy, the pericardiocentesis needle, clamped flush to the skin at the proper depth of penetration, should be left in place. By the time the scrub nurse and anesthetist have completed their preparations, enough time will have elapsed to have selected out those patients with self-sealing stab wounds that can be managed by pericardiocentesis alone. An additional delay *in* the operating room while close monitoring continues will provide assurance that these patients can be safely transferred to an intensive care unit. One should proceed with thoracotomy in patients with gunshot wounds or those with stab wounds who are hemodynamically unstable at this point.

Repeated pericardiocentesis may be required, and the rate of redevelopment of tamponade will soon determine if persistence with the nonoperative approach is justified. Although it has been argued that the mortality from unnecessary thoracotomy will be less than that from pericardiocentesis failures, it remains our impression that most deaths from penetrating heart wounds occur *in spite* of thoracotomy rather than *because* of attempts at pericardiocentesis and that both an unselected policy of routine thoracotomy and overpersistence with pericardiocentesis represent weakness in surgical judgment.

TECHNIQUE OF PERICARDIOCENTESIS. A long large-bore needle (16 to 18 gauge) is attached to a 50 ml. syringe via a three-way stopcock. The needle is passed either to the left of the sternum in the fourth interspace or at a 45-degree angle inward and upward from a point just lateral to the xyphoid (Fig. 13–13). If time permits, as it often does with subsequent aspirations, a precordial electrocardiogram lead will signal contact with the heart and warn of overpenetration. Attaching the lead to the needle itself creates an electrical hazard that may manifest itself by ventricular fibrillation. A "popping" sensation will often be noted as the pericardium is penetrated and the withdrawal of nonclotting blood associated with the relief of the patient's distress will mark the successful pericardiocentesis. The needle should be withdrawn until aspiration stops and then reintroduced slowly until blood returns in the syringe. The proper depth of penetration can be maintained by placing a clamp on the needle flush with the skin. This prevents inadvertent overpenetration and provides a reference for future aspiration.

THORACOTOMY FOR PENETRATING CARDIAC WOUNDS. Ordinarily, an anterior thoracotomy in the left fourth intercostal space will provide adequate exposure. This can be extended across the sternum with ligation of the internal mammary vessels if more exposure is needed. Division of the costal cartilages near their insertion into the sternum can be used to gain room in a cephalic or caudal direction. A sternal splitting incision provides even better exposure but is usually more time-consuming.

The opening of pericardium is usually followed by gushing of blood at a more rapid rate than anticipated as the countereffect of tamponade is broken and the cardiac wound bleeds unopposed. It was because of the difficulty of controlling bleeding from a writhing heart in a gushing pool of blood that Sauerbruch[63] first suggested gripping the heart with the fingers in the transverse sinus. Ordinarily, however, "Sauerbruch's grip" is not necessary. Bleeding can be controlled by finger pressure while 2-0 absorbable sutures are passed deeply through the myocardium in the underlying wound. By crossing and applying gentle traction to these sutures the bleeding usually can be controlled well enough to visualize their placement and to assure that no major coronary artery will be occluded if they are tied. However, even if the initial sutures are poorly placed they provide traction and hemostasis until de-

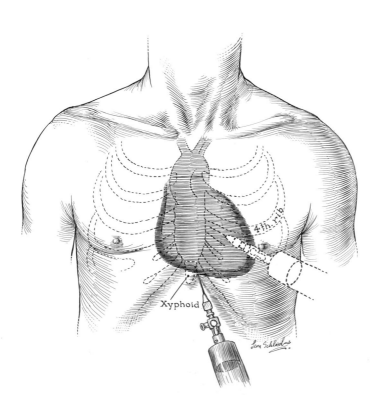

Figure 13–13. The technique of pericardiocentesis as described in the text.

finitive sutures are placed and tied. After satisfactory hemostasis is established, the pericardium is loosely reapproximated with interrupted sutures to allow free drainage of the pericardial space. The thoracotomy is then closed in layers after placement of a dependent or posterolateral thoracotomy drainage tube. The use of prophylactic antibiotics is indicated in this situation.

Myocardial Contusion

This condition should be considered in any patient who has received a severe blow to the chest, particularly a steering wheel injury. Estimates of its frequency have risen steadily with the more frequent use of the electrocardiogram and serum enzyme determinations in evaluating patients with such a history. At least 10 per cent of patients with a steering wheel injury will be found to have some evidence of myocardial contusion. The patient complaining of precordial discomfort after blunt trauma to the thorax may be thought to have a contusion of the chest wall, costochondral separation, or nondisplaced fracture of the anterior ribs or sternum. Patients whose pain arises from such chest wall injuries usually complain of aggravation or discomfort from breathing; the discomfort from myocardial contusion is more independent of respiratory movements. However, this differentiation is frequently complicated by the coexistence of such chest wall injuries. It is a reasonable approach to assume that any blow sufficient to have so injured the chest wall may also have resulted in myocardial contusion and to take steps to investigate this possibility.

Many of the signs and symptoms of myocardial contusion are similar to those of pericarditis with or without an effusion because such patients have a focal area of pericardial irritation. If there has been some bleeding from the contused pericardium, a secondary effusion may result. The electrocardiogram may show T-wave inversion or, in some instances, QRS changes or conduction disturbances. In older patients it may be hard to decide whether there has been a myocardial infarction precipitated by the stress of the accident or a myocardial contusion secondary to the chest trauma. This may not have immediate therapeutic significance since the initial treatment is similar, but from a prognostic and medical-legal standpoint, the differentiation may be quite important. The evolution of a classic infarction pattern on serial electrocardiograms or its failure to appear will usually settle this issue, but it should be remembered that a coronary artery can be damaged by a severe blow to the precordium, and that a severely contused area of myocardium may be virtually indistinguishable from the damage caused by regional coronary occlusion. Generally, however, the myocardial contusion produces milder, more variable electrocardiogram changes that do not fit the distribution patterns classically ascribed to occlusion of the coronary branches.

A myocardial contusion may be missed if serial electrocardiograms and enzyme studies are not done. An elevation of the serum glutamic oxalacetic transaminase (SGOT), creatinine phosphokinase (CPK), or lactic acid dehydrogenase (LDH) may confirm the suspicion of myocardial contusion in cases in which the electrocardiogram shows only fleeting or variable changes. These studies are also helpful in older patients when one does not know whether the EKG abnormalities existed prior to injury. Initial attempts with radionuclide imaging of the myocardium to identify an area of contusion were disappointing, but improvements in technique directed toward the diagnosis of coronary artery occlusive disease may change this assessment. The problem of ready availability to the emergency department may pose a greater limitation.

The outcome of a myocardial contusion depends to a large extent upon its severity and the association of conduction disturbances that may, as in the case of coronary occlusion, lead to fatal arrhythmias. The damage is rarely extensive enough to lead to delayed rupture or ventricular aneurysm, although isolated cases of this have been reported. When rupture does occur it usually results in immediate fatality and, as shown by Parmley and associates' review of the records from the Armed Forces Institute of Pathology,[53] this is the major cause of death from nonpenetrating injury to the heart. Although cardiogenic shock is rarely a problem after myocardial contusion, Pomerantz[57] has shown that acute reductions in cardiac output are not uncommon with this injury. However, it should be kept in mind that the use of anesthetic agents that depress myocardial contractility could make this problem clinically manifest during the operative management of other injuries.

Treatment. The treatment of patients with myocardial contusion consists of restricted activity and continued observation. Patients with arrhythmias should be carefully monitored. Digitalis and antiarrhythmic drugs are given for the usual indications. The patient can be discharged after stabilization of the electrocardiogram and subsidence of symptoms, although restricted activity for a full 6 weeks is usually advisable.

Rarer Cardiac Injuries

Although the following cardiac injuries are encountered too infrequently to warrant detailed discussion, one must be aware of such possibilities. Valvular insufficiency may result from a ruptured cusp (usually aortic) or a torn attachment to a papillary muscle (usually mitral). Atrial or ventricular septal defects may be caused by penetrating wounds and, occasionally, the membranous ventricular septum may be torn after severe blunt trauma. Severe damage to the myocardium may result in ventricular aneurysm, but this is much less likely than myocardial rupture. Hemorrhage into the area of the major conduction pathways is seen in cases of severe hypoxia and shock but also has been reported after blunt trauma. The indications for surgical intervention follow those for similar conditions of a nontraumatic origin, with the exception that the hemodynamic derangements resulting from acute traumatic defects are often not so well tolerated as those acquired more gradually or those that develop under the protection of the maternal circulation.

Foreign Bodies in the Heart

The management of missiles in the heart is a controversial subject that has been fanned by the flames of each of the great wars of this century. In World War I the bolder surgeons favored their removal. Delormé in France cited 13 operations (with

three deaths), including the successful removement of fragments from the right ventricle. In 1918 LeFort reported the first successful removal of a missile from the left ventricle and recorded nine consecutive cardiotomies for removal of foreign bodies with only one death. By the advent of World War II, however, opinion was still divided. Decker reported that the mortality from expectant and from operative treatment were both about 20 per cent but suggested that many more unsuccessful surgical attempts had probably escaped publication. In 1914 Sauerbruch in Germany advised removal of all foreign bodies from the heart to forestall later complications and reported 105 cases, with an operative mortality of 8 per cent. At the same time, in England, Turner still cautioned that "it would seem a good rule to leave the foreign body alone unless the heart continues to rebel against its presence."

American opinions on this subject were expressed by Harken[33] and Swal et al.,[66] who noted that recurrent pericardial effusion and infection were the usual indications for surgical removal. Since that time the development of bolder cardiac operations has been fostered by the use of hypothermia and extracorporeal bypass. This has allowed a more confident approach to the intracardiac missile. However, the consensus still opposes searching for small, scattered foreign bodies that are causing no symptoms.

Bland and Beebe[9] recently reported an enlightening 20-year follow-up of 40 patients with missiles left in the heart after injury sustained in World War II. They noted that pericarditis was a common accompaniment and that an effusion of considerable degree (sometimes delayed) occurred in 25 per cent. Elective removal was later attempted in eight of these 40 patients. It was successful in only three and was abandoned in five, in two of whom the foreign body could not be found. In one the shell fragment lodged first in the left pulmonary artery, and later migrated into the right pulmonary artery where it eroded into and obstructed the bronchus. Although benign clinical courses have been recorded in the remainder of the cases, the psychic strain of living with a missile in the heart has been formidable. All these veterans are generally concerned about the threat of this condition, and five were totally incapacitated by an anxiety neurosis. This experience also suggested that once the foreign body is fixed in the myocardium, subsequent migration was unlikely; erosion or infection was not encountered during the 20-year follow-up period.

Considering these facts and the availability of advanced techniques in open-heart surgery, the following approach is recommended. Barring other complications of the injury that have therapeutic precedence, all missiles of reasonable size in the heart should be carefully localized by fluoroscopic examination. If movement of the missile suggests that it is free in one of the chambers of the heart, immediate plans for its removal by open cardiotomy using cardiopulmonary bypass should be made. At operation these patients should be placed on a table with an x-ray cassette under the chest that will allow portable chest x-ray to be made at the commencement of the procedure and again later if the foreign body cannot be found. After caval drainage catheters are inserted, the aorta and pulmonary arteries should be cross-clamped at the beginning of inflow occlusion to prevent migration of the missile out of the heart. The initial attempt at removal of the missile should be through a wide atriotomy.

If fluoroscopy suggests that the missile is not moving with the contracting myocardium, one should also consider the possibility that it lies free in the pericardium. At the time of exploration the pericardium and great vessels should always be carefully explored before continuing with preparations for open removal.

Occasionally, one may be fortunate to be presented with a foreign body whose surface is visible in the myocardial wound. Unless easy extraction can be expected it is wise to cannulate the cavae and have a vascular clamp ready to close on the great vessels through the transverse sinus before extraction is attempted lest the attempt result in either the loss of the foreign body into the underlying heart chamber or uncontrollable massive bleeding on its removal.

The fact that a missile has penetrated the heart demands careful evaluation for traumatic septal or valve defects. Any murmurs should be thoroughly assessed by cardiac catheterization or angiography before surgical exploration. If the missile is not free in the chamber of the heart, its accurate localization by careful cinefluorometric study will greatly facilitate its localization and removal. All patients with this complication warrant heavy antibiotic coverage.

THE AORTA AND GREAT VESSELS

Penetrating Injuries

A laceration of the aorta or its major branches or the hilar pulmonary vessels is one of the most lethal forms of penetrating chest trauma. Depending on whether the site of vessel injury is intra- or extrapericardial, the trauma may result in cardiac tamponade or exsanguinating hemothorax. Occasionally, if the wounding agent is small, such as an icepick or small missile or if the vessel has been barely nicked, the rate of bleeding may not be very rapid or a false aneurysm may form. Equally rare is the formation of an arteriovenous fistula. In most cases, the patient dies before reaching the hospital and most of those who manage to reach the hospital present the attending physician with the problem of massive hemothorax or rapidly re-forming cardiac tamponade. These patients may survive if a decision for immediate thoracotomy is quickly made.

The first successful outcome of such a penetrating wound of the aorta was recorded by the Russian Dshanelidze in 1922.[24] His patient had an 8 mm. laceration in the aorta 1 cm. above the heart. In 1932 Blalock reported the successful suture of an icepick wound of the intrapericardial ascending aorta. In a subsequent review, Blalock[7] noted that only 13 of 66 patients survived the immediate postinjury period. In a more recent report Beall[4] reported 23 cases; 10 of these patients survived operation and 7 were long-term survivors. In 1959 Perkins and Elchos[55] reported the first successful early repair of a stab wound of the extrapericardial aorta. They pointed out the reasons such wounds carry more serious prognosis than cardiac stab wounds: (1) high pressure is sustained in the aorta, (2) the thinner aortic wall does not seal so well as the myocardium, (3) the easily distensible mediastinum offers less resistance to the egress of blood than the intact pericardium, (4) delayed rebleeding is common, and (5) if the patient survives the initial injury, later problems such as false aneurysm or arteriovenous fistulas remain.

Nonpenetrating Injuries

The most common cause of death among victims of traffic accidents who do not reach the hospital alive is rupture of the aorta (36 per cent). The most common site of rupture in decelerating injuries is near the aortic isthmus just below the origin of the subclavian artery. This is also the most frequent site for crushing injuries; but in falls from great heights, the tear may be near the root of the aorta, resulting in hemopericardium and cardiac tamponade. Although such injuries are usually immediately fatal, it has been pointed out that 15 per cent of these patients survive beyond 1 hour after reaching the hospital and 11 per cent live over 6 hours.[54] Those patients who survive this long do so because the tear has not traversed the full thickness of the aortic wall; instead, the outer layers of the aorta, mediastinum and pleura have contained the egress of blood and a false aneurysm has formed. This damming of the exsanguinating flood may be successful for minutes, hours or weeks. Occasionally, the aneurysm may remain intact indefinitely.

Cammack et al.[15] have estimated that the occupants of cars involved in a 60 mph head-on collision develop a sudden elevation in aortic pressure to about 1250 mm. Hg, or 250 mm. Hg more than required to rupture the aorta. However, Zehnder[77] has estimated that it requires 2000 mm. Hg to rupture the aorta. The frequency of the injury suggests that something more than simple elevation of the intraluminal pressure is involved. The frequent location of this tear at the aortic isthmus just below the origin of the subclavian artery provides the probable clue to the mechanism. This is the point of greatest fixation of the aorta to the chest wall, and it is thought that the sudden forward movement of the aorta above and below this fixed point produces a shearing force that, in combination with the increased intraluminal pressure, causes the injury. Maximum stress occurs at the inner surface of the vessel. The adventitia and external elastic lamella, having a higher elastic limit, withstand the stress best and occasionally, by remaining intact, allow the formation of a false aneurysm. A similar explanation has been postulated for the frequent location of aortic disruption at the root of the aorta following falls from great heights.

Diagnosis. At one extreme the patient may present with exsanguinating hemorrhage into the left chest or a rapidly re-forming pericardial tamponade and, at the other, with an asymptomatic aneurysm of the distal arch of the aorta accidentally discovered by routine x-rays some time after the injury. It is the situation between these two extremes that offers the greatest therapeutic potential — a false aneurysm whose rupture has been temporarily delayed by the adventitia and surrounding tissues. The key to survival in these patients is the recognition of the possible significance of mediastinal widening on the initial chest x-ray (Fig. 13–14A). Other less common radiographic findings are elevation and rightward shift of the left mainstem bronchus and loss of the silhouette of the aortic arch (knob) and descending aorta. These x-ray signs should be specifically sought in any victim of severe blunt trauma to the chest. If such a finding is associated with significant bleeding into the left chest, immediate operation is justified. Otherwise, it is recommended that an aortogram be obtained while the operating theater stands by in readiness. This definitive diagnostic step is required because of two facts: not all mediastinal widening following trauma represents aortic rupture and not all aortic tears occur at, or near enough to, the aortic isthmus to be approached through the same incision. The aortogram may be obtained by retrograde catheterization, but this may not be done without some risk of rupturing the aneurysm. For this reason some have suggested the use of a "forward" aortogram, obtained by injecting a large bolus of dye through a central venous catheter whose tip lies near the heart. However, this often does not provide adequate enough resolution. Therefore, the brachial approach probably should be used even though it is associated with a significantly higher incidence of catheter complications.

MacKenzie et al.[43] have suggested that extravasation of blood into the anatomical

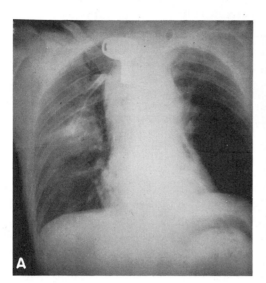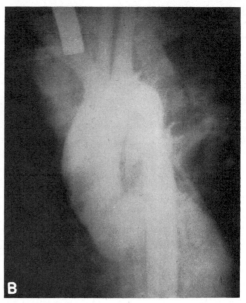

Figure 13–14. *Traumatic rupture of the thoracic aorta. The condition was suspected from the initial antero-posterior chest film (A), which demonstrated a widened mediastinum with loss of definition about the aortic knob. Aortography (B) revealed complete intimal disruption in the descending aorta just distal to the level of the ligamentum arteriosum. An irregularity at the origin of the left subclavian artery suggests its avulsion. (From Blazek, J. V.: Acute traumatic rupture of the thoracic aorta demonstrated by retrograde aortography. Radiology 85:253, 1965.)*

spaces of the neck may be a valuable diagnostic sign of rupture of the great vessels of the thorax. They recommend the use of a minor supraclavicular incision to establish this fact. In an autopsy study of 38 accident victims, 16 of 17 patients with ruptured aorta showed blood within the carotid artery sheath. Blood was found within the sheath of the jugular vein in four patients with rupture of the superior vena cava. Four patients with rupture of the pulmonary arteries bled into the tracheal esophageal compartment in the neck; in 13 in whom there was no great vessel rupture, blood was not found in these cervical spaces. These autopsy observations were confirmed experimentally by the injection of varying amounts of blood around the intrathoracic vessels at the usual site of rupture. Significantly, it required 75 ml. of blood or less to stain the cervical vascular spaces but 400 or more ml. to cause a radiologically visible widening of the mediastinum. Further clinical experience is needed to fully assess the merit of this approach. The aortogram has the important advantage of localizing the site of injury and determining the appropriate thoracotomy exposure,

but the use of a diagnostic supraclavicular incision may have merit when facilities for emergency aortography are not readily available.

Treatment. Intrapericardial injuries to the great vessels will present with hemopericardium, as discussed earlier in this chapter. Extrapericardial injuries usually produce massive bleeding into one hemithorax (usually the left). In such cases, it is hopeless to persist with efforts at transfusion and evacuation of the hemithorax; only prompt recourse to thoracotomy will lead to survival. Unless the location of the site of bleeding has been clearly suggested by the injury itself, a lateral thoracotomy in the fourth or fifth intercostal space should be performed. Bleeding points in a thoracotomy incision should be ignored initially. The hemothorax should be evacuated and the source of bleeding localized. No attempt should be made to control the bleeding directly by clamps; instead, pressure should be applied to control the bleeding site. If the bleeding can be controlled by pressure, the surgeon should gain adequate exposure, proximal and distal control of the bleeding vessel and wait for adequate blood volume replacement before renewing his attack.

Small stab wounds can usually be controlled by direct suture with or without the aid of partial occluding vascular clamps or brief cross-clamping. Patients with larger penetrating wounds are not likely to reach the operating room. The cases of nonpenetrating trauma present more challenging technical problems. Extensive mediastinal hemorrhage and false aneurysm formation make it difficult to evaluate the extent of damage to the aortic wall. There may be a small intimal tear or complete circumferential laceration with discontinuity (Fig. 13–14B). Intramural dissection or intramural hematoma may involve a variable segment of aorta adjacent to the tear. Such injuries must be opened to determine the extent of injury and to assure complete repair. To do this, the involved segment of aorta must be isolated and bypassed. The site of the injury determines whether a temporary (Gott) shunt or left heart bypass is required. Occasionally, such injuries can be repaired with sutures alone; more often than not a segmental replacement is required. The risk of dissecting the false aneurysm and disrupted segment from the vital structures running through the surrounding mediastinal hematoma often dictates that the prosthesis replacement bypass the area or be laid in its bed after it has been opened and collateral bleeding controlled from within.

Most traumatic false aneurysms of the thoracic aorta rupture relatively early. However, it has been shown that if rupture has not occurred by 2 months it rarely does.[65] Because of the technical difficulties involved in excision of an organized false aneurysm and the danger of injury to surrounding structures such as the esophagus, recurrent laryngeal nerve and left stem bronchus, it has been suggested that patients presenting more than 2 months after injury be operated on only because of signs of enlargement or other significant symptoms. However, many of these patients still require thoracotomy for these indications, and a common manner of the late presentation is compression of the left main bronchus. Because of more recent experiences using temporary nonthrombogenic plastic tube bypass (that avoids heparinization and partial cardiac bypass) and laying the graft inside the bed of the aneurysm, this conservative approach to the "older" aneurysms is losing its hold.

REFERENCES

1. Andersen, I., and Halkier, E.: Closed injuries of the thorax. Acta Chir. Scand. Suppl. *332*:32, 1964.
2. Anderson, R. P., and Sabiston, D. C., Jr.: Acquired bronchoesophageal fistula of benign origin. Surg. Gynecol. Obstet. *121*:261, 1965.
3. Avery, E. E., Mörch, E. T., and Benson, D. W.: Critically crushed chests; new methods of treatment and continuous mechanical hyperventilation to produce alkalotic apnea and internal pneumatic stabilization. J. Thorac. Surg. *32*:291, 1956.
4. Beal, A. C., Jr.: Penetrating wounds of the aorta. Am. J. Surg. *99*:770, 1960.
5. Beck, C. S.: Wounds of the heart. Arch. Surg. *13*:205, 1926.
6. Blair, E., Topuzlu, C., and Deane, R. S.: Major Blunt Chest Trauma in Current Problems in Surgery. Chicago, Year Book Medical Publishers, May, 1969.
7. Blalock, A.: Successful suture of a wound of the ascending aorta. J.A.M.A. *103*:1617, 1934.
8. Blalock, A., and Ravitch, M. M.: Consideration of nonoperative treatment of cardiac tamponade resulting from wounds of the heart. Surgery *14*:157, 1943.
9. Bland, E. F., and Beebe, G. W.: Missiles in the heart: A twenty year follow-up report of World War II cases. U. S. Navy Medical News Letter, *48*(No. 3):3, August 12, 1966.
10. Border, J. R., Hopkinson, B. R., and Schenk, W. G., Jr.: Mechanisms of pulmonary trauma: an experimental study. J. Trauma *8*:47, 1968.
11. Boyd, T. F., and Strieder, J. W.: Immediate surgery for traumatic heart disease. J. Thorac. Surg. *50*:305, 1965.
12. Brewer, L. A., Burbank, B., Samson, P. C., and Schiff, C. A.: The wet lung in war casualties. Arch. Surg. *123*:343, 1946.
13. Burford, T. H., and Burbank, B.: Traumatic wet lung; observations on certain physiologic fundamentals of thoracic trauma. J. Thorac. Surg. *14*:415, 1945.
14. Burke, J. F.: Early diagnosis of traumatic rupture of the bronchus. J.A.M.A. *181*:682, 1962.
15. Cammack, K., Rapport, R. L., Paul, J., and Baird, W. C.: Deceleration injuries of the thoracic aorta. A.M.A. Arch. Surg. *79*:244, 1959.
16. Carter, B. N., and Giuseffi, J.: Tracheotomy: Useful procedure in thoracic surgery with particular reference to its employment in crushing injuries of the thorax. J. Thorac. Surg. *21*:495, 1951.
17. Carter, R., Warsham, E. E., and Brewer, L. A.: Rupture of the bronchus following closed chest trauma. Am. J. Surg. *104*:177, 1962.
18. Conn, J. H., Hardy, J. D., Fair, W. R., and Netterville, R. E.: Thoracic trauma: Analysis of 1022 cases. J. Trauma *3*:22, 1963.
19. Cooley, D. A., Dunn, J. R., Brockman, H. L., and

DeBakey, M. E.: Treatment of penetrating wounds of the heart: Experimental and clinical observations. Surgery 37:882, 1955.

20. Daniels, R. A., Jr., and Cate, W. R., Jr.: Wet lung — an experimental study. Ann. Surg. 127:836, 1948.

21. Decancq, J. G.: The treatment of chylothorax in children. Surg. Gynecol. Obstet. 121:509, 1965.

22. Doubleday, L. C.: Radiologic aspects of stab wounds of the heart. Radiology 74:26, 1960.

23. Drinker, C. K., and Warren, M. F.: The genesis and resolution of pulmonary transudates and exudates. J.A.M.A. 122:269, 1943.

24. Dshanelidze, I. I.: Manuskript Petrograd, 1922. Quoted by Lilienthal, H.: Thoracic Surgery. Philadelphia, W. B. Saunders Company, 1925, p. 489.

25. Elkins, D. C., and Campbell, R. E.: Cardiac tamponade: Treatment by aspiration. Ann. Surg. 133:623, 1951.

26. Errion, A. R., Houk, V. N., and Kettering, D. L.: Pulmonary hematoma due to blunt, nonpenetrating thoracic trauma. Am. Rev. Resp. Dis. 88:384, 1963.

27. Fischer, G.: Die Wunden des Herzens und des Herzbeutels. Arch. Klin. Chirurgie 9:571, 1868.

28. Franz, J. I., Richardson, J. D., Grover, F. L., and Trinkle, J. K.: Effect of methylprednisolone sodium succinate on experimental pulmonary contusion. J. Thorac. Cardiovasc. Surg. 68:842, 1974.

29. Garzon, A. A., Seltzer, B., Lichtenstein, S., and Karlson, K. E.: Influence of tracheostomy cannula size on work of breathing. Ann. Surg. 162:315, 1965.

30. Gibson, L. D., Carter, R., and Hinshaw, D. B.: Surgical significance of sternal fracture. Surg. Gynecol. Obstet. 114:443, 1962.

31. Goorwitch, J.: Traumatic chylothorax and thoracic duct ligation: Case report and review of literature. J. Thorac. Surg. 29:467, 1955.

32. Gray, A. R., Harrison, W. H., Jr., Coures, C. M., and Howard, J. M.: Penetrating injuries to the chest. Am. J. Surg. 100:709, 1960.

33. Griffith, J. L.: Traumatic fracture of the left main bronchus. Thorax 4:105, 1949.

34. Harken, D. E.: Foreign bodies in, and in relation to, the thoracic blood vessels and heart. Surg. Gynecol. Ostet. 83:117, 1946.

35. Harrison, W. H., Jr., Gray, A. R., Coures, C. M., and Howard, J. M.: Severe nonpenetrating injuries to the chest. Am. J. Surg. 100:715, 1960.

36. Hershgold, E. J.: Roentgenographic study of human subjects during transverse accelerations. Aerospace Med. 31:213, 1960.

37. Hood, R. M., and Sloan, H. E.: Injuries of the trachea and major bronchi. J. Thorac. Cardiovasc. Surg. 38:458, 1959.

38. Isaacs, J. P.: Sixty penetrating wounds of the heart. Surgery 45:696, 1959.

39. King, O. J., Jr. and Glas, W. W.: Complications of tracheostomy. Rocky Mountain M. J. 57:36, 1960.

40. Lampson, R. S.: Traumatic chylothorax. A review of the literature and report of a case treated by mediastinal ligation of the thoracic duct. J. Thorac. Surg. 17:778, 1948.

41. Laustela, E.: Thorax traumatology. Acta Chir. Scand. Suppl. 332:17, 1964.

42. MacKenzie, M. A.: A Manual of Diseases of the *Throat and Nose*. II. Diseases of the Oesophagus, Nose and Nasopharynx. New York, William Wood & Co., 1884.

43. MacKenzie, J. R., Hackett, M., and Munro, D. D.: Diagnosis of ruptured great vessels of the thorax. A simple and reliable method. Presented to the American Association for the Surgery of Trauma, Santa Barbara, 1966.

44. Mackler, S. A.: Spontaneous rupture of the esophagus, an experimental and clinical study. Surg. Gynecol. Obstet. 95:345, 1952.

45. Mahaffey, D. E., Creech, O., Jr., Boren, H. G., and DeBakey, M. E.: Traumatic rupture of the left main stem bronchus successfully repaired eleven years after injury. J. Thorac. Surg. 32:312, 1956.

46. Maloney, J. V., Jr., and MacDonald, L.: The treatment of blunt trauma to the thorax. Am. J. Surg. 105:404, 1963.

47. Maloney, J. V., Jr., Schmutzer, K. J., and Raschke, E.: Paradoxical respiration and "pendelluft." J. Thorac. Cardiovasc. Surg. 41:391, 1961.

48. Maloney, J. V., and Spencer, F. C.: The nonoperative treatment of traumatic chylothorax. Surgery 40:121, 1956.

49. Maynard, A., Avecilla, M. J., and Naclerio, E. A.: The management of wounds of the heart. Ann. Surg. 144:1018, 1956.

50. Moore, B. P.: Operative stabilization of nonpenetrating chest injuries. J. Thorac. Cardiovasc. Surg. 70:619, 1975.

51. Munnell, E. R.: Fracture of major airways. Am. J. Surg. 105:511, 1963.

52. Paris, F., Tarazona, J., and Blasco, E.: Surgical stabilization of traumatic flail chest. Thorax 30:521, 1975.

53. Parmley, L. F., Manion, W. C., and Mattingly, T. W.: Nonpenetrating traumatic injury of the heart. Circulation 18:371, 1958.

54. Parmley, L. F., Mattingly, T. W., Manion, W. C., and Jahnke, E. J.: Nonpenetrating traumatic injury of the aorta. Circulation 17:1086, 1958.

55. Perkins, R., and Elchos, T.: Stab wound of the aortic arch. Ann. Surg. 147:83, 1958.

56. Petty, T. L.: Intensive and Rehabilitative Respiratory Care. Philadelphia, Lea & Febiger, 1971.

57. Pomerantz, M.: Personal communication. 1973.

58. Randall, H. T., and Glass, A.: Gunshot wounds of the heart. Am. J. Surg. 99:788, 1960.

59. Ransdell, H. T., McPherson, R. C., Haller, J. A., Williams, D. J., and Conner, E. H.: Treatment of flail chest injuries with a piston respirator. Am. J. Surg. 104:22, 1962.

60. Rutherford, R. B., Hurt, H. H., Jr., Brickman, R. D., and Tubb, J. M.: The pathophysiology and treatment of progressive tension pneumothorax. J. Trauma 8:212, 1968.

61. Rutherford, R. B.: Personal communication.

62. Rutherford, R. B., and Valenta, J.: An experimental study of "traumatic wet lung." J. Trauma 11:146, 1971.

63. Sauerbruch, F.: Die Verwendbarkeit des Unterdruchverfahrens bei der herz Chirurgie. Arch. klin. Chirurgie 83:537, 1907.

64. Schramel, R. J., Tyler, J., Kirkpatrick, J. L., Ziskind, M., and Creech, O.: Respiratory function after thoracic injuries. J. Trauma 3:206, 1963.

65. Spencer, F. C.: Treatment of chest injuries. Curr. Prob. Surg. Jan., 1964.

66. Swan, H., Forsee, J. H., and Goyette, E. M.: Foreign bodies in the heart. Ann. Surg. 135:314, 1952.

67. Trinkle, J. K., Richardson, J. D., Franz, J. L., Grover, F. L., Arom, K. V., and Holmstrom, F. M. G.: Management of flail chest without mechanical ventilation. Ann. Thorac. Surg. 19:355, 1975.

68. Valle, A. R.: An analysis of 2,811 chest casualties of the Korean conflict. Dis. Chest 26:623, 1954.

69. Van Waggoner, F. H.: Died in hospital: A three-year study of deaths following trauma. J. Trauma 1:401, 1949.

70. Ware, P. F., and Strieder, J. W.: Spontaneous perforation of the normal esophagus. Dis. Chest 16:49, 1949.

71. Westermark, N.: A roentgenological investigation into traumatic lung changes arising through blunt violence to the thorax. Acta Radiol. (Stockholm) 22:331, 1941.

72. Williams, K. R., and Burford, T. H.: The management of chylothorax related to trauma. J. Trauma 3:317, 1963.

73. Worman, L. W.: Fluid Volume Deficits in the Mediastinum. Paper presented before the Society of University Surgeons, Milwaukee, Wisconsin, Febraury 10, 1966.

74. Worman, L. W., Hurley, J. D., Pemberton, A. H., and Narodick, B. G.: Rupture of the esophagus from external blunt trauma. Arch. Surg. 85:333, 1962.

75. Wren, H. B., Texada, P. J., and Krementz, E. T.: Traumatic rupture of the diaphragm. J. Trauma 2:117, 1962.

76. Yao, S. T., Carey, J. S., Shoemaker, W. C., Weinberg, M., and Freeark, R. J.: Hemodynamics and therapy of acute hemopericardium. J. Trauma 13:36, 1973.

77. Zehnder, M. A.: Delayed posttraumatic rupture of the aorta in a young healthy individual after closed injury Mechanical-etiologic consider ations. Angiology 7:252, 1956.

CHAPTER 14

ABDOMINAL INJURIES

Charles B. Anderson, M.D.
Walter F. Ballinger, M.D.

INTRODUCTION

The management of abdominal injuries has been extensively discussed in the surgical literature, and problems of diagnosis and treatment are well defined. For those interested in the historical aspects of abdominal injuries, Loria's excellent contributions are recommended.[92, 93] Most of the ancient accounts concern penetrating injuries and their well-known mortality. Conservative management was usually adhered to from the time of the Egyptians to the early 1800's. Operative intervention was limited and of no great magnitude during this period. In 1836 Baudens published the results of his experiences in the French-Algerian war and suggested "bold operations" in some cases of gunshot wounds of the abdomen. On the basis of two patients operated on in 1830, one of whom survived, he is probably the first to have performed laparotomy for gunshot wounds of the abdomen. Sims was the first in the United States to advocate surgical intervention; Walter, in 1859, and Kinlock, in 1863, were the first to perform abdominal operations in this country for blunt and gunshot injuries, respectively. In 1887, the American Surgical Association expressed a favorable opinion for operative intervention. Réclus, of France, strongly opposed surgical intervention and showed that 66 of 88 dogs with abdominal bullet wounds recovered without surgery. Controversy between the interventionists and the arch-conservatists continued throughout the nineteenth century. Because of the 75–85 per cent mortality associated with laparotomy, and since 25–75 per cent of penetrating wounds were not associated with visceral injuries, the general policy was to avoid surgical procedures. Nevertheless, the British, at the start of the Boer War in 1899, advocated surgical intervention for penetrating abdominal injuries. The mortality rate, however, was highest among patients treated by laparotomy, and thus the policy of conservatism again ruled until the early part of World War I. Because of the larger caliber missiles and higher velocity weapons used in World War I, the mortality associated with abdominal injuries was inordinately high. This led to the popularization of surgical intervention, which reduced the mortality from 85 per cent to 56 per cent. Controversy in the management of abdominal wounds continues, however, especially with regard to stab wounds, in which some advocate immediate surgical intervention in all cases and others postulate selective management.

Innovations in diagnostic methods have included peritoneal lavage, radioisotope scanning, arteriograms and sinograms. Enthusiastic supporters can be found for each of these modalities.

Improved methods of treating specific organ injuries, particularly those of the vascular system, liver and pancreas, and of managing infections, shock and respiratory insufficiency have significantly reduced the mortality from abdominal injuries.

Loria's series of 478 abdominal wounds between 1927 and 1942 had an overall mortality rate of 55 per cent.[91] Today the mortality rate has decreased to somewhat less than 5 per cent for penetrating wounds of the abdomen.[142] As a comparison, the mortality rates during World War I (53.5 per cent), World War II (25 per cent) and the Korean War (12 per cent) are of interest.[142]

The main problem with all abdominal injuries lies in establishing the correct diagnosis soon enough to prevent death and limit morbidity. Two major life-threatening situations occur following either penetrating or blunt trauma to the abdomen: hemorrhage and hollow viscus perforation with associated chemical and bacterial peritonitis.

Much experience has been gained in time of war regarding the management of injuries to the abdomen. Military surgeons become civilian surgeons, and principles learned during wartime are then applied to the general public. Principles of treating any abdominal injury are operative control of hemorrhage and deterrence of peritoneal contamination. These are applicable to the management of both civilian and military casualties. It is essential, however, that the difference between combat and civilian casualties be understood.[114] Abdominal wounds sustained during combat are more serious and had an associated 10 per cent mortality in the Vietnam war[70] as compared to a 3 per cent mortality rate associated with the usual civilian penetrating abdominal wound.[142] Military injuries are caused by missiles in 60 to 80 per cent of cases and are frequently multiple. The remaining one third of cases are caused by bullets of the high-velocity type. Large areas of destruction necessitate wide debridement and healing of wounds by granulation and skin grafting.

Although civilian weaponry contributes considerably to the high incidence of abdominal wounds seen in large urban emergency departments, an ever-increasing number of nonpenetrating abdominal injuries result from automobile accidents caused by excessive speed on crowded highways. Diagnosis soon after arrival of the patient in the emergency department is often difficult because of the high incidence of serious extra-abdominal injuries and the frequent association of shock. The penetrating wounds most often encountered in civilian life are knife and bullet wounds, and there is an inordinately high incidence of drunkenness among such patients with its attendant stupor and masking of abdominal signs. The soldier — young, healthy, sober and usually efficiently transported — presents no problem in diagnosis of a large shrapnel wound involving the anterior abdominal wall. Immediate therapeutic measures are undertaken with full knowledge of the nature of the injury. In contrast, an elderly man found semicomatose by the side of the road presents a serious problem in quick and efficient diagnosis. A high index of suspicion and repeated examinations are needed to point to the correct diagnosis.

CLASSIFICATION OF INJURIES

Methods of classifying abdominal injuries are, of necessity, artificial and arbitrary. Of major consideration in abdominal injury is the degree of urgency and the chance for survival. Thus, a patient is automatically classified according to the speed with which treatment is required. Some have injuries so severe that there is little chance for survival. Others have massive intra-abdominal hemorrhage and require immediate transfusion and laparotomy. Those who exhibit no evidence of severe internal hemorrhage but display signs of peritoneal irritation will require operative intervention on a less than immediate basis. Finally, some individuals have evidence of abdominal trauma but no indication that there has been visceral injury and consequently may be watched for further developments. In essence, then, individuals with evidence of hemorrhage require urgent treatment, and those with peritonitis may have operation delayed temporarily. Every patient is immediately classified by the physician according to the priority of treatment required. Classifications involving the delay before treatment, the number of organs injured, the association of extra-abdominal injuries, or the particular organ injured are not practical methods of diagnosing or treating abdominal injuries. A classification devised by Farrell[46] identifies abdominal injuries according to the principal manifestations: hemorrhage, peritonitis and injuries such as contusions to the abdominal wall, mesentery or diaphragm. However, *recognition of the two major groups of abdominal injuries — penetrating and nonpenetrating (or open and closed) — is of greater importance for prospective treatment* and has a direct relationship to accuracy and speed of diagnosis, mortality and morbidity. In Table 14–1 is an etiological classification of abdominal injuries that is useful in caring for individuals with abdominal trauma and facilitates discussion of this topic. In addition to the usual classifications of penetrating and nonpenetrating injuries, an iatrogenic classification is added because of the peculiar circumstances and effects associated with these latter injuries.

Penetrating Wounds

In recent years the hand gun has replaced the knife as the most common

TABLE 14–1. Etiological Classification of Abdominal Injuries

PENETRATING
 Stab wounds
 Gunshot wounds (velocity)
 Shotgun wounds (range)
 Other (shrapnel, picket, stake, glass)

NONPENETRATING
 Blunt injury
 Crush injury
 Blast injury
  Air
  Immersion
 Seat belt syndrome
 Ingestion
  Corrosive agents
  Foreign body

IATROGENIC
 Endoscopy (biopsy)
 External cardiac massage
 Paracentesis and thoracentesis
 Peritoneal dialysis
 Inhalation therapy (gastric rupture)
 Barium enema
 Peritoneoscopy
 Liver biopsy
 Radiation therapy
 Other

TABLE 14–2. Frequency of Injury in Penetrating Abdominal Trauma

VISCERA	PER CENT
Liver	37
Small bowel	26
Stomach	19
Colon	16.5
Major vascular and retroperitoneal	11
Mesentery and omentum	9.5
Spleen	7
Diaphragm	5.5
Kidney	5
Pancreas	3.5
Duodenum	2.5
Biliary system	1
Other (uterus, sciatic plexus, bladder, muscle, ovary, vagina, adrenal)	1
Injuries per patient	1.4

weapon used in assaults. Gunshot wounds of the abdomen are now more common than stab wounds in many major trauma centers.[75]

The incidence of organ injury in penetrating wounds of the abdomen is shown in Table 14–2. This represents a compilation of series in the literature that includes 3162 patients with 1623 positive laparotomies.[72, 80, 91, 106, 120, 121, 123, 138, 172] The percentages relate to those patients having sustained at least one intra-abdominal injury. For any individual case, such a list only provides a guide along with the location of the wound, indicating where to look first during exploratory laparotomy. In the selective treatment of abdominal stab wounds, the incidence of liver injuries will decrease because many liver wounds are trivial, require no surgical repair and thus do not require laparotomy. Forty per cent of liver injuries are of no importance when "routine" laparotomy is employed.[121] Although the small bowel is not the organ most frequently injured, there are, on the average, five and a half perforations per patient with bowel injury.[199]

The immediate mortality from penetrating abdominal wounds depends on the injury to major vascular structures and resultant intra-abdominal hemorrhage. Otherwise, mortality is directly correlated with the number of abdominal organs injured. Wilson and Sherman[199] reported the relative lethality associated with particular visceral injuries as follows:

vena cava	33%
biliary tract	33%
duodenum	26%
pancreas	20%
urinary bladder	17%
kidney	15%
vascular	12%
colon	12%
small intestine	11%
spleen	11%
stomach	9%
liver	7%

Penetrating wounds of the thorax can often traverse the diaphragm and result in intra-abdominal injury because of the variable position of the diaphragm during respiration — often reaching the level of the nipple or the fourth intercostal space during exhalation (Fig. 14–1). In high wounds like this, prophylactic insertion of a thoracostomy tube prior to laparotomy, despite the absence of a hemothorax or pneumothorax, is a wise precaution against tension pneumothorax during positive-pressure anesthesia. Involvement of both the thoracic and abdominal cavities occurs in one fourth of patients with penetrating wounds of the abdomen.[52]

Stab Wounds. Knives, screw drivers, scissors, pencils, glass bottles, automobile radio antennae, bicycle spokes and nu-

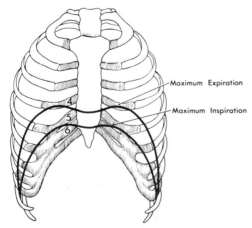

Figure 14–1. *Because of the high position of the diaphragm on forced expiration, penetrating wounds of the lower chest frequently pierce the diaphragm and injure intra-abdominal structures.*

merous other articles are used to inflict stab wounds. The size, shape and length of the instrument are important in estimating the amount of damage that might have been caused. The skin and subcutaneous injury is usually not significant and requires no particular treatment. Simple cleansing and primary closure may be performed. Frequently, a dressing alone suffices. The injury to intra-abdominal viscera is confined to the immediate area of penetration and only limited debridement is required. Multiple stab wounds occur in 20 per cent of cases and the thorax is penetrated in 10 per cent.[106] Whether selective management or mandatory laparotomy is the best method of treating stab sounds is heatedly debated in the literature and is discussed in the following paragraphs.

Gunshot Wounds. Gunshot wounds technically include shotgun injuries, but because of the particular characteristics of the latter they are discussed separately. Civilian gunshot wounds are usually caused by low-velocity pistols, whereas military bullet wounds are of the high-velocity type and result in extensive tissue destruction that requires wide and thorough debridement. The physical factors involve the kinetic energy imparted to the body by the missile. The kinetic energy of a missile is expressed by the formula: $E = mv^2/2g \times 7000$, where E equals kinetic energy in foot pounds, m equals mass of the missile in grains, v equals velocity in feet per second, g equals gravitational acceleration in feet per second and 7000 is a conversion factor. Kinetic energy is thus proportional to the mass of the object and the square of the velocity. Revolver muzzle velocities are in the range of 1000–1500 feet/sec., whereas military rifles have velocities of 2000–3250 feet/sec.[192] It follows that a threefold increase in velocity results in nine times the kinetic energy. The amount of energy imparted to the body is the difference between the kinetic energy of the missile entering minus that when leaving the body. This energy is dissipated by the movement of tissues in a perpendicular direction from the trajectory of the bullet. A high-velocity injury is arbitrarily defined as one in which the wounding missile has a velocity over 2500 feet per second. In high-velocity injuries a large temporary cavity is formed that determines the extent of damage. After passage of the bullet, the tissues collapse and a relatively small tract is left that leads to underestimation of the injury. Low-velocity gunshot wounds require limited debridement because less kinetic energy is imparted to the tissues and consequently the amount of destruction is not as great.

Characteristics of the tissues determine the extent of destruction. Fascia, skin and lung reveal little devitalization when struck by high-velocity missiles, whereas solid tissue such as muscle, bone, liver and spleen are violently disorganized and devitalized.

With few exceptions[143, 122, 172] most agree that gunshot wounds of the abdomen should be explored. Even tangential wounds that have not entered the peritoneal cavity can cause intra-abdominal visceral injury from the "blast effect." Occasionally, low-velocity .22 caliber tangential wounds confined to the right upper quadrant of the abdomen can be observed to determine the need for operative intervention.

Shotgun Wounds. The ballistics and characteristics of shotgun wounds have been described.[33, 104, 160] The term shotgun wound usually implies a pellet load, although slugs of rather heavy weight can be implicated. The amount of powder charge, size of pellets, choke of the gun, and distance to the target all determine the destructive effect. The pattern is the area over which the pellets are dispersed at any given distance. A close pattern concentrates more kinetic energy in a localized region and is thus more destructive than when pellets are widely spread. Usually when a major portion of the charge is concentrated within a wound of entry having a diameter of 15 cm. or less, one can assume that the velocity has been sufficiently high to produce a severe deep wound.[33] In addition, in shotgun blasts, the wad and plastic cups used to separate the powder charge from the shot very often penetrate deeply into the wound. Removal of wadding, clothing and other foreign materials is essential to prevent wound suppuration.

Innumerable combinations of shotgun gauge, shot size, powder load and barrel choke are possible. It is difficult, therefore, to categorize the damage likely at various distances. Usually a No. 6 shot or smaller is used, and a 12-gauge shotgun is the most frequent weapon employed. For example, at 10 yards approximately 95 per cent of No. 6 shot pellets will be within a skin wound 9 inches in diameter if fired from a full-choke barrel, and within an 18-inch diameter if fired from a cylinder bore. At 20 yards wound diameters are doubled.[33] An initial muzzle velocity of 1300 feet/sec. will be reduced 25 per cent to 950 feet/sec. after traveling 20 yards. The unfavorable ballistic characteristics of the pellet (sphere) are responsible for the rapid fall-off of velocity and thus most serious human shotgun injuries occur within a short range. Distance is the most critical factor in determining seriousness of shotgun wound injuries. Sherman and Parrish[160] describe three types of injury. Type I injuries are sustained at long range (a distance of more than seven yards) and result in subcutaneous or deep fascia location of the pellets. Type II wounds are sustained at close range of 3 to 7 yards, and structures beneath the deep fascia are perforated. In Type III massive wounds occur at point-blank range under 3 yards.

The treatment of shotgun injuries sustained at close range requires extensive debridement. Other injuries produce only a few scattered small wounds of minimal significance. A wide spectrum of injury exists between these two extremes and requires careful evaluation and management. An interesting observation by several authors involves the expectant treatment of multiple, widely scattered shotgun injuries that have penetrated the abdominal cavity.[21, 41, 104, 196] Perforations may be legion, thus making it impossible to locate all visceral wounds. Moreover, small holes in the intestine made by the pellets show no pouting of mucosa, no eversion of the wound edges and no significant leakage or soiling. When minimal leakage does occur, the holes usually close spontaneously and with appropriate antibiotic therapy the peritonitis will be limited and the patient will recover. Handling the bowel with innumerable perforations results in milking of the intestinal contents through the perforations and causes serious contamination. Thus it may be reasonable to treat certain selected shotgun wounds by the conservative method of careful observation.

Overall, shotgun wounds of the abdomen have twice the mortality of other gunshot injuries, and those involving the chest lead to 10 times the mortality.[160]

Other Wounds. Fragmentation and secondary missiles from grenades, bombs and antipersonnel mines constitute the most frequent cause of injury in wartime. During the Vietnam conflict only 19 per cent of injuries were due to small-arms fire, whereas 65 per cent were attributed to fragmentation missiles.[73] Shrapnel wounds are usually large and result in extensive destruction of tissues. Impalement on stakes and picket fences occurs and requires innovations of treatment determined by the circumstances of the particular injury. Flying missiles from lawn mowers, explosions, storms and automobile accidents are only a few of the numerous causes of penetrating trauma to the abdomen.

Nonpenetrating Trauma

A comprehensive review of blunt abdominal trauma was published by Griswald and Collier[64] in 1961. Aristotle has been given credit for being the first to describe visceral injury from blunt abdominal trauma by noting that the intestine of the deer was so delicate that it might be ruptured by a slight external blow without injuring the skin. Today the incidence of blunt abdominal trauma is increasing primarily because of soaring automobile accident rates. The automobile is responsible for at least 50 per cent of nonpenetrating abdominal injuries. In a series of 518 cases of blunt abdominal trauma reported by Di Vincenti and associates,[35] auto accidents and pedestrian accidents combined accounted for 74 per cent; blows to the abdomen, 14 per cent; falls, 9 per cent; and other causes, 3 per cent. Three distinct mechanisms of abdominal trauma that occur in children include birth-associated injuries, unrecognized congenital anomalies and the battered child syndrome.[139]

Although blunt abdominal trauma constitutes only 0.1 per cent of all hospital admissions and 1 per cent of all trauma admissions, it is associated with a 20 to 30 per cent mortality rate,[81] much of which is attributable to associated injuries of the head and chest, and fractures of the extremities. DiVincenti's group noted the following:[35]

Ten per cent of patients will die before treatment is instituted; 30 per cent will not be operated on, and 18 per cent of these will die — one third because of other severe injuries and two thirds from error in diagnosis. Diagnostic errors occur either when physicians are distracted from finding the primary injury while treating associated injuries (fractures) or in the absence of a history of trauma. Of the 70 per cent who are explored, 14 per cent will succumb.

The incidence of specific organ injuries is listed in Table 14–3. Griswald and Collier[64] derived these figures by reviewing numerous series in the literature. A 50 per cent mortality occurs with liver injuries, ruptured diaphragms, kidney lacerations and retroperitoneal hematomas. A 25 per cent mortality is seen with ruptured spleens and urinary bladders, while pancreatic injuries and hollow viscus ruptures have a 15 per cent mortality. Naturally, much of this mortality was in association with other injuries.

Mechanisms of blunt visceral injury include crushing, shearing and bursting forces. The first is the crushing of an organ against the posterior abdominal wall, especially the anterior ridge in the midline produced by the vertebral bodies. Second, a sharp shearing force may suddenly be applied to both solid and hollow organs, resulting in tears with perforation or hemorrhage or both. Finally, an intra-abdominal hollow viscus can be burst open by a sudden increase in its intraluminal pressure.

A sudden application of pressure is more apt to rupture solid than hollow viscera, thus accounting for the greater incidence of solid organ injury. The more elastic tissues

TABLE 14–3. Frequency of Injury in Blunt Abdominal Trauma[64]

VISCERA	PER CENT
Spleen	26.2
Kidney	24.2
Intestine	16.2
Liver	15.6
Abdominal wall	3.6
Retroperitoneal hematoma	2.7
Mesentery	2.5
Pancreas	1.4
Diaphragm	1.1

of the young tolerate trauma better than the less resilient tissues of the aged. A strong, firmly muscled abdominal wall constitutes a better barrier than the flaccid, relaxed abdomen of the old or intoxicated.

Blast Injuries. These can occur in air or under water (immersion). Gas-filled cavities such as the lung and intestines are primarily affected, and air blast injuries are not as severe as immersion blasts. Solid organs transmit blast waves better and are therefore less often injured. Indeed, Greaves and associates[63] did not observe pathological changes in solid organ tissues that did not contain air or gas. Observation and treatment are similar to that performed with blunt abdominal trauma.

Crush Injuries. These imply a diffuse and prolonged appliction of great force with all the attendant problems seen in the usual blunt trauma patient.

Seatbelt Injuries. Since Kulowski and Rost[85] in 1956 first attributed a case of intestinal obstruction to a previously incurred seat belt injury, numerous cases of the "seat belt syndrome"[60] have appeared in the literature. Williams and Kirkpatrick[195] collected 87 cases of lap belt injury. Intra-abdominal injuries occurred in 42 of these patients, and 39 had intestinal or mesenteric injuries. Thirty-seven were subjected to surgery with three deaths. Lumbar spine injuries occurred 51 times and in seven instances were associated with intra-abdominal injury as well. Twenty-four patients wearing a shoulder restrainer sustained predominantly skeletal injuries, although intra-abdominal trauma was also noted. Sixty-three individuals wearing the three-point shoulder-lap belt restrainers had primarily fractures of the ribs, clavicle or sternum but intra-abdominal injury was rare. This last device was the most effective in preventing injuries.

The method of injury to the bowel in this syndrome involves direct trauma that results in seromuscular tears and closed-loop obstructions that temporarily increase intraluminal pressure, resulting in intestinal rupture. Shearing and torsion forces are probably also active. Besides the intestines and mesentery, practically all abdominal structures, including the gravid uterus, have been injured by seatbelts. The terminal ileum is the most common location for the intestinal injuries. A correctly worn seatbelt rests low over the anterior iliac spines and should not result in intra-abdominal trauma. However, the seatbelt is often worn improperly above the iliac crests or migrates there during the accident and thus predisposes to injury of the abdomen. Properly worn seatbelts seldom cause serious injury and are definitely effective in reducing mortality and morbidity in automobile accidents.

The "seatbelt sign" consists of a transverse band of contusion, abrasion or ecchymosis across the lower abdomen. It occurs in less than one third of cases of intra-abdominal injury but should always alert the examiner to the possibility that the accident victim may have incurred an abdominal visceral injury or fracture of the lumbar spine or pelvis.

Most seatbelt injuries have had significant delays in diagnosis with increased morbidity and mortality. Deterioration is usually apparent by 12 hours,[195] but delays of up to 65 days are reported.[205] Diagnosis and treatment of these injuries have all the problems and pitfalls of managing other blunt abdominal trauma.

Corrosive Gastritis. Trauma to the abdominal viscera is not limited to blows and bullets. Corrosive gastritis is a form of abdominal injury that requires expert diagnostic and therapeutic acumen. Citron and associates[25] have thoroughly reviewed this problem, and Nicosia and colleagues[124] have stressed the need for a well-planned surgical approach.

The selective effects produced by acid and alkaline corrosives on different parts of the alimentary tract are well documented. Acids spare the esophagus and damage the stomach, whereas alkalis affect primarily the esophagus, causing gastric injury in only 20 per cent of the cases. These findings are attributable to the rapid passage of acid in an esophagus lined with acid-resistant squamous epithelium and to the neutralizing effect of the gastric content on ingested alkali. Concentrated acids produce a coagulative necrosis with subsequent eschar formation but little likelihood of perforation, whereas alkalis cause a liquefying necrosis with deep penetration and increased probability of perforation.

Hydrochloric, nitric, trichloracetic, sulfuric and carbolic acids are the most common causes of corrosive gastritis. The primary effect in the stomach is on the antrum because rapid passage along the lesser curvature magenstrasse and pylorus spasm initiated by the acid causes the corrosive to accumulate in the distal stomach. An empty stomach is more likely to be diffusely involved.

Following ingestion the patient is seized with acute generalized abdominal pain that becomes more localized to the epigastric area. Retching, hematemesis and cardiovascular collapse may ensue. If the patient survives, pyloric outlet obstruction usually develops, requiring surgical intervention.

The emergency management of gastric corrosive injuries involves cautious passage of a large, soft rubber nasogastric tube, taking care to avoid further injury to the already damaged esophagus and stomach, followed by gastric lavage with antacids or specific antidotes. Supportive measures include sedation, antibiotics and appropriate intravenous fluid administration. Anticholinergic agents may be beneficial in relieving spasm.

After the acute period, signs and symptoms of peritonitis may develop. Steigmann[175] has stressed that emergency laparotomy should be avoided at this time because the process is a chemical burn–producing coagulative rather than liquefying necrosis and rarely perforates. Allen and associates,[3] however, recommend immediate laparotomy if signs of perforation or massive bleeding develop. They noted that a total gastrectomy with no anastomosis was the most common procedure performed. No doubt a spectrum of damage to the stomach exists with limited mucosal inflammation at one extreme and frank perforation at the other. Expert judgment is obviously required in deciding if surgery is indicated.

Following this initial period, healing and scarring occur and may result, months later, in pyloric outlet obstruction. Pyloroplasty, gastroenterostomy and subtotal gastrectomy are the usual procedures employed to rectify this problem.

Ingested Foreign Bodies. Swallowed foreign bodies that reach the stomach almost always pass completely through without causing obstruction or perforation. Only 1 per cent of 800 patients treated for ingested foreign bodies at Boston City Hospital had perforations.[71] An almost unending assortment of objects — sharp or dull, pointed or blunt and large or small — have been treated by watchful waiting.

Perforations, when they do occur, commonly result from small objects becoming trapped in the appendix or Meckel's diverticulum. In addition, some pins probably perforate the bowel on their way to the rectum but these wounds heal spontaneously and cause no symptoms. If the object is radiopaque, serial x-rays taken twice a week will insure that the object is not being held up. If the object does become fixed, or if pain, fever, tenderness or signs of peritonitis develop, removal by celiotomy is indicated. Bulk diets are not indicated and cathartics should be avoided.

Iatrogenic Injuries

In Table 14–1 are listed some of the iatrogenic causes of abdominal injury. These represent an assortment of commonly performed diagnostic and therapeutic procedures that can, albeit infrequently, lead to intra-abdominal injury.

Sigmoidoscopy, particularly in conjunction with biopsy, has been associated with perforations of the lower bowel. Extraperitoneal perforations are not nearly as serious as the intraperitoneal perforations. When the perforation occurs, a piece of fat or omentum may be seen plugging the newly made hole. However, perforation is often not diagnosed until signs of peritonitis develop. Immediate laparotomy with primary closure of the perforation is indicated. A diverting colostomy may not be necessary, particularly since most of these patients have had a lower bowel prep prior to the endoscopy and contamination is negligible.

The injuries that may be associated with external cardiac massage can be considerable and become important if the resuscitation is successful. Fractures of the sternum and multiple ribs with hemopneumothorax, flail chest and rupture of the spleen or liver are the most frequent injuries. Often the critical status of the patient distracts the attending physician from recognizing these injuries.

Abdominal paracentesis, performed with a needle, rarely causes significant intra-abdominal injury even if the bowel is perforated. Needle puncture wounds of the intestine quickly seal without leakage, except in the presence of intestinal obstruction. However, laceration of the intestine can occur and will usually require operative repair. Trocar insertion can cause serious laceration or perforation of the bowel, particularly in areas where the bowel is fixed by adhesions. The withdrawal of intestinal contents during paracentesis is diagnostic of this complication. Avoidance of abdominal scars when selecting the site of trocar insertion is important. Trauma to the iliac vessels has also occurred from this maneuver and requires immediate exploration to prevent exsanguination and vascular thrombosis. Insertion of an abdominal catheter for peritoneal dialysis has the same potential for complications as the abdominal trocar paracentesis. Both thoracentesis and tube thoracostomy have been associated with injuries to the liver and spleen. Treatment is determined by the degree and type of injury.

Inadvertent insertion of a nasal oxygen line into the esophagus can cause gastric distention, rupture and even tension pneumoperitoneum with compression of the inferior vena cava and obstruction to venous return to the right heart. Immediate insertion of a large needle into the peritoneal cavity will relieve the pressure, after which laparotomy is indicated to repair the gastric rent.

Perforation of the colon during a barium enema examination introduces a potentially lethal combination of barium and feces into the peritoneal cavity. Biopsy of the rectosigmoid colon, done shortly prior to the barium enema, may at times be a predisposing factor by creating an area of weakness in the bowel wall. Celiotomy with closure of the perforation, a completely diverting proximal colostomy, thorough lavage of the abdominal cavity with large amounts of saline solution and parenteral administration of antibodies for aerobic and anerobic bacteria constitute effective therapy.

The procedure of Fallopian tube interruption by peritoneoscopy has resulted in perforations of the small bowel during electrocoagulation of the tubes. Perforation is not necessarily immediate and symptoms may appear after several days as the necrotic area in the small bowel sloughs, resulting in leakage of intestinal contents. Injury

to the iliac artery resulting in massive hemorrhage can also occur.

Liver biopsies associated with significant hemorrhage or bile leakage are not very common. On the other hand, liver biopsies or percutaneous cholangiograms performed in the presence of obstruction to the common bile duct will usually result in a bile leak. Therefore, if percutaneous cholangiography does demonstrate obstruction, abdominal exploration should be carried out immediately.

Radiation effects on the rectum or the small bowel fixed in the pelvis by adhesions during radiotherapy create problems of irradiation proctitis with bleeding and obstruction and stricture of the small intestine.[155] Symptomatology determines when operative intervention is necessary.

ASSOCIATED CONDITIONS

Other factors that may have an important bearing on the diagnosis, management and prognosis of abdominal injuries deserve comment.

Extra-abdominal Injuries. Such injuries are associated with a higher mortality in patients with abdominal trauma. Fitzgerald and associates[49] reported on 100 patients who arrived dead at the hospital following nonpenetrating abdominal trauma. Extra-abdominal injuries were present in 97 per cent of patients who were dead on arrival but in only 70 per cent of those arriving alive. Seventeen of the patients who arrived alive died before resuscitative measures could be instituted. Another 3 patients died because of failure to recognize intra-abdominal bleeding in the presence of other severe injuries. Of the remaining 80 patients, 50 had extra-abdominal injuries, 78 per cent of whom survived, whereas of the 30 patients with injuries limited to the abdomen 93 per cent survived. These figures emphasize the fact that mortality of abdominal trauma is low if the diagnosis is made early and if there are no extra-abdominal injuries.

Aside from affecting prognosis, associated injuries complicate and hamper the transportation and examination of the injured. A patient with a fractured cervical vertebra or femur with the appropriate splinting and traction devices in place is difficult to transport and almost impossible to position for proper abdominal x-rays.

London[88] reported 58 deaths following laparotomy for abdominal injury, 45 of which occurred in patients with extra-abdominal injuries. Wilson and co-authors[198] indicate that the presence of head injury in association with abdominal injury not only increases the mortality rate by a factor of four but also increases the likelihood of nonpenetrating abdominal trauma being undiagnosed. Only 22 per cent of their patients with combined injuries did not exhibit coma, shock or both (Fig. 14–2). In patients sufficiently reactive to respond to painful stimuli, the presence of abdominal rigidity and tenderness is an important finding and should not be discounted. These authors stress the importance of abdominal paracentesis in such patients and note a diagnostic accuracy of 95 per cent when the procedure yields free blood, bile and air. The most important lesson learned from this reported experience is that preoccupation with other injuries, misinterpretation of obvious clinical signs and avoidance of abdominal paracentesis are the chief factors leading to unnecessary deaths.

Alcohol. Hopson and coauthors[72] noted that 87 per cent of 297 patients with stab wounds of the abdomen had probably been drinking. Maynard and Orapeza,[106] in a series of 569 patients, noted that 35 per cent were obviously intoxicated. The obtunded reactions of inebriated patients make abdominal evaluation difficult. Also, the histories are less accurate, the chances of aspiration greater, and the likelihood of postoperative delirium tremens enhanced. The combative, obnoxious drunk must at times be restrained for his own as well as the attending personnel's protection.

Narcotics and Other Drug Abuses. The recent increase in the use of "hard drugs" has provided yet another set of complicating circumstances in the management of abdominal trauma. Obtunded sensation, lack of response to usual analgesic doses, postoperative withdrawal, the need to continue methadone maintenance therapy, the lack of veins for intravenous infusions because of drug-induced thrombophlebitis, and the higher incidence of hepatitis are a few of the added problems encountered. A 26 per cent incidence of narcotics addiction has been reported in one trauma series.[80]

Treatment Delay. The delay between injury and definitive medical management has a very significant bearing on the outcome. In over 80 per cent of cases, admission to the hospital occurs within 4 hours of the accident. Injuries managed soon after the insult have less mortality and morbidity than when treatment is postponed.[90] Some authors have attempted to show that minor delays in performing laparotomy have no effect on morbidity.[22, 114, 199] Nance and Cohn,[121] in a study on selective management of abdominal stab wounds, reported a 49 per cent complication rate in those operated on in less than 6 hours after injury and a 50 per cent complication rate in those with a delay exceeding 6 hours. However, individuals with continued bleeding or peritonitis will succumb if corrective surgery is *not* performed. Deterioration is a continuous process and it seems unlikely that a definite time interval can be defined during which delay is not harmful.

Shock. That the mortality of patients admitted in shock is greater than those without hypotension is well established. The point that requires emphasis is that *shock in association with abdominal trauma is due to an abdominal injury until proven otherwise*. Other frequent etiologies of shock after trauma include spinal

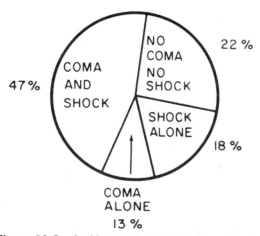

Figure 14–2. *Incidence of coma and shock in 91 patients with combined head and abdominal injuries. (Reproduced with permission from Wilson, C. B., Vidrin, A., Jr., and Rives, J. D.: Unrecognized abdominal trauma in patients with head injuries. Ann. Surg. 161:608, 1965.)*

cord transection, cardiac tamponade, hemothorax, tension pneumothorax, obstructive airway, external blood loss, fractured pelvis, fractured femur and myocardial infarction. *Head injuries do not produce hypotension except in terminal stages.* The possibility of extra-abdominal injuries obviously complicates matters. A 25-year-old patient with hypotension and a single stab wound of the abdomen is certainly less of a diagnostic dilemma than a 60-year-old man who had an accident while driving his car and is admitted unconscious and hypotensive.

Psychosis. Psychotic individuals can be a formidable challenge to the trauma surgeon. Self-inflicted stab and gunshot wounds or ingestion of foreign objects are the most common forms of presentation. Repetitive attempts at self-destruction and an uncooperative attitude may be encountered. Large doses of thorazine in divided doses of up to 400 mg. per day may be required to control such agitated individuals.

DIAGNOSIS

In acute abdominal trauma, the history, physical examination and treatment are integrated and concurrent aspects of total patient care. Of necessity, artificial divisions are employed to facilitate discussion.

History

An accurate history is essential. However, because of urgent requirements for therapy, it may be necessary to gather this information piecemeal. This history may be inaccurate or impossible to obtain. The emotional stress associated with trauma affects both patient and bystanders, especially relatives. Shock, semistupor and drunkenness all tend to prevent a clear recitation of the events leading to hospitalization. Furthermore, a history may be inaccurate because of legal or moral problems raised by the nature of the accident. Therefore, the examiner must always be alert to the possibility of distortion in the history.

Especially pertinent in trauma victims are the time and circumstances of the injury. Knowing the trajectory of the bullet or the direction of a knife thrust can be helpful. The coexistence of systemic diseases should always be sought. General comments that apply to all injured patients will not be discussed further here.

Physical Examination

The physical examination may be complicated by the presence of shock, coma, drunkenness or other conditions that prevent full cooperation on the part of the patient. Associated injuries may mask the presence of abdominal trauma.

The physical examination should be modified to fit the needs of the particular situation. A patient with a gunshot wound of the mid-abdominal region who is in shock does not need a detailed examination of the abdomen in an attempt to document tenderness, guarding or hypoactive bowel sounds since immediate exploration is mandatory; with blunt abdominal trauma, a detailed baseline examination of the abdomen may be critical in making this decision. Repeated examinations by the same observer are often needed to correctly assess the situation. Initially, a cursory examination of the entire patient should be performed to detect any other life-threatening problems. Often, resuscitative measures must be carried out in conjunction with the physical examination. Once the immediate threat to life has been alleviated, a more detailed and methodical examination can be completed.

Location of Wound. In penetrating injuries the location of the wound is of diagnostic importance. Approximately three fourths of all penetrating wounds occur in the upper abdomen.[120] The majority of these are in the left upper quadrant, reflecting the fact that when two assailants face each other, a right-handed opponent is most likely to inflict a left upper quadrant injury.[72, 106] Since many stab wounds are inflicted with relatively short-bladed knives, the location of the wound will help the surgeon to gain a rough idea preoperatively of the extent of the abdominal injury.

Penetrating missiles, such as bullets or bits of wire or stones thrown up from a rotary law mower, may travel in erratic paths through the abdomen, ricochetting from one of the lowermost ribs or vertebral bodies or the inner walls of the pelvis. Nevertheless, knowledge of the wound of entrance, the angle or trajectory of the missile and the wound of exit usually provides significant information as to its intra-abdominal course. If the type of missile used in a shooting assault is known, the surgeon may also know whether to expect a greater or lesser degree of tissue damage. This depends upon whether a rifle, shotgun or pistol was used and whether or not the bullet was soft-tipped and likely to flatten out during tissue penetration.

The back, perineum, rectum and vagina should always be examined for wounds of entrance or exit. The location of the entrance wound, more than its size, may have significant bearing on the decision to perform laparotomy. A tiny puncture wound may have been inflicted by a long, stiletto-like weapon that caused considerable intraperitoneal injury. Patients with stab wounds usually present at the hospital within 4 hours of the time of injury, but a latent asymptomatic period may be present so that there are virtually no physical findings other than a small puncture wound accompanied by minimal tenderness and normal bowel sounds. This fact led to the dictum, practiced by surgeons for many years, that laparotomy is the single most important diagnostic tool in such situations since waiting for the physical signs of hemorrhage or perforation to develop results in higher mortality and morbidity. This concept, however, has been vigorously challenged over the past 12 years by those advocating selective management.

Signs and Symptoms. Physical examination of the abdomen of patients with nonpenetrating injuries presents much greater difficulties. A wide variation in signs and symptoms can occur. A patient may present following an automobile accident with an obvious history of severe blunt abdominal trauma but with virtually no physical findings. At the other extreme is the patient with extensive guarding, rebound tenderness and other strongly suggestive findings with no history of an abdominal blow. The state of consciousness or the presence of other painful injuries may make examination of the abdomen extremely difficult to perform and to evaluate. The presence of profound shock may produce a degree of unresponsiveness in which the injured patient may not complain even during thorough examination.

Discussions in the literature are often devoted to the physical signs resulting from injury to a specific organ. As Fitzgerald and associates[49] have pointed out, such descriptions are necessarily retrospective. When the examiner is confronted with a patient with blunt abdominal trauma, one or more of many organs may have been injured to a greater or lesser degree; the picture is rarely one of a single organ injury. Furthermore, they noted that many descriptions in standard works of reference use classic findings of physical diagnosis more applicable to less acute disease states than external trauma. The signs and symptoms of blunt abdominal trauma result from blood loss, bruising and tearing of solid organs and leaking of irritating juices from hollow abdominal viscera.

Thus, a patient with few or no physical findings may be safely observed or may require laparotomy based upon a high degree of probability of internal injury. Most patients with intra-abdominal injuries exhibit one or more positive signs that aid the examiner. Abdominal rigidity alone warrants exploration in most cases of blunt trauma, despite other known causes for rigidity such as fractured lower ribs or contusions. Rigidity is a variable sign but a dangerous one to ignore. Local infiltration about the fracture site of a broken rib relieves associated pain but does not abolish abdominal guarding or rigidity due to intra-abdominal injury. It may be quite difficult to differentiate intra-abdominal injury from the pain associated with severe contusion of the abdominal wall. Usually the patient with intraperitoneal injury will be able to sit up unassisted and with less abdominal wall pain than the patient with contusion of the subcutaneous tissues and musculofascial planes of the abdomen. When any doubt at all exists, however, it must be assumed that the guarding or rigidity is caused by intraperitoneal injury.

The presence of an abdominal hernia, particularly an umbilical hernia, affords an excellent opportunity to elicit peritoneal signs. We have noted excellent correlation between exquisitely tender umbilical hernias and visceral injuries or blood in the peritoneal cavity.

REFERRED PAIN. Sites of referred pain are frequently helpful in diagnosing intraperitoneal injury. A common site is the shoulder, especially the left shoulder (Kehr's sign) in patients bleeding from a ruptured spleen. Similarly, pain in the right shoulder can result from laceration of the liver. When attempting to elicit shoulder pain, it is useful to place the patient in Trendelenburg's position for a few minutes, thus permitting either blood or chemical irritants from the alimentary canal to collect beneath the diaphragm.

ABDOMINAL MASS. The presence of an abdominal mass following blunt abdominal trauma occurs late in the progression of the clinical picture, as do most physical signs. Such a mass most likely represents a semicontained or subcapsular hematoma of the liver, spleen, mesentery or omentum. The presence of a mass may, however, be an important diagnostic aid in the evaluation of a patient with forgotten or only dimly remembered trauma of days or weeks past.

HEMORRHAGE. Massive intraperitoneal bleeding is associated with shock and demands immediate control. Signs of shifting dullness are late manifestations and not of much help. However, dissection of blood between the leaves of the mesentery or directly into the abdominal wall or retroperitoneal tissues and its eventual appearance in about 3 days as an ecchymosis is a valuable delayed sign. Since such dissection requires a certain period of time to develop, it is usually indicative of slow, steady bleeding or recurrence of bleeding following a period of stability.

AUSCULTATION. Classically, the injured abdomen has been described as silent upon auscultation, and Jarvis,[74] in a review of 128 patients, found no cases of free peritoneal bowel perforation in which peristaltic sounds were audible. Others have noted decreased or absent bowel sounds in 89 per cent of visceral injuries.[72] However, the *presence* of peristaltic sounds is not a reliable sign since it has been demonstrated that normal peristaltic sounds can be heard both in the presence of active intraperitoneal bleeding and following rupture of hollow abdominal organs. Thus, reliance upon the presence of peristalsis as assurance that no intraabdominal injury exists is fallacious and dangerous. However, absence of peristaltic sounds, when carefully sought, should be given serious consideration. Abnormal location of peristaltic sounds has diagnostic importance. Peristaltic sounds heard in the chest in this setting are diagnostic of traumatic diaphragmatic herniation, as discussed in the chapter on chest injuries.

PALPATION. Subcutaneous emphysema of the abdominal wall is most likely the result of an intrathoracic injury. However, rupture of the retroperitoneal duodenum, rupture of any intestine along its mesenteric border or rupture of the distal colon and rectum may produce this finding.

RECTAL AND PELVIC EXAMINATION. Digital examination of the rectum should never be omitted in any patient who has sustained significant trauma. Although the presence of emphysema or gross bleeding is relatively rare, pelvic tenderness may be elicited or the presence of fluid in the pelvis detected. In women, vaginal and bimanual examination are of great aid in detecting the presence of pelvic bleeding or injuries to adjacent viscera following pelvic fracture. Culdocentesis can be helpful in documenting the presence of blood, bile or air in the peritoneal cavity. Other even less common signs of intraperitoneal injury include priapism, which may result from retroperitoneal injuries, especially those involving the spine, or the presence of testicular pain as a sign of retroperitoneal perforation.

INTUBATION. The nasogastric tube and the Foley catheter both serve as important diagnostic and therapeutic aids in the care of the severely traumatized patient. Insertion of a nasogastric tube, or at times a larger Ewald tube, permits decompression of the stomach, removal of gastric contents and prevention of further accumulation of gastrointestinal air or gas. Moreover, the aspirated contents can be checked for blood that, if present, provides a valuable diagnostic clue. The insertion of a Foley catheter into the urinary bladder will provide an immediate specimen of urine that can be examined for blood. A positive test would indicate the need for a cystogram and intravenous pyelography. Instillation of several hundred cubic centimeters of normal saline solution with no return on aspiration would confirm the suspicion of a major bladder rupture, probably in the

dome and communicating with the peritoneal cavity. Following pelvic fractures and
other perineal trauma, the urethra is often
damaged and may be transected. Early insertion of a Foley catheter before the severed urethral ends are displaced will provide an adequate splint and often provide
definitive care of this type of injury.
Undue delay in inserting a Foley catheter
may miss the period when the urethral
ends are still in relatively close approximation. Surgical intervention will then be
necessary to repair the transected urethra.
Aside from its specific diagnostic value,
the use of a Foley catheter enables hourly
monitoring of urine output, which is essential in the management of severely injured patients.

Laboratory Studies

The most valuable laboratory tests in the
evaluation of the patient with abdominal
trauma include a hematocrit and leukocyte
count, urinalysis and serum amylase.
Serum creatinine, glucose and electrolyte
determinations are usually obtained for
baseline values. The diagnosis of massive
hemorrhage is usually fairly obvious and
the hematocrit merely confirmatory. Experience from Vietnam has indicated that
massive hemorrhage of more than 20 per
cent of blood volume is associated with a
rapid plasma refill rate and consequently
early decrease in the hematocrit level.[24] In
cases of hidden massive intraperitoneal
hemorrhage, a low hematocrit early in the
treatment of the patient may, indeed, be
quite significant.

Leukocytosis is commonly associated
with trauma in general, and except for late
evaluation in blunt trauma cases it has little significance. Fifteen thousand cells per
cubic millimeter are commonly seen shortly after injury. Urinalysis will indicate the
presence of bleeding in the genitourinary
tract, the presence of diabetes mellitus or
severe underlying renal disease. The
serum glucose and creatinine are also useful in discovering systemic disease.

Serum amylase values can be normal in
the face of major pancreatic in-
jury,[10, 77, 193, 203] but elevated values give
important information. In the presence of
blunt pancreatic trauma, the serum amylase values are elevated in 48 to 91 per

cent of patients. In the presence of penetrating trauma to the pancreas, the serum
amylase is elevated in 9 to 40 per cent of
cases. Injury to the head of the pancreas is
more commonly associated with elevated
serum amylase than when the tail of the
pancreas is injured. Elevated serum amylase values usually return to normal within
48 hours aftery injury.[193] Elevated amylase
values can also be associated with perforations of the gastrointestinal tract, particularly retroperitoneal ruptures of the duodenum.[15] Gambill and Mason[59] believe
that the determination of the diastase in a
2-hour urine collection is the most reliable
index of pancreatic injury. Increased concentrations of amylase in the peritoneal
fluid following pancreatic injury have
been noted.[82, 138] A peritoneal amylase concentration in the lavage fluid greater than
100 Somogyi units per 100 ml. has been
uniformly diagnostic of injuries to the pancreas or upper small bowel.[138]

Liver function studies are not usually
carried out in patients requiring emergency procedures. However, the presence
of subcapsular hematoma or hematobilia
after injury may require a more sophisticated evaluation. These studies are discussed under liver injury.

Roentgenological Studies. It is necessary to exercise judgment in the use of
roentgenographical aids for the diagnosis
and localization of intra-abdominal injury.
In the presence of shock, resuscitative
measures take precedence over x-ray studies. When laparotomy is clearly indicated,
undue delay caused by unnecessary x-ray
examinations is unwarranted. Nevertheless, when there is adequate time, proper
utilization of x-rays adds much to the precision of diagnosis and planning of therapy.

The basic roentgenographical examination consists of an upright posterior-
anterior chest roentgenogram, an anterior-
posterior supine abdominal film and a left
lateral decubitus abdominal film. If possible, an upright x-ray of the abdomen is
performed, but this often is not feasible in
the seriously injured patient. Careful radiographical technique is essential to provide the proper detail necessary for interpreting subtle findings. Amplification of
these studies by the use of water-soluble
opaque medium often provides important

additional information. X-rays of the pelvis, spine and ribs are obtained as indicated.

A chest x-ray is considered an integral part of the abdominal examination because thoracic injuries are frequently associated with abdominal trauma. Even if no positive findings are demonstrated, the chest x-ray will have provided a valuable baseline study.

A standard approach should be followed in examining roentgenograms in cases of abdominal trauma. The following routine has been useful:

1. Examine the skeletal structures, looking for fractures of the vertebral bodies, transverse processes, pelvis and ribs. Fractures of the transverse process are often associated with retroperitoneal hematomas and left-sided rib fractures with splenic injury.

2. Note any foreign bodies and attempt to determine the trajectory of missiles by correlation with the wound of entrance. The absence of a missile when no exit wound is present connotes peripheral arterial embolization, proximal migration to the right heart and pulmonary artery via the venous system, or entrance into and passage through the gastrointestinal tract.

3. Inspect for free intraperitoneal air, indicative of a ruptured hollow viscus, which may be seen subdiaphragmatically beneath the lateral abdominal wall on a lateral, decubitus film or as the "dome sign," "falciform ligament sign," or the "double wall sign" on a supine film. Both walls of the bowel (inner and outer) stand out sharply when there is air inside and outside of the bowel (Fig. 14–3). Stomach and colon perforations frequently give rise to free air, whereas small bowel perforations only occasionally do so. Positioning the patient for 10 to 15 minutes prior to taking the x-rays will improve the ability to identify free air.

4. Look for the classic "stippling" of retroperitoneal air, usually indicating rupture of the retroperitoneal portion of the duodenum or rectum.

5. Delineate the psoas shadows whose absence may indicate retroperitoneal bleeding.

6. Examine the separation of the gas-filled right or left colon from the properi-

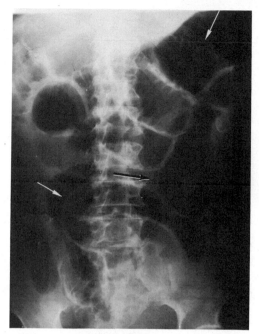

Figure 14–3. *A supine roentgenogram of the abdomen demonstrating the double wall sign. The presence of free intraperitoneal air permits visualization of the small bowel outer wall (arrows).*

toneal fat line, indicating intraperitoneal blood or fluid in the flanks. Also, flotation of the small bowel toward the center of the abdomen, increased space between loops of small bowel and a general ground glass appearance are all compatible with intraperitoneal accumulation of blood. With intraperitoneal bleeding the retroperitoneal structures will remain sharp.

7. Look for enlargement or distortion of the outlines of the spleen, kidneys or liver, indicating a subcapsular hematoma or a hemorrhage confined to that vicinity. A distinctive finding in splenic rupture is medial displacement of the stomach with indentations along its greater curvature caused by hemorrhage into the gastrosplenic ligament (Fig. 14–4). Ingestion of a carbonated beverage with subsequent gastric distension can assist in delineating displacement of the stomach from splenic injury.

Hypaque studies have proven useful in documenting injuries at first suspected on the "routine" films. This applies particularly to perforations of the duodenum. Cystograms and intravenous pyelograms are

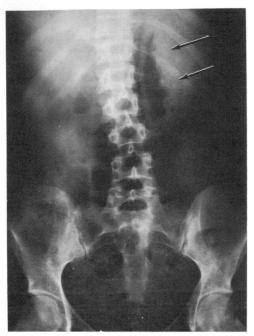

Figure 14–4. *A supine roentgenogram of the abdomen in a patient with rupture of the spleen due to blunt trauma. The arrows indicate medial displacement of the stomach with indentations along the greater curvature due to hematoma in the gastrosplenic ligament.*

needed to assess injuries of the urinary tract. Detailed discussion of these tests is covered in the chapter on genitourinary trauma.

Many experienced observers have noted that roentgenographical examinations provide useful information in less than one third of patients with abdominal injuries.

Nonetheless, any additional information is important, particularly with blunt abdominal trauma where diagnosis is always a difficult challenge. For those interested in a more detailed discussion of diagnostic x-rays in blunt abdominal trauma, McCort's book has a succinct, well-illustrated, pertinent discussion.[111]

Angiography. Norell[127] was the first to use abdominal aortography in blunt abdominal trauma when he diagnosed a splenic rupture by this method in 1957. Since then numerous reports have appeared, with Freeark[51, 55, 56] being the most enthusiastic supporter of this diagnostic approach, encouraging more frequent use of arteriography and emphasizing its usefulness pre-, intra- and postoperatively.

Both false positive and false negative interpretations occur with arteriography, and it has not been effective in the identification or management of injuries to the stomach, small and large intestines or the more peripheral mesenteric vessels. Its primary benefit has been in the evaluation of injuries to the spleen, kidneys, liver, pancreas and duodenum. Selective arteriography provides better visualization and is preferable to mid-stream aortography.[87] Arteriography is indicated in blunt trauma to the abdomen when injuries to the spleen, liver, pancreas, duodenum or kidneys are suspected but the physical examination and the other common diagnostic studies are equivocal. The arteriographic findings are peculiar to each organ injured. For example, splenic injuries display extravasated contrast material (Fig. 14–5), radiolucent

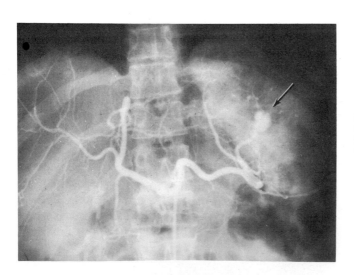

Figure 14–5. *Selective celiac artery arteriogram in a patient with blunt rupture of the spleen demonstrating extravasation of contrast material (arrow).*

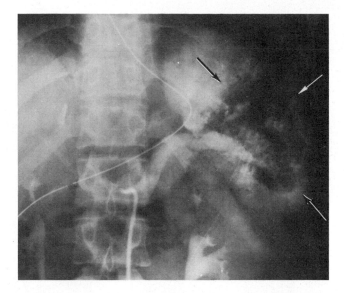

Figure 14–6. *Late phase of a selective celiac arteriogram in a patient with blunt rupture of the spleen. Arrows indicate a filling defect caused by a large intrasplenic hematoma.*

defects due to the hematoma (Fig. 14–6), and arteriovenous shunting manifested by splenic vein opacification 1 or 2 seconds after visualization of contrast material in the splenic artery.

Sinograms. Cornell, Ebert and Zuidema[32] described a method of injecting abdominal stab wounds with water-soluble contrast material in order to determine if the peritoneal cavity had been perforated. At last report, there was one false positive and three false negatives in 192 cases.[207] Sixty-eight demonstrated peritoneal perforation and underwent laparotomy, and 78 per cent of these had significant injuries. Steichen and associates[172] also had success in predicting peritoneal cavity perforation with only one false negative result in 95 patients studied. However, they found that selective management by clinical signs alone resulted in 7.3 per cent "unnecessary" laparotomies, whereas the radiographical technique led to 15.9 per cent laparotomies in which no significant visceral injury was found. Others have reported poor results with frequent false negative tests.[185] The pitfalls in interpreting the study have been discussed.[25] Pain in the area after injection makes it difficult to evaluate abdominal findings, but if the test can be performed with a high degree of accuracy, there is no need for close observation once nonperforation has been demonstrated. The method entails proper antiseptic preparation and draping of the area surrounding the penetrating wound, fol-

lowed by instillation of a local anesthetic. A small (14 F) catheter is inserted through the wound of entry, and the skin edges are tightly secured around the catheter with a purse-string suture. Sixty to 80 ml. of 50 per cent sodium diatrizoate (Hypaque) with 1 ml. of methylene blue added is injected under moderate pressure through the catheter. Recumbent and lateral abdominal roentgenograms will then demonstrate whether the opaque material has passed into the peritoneal cavity (Fig. 14–7) or whether the wound itself was superficial and nonpenetrating. Failure to demonstrate contrast material in the peritoneal cavity is considered reliable evidence that the peritoneum has not been perforated (Fig. 14–8).

Abdominal Paracentesis

A diagnostic study of considerable usefulness, especially in nonpenetrating abdominal injuries, is paracentesis. This examination has been utilized for many years and has proven an invaluable aid in many circumstances. Yurko and Williams[204] indicated that a diagnostic accuracy of 90 per cent can be obtained when needle aspiration of the peritoneal cavity is properly performed. Nonclotting blood withdrawn in the syringe is considered strong evidence of intraperitoneal injury, as is air or bile-stained fluid. In those patients in whom the abdominal paracentesis was positive, the delay between initial examina-

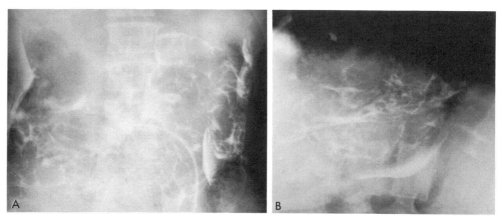

Figure 14–7. A and B, *Injection of 60 ml. of sodium diatrizoate into a stab wound, followed by a roentgenogram in the anteroposterior and lateral positions, reveals penetration of the material into the peritoneal space, outlining the viscera.*

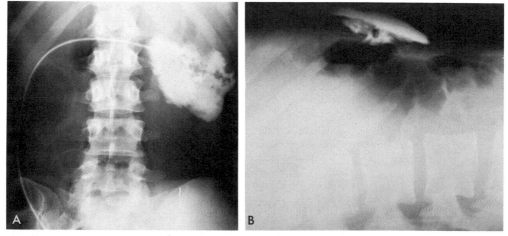

Figure 14–8. A and B, *Injection of the radiopaque material into a stab wound of the left upper quadrant indicates extravasation into the subcutaneous extraperitoneal planes with no intraperitoneal extension.*

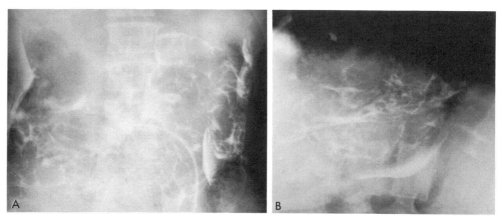

tion and operation was reduced and the need for blood transfusions lowered as compared to patients who did not have paracentesis performed. Others have confirmed these results.[112] All investigators experienced in the technique of abdominal paracentesis have emphasized that *a negative abdominal tap has no diagnostic significance*; that is, one should act as though the study has never been performed.

Certainly, the most useful application of abdominal paracentesis is in patients with other serious injuries, especially craniocerebral ones. These patients, who may be in a coma and have severe respiratory difficulties from flail chest or extensive soft tissue and skeletal injuries, would obviously do better if they could be managed without the extra burden of a laparotomy to rule out intra-abdominal injury. It may be difficult, if not impossible, to determine whether shock is due to other injuries or to occult intraperitoneal bleeding. Paracentesis will usually help the surgeon in making his decision. In some situations abdominal paracentesis may provide the only opportunity to obtain a definitive indication for laparotomy. Wilson and associates[198] not only have emphasized this but also have urged that the paracentesis be repeated throughout the early hours of observation.

The technique for abdominal paracentesis is not difficult. A sterile syringe and a long 18- or 20-gauge spinal needle are the only essential instruments. It is mandatory to have the patient void or to have the bladder emptied by catheterization before needle aspiration. The abdomen is inspected for scars of previous operations or injuries in order to predict and avoid areas where adhesions might be present. The study is contraindicated when the peritoneal space is suspected of being extensively involved with adhesions.

A four-quadrant approach, beginning with the left lower quadrant, is preferred. The sites of penetration are indicated in Figure 14–9. The needle should be introduced lateral to the rectus sheath in order to avoid a hematoma that may easily occur in this muscle because of its close association with the inferior epigastric vessels. Another technique employs aspiration along the lateral gutters to identify the presence of intraperitoneal bleeding.

An initial wheal is made in the skin with 1 per cent Xylocaine using a 25-gauge needle. It is wise to continue infiltration to the level of the peritoneum, including the fascia, if possible. Using a 10-ml. syringe, an 18- or 20-gauge spinal needle with a short bevel is gently inserted through the abdominal wall and peritoneum. It is usually an easy matter to determine whether the peritoneum has been penetrated since there is minimal resistance followed by a slight give to the needle as it enters. At this point, the operator applies gentle suction as the needle is slowly advanced in a lateral direction toward the gutters. Gentle repositioning of the needle within the peritoneal space may permit the withdrawal of a small quantity of fluid. As little as 0.1 ml. of non-

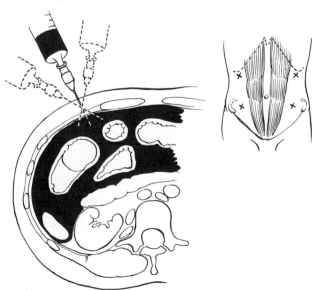

Figure 14–9. *Diagnostic peritoneal tap.*

clotting blood is sufficient evidence of intraperitoneal bleeding. Any nonbloody fluid obtained should be cultured and smeared immediately. The "tap" is repeated in the other quadrants if the first is negative. It is advisable to check the upper abdomen carefully for the presence of either splenomegaly or hepatomegaly prior to paracentesis, which in the upper quadrants should be directed downward to avoid these organs. The authors prefer to aspirate in the following order: left lower quadrant, right lower quadrant, left upper quadrant, right upper quadrant.

If the initial penetration with an 18-gauge needle is negative in the left lower quadrant, some observers prefer to thread a thin polyethylene catheter through the needle into the peritoneal space and then withdraw the needle over the tubing. This permits the catheter to lie either in the left gutter or in the pelvis, and repeated aspiration may be carried out over the subsequent minutes or hours. This has the advantage of permitting continued observation but the disadvantage of not allowing placement of the aspirating tip in different locations. We think it is preferable to aspirate both in different locations and repeatedly, if necessary. The latter is particularly important in patients with multiple-system trauma.

A high degree of accuracy in abdominal paracentesis has not been the experience of all observers. Olsen and Hildreth,[131] in a prospective study comparing abdominal paracentesis versus peritoneal lavage on the same patients, showed that abdominal paracentesis was accurate in diagnosing significant hemoperitoneum in only 21 per cent of cases but that peritoneal lavage was accurate in 100 per cent of cases.

Peritoneal Lavage

Rott first introduced diagnostic peritoneal lavage in 1964.[152-154] In a 5-year experience with 304 patients there were 3 (1 per cent) false positive tests and 9 (3 per cent) false negative tests. The technique involves insertion of a peritoneal dialysis catheter into the pelvis. Under local anesthesia a small lower midline incision is made just below the umbilicus and dissection is carried down to the peritoneum. After carefully securing hemostasis, the peritoneum is opened and the catheter inserted into the peritoneal cavity. If aspiration recovers gross blood, laparotomy is performed. If no blood is recovered, then 1 liter of normal saline solution is infused through the catheter, after which the fluid is siphoned back off into the bottle placed on the floor. In addition to grossly bloody lavage fluid, the following are indicative of a positive tap: more than 500 white blood cells per mm.[3], an amylase over 100 Somogyi units/100 ml., more than 100,000 red blood cells per mm.[3], or bile, bacterial or intestinal contents in the lavage fluid. These additional examinations of the fluid account for 6 per cent of the positive results.

Peritoneal lavage, like paracentesis, is of greatest value in those patients whose physical findings may be difficult to evaluate, when the patient cannot communicate and when there is unexplained hypotension.[138] Its advantages are that it can be quickly performed in bed with the patient in the supine position under local anesthesia with readily available equipment.

Thus, a variety of modalities is available to the examiner to determine whether an intra-abdominal injury is present. The most important tool to the examiner, however, is his awareness of the various injuries that may occur, their potential lethality, as well as the progression of signs and symptoms they produce. A physician suspicious of serious trauma, and prepared to operate if these suspicions are supported by physical examination and the studies described, can at least reduce the consequences of diagnostic error to a minimum.

TREATMENT

Before the treatment of specific individual injuries is discussed, a brief résumé of the prognosis of abdominal injuries and some principles of their initial care will be detailed. Throughout this text it has been repeatedly emphasized that injuries should never be treated as isolated entities, and it has been pointed out that patients with multiple injuries have a higher mortality than those with isolated injuries. Thus, a system of priorities of care should govern the actions of the surgeon who first takes charge of the injured patient in the emergency room. This priority of therapy need not be detailed extensively in this chapter:

cardiorespiratory resuscitation always commands first priority, and relief of airway obstruction is an integral part of these maneuvers; next, control of major hemorrhage must be achieved; and restoration of the intravascular circulating volume follows. Further details are found elsewhere in this text.

Similarly, priority of care of certain types of wounds involving different organ systems is readily established. Aside from rapidly progressive craniocerebral injuries, such as an epidural hemorrhage, or similarly life-threatening situations within the thorax, such as massive continuing hemothorax, *abdominal injuries usually receive highest priority*. There are two reasons for this. First, major hidden hemorrhage is commonly associated with both blunt and penetrating abdominal injury. Second, perforation of the alimentary tract results in peritoneal contamination with all its serious consequences. Confirmation of the degree of severity of the abdominal injury by prolonged observation can be disastrous, but unnecessary celiotomy can be equally calamitous and is never beneficial, especially in those individuals with associated serious injuries. Maturity in judgment, accuracy in diagnosis and therapeutic (surgical) skill are essentials for successful management of abdominal trauma.

Treatment of Penetrating Abdominal Injuries

Gunshot Wounds. With few exceptions[143, 172] most authors agree that gunshot wounds of the abdomen should be explored. It is unusual for a bullet to penetrate the peritoneal cavity and not cause visceral injury.[172] Tangential bullet wounds that apparently miss the peritoneal cavity should usually also be explored, as significant visceral disruption can result from the "blast effect." However, the authors have occasionally observed patients with tangential bullet wounds in the right upper quadrant caused by low-velocity .22 caliber "shorts" and have not had to perform delayed laparotomy. Shotgun injuries manifested by only a few subcutaneous pellets or a widely spread pattern (and probably only scattered single visceral perforations) may be managed conservatively in the absence of signs of bleeding or peri-

tonitis. Otherwise, shotgun wounds are routinely explored.

Nance and associates in a recent review of 1034 patients with gunshot wounds of the abdomen indicated that 5 per cent were managed by observation alone, 13 per cent had negative laparotomies, and 3 per cent had an injury that did not require repair.[122] Thus, theoretically, an operation could have been avoided in 21 per cent of patients. These authors, after a considerable experience with penetrating abdominal trauma, recommend a policy of selective observation. Further confirmatory reports are needed before we can recommend this approach.

Stab Wounds. The present controversy over treating abdominal stab wounds revolves about the "selective management" versus the "routine laparotomy" approach. The 25 to 75 per cent incidence of negative laparotomies has prompted clinicians to develop methods of trying to avoid surgery in those patients without significant injuries. Reports both from those in favor of mandatory exploration for all penetrating injuries[20, 72, 106, 120, 123] and from those proposing more selective management are prevalent in the literature.[31, 57, 105, 114, 121, 143, 148, 158, 168, 172, 173, 176, 183, 194]

Interpretation of the voluminous data available is difficult because case series are often not comparable. Many authors do not distinguish significant from trivial injuries; stab and gunshot statistics are often combined; inclusion of morbidity rates depends on the whim of the investigator; and the incidence of associated injuries varies among series and contributes significantly to the final results. Table 14–4 lists the important points of contention between those advocating routine laparotomy and those proposing more selective methods of management.

Shaftan[158, 159] is credited with popularizing the selective approach to managing penetrating abdominal stab wounds by emphasizing meticulous clinical observation and defining the indications for exploratory laparotomy. Tenderness, rebound, guarding and absent bowel sounds were believed to be the prime indicators for surgical intervention. In his study of 535 patients, 90 per cent of whom had stab wounds, only 28 per cent underwent celiotomy, with a mortality of 7.3 per cent. The nonoperative group had a mortality of 0.5

TABLE 14–4. Points of Contention in the Management of Abdominal Stab Wounds

IMMEDIATE LAPAROTOMY	SELECTIVE MANAGEMENT
75 per cent have visceral injuries.	Only 25 per cent have *significant* visceral injuries.
Delay in treatment is significant.	Minor delays of more than 24 hrs. are probably inconsequential. Most injuries "declare" within 12 hrs.
Negative laparotomy carries a mortality of close to zero.	Negative laparotomy has been associated with a mortality up to 6 per cent.
Morbidity with negative laparotomy is 3 per cent.	Morbidity with negative laparotomy approaches 33 per cent.
Intoxication, drugs and psychosis mask signs and symptoms.	Meticulous clinical evaluation and mature judgment are necessary. Increased risk with general anesthesia.
Lacerations of the diaphragm are often asymptomatic and may lead to herniation.	Late post-traumatic diaphragmatic hernias are not a common problem.
25 per cent of significant injuries initially lack signs of visceral trauma.	Only 5 per cent of those initially observed will require laparotomy.
Medicolegal implications—laparotomy is the accepted mode of therapy.	Minor assaults can become homicides if mortality is associated with negative laparotomy.
0–6 per cent overall mortality.	0–5 per cent overall mortality.

*Those proposing selective management claim that this method keeps the mortality rate the same but decreases the overall morbidity by 50 per cent because of avoiding unnecessary laparotomy.

per cent and the overall mortality was 2.6 per cent. Morbidity of the operated group was 31 per cent versus only 3.3 per cent for those spared operation. He concluded that no deaths could be attributed to delay or failure to recognize the need for abdominal exploration.

Several authors[105, 114, 121] have studied comparable series of "routine" exploration versus selective management, and all document reductions in overall morbidity with the same or improved mortality. Although this approach to managing abdominal stab wounds is a worthy one in terms of decreased morbidity and hospital time, definite risks exist for 5 to 10 per cent of patients with serious abdominal injuries who initially do not present with abdominal findings. Frequent, usually hourly, observations are required. This method lends itself only to situations in which full-time physician coverage is available to fulfill this responsibility. The surgeon who only occasionally treats abdominal trauma will probably serve his patient best by following the approach of routine exploratory laparotomy.

Table 14–5 diagrams the options avail-able in the management of abdominal stab wounds with outcome probabilities. The quoted percentages for the various approaches are approximations derived from numerous publications.

Mandatory indications for immediate laparotomy include:

1. Shock
2. Signs of peritonitis (rebound tenderness, muscle guarding, absent bowel sounds)
3. Gastrointestinal bleeding
4. Free air in the peritoneal cavity
5. Evisceration
6. Massive hematuria

The findings will be present in approximately 20 per cent of all patients with stab wounds admitted to the emergency department. If none of these exists, five alternative avenues of management can be followed:

1. Close observation by the same examiner with laparotomy if evidence of bleeding or peritonitis occurs

TABLE 14–5.   Management of Abdominal Stab Wounds

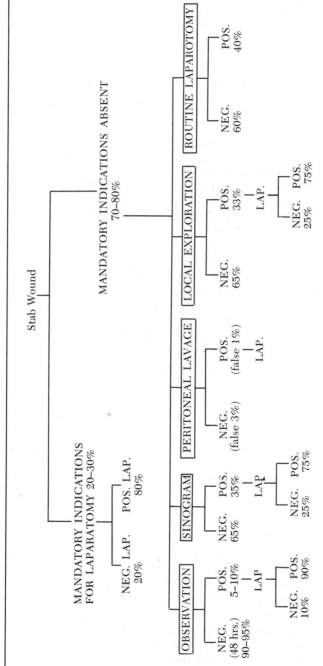

2. Sinogram of the stab wound with laparotomy, if positive

3. Paracentesis, culdocentesis or peritoneal lavage followed by laparotomy, if positive

4. Exploration of the stab wound under local anesthesia proceeding to formal laparotomy, if penetration of the peritoneal cavity is documented

5. Immediate laparotomy

An inflexible approach to managing abdominal stab wounds can be impractical. Each patient's case will involve unique circumstances that must be considered before deciding on the most appropriate diagnostic and therapeutic procedures. A 25-year-old healthy male, who presents 24 hours after a single penknife wound of the abdomen and who is completely asymptomatic and has no abdominal findings, hardly seems suitable for anything other than continued observation. A busy trauma service in a large charity hospital may not have enough personnel either to explore every such patient or to perform hourly examinations; thus, exploration of the wound under local anesthesia might be a reasonable compromise. The surgeon who treats few stab wounds per year and who practices without the support of house staff would probably best manage the healthy young stabbing victim by routine exploratory laparotomy.

An approach to managing abdominal stab wounds that the authors have found useful is as follows:

1. Any patient with mandatory indications for celiotomy (as previously described) undergoes immediate operation.
2. Of the remaining patients:
   a. Those that present within 6 hours of stabbing have exploration of the wound under local anesthesia. If penetration into the peritoneal cavity is confirmed, laparotomy follows.
   b. Those presenting after 6 hours are observed. If questionable abdominal findings are present (a not uncommon circumstance), wound exploration is undertaken.
   c. Any patient who, for reasons of intoxication, narcotic addiction, psychosis or coma, cannot be properly evaluated or observed is also subjected to local wound exploration.
   d. Patients with stab wounds inflicted through the lower rib cage that have probably penetrated the diaphragm are explored because of the risk of herniation through unrepaired diaphragmatic lacerations.
   e. Patients with *multiple* stab wounds seen within the first 12 hours require laparotomy.
   f. Abdominal paracentesis may be done under any of the circumstances dictating local wound exploration but only positive "taps" are accorded any value.

Treatment of Nonpenetrating Abdominal Injuries

The approach to the management of nonpenetrating abdominal injuries is not surrounded with the controversy associated with stab wounds of the abdomen. Nevertheless, there is little question that the early diagnosis and treatment are much more difficult in nonpenetrating injuries. Frequent and repeated examinations of the patient by the same clinician are an absolute prerequisite for good management.

If the patient is not otherwise seriously injured and is alert and cooperative, the physical examination is usually quite reliable in evaluating patients for intra-abdominal trauma. The presence of generalized abdominal pain, rebound tenderness and rigidity usually reflects peritoneal irritation from blood or intestinal contents. These signs or symptoms, when localized to a particular part of the abdomen, indicate damage to subjacent organs. However, similar signs and symptoms may be due to contusions of the abdominal wall or fractured ribs. In blunt abdominal trauma rigidity alone probably warrants exploratory laparotomy. Shock and the suspicion of concealed hemorrhage are usually cause enough for laparotomy. Multiple considerations contribute to the final decision regarding operative intervention. The physical findings, the presence of associated injuries, the time of injury and the results of various diagnostic tests are all integrated into the final decision.

Much of the earlier discussion under diagnosis pertains to blunt abdominal trauma in particular. The discussion in that section of various physical findings and diagnostic procedures will not be detailed again. Although the management of each case must be individualized to fit the circumstances, it is desirable to have a general plan of approach. The basic decision, of course, is whether or not exploratory laparotomy is indicated. The following criteria are formulated to aid in making the decision:

1. Immediate laparotomy is indicated when:
    a. Signs of peritoneal irritation are unequivocal and persist.
    b. X-rays indicate free peritoneal air or rupture of the diaphragm.
    c. Hypotension persists in the absence of other likely causes or is unresponsive to or recurs after appropriate intravenous fluid therapy.
    d. Abdominal paracentesis is positive.
    e. Blood is present within the gastrointestinal tract.
2. Peritoneal lavage is indicated in those:
    a. With equivocal findings.
    b. Who cannot be accurately examined.
3. Scans and arteriograms are performed in those patients without indications for immediate laparotomy but who have findings suggestive of a specific organ injury.
4. Intravenous pyelograms and cystograms are performed routinely in patients with hematuria or flank tenderness and in most patients in whom exploration is planned.
5. All patients are closely followed for the development of new signs and symptoms until the need for operation has been clearly determined. Delayed posttraumatic intestinal obstruction may occur days, weeks or months after blunt abdominal trauma and is the result of cicatricial narrowing of the bowel wall (localized ischemia, intramural hemorrhage, inflammation from bowel perforation), internal herniation or adhesions.[162]

General Measures

Once the decision to operate has been made, the question of timing becomes important. Operations should be delayed as little as possible to prevent deterioration in the clinical situation and an increase in the operative risk. If not already present, a nasogatric tube and a Foley catheter are inserted. Typing and cross-matching of the patient's blood should have been performed by this time, and the responsible surgeon should ascertain that an adequate supply of properly matched blood is available.

If there are associated fractures, it may be necessary to use reasonable, temporary means to immobilize extremities so that the patient may be transported properly to the operating room. It may be necessary to perform a tracheostomy preoperatively in order to assure an adequate airway in patients with severe maxillofacial injuries. Usually, however, an endotracheal tube can be passed quickly, avoiding the necessity of tracheostomy.

If shock ensues, large quantities of fluids are administered rapidly while the blood pressure, pulse pressure pulse rate, central venous pressure and urine output are monitored. Failure of the patient to respond to these resuscitative measures indicates the necessity for operation without delay. Usually, however, a significant response can be obtained. Patients respond better to the trauma of operation, and morbidity and mortality seem to be reduced if reasonable restoration of effective circulating volume can be accomplished preoperatively. One should not hesitate to continue these measures in the operating room in order that the procedure may begin as soon as blood volume replacement seems adequate. This is usually heralded by a rise in the previously subnormal central venous pressure toward normal. The use of a Swan-Ganz catheter to measure pulmonary wedge pressure (indicative of left atrial pressure) is more accurate than central venous pressure in assessing intravascular blood volume, but it is technically more complicated. Both osmotic and loop diuretics should be avoided during the period of volume restoration to treat hypovolemic shock as they interfere with monitoring urine output and may aggravate the hypovolemic state if diuresis ensues.[95] Only if correction of hypovolemia fails to induce adequate urine output should diuretics be used.

Those patients in need of exploration who have a penetrating wound of the thorax should have a thoracostomy tube inserted, regardless of whether or not a hemo- or pneumothorax is present. "Prophylactic" insertion of a chest tube will prevent tension pneumothorax during positive pressure general anesthesia.

Prophylactic Antibiotics

Bowel perforation from external trauma is associated with a high incidence of intra-abdominal abscess, sepsis and wound infection. Indeed, much of the morbidity and mortality from abdominal trauma is the result of infection. Recent appreciation of the normal bowel flora has resulted in a logical use of antibiotics in patients with disruptions of the intestinal tract.[6] The terminal ileum and colon have the highest concentration of bacteria, particularly those of the gram-negative aerobic and anaerobic variety. In the colon the anaerobic bacteria outnumber the aerobes 1000:1, with the anaerobe *Bacteroides fragilis* being the most prevalent.

Experiments have demonstrated that treatment with antibiotics effective against *both* aerobic and anaerobic bacteria decreases the mortality from sepsis and the incidence of intra-abdominal abscess formation in animals challenged with intraperitoneal injections of fecal organisms.[190] Fullen and associates[58] have shown that penicillin and tetracycline started preoperatively significantly decreased the incidence of wound and deep infections after laparotomy for penetrating injuries to the abdomen. Others,[129, 180] using clindamycin and kanamycin or gentamycin in patients with penetrating abdominal trauma, also documented a decrease in wound infection rates.

We use a combination of antibiotics that include clindamycin, which is effective against anaerobes, and gentamycin or kanamycin for the gram-negative rods. Although enterococci are not covered by this regimen, the necessary synergistic relationship for growth of enterococci is effectively inhibited. The antibiotics are immediately administered parenterally to all patients with penetrating abdominal wounds or blunt abdominal trauma when intestinal injury is suspected and a celiotomy planned. Antibiotics are always administered preoperatively to ensure adequate blood levels at the time of operation.

They are continued for an additional 3 to 4 days, unless septic complications ensue and dictate the need for more prolonged treatment.

Operation

In general, endotracheal anesthesia is ideal for allowing as much muscular relaxation as required and permitting the patient to breathe a high percentage of oxygen. The patient is positioned supine with the right side elevated 20 degress if a major liver resection is likely. Placement of a cassette under the patient to allow x-rays to be taken during the operation is worthwhile. While preparing and draping, it is advised to widely expose the chest and groin as well as the abdomen.

Planning the incision and the operative maneuvers is important. Thoroughness, efficiency and controlled speed are the bywords of abdominal exploration for trauma. Patients do not fare well when unduly prolonged operative trauma is superimposed upon their original injuries. Nevertheless, it is important not to miss an intra-abdominal injury. This can occur especially when more than one injury is present.

Midline incisions permit exploration of the entire intraperitoneal contents and management of whatever injuries may be encountered. Occasionally, extension of such an incision upward into the chest may be indicated for the management of injuries to the liver or, less frequently, the spleen. Rarely, a lateral limb to the left or right is needed to improve exposure. The midline incision also has the advantages of rapid execution and less bleeding.

Once the peritoneal space has been entered, one of two alternative situations usually presents itself. First, bleeding may be voluminous and continuing. Any hemorrhage noted to be coming from a specific area should be immediately controlled, but often the abdomen is filled with blood and its source is not obvious. Under these circumstances, *immediate compression of the aorta as it passes through the diaphragm*, either manually or with a sponge stick, can provide those few extra minutes of protection for volume restoration and definitive hemostasis. Otherwise, in the absence of significant hemorrhage, an orderly sequence of abdominal exploration that varies little from patient to patient can be performed so that no injury will remain undetected. It is usually advisable to repeat this exploration at the conclusion of the operation.

The authors prefer to begin this exploration with the left lobe of the liver and the esophageal hiatus. The fundus of the stomach is examined next, followed by the spleen and the splenic flexure of the colon. The left kidney is palpated carefully, and the distal half of the pancreas examined. Next the descending colon, sigmoid colon and cul-de-sac are inspected, as is the mesentery of the sigmoid colon. In women the pelvic organs should be carefully examined. Following inspection of the cecum, ascending colon and hepatic flexure, a careful view of the right lobe of the liver over its dome and the diaphragmatic surface can be carried out. Attention is then directed to the gallbladder and biliary apparatus as well as the undersurface of the right lobe of the liver. The head of the pancreas, the lesser curvature of the stomach, pylorus and proximal duodenum are examined, as is the right kidney. If indicated, a Kocher maneuver is performed to fully examine the duodenum. The surgeon should provide enough exposure so that the foramen of Winslow can be seen. Blood may be seen escaping from the lesser sac into the peritoneal cavity. If this is true or if any doubt of its integrity exists, the lesser sac may be examined by dividing the gastrocolic omentum. There remain the transverse colon and the small intestine to inspect. It is most important to look at the base of the transverse mesocolon as well as the root of the mesentery of the small intestine for possible major vascular injuries. Also, at this juncture, the aorta and inferior vena cava should be carefully examined for small hematomas that may signify partially contained areas of hemorrhage. If these are penetrating injuries of the intestines, the surgeon must assure himself that there is an even number of perforations, or prove that the injury to the intestine is tangential or that the penetrating missile is inside the bowel lumen. Otherwise, a small perforation may be missed. This is extremely important since a small perforation into the mesenteric surface of the small intestine may be easily overlooked. Filling the abdominal cavity with saline and compres-

sion of the small intestine can help identify bowel perforations. After careful inspection of the diaphragm for perforations, the exploration is completed.

Once the intra-abdominal portion of the operation has been concluded, the abdomen is closed. Some surgeons prefer to lavage the peritoneum with large quantities of sterile saline solution. The use of antibiotics, especially neomycin in large doses in the irrigating solutions, has resulted in rapid absorption and respiratory depression in some patients. Smaller doses of neomycin do not appear to cause this, but its usefulness in such situations may be questioned. Cephalothin instillation has not been effective.[145] Two double-blind, randomized clinical studies, one by Noon and associates[125] using kanamycin sulphate and bacitracin and another by Brockenbrough and Moylan[18] using kanamycin only, both show a 50 per cent decrease in infections with the use of these antibiotics. Although a categorical recommendation with regard to the use of antibiotics cannot be made at this time, thorough irrigation of the peritoneal cavity with copious amounts of isotonic saline solution is advised.

The niceties of layer closure are of no advantage following exploration for abdominal trauma. The risk of infection is great, and these patients' abdomens tend to become distended and they can develop respiratory complications that necessitate forced coughing and often tracheal aspiration. Therefore, the linea alba and peritoneum should be closed with a single layer of interrupted figure-of-eight sutures of No. 28 wire. The ends of the cut wire should be turned into the fascia to prevent discomfort to the patient caused by their projection into the subcutaneous tissues. Retention sutures are used in very obese patients when massive contamination has occurred or when very rapid abdominal closure is necessary. The skin is left open and packed with saline-wetted fine-mesh gauze if contamination has occurred.

The use of drains has been thoroughly discussed in the surgical literature on trauma. Recent studies have shown that in 17 of 50 patients with prophylactic drains placed during laparotomy, there were definite skin contaminants on the insides of the drain ends.[126] In general the authors prefer to drain the retroperitoneum when a hematoma has been evacuated or when significant quantities of nonviable tissue have been excised if there has been contamination by spillage from the intestines. However, drainage of the peritoneal space itself is usually not necessary or even advisable. However, drainage is necessary when significant wounds of the liver have required repair or resection. Draining of the left upper quadrant after splenectomy may prevent the accumulation of serum or blood under the left hemidiaphargm, but there may be a greater incidence of subphrenic abscess following drainage. Unless a significant accumulation is expected, the authors prefer not to insert drains following splenectomy. If the pancreas has been injured, drainage is mandatory. The use of soft rubber sump suction catheters for draining the liver or pancreas represents a distinct improvement. Drains should never be placed in contact wih skeletal structures or intestinal suture lines. Separate stab incisions should be used to bring abdominal drains to the outside.

Bullets removed by individuals should be scored by the surgeon with his initials for later identification in court.

ABDOMINAL WALL

Hematoma

Injury to the abdominal wall alone occasionally produces clinical findings that suggest injury to intra-abdominal organs. Pain, anorexia, nausea, vomiting, tenderness, guarding and rigidity may all be associated with a hematoma of the abdominal wall. This hematoma is usually the result of hemorrhage inside the rectus sheath and may be caused by rupture of the rectus muscle or tears of the epigastric vessels. If the hematoma occurs below the line of Douglas, it may dissect through the extraperitoneal tissues of the pelvis and produce signs of pelvic peritoneal irritation.[78] Rarely, the extravasation of blood is sufficient to produce hypovolemia and shock. The fact that the hematoma is limited to the confines of the rectus sheath is of diagnostic help. Also, an abdominal mass that is palpable as the patient sits up and tenses his rectus muscle but that cannot be moved from side to side (Bouchacourt's sign) is more likely to be within the abdominal wall. Bluish discoloration of the skin over the abdominal mass

suggests hematoma; however, the color change is usually not seen for several days after the bleeding, unless the anterior rectus sheath has been disrupted.

A patient may have severe intra-abdominal wounds in addition to an abdominal wall hematoma. In most instances it is safer to explore the peritoneal cavity if the diagnosis is uncertain. If more serious injuries have been excluded and the hematoma is not large, the condition may be treated nonoperatively by rest and heat applications. Since most patients with abdominal wall hematomas require laparotomy for diagnosis, it is usually preferable to evacuate the hematoma and ligate any bleeding points. The rectus sheath may then be repaired and drainage established if necessary.

Penetrating Injuries

Penetrating wounds of the abdominal wall itself are ordinarily relatively easy to manage. Follwing excision or debridement and thorough irrigation, they may be closed primarily, closed over a drain, or simply drained — depending upon the size and nature of the wound. Large defects of the abdominal wall, such as those that result from shotgun blasts at close range, must be adequately debrided and packed. Pedicle flaps of skin and subcutaneous tissue can be used to cover defects, but at times only packing of the defect with later skin grafting on the granulating bowel surface is feasible. If adequate primary closure is not possible without tension, Marlex mesh can be used to close large abdominal wall defects, even in the presence of infection. Once the bowel is fixed in position and covered, the Marlex is removed and skin grafts are applied. At times the wound will properly heal with the Marlex left in place.

DIAPHRAGM

Trauma to the diaphragm is discussed in the chapter on thoracic injuries. However, because diaphragmatic perforations are frequently associated with injuries to intra-abdominal viscera, it is the abdominal surgeon who sees the majority of these injuries.

All perforations require closure because

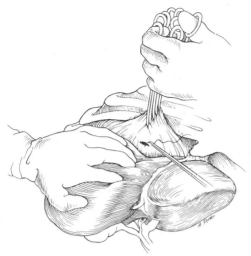

Figure 14–10. *Exposure of the undersurface of the right hemidiaphragm is facilitated by the sequential application of long clamps which mobilize the diaphragm forward.*

of the potential for subsequent herniation and, in conjunction with liver injuries, the risk of a biliary-pleural fistula. Left hemi-diaphragmatic injuries are usually easily identified. Right hemidiaphragm injuries, lying far posteriorly, are identified by palpation and exposure with difficulty. A method of facilitating exposure involves pulling the diaphragm forward by the sequential application of long clamps to the under-surface of the diaphragm (Fig. 14–10). Interrupted sutures of heavy silk are used for closure.

Low-velocity wounds located in the bare area of the liver are not usually explored or repaired. Spillage of intestinal contents through a laceration in the diaphragm requires thorough irrigation of the hemithorax before closure.

SPLEEN

The spleen is the intra-abdominal organ most frequently injured by blunt trauma (Fig. 14–11) and also is often lacerated by penetrating wounds of the left upper quadrant.[64] Massive intra-abdominal hemor-

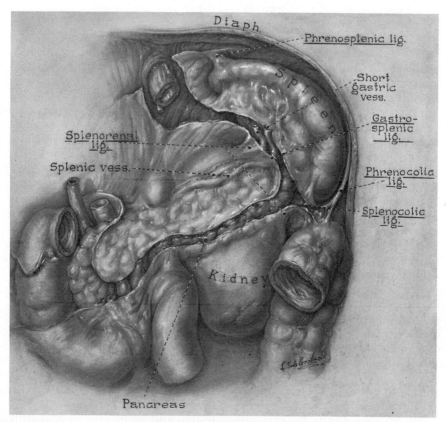

Figure 14–11. *Tears of the friable, vascular spleen occur easily at the sites of ligamentous attachments, especially in the presence of splenomegaly. (From Ballinger, W. F., II, and Erslev, A. J.: Splenectomy. In Current Problems in Surgery, February, 1965. Used by permission of Year Book Medical Publishers.)*

rhage commonly occurs from injuries to this friable, vascular organ. The seriousness of splenic injury is adequately emphasized by the fact that the mortality rate is approximately 10 per cent; in the presence of multiple organ injury, the mortality increases to between 15 and 25 per cent.[12] In one series, isolated splenic injury occurred in only 20 per cent of patients.[138] Delayed diagnosis of a ruptured spleen contributes significantly to the mortality. The treatment of an injured spleen is nearly always splenectomy.

Signs and Symptoms

The signs and symptoms of ruptured spleen are, in general, those associated with intra-abdominal bleeding and vary according to the severity and rapidity of hemorrhage, the presence of other injuries and the time between injury and examination. The responsible injury may have been trivial and forgotten by the patient; this is especially true in children. Usually, however, the patient is seen because of and soon after a specific episode of trauma. Ordinarily, there is a generalized abdominal pain and nausea. The patient may have vomited. Pain localized to the left upper quadrant is noted in about 30 per cent of these patients. The reported incidence of pain at the tip of the left shoulder (Kehr's sign) has varied from 15 to 75 per cent. This sign can often be elicited in patients with ruptured spleens if gentle, bimanual compression of the left upper quadrant is performed after the patient has been in the Trendelenburg position for several minutes. Tachycardia, hypotension, or both, may be present. Palpation of the abdomen usually reveals tenderness and muscle spasm, especially in the left upper quadrant. Rebound tenderness is often greater than direct tenderness in this area. Rarely, a tender mass can be palpated below the left costal margin, and occasionally an area of fixed dullness in this region may be outlined by percussion (Ballance's sign) when a large extra- or subcapsular hematoma or mass of adherent omentum is present.

The white blood cell count rises rapidly after splenic injury, and leukocytosis with white cell counts between 12,000 and 30,000 is the rule rather than the exception. The initial hematocrit level may not

be helpful, but a progressive decrease should suggest intra-abdominal hemorrhage, even though the source of bleeding is not apparent. Many patients with ruptured spleens are first seen during the early period when examination may be relatively unrevealing. These patients may be dismissed, especially when there has been seemingly trivial blunt trauma, only to present later with serious hypovolemia. This error can usually be avoided if asymptomatic patients who have incurred nonpenetrating abdominal injury are observed for at least a period of 4 or more hours during which time careful examination is repeated frequently. Within this period, most patients with ruptured spleens will demonstrate one or more of the following:

1. Tenderness to compression below the left costal margin
2. Left shoulder pain while in the Trendelenburg position
3. Tenderness or guarding in the left flank, and
4. Some abdominal distention.

Any patient in whom one or more of these signs is elicited should be observed further and should have x-ray examinations and abdominal paracentesis. X-ray findings that suggest splenic injury include an increased splenic shadow, and loss of the normal outline of the spleen, the left kidney or the left psoas muscle. The left half of the transverse colon may be depressed or the stomach shifted to the right. The greater curvature of the stomach may be serrated as a result of extravasation of blood into the gastrosplenic ligament (Fig. 14–4). Fractures of the lower left ribs, a bloody left pleural effusion or a hematuria should also arouse suspicion of a concomitant splenic injury.

Diagnosis

Despite precautions, the correct diagnosis is not made in a significant number of patients with this injury. It has been estimated that from 15 to 30 per cent of nonpenetrating splenic injuries result in delayed rupture.[166] The interval between injury and the onset of abdominal hemorrhage is called the latent period of Baudet. About 75 per cent of cases of delayed hem-

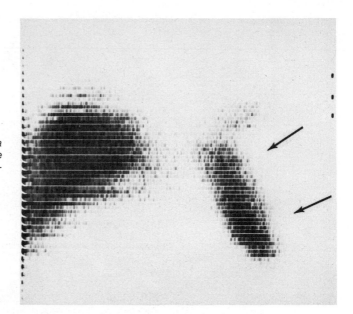

Figure 14-12. *Radioisotope scan of a ruptured spleen demonstrating a large lateral filling defect (arrows) due to the formation of a hematoma.*

orrhage become manifest during the first 2 weeks following injury. Some of the patients with delayed rupture will have forgotten the responsible trauma. This "delayed rupture" may represent more a missed diagnosis than an actual delayed hemorrhage.[132]

Automobile-pedestrian accidents are the most common cause of nonpenetrating splenic injury; abdominal blows during fights and bicycle accidents are also common causes. Spontaneous rupture of the spleen is extremely rare, and even then, it usually occurs in an enlarged, diseased spleen. An apparently slight, forgotten injury almost certainly precedes rupture of a normal spleen.

Splenic puncture is frequently used for measurement of portal pressures and for the injection of radiopaque material into the portal venous system. Occasionally, this results in laceration of the splenic capsule with continued bleeding. Few complications have been reported if the patient remains apneic during the procedure.

Splenic scintiscans[133, 191] (Fig. 14-12) and selective splenic artery angiograms[87] (Figs. 14-5 and 14-6) can provide useful information in a significant portion of individuals with obscure diagnostic features. False negative and false positive results can occur with both methods.

Treatment

If suspicion is high that the spleen has ruptured, operation should not be delayed. Blood and electrolytic solutions are administered intravenously during preparation for laparotomy. A left subcostal incision provides ideal exposure for splenectomy, but if injury to other intra-abdominal organs is suspected, a vertical midline incision is probably preferable (Fig. 14-13). The latter incision also permits more rapid entry into the peritoneal cavity and is therefore advantageous in the hypotensive patient. Once the peritoneal cavity has been entered, the left hand is placed over the diaphragmatic surface of the spleen, gently retracting it downward. If adhesions are present, this maneuver is not possible. The splenocolic ligament is brought anteriorly and divided. This ligament and the splenorenal and splenophrenic folds, which are divided next, are usually avascular and need not be clamped. If portal hypertension or congestive splenomegaly is present, numerous vessels that require ligation may pass through these folds.

When the ligaments have been divided, the spleen is rotated forward and medially and delivered into the wound. In the presence of profuse bleeding from the spleen,

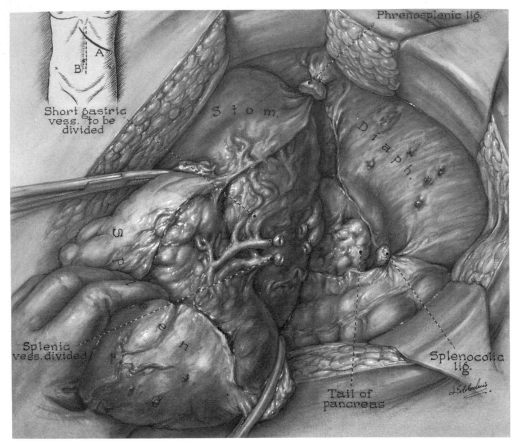

Figure 14–13. *Technique of splenectomy. (From Ballinger, W. F., II, and Erslev, A. J.: Splenectomy. In* Current Problems in Surgery, *February, 1965. Used by permission of Year Book Medical Publishers.)*

these maneuvers are performed rapidly and the vessels of the splenic hilum are controlled by finger compression. The short gastric vessels in the gastrosplenic omentum are divided between clamps and ligated.

The vessels in the hilum of the spleen may then be carefully isolated, clamped, divided and ligated without injury to the tail of the pancreas. The spleen is removed and the entire area inspected again for additional bleeding sites. In patients in whom the damaged spleen is solidly adherent to the diaphragm and the lateral abdominal wall, hemorrhage may be controlled by first compressing and then ligating the splenic artery at the celiac axis or on its course along the superior border of the pancreas. At these sites, the artery can be rapidly exposed by entering the lesser sac through the gastrocolic omentum. It is not necessary to ligate the splenic vein at

this stage. The spleen is then mobilized deliberately by careful division of the diaphragmatic and abdominal wall adhesions. The splenic vessels are individually divided and ligated at the hilum after the spleen has been completely freed of its attachments. Drainage of the splenic fossa is usually not necessary unless there is associated injury to the pancreas. Prolonged prophylactic drainage of the left subphrenic space increases the incidence of abscess formation and drain tract infection.[130] If there is considerable oozing from the diaphragm, sump suction catheters or closed-system vacuum catheters are inserted and then removed after 48 hours.

Complications peculiar to splenectomy itself are few. Postoperative pancreatitis is not uncommon but usually subsides spontaneously. The potential of postoperative thrombocytosis leading to thrombosis has probably been overemphasized, but must not be ignored.[197] Temporary anticoagulation therapy should be considered if the platelet count rises to 1,000,000 or more. Splenic vein thrombosis with extension of the process into the portal vein is a rare complication today.

An interesting complication of splenic injury is "splenosis." This condition is characterized by the finding of numerous nodules of splenic tissue upon various peritoneal surfaces and is thought to represent autotransplantation of small pieces of a ruptured spleen. In 1972, Trimble and Eason[186] were able to find 55 cases in the literature. Although splenosis is usually harmless, intestinal obstruction may occur if implants on adjacent loops of bowel become adherent.[61]

There is clearly an increase in overwhelming sepsis and mortality following splenectomy.[34] This occurs primarily in children less than 3 years old. *Diplococcus pneumoniae* is the most frequently recovered organism (50 per cent of cases). The increased infection rate has been attributed primarily to the underlying pathology leading to planned splenectomy.[45] On the other hand, a controversy presently exists as to whether or not there is an increased incidence of sepsis after splenectomy *for trauma* in children. Infection rates in patients after splenectomy for trauma have been reported to be almost 60 times greater than in controls,[165] with a mortality rate of 70 per cent.[11] This has caused some surgeons to advocate, in selected cases, repair of injured spleens by suture, partial resection or application of microcrystalline collagen powder.[40, 117, 118] Other reports have indicated no relationship between splenectomy for trauma and subsequent sepsis.[43-45, 65, 134]

Our current practice is to attempt salvage of spleens with minimal injury that are not actively bleeding in children less than 4 years in age and to remove all other spleens. With patients younger than 4 years who require splenectomy, prophylactic oral penicillin therapy is administered for 2 years. In asplenic adults oral penicillin or ampicillin is immediately started at the first sign of infection. A possible alternative to long-term prophylactic antibiotics is a pneumococcal vaccine that has recently been used in patients with sickle-cell anemia and splenectomy.[4] Fur-

ther experience is required before this approach can be recommended.

LIVER

Liver injuries encountered in civilian practice today vary from simple superficial lacerations to deep hepatic fractures with massive tissue disruption and destruction. In spite of the protection afforded by the lower ribs, the liver's size, weight, consistency, location and attachments make this organ particularly susceptible to injury from blunt trauma. Its size alone makes it the organ most frequently injured with penetrating injuries to the abdomen (Table 14–2).

In recent years, blunt trauma and gunshot wounds have been more common causes of liver injury than stab wounds. In large series of liver injuries, the mortality rate associated with knife wounds is 3 per cent, gunshot wounds, 18 per cent, and blunt trauma, 30 per cent.[97, 119] The patient's general condition, the number of associated injuries and the delay between injury and treatment influence the results of treatment.

The monograph by Madding and Kennedy[101] is recommended for those interested in a complete and thorough review of the subject of liver injuries. An understanding of the surgical anatomy of the liver is essential for surgeons contemplating major hepatic resections. Several authors have adequately described the details of liver anatomy as it applies to hepatic resection.[65, 119]

Treatment

The major goals in the management of liver trauma are control and prevention of bleeding and bile drainage, removal of all severely damaged and nonviable liver tissue, and adequate wound drainage. Ideally, the operative treatment of liver trauma includes one or a combination of the following: (1) suture, (2) drainage, (3) resection and (4) hepatic artery ligation.

Suture. Cleanly incised, superficial lacerations of the liver, similar to a hepatic biopsy wound, may be treated by suture only. All other hepatic injuries must be adequately drained. Madding[99] has stated that external drainage represents the most important step in the treatment of hepatic injury, and Sparkman and Fogelman[170] have emphasized that the size and appearance of a liver wound are not reliable indications of the probability of subsequent bile drainage. The possibility of preventing bile peritonitis or abscess by adequate drainage seems to make the omission of this simple procedure unwarranted. Lacerations with little surrounding devitalized tissue, such as stab wounds and small bullet wounds that are not bleeding, may be treated with external drainage alone. This can be accomplished with several soft rubber drains leading from the area of injury to the outside through a stab wound in the abdominal wall. Subsequent hemorrhage from simple hepatic wounds that are not bleeding at the time of exploration is unusual, and biliary drainage ordinarily stops after a few days. Suturing nonbleeding wounds is unnecessary and it may cause resumption of bleeding that is difficult to control. Also, the closure of the superficial portion of a deep wound may cause the accumulation of bile or liquefied blood clots and necrotic tissue within the liver and lead to hepatic abscess or hemobilia.

Drainage. Hepatic wounds associated with bleeding that cannot be stopped by individual vessel ligature require either suture or resection in addition to drainage. The combination of suture and generous drainage provides adequate treatment for most liver wounds. When wounds are so situated that hemostasis and closure of raw surfaces can be accomplished by suture, this method is most satisfactory. If possible, bleeding vessels should be individually ligated before wound edges are approximated. Deep lacerations should be closed loosely around a soft rubber drain placed into the depths of the wound. This acts to prevent hematoma and dead space.[170]

The use of biliary decompression by T-tube drainage of the common bile duct, or occasionally cholecystostomy, is controversial. This method was advocated by Merendino et al.[116] for all but the most peripheral liver injuries. They contended that decompression of the common bile duct would decrease biliary fistula formation and intraperitoneal bile collection and prevent lysis of blood clots secondary to bile stasis. Moreover, it provides a method

for checking bile leaks during surgery and permits cholangiograms in the postoperative period when abscess formation, hematobilia or jaundice occurs.

Several authors[50, 94, 97, 137] have criticized routine common bile duct drainage. Lucas and Ledgerwood[96] in a prospective randomized study demonstrated an increase in biliary cutaneous fistula, septic jaundice, cholangitis, intra-abdominal abscess, wound infection and gastric bleeding after T-tube drainage of the common bile duct in patients with major penetrating injuries to the liver. The disadvantages of controlled extrahepatic biliary drainage include the difficulty in inserting T-tubes in normal, small, common bile ducts and the possibility of later stricture formation, plus the increased incidence of stress ulcers as noted by Foster et al.[50] Our recommendation at this time is that common bile duct drainage be reserved for major resections, provided that the common bile duct diameter is larger than 5 mm.

The use of packing, except for temporary intraoperative control of bleeding, is generally condemned. The packing of liver wounds with nonabsorbable material leads to necrosis, prevents bile drainage, is followed by significant bleeding when the packs are removed, and is associated with increased mortality and morbidity. More recently, others have advised avoiding the use of hemostatic agents such as Gelfoam and Oxycel for packing liver defects.[110] These materials also act as foreign bodies and as such predispose to necrosis and infection. The cautious use of small amounts of hemostatic materials in conjunction with various suture techniques to control hemorrhage in difficult situations does not seem unreasonable and is probably more realistic than the absolute condemnation of such substances; also the gauze pack is valuable for the temporary control of bleeding during operation, although it must not be used as definitive treatment. Most hepatic wounds that would require large amounts of packing for control of hemorrhage are better resected or treated with hepatic artery ligation.

Intrahepatic hematomas are best treated by evacuation and adequate drainage. Likewise, it is advisable to explore, in most cases, subcapsular hematomas to locate and secure the site of bleeding. Formidable hemorrhage can occur in these situations, but it is better controlled at that time under direct vision rather than encountered days or weeks later when the abdomen is closed and rupture occurs.

Resection. Some surgeons have advocated the more liberal use of hepatic resection because of the excessive morbidity and mortality following conservative suture and drainage of bursting liver wounds.[22, 109, 144] The techniques of hepatic resection are those outlined by the Quattlebaums, Byrd and McAfee,[23] and McClelland and associates.[109] Exposure through a long vertical laparotomy incision is usually adequate. Depending upon the area of injury, the right or left triangular ligament is divided and the liver retracted inferiorly and medially. If this does not provide satisfactory access, the abdominal incision is extended obliquely into the right chest, usually through the sixth intercostal space. The diaphragm is then opened radially or around its perimeter to avoid injury to major branches of the phrenic nerve. Massive hepatic hemorrhage can be controlled in most instances by temporary packing and occlusion of the portal triad in the hepatoduodenal ligament with the fingers or a padded clamp (Pringle maneuver). The periods of occlusion probably should not exceed 15 minutes unless hepatic hypothermia has been instituted and not more than 5 to 10 minutes in the presence of shock.

If a total lobectomy is required, the porta hepatis is dissected next and the hepatic artery, portal vein and bile duct to the injured lobe are ligated and divided. Opening the common duct and inserting a probe into the appropriate hepatic duct is often helpful in the location and dissection of the lobar structures. Since the common duct will be drained at the end of the procedure, this step is not superfluous. When sublobar resection is to be performed, ligation of the vessels in the porta hepatis is omitted. The line of resection is then chosen, based on the more recent concepts of hepatic anatomy[69] (Fig. 14–14). A plane of resection passing through the falciform ligament should be avoided since branches of the left hepatic artery, portal vein and biliary ducts are especially profuse in this region (Fig. 14–15).

To resect the lateral segment of the left lobe, a line 1 to 2 cm. to the left of the falciform ligament is chosen (Fig. 14–16A). The entire left lobe may be removed by dividing the liver along a plane extending from the left gallbladder margin to a point just to the left of the vena cava (Fig. 14–16B). The plane for total right lobectomy crosses the liver from the right margin of the gallbladder to the right side of the vena cava (Fig. 14–16C). Use of these planes spares the middle hepatic vein in right and left lobectomies.

The so-called extended right lobectomy requires a line of division running from the left gallbladder margin to the right side of the vena cava. Here the middle hepatic vein, which courses in the hepatic tissue beneath the gallbladder fossa and above the vena cava, must be divided near its

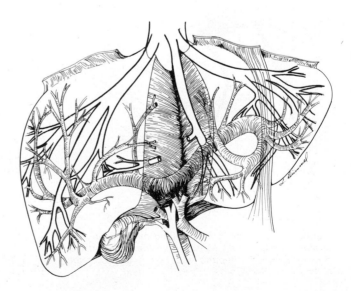

Figure 14–14. *Intrahepatic anatomy. The liver is opened in the interlobar plane. The intrahepatic anatomy of the portal and hepatic venous systems is depicted. The middle hepatic vein lies in the interlobar plane and joins with the left hepatic vein proximal to the vena cava. The umbilical portion of the left portal vein is visualized in the plane of the falciform ligament. This plane is the division between medial and lateral segments of the left lobe. (From Donovan, A. J., Turrill, F. L., and Facey, F. L.: Hepatic Trauma. Surg. Clin. North Am. 48:1313, 1968.*

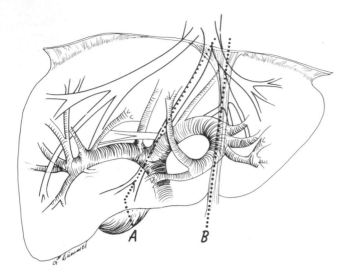

junction with the left hepatic vein, and great care must be taken to preserve the adjacent left hepatic vein. The vena cava usually receives three to five hepatic veins. The portions of these veins between the liver and vena cava are short and thin, and it is difficult to determine the area drained by each. It is therefore safer to divide the veins within the liver rather than at the cava. It is important when exposing the juncture of hepatic veins with the inferior vena cava that undue torsion not be applied for fear of occluding the inferior vena cava and acutely obliterating venous return from the lower portion of the body. After the line of resection has been chosen, long curved needles may be used to place rows of interlocking sutures of heavy chromic on either side of the intended line. Bluntly dissecting the tissues with a knife handle as suggested by the Quattlebaums[144] allows the blood vessels and bile ducts to be individually identified and ligated before division. This substantially reduces blood loss and bile drainage. When the liver has been divided to the depth of the first layer of sutures, a second tier is placed and blunt dissection is continued. These maneuvers are repeated until division is completed. Additional ligatures and sutures are then placed as needed. The raw area of liver can be covered with the falciform ligament or omentum to obliterate dead space. Rubber suction tubes and several soft rubber drains are placed in the bed of the resected liver and adjacent to the remaining raw surface and brought through the abdominal wall via a small subcostal incision. Drains are advanced slowly, beginning about the fifth postoperative day, and are usually out by the tenth day following operation. They are not removed if continued drainage is significant. In addition to anterior drains, McClelland et al.[109] place drains through the bed of the resected twelfth rib, thereby effecting a through-and-through drainage of the area. As mentioned, a T-tube or rubber catheter is placed in the common duct and exteriorized through a separate stab incision.

Inf. vena cava

Middle hepatic v.

R. hepatic v.

L. hepatic v.

R lobe

Left

lobe

c.

b.

a.

Gall bladder Portal v. Falciform lig.

Figure 14–16. Diagram indicating major lobar and sublobar vascular divisions within the liver and the optimal planes for hepatic resection. A, B and C refer to lines of resection described in the text.

Smaller and easily accessible areas of devitalized tissue can be treated by resectional debridement.[141] The area of damage is excised between rows of tiers of interlocking catgut sutures, blunt dissection is used and, if possible, vessels are individually ligated before division. No attempt is made to close the defect and the area is well drained.

A word of caution is needed for those embarking on major liver resections. Despite favorable reports on their use, major hepatic resections are associated with significant risks and mortality and should be reserved for massive destruction or uncontrollable hemorrhage. Morton and associates[119] performed extensive resections in only 3 per cent of cases and noted an overall mortality rate similar to those who performed major resections three times as often. The niceties of an anatomical dissection as described by the Quattlebaums[144] or Madden and Brunschwig[98] are not always practical or feasible under some circumstances. Often simple hand compression of the liver by an assistant with the hepatic and portal blood supply occluded will permit a rapid resection followed by suture ligation of vessels and bile ducts.[48]

Hepatic Artery Ligation. Madding and Kennedy[102] have reviewed the use of hepatic artery ligation in hepatic trauma. Hepatic resection is certainly a formidable undertaking and the easier method of ligating the hepatic artery is often effective in controlling hemorrhage in many cases. The risk of hepatic necrosis is small, especially if the common hepatic artery is ligated proximal to the gastroduodenal or right gastric branches. Ligation of the right or left hepatic arteries probably carries more risk than ligation of the common hepatic artery but less than ligation of the proper hepatic artery. Cholecystectomy is indicated when the right hepatic artery is ligated. Mays[108] has demonstrated that lobar dearterialization is a safe and effective method of securing liver hemostasis. Rearterialization occurs in 7 to 10 days from the uninjured lobe via subcapsular arteries. During this period the patient is fasted and continuous glucose and albumin infusions are administered. Blood glucose and serum sodium levels as well as SGOT, SGPT and LDH values are monitored to detect evidence of liver necrosis. Hepatic arterio-

grams, cholangiograms and scintiscans are also useful in documenting necrosis. If in the postoperative period there is evidence of significant hepatocellular damage and necrosis, re-exploration is indicated for resection of devitalized tissue.

Results of Treatment

Clinical and experimental studies indicate that survival is possible with only 20 per cent of normal hepatic tissue remaining, and the ability of liver to regenerate is remarkable. Liver function tests may be expected to be abnormal for days or weeks after major resection, but hepatic dysfunction rarely poses a serious problem if all devitalized tissue has been removed and drainage is adequate. The two most significant changes are decreases in the blood sugar and albumin. Continuous glucose infusions for several days with careful evaluation of blood sugars thereafter is necessary to prevent sudden, severe hypoglycemia episodes. The hypoproteinemia should be treated by the vigorous administration of serum albumin. The hypoalbuminemia, which may not be affected by the intravenous serum albumin, becomes most severe at 1 week and improves thereafter. Bleeding diathesis is not frequent, despite measurable decreases in multiple clotting factors, and when it occurs is probably due to multiple transfusions with subsequent thrombocytopenia, disseminated intravascular coagulation or pathologic fibrinolysis. Elevated bilirubin levels peak at 2 weeks and then gradually decrease over several weeks.

Pinkerton and associates[140] have stressed the malnutrition and gastrointestinal hemorrhage that follow major hepatic resection, and advocate parenteral hyperalimentation and early instillation of antacids into the stomach.

Abscess and hemorrhage require reoperation and must be watched for carefully. Hemobilia is easily detected if a catheter has been left in the common duct. If it has not, episodes of crampy abdominal pain and gastrointestinal bleeding with or without jaundice indicate the presence of this complication, which may occur from a few days to weeks after the injury. It is almost always associated with an intrahepatic abscess or cavity that has eroded blood vessels and biliary ducts. Hepatic scans[169] and arteriograms are helpful in locating the cavity, which must be resected or drained. Other significant complications include subphrenic abscess and bile peritonitis. Cholangiograms performed through the T-tube are helpful in diagnosing subphrenic and intrahepatic abscesses in the early postoperative period.[22]

Vena Cava and Hepatic Veins

Injuries to the juxtahepatic vena cava and hepatic vein tributaries are notoriously difficult to control and repair. Control of hemorrhage is at times unsuccessful and exsanguination results. Air embolus and, more rarely, hepatic tissue embolus are a danger.[140] Major injury to the liver may be associated with massive bleeding due to retrograde flow through injured hepatic veins that is not stopped by occlusion of the hepatic artery and portal vein.

Recently, several techniques have been suggested to solve this problem.[1, 16, 19, 163, 202] A variety of tubes, with and without balloons, for insertion into the vena cava both above and below the diaphragm, have been proposed. The main objective is to stop the bleeding yet permit the inferior vena cava blood to return to the right heart and thus avoid precipitous decreases in cardiac output. All methods include the Pringle maneuver to prevent inflow of portal vein and hepatic artery blood into the liver.

The fastest method to gain control, as demonstrated by Yellin and associates,[202] is to place four vascular clamps — one across the porta hepatis, one across the aorta above the celiac axis, another across the supradiaphragmatic inferior vena cava via a pericardiotomy incision, and the last above the renal veins. In those patients who cannot tolerate complete inferior vena cava occlusion, a shunt will have to be inserted.

Shunts inserted downward from above the diaphragm are secured by placing a purse-string suture around the right atrial appendage, excising the appendage and inserting either a No. 36 plastic chest tube or an endotracheal tube through the appendage into the inferior vena cava with the tip located at the level of the renal veins (Fig. 14–17). Side holes are cut at the appropriate level to permit the blood flowing up the tube to exit into the right

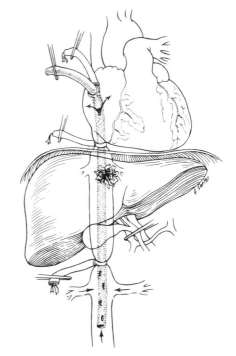

Figure 14–17. *Diagram demonstrating a method of inserting a shunt via the right atrial appendage to bypass the retrohepatic inferior vena cava.*

atrium. A tourniquet is tightened around the intrapericardial inferior vena cava. When the endotracheal tube is used, the cuff is inflated as it lies above the renal veins. In the case of the chest tube, a second tourniquet must be placed and tightened around the suprarenal inferior vena cava. Along with the Pringle maneuver, this then effectively secures all blood flow to the juxtahepatic inferior vena cava.

Shunts inserted upward from below the diaphragm have included Foley catheters and straight pieces of plastic tubing. Both are placed via an incision in the infrarenal inferior vena cava. The straight tube is completely inserted within the inferior vena cava with a suture secured to the caudal end for later removal. Tourniquets above and below the retrohepatic inferior vena cava are required. The Foley catheter is inserted with the balloon placed cephalad (Fig. 14–18). The side arm for inflating the balloon is brought out of the incision in the inferior vena cava. The balloon is inflated in the supradiaphragmatic inferior vena cava and a tourniquet placed around the inferior vena cava above the renal veins. Tubes with sausage-shaped balloons have

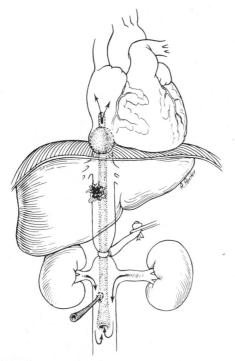

Figure 14–18. *Diagram demonstrating a method of inserting a Foley catheter in the infrarenal inferior vena cava to bypass the retrohepatic vena cava.*

been designed to eliminate the need for tourniquets and are inserted through the right atrium.[107] Despite these innovations, juxtahepatic inferior vena caval and hepatic vein injuries remain a formidable challenge.

Hepatoduodenal Ligament and Gallbladder

Structures contained within the hepatoduodenal ligament are infrequently injured. The most common injuries are those sustained during biliary tract surgery.

Blood or bile found in the subhepatic space at laparotomy suggests injury to the structures in the hepatoduodenal ligament and requires thorough exploration of the hepatic artery, portal vein and extrahepatic bile duct. All clots should be removed, but this may restart substantial bleeding. Hemorrhage from wounds of the hepatic artery or portal vein can usually be controlled temporarily by digital compression of the hepatoduodenal ligament. Vascular or rubber-shod clamps may be applied for this purpose. Hepatic blood flow should not be completely interrupted more than 15 min-

utes at a time unless hepatic hypothermia is induced. The components of the portal triad are carefully dissected and exposed. Once the vascular injury has been located, it is isolated between vascular clamps and repaired by an appropriate technique of vascular surgery. Successful reconstruction of the common hepatic artery with an autogenous saphenous vein graft has been reported.[86] This technique warrants trial for hepatic artery and portal vein injuries that cannot be repaired directly.

If all attempts at repair of the hepatic artery or one of its branches fail, the artery must be ligated. Survival of patients with normal livers may be anticipated following hepatic artery ligation if the remaining hepatic inflow and oxygenation are not further reduced by shock, anoxia or high fever.[17, 102] The common hepatic artery can usually be safely ligated proximal to the gastroduodenal artery since the latter vessel will provide adequate collateral flow. Massive doses of antibiotics should probably be employed if hepatic artery ligation is required, although the efficacy of this has not been demonstrated in humans. Glucagon may be given at 2 mg. per hour intravenously for 3 to 4 days because of evidence that it increases portal venous flow.[100]

Portal vein injuries are usually fatal before repair can be accomplished. Hemorrhage during repair is significant and the application of vascular clamps difficult. Fogarty catheters inserted distally and proximally can be used to secure hemostasis. Primary repair or portacaval anastomosis may be used to rectify the injury. Often repair is not possible, in which case ligation is performed with the full expectation that a good result will be obtained. Child[26] has shown that acute portal vein occlusion in humans with normal livers is well tolerated.

Trauma to the extrahepatic biliary system is fortunately unusual but often leads to death if unrecognized. Although there was an 85 per cent mortality in a group of patients with bile peritonitis reported by Means,[115] the clinical course of patients with rupture of the bile duct is often surprisingly prolonged.[66] In isolated hepatic duct injuries, Zollinger et al.[206] reported an average delay of 2 weeks between injury and diagnosis. If hepatic duct injury was missed at the initial laparotomy, the delay was 3 weeks. Bile peritonitis resulting from a ruptured bile duct may manifest itself by jaundice, ascites, acholic stools and general deterioration in a patient who has suffered recent abdominal trauma. It can be particularly perplexing postoperatively if the biliary duct rupture was not recognized at laparotomy. During exploration for nonpenetrating abdominal wounds, the duodenum should be mobilized by a Kocher maneuver and the entire extrahepatic biliary system inspected. Bile straining without a demonstrable source is an indication for an operative cholangiogram.

Injuries of the gallbladder and cystic duct are best treated by cholecystectomy, although primary repair and cholecystostomy are effective when the wound is simple and may be preferred in patients with multiple other injuries or who are in shock.[167] Lacerations of the major bile duct should be carefully closed over one arm of the T-tube inserted into the common duct through an incision above or below the wound. When the common duct is completely transected, the distal end may retract behind the duodenum and be difficult to find. Duodenal mobilization, duodenotomy and retrograde probing of the common duct will facilitate the location of the distal end.[184] Using a catheter as a stent, end-to-end anastomosis with interrupted 4–0 silk sutures can then be performed. Necessary wound debridement of the injury itself may result in loss of tissue sufficient to prevent anastomosis, despite extensive duodenal mobilization. Cholecystoduodenostomy, cholecystojejunostomy, choledochoduodenostomy and choledochojejunostomy are all acceptable methods of bypass; the one preferable will depend upon individual considerations. However, the complication of anastomotic leak is more serious if the duodenum rather than the jejunum has been used to receive the bile. A very satisfactory procedure is the two-layer anastomosis of the common bile duct to a Roux-en-Y limb or simple loop of jejunum. The end of the Roux-en-Y limb should be closed and the bile duct implanted 2 to 3 cm. from this end. If the simple jejunal loop is used, an additional enteroenterostomy is advantageous in reducing reflux of intestinal contents into the biliary tract. In either instance, it is helpful to make the anastomosis over one arm of the T-tube placed through a separate incision in the common duct. The tube may be removed 3 to 4 weeks postoperatively.

PANCREAS

As surgeons throughout the country encounter an increasing number of patients with upper abdominal trauma, the treatment of pancreatic injuries has become a subject of considerable interest and controversy.[10, 39, 54, 76, 178, 181, 182] Reviews of the literature have clarified some of the details regarding pancreatic injuries and their management.[128, 179] Pancreatic injuries account for only 1 to 2 per cent of all abdominal trauma with penetrating trauma responsible for two thirds of the injuries. The mortality rates (8 per cent for stab wounds, 25 per cent for gunshot wounds, and 50 per cent for shotgun wounds and blunt trauma) primarily reflect injuries to associated organs. Injuries to the head of the pancreas have twice the mortality of those to the body or tail.

The major complications of pancreatic injury are pancreatic fistulas (19 per cent), pseudocyst formation (12 per cent), pancreatic abscesses (5 per cent) and recurrent hemorrhage and pancreatitis (3 per cent). Pseudocyst and abscess formation are more common after blunt trauma and are probably indicative of inadequate drainage. A pancreatic fistula is not necessarily a complication but is the desired result in many cases of severe pancreatic injury.[128] Spontaneous closure of these fistulas is the rule and surgical intervention is rarely required. Even complicated pancreaticoduodenal fistulas have closed spontaneously with the aid of parenteral hyperalimentation.[42]

Diagnosis

Signs and symptoms are characteristically slow to appear following isolated blunt trauma to the pancreas. Some patients may have been asymptomatic for years when a pseudocyst appears. At the other extreme, some injuries present with severe and persistent pain that suggests the need for immediate celiotomy. Ninety per cent of patients with blunt pancreatic trauma have elevated amylase, but it might not be elevated initially owing to transient secretory inhibition. Elevations seldom exceed 500 Somogyi units. Serial values are of prognostic importance because persistently elevated values beyond 6 days usually signal the development of a pseudocyst. A ruptured duodenum, among other causes, can account for an elevated amylase; therefore, if surgery is not planned but the amylase is elevated, hypaque duodenography is indicated.

The pancreas must be thoroughly examined in all patients operated on for trauma. The body and tail of the pancreas can be adequately exposed by dividing the greater omentum just below the greater curvature of the stomach and entering the lesser sac. Exposure of the head of the pancreas may be obtained by reflecting the right colon and mobilizing the duodenum. These maneuvers also allow inspection for injuries of the duodenum and the vena cava, aorta, renal and superior mesenteric vessels. Upper abdominal retroperitoneal hematomas should be considered presumptive evidence of pancreatic or other significant injury and therefore explored. Division of the ligament of Treitz will facilitate exposure of the third and fourth portions of the duodenum.

Treatment

The objectives in treating pancreatic injuries are control of hemorrhage, control of exocrine secretions and conservation of pancreatic function. The last consideration is the least important. In all the cases of pancreatic trauma reported in the literature, only two instances of exocrine and endocrine insufficiency are recorded.[128] Resections of traumatized pancreatic tissue can therefore be performed without fear of pancreatic insufficiency.

Control of hemorrhage, debridement of devitalized tissue, and adequate drainage constitute the basis for effective surgical treatment. Minor lacerations may be sutured superficially with silk, being careful to avoid the main pancreatic ducts. Sump drainage is more effective than Penrose drainage in preventing the complications of pancreatic trauma, 6 per cent versus 29 per cent, respectively.[10, 177] The best form of drainage is a combination of both sump catheters and Penrose drains.[5] Soft rubber sump drains should be left in place for at least 2 weeks as drainage is frequently prolonged and may not become significant until after 7 to 10 days. Penrose drains should always be placed alongside the sump drains. The Penrose drains are slowly removed during the first 2 weeks, breaking up loculations.

Contusion of the pancreas with an intact capsule is best treated with drainage alone. Decompressive procedures on the biliary tract are not indicated. Lacerations without major ductal disruption should be sutured and well drained. Major ductal disruptions in the neck, body or tail are best managed by distal resection rather than intestinal pancreatic anastomosis[128, 178, 179] because: (1) exocrine or endocrine insufficiency is extremely rare, (2) resection is faster in critically ill patients, (3) bacterial contamination occurs with bowel anastomosis, (4) pancreatic enzymes are activated in the presence of bowel contents, (5) there is a 25 per cent incidence of fistulas with pancreatic intestinal anastomosis. If, however, major duct disruption is located in the head but is not complete, then an onlay Roux-en-Y limb can be sutured over the rent.[54] A complete transection may be treated by carefully closing the proximal end with nonabsorbable suture and anastomosing the distal end into a Roux-en-Y limb of jejunum. However, distal resection is preferred.

Combined injuries to the pancreas and duodenum result in a much higher mortality rate than either injury alone. The morbidity is also increased with this injury and the treatment is much more difficult. Anderson and associates[7] claimed satisfactory management of this type of injury with debridement, suture closure of the duodenum and pancreas and wide adequate drainage. Berne and associates[15] advocate antral exclusion by closing the duodenal perforation, drainage of the pancreas, antrectomy, gastrojejunostomy, vagotomy, biliary decompression and duodenal tube decompression. Pancreaticoduodenectomy is indicated when there is extensive injury to the duodenum and head of the pancreas or distal common bile duct. Sound surgical judgment is required in making a decision to perform a Whipple procedure for traumatic indications because of the significant risk involved in patients already seriously stressed by their original injuries. Thirty-four cases of pancreaticoduodenectomy have been reported with an overall mortality of 30 per cent.[7] To summarize, blunt abdominal trauma and penetrating injuries in the vicinity of the pancreas require extensive mobilization and thorough examination of the extrahepatic bile ducts, pancreas, duodenum and other retroperitoneal structures in this area. Once hemostasis is obtained, the degree of pancreatic injury is assessed and the method of treatment is decided upon. Simple wounds may be sutured and drained externally. Distal pancreatectomy is used for extensive damage to the body and tail. Crushing injuries of the head of the pancreas are debrided and the open end of a jejunal Roux-en-Y limb sutured around the circumference of the injured area. Complex injuries of this area that involve the duodenum and common bile duct as well as the pancreatic head occasionally require pancreaticoduodenectomy, but usually more conservative measures suffice. If the patient's condition deteriorates rapidly during laparotomy, it may be necessary to confine treatment to achievement of hemostasis and establishment of external drainage. Such patients should have reoperation and definitive repair carried out as soon as their general condition permits. Regardless of the type of repair, all pancreatic injuries require external drainage, preferably with sump suction. Several Penrose drains in addition to the sump drain are placed in the area of the pancreas through a stab incision in the abdominal wall. The sump is connected to suction and the drains are not removed before the fourteenth postoperative day since drainage is frequently prolonged or becomes significant only after 7 to 10 days.

DUODENUM

Diagnosis

Duodenal wounds range from simple stab wounds to bursting or crushing injuries resulting from nonpenetrating trauma. The latter is frequently associated with complex wounds of the pancreas, liver and extrahepatic biliary systems. Such combined injuries in the right upper quadrant provide one of the major challenges for today's surgeon. The mortality and morbidity associated with complex wounds in this area remain high despite advances in resuscitation and surgical technique.[82, 188] Delay in treatment contributes to the high mortality. A delay of 24 hours before surgery is associated with a 65 per cent mortality. Those operated on in less than 24 hours from the time of injury have a 5 per cent mortality.[149]

Blunt duodenal injuries usually occur in the second and third portions and are often associated with fever, jaundice, signs of high intestinal obstruction and third-stage fluid loss, especially when there is a prolonged delay between injury and examination. X-ray stippling of the retroperitoneal space, hyperamylasemia, hyperbilirubinemia and extravasation seen on intestinal roentgenographic contrast studies are all indicative of duodenal perforation.

Experience has shown that extensive duodenal mobilization, allowing adequate exposure and thorough examination of it and the adjacent organs, is essential when dealing with wounds of the pancreaticoduodenal area. Penetrating wounds in this region, bile staining of adjacent tissues, retroperitoneal hematoma and crepitation are all indications for painstaking examination of the entire pancreaticoduodenal area. The necessary exposure may be obtained by incising the peritoneum lateral to the right colon and retracting the right colon and the right half of the transverse colon to the left. This provides exposure of the retroperitoneal structures from the right side of the abdominal wall to the spine. The duodenum is then reflected to the left after incision of its lateral peritoneal reflection (Kocher maneuver). If necessary, the ligament of Treitz may be divided and the terminal duodenum retracted to the right beneath the mesentery and superior mesenteric vessels. A thorough examination of the duodenum, common bile duct, pancreas and the major vessels of the retroperitoneum may then be carried out.

Treatment

Several operative procedures have been prepared for the management of duodenal injuries.[29, 38, 181] Most authors agree that simple lacerations of the duodenum may be closed primarily, but severe duodenal wounds or combined pancreaticoduodenal injuries require procedures that provide duodenal defunctionalization in addition to repair. Cleveland and Waddell[29] listed a number of alternative procedures that may be used in the treatment of such injuries. Included in these was transection of the duodenum at the site of injury, closure of both duodenal ends and gastrojejunostomy or duodenojejunostomy. Thal and Wilson[181] have recommended pancreaticoduodenectomy, and recently Donovan and Hagen[38] have proposed wound closure combined with vagotomy, antrectomy, duodenostomy and gastrojejunostomy for pancreaticoduodenal or severe duodenal injury. Serosal patch repair has been recommended for closure of duodenal wounds in which primary repair would produce stenosis.[84, 113, 201] All these procedures have merit and are satisfactory in some instances but not in others. None is applicable in all situations, and the difference between a favorable and an unfavorable outcome often depends upon the surgeon's ability to decide which procedure is best suited for a particular situation.

It is helpful to consider not only the type and severity but also the location of the wound. Vagotomy, antrectomy and gastrojejunostomy are especially applicable in wounds of the first part of the duodenum where the injured portion of bowel may be resected along with the antrum. Tube duodenostomy is added if stump closure is difficult or insecure. Similarly, it may be possible to treat severe wounds of the fourth part of the duodenum by a resection of the distal duodenum and duodenojejunostomy of some type, end-to-end, end-to-side or side-to-side. The anastomosis must be made only to uninjured bowel. In conjunction with this, distal pancreatectomy and splenectomy may be employed for combined injuries of the body and tail of the pancreas. The major problem in the operative management of duodenal trauma arises in deciding what to do for severe injuries to the second and third part of the duodenum, particularly if combined with injury to the head of the pancreas. Primary closure of extensive wounds in these portions of the duodenum is frequently complicated by lateral duodenal fistula, postoperative hemorrhage and sepsis, which all too often lead to death of the patient.

Although it is relatively easy to transect the duodenum at the site of injury and perform a gastroenterostomy (preferably combined with a vagotomy), this leaves a long, blind, proximal duodenal loop that receives the bile and pancreatic juices. These secretions must move against the forces of peristalsis in order to decompress the proximal duodenum. Stasis and distention are therefore likely in the blind proximal duodenal limb and may contribute to the occurrence of a duodenal fistula. There is a distinct advantage in allowing the duodenum to drain in an isoperistaltic manner,

and the recent report of Donovan and Hagen supports this concept.[38]

If a duodenal laceration can be approximated without tension following adequate debridement, and the associated injury to the head of the pancreas is not extensive, it may be closed with two layers of interrupted inverting silk sutures and antrectomy, vagotomy and gastrojejunostomy performed. The duodenal stump is closed over a sump-type drainage tube. If the duodenal wound is extensive and *cannot* be easily closed following adequate debridement, if the associated pancreatic damage is severe or if the common bile duct and pancreatic ducts have been avulsed from the duodenum, pancreaticoduodenectomy is the procedure of choice. By this means, all devitalized tissue can be resected and all anastomoses performed between tissues with good blood supply. If not severely damaged, the distal pancreas is preserved and the pancreatic capsule sutured to the circumference of the open end of the jejunal loop. The pancreas is further invaginated into the jejunum by additional layers of sutures placed between the pancreatic capsule and the jejunal serosa. Anastomoses are then made between the side of the jejunal loop and the common bile duct and stomach. The biliary anastomosis is made over a T-tube inserted into the bile duct through a separate incision above the anastomosis.

Regardless of the method of treatment, the area must be thoroughly drained to the outside and the gastrointestinal tract decompressed postoperatively. A sump drainage tube is laid along the pancreas and, in addition, several Penrose drains are placed in the area of injury and near, but not against, the anastomoses. Gastrointestinal decompression is achieved with nasogastric, gastrostomy or jejunostomy tubes, depending upon the surgeon's preference and the procedure performed. Combined decompressing and feeding jejunostomies are advantageous in these patients since they allow the patient to be fed distally while decompression is maintained proximally in the areas of injury and anastomoses. This approach is almost indispensable if a duodenal fistula or other regional complications occur and the patient cannot take food orally for perhaps several weeks.

The discussion of duodenal trauma must

include some comment on two special forms of duodenal injury — retroperitoneal duodenal rupture and intramural hematoma.

Retroperitoneal Duodenal Rupture

This condition has been the subject of review by Cocke and Meyer.[30] Retroperitoneal duodenal rupture usually follows some type of blunt abdominal trauma, commonly a blow to the body received during athletics, fights or falls. Cocke and Meyer postulate that the mechanism responsible for this injury is the rapid increase in the intraluminal pressure of a loop of duodenum closed betwen the pylorus and the ligament of Treitz. Under proper circumstances, a relatively minor force may produce a blowout injury of the duodenal wall. Since anatomical factors necessary to produce a closed loop in the duodenum exist in only a small number of people, retroperitoneal duodenal rupture differs from other types of duodenal wounds resulting from blunt abdominal trauma in that associated organ injuries are rare and the duodenal damage is usually not severe. Diagnosis is often difficult. The patient may give a vague history of trauma and have little pain and no significant physical, laboratory or x-ray findings; most patients, however, complain of pain in the epigastrium or right lower quadrant and give a definite history of trauma. Frequently, nausea, vomiting and even hematemesis have occurred. Signs range from mild epigastric or right-sided tenderness to those typical of a perforated viscus, including shock. Roentgenograms may be helpful but frequently are not. Intraperitoneal and retroperitoneal air and blurred psoas outlines should be sought; if the plain films are not diagnostic, administration of a water-soluble contrast material may demonstrate an intestinal perforation. When the diagnosis of retroperitoneal duodenal rupture has been made, laparotomy should be performed without delay. Ordinarily, simple two-layer closure of the duodenal tear is sufficient. The mortality and morbidity of this injury should be low, provided the diagnosis is made early and closure carried out promptly. Cocke and Meyer[30] point out that the duodenal rupture was not operated upon or recognized at laparotomy in 15 per cent of the reported cases, and among these patients the mortality was 71 per cent. They again emphasized the necessity for complete duodenal mobilization and examination in patients explored for abdominal trauma.

Intramural Hematoma

Traumatic intramural hematoma is another entity caused by nonpenetrating abdominal trauma; it is unusual but has been encountered more frequently in recent years.[9, 83] Patients exhibit clinical findings of upper gastrointestinal obstruction; occasionally the common bile and pancreatic ducts are also occluded. The diagnosis is frequently delayed but can often be made from a contrast study of the upper gastrointestinal tract, which presents a typical appearance. Optimal treatment consists of laparotomy, complete assessment of the duodenal damage and a search for associated injuries. Since the bowel wall is intact in most instances, incision of the serosa over the hematoma and evacuation of all blood clots are sufficient in most of these patients. Duodenal decompression is maintained for several days. Gastrostomy and jejunostomy may be helpful during this period, but gastroenterostomy appears unnecessary in the management of intramural duodenal hematoma.

STOMACH

Gastric lacerations are encountered rather frequently in laparotomy for penetrating wounds of the upper abdomen and lower thorax. On the other hand, blunt abdominal trauma is seldom the cause of significant stomach injury; this is probably because of the protective location and the mobility of the organ. Bloody aspirate can usually be obtained from a nasogastric tube when the stomach has been injured. If a wound of the anterior wall is found or there is other reason to suspect gastric injury, the gastrocolic omentum must be divided and the posterior wall of the stomach thoroughly examined. In one third of cases, both walls of the stomach are perforated. The stomach along the greater and lesser omental attachments should be carefully inspected since the fat in these areas hides wounds easily. All lacerations of the stomach should be closed with two layers of sutures; small perforations due to high-velocity missiles are excised and converted into linear closures; bleeding vessels are ligated. A continuous inverting 2–0 chromic catgut suture through the entire stomach wall is recommended for the first layer. This provides hemostasis in the highly vascular submucosa of the stomach. Interrupted Lambert sutures of 3–0 silk may then be used for the second layer of the closure. Purse-string sutures are not used because they are not as effective for the control of gastric wall bleeding. Resections of portions of the stomach should be carried out if necessary for debridement of devitalized tissue and, occasionally, partial gastrectomy is required for extensive injury. Removal of spilled gastric contents from the peritoneal cavity and copious lavage of the lesser sac and subhepatic spaces may decrease later abscess formation. As in the treatment of perforated peptic ulcer, the peritoneal cavity need not be drained if only the stomach has been injured.

MESENTERY AND SMALL INTESTINE

Injuries to the mesentery are often encountered in patients with abdominal trauma, and possible compromise of the intestinal blood supply makes correct appraisal and treatment of mesenteric damage necessary.

Blunt trauma to the intestine may be caused by shearing, crushing, tearing or compressive forces. Injuries to the proximal jejunum and distal ileum (points of relative fixation) are most common. Similarly, when adhesions are present, they may predispose to and localize intestinal tears. The mechanics of seat-belt injuries have been discussed previously. Penetrating injuries may occur anywhere and are commonly multiple, averaging five holes per injury.

The pH of the distal small bowel is often near neutral and produces less chemical irritation and thus an apparently milder, more delayed presentation is seen with lower ileal injuries when compared to those of the upper jejunum. The hazards of bacterial contamination are theoretically greater for more distal wounds in the small bowel because of the increasing bacterial

flora in the caudal small intestine. Thus, it may be advantageous to close distal perforations first.

Methodical inspection of the small intestine, examining both sides including the mesentery, is essential. The ligament of Treitz is taken down and the large vessels at the root of the mesentery are inspected. Hematomas of the mesentery are evacuated, and bleeding vessels are identified and ligated. Hematomas on the mesenteric border of the intestine should be carefully inspected in case they represent perforation in this area. An even number of perforations should be found or a tangential wound identified.

Small contusions or perforations may be closed with interrupted silk. Linear lacerations should be closed in a transverse direction with a double layer of inverting sutures. High-velocity injuries require extensive debridement prior to closure, low-velocity injuries a little and knife wounds practically none. Adequate bleeding from the wound edges should be noted prior to closure.

Criteria for resection of bowel include:

1. Injuries that cannot be closed without significantly narrowing the bowel lumen
2. Large or irregular wounds
3. Short segments containing multiple perforations
4. Areas that are infarcted or crushed
5. Bowel with injury in the leaves of the mesentery
6. Large hematomas at the mesenteric border
7. Large intramural hematomas
8. Avulsion of the mesentery
9. Large transverse tears of the mesentery
10. Long linear lacerations of the bowel.

In most cases in which doubt as to viability exists, cover the area with warm packs and reinspect it later, prior to abdominal closure. End-to-end anastomoses are made only with bowel of unquestionable viability.

Injuries of the major mesenteric vessels are rare and usually require repair to prevent infarction. Ligation of large veins is better tolerated than that of arteries because of the more extensive collateral pathways. Intestines perfused by the injured vessels should be inspected prior to closure and resected if their circulation appears inadequate. When thrombosis of the superior mesenteric vessels occurs secondary to contusion, it usually involves the vein. Progression of the thrombus into the entire portal venous system may occur slowly over days or weeks with fatal results. There are probably many instances of minor mesenteric vessel thrombosis due to abdominal trauma that require no specific therapy and that resolve undetected. It has been suggested that some instances of idiopathic or spontaneous portal and superior mesenteric vein thrombosis are actually the result of previous unremembered abdominal trauma.[83] In any case, contusion of the superior mesenteric vessels may lead to bowel necrosis, which will require resection either initially or sometime following the responsible trauma.

COLON, RECTUM, AND PERINEUM

The operative management of injuries of the large bowel may be outlined as follows:

1. Primary closure
2. Resection and primary anastomosis
3. Primary closure with proximal colostomy
4. Resection with colostomy
5. Exteriorization.

During World War II the routine use of exteriorization of colon wounds by combat surgeons was associated with such a striking reduction in the mortality and morbidity that this procedure was used extensively in civilian practice following the war. The further reduction in complications attending the treatment of colon injuries observed during the Korean conflict appeared to confirm the efficacy of exteriorization in the treatment of colon injury.[156] However, several factors were responsible for the improved results. Among these were the decreased time between injury and definitive treatment, rapid replacement of blood loss, extensive use of antibiotics and intravenous fluid therapy, and the availability of well-trained anesthesia and surgical personnel. As war

wounds are usually the result of fragmentation of high-velocity missiles, they differ significantly from the majority of wounds seen in civilian practice. It is now recognized that many civilian colon injuries can be treated definitively in one stage since these wounds often involve little tissue destruction and are encountered soon after injury.[14, 68, 150, 187, 201] Others have experienced excessive complication rates with primary repair.[27] Therefore, patients treated by primary closure or resection and anastomosis must be selected very carefully. Integral steps in all methods of managing colon injuries include thorough irrigation of the abdominal cavity with copious volumes of saline solution, the meticulous removal of all feculent material from the abdominal cavity, irrigation of the colon to remove retained feculent material and administration of antibiotics effective against both aerobic and anaerobic bacteria.

Types of Injuries

High-Velocity and Blunt Injuries. There is little disagreement that injuries to the colon from high-velocity missiles, shotgun blasts or blunt trauma should be treated by exteriorization or resection and colostomy. Right colon injuries under these circumstances are probably best treated by a matured ileostomy and mucous fistula.

Low-Velocity and Stab Injuries. If primary repair of the colon can be accomplished in selected patients without increased mortality or morbidity, those individuals are spared the time, risk and expense of a second hospitalization for closure of the colostomy. In deciding about primary repair, several factors must be considered. These include the etiological agent, the location and extent of injury, the time since injury, the amount of peritoneal soiling, the number of associated injuries and the general condition of the patient. A young, healthy individual with a stab wound of the transverse colon measuring 2 cm., seen 2 hours after injury with no significant peritoneal soiling and no associated injuries, would be an exemplary candidate for primary closure.

Areas Affected

Right Colon. Stab wounds of the cecum may be treated by converting it into a tube cecostomy. Other penetrating injuries may be treated by primary repair and may or may not need a venting cecostomy performed. More extensive injuries will require resection of the right colon and ileocolostomy. If there is significant soiling, contamination or multiple visceral injuries, exteriorizing colostomy or resection with a proximal ileostomy and distal mucous colonic fistula is advisable. The patient will be better able to cope with this temporary ileostomy than an anastomosis leak and abscess of fistula formation.

Transverse Colon. Primary repair, exteriorization, resection and primary anastomosis or resection with colostomy are all acceptable procedures, depending on the degree of injury. Exteriorization is reserved for injuries of the transverse and sigmoid colon in patients in whom primary repair or resection with anastomosis is considered unwise. The right and left colon are ordinarily difficult to exteriorize and are more easily managed by resection and colostomy. Exteriorization may be advantageous when the viability of a segment of colon and the necessity for resection are uncertain.

Left Colon. Exteriorization or the formation of a colostomy is difficult with this portion of the bowel. Therefore, in primary repair that is insecure, a completely diverting proximal colostomy is necessary. Those lesions with more destruction require resection and colostomy with mucous fistula formation. Rarely are resection and primary anastomosis advised.

Sigmoid Colon. If primary repair is not secure or if there is extensive destruction, then resection and colostomy with a mucous fistula should be done. There seems to be little reason to anastomose the colon primarily and then perform proximal colostomy. If primary anastomosis seems to be unwarranted following resection, the remaining bowel ends should be mobilized only enough to place them on to the abdominal wall as colostomies. The dissection required to bring the ends of colon together is better reserved for the second-stage operation when circumstances hopefully will be more favorable. The terminal colon may be too short to bring easily onto the abdominal wall following some resections of the distal large bowel; in these instances, it may be closed and left within the peritoneal cavity. The proximal colon is used for a colostomy.

Rectum. The treatment of injuries of the intraperitoneal rectum is the same as that for colon wounds. Damage to the rectum below the peritoneal reflection should be treated by primary repair if possible, drainage of the retroperitoneal space adjacent to the wound, complete diverting colostomy and irrigation of the rectum to remove retained feces.[2, 8] Access to the retroperitoneal space can be accomplished through an incision lateral to the coccyx or by coccygectomy. The second procedure gives the advantage of generous exposure of the distal rectum and thereby permits control of pelvic hemorrhage and repair of wounds that are otherwise inaccessible. If necessary, rectal resection with preservation of the anal sphincter can be performed through an abdominoperineal approach.[37] The repair of all but the smallest rectal wounds should be protected by a completely diverting proximal colostomy, preferably in the transverse colon, away from the area of damage where additional surgery may be required.[189] Irrigation of the rectum is indicated when massive fecal residue is present. In all wounds of the anorectum, the anal sphincter muscles should be carefully repaired if at all possible and adequate drainage established. Perineal wounds must be widely debrided; if large and grossly contaminated, they are left open. Smaller wounds that have been well debrided may be closed with drainage. Extensive perineal injury requires a colostomy.

RETROPERITONEUM AND VASCULAR STRUCTURES

Retroperitoneal Hematoma

Retroperitoneal hematoma does not usually receive consideration as a primary diagnosis, except in the presence of pelvic fractures but rather is a finding seen at laparotomy for blunt or penetrating abdominal trauma. The retroperitoneal space can accommodate up to 4 liters of blood, pushed into it under arterial pressure. It is possible, therefore, for hypotension to be secondary to a retroperitoneal hematoma alone. Abdominal pain, back pain, hypoactive bowel sounds (adynamic ileus), a tender abdominal or rectal mass and later bluish discoloration of the flanks are all possible symptoms and signs caused by this entity. A falling hematocrit and oblit-

eration of the psoas signs on abdominal
x-rays are additional findings.

Blunt Trauma. When retroperitoneal
hematoma is associated with blunt trauma,
the most frequent source of bleeding is
fractures of the pelvis or spine (50–60 per
cent).[135] Less often, wounds of the kidney,
bladder, pancreas and duodenum, and
rarely injuries of the aorta or vena cava, are
responsible for the retroperitoneal bleeding. Evidence of major blood loss in the
presence of pelvic fractures is due most
often to a retroperitoneal hematoma. The
bleeding will cease spontaneously in most
circumstances, but in some situations over
20 units of blood may be given and the
problem of stemming continued blood loss
arises. The success of treatment by internal iliac artery ligation has been varied.
Ravitch[146] has concluded that the mortality
from operative intervention exceeds the
risk of nonoperative management with
continued blood replacement. Arteriography has been helpful in identifying major
vascular injuries and in two cases selective
injection of autologous clot into the anterior division of the internal iliac artery
was successful in controlling bleeding
from lacerated obturator arteries.[103] Continued need for blood replacement beyond
10 units is probably a reasonable point at
which to intervene surgically. At the time
of surgery, the pelvic wall is explored with
attention paid to the iliac vessels. If no
definite source of bleeding is found, bilateral hypogastric artery ligation is performed.[157]

Other indications for operation with pelvic fractures are any findings compatible
with intra-abdominal visceral injury, particularly a positive paracentesis or peritoneal lavage, or rupture of the bladder.

Retroperitoneal hematomas discovered
at the time of laparotomy that are mainly
situated in the pelvic area, associated with
pelvic fractures and not expanding do not
ordinarily need to be explored. However,
tears in the peritoneum with continued
blood loss or expanding hematomas and
unstable vital signs after blood replacement may require exploration.

Upper abdominal retroperitoneal hematomas all require exploration because of
the high incidence of injury to associated
structures, particularly the kidney, pancreas and duodenum. Rupture of the aorta

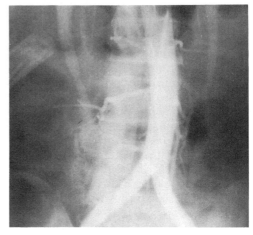

Figure 14–19. *Arteriovenous fistula between lumbar
artery and inferior vena cava caused by a gunshot
wound. The right ureter was damaged and can be
seen entering area of massive retroperitoneal hematoma. The aortogram reveals filling of the inferior
vena cava via the right lumbar artery next to the
bullet, which is embedded in the vertebral body.*

from blunt trauma with successful repair
has been reported.[164]

Penetrating Trauma. Retroperitoneal
hematomas caused by penetrating wounds
must be explored to determine the source
of bleeding. Some have advised leaving
undisturbed those hematomas that are not
actively bleeding.[136] However, the problems of rebleeding, false aneurysms, arteriovenous fistulas (Fig. 14–19) and possible injury to the main vessels, pancreas,
duodenum or kidney dictate that exploration is the wiser choice after insuring that
adequate preliminary precautions have
been taken.[171] Large amounts of blood and
a means for its rapid administration should
be available. If possible, control of vessels
proximal and distal to the hematoma
should be obtained. When these preparations have been made, the hematoma may
be opened and the retroperitoneal structures explored.

Aorta and Inferior Vena Cava

Penetrating wounds account for the vast
majority of injuries to the aorta and inferior
vena cava. Patients with these injuries
often arrive in the emergency room moribund and only immediate celiotomy and
compression of the aorta at the diaphrag-

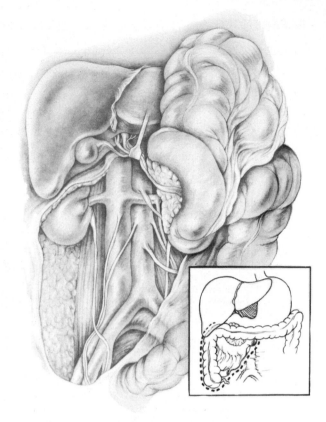

Figure 14–20. *Exposure of the major retroperitoneal vascular structures by reflecting the right colon, root of the small bowel mesentery, duodenum and head of the pancreas superiorly and to the left.*

matic hiatus or direct pressure on the bleeding point will provide any chance for survival. The treatment of injuries to the juxtahepatic inferior vena cava has been previously covered in the section on liver injuries. Exposure of the aorta and inferior vena cava is provided by reflecting the right colon and the root of the small bowel mesentery superiorly and medially as well as mobilizing the duodenum and head of the pancreas medially (Fig. 14–20).

Control of either the aorta or inferior vena cava will require not only proximal and distal clamps but pressure applied medially and laterally by sponge sticks or an assistant's finger to control the lumbar vessels. Wounds are often through both the anterior and posterior walls, and at times transluminal repair of the posterior laceration will be required.[47] Most aortic injuries can be repaired by primary closure. Occasionally, a patch or circumferential graft is required. The use of prosthetic grafts should be avoided because of the high incidence of infection in these wounds. The experience in Vietnam demonstrated that

a 75 per cent failure rate can be expected when prosthetic material is used in repair of the aorta or iliac vessels under these conditions.[147] A saphenous vein or an opposite internal iliac artery graft can be used in repairs of the iliac vessels when debridement and end-to-end suturing is not possible.

Inferior vena caval injuries are at best difficult and at times impossible to repair and in these circumstances the inferior vena cava may have to be ligated below the renal veins. Nevertheless, by doggedly gaining proximal and distal control and adequate exposure, repair of caval lacerations is usually possible, although occasionally only with the aid of massive blood transfusions. Iliac vein injuries may also require ligation and can be done with minimal morbidity. It is essential that suprarenal injuries be repaired.

Bullets not accounted for in vascular injuries must have appropriate x-rays to rule out peripheral or central embolism.[13] Combined arteriovenous injuries should be noted because of later fistula formation.

REFERENCES

1. Albo, D., Christensen, C. Rasmussen, B. L., and King, T. C.: Massive liver trauma involving the suprarenal vena cava. Am. J. Surg. *118*:960, 1969.
2. Allen, D. B.: Penetrating wounds of the rectum. Tex. Med. *69*:77, 1973.
3. Allen, R. E., Morton, J., Thoskinsky, R., Stallone, J., and Hunt, T. K.: Corrosive injuries of the stomach. Arch. Surg. *100*:409, 1970.
4. Ammann, A. J., Addiego, J., Wara, D. W., Lubin, B., Smith, W. B., and Mentzer, W. C.: Polyvalent pneumococcal-polysaccharide immunization of patients with sickle-cell anemia and patients with splenectomy. N. Engl. J. Med. *297*:897, 1977.
5. Anderson, C. B., Connors, J., Mejia, D. C., and Wise, L.: Drainage methods in the treatment of pancreatic injuries. Surg. Gynecol. Obstet. *138*:587, 1974.
6. Anderson, C. B., Marr, J. J., and Ballinger, W. F.: Anaerobic infections in surgery: Clinical review. Surgery *79*:313, 1976.
7. Anderson, C. B., Weisz, D., Rodger, M. R., and Tucker, G. L.: Combined pancreaticoduodenal injury. Am. J. Surg. *125*:530, 1973.
8. Armstrong, R. G., Schmitt, H. J., and Patterson, L. T.: Combat wounds of extraperitoneal rectum. Surgery *74*:570, 1973.
9. Bailey, W. C., and Akers, D. R.: Traumatic intramural hematoma of the duodenum in children. Am. J. Surg. *110*:695, 1965.
10. Baker, R. J., Dippel, W. F., Freeark, R. J., and Strohl, E. L.: The surgical significance of trauma to the pancreas. Arch. Surg. *86*:1038, 1963.
11. Balfanz, J. R., Nesbit, M. E., Jr., Jarvis, C., and Krivit, W.: Overwhelming sepsis following splenectomy for trauma. J. Pediatr. *88*:458, 1976.
12. Ballinger, W. F., II: Splenectomy. Curr. Probl. Surg. February, 1965.
13. Bartlett, H., Anderson, C. B., and Steinhoff, N. G.: Bullet embolism to the heart. J. Trauma *13*:476, 1973.
14. Beall, A. C., Jr., Crosthwait, R. W., and DeBakey, M. E.: Injuries of the colon including those incident to surgery upon the aorta. Surg. Clin. N. Am. *45*:1273, 1965.
15. Berne, C. J., Donovan, A. J., and Hagen, W. E.: Combined duodenal pancreatic trauma. The role of end-to-side gastrojejunostomy. Arch. Surg. *96*:712, 1968.
16. Bricker, D. L., Morton, J. R., Okies, J. E., and Beall, A. C., Jr.: Surgical management of injuries to the vena cava: changing patterns of injury and newer techniques of repair. J. Trauma *11*:725, 1971.
17. Brittain, R. S., Marchioro, T. L., Germann, G., Waddell, W. R., and Starzl, T. E.: Accidental hepatic artery ligation in humans. Am. J. Surg. *107*:822, 1964.
18. Brockenbrough, E. C., and Moylan, J. A.: Treatment of contaminated surgical wounds with a topical antibiotic: A double blind study of 240 patients. Am. Surg. 35:789, 1969.
19. Brown, R. S., Boyd, D. R., Matsuda, T., and Lowe, R. J.: Temporary internal vascular shunt for retrohepatic vena cava injury. J. Trauma *11*:736, 1971.
20. Bull, J. C., Jr., and Mathewson, C., Jr.: Exploratory laparotomy in patients with penetrating wounds of the abdomen. Am. J. Surg. *116*:223, 1968.
21. Bunch, G. H.: Shotgun wounds of the abdomen. Trans. South. Surg. Assoc. *41*:38, 1928.
22. Burne, R. V.: The surgical repair of major liver injuries. Surg. Gynecol. Obstet. *119*:113, 1964.
23. Byrd, W. M., and McAfee, D. K.: Emergency hepatic lobectomy in massive injury of the liver. Surg. Gynecol. Obstet. *113*:103, 1961.
24. Carey, L. C., Lowery, B. D., and Cloutier, C. T.: Hemorrhagic shock. Curr. Probl. Surg. January, 1971.
25. Carter, J. W., and Sawyers, J. L.: Pitfalls in diagnosis of abdominal stab wounds by the contrast media injection. Am. Surg. 35:107, 1969.
26. Child, C. G., III: Liver and Portal Hypertension. Philadelphia, W. B. Saunders Co., 1964, p. 23
27. Chilimindris, C., Boyd, D. R., Carlson, L. E., Folk, F. A., Baker, R. J., and Freeark, R. J.: A critical review of management of right colon injuries. J. Trauma *11*:651, 1971.
28. Citron, B. P., Pincos, I. J., Geokas, M. C., and Haverback, B. J.: Chemical trauma of the esophagus and stomach. Surg. Clin. N. Am. *48*:1303, 1968.
29. Cleveland, A. C., and Waddell, W. R.: Retroperitoneal rupture of the duodenum due to nonpenetrating trauma. Surg. Clin. N. Am. *43*:413, 1963.
30. Cocke, W. M., Jr., and Meyer, K. K.: Retroperitoneal duodenal rupture. Am. J. Surg. *108*:834, 1964.
31. Cornell, W. P., Ebert, P. A., Greenfield, L. J., and Zuidema, G. D.: A nonoperative technique for the diagnosis of penetrating injuries to the abdomen. J. Trauma 7:307, 1967.
32. Cornell, W. P., Ebert, P. A., and Zuidema, G. D.: X-ray diagnosis of penetrating wounds of the abdomen. J. Surg. Res. 5:142, 1965.
33. DeMuth, W. E., Jr.: The mechanism of shotgun wounds. J. Trauma *11*:219, 1971.
34. Dickerman, J. D.: Bacterial infection and the asplenic host: A review. J. Trauma *16*:622, 1976.
35. DiVincenti, F. C., Rives, J. D., LaBorde, E. J., Fleming I. D., and Cohn, I., Jr.: Blunt abdominal trauma. J. Trauma 8:1004, 1968.
36. Doersch, K. B., and Dozier, W. E.: The seatbelt syndrome. The seatbelt sign, intestinal and mesenteric injuries. Am. J. Surg. *116*:831, 1968.
37. Donaldson, G. A., Rodkey, G. V., and Behring, G. E.: Resection of the rectum with anal preservation. Surg. Gynecol. Obstet. *123*:571, 1966.
38. Donovan, A. J., and Hagen, W. E.: Traumatic perforation of the duodenum. Am. J. Surg. *111*:341, 1966.
39. Doubilet, H., and Mulholland, J. H.: Some observations on the treatment of trauma to the pancreas. Am. J. Surg. *105*:741, 1963.
40. Douglas, G. J., and Simpson, J. S.: The conservative management of splenic trauma. J. Pediatr. Surg. 6:565, 1971.

41. Drye, J. C., and Schuster, G.: Shotgun wounds. Am. J. Surg. 85:438, 1953.
42. Dudrick, S. J., Wilmore, D. W., Steiger, E., Mackie, J. A., and Fitts, W. T., Jr.: Spontaneous closure of traumatic pancreatoduodenal fistulas with total intravenous nutrition. J. Trauma 10:542, 1970.
43. Ein, S. H., Shandling, B., Simpson, J. S., Stephens, C. A., Bandi, S. K., Biggar, W. D., and Freedman, M. H.: The morbidity and mortality of splenectomy in childhood. Ann. Surg. 185:307, 1977.
44. Eraklis, A. J., and Filler, R. M.: Splenectomy in childhood.: A review of 1413 cases. J. Pediatr. Surg. 7:382, 1972.
45. Eraklis, A. J., Kevy, S. V., Diamond, L. K., and Gross, R. E.: Hazards of overwhelming infection after splenectomy in childhood. N. Engl. J. Med. 276:1225, 1967.
46. Farrel, J. J.: Nonpenetrating abdominal trauma. J. Florida Med. Assoc. 43:1104, 1957.
47. Field, S. B.: Transluminal repair of penetrating injury of the inferior vena cava. Ann. Surg. 31:6, 1965.
48. Fischer, R. P., Stremple, J. F., McNamara, J. J., and Guernsey, J. M.: The rapid right hepatectomy. J. Trauma 11:742, 1971.
49. Fitzgerald, J. B., Crawford, E. S., and DeBakey, M. E.: Surgical considerations of nonpenetrating abdominal injuries. Am. J. Surg. 100:22, 1960.
50. Foster, J. H., Lawler, M. R., Jr., Welborn, M. B., Holcomb, G. W., Jr., and Sawyers J. L.: Recent experience with major hepatic resection. Ann. Surg. 167:651, 1968.
51. Freeark, R. J.: Role of angiography in the management of multiple injuries. Surg. Gynecol. Obstet. 128:761, 1969.
52. Freeark, R. J.: Penetrating wounds of the abdomen. N. Engl. J. Med. 291:185, 1974.
53. Freeark, R. J., Corley, R. D., Norcross, W. J., and Strohl, E. L.: Intramural hematoma of the duodenum. Arch. Surg. 92:463, 1966.
54. Freeark, R. J., Kane, J. M., Folk, F. A., and Baker, R. J.: Traumatic disruption of the head of the pancreas. Arch. Surg. 91:5, 1965.
55. Freeark, R. J., Love, L., and Baker, R. J.: The role of aortography in the management of blunt abdominal trauma. J. Trauma 8:557, 1968.
56. Freeark, R. J., Shoemaker, W. C., and Baker, R. J.: Aortography in blunt abdominal trauma. Arch. Surg. 96:292, 1968.
57. Friedmann, P.: Selective management of stab wounds of the abdomen. Arch. Surg. 96:292, 1968.
58. Fullen, W. D., Hunt, J., and Altemeier, W. A.: Prophylactic antibiotics in penetrating wounds of the abdomen. J. Trauma 12:282, 1972.
59. Gambill, E. E., and Mason,H. L.: One hour value for urinary amylase in 96 patients with pancreatitis. J.A.M.A. 186:130, 1963.
60. Garrett, J. W., and Braunstein, P. W.: The seat belt syndrome. J. Trauma 2:220, 1962.
61. German, J. D., and Davis, W. C.: Peritoneal splenosis following traumatic rupture of the spleen. Am. Surg. 32:329, 1966.
62. Goldsmith, N. A., and Woodburne, R. T.: The surgical anatomy pertaining to liver resection. Surg. Gynecol. Obstet. 105:310, 1957.
63. Greaves, F. C., Draeger, R. H., Brines, O. A., Shaver, J. S., and Coreys, E. L.: Experimental study of underwater concussion. U.S. Nav. Med. Bull, 41:33, 1943.
64. Griswold, R. A., and Collier, H. S.: Blunt abdominal trauma. Int. Abstr. Surg. 112:309, 1961.
65. Haller, J. A., and Jones, E. L.: Effect of splenectomy on immunity and resistance to major infections in early childhood. Clinical and experimental study. Ann. Surg. 163:902, 1966.
66. Hartman, S. W., and Greaney, E. M., Jr.: Traumatic injuries to the biliary system in children. Am. J. Surg. 108:150, 1964.
67. Harvey, E. N., Korr, I. M., Oster, G., and McMillen, J. H.: Secondary damage in wounding due to pressure changes accompanying the passage of high velocity missiles. Surgery 21:218, 1947.
68. Haynes, C. D., Gunn, C. H., and Martin, J. D., Jr.: Colon injuries. Arch. Surg. 96:944, 1968.
69. Healey, J. E., Jr.: Clinical anatomic aspects of radical hepatic surgery. J. Int. Coll. Surg. 22:542, 1954.
70. Heaton, L. D., Hughes, C. W., Rosegay, H., Fisher, G. W., and Feighny, R. E.: Military surgical practices of the United States Army in Vietnam. Curr. Probl. Surg. November, 1966.
71. Henderson, F. F., and Gaston, E. A.: Ingested foreign body in the intestinal tract. Arch. Surg. 36:66, 1938.
72. Hopson, W. B., Sherman, R. T., and Sanders, J. W.: Stab wounds of the abdomen. Am. Surg. 32:213, 1966.
73. Howard, J. M., and Brown, R. B.: Military Surgery, In Rhoads, J. E., Allen, J. G., Harkins, H. N., and Moyer, C. A. (eds.): Surgery: Principles and Practice, 4th Ed. Philadelphia, J. B. Lippincott Co., 1970, p. 601.
74. Jarvis, F. J., Byers, W. L., and Platt, E. V.: Experiences in the management of abdominal wounds of warfare. Surg. Gynecol. Obstet. 82:174, 1946.
75. Jett, H. H., Van Hoy, J. M., and Hamit, H. F.: Clinical socioeconomic aspects of 254 admissions for stab and gunshot wounds. J. Trauma 12:577, 1972.
76. Jones, R. C., and Shires, G. T.: The management of pancreatic injuries. Arch. Surg. 90:502, 1965.
77. Jones, R. C., and Shires, G. T.: Pancreatic trauma. Arch. Surg. 102:424, 1971.
78. Jones, T. W., and Merendino, K. A.: The deep epigastric artery: rectus muscle syndrome. Am. J. Surg. 103:159, 1962.
79. Jordan, J. S., and McAfee, D. K.: Wounds of the jejunum and ileum. Am. Surg. 29:630, 1963.
80. Kazarian, K. K., DiSpaltre, F. L., McKinnon, W. M. P., and Mersheimer, W. L.: Stab wounds of the abdomen: An analysis of 500 patients. Arch. Surg. 102:465, 1971.
81. Kennedy, R. H.: Presidential address: Problem areas in surgery of trauma. Am. J. Surg. 91:457, 1956.

82. Kerry, R. L., and Glas, W. W.: Traumatic injuries of the pancreas and duodenum. Arch. Surg. 85:813, 1962.

83. Killen, J. A.: Injury of superior mesenteric vessels secondary to nonpenetrating abdominal trauma. Am. Surg. 30:306, 1964.

84. Kobold, E. E., and Thal, A. P.: A simple method for the management of experimental wounds of the duodenum. Surg. Gynecol. Obstet. 116:340, 1963.

85. Kulowski, J., and Rost, W. B.: Intraabdominal injury from safety belts in auto accidents. Arch. Surg. 73: 970, 1956.

86. Lenyenwegen, F.: Hepatic artery reconstruction. Lancet. 1:21, 1965.

87. Lim, R. C., Jr., Glickman, M. G., and Hunt, T. K.: Angiography in patients with blunt trauma to the chest and abdomen. Surg. Clin. N. Am. 52:551, 1972.

88. London, P. S.: The management of persons with multiple injuries. In Rob, C., and Smith, R. (eds.): Operative Surgery. Philadelphia, F. A. Davis Co., 1964.

89. Longmire, W. P., Jr., and Cleveland, R. J.: Surgical anatomy and blunt trauma of the liver. Surg. Clin. N. Am. 52:687, 1972.

90. Loria, F. L.: Prognostic factors in abdominal gunshot wounds. New Orleans Med. Surg. J. 83:393, 1930.

91. Loria, F. L.: Abdomino-thoracic gunshot injuries. New Orleans Med. Surg. J. 95:105, 1942.

92. Loria, F. L.: Collective Review — Historical aspects of penetrating wounds of the abdomen. Int. Abst. Surg. 87:521, 1948.

93. Loria, F. L.: Historical Aspects of Abdominal Injuries. Springfield, Ill., Charles C Thomas, 1968, Chap. XI, pp. 134–138.

94. Lucas, C. E.: Prospective clinical evaluation of biliary drainage in hepatic trauma: an interim report. Ann. Surg. 174:830, 1971.

95. Lucas, C. E.: Resuscitation of the injured patient: The three phases of treatment. Surg. Clin. North Am. 57:3, 1977.

96. Lucas, C. E., and Ledgerwood, A. M.: Controlled biliary drainage for large injuries of the liver. Surg. Gynecol. Obstet. 137:585, 1973.

97. Lucas, C. E., and Walt, A. J.: Critical decisions in liver trauma. Arch. Surg. 101:277, 1970.

98. Madden, J. L., and Brunschwig, A.: Right hepatic lobectomy. In Madden, J. L.: Atlas of Technics in Surgery. New York, Appleton-Century-Crofts, 1964, pp. 468–473.

99. Madding, G. F.: Wounds of the liver. Surg. Clin. N. Am. 38:1619, 1958.

100. Madding, G. F., and Kennedy, P. A.: The effects of glucagon on hepatic blood flow. J.A.M.A. 212:482, 1970.

101. Madding, G. F., and Kennedy, P. A.: Trauma to the liver. In Dunphy, J. Englebert. (ed.): Major Problems in Clinical Surgery. Vol. II, 2nd Ed. Philadelphia, W. B. Saunders Co., 1971.

102. Madding, G. F., and Kennedy, P. A.: Hepatic artery ligation. Surg. Clin. N. Am. 52:719, 1972.

103. Margolies, M. N., Ring, E. J., Waltman, A. C., Kerr, W. S., Jr., and Baum, S.: Arteriography in the management of hemorrhage from pelvic fractures. N. Engl. J. Med. 287:317, 1972.

104. Martin, J. B.: The management of shotgun wounds. J. Trauma 11:522, 1971.

105. Mason, J. H.: The expectant management of abdominal stab wounds. J. Trauma 4:210, 1964.

106. Maynard, A. de L., and Ordeza, G.: Mandatory operation for penetrating wounds of the abdomen. Am. J. Surg. 115:307, 1968.

107. Mays, E. T.: Complex penetrating hepatic wounds. Ann. Surg. 173:421, 1971.

108. Mays, E. T.: Lobar dearterialization for exsanguinating wounds of the liver. J. Trauma 12:397, 1972.

109. McClelland, R., Shires, T., and Poulos, E.: Hepatic resection for massive trauma. J. Trauma 4:282, 1964.

110. McClelland, R. N., and Shires, T.: Management of liver trauma in 259 consecutive patients. Ann. Surg. 161:248, 1965.

111. McCort, J. J.: Radiographic Examination in Blunt Abdominal Trauma. Philadelphia, W. B. Saunders Co., 1966.

112. McCoy, J., and Wolma, F. J.: Abdominal tap: indication, technic and results. Am. J. Surg. 122:693, 1971.

113. McKittrick, J. E.: Use of a serosal patch in repair of a duodenal fistula. Calif. Med. 103:433, 1965.

114. McNabney, W. K., and McCanse, A.: Management of abdominal stab wounds. Am. J. Surg. 114:726, 1967.

115. Means, R. L.: Bile peritonitis. Am. Surg. 30:583, 1964.

116. Merendino, K. A., Dillard, D. A., and Cammock, E. E.: The concept of surgical biliary decompression in the management of liver trauma. Surg. Gynecol. Obstet. 117:285, 1963.

117. Mishalany, H.: Repair of the ruptured spleen. J. Pediatr. Surg. 9:175, 1974.

118. Morgenstern, L.: Microcrystalline collagen used in experimental splenic injury. A new surface hemostatic agent. Arch. Surg. 109:44, 1974.

119. Morton, J. R., Roys, G. D., and Bricker, D. L.: The treatment of liver injuries. Surg. Gynecol. Obstet. 134:298, 1972.

120. Moss, L. K., Schmidt, F. E., and Creech, O.: Analysis of 550 stab wounds of the abdomen. Am. Surg. 28:483, 1962.

121. Nance, F. C., and Cohn, I., Jr.: Surgical judgment in the management of stab wounds of the abdomen. Ann. Surg. 170:569, 1969.

122. Nance, F. C., Wennar, M. H., Johnson, L. W., Ingram, J. C., and Cohn, I., Jr.: Surgical judgement in management of penetrating wounds of the abdomen: Experience with 2212 patients. Ann. Surg. 179:639, 1974.

123. Netterville, R. E., and Hardy, J. D.: Penetrating wounds of the abdomen. Analysis of 55 cases with problems in management. Ann. Surg. 166:232, 1967.

124. Nicosia, J. F., Thornton, J. P., Folk, F. A., and Saletta, J. D.: Surgical management of corrosive gastric injuries. Ann. Surg. 180:139, 1974.

125. Noon, G. P., Beall, A. C., Jr., Jordan, G. L., Jr., Riggs, S., and DeBakey, M. E.: Clinical

evaluation of peritoneal irrigation with antibiotic solution. Surgery 62:73, 1967.

126. Nora, P. F., Vanecko, R. M., and Bransfield, J. J.: Prophylactic abdominal drains. Arch. Surg. 105:173, 1972.

127. Norell, H. G.: Traumatic rupture of the spleen diagnosed by selective arteriography. Acta Radiol. 48:449, 1957.

128. Northrup, W. R., III, and Simmons, R. L.: Pancreatic trauma: a review. Surgery 71:27, 1972.

129. O'Donnell, V. A., Lou, M. A., Maxwell, T. M., Mandal, A. K., and Alexander, J. L.: Penetrating wounds of the abdomen. J. Natl. Med. Assoc. 67:155, 1975.

130. Olsen, W. R., and Beaudoin, D. E.: Wound drainage after splenectomy. Am. J. Surg. 117:615, 1969.

131. Olsen, W. R., and Hildreth, D. H.: Abdominal paracentesis and peritoneal lavage in blunt abdominal trauma. J. Trauma 11:824, 1971.

132. Olsen, W. R., and Polley, T. Z., Jr.: A second look at delayed splenic rupture. Arch. Surg. 112:422, 1977.

133. O'Mara, R. E., Hall, R. C., and Dombroski, D. L.: Scintiscanning in the diagnosis of rupture of the spleen. Surg. Gynecol. Obstet. 131:1077, 1970.

134. Orlando, J. C., and Moore, T. C.: Splenectomy for trauma in childhood. Surg. Gynecol. Obstet. 134:94, 1972.

135. Orloff, M. J., and Charters, A. C.: Injuries of the small bowel and mesentery and retroperitoneal hematoma. Surg. Clin. N. Am. 52:729, 1972.

136. Ochsner, J. L., Crawford, E. S., and DeBakey, M. E.: Injuries of the vena cava caused by external trauma. Surgery 49:397, 1961.

137. Payne, W. D., Terz, J. J., and Lawrence, W., Jr.: Major hepatic resection for trauma. Ann. Surg. 170:929, 1969.

138. Perry, J. F., Jr.: Blunt and penetrating abdominal injuries. Curr. Probl. Surg. May, 1970.

139. Philippart, A. I.: Blunt abdominal trauma in childhood. Surg. Clin. North Am. 57:151, 1977.

140. Pinkerton, J. A., Sawyer, J. L., and Foster, J. H.: A study of the postoperative course after hepatic lobectomy. Ann. Surg. 173:800, 1971.

141. Poulos, E.: Hepatic resection for massive liver injuries. Ann. Surg. 157:525, 1963.

142. Pridgen, J. E., Herff, A. F., Jr., Watkins, H. O., Halbert, D. S., D'Avila, R., Crouch, D. M., and Prud'Homme, J. L.: Penetrating wounds of the abdomen: analysis of 776 operative cases. Ann. Surg. 165:901, 1967.

143. Printen, K. J., Freeark, R. J., and Shoemaker, W. C.: Conservative management of penetrating abdominal wounds. Arch. Surg. 96:899, 1968.

144. Quattlebaum, J. K., and Quattlebaum, J. K., Jr.: Technic of hepatic lobectomy. Ann. Surg. 149:648, 1959.

145. Rambo, W. M.: Irrigation of the peritoneal cavity with cephalothin. Am. J. Surg. 123:192, 1972.

146. Ravitch, M. M.: Hypogastric artery ligation in acute pelvic trauma. Surgery 56:601, 1964.

147. Rich, N. M., and Hughes, C. W.: The fate of prosthetic material used to repair vascular injuries in contaminated wounds. J. Trauma 12:459, 1972.

148. Richter, R. M., and Zaki, M. H.: Selective conservative management of penetrating abdominal wounds. Ann. Surg. 166:238, 1967.

149. Roman, E., Silva, Y. J., and Lucas, C.: Management of blunt duodenal injury. Surg. Gynecol. Obstet. 132:7, 1971.

150. Roof, W. R., Morris, G. C., Jr., and DeBakey, M. E.: Management of perforating injuries to the colon in civilian practice. Am. J. Surg. 99:641, 1960.

151. Root, H. D.: When to explore the abdomen with penetrating wounds. In Pridgen, J. E., Aust, J. B., and Fisher, G. W. (eds.): Penetrating Wounds of the Abdomen. Springfield, Ill., Charles C Thomas, 1970.

152. Root, H. D., Hauser, C. W., McKinley, C. R., LaFave, J. W., and Mendiola, R. P., Jr.: Diagnostic peritoneal lavage. Surgery 57:633, 1965.

153. Root, H. D., Keizer, P. J., and Perry, J. F., Jr.: The clinical and experimental aspects of peritoneal response to injury. Arch. Surg. 95:531, 1967.

154. Root, H. D., Keizer, P. J., and Perry, J. F., Jr.: Peritoneal trauma, experimental and clinical studies. Surgery 62:679, 1967.

155. Roswit, B., Malsky, S. J., and Reid, C. B.: Severe radiation injuries of the stomach, small intestine, colon and rectum. Am. J. Roentgenol. Radium Ther. Nucl. Med. 114:460, 1972.

156. Sanders, R. J.: The management of colon injuries. Surg. Clin. N. Am. 43:457, 1963.

157. Seavers, R., Lynch, J., Ballard, R., Jernigan, S., and Johnson, J.: Hypogastric artery ligation for uncontrollable hemorrhage in acute pelvic trauma. Surgery 55:516, 1964.

158. Shaftan, G. W.: Indications for operation in abdominal trauma. Am. J. Surg. 99:657, 1960.

159. Shaftan, G. W.: Selective conservatism in penetrating abdominal trauma. Surgery 59:650, 1966.

160. Sherman, R. T., and Parrish, R. A.: Management of shotgun injuries. J. Trauma 3:76, 1963.

161. Shirkey, A. L., Wukasch, D. C., Beall, A. C., Jr., Gordon, W. B., and DeBakey, M. E.: Surgical management of splenic injuries. Am. J. Surg. 108:630, 1964.

162. Shively, E., Pearlstein, L., Kinnaird, D. W., Roe, J., and Jones, C. E.: Post-traumatic intestinal obstruction. Surgery 79:612, 1976.

163. Shrock, T., Blaisdell, F. W., and Mathewson, C.: Management of blunt trauma to the liver and hepatic veins. Arch. Surg. 96:698, 1968.

164. Sinclair, T. L., and Stephenson, H. E., Jr.: Survival following abdominal aortic rupture from blunt trauma. Missouri Med. 69:271, 1972.

165. Singer, D. B.: Postsplenectomy sepsis. Perspect. Pediatr. Pathol. 1:285, 1973.

166. Sizer, J. S., Wayne, E. R., and Frederick, P. L.: Delayed rupture of the spleen. Arch. Surg. 92:362, 1966.

167. Smith, S. W., and Hastings, T. N.: Traumatic rupture of the gallbladder. Ann. Surg. 139:517, 1954.

168. Sorour, V. E., and Bijlsma, P. J.: Stab wounds of the abdomen. S. Afr. J. Surg. *4*:85, 1966.
169. Sparkman, P. S.: Massive hemobilia following traumatic rupture of the liver. Ann. Surg. *138*:899, 1953.
170. Sparkman, R. S., and Fogelman, M. J.: Wounds of the liver. Ann. Surg. *139*:690, 1954.
171. Starzl, T. E., Kaupp, H. A., Beheler, Z. M., and Freeark, R. J.: Penetrating injuries of the inferior vena cava. Surg. Clin. N. Am. *43*:87, 1963.
172. Steichen, F. M.: Penetrating wounds of the chest and the abdomen. Curr. Probl. Surg. August, 1967.
173. Steichen, F. M., Efron, G., Pearlman, D. M., and Weil, P. H.: Radiographic diagnosis versus selective management in penetrating wounds of the abdomen. Ann. Surg. *170*:978, 1969.
174. Steichen, F. M., Pearlman, D. M., Dargan, E. L., Prommas, D. C., and Weil, P. H.: Wounds of the abdomen: Radiographic diagnosis of intraperitoneal penetration. Ann. Surg. *165*:77, 1967.
175. Steigmann, F., and Doleheck, R. A.: Corrosive (acid) gastritis. N. Engl. J. Med. *254*:981, 1956.
176. Stein, A., and Lissoos, I.: Selective management of penetrating wounds of the abdomen. J. Trauma *8*:1014, 1968.
177. Stone, H. H., Stowers, K. B., and Shippey, S. H.: Injuries to the pancreas. Arch. Surg. *85*:525, 1962.
178. Sturim, H. S.: Surgical management of traumatic transection of the pancreas. Ann. Surg. *163*:399, 1966.
179. Sturim, H. S.: The surgical management of pancreatic injuries. Surg Gynecol. Obstet. *122*:133, 1966.
180. Thadepalli, H., Gorbach, S. L., Broido, P. W., Norsen, J., and Nyhus, L.: Abdominal trauma, anaerobes, and antibiotics. Surg. Gynecol. Obstet. *137*:270, 1973.
181. Thal, A. P., and Wilson, R. F.: A pattern of severe trauma to the region of the pancreas. Surg. Gynecol. Obstet. *119*:773, 1964.
182. Thompson, R. J., and Hinshaw, D. B.: Pancreatic trauma. Ann. Surg. *163*:153, 1966.
183. Tobias, S., DeClement, F. A., and Cleveland, J. C.: Management of abdominal stab wounds: Roentgenographic technique for diagnosis of peritoneal penetration. Arch. Surg. *95*:27, 1967.
184. Tolins, S. H.: Complete severance of the common bile duct due to blunt trauma. Ann. Surg. *140*:61, 1959.
185. Trimble, C.: Stab wound sinography. Surg. Clin. N. Am. *49*:1217, 1969.
186. Trimble, C., and Eason, F. J.: A complication of splenosis. J. Trauma *12*:358, 1972.
187. Vannix, R. S., Carter, R., Hinshaw, D. B., and Joergenson, E. J.: Surgical management of colon trauma in civilian practice. Am. J. Surg. *106*:364, 1963.
188. Webb, H. W., Howard, J. M., Jordan, G. L., and Vowles, D. J.: Surgical experiences in the treatment of duodenal injuries. Int. Abstr. Surg. *106*:105, 1958.
189. Weckesser, E. C., and Putnam, T. C.: Perforat-

ing injuries of the rectum and sigmoid colon. J. Trauma *2*:474, 1962.
190. Weinstein, W. M., Onderdonk, A. B., Bartlett, J. G., et al.: Antimicrobial therapy of experimental intraabdominal sepsis. J. Infect. Dis. *132*:282, 1975.
191. Werner, L.: Scintiscan diagnosis of splenic hematoma. Surg. Gynecol. Obstet. *134*:430, 1972.
192. Whelan, T. J., Burkhalter, W. E., and Gomez. A.: Management of war wounds. *In* Claude E. Welch (ed.): Advances in Surgery. Vol. 3, Chicago, Year Book Medical Publishers, 1968, pp. 227–350.
193. White, P. H., and Benfield, J. R.: Amylase in the management of pancreatic trauma. Arch. Surg. *105*:158, 1972.
194. Wilder, J. R., Habermann, E. T., and Schachner, S. J.: Selective surgical intervention for stab wounds of the abdomen. Surgery *61*:231, 1967.
195. Williams, J. S., and Kirkpatrick, J. R.: The nature of seatbelt injuries. J. Trauma *11*:207, 1971.
196. Willis, B. C.: Shotgun wounds of the abdomen. Am. J. Surger. *28*:407, 1935.
197. Willox, G. L.: Nonpenetrating injuries of abdomen causing rupture of spleen. Arch. Surg. *90*:498, 1965.
198. Wilson, C. B., Vidrine, A., Jr., and Rives, J. D.: Unrecognized abdominal trauma in patients with head injuries. Ann. Surg. *161*:608, 1965.
199. Wilson, H., and Sherman, R.: Civilian penetrating wounds of the abdomen. I. Factors in mortality and differences from military wounds in 494 cases. Ann. Surg. *13*:639, 1961.
200. Wolfman, E. F., Jr., Trevino, G., Heaps, D., K., and Zuidema, G. D.: An operative technic for the management of acute and chronic lateral duodenal fistulas. Ann. Surg. *159*:563, 1964.
201. Wolma, F. J., and Williford, F., III: Treatment of injuries to the colon. Am. J. Surg. *110*:772, 1965.
202. Yellin, A. E., Chaffee, C. B., and Donovan, A. J.: Vascular isolation in treatment of juxtahepatic venous injuries. Arch. Surg. *102*:566, 1971.
203. Yellin, A. E., Vecchione, T. R., and Donovan, A. J.: Distal pancreatectomy in trauma to the pancreas. Am. J. Surg. *124*:135, 1972.
204. Yurko, A. A., and Williams, R. D.: Needle paracentesis in blunt abdominal trauma: A critical analysis. J. Trauma *6*:194, 1966.
205. Zacheis, H. G., and Condon, R. E.: Seat belts and intraabdominal trauma: report of two unusual cases. J. Trauma *12*:85, 1972.
206. Zollinger, R. M., Keller, R. T., and Hubay, C. A.: Traumatic rupture of the right and left hepatic ducts. J. Trauma *12*:563, 1972.
207. Zuidema, G. D.: In discussion of Nance, F. C., and Cohn, I.: Surgical judgement in the management of stab wounds of the abdomen: A retrospective and prospective analysis based on a study of 600 stabbed patients. Ann. Surg. *170*:569, 1969.

CHAPTER 15

OBSTETRICAL AND GYNECOLOGICAL INJURIES

James J. Delaney, M.D.

GENERAL CONSIDERATIONS

Women are subject to the same traumatic situations that men face. They spend as much time as men do behind the wheel of an automobile and, therefore, are at least as apt to be involved in automobile accidents as are men. They may be subject to beatings either by jealous mates or boyfriends or as the victims of sexual assault. As more women enter the labor market, they will become subject to more industrial accidents. The general principles involved in managing all these types of trauma are discussed elsewhere in this book. The purpose of this chapter is to discuss those traumatic injuries that are more or less specifically limited to the female pelvis and reproductive organs. This includes perineal trauma, trauma associated with sexual activity and assault, induced abortion and trauma resulting from automobile accidents and blunt or penetrating injuries.

Anatomical Principles

The perineum is that area of the torso covering the pelvic outlet. It is well protected from most incidental traumatic injuries by its anatomical position. It becomes exposed only when the thighs are abducted. The anterior boundary is the symphysis pubis; the lateral boundaries are the ischial pubic rami, ischial tuberosities and the sacrosciatic ligaments; and the posterior boundary is the coccyx. The pelvic viscera include the urinary bladder and urethra, the vagina, uterus and tubes, ovaries and rectum. These organs are protected anteriorly, posteriorly and laterally by the bony pelvis and inferiorly by the pelvic diaphragm, which is made up of a series of fascial and muscular planes. Careful examination of Figures 15–1 and 15–2 will help clarify this anatomy. There are eight planes and a knowledge of the limits of these planes will enable one to understand how hematomas and/or sepsis will be confined or the extent to which they may spread. Superiorly to inferiorly, the planes are as follows: The first plane consists of parietal peritoneum, which is reflected over all the pelvic organs. The second plane consists of a layer of adipose tissue in which the blood vessels and nerves of the pelvis, lower extremities and the uterus are found. The clinical significance of this plane is that hematomas or infections arising in this plane may spread into the retroperitoneal space. This extension may occur posteriorly and superiorly to the diaphragm and laterally and anteriorly to the anterior abdominal wall. The third plane consists of the endopelvic or superior fascia of the levator ani muscles. The fourth plane consists of the levator ani musculature made up of the iliococ-

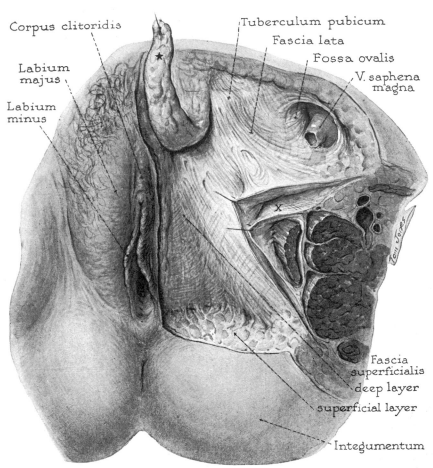

Figure 15–1. *Female perineum. Subcutaneous layers; specimen I. On the (observer's) right side the superficial layer of the superficial fascia has been removed to expose the deep (Colles') layer in the anterior (urogenital) part of the perineum; in the posterior (anal) part of the perineum the superficial layer, locally thickened and adipose, remains intact behind the line of cut, i.e., in the ischiorectal fossa. The sleeve of fascia lata, shown by transecting the thigh, has been freed from the muscle fascia; the latter is shown as it invests the sartorius (at x) and the adductors, freed from the muscles and retracted. The diverticular process has been mobilized and lifted (marked with star). (From Curtis, A. H., Anson, B. J., and Ashley, F. L.: Further studies in gynecological anatomy and related clinical problems. Surg. Gynecol. Obstet. 74:709, 1942.)*

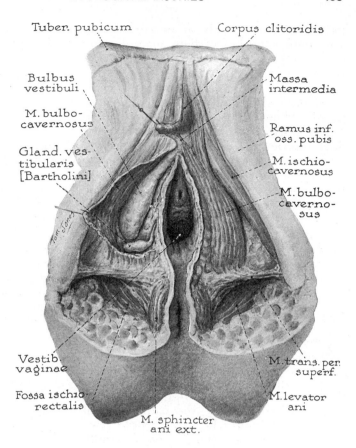

Figure 15–2. *In the anal part of the perineum the levator ani and external and sphincter muscles of each side are shown by removal of the superficial fatty tissue. In the urogenital part of the perineum, on the right side, by cutting away the muscle fascia, the ischiocavernosus, superficial transverse perineal, and bulbocavernosus muscles have been brought into view. On the left side the bulbocavernosus muscle has been reflected to expose the bulb of the vestibule and greater vestibular (Bartholin's) gland and duct. Anteriorly are seen the glans, body, and intermediate mass of the clitoris. (From Curtis, A. H., Anson, B. J., and Ashley, F. L.: Further studies in gynecological anatomy and related clinical problems. Surg. Gynecol. Obstet. 74:709, 1942.)*

cygeus, pubococcygeus and coccygeus muscles. The fifth plane consists of the inferior fascia of the levator ani musculature. The sixth plane is divided into an anterior and posterior compartment by the superficial transverse perineal muscle. The anterior compartment is relatively small and bounded by the symphysis anteriorly and pubic rami laterally. This compartment contains the ischiocavernosus and bulbocavernosus muscles and the vestibular bulb made up of vascular erectile tissue. The posterior compartment is called the ischiorectal fossa and primarily contains adipose tissue. The lateral boundaries are the arcuate tendons of the levator musculature and the posterior boundary is the sacrum and coccyx. The clinical significance of the two compartments of this sixth plane is that a hematoma or infection in the anterior compartment will be localized in a small area. It cannot spread across the midline superiorly or posteriorly. On the other hand, an infection or hematoma in the posterior compartment will not spread anteriorly and can be at least five times as large as in the anterior compartment. The seventh plane consists of the superficial and deep (Colles') fascia. The eighth plane consists of the subcutaneous tissue and skin. This diaphragm is pierced by the rectum, vagina and urethra. Muscle fibers from the levator ani surround these orifices, forming sphincters of which the anal sphincter is most easily identified.

Trauma to the bony pelvis may spare the pelvic viscera. The female urethra is relatively short and much less apt to be transected than the male urethra. Pressure transmitted to the bladder from blunt trauma may cause the bladder to burst, but more often than not, such force will spontaneously empty the bladder without damage. This is probably caused by the fact that the female urethra is relatively short. The diagnosis and treatment of urinary tract injuries are discussed in Chapter 16. In trauma-producing pelvic fractures, the femoral and obturator vessels and nerves are more apt to be damaged than are the pelvic organs, vessels or nerves. Extensive, concealed hemorrhage may occur in the retroperitoneal space as a result of a pelvic fracture.[6, 30]

Perineal and vaginal trauma is most commonly obstetrical in origin. The majority of perineal and pelvic lacerations and hematomas result from vaginal delivery. Such injuries may be associated with spontaneous deliveries, with forceps or with extraction deliveries. Most uterine ruptures are associated with obstetrical manipulation, although rupture may occasionally result from severe abdominal trauma.[5, 15, 21, 25, 27, 29] The reader is referred to standard textbooks on obstetrics for a discussion of trauma associated with obstetrical procedures.[13, 38]

Psychological Factors

Each and every part of the body has significant meaning to a patient and her family, but injuries involving the pelvis produce special anxiety. When it is apparent that the injury will not impair reproduction or sexual activity, the patient and/or her parents should be immediately reassured. In cases involving sexual assault, criminal abortion or pregnancy loss, extensive psychological support may be necessary, including psychiatric care. The physician must be careful not to make dogmatic statements regarding reproductive function or sexual activity in cases where either may be impaired. In doubtful cases, cautious optimism should be expressed. An unconcerned attitude or a rough or painful examination by the physician may seriously aggravate any associated emotional trauma.

Foreign Bodies

Occasionally a sadistic attacker or a woman herself may place a foreign body in the urethra, vagina or rectum; a curious child who has done this may be brought in for treatment. Trauma may or may not have resulted, depending on the type of object and manner in which it is placed. Women will frequently consult a physician, claiming they have "lost" a tampon or diaphragm. In almost all such cases, the "lost" object has been lost in the toilet and the only treatment necessary is an inspec-

tion of the vagina and reassurance that the object is not present and has not been "lost" above the vagina. The problem of foreign bodies in small girls is usually one of infection rather than trauma, although perineal or vaginal lacerations may also have been produced. Because of the sensitivity of the vagina of a child, sedation or anesthesia may be necessary to adequately inspect the area and remove the foreign body.

Occasionally, severe trauma will be seen from a foreign body inserted into the vagina by a sexual pervert. Such an object may be driven through the cul-de-sac into the peritoneal cavity by a kick or other heavy blow. An exploratory laparotomy is indicated in such cases.

A woman or her sexual partner may place a foreign body in the vagina, urethra or rectum for the purpose of stimulating venereal pleasure. The trauma caused by such a practice will depend on the object used, where it is placed and what forces were used to place it. If the patient is unable to remove the object, the examining physician should have no trouble making the correct diagnosis. Treatment obviously consists of removing the object and repairing any lacerations that may be bleeding.

PERINEAL INJURIES

Straddle Injuries

Very little is written in standard textbooks of obstetrics and gynecology regarding perineal injuries, especially straddle injuries. As the term suggests, such injuries are caused by falling on an object with the legs on either side of an object so that the perineum absorbs most of the impact. These injuries are most often seen in girls who fall while playing. With the increasing popularity of cycling and the preference by girls for the so-called boy's bike, we will undoubtedly see more straddle injuries.

Management.   In this type of injury, the main concern of most girls and their parents is whether or not reproduction or sexual function will be impaired. In almost all cases, they can be reassured following a brief examination. Following initial inspection of the injury to determine its extent, treatment should begin by relieving any pain that may be present. This may require anything from oral analgesics to general anesthesia. It is usually impossible to perform an adequate vaginal examination on a prepubescent child without anesthesia. The extent of the examination will depend on the type of injury. Most straddle injuries produce blunt trauma and result in contusions or hematoma formation. Occasionally, the object may be sharp, resulting in lacerations or a puncture wound. Unless the injury is obviously minor, a digital vaginal or rectal examination should be done to determine the presence or absence of hematoma formation above the pelvic diaphragm. Hematomas can usually be treated nonoperatively. A hematoma should be evacuated only if it is growing or is excessively painful. If a hematoma is evacuated, usually no active site of bleeding will be found. If generalized bleeding is apparent, hemostatic sutures may be necessary using absorbable suture. If the bleeding is not brisk, a firm pack should be placed either in lieu of the sutures or in addition to the sutures. The pack should be removed in 24 hours. Prophylactic antibiotics should also be administered. Lacerations and puncture wounds should be treated the same as in any other area of the body. If there is a question of a rectal injury, the principles of managing bowel injuries, as described in Chapter 14, should be followed.

TRAUMA RESULTING FROM SEXUAL ACTIVITY

Trauma may result from either voluntary or involuntary sexual activity.[40] These injuries may be the result of normal heterosexual activity, homosexual activity, perverted activity or masturbation. The most common injury is a laceration and the most common presenting complaint is abnormal vaginal bleeding. Because of embarrassment, intoxication or fright, an accurate history may not be obtained, so trauma from sexual activity should always be considered in cases of acute onset of vaginal bleeding. Certain factors may render a woman susceptible to injury from sexual activity. These include a lack of estrogen effect (which normally produces a well-cornified vaginal epithelium and distensible vagina), pregnancy and recent vaginal surgery. The true incidence of such injuries is unknown, as most patients with these injuries probably do not seek care unless there is significant bleeding or pain. Wilson and Swartz[40] report only 37 cases of vaginal trauma from sexual activity over a 10-year period at the Harlem Hospital Center. Death has resulted from such trauma,[4] but is almost inexcusable with appropriate therapy.

Management. Careful inspection of the vagina should be carried out to make sure that there are no multiple lacerations. If a bivalve speculum is used, the speculum should be rotated laterally so that both the anterior and posterior walls of the vagina can be seen as well as the lateral walls. The presence of perineal lacerations should not prevent inspection of the vagina. A gentle bimanual rectovaginal examination should also be carried out to make sure there are no retroperitoneal hematomas developing as a result of the trauma. If the laceration is actively bleeding, fairly extensive or on the perineum, the best method of management is repair with absorbable suture. Packing should be utilized to control hemorrhage only when the trauma is too extensive to repair primarily. If a pack is placed, it should be soaked in Furacin or other antibiotic cream and packed tightly into the vagina. It should be removed in 12 to 24 hours. There are practically no residual complications from vaginal lacerations once the bleeding has been controlled. If the introitus has been injured, the repair may occasionally lead to a decrease in size of the introitus or it may result in some fibrous scar tissue which might make intercourse moderately painful in the future. However, this complication is only rarely seen and is more commonly associated with the repair of an episiotomy.

Assault and Molestation

Any female, regardless of age, may be the victim of an unprovoked sexual attack. The physician involved in caring for such patients must be cognizant of the individual needs of the patient as well as the potential legal ramifications of a particular case. Many physicians are reluctant to treat patients who have been the objects of assault because of the fear of getting involved with the legal aspects of the case. This reluctance to act is usually based on ignorance of what may be expected of the physician.

Legal Aspects. In most cases, the physician should have no fear of legal repercussions because he has cared for the victim of a sex crime. He should understand that state statutes regarding assault and molestation merely define what acts are illegal and prescribe a penalty for any individual convicted of having committed the defined offense. Rape is generally considered to have occurred if a woman is forced to submit to coitus without consent. Statutory rape is defined as coitus with a female below the age of consent. The age of consent varies from state to state, and it should be noted that consent is not a consideration in a statutory rape. Sexual molestation is usually considered to have occurred if noncoital sexual contact has occurred in an individual below the age of consent.

Institutions such as large city or community hospitals that deal with these problems on a fairly frequent basis should have a recommended standard procedure to which physicians can refer in such cases. The American College of Obstetricians and Gynecologists has published a technical bulletin covering most of the problems related to rape, which suggests a procedure to be followed.[1] The reader is also referred to other articles dealing with the problems involved in cases of sexual assault.[16, 19, 20, 26, 32]

The assessment and management of a victim of sexual assault can be divided into three considerations: (1) treatment of physical and psychological trauma, (2) collection and processing of evidence, and (3) prevention of pregnancy and venereal disease. These three are interrelated and can be carried out best if the individual or team caring for these patients has received special training.

If the criminal and judicial processes are understood, proper care of the patient will be facilitated. It must be remembered that the victim of a sexual assault is only a witness to a crime. In order for an assailant to be charged and convicted, he must be apprehended and the alleged crime proven in court. The physician's role is to assure the collection and preservation of all evidence that may help to convict the assailant. A detailed history obtained from the patient regarding the assault cannot be used in court; therefore, only information that will be useful in treating the patient need be obtained. If the alleged assailant is accused of the crime and brought to trial, he may either deny that he assaulted the patient or admit that he had sexual relations with the patient but with her consent. If the chain of physical evidence can be successfully challenged in court, the chances of securing conviction are slim even if other evidence is overwhelming. Therefore, a standard procedure for collecting and processing this evidence should be established in every emergency department or health care facility dealing with sexual assault. In conjunction with the Colorado Bureau of Investigation, we have developed a "Rape Kit" that has been distributed and used throughout the state outside of metropolitan Denver to assure the adequate collection and processing of evidence.

Initial Evaluation. The patient may be brought in by a member of a local law enforcement agency, may come in of her own volition, or be brought in by a parent or spouse. If the alleged attack has not been formally reported, the patient should be urged to report it to the proper authority. The patient should be given the benefit of care even if she refuses to report the assault; however, there is no need to collect evidence that will not be processed.

The initial professional evaluation should be done by the same individual who will be responsible for the entire care of the patient. It is inappropriate for one individual to do a general evaluation and another to evaluate the pelvic findings. The patient should not be disrobed until after being seen by the professional evaluator and being told what the evaluation will entail.

The medical record should be dictated and typed if possible. It should contain the following information:

Background Data:
  Age.
  Marital status.
  Brought in by whom.
  State of consciousness.
  Ability to give reliable history.

Method of birth control, if any.
Last normal menstrual period.
Frequency of intercourse. Last intercourse prior to alleged assault.

History:
When and where did alleged assault occur?
What was patient doing?
Did she resist?
Did penetration occur?
Has patient bathed or douched since attack?
Has she changed clothes?

Objective evaluation:
Vital signs.
Statement regarding appearance (clothed *and* unclothed) and mental status.
Recording of general physical findings.
Description of signs of trauma, including trunk, extremities, head, perineum and pelvis.

The Collection of Evidence. Our "Rape Kit" consists of two large manila envelopes with instructions printed on each envelope. One envelope, containing the supplies needed to collect evidence is placed inside the first envelope, which is then sealed. The instructions for using the kit, printed on the outside of the first envelope, are as follows:

The Collection of Evidence for Victims of Sexual Assault

Contents:
5 labeled small clean white envelopes, each with a folded packet of white paper to collect pubic and head hair and nail scrappings.
1 clean comb
6 sterile packets of cotton swabs
1 wooden stick swab (to collect fingernail scrappings)
6 clean glass slides with slide holder
5 vacuum test tubes
2 labeled "Serology"
1 labeled "Acid phosphatase"
1 labeled "Saliva swabs"
1 labeled "Vaginal swabs"
1 large manila envelope to hold evidence

Instructions:
Before opening, write your name and the time and date across the seal, then break seal and use its contents for collecting evidence. Retain this envelope as evidence.

The instructions for collecting the evi-

dence, printed on the second envelope, are detailed:

Instructions for Collecting Evidence

1. Clothes:
Each article of the patient's clothing should be placed in a separate paper bag, which is sealed and initialed.
2. Head hair—standard:
Pluck with fingers 20-30 head hairs from different parts of the head. Place hairs in packet and envelope labeled "Head Hair." Seal and initial.
3. Foreign hair:
Comb pubic area with comb and place comb and collected hair in envelope labeled "pubic hair, combed." Seal and initial.
4. Pubic hair—standard:
Pluck with fingers 10-20 pubic hairs from different parts of pubic area. Place hairs in packet and envelope labeled "Pubic hairs, plucked." Seal and initial.
5. Sperm presence and motility:
Using 2 separate swabs and slides, obtain and examine specimens from endocervix and vaginal pool. Record presence or absence of sperm and comment on motility if sperm are present. (These slides need not be saved. The presence or absence of sperm neither proves nor disproves anything, but the information may be valuable when the history and other evidence are compared.)
6. Sperm presence:
Make slides as in (5) above. Label source and place in slide containers. If fellatio or sodomy are alleged, make slide specimens from mouth or rectum, respectively.
7. Acid phosphatase determination:
Place swabs from (6) above in clean test tube and label tube(s).
8. Semen typing:
Take 2 swabs of vaginal contents and place in clean test tube and label.
9. Saliva for secretor status:
Have patient suck on 2 swabs to saturate them with saliva. Place in test tube and label.
10. Fingernails:
Break wooden stick-swab and scrape beneath nails of one hand. Place stick and contents in labeled envelope. Seal and initial. Repeat for other hand.
11. Blood:
Fill 2 tubes with venous blood; send one for serology and retain the other for typing.
Labeling:
Be sure all specimens are labeled, sealed, and initialed by examiner. Place all speci-

mens in envelope. Seal, date, and initial over seal. Place envelope and clothing in cardboard box-seal; label and date. Give box to investigating police officer.

A written "Medical Encounter" sheet should be filled out in addition to the dictated note. It should contain the following information:

Patient's name, address and phone number

Date and time seen

Brought in by whom

Seen by whom

Dictation: Date, time, and number of dictating machine or phone summary of treatment instructions for follow-up. Copies should be sent to appropriate police authority, placed in the medical chart, and retained for the records of the primary examiner.

Note: In recording one's assessment of the patient, "rape" is an inappropriate diagnostic term. "Evidence of recent sexual activity" with or without "evidence of trauma" is more appropriate.

Processing of Evidence.   All specimens should be collected, labeled with the initials of the examiner and placed in the manila envelope. The examiner's name or initials should be written over the seal. Individual pieces of clothing should be placed in clean paper bags, sealed and initialed by the examiner. All evidence should be placed in a cardboard box and sealed with tape. The name or initials of the examiner should be written across the seal. The box should be given to the investigating law enforcement officer and the officer should be instructed to deliver it to the appropriate laboratory for analysis.

If the patient is a child, she should not be subjected to a pelvic examination without sedation, and serious consideration should be given to doing such an examination under anesthesia. Obviously, any severe trauma should be treated as soon as possible, but not before a complete examination has been performed.

Sedation may be necessary as a form of management but preferably should not be given prior to obtaining an accurate history. Hospitalization may or may not be required, depending upon the severity of injuries and the psychological state of the patient. Emotionally unstable patients should be kept in the hospital for observation. Psychiatric consultation may or may not be necessary, depending upon the psychological state of the patient. Victims of an assault may have been forced to submit to unnatural sexual activity as well as so-called natural activity, which may aggravate their anxiety. Some arrangements for follow-up should be made with the patient given a return appointment within a week.

Pregnancy Prevention.   It is extremely unlikely that a pregnancy will result from criminal assault, but there is no excuse for not acting to prevent such a pregnancy in any woman who is in the first half of her menstrual cycle. As part of the history, the date of the last normal menstrual period should be obtained and information regarding contraceptive practices should also be included. If the patient is using oral contraceptives or an intrauterine device, it can be assumed that pregnancy will not result from the assault. This is likewise true of a woman who is past the menopause or of a prepubescent girl. If the woman is past midcycle and she has a cellular effect as seen in her cervical mucus smear, it can be assumed that she has ovulated and will not become pregnant as a result of the assault. The patient may already be pregnant. If there is a possibility of an existing pregnancy, this should be documented by appropriate examination and pregnancy test. This is necessary both to assure the patient that a developing pregnancy was not the result of the assault and to be sure that no sex steroids, which are usually given to prevent an unwanted pregnancy, are given that might have an adverse effect on an existing pregnancy. If a state of pregnancy already exists, the patient should be reassured that the assault did not endanger her pregnancy. If the patient is in the first half of her cycle and has not been taking oral contraceptives, it is desirable to act to prevent a possible pregnancy. The use of relatively high doses of estrogen within 48 hours of the assault will prevent pregnancy.[24] The mechanism for action of this therapy is not known. The estrogen must somehow act by either preventing fertilization or implantation since an existing early pregnancy will not be terminated. One of the standard regimens has been to give 25 mg of diethylstilbestrol daily for 3 days. However, because of the recent controversy over the delayed carcinogenic effect of diethylstilbestrol in the young female offspring of women who have been treated with stilbestrol, this drug is no longer used as often for the prevention of pregnancy. It would appear on the basis of current experience that conjugated estrogens may also be effective in preventing pregnancy. A regimen consisting of 40 mg. of conjugated estrogen (Premarin) given intravenously following the examination followed by 5 mg. orally 3 times a day for 7 days will most likely prevent any pregnancy. Ten mg. of Provera should be given during the last 5 days. The reason for giving estrogen and progesterone is to assure that there will be an adequate slough of the endometrium following hormonal therapy. Giving estrogen alone may lead to an incomplete slough of the endometrial lining and cause irregular bleeding. It should be stressed that there are currently no published data available documenting the effectiveness of conjugated estrogens in preventing pregnancy.

Venereal Disease Prophylaxis. Antibiotic therapy should probably be instituted to prevent the possible development of either gonorrhea or syphilis. Penicillin still is the drug of choice for treating these diseases; however, because of the recent controversies over the emergence of resistant strains of *Neisseria gonorrhoeae*, some consideration may be given to treating the patient with an alternative drug such as tetracycline.[34] The choice of prophylactic antibiotic therapy to prevent venereal disease is an individual one. It seems inappropriate to subject the victim of an assault to painful parenteral therapeutic doses of penicillin to prevent possible infection. A reasonable compromise would be to give 250 mg. of ampicillin or tetracycline every 6 hours for 5 days. The patient should be advised to have a repeat vaginal culture after her next menstrual period and to have repeat serology in 6 weeks.

Children who are the victims of molestation should be evaluated in a manner similar to rape cases. However, the physician must be even more careful in dealing with a child to prevent unnecessary pain and psychic trauma.

ABORTION

Induced Abortion

Not too many years ago a woman who found herself unexpectedly pregnant had three alternatives. She could keep the child, give it up for adoption or seek a criminal abortion. If she chose the third option, more often than not, she would eventually end up in the hospital suffering from one or more of the potential complications of the procedure. Sepsis and/or bleeding were the most commonly seen complications and often existed simultaneously. The illegal abortionist would often prescribe or administer an antibiotic that was just effective enough to delay or mask some of the signs of sepsis, thus delaying an accurate diagnosis and the onset of appropriate treatment.

During the last few years, the change in public attitude has led to a change in our laws and consequently a change in physicians' attitudes toward induced abortion. An unknown number of "legal" abortions are now being performed by licensed physicians. This practice has led to a marked decrease in the number of criminal abortions performed but has not completely eliminated them. This in turn has led to a decrease in the number of complications resulting from illegal abortions. The types of complications seen have changed considerably and most of these complications are managed by the people performing the abortions. However, since many patients travel elsewhere to be aborted and because criminal abortions are still performed, it is important for physicians to understand how to manage these traumatic complications.

A viable pregnancy is relatively difficult to terminate. The cervix, especially in a nulligravida, is firm and tightly closed, rendering it subject to laceration upon forced dilatation. The trophoblastic tissue of the developing placenta burrows directly into the myometrium, exposing large blood vessels. This tissue is removed only with difficulty, and considerable bleeding results. The relatively thin wall of the uterus at the site of implantation may be perforated by a relatively sharp instrument. The uterine cavity with its vascular lining, the endometrium, may serve as a favored site for the proliferation of bacteria.

Management. In the past, because of the criminal nature of these procedures, it was often difficult to obtain an adequate history from a patient. To some extent, this may continue to be the case because of the stigma that is still attached to abortion, but a woman may be much more likely to state that she has had an induced abortion and to think that her problem may be related to this procedure. It is important to obtain from the patient information regarding the method used to induce the abortion and the date of her last normal menstrual period so that an accurate gestational age can be calculated. In addition to a general physical examination with special attention to vital signs and abdominal signs, a careful pelvic examination should be carried out. At the time of pelvic examination, the amount of bleeding should be noted and the vagina should be inspected for the presence of lacerations. The cervix should be inspected and a bimanual examination should be done with special emphasis on determining the size of the uterus. If the uterus is compatible with the calculated gestational age or larger, it is probable that the abortion has not been completed and that products of conception most likely still remain in the uterus. Following the bimanual examination, either a sterile ring forceps or a Hegar dilator should be passed into the cervix to determine if the internal cervical os is opened or closed. If the uterus is 16 weeks' size or larger the presence or absence of fetal heart tones should also be determined, but this usually requires the use of a Doppler ultrasound instrument.

After a complete examination has been performed, appropriate treatment should be instituted. A complete blood count should be obtained. The hematocrit and hemaglobin values will serve as a reference for circulating blood volume. The white blood count can serve as a reference for the severity of infection. It should be remembered that every pregnant patient will have a slightly elevated white blood count and an elevated sedimentation rate. Therefore, a white blood count up to 14,000 cells per ml. may be seen in the absence of infection. If there is minimal bleeding, if the uterus is 8 weeks' size or less and is firm and nontender, and if the CBC is essentially normal

and the cervix is either closed or open with no tissue present, the patient should be observed. If the uterus is larger than 8 weeks' size and fetal heart tones are present, the patient should also be observed. If the patient has signs of hypovolemia or frank shock, vigorous intravenous fluid therapy should be initiated to restore effective circulating volume. An indwelling Foley catheter should be used to accurately measure urine volume, and a central venous pressure catheter should be introduced to monitor the response to this therapy. The management of hypovolemic shock is discussed in further detail in Chapter 4. If there is evidence of infection, large doses of broad spectrum antibiotics should be given intravenously.

The decision regarding surgical intervention should be made on the basis of whether residual products of conception are still present in the uterus or perhaps have been expelled into the pelvis from a uterine perforation. If fetal heart tones are present, the decision to intervene may be difficult to make. In spite of sepsis and excessive bleeding, it is well established that such pregnancies can continue to term with the delivery of a normal, healthy infant. In such cases, the blood volume has been replaced by transfusion and the sepsis eliminated by the use of antibiotics.

In most cases, surgical intervention should be delayed until appropriate supportive measures have been carried out. If there is no evidence of sepsis, which is rare, the patient may be taken to the operating room when effective circulating blood volume is sufficiently restored to allow the administration of anesthesia with safety. On rare occasions, bleeding may be so profuse that the maintenance of blood volume by transfusion may be impossible, in which case early surgical intervention is indicated to control the hemorrhage. If sepsis is present, as it usually is, the patient should ideally be treated with antibiotics for 6 to 12 hours before any surgery is performed. In most cases, the only surgical procedure necessary is a curettage of the uterus. The cervix is usually already dilated and will readily admit a curette. The uterus should first be sounded with a dull probe to accurately determine its size and to rule out a possible perforation. The uterine cavity should then be gently curetted with either a sharp curette or a suction curette. Great care should be taken not to perforate the uterus during this procedure. The suction curette should not be used if a uterine perforation is thought to be present. However, a sharp curettage should be done to attempt to remove all the products of conception. An exploratory laparotomy should be performed if there is reason to believe that products of conception have been expelled into the abdominal cavity or if there is a probability that a bowel injury has occurred. Bowel may be sucked through a uterine perforation by the suction curette. When an exploratory laparotomy is performed and a uterine perforation is found, no attempt should be made to close the perforation. Any products of conception that are present should be removed, the bowel should be inspected for injury and the cul-de-sac should be drained either into the vagina or laterally in either lower quadrant. In most cases, the uterine perforation will heal and be of no concern if a subsequent pregnancy occurs. In cases of massive pelvic infection, a total abdominal hysterectomy and bilateral salpingo-oophorectomy may be necessary.

The complications arising from abortions induced by amniocentesis are usually so acute that the person performing the abortion is aware of the problem and must manage it. Probably in all amniocentesis-induced abortions, regardless of the solution used, the patients develop signs of intravascular coagulation. The reason for this is unknown, but one possibility is the release of placental thromboplastin into maternal circulation.[35] Fortunately, most cases are mild and require no treatment.

Miscellaneous Problems. For a variety of reasons, a woman may not seek legal termination of an unwanted pregnancy, preferring instead to seek some other avenue of terminating her pregnancy. She may take some form of medication. Quinine-containing drugs have frequently been used to this end. The side effects of excessive quinine may include nausea, vomiting, vertigo, tinnitus and diarrhea. Fortunately, these side effects are self-limiting. Other drugs may be ingested, so the physician must use common sense and consult a toxicology reference in managing any complications that arise.

A woman may also seek to terminate her pregnancy by introducing an irritating substance or foreign body into the vagina or uterus. Potassium permanganate tablets have been used for this purpose. These tablets react with the vaginal mucosa, resulting in ulceration and subsequent vaginal bleeding that may be extensive. Lye-containing substances have also been used with similar results. Treatment consists of vaginal irrigation, blood replacement when necessary, control of the bleeding with a vaginal pack saturated with a steroid cream and frequent follow-up to assure that healing occurs. Extensive burns may result in extensive scarring with vaginal stenosis. The use of a foreign body may produce vaginal or cervical lacerations and perforation of the cul-de-sac or uterus. Management of these complications was discussed previously in this chapter.

Spontaneous Abortion

Perhaps it is improper to discuss the management of spontaneous abortion in a book on trauma, but occasionally it is difficult to differentiate between a spontaneous abortion and an induced abortion, and the principles of management are similar. The subject is mentioned here only to remind the physician that spontaneous abortion may lead to excessive blood loss so that when the patient presents in the office or in the emergency department, general principles of management expressed in this book are applicable.

Summary

Any woman of childbearing age who presents with any of the symptoms of lower abdominal or pelvic pain, vaginal bleeding and/or infection should be evaluated for the possibility of the complications of abortion. At the time of the physical examination, special attention should be directed toward the presence or absence of lacerations of the vagina, lacerations of the cervix, the size of the uterus and the intactness of the uterine cavity. In most instances, supportive measures such as blood transfusions and antibiotics should be instituted before a patient is taken to the operating room. A curettage of the uterus should always be performed if there is any question of retained products of conception. Exception to this would be cases in which fetal heart tones are detectible, the amount of bleeding is not significant and the evidence of excessive blood loss is not present. In such cases, even if an induced abortion has been attempted, the pregnancy may continue to viability.

A uterus that has been perforated should not be repaired. In the absence of massive infection, the perforation will heal spontaneously and will not jeopardize future childbearing. On the other hand, if widespread pelvic sepsis is present, the only treatment may be total hysterectomy and bilateral salpingo-oophorectomy.

Fetal red blood cells are present by the twenty-first day of embryological development and consequently the potential for sensitization exists in an Rh-negative woman. There is currently considerable debate regarding the risk of Rh sensitization in a woman who has either induced or spontaneous abortion. Mini doses of Rhogam are now available and do not require cross matching. Therefore, a mini dose of Rhogam should probably be given to any Rh-negative woman after abortion or after ectopic pregnancy.

TRAUMA IN PREGNANT WOMEN

In cases of trauma involving a pregnant patient, there are certain additional therapeutic considerations of which the examining physician must be aware. He must consider the well-being of the infant as well as that of the mother. He must also be aware of the potential late complications resulting from trauma and may often be asked in court if termination of the pregnancy occurred as a result of the traumatic incident. Finally, the size of the pregnant uterus may actually serve as a protection to more severe trauma to a woman, especially in cases of penetrating trauma.

General Principles

For all practial purposes, the developing infant is extremely well protected within the confines of the uterine cavity. The amniotic fluid acts as an excellent shock absorber and it is unusual for a fetus to experience physical trauma as a result of anything but direct penetrating trauma. During the first trimester, the uterus is protected by the

bony pelvis, while in the last two trimesters, the enlarging uterus distends the abdominal wall and at the same time displaces the bowel superiorly. Such an anatomical arrangement, although making the infant more susceptible to trauma during the last two trimesters, actually protects the major blood vessels and the intestines of the mother from damage from penetrating trauma, such as in the cases of knife wounds, bullet wounds or shrapnel wounds.

In cases of blunt trauma involving the abdomen, the major risk to the fetus is placental abruption. In such cases, the abruption may be either partial or total and vaginal bleeding may or may not be present. In cases of complete abruption, the infant will be dead at the time of the examination, but in cases of partial abruption, the infant may survive only to suffer intrauterine malnutrition from an incomplete placental circulation. Fetal skull fractures have been reported to result from blunt trauma.[33] The infant usually dies, but it may survive without damage.

In evaluating injured women in the childbearing age, pregnancy should be considered possible until ruled out by examination. The risk to the mother and the prognosis of the pregnancy will vary, depending upon the type of trauma and the gestational age at the time the trauma occurred.[12, 17, 31] The physician must also consider the late sequelae of this trauma in regard to future pregnancy. A pelvic fracture may lead to a contracture, which will necessitate a cesarean section. It is also possible, but unlikely, that a traumatic incident may produce sterility.

Fetal risks from diagnostic radiological procedures necessitated by trauma are a concern to both the patient and the managing physician. There appears to be *little* if any risk of fetal defects developing as a result of diagnostic radiological procedures regardless of the gestational age when the procedure(s) are performed. The American College of Obstetricians and Gynecologists has issued a policy statement regarding the risks of diagnostic x-ray procedures.[2] Intrauterine exposure to diagnostic radiation is not an indication for interruption of a pregnancy. This statement does not imply that there is *no* risk to an infant exposed to intrauterine radiation. There is some suggestion that an infant exposed to intrauterine radiation is at some risk of developing a childhood malignancy.[7] On the basis of current information no pregnant woman should be subjected to unnecessary radiological procedures. On the other hand, necessary radiological procedures should not be withheld because a woman is known to be, or thought to possibly be, pregnant. Prudence would seem to suggest appropriate screening with lead apron when and where appropriate.

Premature Labor

Women who undergo major surgical procedures, especially exploratory laparotomy, when pregnant may be at risk of premature labor. The mechanism(s) that initiate labor are not known, but it has been observed that progesterone seems to inhibit uterine contractions. For this reason, many women are treated with progesterone to prevent the onset of premature labor. Whenever an exploratory laparotomy is performed or whenever a pregnant woman has been subjected to some form of trauma, it is probably a good idea to treat her with progesterone. The dosage is empirical. One hundred mg. of progesterone in oil should be given intramuscularly to give immediate elevated blood levels of progesterone. At the same time, 500 mg. of hydroxyprogesterone caproate (Delalutin) should be given intramuscularly and repeated in 2 to 3 days. The longer-acting hydroxyprogesterone acetate (Depo-Provera) should not be administered because of prolonged action and unpredictable effect on future menstrual normality. There are no known side effects from progesterone administered as recommended.

Deliberate termination of a pregnancy in a woman who has been subjected to trauma is indicated in only two instances. The first indication is excessive bleeding from the uterus, which is usually caused by a severe placental abruption, and the second is evidence of fetal distress (fetal heart rate less than 110) in a potentially salvageable pregnancy (30 weeks or more).

Nontraumatic Surgical Diseases

The pregnant patient may require surgery for the same reasons as the nonpregnant patient. The pregnancy should not be terminated in such cases because its prognosis is excellent.[31] Progesterone may be used in the dosage recommended earlier in the discussion.

Automobile Injuries

In the past there has been controversy over whether pregnant women should wear restraining harnesses or seatbelts when traveling in automobiles. The reason for this concern had to do with the transmission of forces on impact from the restraints to the fetus. There now seems to be sufficient information to resolve this controversy.[9] Crosby and his co-workers have shown conclusively that the use of lap belts *with* or *without* shoulder harnesses has saved more fetal and maternal lives than has failure to use them.[10, 11] The leading cause of fetal mortality from automobile accidents is maternal mortality. In cases in which the mother survives, the primary risk to the infant is from abruption of the placenta. This may occur at the time of the accident or may be delayed several days.

Management. Any woman involved in an automobile accident should undergo a thorough examination including a pelvic examination. Information regarding her last normal menstrual period should be recorded in the history, and all physical findings, including those noted at the time of pelvic examination, should be accurately recorded. There are two reasons for this: (1) to determine whether a pregnancy is present so that its continuation can be closely monitored and (2) because of the possible litigation that may occur if a pregnancy is lost as a result of the accident. If a pregnancy does exist, the management of the patient will depend in part on the gestational age of the fetus. The management of airway problems, hemorrhage, central nervous system injuries and fractures takes precedence over the management of the pregnancy unless bleeding from an abrupted placenta or ruptured uterus is contributing to uncontrolled hemorrhage.

As mentioned earlier, the only indication for terminating a pregnancy is excessive uterine bleeding or evidence of fetal distress in a potentially salvageable pregnancy. If the gestational age is less than 20 weeks, usually no treatment is necessary. However, progesterone may be given in the dosage recommended. If a spontaneous abortion subsequently occurs, the products of conception should be examined to attempt to determine the etiology of the abortion. If the fetus is well formed and the abortion resulted from the accident, placental hemorrhage should be evident. On the other hand, if an identifiable fetus is not present, the abortion could not possibly have been caused by the accident; it would have occurred spontaneously in any event. In more advanced pregnancies, especially those pregnancies beyond 25 weeks, the presence or absence of fetal heart tones should be determined as soon as practical. If fetal heart tones are absent, nothing can be done to salvage the pregnancy. The usual cause of this is complete abruption of the placenta. Management in such cases is to observe the patient for the development of shock or abnormal bleeding. If there is no sign of shock and no other evidence of serious injury, the patient may be observed and spontaneous labor will undoubtedly occur within a short period of time. Occasionally, a delay of several days may occur.

Sometimes the uterus is ruptured in a severe accident and the infant is expelled into the abdominal cavity. In such cases, the infant will die from a lack of placental perfusion and the uterus will contract sufficiently to prevent continued hemorrhage. The diagnosis of a ruptured uterus may be difficult to make, but as long as the patient is not in shock or the shock can be prevented, the patient can be observed until a definitive diagnosis can be made. Once the diagnosis has been made, an exploratory laparotomy should be performed and the uterine defect repaired. A subsequent pregnancy should be terminated by cesarean section.

If fetal heart tones are present, these heart tones should be monitored, preferably with an external monitoring device for 24 to 48 hours. There are cases of partial abruption in which the infant does not die immediately, but there is insufficient placental circulation to maintain growth and development. This failure to grow can be documented by measuring the fundal height in centimeters. The height should equal the weeks of gestation between 20 and 32 weeks. Even if there are no significant physical injuries present in severe automobile accidents, it is advisable to hospitalize the patient and, if an external fetal

monitor is available, to monitor fetal heart tones for a period of 24 to 48 hours. If a partial abruption of the placenta has occurred, evidence of fetal distress will eventually be noted and the pregnancy should then be terminated by cesarean section, as long as the patient's condition is stable enough to tolerate this procedure.

The delayed complications of pregnancy resulting from automobile trauma are specifically related to pelvic fractures that may produce pelvic dystocia and result in the need for abdominal delivery. It is extremely difficult to predict which patient will require abdominal delivery and which will be able to deliver vaginally on the basis of either clinical or x-ray pelvimetry. Any obstetrician who has had experience with patients with pelvic contractures realizes that the real proof of pelvic dystocia must await a trial of labor. As long as there is no complication of the pregnancy and no contraindication to allow a trial of labor (such as a previous cesarean section), every patient should be given an opportunity to deliver vaginally. However, no heroic efforts such as Pitocin stimulation should be carried out in an attempt to force an infant through a contracted pelvis. Dyer[12] and Spear[37] reported that four out of five patients who sustained pelvic fractures at the time of an automobile accident subsequently delivered vaginally without difficulty.

MISCELLANEOUS TRAUMA

Penetrating Injuries. Penetrating abdominal or pelvic injuries in the nonpregnant woman should be managed as described elsewhere in this book, and penetrating injuries to the abdomen of pregnant women should be managed in a manner similar to that of nonpregnant women. Occasionally, if there is no evidence of shock, excessive blood loss or evidence of a ruptured hollow viscus, the patient may be observed closely in the hospital. The decision to do an exploratory laparotomy should be based upon the extent of trauma, the type of trauma involved and the condition of the patient at the time she is evaluated. As a general rule, all patients with penetrating abdominal wounds should be explored. If an exploratory laparotomy is performed, there is no justification for doing a cesarean section just to deliver the infant at that time. More often than not, these infants will die of the complications of prematurity, and the potential postoperative complications from the cesarean section may make management of the patient's other injuries more complicated than need be. Even if the fetus is dead, there is no indication for immediate termination of the pregnancy.

In advanced pregnancy, the uterus will probably be entered by the penetrating trauma. Because of the muscular wall, damage to the uterus may be slight. The fetus may or may not be injured in such cases. There have been reports of fetuses surviving such trauma, including gunshot, stab and shrapnel injuries.[3, 14, 18, 22, 23, 41] In such cases, the only indication for terminating the pregnancy is excessive bleeding or a large defect, in which case the infant will not have survived and may have been expelled through the defect. The uterine defect should be closed by suturing. Debridement, if necessary, should be done prior to the repair.

Blunt Trauma. Most blunt trauma sufficient to cause maternal injury or place the fetus in jeopardy results from automobile accidents. Occasionally, a woman may be subjected to a severe beating, fall from a considerable height or be crushed by a heavy object.[15, 17] The principles of management in these cases are the same as those discussed under nonpenetrating abdominal injuries secondary to automobile accidents (Chapter 14). In this regard, peritoneal lavage may be extremely useful in deciding whether to do an exploratory laparotomy in a pregnant accident victim. It is *not* contraindicated in pregnancy.[33]

One other problem that the physician should be aware of is the traumatic or spontaneous rupture of an epigastric vessel, which may simulate an acute abdomen or concealed placental abruption. The signs and symptoms usually are evidence of hidden blood loss, abdominal pain and uterine irritability. Treatment in such cases is blood transfusion and operation to ligate the ruptured vessel.

Spontaneous or traumatic rupture of the liver and spleen has been reported to occur in pregnancy.[8, 28, 36] The management of these problems is the same as it would be in the nonpregnant state. Termination of the

pregnancy is no more indicated in such cases than it is in any of the other traumatic problems previously discussed.

Thermal Injuries. A pregnant woman suffering burns should be treated no differently from a nonpregnant one. A recent review of 19 pregnant burn casualties treated at Brooke Medical Center[39] led to several conclusions. Pregnancy does not alter maternal outcome. Maternal survival usually results in fetal survival, but if the burns are lethal, the infant will die before maternal death occurs. Obstetrical intervention therefore is indicated only in presumptive terminal maternal cases when the chance of fetal survival is reasonable (28 weeks or greater).

Secondary Effects of Trauma on Pregnancy

There will always be concern regarding the long-term indirect effects on the outcome in a severely traumatized patient's pregnancy. There will be questions regarding the effect on the fetus of shock, hypoxia, anesthesia, extensive surgical procedures, blood transfusions, acidosis and renal failure. None of these concerns can be allayed easily. However, it seems reasonable to be optimistic about the outcome of pregnancy as long as the mother survives, the infant is not injured as a direct result of the trauma and the mother does not abort or deliver an immature infant that cannot survive. The oxygen disassociation curve for fetal hemoglobin is shifted to the left, suggesting that a fetus can tolerate hypoxia relatively better than the mother. Anesthesia techniques in trauma cases currently are directed at maintaining as high an O_2 concentration as possible, so there should be no concern about adverse fetal effects from anesthesia. if renal function is impaired, azotemia may be fatal to the unborn child, but patients have delivered healthy infants after dialysis. However, the prospect of intrauterine fetal death increases as the BUN rises. Dialysis should probably be instituted in the pregnant woman before the BUN reaches 50 mg. per cent. Little is known about the effects of electrolyte imbalance on the fetus. It is known that ketoacidosis in pregnant diabetics is almost always fatal to the fetus, but whether acidosis of a different origin is likely to be lethal is not clear. In any event, fluid and electrolyte imbalances should be corrected as quickly as possible. Little else can be done in this situation. Patients receiving blood may become sensitized; therefore, any pregnant patient should be followed for the development of antibodies and the infant evaluated for erythroblastosis if maternal antibodies are detected. Modern blood bank techniques can predict whether or not the sensitizing antigen is likely to produce erythroblastosis.

At this writing, there have been two well-publicized cases of pregnant women suffering fatal central nervous system damage. Both women had nonviable pregnancies and there was much speculation about the possibility of supporting maternal vital functions until the pregnancies could reach viability, thus salvaging the unborn infants. In both cases the women died within a short period of time and both fetuses died before the mothers were removed from life-support machines. These problems will undoubtedly continue to confront physicians who manage patients with severe trauma. Each case must be handled according to its individual circumstances. The greater the length of gestation the more likely the chances of delivering a child that will survive. If the gestational age is greater than 30 weeks and the infant is alive at a time when clinical evaluation indicates that maternal survival is unlikely, the infant should probably be delivered by cesarean section. Between 24 and 30 weeks, fetal survival in this setting is questionable. Prior to 24 weeks there is essentially no chance of survival.

SUMMARY

Some common principles regarding trauma to the external genitalia, pelvis and abdomen of women, both in the pregnant and nonpregnant states, have been discussed. The principles involved in managing these cases are similar to those involved in managing any case of trauma. All of the patient's organ systems should be evaluated when appropriate and antibiotics used in the face of infection. Good common sense and reassurance are essential in managing these problems.

The treating physician should be cognizant of the potential litigation that may result from the traumatic episode, but the fear of having to testify in court regarding a particular case should not in any way prevent him from treating the patient in an appropriate manner. By recording objective findings, saving potential evidence and not recording subjective impressions, the physician should have no problem if litigation results from a case of trauma. There are two different potential legal problems. The most common situation is the one in which the victim of the trauma sues the instigator of the trauma or the instigator is prosecuted for a felonious act, such as rape. In these situations, the only information requested is an accurate description of the physical findings at the time the patient was treated. The second problem, the one most feared by physicians, is that the patient may have a bad result or be unhappy with the treatment she received from the physician and bring suit against him for malpractice. Most such cases can be avoided by following the principles described in this book and seeing that the patient has competent follow-up treatment. Hopefully, the fear of a malpractice suit will not prevent any physician from treating a patient who has been the victim of trauma.

REFERENCES

1. American College of Obstetricians and Gynecologists: Suspected rape. Am. Coll. Obstet. Gynecol. Tech. Bull. No. 14, July 1970.
2. American College of Obstetricians and Gynecologists: Statement of Policy. Guidelines for diagnostic x-ray examination of fertile women, May 1977.
3. Beattie, J. F., and Daly, F. R.: Gunshot wound of the pregnant uterus. Am. J. Obstet. Gynecol. 80:771, 1960.
4. Blair, R.: A fatal injury of the vagina. Br. Med. J. 1:828, 1925.
5. Bochner, K.: Traumatic perforation of the pregnant uterus. Obstet. Gynecol. 17:520, 1961.
6. Braunstein, P. W., Skudder, P. A., McCarroll, J. R., Musolino, A., and Wade, P. A.: Concealed hemorrhage due to pelvic fracture. J. Trauma 4:832, 1964.
7. Bross, I. D. J., and Natarajan, N.: Leukemia from low-level radiation. N. Engl. J. Med. 287:107, 1972.
8. Cairns, J. D., Woods, J. M., and Sladen, J. G.: Traumatic rupture of the spleen with delayed intraperitoneal hemorrhage during pregnancy. J. Can. Med. Assoc. 90:30, 1964.
9. Committee on Medical Aspects of Automobile Safety: Automobile safety belts during pregnancy. J.A.M.A. 221:20, July 3, 1972.

10. Crosby, W. M., and Costilloe, J. P.: Safety of lap belt restraint for pregnant victims of automobile collisions. N. Engl. J. Med. 284:632, 1971.
11. Crosby, W. M., King, A. I., and Stout, A. C.: Fetal survival following impact: Improvement with shoulder harness restraint. Am. J. Obstet. Gynecol. 112:1101–1107, April 15, 1972.
12. Dyer, I., and Barclay, D. L.: Accidental trauma complicating pregnancy and delivery. Am. J. Obstet. Gynecol. 83:907–929, April 1962.
13. Eastman, J. J., and Hellman, L. M.: Williams Obstetrics (15th Ed). New York, Appleton-Century-Crofts, 1976.
14. Eckerling, B., and Teaff, R.: Obstetrical approach to abdominal war wounds in late pregnancy. J. Obstet. Gynecol. Br. Emp. 57:747, 1950.
15. Elias, M.: Rupture of the pregnant uterus by external violence. Lancet 2:253, 1950.
16. Evrard, J. R.: Rape: The medical, social and legal implications. Am. J. Obstet. Gynecol. 111:197, 1971.
17. Fort, A. T., and Harlin, R. S.: Pregnancy outcome for noncatastrophic maternal trauma during pregnancy. Obstet. Gynecol. 35:912, June 1970.
18. Geggie, N. S.: Gunshot wound of the pregnant uterus with survival of the fetus. J. Can. Med. Assoc. 84:489, 1961.
19. Hayman, C. R., and Lanza, C.: Sexual assault on women and girls. Am. J. Obstet. Gynecol. 109:480, February 1, 1971.
20. Hayman, C. R., Lanza, C., Fuentes, R., and Algor, K.: Rape in the District of Columbia. Am. J. Obstet. Gynecol. 113:91, May 1, 1972.
21. Keifer, W. S.: Rupture of the uterus. Am. J. Obstet. Gynecol. 89:335, 1964.
22. Kobak, A. J., and Hurwitz, C. H.: Gunshot wounds of the pregnant uterus. Obstet. Gynecol. 4:383, 1954.
23. Kracke, A. D.: Congenital paraplegia from intrauterine injury. J. Pediatr. 63:1184, 1963.
24. Kuchera, L. K.: Postcoital contraception with diethylstilbestrol. J.A.M.A. 218:28, 1971.
25. Lazard, E. M., and Kliman, F. E.: Traumatic rupture of the uterus in advanced pregnancy. Cal. West. Med. 45:482, 1936.
26. Massey, J. B., Garcia, G. R., and Emich, J. P., Jr.: Management of sexually assaulted females. Obstet. Gynecol. 38:29, July 1971.
27. McClure, J. N., Jr.: Rupture of the pregnant uterus due to non-penetrating abdominal trauma. Surgery 35:487, 1954.
28. O'Brien, S. E.: Spontaneous rupture of the spleen in pregnancy. J. Can. Med. Assoc. 89:667, 1963.
29. O'Rourke, C. A.: Rupture of the pregnant uterus due to non-penetrating external trauma. Med. J. Australia 2:496, 1963.
30. Quast, D. C., and Jordan, G. L., Jr.: Traumatic wounds of the female reproductive organs. J. Trauma 4:839, 1964.
31. Radman, H. M.: Pregnancy complicated by non-obstetric surgical disease. Arch. Surg. 88:279, 1964.
32. Robinson, H. A., Jr., Sherrod, D. B., and Malcarney, C.: Review of child molestation and alleged rape cases. Am. J. Obstet. Gynecol. 110:405, June 1971.
33. Rothenberger, D. A., Quattelbaum, F. W., Zabel, J., and Fischer, R. P.: Diagnostic peritoneal lavage for blunt trauma in pregnant women. Am. J. Obstet. Gynecol. 129:479, 1977.
34. Schroeter, A. L., and Lucas, J. B.: Gonorrhea — Diagnosis and treatment. Obstet. Gynecol. 39:174, 1972.
35. Schwartz, R., Greston, W., and Kleiner, G. J.: Defibrination in saline abortion. Obstet. Gynecol. 40:728, 1972.
36. Sparkman, R. S.: Rupture of the spleen in pregnancy. Am. J. Obstet. Gynecol. 76:587, 1958.
37. Speer, D. P., and Peltier, L. F.: Pelvic fractures and pregnancy. J. Trauma. 12:474, June 1972.
38. Taylor, E. S.: Beck's Obstetrical Practice. (9th Ed.) Baltimore, Williams & Wilkins, 1971.
39. Taylor, J. W., Plunkett, G. D., McManus, W. F., and Pruitt, B. A., Jr.: Thermal injury during pregnancy. Obstet. Gynecol. 47:434, 1976.
40. Wilson, F., and Swartz, D. P.: Coital injuries of the vagina. Obstet. Gynecol. 39:182, 1972.
41. Wright, C. H., Posner, A. C., and Gilchrist, J.: Penetrating wounds of the gravid uterus. Am. J. Obstet. Gynecol. 67:1085, 1954.

CHAPTER 16

TRAUMA OF THE GENITOURINARY SYSTEM

Rainer M. E. Engel, M.D.

Motor vehicle accidents as etiological factors of urinary tract injury by far outnumber others, such as industrial accidents, bullet wounds, stab wounds, the occasional iatrogenic trauma or the rare self-inflicted injury. The victims of such accidents usually sustain compound injuries that involve multiple organ systems in addition to the genitourinary tract, namely, skeletomuscular (e.g., fractures), gastrointestinal (e.g., perforated viscus) or vascular (e.g., hemorrhage) trauma. It is obvious that some of these injuries might be life-threatening, whereas others might not necessarily require immediate intervention. Thus, a rapid diagnostic evaluation to assess priorities in treatment is of utmost importance. Usually, genitourinary injury is of secondary importance. It is our strong conviction that, in the best interest of the severely injured patient, one individual, preferably a general surgeon, be charged with the overall care of the patient.

Team discussion and cooperation decide the priorities of treatment that has to be directed to life-threatening problems: restoration and maintenance of an adequate airway and pulmonary function, restoration of blood loss, control of hemorrhage, closure of perforations in various organ systems and stabilization of fractures.

In injuries that are limited to the genitourinary tract, such intense teamwork is not necessary. Clinical evaluation in this group may be primarily directed toward the genitourinary tract, whereas in the patient with complex injuries, full urological evaluation often has to wait until the overall condition of the patient has been stabilized or improved.

RENAL INJURIES

Injuries to a kidney can be classified by the causative factor into *penetrating* and *nonpenetrating* injuries, or, as we have found useful, on the basis of clinical symptomatology, into *minor, major* and *critical* injuries.

The adult kidney is extremely well protected by the rib cage posteriorly and posterolaterally and the abdominal viscera anteriorly. In addition, it is suspended in a fatpad confined by Gerota's fascia, which serves as a buffer. Renal injuries in the pediatric age group are somewhat more common since the kidney has not reached its protected position in the lower part of the rib cage, and because the pararenal and perirenal fatpad is not as well developed as in the adult. Thus, the renal parenchyma in children is somewhat more prone to contusions and lacerations. Also, the ureteropelvic junction has been seen to shear off, probably also due to the lack of "buffering suspension" supporting the kidney.

It is worthwhile to remember that pre-existing renal disease may predispose to severe renal damage in even minor trauma. This is particularly true for hydronephrosis but also for cystic disease, chronic infection or malignant degeneration.[6, 50, 54]

Malpositioning of the kidney, particularly over bony prominences, such as the spine or sacrum, can also lead to significant damage with minor injuries.

Renal injuries account for approximately one half of all injuries to the genitourinary tract. Waterhouse and Gross[61] found, in a series of 251 patients with genitourinary injuries, 116 renal injuries, 38 injuries to the bladder and 23 injuries to the urethra; the remainder were injuries to the external genitalia. The incidence of renal injuries in association with other trauma is difficult to assess from the literature as most authors do not state such figures. However, Scott et al.[53] report that in a total of 2525 patients with penetrating wounds of the abdomen, 7 per cent (181 patients) had associated renal injuries. This incidence

was essentially equal for both gunshot wounds and stab wounds. Waterhouse[61] reports on 9660 patients who were admitted to the Trauma Service of King's County Hospital Center, of whom 251 patients (2.5 per cent) had injuries to the genitourinary tract. The incidence of renal injury is highest in the second and third decades and involves predominantly male patients.[13, 50, 61] (See also Table 16–1.)

Abdominal rigidity as a sign of renal trauma is often difficult to assess since many of these patients have sustained other abdominal injuries; shock may be due to blood loss from renal causes.

The diagnosis of a renal injury may at times be difficult. We have adopted and, with modification, still adhere to the diagnostic outline presented by Orkin[41] for the diagnosis of trauma to the genitourinary tract (Table 16–2).

Use of a Proper Stretcher. Immediately upon arrival in the accident room, the patient is placed on a radiolucent stretcher. These stretchers are equipped with a Bucky and can be wheeled under a stationary x-ray machine. Films obtained in this manner are far superior to those obtained in bed with portable equipment.

TABLE 16–1. Renal Injuries

	Scott (1)	Scott (2)	Glenn	Scholl	Number	Per Cent
					TOTALS	
No. of Patients	111	181	84	478	854	
Etiology						
Gunshot Wounds		127	1	56	238	28 %
Stab Wounds		54				
Motor Vehicles	59 (52%)		34	264	357	42 %
Falls	26 (24%)		27	88	141	16.5%
Sports	26 (24%)		16	62	104	12 %
Other			6	8	14	1.5%
Sex { Male			66	382	448/562	79.8%
Female			18	96	114/562	21.2%
Pain { Flank or	94 (85%)		74	359	567/673	78.3%
Mass { Abdominal		170	11	88	269/743	36.2%
Hematuria { Gross	92 (83%)	140 (71%)	44	427	757/854	88.5%
Micro	111 (100%)		35			
Associated Injury		>80%	36	334	370/562	65.8%

TABLE 16–2. Route for Detection of Urological Trauma in the Presence of Other Injuries*

1. Transfer to proper stretcher.	6. Infusion intravenous pyelography.
2. Urological history.	7. Retrograde cystourethrography.
3. Evaluation of symptoms.	8. Retrograde cystoscopy and retrograde pyelography.
4. Physical examination.	9. Arteriography.
5. Initial x-ray examination.	10. Catheter drainage.

*Modified from Orkin.[41]

The stretcher allows not only rapid x-ray examination but also proper physical evaluation and emergency treatment.

Urological History. A careful urological history is of utmost importance. The area of the greatest blow may direct attention to the injured organ in patients with blunt trauma. The patient will usually know the time of last micturition and whether or not the urine was bloody. A past history of urological diseases, instrumentation and, particularly, surgery should be asked for. Some of this information may be gathered from relatives if the patient is unconscious. In particular, previous surgical removal of a kidney has to be ruled out.

Evaluation of Symptoms. The diagnosis of renal injury may at times be difficult. Hematuria, either gross or microscopic, is the most frequent finding of renal injury. However, our opinion is at variance with that of Scott et al.[52] who state, ". . . Indeed, microscopic hematuria was a required criterion of renal injury." It is evident from the literature that the absence of hematuria does not exclude even major renal injury since, in some injuries, occlusion or severance of the vascular pedicle or complete disruption of the ureter may prevent the passage of urine and blood into the lower urinary tract. Gross hematuria is seen in more than one half of patients with renal injuries, and only 5–10 per cent do not exhibit microscopic hematuria. Hematuria may be transient and cease after a few hours or may continue for days. Gross hematuria usually clears within a matter of hours, but we have seen an occasional patient who has bled intermittently for weeks following renal trauma. It is impor-

tant to point out that cessation of hematuria is not identical with healing of the injury since clots may obstruct the source of bleeding or the injured kidney may actually decrease its output and finally cease to function.

Localizing flank or abdominal pain is seen in 80–85 per cent of all patients. Since up to 80 per cent of patients with renal trauma have associated injuries, the symptomatology from the involvement of other organ systems may mask renal injury. The absence of flank mass does not exclude the possibility of even major renal trauma, as shown by Scott.[52, 53] Therefore, only a high degree of suspicion will lead to the early and correct diagnosis. Pain may be only slight but can be severe and agonizing. Typical renal colic can be seen with radiation from the flank into the groin, external genitalia and inner aspect of the thigh. Such colicky pains may be due to the passage of blood clots.

X-ray Examination. A plain film of the abdomen is obtained. Fractures of the lower ribs or the dorsolumbar transverse processes are suggestive of associated renal trauma. Obliteration of the psoas shadow or the renal shadow may direct the attention of the attending physician toward renal trauma but is not reliable. Scott[52] reports 28 per cent of blunt nonpenetrating renal trauma to show such radiological signs, but Glenn[13] found them in only 13 per cent of his patients. Thus, the absence of these findings is *inconclusive*, whereas their presence makes renal trauma highly likely.

Excretory urography is performed with infusion pyelography. There is significant discrepancy among the various authors concerning the percentage in which excretory urography is diagnostic of renal injury. Glenn[13] reports this figure as 50 per cent; Scott reports the incidence of diagnostic intravenous pyelograms as slightly over 60 per cent in patients with penetrating renal injuries[53] and slightly less than 40 per cent in patients with nonpenetrating renal injuries.[54] Rieser[47] reports this figure to be as low as 25 per cent of his cases. In patients who are in shock, renal perfusion is inadequate to permit adequate excretion of the dye and thus, insufficient visualization of the kidneys results.

The extent and exact localization of renal trauma is best visualized by other radiographical methods. The major value of excretory urography may well be in establishing the presence and adequate function of the contralateral kidney.

Retrograde pyelography, in the absence of significant lower urinary tract trauma, may be performed to visualize the extent of the injury. Retrograde pyelography, however, continues to be a subject of controversy. It is diagnostic in approximately 20 per cent of cases.[13] Other radiographical methods may provide more accurate information. The possibility of introducing infection is frequently mentioned, but this risk is extremely small in our experience.

Nephrotomography has been advocated, but selective renal *angiography* by the percutaneous femoral route is preferable and has received wide acceptance in the study of renal trauma. Many centers are now equipped to perform excellent emergency renal arteriography. The renal arterial supply and its arborization within the parenchyma are concisely illustrated by the arterial phase of the angiogram as well as any thrombosis or rent with extravasation within the perfused area. Simultaneous injection of the celiac axis may help in delineating injuries to the spleen or liver.

Sonography has been utilized extensively to assess extent and location of any possible extravasation. Gray scale sonography with its high gain is now almost exclusively used for these studies, which have shown their value not only in the initial assessment of extravasation but also in the follow-up of such problems. As the procedure is noninvasive, does not require any preparation and can be performed easily and quickly, it has become a most helpful tool to us, both in the acute phase of the trauma case and its clinical recovery phase.

As mentioned previously, renal injuries may be classified into minor, major and critical trauma, as illustrated in Figure 16–1. This classification has much practical value in determining the indications for an aggressive surgical approach as opposed to "watchful waiting."

Minor Trauma

Patients with minor trauma have suffered some damage to the renal parenchyma, which is contused. There is no rupture of the renal capsule or any tear into the collecting system. Unless other significant injury is present, such patients do not exhibit significant blood loss or shock. Hematuria may be apparent initially but usually subsides rapidly. Pain and tenderness in the involved flank may be marked shortly after injury but also subside quick-

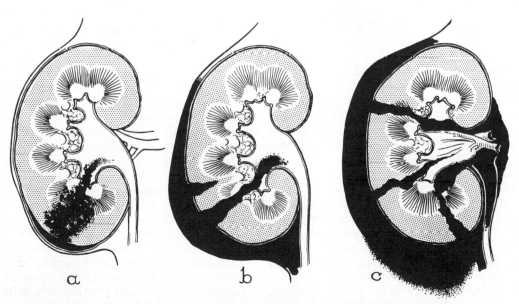

Figure 16–1. *Classification of renal injuries. A, minor; B, major; C, critical.*

ly. A flank mass is not palpable. Radiographically, no extravasation of dye can be demonstrated by intravenous pyelogram or retrograde urography. Excretion may be slightly decreased in such a kidney, and the nephrographic phase may show a subcapsular hematoma.

Fortunately, most renal injuries fall into this minor group. The incidence is cited by various authors as over 80 per cent of all renal injuries.[9, 13, 14, 18, 20, 24, 28, 50, 52, 53]

Treatment of this minor trauma type of renal injury consists of nothing but rest and observation. Full and uncomplicated recovery is almost always the case, and late complications of this type of renal injury have not been reported.

Repeated minor trauma may produce a distinctive lesion characterized by pericalyceal and peripelvic proliferations with distortions of the calyces. This is a very frequent finding in professional athletes (up to 50 per cent), producing microhematuria, pyuria, proteinuria and casts.[25] Treatment includes adequate rest, and stringent follow-up is necessary to prevent progressive renal deformity.

Major Injuries

The anatomical lesion in major renal trauma is, in addition to a marked degree of parenchymal laceration, a continuation of this laceration through the renal capsule and also into the pelvis. Although it is possible that a capsular and parenchymal tear may occur without extension of this laceration into the collecting system, this is rare. This laceration, extending from the collecting system through the parenchyma and through the renal capsule, allows free mixture of blood and urine not only within the collecting system but also in the space surrounding the kidney. Usually, this is confined by Gerota's fascia. This collection of blood and urine may present, on physical examination, as a palpable, either stable or expanding, flank mass.

Major injury may be caused by blunt trauma or by perforating or penetrating injuries. Approximately 15 per cent of all renal injuries fall into this group. Uncontrollable bleeding may also occur in 0.1 per cent of renal needle biopsies.[3, 51]

Physical findings may be misleading. Shock may exist initially, or it may develop later. Pain, tenderness and splinting may be due to the renal injury; however, the usually present concomitant injuries may well mask the renal trauma initially. Hematuria, again, may not be proportional to the degree of trauma; however, symptoms and signs usually become worse with time, contrary to the gradual improvement seen in minor trauma.

Radiographical demonstration of extravasation of contrast medium is the diagnostic criterion for major renal trauma (Fig. 16–2). Intravenous pyelography, drip-infusion pyelography or retrograde pyelography may show this extravasation. Their advantages and disadvantages have been presented earlier in this discussion, but it is important to stress that intravenous pyelography, even in penetrating renal trauma, may be normal in over 30 per cent of such patients.[53] The most reliable radiological evaluation is performed with arteriography (Fig. 16–3), which, however, is not always possible in an acutely ill patient who may require urgent operation.

Severe blunt trauma may also lead to renal artery thrombosis, probably on the basis of intimal and intramural vascular damage. This lesion is well known in both pediatric[19] and adult[45] age groups. Hematuria is usually absent, but proteinuria may be present. Physical examination does not offer any significant findings. On excretory urography, the kidney shows no function, and retrograde pyelography will demonstrate a normal collecting system. Renal arteriography accurately demonstrates the site and nature of this lesion. Prompt thrombectomy is required to salvage renal function.

Treatment of major renal injuries depends largely on the extent of the renal injury. Most urologists will adopt an expectant policy as to the management of such patients and will not intervene surgically as long as vital signs are stable, no significant blood loss occurs and the flank mass is not expanding. Surgical intervention in the early post-trauma period has all too frequently resulted in nephrectomy for otherwise salvageable kidneys, simply because the extent of the perirenal hematoma and the continuous bleeding after release of the tamponade by opening of Gerota's fascia made it extremely difficult to identify and ligate any bleeding vessels.

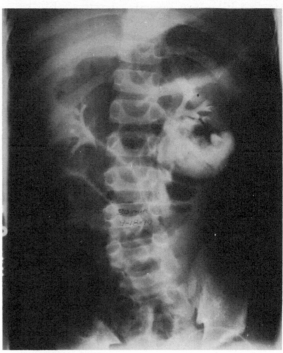

Figure 16-2. An eight-year-old boy was hit by a car. Back pain and persistent gross hematuria necessitated admission. On follow-up intravenous pyelogram 3 days later, marked extravasation of dye can be seen surrounding the lower pole and the upper ureter. At operation, complete transection of the lower pole was found for which a heminephrectomy was performed.

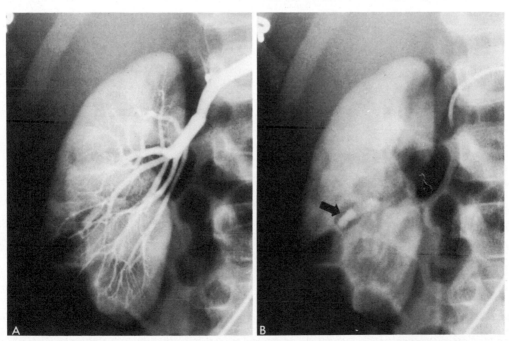

Figure 16-3. Young boy with intermittent gross total hematuria following a car accident injuring his right flank. A, Arteriogram shows collection of contrast material outside the calyceal structures, which becomes more evident on (B) the delayed film (see arrow).

However, with the advent of angiography and thus the possibility of exact localization of bleeding vessels, it is possible to repair such kidneys during the acute phase of the trauma. In nonpenetrating renal injuries, surgical intervention is still limited to those patients with life-endangering hemorrhage. But with penetrating renal trauma, the following plan is proposed:[52]

1. Delineation of location and extent of injury
2. Control of renovascular pedicle prior to mobilization of kidney
3. Debridement of severely damaged parenchyma
4. Meticulous hemostasis
5. Primary approximation of the parenchymal margins
6. Extraperitoneal drainage of the renal fossa.

With this approach, over 35 per cent of such kidneys may be saved.[28, 52, 53] Severe injuries in this category may require nephrectomy. Drainage only may be instituted in small lacerations. Debridement and primary closure are possible in those cases in which vascular injury to the involved part of the kidney has not been so extensive as to devitalize this part of the parenchyma. Should a part of the kidney appear to be viable, then a partial nephrectomy may be the procedure of choice. This may be done sharply or with a guillotine technique (Figs. 16–4 and 16–5).

Exploration of the injured kidney is best performed through an anterior transperitoneal approach, which yields quick access to the renal pedicle (Fig. 16–6). Non-crushing vascular clamps are applied to the pedicle as in surgery for renovascular hypertension. The kidney itself can then be approached through the paracolonic gutter after the colon has been reflected medially. The hematoma is evacuated and intermittent release of the pedicle clamp will allow accurate visualization of any bleeding vessels, which can be suture-ligated. Watertight closure of the torn pelviocalyceal system is important. This is followed by approximation of the renal parenchyma and closure of the renal capsule. Deep mattress sutures through the renal capsule, over a free fatpad or a peritoneal graft, may aid in covering a capsular defect. Should a heminephrectomy be required, it is advantageous to strip the renal capsule off the devitalized parenchyma prior to its removal. This capsule can

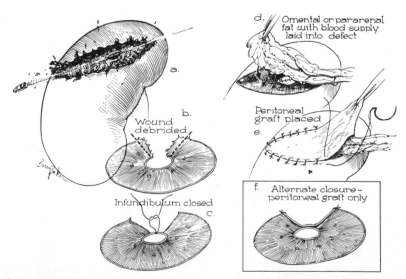

Figure 16–4. *A transcapsular laceration. All larger vessels are suture-ligated. A watertight closure is used for the collecting system. The capsule is closed with running or interrupted sutures. Diverting pyelostomy is performed for clots in the renal pelvis. A and B, All devitalized renal tissue is debrided. C, Collecting system is then closed. D, E and F, It is desirable to place a patch of fat, omentum or peritoneum over defect. (Reprinted by permission. From Scott, R., Jr., Carlton, C. E., and Goldman, M.: Penetrating injuries of the kidney: An analysis of 181 patients. J. Urol. 101:247–253, [March] 1969. © 1969, The Williams & Wilkins Co., Baltimore.)*

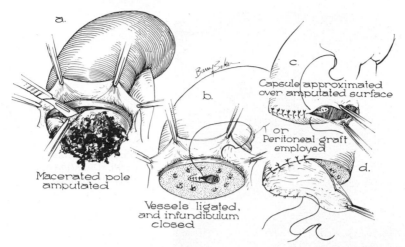

Figure 16–5. *Partial nephrectomy for renal trauma. A, Amputation of injured renal parenchyma. B, Suture ligation of bleeding vessels is followed by watertight closure of the transsected calyces. C and D, A flap of renal capsule, which is seen reflected in (A), or a peritoneal graft, is used to cover the exposed renal surface. (Reprinted by permission. From Scott, R., Jr., Carlton, C. E., and Goldman, M.: Penetrating injuries of the kidney: An analysis of 181 patients. J. Urol. 101:247–253, [March] 1969. © 1969, The Williams & Wilkins Co., Baltimore.)*

then readily be used to oversew the amputated renal surface (Figs. 16–4, 16–5 and 16–6.)

Recent reports in the literature[2, 22, 23, 48] and further experience of our angiography department may well initiate a new phase in the treatment of traumatic renal hemorrhage, whether this hemorrhage is postoperative from a needle biopsy or other surgery, or due to an accident. Arterial embolization with autologous blood clots has been proven to be a method that not only can stop significant renal hemorrhage but does so without need for general anesthesia and without major open surgery. In addition, it may be used to salvage more renal parenchyma than can be hoped for with open surgery and ligation of the bleeding vessels (Figs. 16–7 to 16–10).

Critical Injuries

Fragmentation of the kidney or an extension of the injury into the renal pedicle

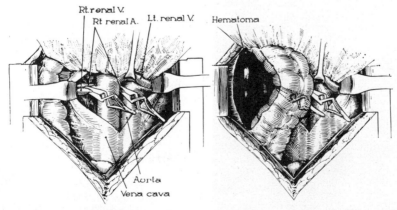

Figure 16–6. *Vertical incision across the aorta at the renal hilum allows access to both renal pedicles. The renal artery of the injured kidney is clamped with noncrushing clamps before reflecting the colon and opening Gerota's fascia. (Reprinted by permission. From Scott, R., Jr., Carlton, C. E., and Goldman, M.: Penetrating injuries of the kidney: An analysis of 181 patients. J. Urol. 101:247–253, [March] 1969. © 1969, The Williams & Wilkins Co., Baltimore.)*

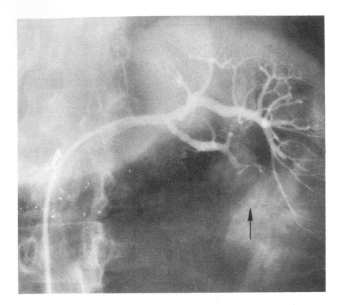

Figure 16–7. Patient with solitary left kidney. Intraoperative injury to lower branch of renal artery. Note jetlike efflux of contrast (arrow) with surrounding circular extravasate. (Courtesy of Dr. C. Barth, Department of Radiology, Johns Hopkins Hospital.)

places such a patient in the group of critical renal trauma. Renal pedicle trauma is more frequent in penetrating renal injuries (29 of 181) than in nonpenetrating injuries (7 in 111).[43, 52, 53] Blood loss in such injuries is apt to be severe and may be fatal in a short time.

A progressively expanding flank mass associated with early and profound shock as well as other evidence of massive hemorrhage readily points out the severity of this lesion. The primary value of the preoperative evaluation is to establish adequate function of the contralateral kidney. However, hemorrhagic shock with subsequent low renal perfusion may prevent adequate visualization of even a normal contralateral kidney.

Rapid intervention in such trauma is indicated to control hemorrhage and save the patient's life. In blunt trauma with destruction of the renal parenchyma and extension of the injury into the renal pedicle, ligation of the renal pedicle is the only possible treatment. However, in penetrating injuries with less damage to the parenchyma, and predominantly vascular pedicle injury, primary repair is possible in approximately 15 per cent.[53]

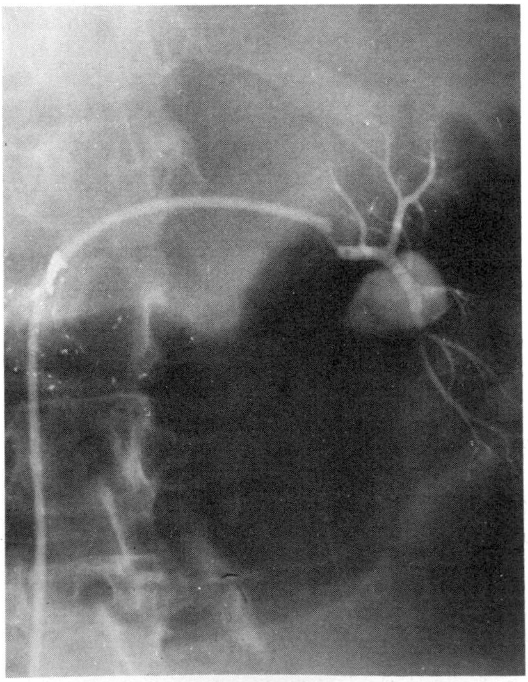

Mortality

Various authors have reported mortalities in their experience of renal trauma.[13, 18, 28, 43, 49, 53] It becomes apparent from the literature that most of these injuries are due to associated injuries. Rarely is the renal trauma itself the cause of death.

Figure 16–8. Selective angiogram of lower branch of renal artery. Pooling of contrast now distinct. (Courtesy of Dr. C. Barth, Department of Radiology, Johns Hopkins Hospital.)

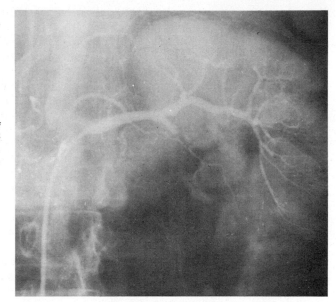

Figure 16–9. *Angiogram after injection of 0.4 ml. of thrombin-enhanced autologous clot. Lower vessel effectively sealed. (Courtesy of Dr. C. Barth, Department of Radiology, Johns Hopkins Hospital.)*

Early Complications

Early complications include those of persistent urinary drainage with the possibility of pararenal abscess formation. Gradual loss of function of the injured kidney, leading to "silent death," has been seen, but no data are available on the incidence of this complication. Organization of a large hematoma may lead to obstruction at the level of the ureter or ureteropelvic junction and thus predisposes to hydronephrosis. Persistent leakage of urine into the perirenal area may lead to the forma-

tion of a pararenal pseudocyst. The last two complications may have to be corrected surgically to prevent progressive renal attrition, infection and stone formation.

Late Complications

Patients with renal trauma should be followed routinely up to 2 years following their trauma to assess renal function and the possibility of renal hypertension. This is reported to occur in as many as 6 per cent of cases.[13, 64] Hypertension is be-

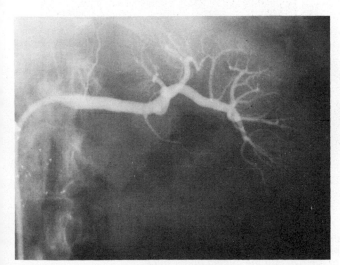

Figure 16–10. *Follow-up study 2 months after embolization. (Courtesy of Dr. C. Barth, Department of Radiology, Johns Hopkins Hospital.)*

lieved to occur as a result of arterial constriction during the healing process with resultant ischemic renal tissue which produces a Goldblatt kidney. Heminephrectomy or nephrectomy is necessary to cure this complication.

URETERAL INJURIES

Incidence

The ureter is rarely the site of urinary tract injury. Throughout its entire course, the ureter is well protected from blunt external trauma by abdominal contents anteriorly and the ileopsoas muscle posteriorly. Approximately 2 per cent of all patients with genitourinary tract trauma sustain ureteral injury, and most of these injuries are secondary to penetrating wounds of the abdomen.[8, 49, 55, 56, 60]

Ureteral injury due to blunt trauma is frequently associated with fracture of one or more transverse processes of the lumbar vertebrae on the ipsilateral side.

Surgical injury of the ureter occurs more often than is apparent. The close relation of the ureter to rectosigmoid and female reproductive tract renders the ureter vulnerable during radical surgery on these organs.

Ureteral instrumentation with catheters, particularly with stylets or stone extraction baskets, has also produced a number of ureteral perforations. However, over the past decade, this type of trauma has drastically decreased in incidence.

Wertheim[62] reported an incidence of 10 per cent ureteral injuries in 500 radical hysterectomies. The incidence with this procedure today is still the same. With hysterectomies for benign diseases, the incidence is less than 0.5 per cent.[17, 49, 55]

The incidence of injuries due to radical general surgical procedures is much lower and is quoted to be as low as 1 per cent in abdominal perineal resections.[17, 55] Ureteral injury during other intraperitoneal surgery is rare indeed, as is the occasional trauma to the ureter during spinal surgery. It may occur as a delayed complication following radiotherapy for carcinoma of the cervix[1] (Fig. 16–11). The high incidence of over 80 per cent in women is directly related to the risks of hysterectomy. Even with modern techniques, this risk has not been reduced. Important, however, is prompt repair. Higgins stated, "The venial sin is injury to the ureter, but the mortal sin is failure of recognition."[17] Parenthetically, it is a well-accepted surgical procedure to insert ureteral catheters

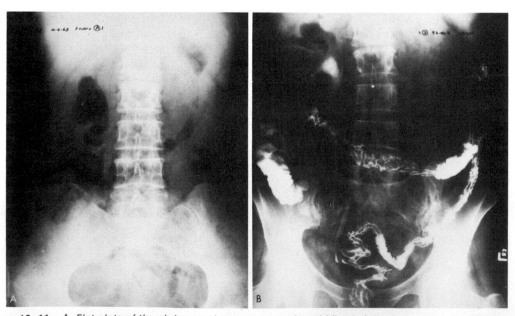

Figure 16–11. A, Flat plate of the abdomen shows a ureterosigmoid fistula following radium therapy for cervical carcinoma 8 years previously. Right ureter and pelvis are filled with gas. B, Gastrografin enema demonstrates the ureterosigmoid fistula with reflux of the dye into the dilated upper tract.

into both ureters prior to radical pelvic surgery. This may well make identification of the ureters during such surgery much easier.

Symptoms and Signs

Localizing symptoms and signs of ureteral injury following surgical trauma may initially be overlooked. Flank discomfort or fever of unknown origin in a patient who has undergone radical pelvic surgery should alert one to the possibility of ureteral injury. Hematuria may be absent in cases of complete transsection of the ureter; in partial transsection of the ureter, microhematuria is usually found. Complete or partial ligation by a suture or inadvertent application of hemostats, which compromises ureteral blood supply and may later result in necrosis and slough, is among the most frequent types of iatrogenic ureteral injury. In these patients, hematuria is usually *not* seen, but the signs of upper tract obstruction with flank discomfort, vague abdominal distress and possibly fever point toward the obstructed kidney. Unless such conditions are relieved early, this kidney may succumb to a "silent death." Urinary sepsis will occur in approximately half of the patients whose upper tract has been obstructed through a surgical mishap. In patients with insufficient renal function of the contralateral side, or those with bilateral ureteral injury, azotemia and uremia may supervene. This makes it obvious that early and accurate diagnosis is important so that the necessary surgical treatment can be promptly instituted.

In patients with ureteral ligation, immediate release in the first 24 to 48 hours, or best at time of injury, is the proper course. Delayed release can make successful reconstruction of the ureteral continuity impossible, and nephrectomy may be necessary in 30 per cent of such patients.[16]

Urinary extravasation, if intraperitoneal, is dramatic. Acute peritoneal irritation and sepsis occur with marked urinary leakage, whereas mild spillage may simply lead to low-grade fever, leukocytosis and prolonged ileus. Extraperitoneal extravasation in patients with stab wounds will usually lead to a retroperitoneal urinoma that may be silent but can, not infrequently, be demonstrated on a flat film of the abdomen as a mass of "ground glass" appearance. Since the majority of ureteral injuries occur with radical gynecological pelvic surgery, ureterovaginal fistulas are very common. Continuous dribbling of urine in patients who have an otherwise normal voiding pattern is characteristic for such a lesion.

Diagnosis

Excretory urography may be helpful in the diagnosis of ureteral trauma, but the most helpful diagnostic procedure is retrograde pyelography. In cases of disruption of the ureter, extravasation will pinpoint the exact location and extent of the ureteral injury. In patients with a ligated ureter, a varying degree of delayed function and hydronephrosis may be the result of this obstruction. This will be evident on excretory pyelography. Delayed films may be helpful in delineating the entire ureter down to the point of obstruction. Retrograde pyelography in conjunction with excretory urography will then visualize the lower segment of the ureter, and the nonvisualizing gap delineates the extent of obstruction. Sonography can demonstrate extent and stability or progression of extravasation on subsequent examinations.

Treatment

Much of the treatment of ureteral injuries is based on the concept of ureteral regeneration, which was pioneered by Davis.[7] Briefly, the ureter will regenerate its entire wall, epithelial lining and muscular coat along a narrow strip of ureteral wall bridging a gap. However, this regeneration does not occur across a transverse division unless the ends are directly approximated. The reasons for this extremely selective behavior of the ureter are still unknown.

The surgical procedure to be employed for repair of ureteral trauma depends in large measure on the extent of trauma. A simple transsection, if recognized early enough, can be primarily reanastomosed with an end-to-end anastomosis, preferably with spatulation of both ureteral ends. A urinary diversion with nephrostomy is usually not required in a primary repair but may be necessary in delayed repairs when the renal function has become impaired or the patient's general status has deteriorated owing to urinary sepsis and azotemia.

Gunshot wounds of the ureter may be deceiving since the tissue necrosis may frequently involve tissue that at first sight appears viable. Approximately one-half centimeter of healthy-appearing tissue on both ends of the ureter should be removed prior to reanastomosis. If end-to-end anastomosis is not possible, some other method of establishing ureteral continuity has to be employed.

In long strictures secondary to ureteral ligation, we have successfully utilized the Davis intubated ureterotomy, which is based on the principle of ureteral regeneration. In such ureters, the stricture is opened longitudinally and a catheter of inert material such as silicone, slightly smaller than the normal lumen of the ureter, is used as a splint. This splint must be kept in place long enough to accomplish its purpose of allowing ureteral regeneration around its circumference, usually 4 to 6 weeks, at which time it can be withdrawn through the bladder. However, for the success of the Davis intubated ureterotomy, a continuous strip of mucosal surface bridging this gap is mandatory. Ureteral regeneration will not occur across a mucosal gap.

Fortunately, an obstructed ureter will usually dilate and elongate and thus make anastomosis possible even if several centimeters of the injured or obstructive segment cannot be utilized. A diverting nephrostomy is usually not necessary in patients in whom ureteral repair is performed immediately after injury but is advisable in cases of delayed surgical correction. An alternate method of diversion proximal to the site of injury is a ureterotomy.[15] The urine will drain along a Penrose drain placed at this ureterotomy. When normal peristalsis resumes across the suture line, this ureterotomy will close in a similar fashion to those after ureteral lithotomy. There is, however, some evidence[4] that urinary extravasation surrounding the ureter may lead to stricture formation. Carlton et al.[4] describe a circular, watertight anastomosis associated with a much lower secondary complication rate than those of classical ureteral repairs.

In patients with avulsion of the ureter at the renal pelvis, primary anastomosis may be successful; however, a pyeloplasty utilizing a pelvic flap is probably better. Patients with ureteral avulsion at the ureterovesical junction require a ureteral reimplantation,[57] for which the Politano-Leadbetter method probably gives the best results. An alternate surgical procedure has to be employed if primary anastomosis of the distal and proximal ureteral ends cannot be accomplished without stress on the suture line.[8, 11, 28, 49]

Prostheses of polyethylene, silicone or Teflon have not been successful. Homologous ureteral grafts, veins and arteries have also failed as ureteral substitutes.

A bladder tube flap, as described by Boari, can bridge a substantial ureteral defect. It is important that the anastomosis of ureter to this tube flap be performed with a submucosal tunnel technique to prevent the otherwise occurring reflux. In longer defects, substitution with segments of ileum has been described and used by us with good results. The use of intestine as substitute for portions of the urinary conduit is well known in urology. Transuretero-ureteral anastomosis employs the transfer of the remaining segment of one ureter into the intact ureter of the contralateral side. However, if the kidney on the injured side shows chronic pyelonephritic changes, one might have to expect possible damage and ascending pyelonephritis to the contralateral good kidney.

A promising method[59] has been described that employs a posterior vesical flap with incorporation of the intact ureterovesical junction. This flap may permit advancement of the intact ureterovesical junction for about 5 cm., which will allow bridging of an equidistant deficit in the ureter without tension. Another method frees the bladder from its lateral and posterior attachments on the side of the ureteral defect. This also includes ligation of the superior vesical artery and vein. The bladder is then pulled up on this side and, with an anchoring suture, fixed to the psoas muscle. This procedure allows a significant superior advancement of the ureterovesical junction and thereby permits bridging a long ureteral gap without tension.

At times, urinary diversion is the only possible method of salvaging the upper tracts. If one deals with a solitary kidney and a dilated ureter, a ureterocutaneous anastomosis is the preferred method. Normal ureters have a high tendency to stricture if anastomosed to the skin. This complication is rarely seen in patients with dilated ureters. Diversions utilizing indwelling catheters should, if possible, be avoided unless they are temporary.

Indwelling catheters in the urinary tract carry with them the risk of chronic infection, ascending pyelonephritis and stone formation. Ureterosigmoidostomy has been utilized as urinary diversion in patients with significant injury to the ureters. We prefer the bilateral ureteroileocutaneous urinary diversion, or ileal loop, as permanent urinary diversion. This procedure in our hands has given the best long-term results and has undoubtedly saved many a kidney that otherwise would have been doomed to chronic failure. An alternative to the ileal loop is the colonic loop, which allows construction of a nonrefluxing ureteral anastomosis and thus affords added protection of the upper tracts.

BLADDER TRAUMA

Bladder trauma is less common than injury to the upper urinary tract,[61] and is usually secondary to external force, either blunt or penetrating. By far, the majority are caused by blunt external trauma, usually car accidents, which account for approximately 80 per cent of bladder trauma.[21, 39, 40, 61] Industrial crush accidents are less frequent today but still occur, particularly in the mining industry. Penetrating injuries by gunshot wounds or knives injuring the bladder are much less frequent than those afflicting the kidney. They usually are iatrogenic and are caused by instruments such as urethral sounds, wire catheter guides and resectoscopes.

Incidence

Clark and Prudencio,[5] tabulating about 2500 cases of pelvic fracture, come to the conclusion that 14.5 per cent of pelvic trauma is associated with injury to the lower urinary tract. Of these cases, 32 per cent involve the bladder alone, 10 per cent bladder and urethra and 58 per cent only the urethra.

Anatomy

Bladder perforation in pelvic trauma occurs usually with fractures involving the pubic arch. Fractures of the posterior aspect of the pelvic girdle rarely cause perforation of the bladder but may displace the bladder through hematoma formation. In its resting state, the bladder is fairly well protected from direct injury (Fig. 16–12), but becomes more vulnerable with increased filling. Also, the severity of the injury increases with progressive distention. Most cases of intraperitoneal rupture of the bladder occur from a direct blow to the filled bladder.

Bladder Contusion

Up to one third of patients with fractures of the pelvis, without demonstrable genitourinary trauma, may present with hematuria. This is thought to be due to a contusion of the bladder, in which minor damage has been sustained by the bladder wall. A number of these injuries can be caused by the snubbing action of the seatbelt in car collisions.[12] The diagnosis is made by exclusion of penetrating injury to the urinary tract. No specific treatment is required.

Extraperitoneal Rupture

In their review of 1798 cases of pelvic fractures, Prather and Kaiser[44] report on 181 bladder ruptures, of which 82 per cent were of the extraperitoneal type. Extraperitoneal bladder rupture usually occurs with fractures of the pelvic girdle below the pelvic brim, particularly those of the pubic rami and symphysis. They are usually found, as Morehouse and MacKinnon[35] state, "on the anteriolateral wall rather close to the vesical neck." Urinary extravasation into the pre- and perivesical space occurs and may gradually, following fascial planes, ascend the anterior wall or, in the retroperitoneal space, may reach the kidneys. Extravasation can also extend via the inguinal canal into the scrotal compartment, through the obturator foramen to the

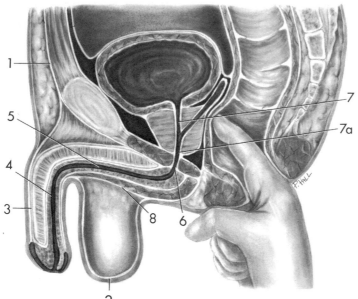

Figure 16–12. Sagittal section of the male lower urinary tract, demonstrating the relationship of the prostate to the rectum: (1) Scarpa's fascia, (2) dartos fascia, (3) Buck's fascia, (4) pendulous urethra, (5) bulbous urethra, (6) membranous urethra, (7) prostatic urethra, (7a) supramembranous urethra, and (8) Colles' fascia. (Reprinted by permission. From Clark, S. S., and Prudencio, R. F.: Lower urinary tract injuries associated with pelvic fractures: Diagnosis and management. Surg. Clin. North Am. 52[1]: 183–201, [Feb.] 1972.)

thigh and through the greater sciatic notch into the buttocks. It may also spread under Colles' fascia, upward in the abdominal wall (Fig. 16–13).

Intraperitoneal Rupture

Intraperitoneal rupture usually occurs in direct trauma to a distended bladder. It involves not only complete penetration of the bladder wall but also a rupture of the visceral peritoneum covering the dome of the bladder. Urinary extravasation will pool in the peritoneal cavity (Fig. 16–13). This type of injury occurs with somewhat higher frequency in children, whose bladders are still largely intraperitoneal and thus more vulnerable to this type of rupture.[10, 44]

Figure 16–13. Routes of extravasation of urine and blood in (1) bulbomembranous urethral rupture with the hematoma appearing in the scrotum and beneath Scarpa's fascia, (2) extraperitoneal perforation with accumulation into the perivesical space, and (3) intraperitoneal perforation with extravasation into the peritoneal cavity. Rectal examination outlines the prostate in its usual position in any of these injuries. (Reprinted by permission. From Clark, S. S., and Prudencio, R. F.: Lower urinary tract injuries associated with pelvic fractures: Diagnosis and management. Surg. Clin. North Am. 52[1]:183–201, [Feb.] 1972.)

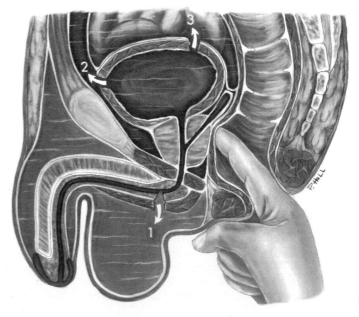

Combined Intra- and Extraperitoneal Rupture

This condition is usually associated with severe crush injuries of the pelvis. It is also associated with a significantly higher number of injuries to adjacent organs, notably the rectum. The severity of the injury, plus the free mixture of blood, urine and contaminated feces, carries with it a very high mortality for this type of injury.

Crush trauma to the pelvis in a child will result in a different type of injury than in the adult patient group. The developing bony pelvis is less rigid than the mature pelvis. A crushing force applied to a child's pelvis may easily disrupt this at both symphysis pubis and the sacroiliac joints. After the force has been removed, the pelvis springs back into a relatively normal position while the soft tissues, on the other hand, are compressed and rapidly decompressed, resulting in total disruption of the rectum and urinary tract, with ensuing contamination of the pelvis with feces and urine.[5] Such a "sprung" or "exploded" pelvis may show remarkably few radiological changes, whereas the damage to the lower urinary tract is enormous.

Diagnosis

Every pelvic fracture should lead one to suspect bladder trauma until proved otherwise. Examination should be done with the patient completely disrobed so that the suprapubic area and perineum as well as the external genitalia can be inspected and examined in detail.

Hematuria, microscopic or macroscopic, is usually present but may be absent in complete disruption of the urethra. Suprapubic tenderness and a "doughy" swelling may be palpated in patients with *extraperitoneal* bladder rupture and extravasation into the space of Retzius. Extravasation into scrotum, buttocks or perineum has to be sought. *Intraperitoneal* extravasation will rapidly lead to the classical signs of peritoneal irritation. Shock may accompany many pelvic fractures without bladder trauma. Blood loss in pelvic trauma can be severe, and 60 per cent of patients who succumb as a result of injury to the bony pelvis die of blood loss.[26, 29, 36] The iliac veins and the prostatic venous plexus of Santorini are the two most vulnerable vascular areas. In children, not only the major vessels but also the sciatic nerves in their courses overlying the sacroiliac joint are particularly vulnerable to trauma.[46] Absence of a femoral pulse and loss of sciatic nerve function is an ominous sign in this type of injury. Local tenderness is not a reliable sign in bladder rupture as the usually associated pelvic fracture masks any discomfort due to bladder trauma. In both intra- and extraperitoneal bladder rupture, the attempt to void will increase a patient's pain, and in intraperitoneal rupture in particular he may be unable to void.

The diagnosis in both intra- and extraperitoneal bladder rupture is made by a cystogram. An excretory urogram may show the typical "teardrop" deformity of the bladder, which is due to a mixture of blood and urine compressing and elevating the bladder. However, concentration of dye in the bladder on such a film is usually inadequate to visualize a small rent. Retrograde injection of Renografin-60 into the bladder is the preferred diagnostic method. To avoid compounding a possible urethral injury, no catheter is used at this point; rather, the contrast material is injected into the urethra through a Brodney clamp or a Chetwood syringe. After obtaining adequate filling films of the bladder, an evacuation film is taken which will show the location and extent of extravasation. Not infrequently, a bladder perforation may be completely missed if a postevacuation film is not obtained. Also, oblique or lateral films may be helpful in establishing the diagnosis. With intraperitoneal rupture, the contrast medium may coat the intestinal loops and outline them, and it will pool in the most dependent portions of the abdominal cavity, usually the paracolic gutter (Fig. 16–14A). Extraperitoneal extravasation usually presents as an ill-defined, hazy, irregular contrast shadow that remains fixed with position changes of the patient (Fig. 16–14B).

Treatment

All intraperitoneal bladder ruptures require prompt surgical closure. The rent can usually be identified, the bladder wall closed, and the peritoneal tear closed in a

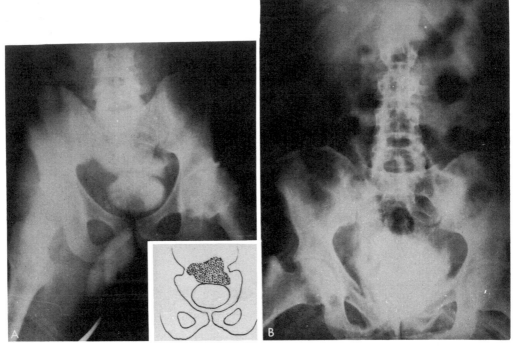

Figure 16–14. A, *Retrograde cystogram and diagrammatic sketch illustrating intraperitoneal extravasation of dye from a bladder rupture. B, Retrograde cystogram shows extravasation of dye from an extraperitoneal bladder rupture.*

separate layer. A number of surgeons prefer to drain such a bladder suprapubically.[26, 27, 39] Our preference is for urethral catheter drainage. The mortality rate with intraperitoneal rupture remains high.

Small extraperitoneal bladder perforations need not necessarily be closed. Transurethral catheter drainage for a week usually suffices in allowing adequate healing of small tears, particularly in patients who sustained such a tear from electroresection of a bladder tumor or false passage of a sound. However, if the prevesical extravasation is significant, and in all patients with infected urine, it is advisable to approach the bladder through a suprapubic incision, close the bladder perforation anteriorly and place a suprapubic Penrose drain until a day after the catheter has been removed and the drainage from the Penrose drain site has ceased.

INJURIES OF THE URETHRA

As pointed out earlier, more than half the injuries to the lower urinary tract in-

volve the urethra, either alone (58.3 per cent) or in conjunction with bladder injuries (9.4 per cent).[44] Virtually all of these injuries occur in males. For the understanding of the mechanism of trauma to the urethra, a brief review of the anatomy is in order: The prostatic urethra, usually 2.5 to 3 cm. long in the adult, courses through the prostate along its longitudinal axis. Just below the apex of the prostate, the urethra traverses the urogenital diaphragm. This portion of the urethra is called the membranous urethra and is approximately 1.0 cm. long. It is firmly attached to the urogenital diaphragm and allows very little mobility. Following this begins the bulbous urethra, which lies within the superficial perineal space and extends in an S-shaped curve into the scrotal and pendulous urethra (Fig. 16–12).

The membranous urethra allows little mobility, as just pointed out. The prostatic urethra likewise is fixed to the surrounding structures by the prostate that, in turn, is attached at its anterior surface, through the puboprostatic ligaments, to the posterior surface of the pubic symphysis. The prostatic base, joining the bladder at the bladder neck, is less restricted through its ligaments to the bony pelvis.

The female urethra, on the other hand, has no such firm and restricting attachments and, owing to its much greater mobility, almost always escapes trauma.

The cause of trauma to the urethra is usually a pelvic fracture, most often due to motor vehicle accidents. However, a significant number of such injuries are caused by industrial accidents. Falls resulting in straddle injuries, such as occur in the roofing or construction industries, are not infrequent. The compression of the perineum against the pubic arch may result in a crush injury of the urethra or an actual disruption of the urethra, usually at the urogenital diaphragm. Pelvic fractures that involve the pubic arch will traumatize the prostatic and bulbomembranous urethra in almost 70 per cent of such accidents.[35, 39, 44, 54] Not infrequently, fractures in this area also disrupt the periprostatic venous plexus, resulting in a large hematoma that may displace the prostate cephalad. Transsections of the urethra below the level of an intact external urinary sphincter usually do not result in extravasation of urine, and thus the ensuing hematoma usually is not contaminated with urine. Disruption above the level of the sphincter leads to unrestricted urinary extravasation.

Diagnosis

Symptoms and signs of urethral trauma, again, may be masked by the accompanying pelvic fractures. A suprapubic mass may be the distended urinary bladder or a large hematoma resulting from injury above the urogenital diaphragm. Such a hematoma may extend underneath the inguinal ligament to the upper thigh.

A hematoma or urinary extravasation from trauma below the urogenital diaphragm will present itself as a swelling in the perineum, scrotum and penis (Fig. 16–13). It may continue to extend underneath Colles' and Scarpa's fasciae and ascend on the anterior abdominal wall. If the urine is infected, cellulitis will rapidly supervene. This may lead to skin necrosis and gangrene of the genitalia.

Hematuria may be an initial or terminal sign in cases of urethral trauma, and if the injury occurs below the external sphincter,

a constant dripping of bright red blood from the external meatus can frequently be observed. With disruption of the urethra, the patient will be unable to void spontaneously.

Rectal examination is an essential part of diagnosis. Frank blood per anum may well indicate a concomitant trauma to the rectosigmoid. In patients with urethral trauma above the urogenital diaphragm, such examination allows assessment of the expansion of a pelvic hematoma or the possible elevation of the prostate gland in complete disruption of the urethra. At times, the prostate may be displaced so high that it cannot be reached by the palpating finger; at other times, it can be freely ballotted (Fig. 16–15). Subsequent rectal examinations allow for follow-up of the resolution of the hematoma.

Following an excretory urogram (which preferably is done with an infusion drip after the blood pressure has been stabilized), further radiological examinations are necessary. The excretory urogram is primarily indicated to assess function and integrity of the upper urinary tract. Films of the bladder, when filled and after evacuation, may be helpful in ascertaining the diagnosis of urethral injury in the posterior urethra since elevation of the bladder may be seen in complete transsection. However, we prefer retrograde cystourethrography as the diagnostic maneuver (Fig. 16–16). It is best *not* to insert a catheter for such a procedure since the necessary manipulation may convert an incomplete transsection of the urethra into a complete one. Twenty to thirty ml. of Renografin-60 are injected with a Brodney clamp through the external meatus. A complete transsection of the urethra at any level will show extravasation and usually no filling of the urethra above the level of transsection. This study will show the site and degree of laceration, with one continuous wall in one projection, and filling above the level of trauma. In suspected trauma of the urethra, the catheter should be passed only by one who is best suited to do so, namely, a urologist.

Treatment

Trauma to the posterior urethra may lead to significant long-term morbidity.[37, 42] Exact figures on the various compli-

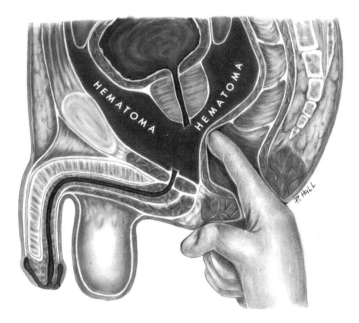

Figure 16–15. *Transection of the posterior urethra with hematoma elevating the prostate and bladder. A finger in the rectum may not feel the prostate. (Reprinted by permission. From Clark, S. S., and Prudencio, R. F.: Lower urinary tract injuries associated with pelvic fractures: Diagnosis and management. Surg. Clin. North Am. 52[1]:183–201, [Feb.] 1972.)*

cations are unknown, but incontinence, stricture formation and impotence are high. Some authors[33, 34, 63] suggest that conventional management may actually increase the incidence of these complications.

Conventional management consists of reapproximating the transsected urethra via Davis interlocking sounds. These

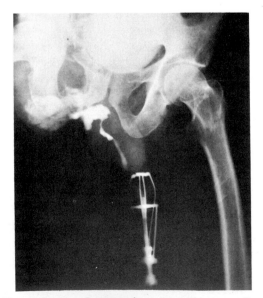

Figure 16–16. *Retrograde cystourethrogram. Rupture of the posterior urethra is shown by the marked gap between the torn end of the urethra and the bladder base.*

sounds are passed antegrade and retrograde until, with gentle manipulation, their tips meet and interlock. Rectal palpation by an assistant significantly aids in this maneuver. The sounds are then passed through the entire urethra, a catheter is tied to the tip of one of these sounds and then pulled into the bladder. After the balloon is inflated, traction is applied to the catheter to pull down the transsected segment of the urethra and approximate it to the distal end. Some authors[32, 37, 42, 63] have preferred to simultaneously evacuate the periurethral hematoma and perform a primary suture anastomosis of the transsected ends of the urethra through a perineal or retropubic approach. Clark and Prudencio[5] and Morehouse and MacKinnon[33, 34, 35] strongly advocate simply diverting the urine suprapubically at the time of injury and leaving the hematoma and transsected posterior urethra undisturbed. Two to four months later, after the hematoma has been absorbed and the posterior urethra has returned to near normal position, a two-stage urethroplasty is performed to bridge the gap between proximal and distal segments. The methods of Johanson and of Turner-Warwick[58] are well suited for this purpose. Morehouse and MacKinnon[35] report on 11 patients who were managed this way. As of the report, all 11 were voiding with good stream; they did not require dilation; all of them had normal urinary control, and nine had normal erection and ejaculation. While these reports are very promising, more experience with this method is needed before the procedure can be properly judged.

Trauma to the urethra below the urogenital diaphragm usually does not result in transsection, but rather laceration. Suprapubic urinary diversion may be performed. We prefer to let such a traumatized urethra heal over a medically inert silicone catheter. Extravasation of urine into the confines of Colles' and Scarpa's fasciae must be incised adequately to prevent necrotizing cellulitis.

INJURIES TO THE EXTERNAL GENITALIA

The external genitalia of the female are rarely involved in direct injury. In the male, the genitalia also usually escape trauma but are not infrequently involved in urinary extravasation secondary to lacerations or fistulas forming below the urogenital diaphragm. Trauma to the external genitalia accounted for roughly one third of injuries to the genitourinary tract in the series by Waterhouse and Gross,[61] but this incidence is significantly higher than the experience in other centers.[28, 54] They are secondary to motor vehicle accidents, industrial accidents, bullet or stab wounds or self-inflicted trauma.

Abrasions, hematomas and minor lacerations constitute the bulk of genital injuries. These injuries will heal quite well with debridement and local treatment. Primary suture of lacerations is necessary. Small hematomas do well if left alone. Large hematomas will require incision and drainage, as do those that are complicated by infection.

Industrial accidents frequently are associated with significant skin loss that may require isolation of flaps from scrotum or thigh. Usually, penile skin deficits can be covered by temporarily burying the penile shaft under the scrotum or suprapubic skin. In a second-stage procedure, after complete wound healing, the penis is freed from its site of temporary implantation.

In deeper injuries that involve the penile shaft, as much of the penile body as possible should be preserved. If the urethra is involved in the injury, temporary urinary diversion with a perineal urethrostomy or suprapubic cystostomy is recommended. Strangulation with amputation in young boys who "dare each other," or self-amputation by psychiatric patients, has been reported.[30, 31] Treatment for these patients usually consists of oversewing the stump. Complete restoration to obtain anatomic and functional results is rarely possible. Prompt psychiatric treatment is important.

Testicular injuries can be divided into those that do not involve rupture of the tunica albuginea and those that do. Testicular trauma is frequently characterized by severe pain that may radiate into the groin and flank, producing nausea, vomiting and at times even shock. Blunt trauma that results in contusion or hematoma of the testis is best treated by analgesics, elevation of the scrotum, icepacks to reduce the swelling and discomfort, and rest. Surgical intervention is rarely indicated. A lacerated tunica albuginea, however, should be repaired. Testicular tissue outside the testis should be removed to prevent the formation of a sperm granuloma. As the testes are the site of androgen production, preservation of even the smallest amount of testicular tissue is worthwhile.

In patients with complete loss of their testes, replacement therapy with testosterone is required.

Herniorrhaphy in the young infant is associated with 1 to 2 per cent incidence of transsection of the vas deferens. At present, it is not known whether repair at a later age will allow transport of fertile sperm across the anastomosis into the ejaculate of such a patient.

Vasectomies, which are performed with continued frequency today, also have a number of surgical complications. Hematomas of significant extent occur in less than 1 per cent. These should be surgically evacuated. The spermatic artery may accidentally be ligated. Should this occur bilaterally, testicular atrophy will occur, which again requires testosterone replacement therapy. As with all iatrogenic trauma, it is extremely important from a medicolegal standpoint to inform the patient of such incidents as ureteral transsection or ligation. Many legal problems can be prevented or ameliorated through complete honesty.

REFERENCES

1. Alfert, H. J., and Gillenwater, J. Y.: The consequences of ureteral irradiation with special reference to subsequent ureteral injury. J. Urol. *107*:369, 1972.

2. Bookstein, J. J., and Goldstein, H. M.: Successful management of postbiopsy arteriovenous fistula with selective arterial embolization. Radiology *109*:535, 1973.

3. Cangiano, J. L., and Kest, L.: Use of a G-suit for uncontrollable bleeding after percutaneous renal biopsy. J. Urol. *107*:360, 1972.

4. Carlton, C. E., Guthrie, A. G., and Scott, R., Jr.: Surgical correction of ureteral injury. J. Trauma 9:457, 1969.

5. Clark, S. S., and Prudencio, R. F.: Lower urinary tract injuries associated with pelvic fractures. Surg. Clin. N. Am. 52:183, 1972.

6. Cohen, S. G., and Pearlman, C. K.: Spontaneous rupture of the kidney in pregnancy. J. Urol. *100*:365, 1968.

7. Davis, D. M.: The process of ureteral repair: Recapitulation of the splinting question. J. Urol. 79:215, 1958.

8. Del Villar, R. G., Ireland, G. W., and Cass, A. S.: Ureteral injury owing to external trauma. J. Urol. *107*:29, 1972.

9. Del Villar, R. G., Ireland, G. W., and Cass, A. S.: Management of renal injury in conjunction with the immediate surgical treatment of the acute severe trauma patient. J. Urol. *107*:208, 1972.

10. Ezell, W. W., Smith, I. E., McCarthy, R. P., Thompson, I. M., and Habib, H. N.: Mechanical traumatic injury to the genital tract in children. J. Urol. *102*:788, 1969.

11. Funkhouser, J. J., and Sacher, E. C.: The contiguous helix ureteral lengthening flap for repair of distal ureteral injury. J. Urol. *107*:567, 1972.

12. Garrett, J. W., and Braunstein, P. W.: The seat belt syndrome. J. Trauma 2:220, 1962.

13. Glenn, J. F., and Harvard, B. M.: The injured kidney. J.A.M.A. *173*:1189, 1960.

14. Graham, W. H.: Injuries to the urogenital tract. Proc. Roy. Soc. Med. *61*:477, 1968.

15. Hamm, F. C., and Weinberg, S. R.: Management of the severed ureter. Trans. Am. Assoc. GU Surgeons 48:130, 1956.

16. Herman, G., Guerrier, K., and Persky L.: Delayed ureteral deligation. J. Urol. *107*:723, 1972.

17. Higgins, C. C.: Ureteral injury during surgery. J.A.M.A. *199*:82, 1967.

18. Hodges, C. V., Gilbert, D. R., and Scott, W. W.: Renal trauma: Study of 71 cases. J. Urol. 66:627, 1951.

19. Jevtich, M. J., and Montero, G. G.: Injuries to renal vessels by blunt trauma in children. J. Urol. *102*:493, 1969.

20. Jones, R. F.: Surgical management of transcapsular rupture of the kidney: 24 cases. J. Urol. 74:721, 1955.

21. Kaiser, J. H., and Farrow, F. C.: Injury of the bladder and prostatomembranous urethra associated with fracture of the bony pelvis. Surg. Gynecol. Obstet. *120*:99, 1965.

22. Kalish, M., Greenbaum, L., Silber, S., and Goldstein, H.: Traumatic renal hemorrhage treatment by arterial embolization. J. Urol. *112*:138, 1974.

23. Kaufman, S. L., Freeman, C., Busky, S. M., and White, R. I., Jr.: Management of postoperative renal hemorrhage by transcatheter embolization. J. Urol. *115*:203, 1976.

24. Kazmin, M. H., Brosman, S. A., and Cockett, A. T. K.: Diagnosis and early management of renal trauma: Study of 120 patients. J. Urol. *101*:783, 1969.

25. Khonsari, H., Morehouse, D. D., and MacKinnon, J. K.: Pararenal pseudocysts. Br. J. Urol. 43:164, 1971.

26. Levine, J. I., and Crampton, R. S.: Major abdominal injuries associated with pelvic fractures. Surg. Gynecol. Obstet. *116*:223, 1963.

27. Lewis, L. G.: Treatment of wounds of the bladder and urethra. Surg. Clin. N. Am. 24:1402, 1944.

28. Lucey, D. T., Smith, M. J. V., and Koontz, W. W., Jr.: Modern trends in the management of urologic trauma. J. Urol. *107*:641, 1972.

29. McLaughlin, A. P., III, McCullough, D. L., Jerr, W. S., and Darling, R. C.: Use of external counterpressure (G-suit) in the management of traumatic retroperitoneal hemorrhage. J. Urol. *107*:940, 1972.

30. McRoberts, J. W., Chapman, W. H., and Ansell, J. S.: Primary anastomosis of the traumatically amputated penis: Case report and summary of the literature. J. Urol. 97:105, 1967.

31. Mendez, R., Kiely, W. F., and Morrow, J. W.: Self-emasculation. J. Urol. *107*:981, 1972.

32. Moore, C. A.: One-stage urethroplasty: A new one-stage anterior urethroplasty. J. Urol. 90:203, 1963.

33. Morehouse, D. D.: Injuries to the bladder and urethra. Lawyer's Med. J. 7:141, 1971.

34. Morehouse, D. D., Belitsky, P., and MacKinnon, K.: Rupture of the posterior urethra. J. Urol. *107*:255, 1972.

35. Morehouse, D. D., and MacKinnon, K. J.: Urological injuries associated with pelvic fractures. J. Trauma 9:479, 1969.

36. Motsay, G. J., Manlove, C., and Perry, J. F.: Major venous injury with pelvic fracture. J. Trauma 9:343, 1969.

37. Myers, R. P., and DeWeerd, J. H.: Incidence of stricture following primary realignment of disrupted proximal urethra. J. Urol. *107*:265, 1972.

38. National Safety Council, Statistics Division: Accident Facts. Chicago, The National Safety Council, 1972.

39. Newland, D. E.: Genitourinary complications of pelvic fractures. J.A.M.A. *152*:1515, 1953.

40. Ochsner, T. G., Busch, F. M., and Clarke, B. G.: Urogenital wounds in Vietnam. J. Urol. *101*:224, 1969.

41. Orkin, L. A.: Diagnosis of urologic trauma in the presence of other injuries. Surg. Clin. N. Am. 33:1473, 1953.

42. Pierce, J. M.: Management of dismemberment of the prostatic-membranous urethra and ensuing stricture disease. J. Urol. *107*:259, 1972.

43. Potempa, J., and Wenz, W.: Die Indikationsstellung zur konservativen und operativen Behandlung geschlossener Nierenverletzungen. Langenbeck's Arch. Klin. Chir. *321*:149, 1968.

44. Prather, G. C., and Kaiser, T. F.: The bladder in fracture of the bony pelvis; the significance of a "tear drop bladder" as shown by cystogram. J. Urol. *63*:1019, 1950.
45. Prince, J. C., and Pearlman, C. K.: Thrombosis of the renal artery secondary to trauma. J. Urol. *102*:670, 1969.
46. Quinby, W. C., Jr.: Fractures of the pelvis and associated injuries in children. J. Pediatr. Surg. *1*:353, 1966.
47. Rieser, C.: Diagnostic evaluation of suspected genitourinary tract injury. J.A.M.A. *199*:714, 1967.
48. Rizk, G. K., Atallah, N. K., and Bridi, G. I.: Renal arteriovenous fistula treated by catheter embolization. Br. J. Radiol., *46*:222, 1973.
49. Rusche, C., and Morrow, J. W.: Injury to the ureter. *In* Campbell, M. F. (ed.): Urology. (2nd Ed.) Philadelphia, W. B. Saunders Co., 1963.
50. Scholl, A. J., and Nation, E. F.: Injuries of the kidney. *In* Campbell, M. F., and Harrison, J. H. (eds.): Urology. (3rd Ed.) Philadelphia, W. B. Saunders Co., 1970.
51. Schreiner, G. E.: The nephrotic syndrome. *In* Strauss, M. B., and Welt, L. G.: Diseases of the Kidney. Boston, Little, Brown & Co., 1963.
52. Scott, R., Jr., Carlton, C. E., Ashmore, A. J., and Duke, H. H.: Initial management of nonpenetrating renal injuries: Clinical review of 111 cases. J. Urol. *90*:535, 1963.
53. Scott, R., Jr., Carlton, C. E., Jr., and Goldman, M.: Penetrating injuries of the kidney: Analysis of 181 patients. J. Urol. *101*:247, 1969.
54. Scott, W. W., and Engel, R. M.: Management of urinary tract trauma. Lawyer's Med. J. 2, Second Series (2):81, May, 1973.
55. Snyder, W. J., Jr.: The surgically traumatized ureter: Surgeon's viewpoint. Western Med. Surg. *3*:180, 1949.
56. Stone, H. H., and Jones, H. Q.: Penetrating and non-penetrating injuries to the ureter. Surg. Gynecol. Obstet. *114*:52, 1962.
57. Thompson, I. M., Karow, W. F., and Ross, G., Jr.: Long-term results of ureteral reimplantation for trauma. J. Urol. *102*:308, 1969.
58. Turner-Warwick: The repair of urethral strictures in the region of the membranous urethra. J. Urol. *100*:303, 1968.
59. Vargas, A. D., and Silva, E. I.: Mobilization of the ureter by a posterior vesical flap in dogs: Preliminary report of a new technique. J. Urol. *107*:742, 1972.
60. Walker, J. A.: Injuries of the ureter due to external violence. J. Urol. *102*:410, 1969.
61. Waterhouse, K., and Gross, M.: Trauma to the genitourinary tract: A 5-year experience with 251 cases. J. Urol. *101*:241, 1969.
62. Wertheim, E.: Ein neuer Beitrag zur Frage der Radikaloperation beim Uletuskrebs. Arch. Gynäk. *65*:1–39, 1901.
63. Wiggishoff, C. C., and Kiefer, J. H.: Pull-through reconstruction of the posterior urethra. J. Urol. *93*:233, 1966.
64. Zimmerman, S. J., and Radding, R. S.: Hypertension due to trauma of the kidney. N. Engl. J. Med. *264*:238, 1961.

CHAPTER 17

SOFT TISSUE INJURIES OF THE EXTREMITIES

John E. Hoopes, M.D.
G. Patrick Maxwell, M.D.

Statistics indicate that approximately three fourths of all trauma involves the extremities. This information, coupled with the fact that extremity injuries produce significantly greater incapacity in terms of time lost from productive activities than trauma to other regions, provides some measure of the magnitude of the problem. The economic devastation attendant upon weeks and months of inability to work is literally inconceivable. The nature of permanent functional impairment frequently precludes return to the level of employment previously enjoyed.

The degree of functional recovery obtained directly reflects the attention to minute detail and basic surgical principles observed in initial management. Casual or misguided treatment adds insult to injury and assigns the patient permanently to the role of a relative cripple.

SURGICAL ANATOMY

A thorough knowledge of functional anatomy is essential in dealing with extremity injuries. Adequate diagnosis is based almost entirely on functional evaluation of the part distal to the site of injury. No attempt will be made to review morbid anatomy; rather, a concise guide to surgical anatomy is presented (Fig. 17–1).

Upper Arm. The upper arm is divided into anterior and posterior compartments by the lateral and medial intermuscular septa. The anterior compartment contains the coracobrachialis, biceps brachialis and brachioradialis muscles. The posterior compartment contains the triceps muscle. The brachial artery extends from the lower border of the teres major muscle to the antecubital fossa, at which point it bifurcates into the radial and ulnar arteries opposite the neck of the radius. The artery lies anterior to the medial intermuscular septum beneath the medial border of the biceps and enters the antecubital fossa beneath the lacertus fibrosis medial to the biceps tendon. The radial nerve progresses distally and laterally beneath the long head of the triceps muscle and, after supplying the triceps, penetrates the lateral intermuscular septum at the junction of the proximal and middle thirds of a line joining the deltoid insertion with the lateral epicondyle. The nerve divides into superficial (sensory) and posterior interosseus (motor) branches anterior to the lateral epicondyle. The musculocutaneous nerve diverges from the axillary artery to pass through the coracobrachialis and progress distally between the biceps and brachialis muscles; it supplies all the muscles of the anterior compartment. The median nerve accompanies the brachial artery, first on its lateral and then on its medial surface, crossing the brachial artery at the middle of the arm. The ulnar nerve accompanies the brachial artery on its medial

522

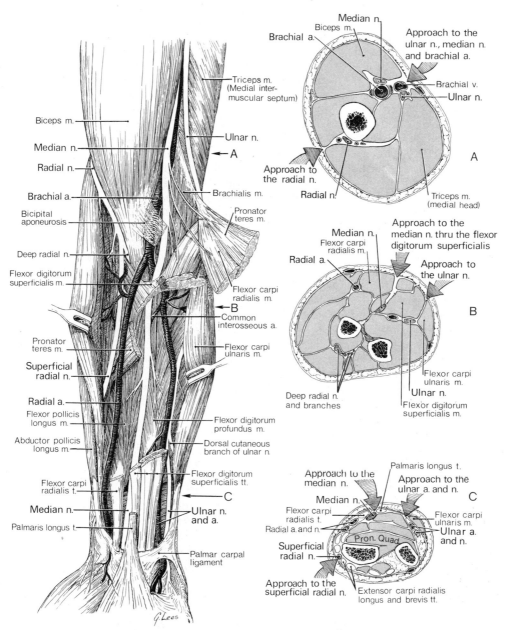

Figure 17–1. *Soft tissue injuries of the extremities.*

surface in the proximal half of the arm and then penetrates the medial intermuscular septum to pass posterior to the medial epicondyle of the humerus.

FOREARM. The forearm musculature is divided into a volar-medial or flexor-pronator group and a dorsal-lateral or extensor-supinator group. The muscles of the flexor-pronator group all arise, at least in part, from the medial epicondyle of the humerus and are divided into superficial and deep layers. Progressing from lateral to medial, the superficial group consists of the pronator teres, flexor carpi radialis, palmaris longus, flexor digitorum superficialis and flexor carpi ulnaris muscles. The deep layer includes the flexor digitorum profundus, flexor pollicis longus and pronator quadratus muscles. All the muscles of the flexor-pronator group except the flexor carpi ulnaris and the flexor digitorum profundi of the ring and little fingers are supplied by the median nerve; these two exceptions are supplied by the ulnar nerve.

The musculature of the extensor-supinator group is divided into radial and dorsal divisions, the dorsal division being divided into superficial and deep groups. All the muscles of the radial and superficial portion of the dorsal group arise from the lateral epicondyle and are supplied by branches of the main trunk of the radial nerve. The deep muscles of the dorsal group arise from the dorsal surface of the radius and ulna and are supplied by the posterior interosseous branch of the radial nerve. The radial group of muscles includes the brachioradialis and the extensor carpi radialis longus and brevis.

The superficial division of the dorsal group contains the extensor digitorum communis, extensor digiti quinti proprius and extensor carpi ulnaris muscles; the deep division consists of the abductor pollicis longus, extensor pollicis brevis, extensor pollicis longus and extensor indicis proprius muscles.

The ulnar artery descends through the anterior surface of the proximal forearm on the surface of the flexor digitorum profundus between the flexor carpi ulnaris and flexor digitorum sublimis. In the distal half of the forearm it lies beneath the flexor carpi ulnaris and passes into the hand superficial to the transverse carpal ligament on the radial side of the pisiform bone.

The radial artery passes laterally on the surface of the supinator muscle beneath the brachioradialis and comes to lie between the brachioradialis and flexor carpi radialis in the distal half of the forearm. The distal third of the radial artery is subcutaneous and lies on the radius and the flexor pollicis longus muscle. The superficial branch of the radial nerve progresses distally beneath the brachioradialis on the lateral aspect of the radial artery; it pierces the deep fascia to become subcutaneous at the junction of the proximal and distal thirds of the forearm. The posterior interosseous branch of the radial nerve passes around the lateral aspect of the neck of the radius and through the supinator muscle to enter the interspace between the superficial and deep muscles of the dorsal group.

The median nerve passes between the superficial and deep heads of the pronator teres to lie between the flexor digitorum profundus and sublimis and progresses distally on the radial aspect of the palmaris longus. The ulnar nerve enters the forearm between the two heads of the flexor carpi ulnaris and descends on the ulnar surface of the flexor digitorum profundus beneath the flexor carpi ulnaris; it accompanies the ulnar artery into the hand on its radial deep surface.

Thigh. The musculature of the thigh is divided into three osteofibrous compartments: an anterior or extensor group consisting of the sartorius and quadriceps femoris muscles supplied by the femoral nerve; a posterior or flexor group including the biceps femoris, semimembranous and semitendinous muscles supplied by the sciatic nerve; and a medial or adductor group consisting of the adductor, pectineus and gracilis muscles supplied by the obturator nerve. The femoral artery enters the thigh beneath the inguinal ligament and is relatively superficial in the femoral triangle. It passes distally in the adductor canal beneath the sartorius to enter the popliteal fossa through a tendinous ring in the adductor magnus muscle. The profunda femoris branch leaves the common femoral artery approximately 4 cm. inferior to the inguinal ligament, passes lateral and posterior to the superficial femoral artery beneath the adductor longus muscle to gain the posterior surface of the shaft of the femur, and enters the popliteal fossa through the adductor magnus muscle. The femoral nerve enters the thigh beneath the inguinal ligament on the lateral aspect of the femoral artery and accompanies the superficial femoral artery in the adductor canal. The sciatic nerve descends between the greater trochanter of the femur and the tuberosity of the ischium beneath the long head of the biceps and terminates in the middle third of the thigh by dividing into the common peroneal and tibial nerves. The obturator nerve enters the thigh through the obturator canal and descends in two branches posterior to the pectineus muscle.

Lower Leg. The musculature of the leg is divided into anterior, lateral and posterior compartments. The anterior compartment contains the tibialis anterior, extensor digitorum longus, extensor hallucis longus and peroneus tertius muscles, all of which are supplied by the deep peroneal nerve. The tibialis anterior arises from the upper two thirds of the lateral surface of the tibia and inserts into the medial aspect of the base of the first metatarsal. This muscle dorsiflexes and inverts the foot.

The lateral compartment consists of the peroneus longus and brevis muscles supplied by the superficial peroneal nerve. The tendons of both muscles pass posterior to the lateral malleolus. The brevis inserts into the lateral aspect of the base of the fifth metatarsal, and the longus crosses the sole of the foot to insert on the lateral aspect of the base of the first metatarsal. They permit plantar flexion, abduction and eversion of the foot.

The posterior compartment contains a superficial group of muscles consisting of the gastrocnemius, soleus and plantaris and a deep group consisting of the flexor digitorum longus, flexor hallucis longus and tibialis posterior muscles, all of which are supplied by the tibial nerve. The popliteal artery bifurcates into anterior and posterior tibial branches at the lower border of the popliteus muscle. The anterior tibial artery enters the anterior compartment through the upper part of the interosseous membrane. The posterior tibial artery descends in the interspace between the superficial and deep muscles of the posterior compartment to become subcutaneous between the medial malleolus and calcan-

eus. The peroneal artery is the largest branch of the posterior tibial; it progresses distally on the posterior surface of the fibula. The tibial nerve passes through the posterior compartment in close association with the posterior tibial artery. The common peroneal nerve divides into superficial and deep branches within the lateral compartment on the lateral aspect of the neck of the fibula. The superficial peroneal nerve descends immediately behind the anterior intermuscular septum between the fibula and peroneus longus. The deep peroneal nerve descends through the anterior compartment in association with the anterior tibial artery.

FIRST AID

The principles of the first aid management of injured extremities are as applicable in the large hospital emergency department as at the scene of the accident. Preparation of injured patients for transportion to medical facilities demands that hemorrhage be controlled and fractures adequately splinted. This should be equally obvious at the time of initial evaluation in the emergency department, but all too commonly patients are referred for extensive radiological evaluation or other diagnostic studies without due regard for protection from further injury. Hemorrhage is controlled by elevation and pressure, not by tourniquets and clamps. Improperly applied tourniquets readily produce peripheral nerve injuries; tourniquets properly applied but left unattended result in irreparable ischemia. Clamps applied directly to severed vessels preclude restoration of continuity; clamps indiscriminately plunged into the wound not infrequently incorporate vital structures. Adequate immobilization of fractures is imperative. Conversion of unsplinted closed fractures into compound fractures occurs readily, not to mention the tissue damage and blood loss associated with instability at the fracture site. Open wounds should be covered with sterile dressings. The physician may proceed with more leisurely evaluation only after assuring himself that his patient is comfortable, protected and free from danger.

INITIAL EVALUATION

All injured patients deserve a thorough physical examination before attention is focused on their outstanding injury. Complete, systematic evaluation is essential to the avoidance of catastrophe from come unsuspected injury. With thoughtfulness and a little practice, the physician quickly develops a routine that allows him to complete a truly thorough examination within a matter of minutes. The importance of developing such a routine cannot be overemphasized.

Preliminary preparations toward definitive operative management are made during or immediately following the initial physical examination. A route of intravenous fluid administration is secured as rapidly as possible in all severely injured patients and in all patients in whom it is anticipated that treatment will require the use of the operating room. Blood for baseline studies and for typing and crossmatching is obtained at the time intravenous fluids are begun. The intravenous line should be placed in a site other than the involved extremity. Occlusive sterile dressings are applied to open wounds. The nursing personnel are instructed to record the vital signs at appropriate intervals.

Having accomplished these steps in a rapid and efficient manner, the physician is prepared to proceed with a more thorough evaluation of the total patient and his specific injury. A complete history is obtained, and emphasis is given to the specific circumstances of the injury. Minute details serve as valuable guides during the physical examination in pointing to the particular structures that might be injured. Victims of automobile accidents are questioned regarding loss of consciousness, chest and abdominal trauma, and so forth. Patients with injuries sustained at work are asked to describe in detail the machinery with which they were working and the exact nature of the accident. Patients with missile and sharp instrument injuries who have been victims of assault are questioned regarding the relative position of their assailant in an effort to determine the trajectory of the injuring agent. Knowledge of the time elapsed from injury to treatment is critical in evaluation of all wounds.

Facilities for the adequate evaluation of extremity injuries should be available in all receiving wards. Ideally, such facilities consist of the set-up usually found in a well-appointed minor surgery operating room: caps and masks, scrub sinks, operating room table with arm board, operating room light and sterile instruments and drapes. The facilities must permit a thorough, unhurried examination in peace and quiet.

Integument. As emphasized previously, the dressing of open wounds is an integral part of first aid treatment. Ordinarily, examination of the wound is deferred until completion of functional examination of the extremity distal to the site of injury. Aseptic technique is observed strictly. Examination of the wound is utilized as an opportunity to secure initial cleansing of the affected part. No solution other than sterile normal saline solution may be applied to the wound itself. The surrounding intact skin may be cleansed with a mild detergent such as Septisol or pHisoHex. Antiseptic solutions have no role in the management of open, traumatic wounds as most are cytotoxic; however, the newer organic bound iodine preparations are much less so than the alcohol solutions. Gentle but thorough scrubbing with a surgical brush may be required to remove the accumulated dirt and grease from a working man's extremities and the imbedded foreign material associated with automobile accidents. Pulsating water jet lavage can help remove foreign debris.[8] Hydrogen peroxide, diluted to a 0.5 per cent to 1 per cent solution with saline, can assist in cleansing, particularly in removing old blood and tiny particles (Fig. 17–2).

The major purposes of this portion of the initial evaluation are assessment of the soft tissue wound and determination of the injuring forces and whether inpatient hospital or operating room care is required. Assessment is made of the extent of soft tissue loss and of the viability of remaining tissue. Knowledge of topographical anatomy allows one to anticipate the subfascial structures involved on the basis of the location of the injury. Knowledge of the type of forces involved in producing the injury provides an index of the degree of soft tissue destruction and also of the possibility of subfascial injury, namely, abrading,

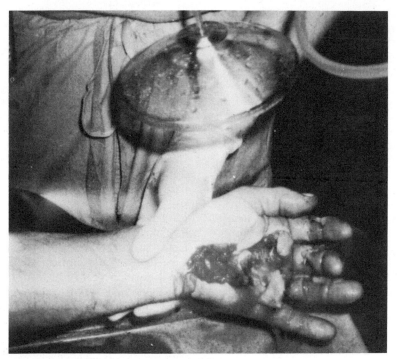

Figure 17–2. Soft tissue irrigation with pulsating water jet lavage is helpful in removing foreign debris.

lacerating, avulsing, crushing and missile injuries. The deep structures are evaluated insofar as is possible without the benefit of dissection. Probing of wounds is of no value; suspicion of significant deep injury demands definitive surgical exploration. Following the examination, the wound is appropriately redressed if definitive repair is to be accomplished in the operating room.

Skeleton. Clinical suspicion of fractures is aroused by the usual signs of pain, swelling, crepitation, abnormal posture and abnormal motion. Confirmation is provided by radiological evaluation. Fracture management is discussed in detail elsewhere. The presence of a compound injury is of considerable concern to the orthopedist and plastic surgeon alike in that adequate soft tissue coverage is absolutely essential to bony union. Initial evaluation must include deliberate consideration of means of securing reliable soft tissue coverage over a compound fracture.

Muscles and Tendons. Evaluation of dynamic function precedes direct inspection of the wound. Again, the importance of an all-encompassing routine of system-

atic examination cannot be stressed adequately. The location and appearance of the skin wound may be grossly misleading regarding the extent of subfascial injury. In addition, the presence of a severe skin wound does not exclude the possibility of injury proximal to this site. The full range of active and passive motion of all joints in a given extremity is elicited, following which the actions of specific muscle groups and tendons are tested. Differentiation between loss of function resulting from tendon injury and that resulting from nerve damage is not difficult.

The shoulder is tested for flexion, extension, abduction, adduction and circumduction. Point tenderness anteriorly and severe pain on all movements of the joint is indicative of a tear in the articular cuff. Inability to initiate abduction but the ability to complete abduction if the initial 15 degrees of movement is assisted passively is pathognomonic of rupture of the supraspinatus tendon.

Flexion, extension, pronation and supination are evaluated at the elbow joint. Severe injury to the triceps prevents extension against gravity. Division or rupture of the biceps tendon prevents flexion with the forearm in supination and prevents supination with the elbow in flexion.

Simple observation of the attitude of the wrist and hand provides valuable information regarding possible tendon injury. In the normal hand at rest, the thumb is held in moderate opposition and flexion, and the fingers are held in progressively increasing flexion from the index to the little finger. Relative extension of one or more digits immediately suggests flexor tendon injury. Injury to the extensor tendons in the forearm results in increased flexion at the wrist and metacarpophalangeal joints.

In testing individual tendon function, it is exceedingly important that the effect of gravity be eliminated and that the part under examination be positioned so as to exclude substitution movements.

The flexor and extensors of the wrist are easily palpable when acting against resistance, making the diagnosis of division of these tendons relatively straightforward. It is well to remember that the palmaris longus tendon is absent in the hands of 10 per cent of people. Injury of the flexor carpi ulnaris tendon immediately raises suspicion of injury to the ulnar nerve. Laceration of the palmaris longus tendon renders imperative the exclusion of median nerve damage.

Accurate evaluation of injury to the long flexor and extensor tendons of the fingers is made somewhat difficult by the fact that discrete, dissociated movements of these structures disappear progressively at more proximal levels in the forearm. The flexor superficialis tendons are tested by mechanically blocking flexion at the distal interphalangeal joints of the other fingers and requesting that the proximal interphalangeal joints be flexed. The flexor profundus tendons are evaluated by mechanically blocking the proximal interphalangeal joints and requesting flexion at the distal interphalangeal joints. The long extensor tendons of the fingers act almost entirely at the metacarpophalangeal joints and are tested by requesting extension against resistance at this level. Injury significantly proximal to the extensor retinaculum of the wrist will usually include all extensor digitorum communis tendons. Injury to the superficialis tendon alone in the palm or the profundus tendon alone in the

finger is seen commonly; forearm injuries involve either the superficialis alone or the superficialis and profundus. In evaluating tendon injuries, it is good practice to demonstrate clearly to the patient the action desired.

Tendon rupture is observed as a closed injury occurring "spontaneously" and attributed by the patient to a single, strenuous physical action. It is seen only rarely in association with other types of extremity trauma. The tendons most commonly ruptured in the upper extremity are the supraspinatus, biceps and extensor pollicis longus ("drummer's palsy"). In the lower extremity, Achilles and plantaris ("tennis leg") ruptures are seen. Tendons that rupture are usually abnormal and have been weakened by chronic trauma or disease.

Nerves. In evaluating motor and sensory loss, serious consideration must be given to the fact that the upper extremity represents an extension of the opposite cerebral cortex. Absence of motor function of cerebral etiology presents as a spastic paralysis without associated sensory disturbance. Cervical cord lesions produce a flaccid paralysis of structures innervated at the level of the lesion and a spastic paralysis below this level. Injury to the trunks of the brachial plexus results in functional impairment of segmental distribution; injury to the cords of the plexus exhibits a peripheral nerve-type distribution.

Subjective impressions of sensory changes usually are quite reliable guides in evaluating peripheral nerve injury. The majority of patients will remark somewhat quizzically that a certain area "feels peculiar" or is "dead." Almost invariably, such patients will prove at exploration to have a significant nerve injury. The same degree of reliability does not apply to motor function in that the majority of patients with peripheral nerve injuries are inexplicably unaware of their motor impairment. Motor function must be tested thoughtfully and specific defects carefully elicited. While sensory loss and muscle malfunction are symptoms of nerve injury, their elucidation requires patient cooperation — not always easily obtained. It is well to remember that the only sign of peripheral nerve injury is the loss of sudomotor function reflected in the absence of sweating. Sweating ceases within minutes of nerve division; with magnification (surgical loupes or ophthalmoscope) its absence is obvious and a reliable sign of nerve injury.

Certain principles must be observed in evaluating peripheral nerve function. The ability to perceive light touch, as with a wisp of cotton, and pinprick is of very little value in the assessment of the relation between the degree of sensation and useful function, but is quite helpful in mapping out areas of sensory loss associated with acute injury. Caution must be exercised not to move the part being evaluated because this will be interpreted as "touch" due to proprioception originating from tendons proximal to the site of injury. Areas tested must be unequivocal in their specificity because of the marked overlapping of peripheral nerve innervation, both motor and sensory. All degrees of hypesthesia are seen with peripheral nerve injuries; complete anesthesia is exceedingly limited in extent. While complete division produces a characteristic sensory and motor loss, partial division or injury may not be as evident on routine examination. The examiner performing sensory evaluation must appreciate subtle alterations.

RADIAL NERVE. Sensory evaluation is of little real value in the diagnosis of division of the radial nerve or its superficial branch because of the overlap provided by the median and ulnar nerves. At most, anesthesia is limited to a half-dollar-sized area overlying the proximal portion of the first dorsal interosseous muscle. Damage to the nerve proximal to the point where it enters the supinator muscle causes wrist drop from paralysis of all the extensors of the wrist and fingers. The hand cannot be extended at the wrist and the fingers cannot be extended at the metacarpophalangeal joints. With support of the wrist and metacarpophalangeal joints in extension, the interphalangeal joints of the fingers can be extended by the intrinsic muscles of the hand. Division of the superficial branch produces no motor impairment and insignificant sensory loss; it is, however, the most common site of painful neuromata. Injury to the deep dorsal interosseous branch paralyzes the extensor pollicis brevis and longus and the abductor pollicis longus. The patient is unable to abduct or extend the thumb and holds the digit in a moderately adducted position.

MEDIAN NERVE. Sensory examination is essential to accurate diagnosis and reveals anesthesia of the radial two thirds of the palm, the volar aspect of the thumb, index, long and radial half of the ring fingers, and the dorsum of the distal phalanges of the thumb, index and long fingers. The degree of peripheral nerve overlap varies considerably. Because of radial nerve overlap, the area of demonstrable anesthesia associated with median nerve division may be significantly smaller than that outlined. The innervation of the tip of the index finger is most frequently and entirely contained in the median nerve and is thus the best "absolute" area in which to test for median nerve integrity. Diagnosis of median nerve injury on the basis of motor function is demonstrated by lack of opposition of the thumb: with the hand flat on a table palm up, the patient is unable to point the thumb directly toward the ceiling; classically, the patient is unable to bring the thumb into true opposition with the fingertips. In addition, division above the elbow results in inability to flex the index and long fingers: with the hand flat on a table palm down, the patient is unable to scratch the table top with the tip of the index finger.

ULNAR NERVE. Sensory examination reveals anesthesia of the ulnar third of the hand, the little finger and the ulnar half of the ring finger. The tip of the little finger is the zone of the hand most frequently and entirely ulnar-innervated and thus the best single area to test. Motor demonstration of ulnar nerve palsy consists of inability to adduct and abduct the fingers. In performing this test, it is important that the metacarpophalangeal and interphalangeal joints not be flexed; the fingers normally converge on flexion and are adducted by the long extensors. With injury to the ulnar nerve above the elbow, the patient is unable to scratch the table top with the tip of the little finger with the hand held palm down on the table. In attempting to produce a strong pinch between the thumb and index finger, the metacarpophalangeal joint of the thumb falls into hyperextension (Froment's sign). "Clawing" of the ring and little fingers, hyperextension at the metacarpophalangeal joints and flexion at the interphalangeal joints are most pronounced when the ulnar nerve is divided in the distal half of the forearm; paralysis of the intrinsics allows the long extensors to hyperextend the metacarpophalangeal joints, and the still-innervated profundus tendons pull the interphalangeal joints into flexion.

MEDIAN AND ULNAR NERVES. The sensory loss is that of the combined distribution of the two nerves. The attitude assumed by the hand is determined by the radial innervated musculature; i.e., the wrist is slightly extended and supinated, the metacarpophalangeal joints are hyperextended. The thumb is abducted and extended into the plane of the hand, and the longitudinal and transverse metacarpal arches are flattened. Injury distal to the innervation of the forearm muscles produces extreme "clawing."

SCIATIC NERVE. The sensory loss following division of the sciatic nerve encompasses the posterolateral aspect of the thigh, all the leg except a narrow area on its most medial aspect supplied by the saphenous nerve, and the entire foot. The hamstring muscles and all the muscles of the leg are paralyzed. Division of the tibial nerve produces paralysis of all the muscles of the posterior compartment of the leg with resultant inability to plantarflex the foot. Damage to the common peroneal nerve paralyzes the musculature of the lateral and anterior compartments and is manifested by inability to dorsiflex the foot.

Vasculature. The integrity of vascular supply to the extremity is best judged on the basis of color and temperature of the part. Arterial pulsation, studied by digital palpation or in hypotensive states by Doppler instrumental amplification of blood flow, is useful in monitoring main artery patency. Arteriography, however, is the most definitive means of evaluation and should always be obtained in situations of doubt. The rate of capillary filling in the nail beds, venous filling and rate of drainage are observed. Patency of the radial and ulnar arteries is established by the simple test of elevating the upper extremity, occluding both arteries, and then releasing them in turn. Immediate flushing on release of one artery with the other occluded demonstrates patency.

Special Diagnostic Methods

The logical step following a thorough physical evaluation is the consideration of diagnostic aids. It is assumed that the requisite basic laboratory data are obtained in all cases. The indications for radiography are self evident. A baseline chest x-ray is obtained in all trauma victims who are to receive a general anesthetic.

Angiography provides precise information regarding the status of the circulation and is indicated in highly specific, complex situations. Usually, the nature, location and extent of vascular injury are apparent and do not require refined techniques for elaboration. The Doppler instrumental amplification of blood flow is a useful technique to study the integrity of actual flow.

Selective nerve blocks may be of value in resolving equivocal findings with respect to peripheral nerve injuries. Anesthetizing the ulnar nerve at the elbow or the median nerve at the wrist abolishes overlap and anomalous innervation, allowing clearer definition of the nerve injury in question. Electromyography and more sophisticated methods of testing are not utilized in the usual traumatic situation.

INFECTION

The importance of infection in traumatic injuries is pointed up by the fact that it is the second leading cause of death among patients surviving the initial trauma, with its lethalness exceeded only by that of hemorrhage. In the extremity, infection can lead to further soft tissue loss or osteomyelitis or result in increased edema, scarring, fibrosis and loss of function of the extremity. All measures to minimize the threat of infection become keystones in the management of soft tissue injuries. Minimizing additional contamination in traumatic wounds is crucial. When patients are initially seen, application of sterile dressings and subsequent use of sterile techniques in all examinations and manipulations are vital to prevent or minimize any additional contamination. The decision to treat the wound by primary closure or by delayed primary or secondary closure is vital. The nature of the initial injury serves as a useful indicator of initial contamination: a knife laceration obtained in emptying a dishwasher is obviously different from that sustained from a glass laceration outdoors. The interval from injury to proposed wound closure affords some index of probable bacterial isolation and replication in the wound to levels assuring infection. By 6 hours following most injuries, bacterial incorporation and isolation within the fibrin of the wound, endolymphatic dissemination to adjacent tissues and bacterial proliferation are well along, making primary closure of such a wound risky. Following debridement of any injured nonvital tissue even with vital deeper structures exposed, temporary closure of the wound with porcine heterograft in no way impairs the viability of deeper exposed tissues and allows for a period of antibiotic administration, repeated examination of the wound and closure when subsequent infection is less likely. While obtaining a closed wound as soon as possible is crucial in the management of extremity trauma, injudicious closing of a badly contaminated wound in no way expedites restoration and rehabilitation of the injured extremity. Sepsis, which puts survival of other tissue at risk and can result in increased edema and subsequent stiffness, can follow injudicious closing of such a wound.

Appropriate antibiotic therapy is instituted preoperatively in the management of all such patients. The drug of choice against gram-positive cocci should be instituted preoperatively and continued for a minimum period of 5 days.[4]

All patients receive tetanus prophylaxis: 0.5 ml. of tetanus toxoid if previously immunized or 4500 units of tetanus antitoxin in the absence of immunization. It must be emphasized that all patients receiving antitoxin also must receive a course of active immunization. Gas gangrene prophylaxis has been demonstrated to be of little or no value.

Clostridial cellulitis and myositis are the most dreaded complications, and massive debridement is indicated. Hyperbaric oxygen may additionally be effective, but many patients will be salvaged only by amputation.[64]

OPERATIVE MANAGEMENT
Type of Management

A decision must be made as to whether the wound can be treated adequately in the emergency department on an ambulatory basis or whether operating room repair and inpatient management are indicated.

Emergency Department. Treatment in the emergency department is reserved for uncomplicated abrasions and lacerations involving only the skin and subcutaneous tissue. Penetration of the fascia is not in itself an indication for formal exploration; repair in the emergency unit is permissible provided the functional examination is unquestionably within normal limits.

Basic principles of wound care are applicable here: thorough wound irrigation, debridement and primary versus secondary closure have already been stressed. Local anesthesia is generally adequate although regional blocks (digital block) may be used. One per cent xylocaine without epinephrine is usually the agent of choice. Sterile technique must be strictly observed. The need for wound drainage must be considered. Layered suture closure is preferable. The muscular fascia is closed with interrupted simple sutures of absorbable chromic catgut or polyglycolic acid. Subcutaneous tissue may be approximated in a similar fashion, taking care to bury the knots. At this point ragged skin edges may be excised with a sharp knife. There is basically no redundant skin in the extremities so only minimal cutaneous tissue can be excised. Interrupted simple or mattress skin sutures should be placed under minimal tension; 5–0 nylon is usually the suture of choice. A sterile dressing is then applied. Gentle circumferential pressure is often helpful in keeping edema at a minimum. Elevation of the extremity is an absolute necessity.

Operating Room. Complex injuries demand operating room repair by qualified surgeons. All tendon and nerve repairs, including isolated extensor tendon injury and digital nerve injury, are performed in the operating room. Crushing injuries, which invariably are followed by extensive hemorrhage and edema, demand hospitalization for purposes of observation if not for operative management.

All the usual adjuncts are employed in the operative management of extremity injuries. The pneumatic tourniquet is employed routinely except in patients exhibiting severe arterial insufficiency. In addition to its obvious benefits, the tourniquet provides an excellent method for assessing viability, that is, the presence or absence of post-tourniquent hyperemia. The tourniquet is inflated to a pressure of 280 to 300 mm. of mercury on the upper extremity and 450 to 500 mm. of mercury on the lower extremity; it may be left inflated for a period not exceeding 2 hours, following which it must be released to permit adequate flushing of the extremity. Provided the tourniquet is released for at least 15 minutes during each 2 hours, tourniquet ischemia may be utilized for as long as is necessary. The pneumatic cuff must be applied sufficiently loosely to prevent it from acting as a venous tourniquet; prior to inflation, the extremity must be drained as completely as possible either by elevation or the application of an elastic bandage. The Boyes' hand table is utilized for all upper extremity repairs. No antiseptic solutions are used in preparation of the operative field. Intact skin is cleansed with detergent solutions; open wounds are prepared by irrigation with large volumes of saline solution. Regardless of the extent of injury the entire extremity is prepared and draped into the operative field.

General Considerations

In order of priority, consideration is given to the repair of vascular injury threatening loss of viability, the integument, skeletal structures, muscles and tendons, and nerves. In the face of serious question regarding viability of the injured member, definitive repair of all structures is delayed for a period of 48 to 72 hours. Soft tissue coverage of subfascial structures must receive thoughtful attention. Consideration must be given to proper positioning and immobilization of fractures prior to embarking on tendon and nerve repair. Divided tendons retract and are, therefore, repaired in preference to nerves if a choice must be made. Delayed repair of nerve injuries is not only feasible but possibly desirable.

Conservation of all usable structures is the most basic of the surgical principles applicable to the management of extremity injuries. Structures that are in themselves irreparably damaged frequently prove of inestimable value in salvaging other structures. Injudicious sacrifice of tissue may effectively block subsequent reconstruction.

Amputation is considered only if the situation appears entirely hopeless in terms of restoration of function. Irreparable damage to any three of the five major structures comprising an extremity (skin and subcutaneous tissue, artery, bone, tendon and nerve) generally is indication for amputation. The concept of "sites of election" of amputation has become obsolete as a result of technical advances in the art of prosthesis manufacture.[28] As much length as possible is preserved in all cases.

Repair of Specific Areas

Integument. Extremity skin and subcutaneous tissue will not tolerate tension. To close a wound of questionable integrity overlying a compound fracture is to court osteomyelitis; exposed tendon and nerve repairs are doomed to failure. Wound margins are excised routinely to prevent traumatic tattooing and to provide nonbeveled, viable margins for suturing. Unlike the face, tissues of questionable viability in the extremities almost certainly will become frankly necrotic. Debridement, therefore, must be adequate. Healthy tissue will successfully resist a significant degree of contamination; ischemic tissue almost invariably will become infected.

The surgeon must especially be wary of the avulsed flap or degloving injury and not fall prey to the tendency to suture the tissue back into its original place. This will consistently lead to necrosis. Determining the location at which this tissue will demarcate has long been a dilemma. The intravenous administration of fluorescein dye has taken most of the guesswork out of this.[30, 40] Fluorescein is resorcinolphthalein: a water-soluble, nontoxic dye that diffuses rapidly through the capillary wall into the extracellular space. Its clinical usefulness is based on two facts: it gains access only to viable cells and it is strongly fluorescent. (It absorbs light of one wavelength and emits it at another.) It absorbs ultraviolet light (maximum absorption of 3600 Ångströms) and emits it in the visible range—the color varying from yellow to green, depending on the pH. Thus vascularized tissue contains dye and appears bright yellow to chartreuse in color while areas without capillary blood flow reflect all of the ultraviolet light and appear dark blue. The patient is given 1 to 3 gm. intravenously (approximately 20 mg./kg. for whites and 40 mg./kg. for blacks) after which the lights are turned off and a Woods lamp is used to study the fluorescence. If a clear line of demarcation is present, this is marked. The flap is then excised at this mark; the proximal portion will survive while the distal portion will not. The excised segment may be defatted to become a full-thickness skin graft or a split-thickness graft may be taken from it with a dermatome. This is reapplied to the wound either primarily or in a delayed primary fashion.

Definitive wound closure at the time of the primary procedure is preferable, but when tissue viability or wound contamination is of great concern, a sterile dressing or biological cover should be applied and wound closure deferred. When there is missing tissue, skin grafts are the preferred mode of coverage (Fig. 17–3). Split-thickness grafts can be easily harvested with a drum or electric dermatone. They may be meshed when their expansion is desirable. There is seldom a need for full-thickness skin grafts in primary extremity coverage.

In certain situations skin graft coverage is not adequate. Fractures lacking adequate muscle coverage, bone devoid of periosteum, exposed tendon, nerve and vascular repairs and sites of future reconstructive procedures all demand flap coverage. Flaps from adjacent tissue are preferable to those from distant locations, but the exceedingly precarious blood supply of extremity skin limits their use.

Upper extremity flap coverage generally

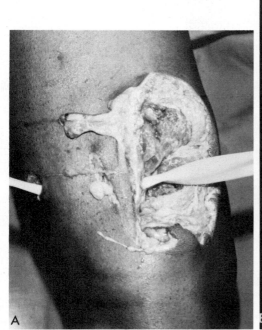
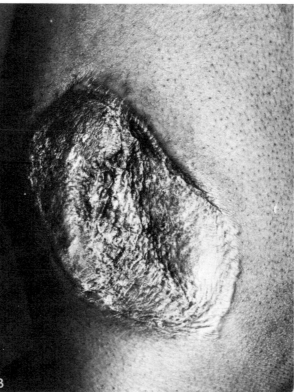

Figure 17–3. *Split-thickness skin grafts are the simplest means of covering open wounds with tissue loss. An avulsive soft tissue wound (A) was covered with a meshed skin graft as shown in (B).*

necessitates a flap from the trunk. The groin flap and the thoracoabdominal flap are reliable for upper extremity coverage. A random flap from the chest or abdomen may also be utilized. The groin flap, described by McGregor and Jackson,[41] is based on the superficial circumflex iliac artery, a small lateral branch from the common femoral artery. The central axis of the flap lies nearly parallel to the inguinal ligament, 2.5 cm. inferior to it and the anterior superior iliac spine. The flap can be extended well around the flank onto the back. This length of pedicle allows early motion of the wrist and joints of the hand. The groin flap is excellent coverage for the lower arm, wrist and hand (Fig. 17–4).

The transverse thoracoabdominal flap[8] is based on the perforators from the rectus abdominis muscle. It is a medially based flap 10 to 15 cm. wide, the superior margin at the inframammary fold, and can extend well onto the back. It provides good coverage of the forearm and antecubital fossa (Fig. 17–5). Random flaps from the chest or abdomen may be used. Pectoral flaps are preferred to abdominal flaps on the basis of the lesser quantity of subcutaneous tissue and the more acceptable position of the upper extremity from the standpoints of joint immobilization and ease of patient care. Flaps having a length to width ratio not exceeding 1:1 may be raised with impunity from any area on the chest or abdomen, may be based superiorly or inferiorly and may cross the midline. Oblique and transverse flaps are based laterally and in general should not cross the midline.

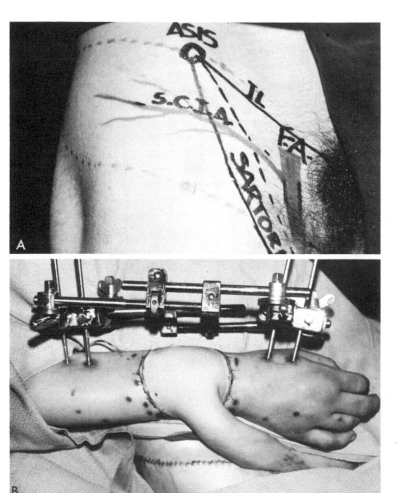

Figure 17–4. The anatomical landmarks of the groin flap are depicted in A. ASIS, anterior superior iliac spine; IL, inguinal ligament; SCIA, superficial circumflex iliac artery; FA, femoral artery; SARTOR, sartorius muscle. In B, the flap has been applied to the wrist with a tubed proximal pedicle.

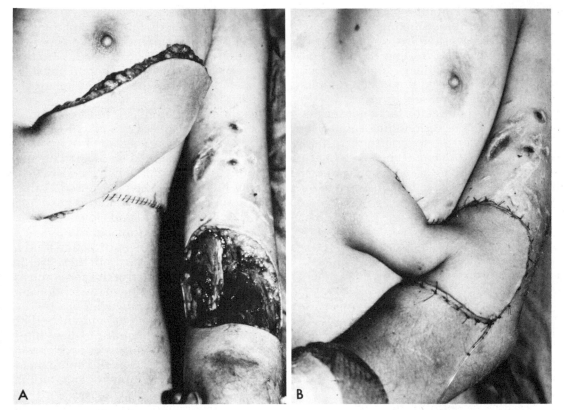

Figure 17–5. A, *Elevated thoracoabdominal flap and antecubital wound.* B, *The flap has covered the wound and the base has been tubed.*

As always, the rule applies that the defect is adjusted to fit the flap and not the flap to fit the defect. Flap donor areas are covered immediately with split-thickness skin grafts; care is taken to extend the graft over the exposed area of the pedicle. A completely closed wound allowing a reasonable degree of mobility of the extremity is achieved. All patients undergoing flap transfer to the extremities are instructed in active exercises to the extent permitted by the specific situation. Flap pedicles are left intact for a period of 3 weeks; ordinarily, a delay procedure need not precede division. By placing an occlusive tourniquet around the base of the flap and administering intravenous fluorescein, one may find that the flap can be divided sooner.

Muscles and Tendons. Determination of viability of traumatized muscle demands considerable judgment based on clinical experience. The color of frayed, contused, lacerated muscle is not a good index of viability, and the use of intravenous fluore-

scein has not proved helpful here. The "pinch test" is a reliable guide: viable muscle fibers contract locally when stimulated by pinching. Bright red blood from the cut muscle edge is probably the best indication of muscle viability. Adequate debridement is imperative for the avoidance of serious infection, particularly clostridial myositis. Uncertainty concerning muscle viability is an indication for delayed primary closure at a later date. Quite extensive sacrifice of muscle mass may result in surprisingly little functional impairment.

Muscle fibers do not hold sutures, and repair is accomplished by meticulous approximation of the enveloping fascia. Division of multiple, discrete muscle groups requires anatomical approximation of all the intermuscular septa. Simple closure of the enveloping fascia of the extremity is adequate in most cases.

Successful tendon repair requires an understanding of tendon anatomy and healing. Tendon is composed of longitudinally oriented parallel bundles of collagen fibers with frequent cross-linking of adjacent bundles. Inactive fibrocytes, incapable of participating in the healing process, constitute the only cellular element. Blood supply is derived from three sources: muscular branches; vessels present in the periosteum of bone at the tendon insertion; and vessels in the surrounding connective tissue that enter the tendon through peritenon, mesotenon and vinculae. The vinculae provide the most important source of blood supply and have been likened to the vessels in the intestinal mesentery.[57]

The basic principle of "one wound —one scar" has been emphasized;[47] the difficulty of producing an anastomosis that possesses both tensile strength and gliding function accounts for the surgeon's dilemma in tendon surgery.

The initial cellular reaction phase of tendon healing entails fibroblast invasion of the anastomosis from surrounding tissues. The fibroblasts synthesize and discharge monomeric collagen and the various mucopolysaccharides necessary for scar synthesis. The monomeric subunits rapidly polymerize into discernible fibril and finally into dense scar. Remodeling of the scar along lines of tension is critical to the development of the thin, filmy adhesions that subsequently permit gliding ability. Short, thick adhesions doom the repair to functional failure if the anastomosis is allowed to remain motionless during the remodeling phase.

Fibroblasts appear in the wound as early as the third day, and collagen synthesis begins immediately. A dynamic process of synthesis and degradation achieves equilibrium on approximately the seventeenth day. A progressive increase in tensile strength allows initiation of active and passive motion shortly after this time.[29] Motion provides the dynamic stresses promoting reorientation of the collagen fibrils.

The blood supply to lacerated tendon ends is primarily through the mesotenon, which is located on the deep surface of the tendon and must be protected. Trauma to the tendon by the careless use of instruments or sutures produces local wounds that will be invaded by fibroblasts and subsequently bound by adhesions.[48] Suture material must be noninflammatory and securely placed to maintain union during the

period when the fresh collagen has minimal tensile strength. Proper splint immobilization is all-important during this period. A careful program of guarded and progressive active and passive motion must be instituted during the proper phase of wound healing.

Tendon lacerations are most commonly repaired by means of the classic Bunnell buried crisscross suture of 4-0 synthetic material. Experimental studies of intrinsic tendon micro circulation have, however, shown the Mason-Allen peritendon suture technique to be the least disruptive of tendon vascularity. Wire tends to cut into tendon, and the minute kinks at the points at which the suture changes direction tend to straighten out with time; both these factors contribute to separation of the anastomosis, with resultant elongation of the tendon and decrease in function. Division of a tendon at its site of origin from the muscle belly is repaired either with multiple fine interrupted sutures or by means of overlapping the muscle and its tendon and approximating the two with continuous longitudinal sutures separated by 180 degrees. Pull-out sutures are not indicated proximal to the wrist or ankle. Wire pull-out sutures-at-a distance are helpful in the lower extremity in relieving tension at the anastomosis.

Considerable local scarring inevitably follows tendon repair. The anastomosis should be surrounded insofar as possible with available soft tissue, either muscle or fat. This principle is particularly applicable when dealing with combined tendon and nerve injuries. Opinions differ regarding the wisdom of primary repair in the management of complex injuries. It can be argued that multiple tendon repairs jeopardize an associated major nerve anastomosis and produce scarring sufficient to compromise function in all tendons. On this basis, many surgeons would advocate repair of only the profundus tendons in dealing with a complex wound of the forearm. It is our feeling that total repair of all injured structures should be accomplished if at all possible, because this approach preserves the greatest number of motors for subsequent utilization as transfers.

Nerves. As clearly elucidated by Seddon,[53] there exist three discrete types of nerve injury, which differ in etiology, pathophysiology, management and prognosis.

Neurotmesis is defined as destruction of all the essential parts of a nerve, as is produced by complete division. Axonotmesis consists of interruption of the axons with preservation of all the supporting structures, as is seen most commonly in association with blunt trauma. Neurapraxia is defined as functional interruption of the nerve without loss of integrity; there is no axonal degeneration, but there may be localized degeneration of the myelin sheath. Neurapraxia usually is the result of a traction-type injury and is the nerve injury most commonly associated with displaced fractures. Spontaneous recovery of excellent function is to be anticipated with neurapraxia. Recovery of normal function probably never occurs following neurotmesis. Axonotmesis carries an intermediate prognosis.

The physiological processes involved in repair following nerve injury are well understood and adequately documented.[70] To review briefly, the stages that must be traversed sequentially for a successful outcome are: (1) closure of the gap between the severed nerve ends, mainly by the outgrowth of Schwann cells; (2) retrograde degeneration; (3) progression of axons across the scar; (4) disintegration of the axons and myelin in the distal segment and removal by macrophages; (5) multiplication of the nuclei and increase in the volume of the cytoplasm of Schwann cells to make Schwann bands that fill the old sheaths; (6) arrival of the growing axons at the end organs; and (7) increase in diameter and degree of myelination of the fibers. It is readily appreciated that the majority of factors influencing the ultimate result lie distal to the point of injury. The two critical areas are the neurorrhaphy and the end organ. The final size reached by regenerating nerve fibers is directly dependent upon their connection with an end organ; proper connection results in an increase in size and a decrease in number of fibers in the distal segment.[1] The number of fibers available for connection with end organs is determined by the quality of the neurorrhaphy.

A perfect neurorrhaphy precisely approximates all the funiculi within the nerve and is probably not obtainable. Sunderland's[59] classic studies of intraneural topography demonstrate a constantly changing funicular pattern as one progresses peripherally in a nerve; cross-sectional areas separated by only a few millimeters exhibit grossly dissimilar patterns. In addition, the course of regeneration following suture is greatly influenced by the size, number and composition of component funiculi and the total area occupied by the fibers of the individual branches within the nerve. A good result can be anticipated if the funiculi are large and few in number. If there are numerous small funiculi or if there are few large funiculi proximal to the neurorrhaphy and multiple small funiculi distally expectations are more guarded.

Acceptable performance of a nerve repair demands the utmost in technical ability. Consideration of the multiple factors determining success leads clearly to the conclusion that anything less than a perfect union is doomed to failure. The technique to be described has proved most satisfactory. A proper neurorrhaphy should always be performed with magnification, using either loupes or a microscope. A pneumatic tourniquet should be employed if at all possible; this may not be feasible with proximal injuries or in the presence of an arterial repair.

Most injuries resulting in nerve division produce fraying of the severed ends. If the divided nerve ends are found to be sharp and clean under microscopic examination, they may be repaired without resection. If there is fraying or contusion, the nerve ends must be resected. The amount resected should be as limited as possible, as the orientation of the spiraling funicular pattern will be adversely altered. The procedure is accomplished by supporting the nerve on a wet tongue depressor; resection is done with the sharpest instrument available, usually a fresh double-edged razor blade. Sufficient dissection of the nerve proximally and distally is carried out to permit a tension-free neurorrhaphy. Lack of tension at the site of repair is, next to precision of repair, the most important factor in successful reconstructive nerve surgery. All possible guides to exact approximation are used — the position of the perineural vessels, the funicular pattern in the proximal and distal ends, and so forth. The slightest degree of relative rotation must be avoided. The finest suture material at hand, not larger than size 8–0, is used for the repair. The two accepted types of neurorrhaphy are epineurial repair and funicular repair. Although there is some experimental evidence to suggest that funicular repair is superior, there is no clinical documentation available. For an epineurial repair, approximation is begun by placing two guide sutures through the epineurium 180 degrees apart. The neurorrhaphy is completed with multiple interrupted epineurial sutures. A funicular repair is performed by first incising the epineurium and removing it for a short distance proximally and distally. The funiculi with their surrounding perineurium are separated by a microsurgical dissection. One or two 10-0 nylon sutures are placed through the perineurium of each funicular group and accurately approximated. The neurorrhaphy must be absolutely tension free.[35] Monofilament nylon is the usual material chosen because of its availability. The tissues are moistened repeatedly with Tis-U-Sol or normal saline solution throughout the procedure. Minimal manipulation of the nerve is observed. Forceps are never used to grasp any portion of the nerve; retraction and support are accomplished as needed by means of fine sutures through the perineurium or epineurium. The level of injury and ability of the surgeon will determine the technique employed. Reports to date do not indicate a clear preference for funicular versus epineurial sutures so long as precise technique is utilized.

A nerve that is partially severed is not completely divided and repaired; rather, the defect is approximated meticulously with as few sutures as possible. The incidence of neuroma-in-continuity and causalgia is greater than that following repair of a completely divided nerve, but the functional result is improved by not disturbing the intact fibers.

Microsurgical techniques have proved a valuable adjunct in the technical performance of neurorrhaphy. As pointed out by Edshage,[9] the intraneural topography following primary suture in the usual fashion is so bad that it is surprising that the results are not worse. Histological examination of nerves repaired by microsurgical technique has demonstrated less inflammatory reaction at the site of the anastomosis and a markedly improved funicular pattern distal to the anastomosis as compared with standard methods.[56] Microsurgical technique is advocated for all repairs.

Whether nerve suture performed at the time of injury (primarily) or several weeks later (secondarily) produces the better result cannot be answered. Experience clearly has substantiated the superiority of secondary suture in war wounds. Entirely satisfactory results have, however, been reported with primary suture in many series of civilian injuries. Considerable judgment is required in all cases, but it is thought that primary repair should be performed if at all feasible. Secondary suture is reserved for those instances in which an adequately trained surgeon is not available at the time of injury or in which the wound situation militates against definitive repair; i.e., delay in excess of 6 to 8 hours following injury, crushing injury with questionable tissue viability, and so forth. In such instances, the nerve ends are tagged with suture material for ready identification at the time of the definitive procedure.

Direct approximation is far superior to other methods of restoring continuity, provided the repair is tension free. Gaps in the medial and ulnar nerves can be overcome by proximal and distal mobilization of the nerves, optimal positioning of joints or nerve grafting.

Interfunicular nerve grafting has become increasingly popular in recent years.[34] It has the advantage of allowing tension-free neurorrhaphy in the nonflexed extremity. It has the disadvantage of two nerve repair sites that must be bridged by the regenerating nerve and the morbidity of the graft donor site. The sural nerve (35 cm.), the superficial radial nerve (20 cm.) and the antebrachial cutaneous nerve of the forearm (12 cm.) are the usual donor nerve sites.[23] The funiculi of the proximal and distal nerve ends are carefully dissected using the microscope. Nerve grafts are then placed from proximal to distal funicular group with tension-free microscopic suturing. Only one or two sutures are necessary for each funicular-graft neurorrhaphy. Millesi has the most extensive experience and best results with this technique (Fig. 17–6).

Alternatively, nerve mobilization may be employed. Simple flexion of the wrist and elbow provides an additional 1 to 2 in. of relative length. Considerable length can be

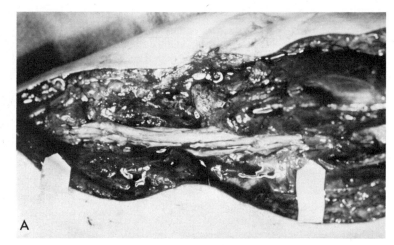

Figure 17-6. A, *Interfunicular technique shown with sural nerve grafts spanning a 10 cm. median nerve gap at the elbow.* B, *This is demonstrated by diagram.*

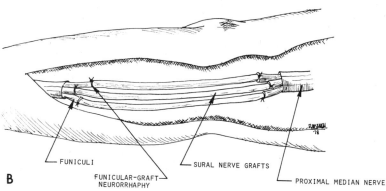

FUNICULI   SURAL NERVE GRAFTS

B   FUNICULAR-GRAFT NEURORRHAPHY   PROXIMAL MEDIAN NERVE

gained with the ulnar nerve by removing the nerve from the fibroosseous tunnel posterior to the medial humeral epicondyle and transposing it to a subcutaneous position in the antecubital fossa. The procedure is accomplished by splitting the two heads of origin of the flexor carpi ulnaris; detachment and replacement of the medial humeral condyle, as formerly practiced, is a crippling procedure. The ulnar nerve branches to the elbow joint are divided, but the motor branches to the flexor carpi ulnaris and flexor profundus muscles are preserved by carefully stripping them away from the main trunk with the back edge of a knife blade. The available length of the median nerve is increased by placing the nerve superficial to the antecubital fascia and the transverse carpal ligament. If lengthening procedures are required, the position of the extremity at the time of anastomosis is maintained for a period of approximately 6 weeks, following which the joints are progressively extended over a several-week period. Loss of continuity over a distance exceeding 9 cm. precludes direct approximation.

Not uncommonly, one must deal with a nerve that is obviously traumatized but in continuity (axonotmesis). Resection of the involved segment is contraindicated as a primary procedure since a majority of such nerves spontaneously recover a satisfactory level of function. Neurolysis, either internal or external, is reserved for those few patients who fail to exhibit satisfactory recovery and is not considered for a minimum period of 3 to 4 months after injury. Internal neurolysis is performed either by meticulous blunt teasing apart of the fascicles with the back edge of a knife blade or by mechanical separation of the fibers by means of distending the nerve with injection of saline solution through an extremely fine-gauge needle. The results obtainable with neurolysis recommend this procedure over excision and anastomosis.

Nerve palsies seen with blunt trauma, with or without associated fracture, almost invariably disappear (neurapraxia). Operative intervention is indicated only if there is no evidence of recovery during an appropriate period of observation, usually not less than 6 months.

SPECIFIC INJURIES

Wringer Injuries. Washing machine wringers account for approximately 100,000 accidents per year in children under the age of 15 years; there are an equal number in adults.[49] The frequency with which these injuries are seen in the receiving ward of a large hospital leads to an attitude of relative complacency. Such injuries must be treated with utmost respect if catastrophe is to be avoided.

The injury produced is the result of a variety of forces, each of which must be given serious consideration in evaluating the extent of damage: compression, contusion, heat due to friction and avulsion.[10] The picture is one of a crushing injury with the usual anticipation of subsequent edema and hemorrhage.

Important features to be elicited in the history are the age of the machine and the status of the wringers, the level to which the extremity entered the wringer, the duration of exposure and the measures taken to extricate the extremity. Prolonged exposure results in deep burning of the skin and subcutaneous tissue and severe contusion of the underlying musculature. Strong countertraction produces avulsion and an increased incidence of peripheral nerve damage.

The most common sites of severe injury are the dorsum of the hand, the dorsum of the wrist, the flexor surface of the elbow and the medial aspect of the brachium of the axilla, representing the areas at which the wringers are most likely to stop (Fig. 17–7). A tear in the web space at the base of the thumb is seen frequently. Separation of the skin and subcutaneous tissue from the underlying fascia results in large areas of hematoma accumulation. Severe pain on passive extension of the fingers indicates significant muscle damage and subfascial hematoma. Peripheral nerve damage usually is of the neurapraxia type, and spontaneous recovery can be anticipated. Fractures occur uncommonly (less than 5 per cent of patients) and usually involve the

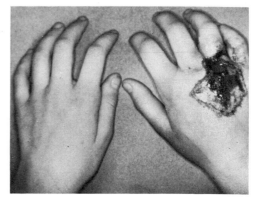

Figure 17–7. *Full-thickness loss over the dorsum of the hand secondary to a washing machine wringer injury. The true degree of soft tissue damage was initially indeterminate.*

proximal phalanx or metacarpal of the thumb. Thorough radiological evaluation is obtained routinely.

Whether to treat a given patient on an inpatient or ambulatory basis is a difficult decision and must be individualized. It is our strong feeling that the majority of patients should be hospitalized for a minimum 48-hour period of observation on the basis that delayed edema and swelling due to an expanding hematoma constitute the major threats. Wringer injuries are exceedingly deceptive, and accurate appraisal of the extent of damage may be impossible initially.

Initial management consists of thorough cleansing of the entire extremity with a mild detergent solution using aseptic technique. Obvious subcutaneous and subfascial hematomas are drained as an operating room procedure. Abraded areas and open wounds are dressed with Xeroform gauze. A bulky, immobilizing pressure dressing is applied from the fingertips to well above the most proximal extent of injury. Tetanus antitoxin is given, and antibiotic therapy is instituted. In the usual case, the patient is then admitted to the hospital, the extremity is elevated, and the nursing personnel are instructed to observe the fingertips frequently and to record the circulatory status. Definitive treatment of areas of full-thickness loss is deferred until resolution of the swelling.

The dressing is changed and the extremity re-evaluated 48 hours after injury. At this time, preparations are made for grafting areas of full-thickness loss; approximately 10 to 20 per cent of patients will require grafting.[10, 26] A careful search is made for undrained hematomas. These will produce diffuse fibrosis with resultant irretrievable loss of function if left untreated. In the absence of complications, the patient may be discharged at 48 hours with a well-applied pressure dressing and a sling in place. Antibiotics are continued for at least 5 days. The dressing is changed at 48- to 72-hour intervals for a total period of 10 days to 2 weeks post-injury, at which time the patient is allowed to gradually resume normal activity.

Missile. The gunshot and shotgun injuries encountered in civilian practice do not present the extensive soft tissue destruction seen with military wounds. Muzzle velocities of 850 ft./sec. (0.38 caliber) and 1150 ft./sec. (0.22 caliber long rifle) do not compare with the muzzle velocities in excess of 3500 ft./sec. produced by military weapons. The muzzle velocity of a shotgun is in the same range as that of a civilian pistol. Massive debridement is, therefore, not a consideration in the management of these wounds.

Gunshot wounds are not by definition "dirty" and are treated as clean wounds. All wounds are cleansed thoroughly with a mild detergent solution, the wound edges are debrided minimally, and a sterile dressing of Xeroform gauze is applied. A concerted effort is made to remove powder burns by means of scrubbing with a surgical brush to prevent permanent tattooing. The wounds are explored only on the basis of specific indications. Major vascular and peripheral nerve injury demand exploration and repair; no attempt is made to remove the missile if it is not easily accessible. Missiles that are easily palpable subcutaneously are commonly painful and subject to external trauma and are removed. All joint injuries are explored. Fractures are treated as closed injuries, with the usual indications for open reduction.

Shotgun wounds are responsible for a greater percentage of deaths than those from any other type of firearm. The single most important factor determining the magnitude of damage is the distance from which the injury was received.[55] Wounds received from greater than 7 yards seldom cause significant injury, whereas wounds inflicted at less than 3 yards produce massive tissue loss. Perforating injuries of subfascial structures are seen with injuries received from an intermediate range. The wounds are more "dirty" than other gunshot wounds because of the quantity of foreign material introduced in the form of wadding, bits of clothing, and so forth. Soft tissue destruction is due to direct damage by the injuring agent and not to a compression wave as is associated with high-velocity missiles.

Debridement consists of thorough irrigation with large volumes of saline solution, meticulous removal of all foreign material and resection of nonviable tissue. Contused muscle may be expected to survive. Inadequate debridement courts the ever-present threat of clostridial infection. Pellets are removed only if readily accessible within the wound. Major structures are repaired as indicated. Simple wounds of entry secondary to close-range injury often may be closed primarily. Skin graft or pedicle flap coverage of larger wounds is secured at the primary procedure if at all possible (Fig. 17–8). Definitive closure is delayed for a period of 48 to 72 hours in the face of massive muscle injury with questionable tissue viability. Multiple small pellet wounds in the skin are dressed with Xeroform gauze. Adequate tetanus prophylaxis and antibiotic coverage are instituted preoperatively.

Impaling Injuries. Impaling injuries are seen infrequently and are usually the result of industrial accidents. Necessary measures are taken to carefully dismantle the machinery and extricate the victim together with the impaling agent. First aid treatment is directed toward immobilizing the involved extremity and stabilizing the impaling agent. Removal of the impaling agent is accomplished as an operating room procedure with provision having been made for possible massive bleeding. Misguided efforts to shorten the impaling agent prior to removal result in increased soft tissue damage; it should be thoroughly cleaned and carefully withdrawn along the path of entry.[50] Repair is undertaken as indicated.

Massive Crush. Severe crushing injuries differ from other types of injuries in several basic respects: massive edema and

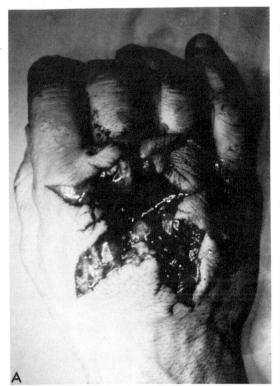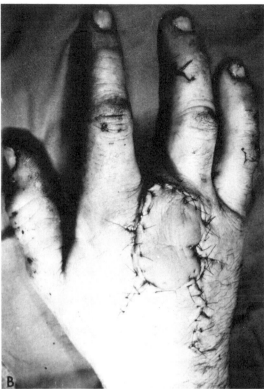

Figure 17–8. A, *Shotgun exit on dorsum of the hand. Bony destruction of the third metacarpal rendered the middle digit of little use, thus a neurovascular island flap was taken from the amputated digit to cover the wound (B).*

interstitial hemorrhage, extensive damage to a multiplicity of structures and highly questionable tissue viability. All these factors combine to render the true extent of injury initially indeterminate. The information obtainable by physical examination is only grossly reliable in determining the structures involved and the nature of their injury. Arterial insufficiency may be caused by vascular spasm, occlusion or division. Nerve deficits may represent neurotmesis, axonotmesis or neurapraxia. Loss of tendon function may be due to division or rupture of the tendons or may be secondary to massive hematoma formation within their muscle bellies. Accurate assessment of soft tissue viability is impossible on the basis of simple inspection and is exceedingly difficult at best at the time of formal exploration. Radiographical evaluation is obtained routinely. Arteriograms and other diagnostic adjuncts are of little value.

Exploration is performed without benefit of tourniquet ischemia. The major goal is to restore adequate circulation, and the entire armamentarium of vascular techniques is used to accomplish this end: vascular anastomoses, flushing of occluded vessels with heparin-saline solution, periarterial sympathectomy, and so forth. All nonviable skin, subcutaneous tissue and muscles are resected, and a meticulous anatomical survey is made of the remaining structures. All too frequently, severe shredding and avulsion result in considerable loss of continuity of tendons and nerves. Anastomoses are performed only if normal tissue can be approximated without tension and covered with viable skin. Tendon and nerve ends that cannot be approximated are tagged with wire for easier identification at subsequent procedures.

Fasciotomy may be one of the most useful adjuncts in the care of such extremities and should be employed freely in the management of wounds resulting from crush, high-velocity missiles or ischemia. Transcutaneous intracompartmental pressure determination, as for a lumbar puncture, is helpful and if found to exceed diastolic pressure indicates the need for decompression by fasciotomy to avoid ischemic necrosis. The fascia may be incised widely under direct vision in the presence of an open wound. Multiple small incisions should be employed in closed injuries. There must be no doubt regarding the adequacy of fasciotomy at the termination of the procedure. Fascial decompression should be considered for all wounds involving the regions of the intrinsic muscles, the volar carpal ligament, the forearm and upper arm, and the thigh and lower leg. It must be recalled that the anterior tibial compartment is anatomically discrete and receives no decompression from posterior or medial incisions.

It is doubtful whether these wounds should ever be closed at the time of the primary procedure: one can never be confident that the debridement was adequate; closure does not allow for the massive edema that inevitably follows these injuries. Porcine heterograft is a useful interim dressing. Skin flaps that are clearly viable at the time of closure may be compromised severely by subsequent swelling; edema within a closed compartment may reduce an already tenuous circulation to a critical level. Following debridement and repair of the deep structures to the extent possible, a bulky, immobilizing pressure dressing is applied. The patient is returned to the operating room for formal re-exploration and closure at the end of a 48- to 72-hour period.

Postoperative management is directed almost entirely at reduction of edema and preservation of viability. In the initial postoperative phase, elevation and pressure dressings are utilized. The Jobst pneumatic bandage provides an excellent method for both splinting and pressure. Stellate ganglion block, continuous axillary block by indwelling axillary catheter, low molecular weight dextran, dimethyl-sulfoxide and local hypothermia, although not of proven clinical value, probably should be given a trial in cases demonstrating circulatory impairment threatening the limb. These measures must be instituted within 4 hours and probably are not beneficial beyond 24 hours. Interstitial precipitation of protein, brawny induration and diffuse fibrosis inexorably follow in the wake of persistent edema; the extremity literally becomes a coagulum.

All patients with severe crushing injuries require staged reconstructive procedures to a greater or lesser degree. Tendolyses and neurolyses are required to extricate these structures from a bed of dense scar. Complications in the form of indolent soft tissue wounds and chronic osteomyelitis are not uncommon. The economic devastation resulting from a 2- to 3-year period of unemployment is obvious.

Limb Replantation

In 1887, William Halsted[13] began experimental work on limb replantation. In the past 15 years of this century the replacement of completely severed limbs has passed from the experimental workshop to clinical reality. Malt[27] first successfully replanted a severed upper extremity above the elbow in 1962, and the first partially successful digital replantation was achieved in China in 1964.[3] Improvement in microscopic instrumentation and technique has paved the way for dramatic clinical advances (Fig. 17–9).

The factors that have proved most important in terms of successful replantation are the duration of warm ischemia time of the amputated part, the amount of trauma inflicted upon the amputated part, and the microsurgical expertise and experience of the surgical team. The more muscle present in the amputated specimen, the less its ability to withstand anoxia. Thus, the higher the level of amputation, the less the duration of warm ischemia that will be tolerated. Major limb replantations probably must be done within 10 hours from the time of amputation, whereas successful digital replantations have been reported as late as 20 hours.[43] Replantation surgeons are becoming increasingly aware of the importance of the mechanism of amputation and the amount of trauma inflicted upon the amputation patient. Clean guillotine amputations inflict the least trauma on the specimen; avulsive or crush wounds may cause such damage to the local vessels or the distal capillary bed that successful replantation is impossible.

The immediate first aid care administered to the amputation victim may determine whether or not replantation will be successful. The public in general and emergency medical personnel in particular must be informed as to the importance of their initial actions. Every amputated part

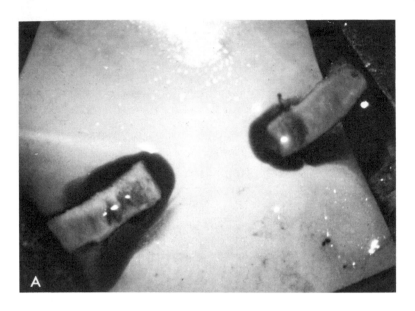

Figure 17–9. *A, Microscopic appearance of 1.0 mm. vessel ends shown before anastomosis. B, The completed anastomosis before release of the microvascular clamps. C, The patent anastomosis. EKG paper depicts 1.0 mm. marks.*

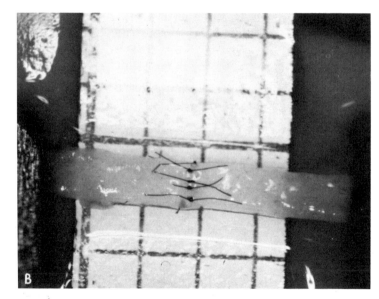

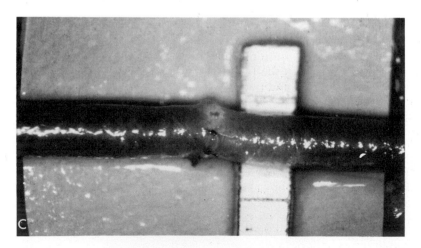

seen outside of the replantation hospital must be considered a potential replantable specimen. After assessing the patient's overall status, the wound should be flushed with lactated Ringer's solution. No scrubbing or debridement should be carried out. A dry sterile dressing should be applied, then a mild pressure gauze wrap, and the extremity elevated. The amputated part should be flushed with lactated Ringer's solution and wrapped in a dry sterile gauze or towel and placed in a plastic bag or container. The part is then put in another container and cooled by a separate plastic bag containing ice. Dry ice should not be used. The patient and the amputated part should then be transferred to the replantation hospital as soon as possible or as determined by the patient's overall condition.

The replantation surgeon, in conjunction with the patient and his family, makes the final decision concerning replantation. Patient selectivity is proving to be an increasing important factor. The patient's general condition, age, hand dominance, occupation, motivation, and his own desires must all be weighed.[44] The nature of injury, the level of the injury, and the quality of the wound and amputated part must then be weighed against these other factors.

The surgical procedure is far more than a vascular operation. Tissue debridement, bone shortening and fixation, muscle and tendon repair, nerve repair and skin closure must all be given equal attention. Bone shortening should probably be carried out in every major limb replantation. This allows not only debridement of traumatized bone but more importantly allows for more soft tissue in the trauma-

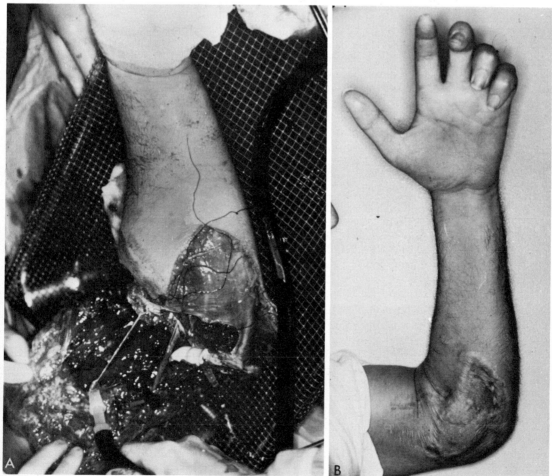

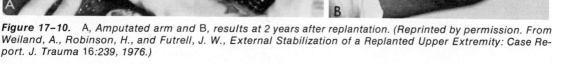

Figure 17–10. A, Amputated arm and B, results at 2 years after replantation. (Reprinted by permission. From Weiland, A., Robinson, H., and Futrell, J. W., External Stabilization of a Replanted Upper Extremity: Case Report. J. Trauma 16:239, 1976.)

tized area to be removed, resulting in the apposition of more normal neural and vascular structures for repair. Microsurgical principles must be adhered to in the performance of the vascular anastomosis. Only normal vessels should be sutured to each other. The donor artery should have an immediate forceful pulsatile flow. If the vessel either does not appear normal or does not spontaneously produce pulsatile flow, it should be further shortened. Tension will not be tolerated in these small vessel repairs, and the necessity of interposition vein grafts has become increasingly apparent.[2] Nerve repairs should be performed if at all possible, using nerve grafts if necessary. Skin coverage may be obtained primarily or skin grafts or biological dressings may be used. The indications for limb perfusion and anticoagulation remain uncertain.[15]

As with digital replantation, major limb replantation is producing increasingly good results as replantation surgeons gain more experience and patient selectivity becomes better defined.[37, 67] Replantations below the mid-forearm especially may be expected to do well, while those above the elbow may not yield as good a functional result. Lower limb replants have been performed less frequently because of the paucity of nerve regeneration and the quality of lower limb prostheses (Fig. 17–10).

LOWER EXTREMITY INJURY

The basic principles applicable to surgery of the lower extremity differ from those for other anatomical regions to such an extent that separate discussion is warranted. The primary reasons for this difference are the somewhat unique vasculature of the lower extremity, and the essentially complete absence of "spare" skin.

The tissues of the lower extremity are relatively ischemic in comparison with the soft tissue of the face. Special features of the vasculature of the lower extremity include a primarily longitudinal orientation of blood vessels; blood vessel innervation by vasoconstrictor fibers only, resulting in a considerable degree of tone; and the superimposition of the hydrostatic pressure of a column of blood the length of the extremity.[51] Objective demonstration of the significance of this particular vascular pattern consists of a progressively decreasing skin temperature gradient below the knee. The skin derives its blood supply from a longitudinally oriented dermal plexus supplied by vessels perforating the fascia. Each perforating vessel nourishes an area of skin approximately 3 in. in diameter; very little overlap is provided by the dermal plexus.

Langer's lines are longitudinal in the lower extremity. The relationship between the deep fascia and the overlying soft tissue is such that no "spare" skin is available by undermining.

Surgeons assuming responsibility for lower extremity injuries must do so with these principles firmly in mind and must observe certain inviolate rules if primary healing and a stable scar are to be obtained: debridement must be stringent, wound closure must be absolutely tension-free, joints must be immobilized and dependency and ambulation are prohibited. The rules are enforced rigidly for all but exceedingly minor injuries, that is, small clean lacerations involving only skin and subcutaneous tissue.

Soft Tissue Injuries. Longitudinal lacerations with minimal skin loss can be closed primarily. Even without skin loss transverse lacerations often demonstrate superficial necrosis along the distal margin of the suture line. Debridement in the lower extremity must not err on the side of conservatism. Wound margins are excised routinely. Tissue of questionable viability is sacrificed without hesitation, with the realization that necrosis on the basis of vascular insufficiency is a foregone conclusion. The use of intravenous fluorescein (discussed earlier) is especially applicable in the lower extremity and its routine use in degloving and avulsive injuries is encouraged. Wound closure is accomplished in two layers. Minute approximation of the skin margins is performed only if the tissues are unquestionably healthy. Skin sutures will produce necrosis of the wound margins in the presence of tension. In equivocal situations, meticulous skin closure is disregarded or accomplished by means of multiple adhesive straps applied transversely. Biological dressings such as porcine xenograft are frequently useful. The dressing incorporates a posterior plaster splint immobilizing the proximal and distal joints in functional positions, that is, moderate flexion of the knee and neutral position of the ankle. Neither dependency of the extremity nor ambulation is permitted for 3 weeks. The period of immobilization may be varied within narrow limits in adaptation to specific situations.

Categorically, wounds distal to the knee exhibiting more than a minimal amount of skin loss require the introduction of additional tissue for adequate closure.

The management of peripheral nerve injuries entails no specific features.

Tendon repairs in the leg and foot are immobilized for significantly longer periods than those in the upper extremities. The cast is left in place for 6 weeks; a walking heel may be applied at 3 to 4 weeks after injury.

Plantar Injuries. The resurfacing of weight-bearing areas presents certain problems peculiar to their functional needs. The tissue utilized for cover must have protective sensibility and be able to withstand repeated trauma. Contrary to popular belief, split-thickness skin grafts prove surprisingly serviceable and in many instances are preferable to flap coverage. As an extreme example, skin grafts applied directly to the plantar surface of the calcaneus have been known to do well over long periods. The grafts develop protective sensibility; the wound becomes concave with healing, thereby offering some protection to the graft. Full-thickness grafts obtained from the instep of the involved foot may be utilized when available. Local rotation flaps of generous proportions may be utilized to cover limited defects of the heel. Small defects in the region of the metatarsal heads may be closed with a local flap taken from the area of the proximal flexion crease of the toes, thus transferring the skin graft to a nonweight-bearing position. A filleted toe transferred on a neurovascular pedicle provides excellent cover for defects of intermediate size and will reach almost any area of the sole (Fig. 17–11). Local muscle flaps or the dorsalis pedis flap may be helpful in plantar coverage (see below). There are some disadvantages inherent in distant flap coverage: because of the quantity of subcutaneous fat, patients complain of instability of the flap, which

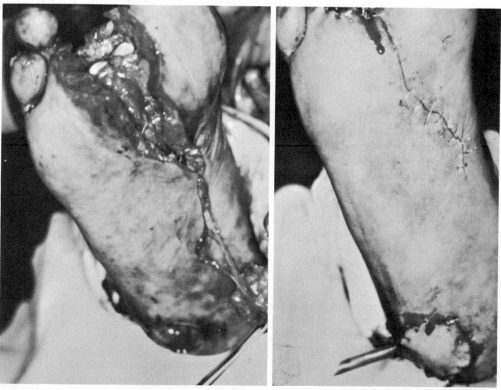

Figure 17–11. *Utilization of a filleted toe transferred on an intact neurovascular pedicle to resurface a full-thickness defect on the weight-bearing area of the heel.*

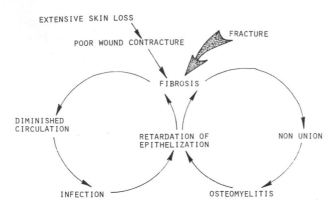

Figure 17–12. Factors affecting the course of compound wounds of the lower extremity. (Reprinted by permission. From Maxwell, G. P. and Hoopes, J. E., Plast. Reconstr. Surg. 63:176, 1979.)

they graphically describe as "walking on a pillow"; there is usually lack of sensation.

Compound Fractures. A historical review of the treatment of compound fractures provides a fascinating chronicle of emergency war surgery in general.[6] The trend in therapy has been toward earlier definitive wound closure. Fortunately, we have progressed beyond the open wound, "closed plaster" method of Trueta,[62] beyond awaiting a clean, granulating wound, and partially beyond delayed primary closure on the fourth to sixth day post-injury. Adequate soft tissue debridement and provision for adequate skin cover are essential to bony union and prevention of osteomyelitis. When wound closure is not accomplished in face of a fracture, a vicious circle is set in motion (Fig. 17–12). The use of external fixation appliances such as the Hoffmann apparatus is extremely useful not only in stabilizing the fracture but also in allowing access to the wound for dressing changes, hydrotherapy or operative reconstruction. Extreme conservatism is observed regarding sacrifice of bone. Obviously devitalized small fragments without periosteal attachment are discarded; all questionable bone is preserved. Closure is accomplished in accordance with the previously outlined principles. Adequate muscle closure allows utilization of a free graft. Massive soft tissue loss with exposed bone demands flap coverage. Failure of healing per primam is managed by conservative treatment designed to produce a granulating wound satisfactory for grafting; the graft is not considered definitive cover. Small areas of exposed, nonviable bone may be

disregarded during this phase of management. Definitive flap coverage is undertaken as an elective reconstructive procedure following wound healing. Nonunion responds dramatically to the introduction of healthy, blood-bearing tissue.

Types of Repair

Grafts. Skin grafts provide the most expedient means of obtaining a clean, healed wound and on this basis are utilized whenever feasible at the time of the primary procedure. The graft can be applied directly to subcutaneous tissue, muscle and periosteum. Skin grafts do not survive well on cortical bone devoid of periosteum but may suffice on cancellous bone. Failure of hemostasis and questionable viability are the only indications for delaying grafting 48 to 72 hours post-injury.

Elevation and immobilization of the extremity for 3 weeks is mandatory. A graft that appears to be healing satisfactorily at 7 to 10 days is readily lost by allowing the extremity to become dependent.

As noted previously, the graft may or may not be intended as definitive cover; its major function lies in securing a healed wound as rapidly as possible in situations in which flap coverage is unavailable or inappropriate. Perfect "take" of the graft is desirable but not essential. Small areas of exposed bone or tendon sequestrate with little or no local reaction.

Skin grafts around the ankle tend to be unstable. The technique of overgrafting[66] may provide a sufficient dermal layer to prevent recurrent ulceration; i.e., in multiple stages the epidermis is removed from previously applied skin grafts by means of dermabrasion and new grafts are applied to the residual dermis. Flap coverage may be required.

Flaps. Skin flap coverage may be utilized as a primary procedure, as a planned delayed procedure within the first week following injury or as a completely elective reconstructive procedure. The usual indications for flap coverage include exposure of important major structures such as bone, joints, tendons and nerves, and the necessity for subsequent reconstructive procedures on these structures. Adequate coverage of the acute wound may well determine whether deep structures survive or perish; if flap coverage is indicated, its accomplishment as a primary or delayed primary procedure is highly desirable.[22, 30] Flap coverage is performed as a planned delayed procedure when the superimposition of additional surgical trauma is inadvisable and when the wound is indeterminate in terms of tissue viability.

Skin flaps may be of either local or distant origin. The limited applicability of random local rotation flaps because of their exceedingly precarious blood supply has been stressed previously. The only arterial flaps of the lower extremity are the groin flap[41] and the dorsalis pedis flap. The former provides local coverage in a limited area of the proximal thigh and is of little use in lower extremity coverage. The dorsalis pedis flap was described by McCraw and Furlow in 1975.[38] Based on the dorsalis pedis artery and its accompanying vein, this flap may be raised with its pedicle intact or as an island flap. Sensation may be preserved in the flap. It will cover the lateral and medial malleoli, the lowest portion of the tibia and a portion of the sole of the foot.

Traditionally, the distant flap most used for lower extremity coverage has been the cross leg (or thigh) flap, first described by Hamilton in 1854.[14] Gross extremity flaps may be based on the opposite leg, thigh or knee. The primary consideration is a purely mechanical one relating the defect to the opposite extremity in the most comfortable position for the patient. The cross-thigh flap is of limited value and is usually reserved for females who wish to avoid creation of a secondary deformity on the opposite leg. The geniculate circulation about the knee allows the designing of retrograde flaps (based distally) with considerable safety; such flaps serve admirably for limited defects involving the distal third of the leg. The cross-leg flap is most commonly used because of the frequency of compound fractures of the tibia and power mower injuries of the foot. The cross-leg flap usually is based anteriorly and elevated from the posteromedial aspect of the calf. Provision is made for as broad a base as possible; the length to width ratio of the flap preferably is maintained close to 1:1 and should not exceed 1.5:1.

Precise preoperative planning is absolutely essential to success and consists of substantial time spent in testing the relative position of the extremities, determining the dimensions of the flap and accurately mapping the location of the flap on the donor leg. Application of casts preoperatively hinders rather than helps the operative procedure. External appliances may be a useful means of fixation. Properly designed cross-leg flaps are elevated and transferred without previous delay procedures. The pedicle is severed, usually without a delay procedure, at 21 days.

Abdominal jump flaps have been reserved entirely for the elective resurfacing of extensive defects requiring more tissue than can be provided by cross-extremity transfer. Their use has been lessened by the advent of muscle flaps, myocutaneous flaps and free flaps (Fig. 17–13).

Muscle Flaps. The use of muscle flaps for coverage of lower extremity wounds was described in 1946, but not until Ger's work in the late 1960s did their use become widespread.[13] Muscle flap transposition offers an additional group of locally available tissues in the lower extremity for wound coverage. The anatomy of the particular muscle and its dominant vascular supply must be known. The muscle flap may be used in a primary, delayed primary or secondary fashion. Likewise, skin graft coverage of the muscle may be done primarily or delayed.[63]

The rectus femoris, vastus lateralis and biceps femoris muscles of the upper leg can survive on dominant vascular pedicles and are useful for wound coverage in this area. The lateral and medial gastrocnemius muscles provide good coverage of the distal upper leg, knee and proximal tibia. They likewise can survive on single vascular pedicles. The soleus muscle offers the best coverage of the mid-tibial area. The flexor digitorum longus can be added to this for

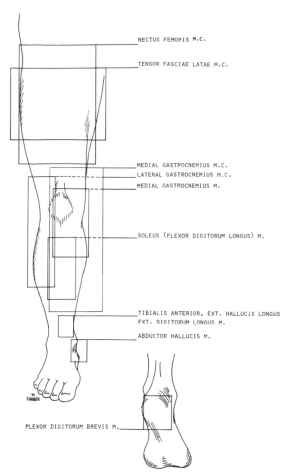

RECTUS FEMORIS M.C.

TENSOR FASCIAE LATAE M.C.

MEDIAL GASTROCNEMIUS M.C.
LATERAL GASTROCNEMIUS M.C.
MEDIAL GASTROCNEMIUS M.

SOLEUS (FLEXOR DIGITORUM LONGUS) M.

TIBIALIS ANTERIOR, EXT. HALLUCIS LONGUS
EXT. DIGITORUM LONGUS M.

ABDUCTOR HALLUCIS M.

FLEXOR DIGITORUM BREVIS M.

Figure 17–13. *Muscle and myocutaneous flaps for coverage of lower extremity wounds are shown above. M, muscle flap; MC, myocutaneous flap.*

larger wounds. The lower third of the tibia is difficult to cover with muscle flaps but small areas may be covered with the tibialis anterior, extensor hallucis longus, or extensor digitorum communis if one of these has adequate distal muscle bulk and patency of segmental vascular perforators in the patient. The abductor hallucis muscle will cover the lower portion of the medial malleolus (Fig. 17–14), and the flexor digitorum longus is helpful in calcaneal coverage.

Possible functional loss from use of the individual muscles must be considered. Extensive infection or traumatic injury to the muscle or its vascular pedicle are relative contraindications to use of muscle flaps.

Myocutaneous Flaps. The concept that muscle provides vascular nourishment to its overlying skin is relatively new.

Owens[45] was the first to exploit this with the sternomastoid compound flap in 1955. Others have contributed to this area, but McCraw was the first to appreciate the significance of the primary myocutaneous unit and adapt it for use in the entire body.[39] A myocutaneous flap is a composite of muscle with its overlying skin and subcutaneous tissue supplied by one or more dominant vascular or neurovascular pedicles.[31] Certain muscles may be isolated on a singular vascular pedicle as an island myocutaneous flap. Since muscle is segmentally supplied by various vascular perforations, knowledge of the anatomy of the particular muscles and those that will survive on dominant vascular pedicles is essential. The cutaneous portion of the flap may usually be larger than the muscle, and a delay procedure may increase the cutaneous area if necessary. As with muscle flaps, one must consider the possible functional loss associated with transfer of the muscle.

In the lower extremity the rectus femoris, gracilis, biceps femoris and tensor fasciae latae myocutaneous flaps are excellent for coverage of upper thigh defects. The rectus femoris and tensor fasciae latae flaps are the largest and probably most reliable of the group, both deriving their blood supply from the lateral femoral circumflex artery. The medial gastrocnemius myocutaneous flap is the workhorse of the lower leg (Fig. 17–15). Based on the sural branch of the popliteal artery, this flap can be taken to approximately 6 cm. above the medial malleolus primarily or longer with delay. The flap will cover the distal aspect of the upper leg, the knee, and the upper two thirds of the lower leg. It may be used as a cross leg flap when the ipsilateral gastrocnemius cannot be utilized (Fig. 17–16). The lateral gastrocnemius muscle is smaller and will not support as large a flap, but this flap is useful for coverage of the lateral knee or lateral upper aspects of the leg.

Free Flaps. As with replantation, the improvement in microscopic instrumentation and technique has brought the elective free tissue transfer via microvascular anastomosis (free flap) into clinical reality. The first successful free flap was performed in 1973 by Daniel and Taylor,[7] and Harii[19] has reported his experience with over 200 such procedures. The advantage of this technique is that a one-stage procedure is performed with the avoidance of prolonged

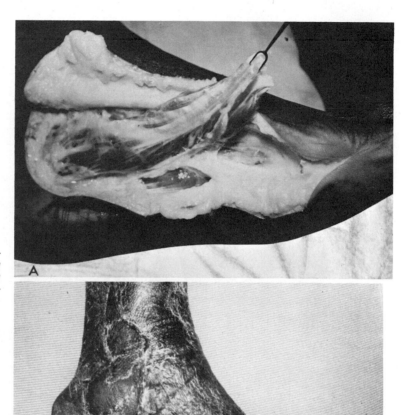

Figure 17–14. A, *Abductor hallucis muscle flap is mobilized and rotated to cover medial malleolar defect. B, One-year follow-up.*

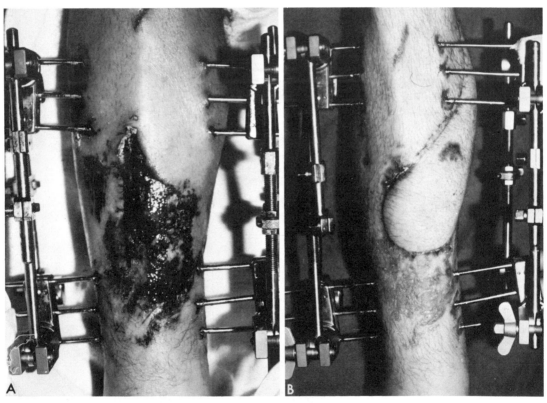

Figure 17–15.   A, A compound tibial fracture closed primarily with ischemic wound edges. This resulted in an open fracture that was covered by a medial gastrocnemius myocutaneous flap, B.

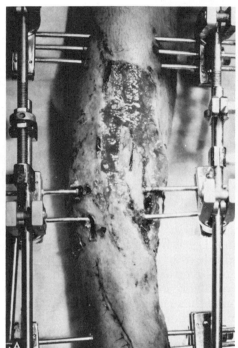

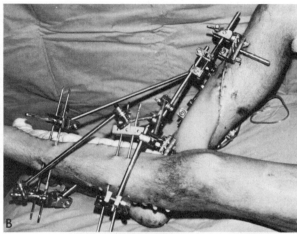

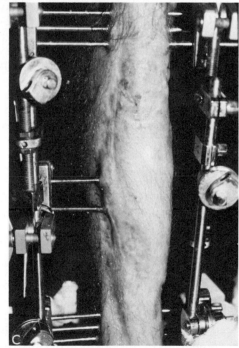

Figure 17–16.   *Medial gastrocnemius myocutaneous flap is transferred as a crossleg flap to cover a large wound exposing a tibial fracture. (Reproduced by permission from Maxwell, G. P., and Hoopes, J. E., Plast. Reconstr. Surg. 63:176, 1979.)*

operating time. Microsurgical expertise would obviously be required of the surgeon.

The lower extremity in particular has been a site frequently used for transfer of free flaps. Increasing experience has shown that the recipient vessels must be shortened sufficiently from the area of trauma so that the microvascular anastomosis is performed on relatively normal vessels. The use of interposition vein grafts has been helpful in this area.

The groin flap is the most popular flap for free transfer to the lower extremity. This flap is isolated on the superficial circumflex iliac vessels. Maxwell et al.[32] have recently advocated the transfer of the latissimus dorsi myocutaneous flap via microvascular anastomosis. This flap has proven to be one of the most reliable local myocutaneous flaps. It can be isolated on the thoracodorsal vascular stalk, producing an extremely long vascular pedicle and vessels of good diameter. This flap may be particularly useful in lower extremity coverage as its size may be quite large and the length of its vascular pedicle may obviate the need for vein grafts (Fig. 17–17). The tensor fasciae latae myocutaneous flap also offers some of these advantages in free transfer.

The statement by Hayhurst relative to indications for free flaps is particularly pertinent: "Each surgeon will develop his own indications for the use of microvascular flaps. These indications will be greatly influenced by past training experience and technical skills. As a surgeon gains facility with the use of the microvascular flap, his indications will likely expand."[20]

POSTOPERATIVE MANAGEMENT

The edema inevitably associated with extremity injuries is the major deterrent to recovery of normal function. Edematous tissues thicken and shorten and eventually become fixed in this position because of the deposition of protein and fibrin. Ligaments shorten, joints stiffen, muscles contract and tendons and nerves become encased in a dense fibrous sheath. Immobilization superimposed on edema and maintained for longer than absolutely necessary completes petrification of the extremity.

Attention during the immediate postoperative period is directed toward reduction of edema, preservation of viability and splinting of the wound. Almost without exception, extremity injuries are managed initially by means of elevation and pressure dressings. Elevation of the upper extremity is accomplished by means of an "arm bag" consisting of a canvas bag enclosing the entire upper extremity and suspended from an intravenous pole; the brachium and elbow rest horizontally on the bed, and the forearm and hand are suspended vertically. The lower extremity is elevated 15 degrees above the horizontal on pillows with care being taken not to exert pressure on the popliteal fossa. The extremities are not permitted to become either elevated or dependent in cases demonstrating severe arterial insufficiency.

Pressure dressings extend from the most distal part of the extremity to well above the area of injury; the toes and fingertips are exposed routinely for evaluation of circulation. Circumferential dressings applied to limited areas produce massive distal edema. Local hypothermia, low molecular weight dextran and stellate ganglion block are employed as therapeutic adjuncts in the face of severe vascular insufficiency. Institution of these measures as soon as feasible following trauma is essential; delay for more than 4 to 6 hours renders them useless. Elevation and complete immobilization of upper extremity injuries is maintained for a minimum period of 48 hours, following which ambulation with the extremity in a sling is allowed. Elevation and immobilization of severe lower extremity injuries is maintained for a minimum period of 3 weeks. Sutures are left intact and dressings continued for a period of 2 weeks.

Volkmann's ischemic contracture is a catastrophe that must be guarded against constantly, especially when dealing with casts and compression bandages. Although the etiology in the majority of cases is an unreduced supracondylar fracture of the elbow, the condition is seen with damage to the brachial or axillary artery and with massive subfascial hematoma secondary to crushing trauma of the forearm. Symptoms of impeding ischemia consist of constant pain exaggerated by forced extension of the fingers and hypesthesia and paresthesia of the hand, usually in the median nerve distribution. Examination reveals marked swelling of the hand and forearm, pale cyanosis,

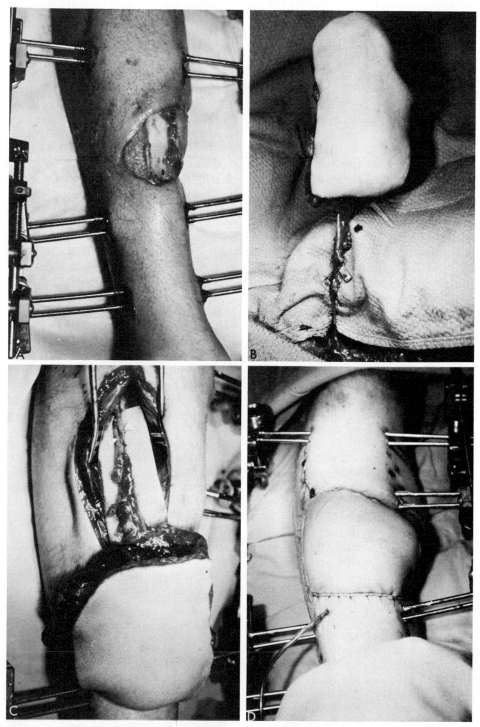

Figure 17–17. *A free latissimus dorsi myocutaneous flap is shown in this group. The flap was transferred end to end into the traumatically severed anterior tibial vessels to cover a compound tibial fracture. (Reproduced by permission from Maxwell, G. P., and Hoopes, J. E., Plast. Reconstr. Surg. 63:176, 1979.)*

partial intrinsic paralysis and an absent radial pulse. Progression to this stage is prevented by repeated evaluation of the circulatory status of the toes and fingertips and repeated questioning of the patient. Damage occurs within 6 to 48 hours of trauma or the application of an excessively tight dressing. The presence of these findings demands immediate removal of the dressings. Fasciotomy and sympathetic block are indicated if symptoms do not improve immediately. At exploration, the problem is found to be limited to the volar fascial space; findings consist of muscles that are either pale or blue-black from extravasation of blood, occlusion of all of the veins in the antecubital fossa and rupture or thrombosis of the brachial artery.

Indolent wounds wreak havoc on the *entire* extremity by producing persistent edema and prolonging the period of inactivity. Postoperative management is not complete until a healed wound has been secured.

REHABILITATION

All except the most minor extremity injuries require organized effort directed specifically at restoration of normal function. Immobilization results in stiff joints that must be overcome by all means available. All surgeons assuming responsibility for extremity injuries must have a thorough working knowledge of static and dynamic splinting[46] and of the methods utilized in an organized program of physiotherapy.

All major peripheral nerve injuries require dynamic splinting until obviated by satisfactory recovery of motor function or the decision to proceed with muscle transfers, the goal being to prevent the creation of deformity by unopposed muscle groups. Dynamic splints are designed to provide the action of the paralyzed muscle groups, thereby offering resistance for the uninvolved muscles to work against. Construction of such splints by the surgeon caring for the patient serves two major purposes: the splint is custom designed to fit properly and to accomplish precisely the desired end; and the physician, of necessity, learns a great deal about the functional anatomy of the hand. One needs only the usual material required in applying a cast plus some ⅛ in. welding rods and leather working tools in order to construct a perfect dynamic splint. The splints are worn for increasingly longer periods as tolerated by the patient; night splints are utilized to overcome contraction of ligaments and tendons. Dynamic transfers are deferred until sufficient time has elapsed to judge the quality of the nerve repair.

The patient with a radial nerve palsy requires a static splint that maintains the wrist and metacarpophalangeal joints in extension; i.e., a volar thin plaster slab held in position by means of wrapping with an elastic bandage. A surprising degree of function is possible with the splint in place provided it does not extend beyond the proximal interphalangeal flexion crease. Such splints usually incorporate a dorsal outrigger with elastic traction producing extension of the thumb. The dynamic splint used in ulnar nerve palsy consists of a "knuckle-bender" component and a dorsal outrigger with elastic traction producing extension of the ring and little fingers (Fig. 17–18). The patient with a median nerve injury requires a splint designed to produce dynamic (elastic) opposition of the thumb. The need for dynamic splinting is increased markedly with median and ulnar nerve injuries distal to the site of innervation of the forearm musculature.

The importance of precise follow-up records to the proper management of extremity injuries cannot be overemphasized. Treatment methods must be altered constantly to achieve maximal progress, and this is not possible if progress is not objectively measurable. Clinic notes such as "sensation improved" and "less flexion deformity" are totally worthless to the individual patient, and have no possible value

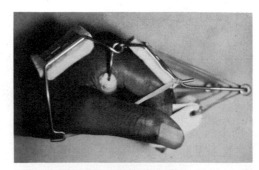

Figure 17–18. *The proper "knuckle-bender" splint with extension outrigger to be utilized in the rehabilitation of median and ulnar nerve palsy.*

in surveying the results of different methods of treatment. Measurements must be repeated sequentially and must be as objective as possible. Joint motion is recorded in degrees as measured with a protractor. The range of passive motion provides a good index of joint function, and the relation between this measurement and that of active motion gives valuable information in terms of tendon and muscle function. Sensory and motor return following peripheral nerve injury is best documented by the method of Nicholson and Seddon[42] (to be discussed later).

Sensory evaluation may be performed by a variety of methods, only a few of which are of real value. Coarse touch is the first sensation to return following peripheral nerve injury and is followed in order by perception of pinprick and light touch, the development of Tinel's sign and, finally, by stereognosis. Mohberg[36] and other investigators[11] have demonstrated clearly the rather gross correlation between the usual tests of sensibility and the degree of functional usefulness of the hand. Response to pinprick and light touch is of no value in predicting the degree of *functional sensibility* of the hand. On this basis, the authors advocate utilization of the Weber two-point discrimination test,[65] the ninhydrin printing test and measurement of "tactile gnosis" by means of the Seddon coin test and the Mohberg pick-up test. Two-point discrimination of 12 mm. or less on the volar aspect of the distal phalanx represents a high degree of recovery; patients with this degree of recovery have little measurable functional impairment.

The ninhydrin printing test is based on Mohberg's excellent demonstration of correlation between sudomotor activity and functional sensibility. It consists of staining by ninhydrin of the amino acids normally present in sweat and is demonstrated by fingerprinting. The hand is applied to a sheet of glazed white paper that is then stained with a 1 per cent solution of ninhydrin in acetone acidified with 5 drops of glacial acetic acid per 10 ml. of solution. After a period of 2 to 3 days, the print is fixed in a 1 per cent solution of copper nitrate in 95 per cent methyl alcohol acidified with a few drops of nitric acid. Unstained areas have no functional sensibility.

An index of tactile gnosis is obtained by requesting the patient to manipulate a group of small and varied objects. As utilized by Seddon, this consists of asking the blindfolded patient to identify a variety of coins; Mohberg provides the patient with a variety of common small objects and requests that they be transferred from the table to a cup with and without the aid of vision.

Tinel's sign is of value primarily in judging the progress of recovery prior to reinnervation. Gentle tapping over the course of the nerve distal to the site of injury elicits paresthesia over the growing axons; this paresthesia is referred to the normal area of innervation of the nerve. In performing the tests, it is important that vibration of the soft tissue proximal to the point of tapping be prevented. Tinel's sign is demonstrable 4 to 6 weeks following nerve suture and persists for a period of 18 to 24 months, i.e., until the regenerated axons have become myelinated.

Muscles return to function in the anatomical order of their innervation. A variable degree of irreversible atrophy may be anticipated and depends upon the time required for nerve regeneration.

Although nerve regeneration proceeds at a rate of approximately 1.5 mm. per day,[54] a considerably longer period of time than might be predicted on this basis is required for significant return of sensory and motor function. Beginning return of sensation may be appreciated within 4 to 6 weeks following nerve injury in the hand. Evidence of sensory return is not seen for a period of 2 to 3 months following nerve injury proximal to the level of the wrist, and motor return may not be appreciated for 6 to 8 months. Function continues to improve slowly over a rather prolonged period of time in association with maturation of the regenerated nerve in terms of myelination and increase in fiber size. Recovery cannot be considered maximal for at least 3 years following major peripheral nerve injury.

The method of evaluation proposed by Nicholson and Seddon[42] should be used as a standard in recording results following peripheral nerve injury:

Sensory:

   (S:O) Absence of sensibility in the cutaneous zone supplied exclusively by the nerve concerned (autonomous zone).

(1) Recovery of deep cutaneous pain.
(2) Recovery of some degree of superficial pain and tactile sensibility.
(2+) Return of tactile and pain sensibility throughout the autonomous zone but with persistent overreaction.
(3) Return of superficial pain and tactile sensibility throughout the autonomous zone with the disappearance of overreaction.
(3+) Return of superficial pain and tactile sensibility throughout the autonomous zone with the disappearance of overreaction, and good localization of stimuli with some return to two-point discrimination.
(4) Complete recovery.

Motor:

(M:O) No contraction.
(1) Return of perceptible contraction in the forearm muscles.
(1+) Median: Forearm muscles able to contract against gravity but paralysis of the thenar muscles.
    Ulnar: Forearm muscles able to contract against gravity but paralysis of the ulnar intrinsic muscles of the hand.
(2) Median: Forearm muscles able to contract against gravity and weak action in the thenar muscles.
    Ulnar: Forearm muscles able to contract against gravity and some power in the hypothenars but little or none in the interossei.
(2+) Ulnar: Forearm and hand muscles all active but the first dorsal interosseous muscle unable to contract against resistance.
(3) Median: Forearm and thenar muscles able to contract against resistance.
    Ulnar: Forearm, hypothenars and first dorsal interosseous muscles able to contract against resistance.
(4) Median: All muscles able to contract against strong resistance with some independent action.
    Ulnar: All muscles able to contract against resistance with some independent lateral movement of fingers.
(5) Full recovery in all muscles.

Patients with return of function to the S:3, M:3 level are classified as having a good result; those with return to the S:4, M:4 or 5 level are classified as having an excellent result. Combined data indicate that not more than 50 or 60 per cent of patients achieve a good or excellent result and that few, if any, patients regain completely normal function.[5, 25, 52, 58, 69] Results with mixed nerve injuries are poorer than those with injuries just to sensory or motor nerves; digital and radial nerve repairs are almost uniformly successful; ulnar repairs provide the least satisfactory results; and median nerve repairs are intermediate in results. Children uniformly obtain a better result than adults and often demonstrate relatively normal sensation after a 2-year period.[25, 52, 58]

Electromyograph and nerve conduction velocity studies provide a more sophisticated measure of the extent of recovery following peripheral nerve damage. Many studies[21, 33] indicate that the conduction velocity never returns to normal following nerve suture; in the usual case, it probably does not exceed 60 to 70 per cent of normal. The electromyogram may be of considerable prognostic value.

The results presently being obtained leave much to be desired. Intensive effort must be directed toward the improvement of repair techniques.

RECONSTRUCTION

It is not our purpose to elaborate upon the complex techniques utilized in restoring function to a badly crippled extremity. It is sufficient to say that the hand is totally dependent on a finely balanced mechanism for functional integrity, and all possible efforts must be directed toward restoring this balance.

REFERENCES

1. Aitken, J. T., Scharman, M., and Young J. Z.: Maturation of regenerating nerve fibers with various peripheral connections. J. Anat. 81:1, 1947.
2. Alpert, B. S., Buncke, H. J., and Brownstein, M.: Replacement of damaged arteries and veins with vein grafts when replanting crushed, amputated fingers. Plast. Reconstr. Surg. 61:17, 1978.

3. Altemeier, W. A., and Alexander, J. W.: Surgical infections and choice of antibiotics. *In* Sabiston, D.C. (ed.): Textbook of Surgery. Philadelphia, W. B. Saunders Co., 1977.

4. American Replantation Mission to China: Replantation surgery in China. Plast. Reconstr. Surg. 52:476, 1973.

5. Benvenuto, R.: Peripheral nerves. Int. Abstr. Surg. 115:528, 1962.

6. Brown, R. F.: The management of traumatic tissue loss in the lower extremity, especially when complicated by skeletal injury. Br. J. Plast. Surg. 18:26, 1965.

7. Daniel, R. K., and Taylor, I. G.: Distant transfer of an island flap by microvascular anastomosis. Plast. Reconstr. Surg. 52:111, 1973.

8. Davis, W. M., McCraw, J. B., and Carraway, J. H.: Use of a direct, transverse, thoracicoabdominal flap to close difficult wounds of the thorax and upper extremity. Plast. Reconstr. Surg. 60:526, 1977.

9. Edshage, S.: Peripheral nerve suture, a technique for improved intraneural topography. Evaluation of some suture materials. Acta Chir. Scand. (Suppl.) 331:1, 1964.

10. Entin, M. A.: Roller and wringer injuries: clinical and experimental studies. Plast. Reconstr. Surg. 15:290, 1955.

11. Flynn, J. E., and Flynn, W. F.: Median and ulnar nerve injuries. Ann. Surg. 156:1002, 1962.

12. Freeman, B. S.: Adhesive neuroanastomosis. Plast. Reconstr. Surg. 35:167, 1965.

13. Ger, R.: The technique of muscle transposition in the operative treatment of traumatic and ulcerative lesions of the leg. J. Trauma 11:502, 1971.

14. Grabb, W. C., Bement, S. L., Koepke, G. H., and Green, R. A.: Comparison of methods of peripheral nerve suturing in monkeys. Plast. Reconstr. Surg. 46:31, 1970.

15. Gross, A., Cutright, D. E., and Blaskar, S. N.: Effectiveness of pulsating water jet lavage in treatment of contaminated crush wounds. Am. J. Surg. 124:373, 1972. Plast. Reconstr. Surg. 63:176, 1979.

16. Halsted, W. S., Reichert, F. L., and Reid, M. R.: Replantation of entire limbs without suture of vessels. Trans. Am. Surg. Assoc. 140:160, 1922.

17. Hamilton, F.: Old ulcers treated by anaplasty. N.Y. Med. J. 13:165, 1854.

18. Harashina, T., and Buncke, H. J.: Study of washout solutions for microvascular replantation and transplantation. Plast. Reconstr. Surg. 56:542, 1975.

19. Harii, K., et al.: Free skin flap transfer: Our five year clinical survey. Presented before the American Society of Plastic and Reconstructive Surgeons. San Francisco, 1977.

20. Hayhurst, J.: Reconstructive Plastic Surgery. Philadelphia, W. B. Saunders Co., 1977.

21. Hodes, R., Larrabee, M. G., and German, W.: The human electromyogram in response to nerve stimulation and the conduction velocity of motor axons. Studies on normal and injured peripheral nerves. Arch. Neurol. Psychiatr. 60:340, 1948.

22. Hueston, J. T., and Gunter, G. S.: Primary cross leg flaps. Plast. Reconstr. Surg. 40:58, 1967.

23. Kilgore, E. S., and Graham, W. D.: The Hand: Surgical and Nonsurgical Management. Philadelphia, Lea and Febiger, 1977, 219.

24. Kline, D. G.: The use of a resorbable wrapper for peripheral nerve repair, experimental studies in chimpanzees. J. Neurosurg. 21:737, 1964.

25. Lindsay, W. K.: Traumatic peripheral nerve injuries in children; results of repair. Plast. Reconstr. Surg. 30:462, 1962.

26. Lindsay, W. K., Thomson, H. S., and Farmer, A. W.: The wringer injury. Can. J. Surg. 1:189, 1957.

27. Malt, R. A.: Replantation of severed arms. J.A.M.A. 189:716, 1964.

28. Marmor, L., and Sollars, R. E.: Amputation levels in severely traumatized extremities, with appropriate prostheses. J. Trauma 2:585, 1962.

29. Mason, M. L., and Allen, H. S.: The rate of healing of tendons: An experimental study of tensile strength. Ann. Surg. 113:424, 1941.

30. Maxwell, G. P., and Hoopes, J. E.: Management of compound wounds of the lower extremity. Plast. Reconstr. Surg. 63:176, 1979.

31. Maxwell, G. P., and Bosley, J. H.: Myocutaneous flaps: Clinical conferences at the Johns Hopkins Hospital. Johns Hopkins Med. J. 141:258, 1977.

32. Maxwell, G. P., Stueber, K., and Hoopes, J. H.: The latissimus dorsi myocutaneous free flap. Plast. Reconstr. Surg. 62:462, 1978.

33. Mayer, R. F.: Nerve regeneration in replanted canine limbs. Am. J. Physiol. 206:1415, 1964.

34. Millesi, H.: The interfascicular nerve graft. J. Bone Joint Surg. 53A:813, 1971.

35. Millesi, H.: The interfascicular nerve-grafting of the median and ulnar nerves. J. Bone Joint Surg. 54A:727, 1972.

36. Mohberg, G. E.: Objective methods for determining the functional value of sensibility in the hand. J. Bone Joint Surg. 40B:454, 1958.

37. Morrison, W. A., O'Brien, B. M., and Macleod, A. M.: Major limb replantation. Orthopedic Clinics of N. Am. 8:343, 1977.

38. McCraw, J. B., and Furlow, L. T., Jr.: The dorsalis pedis arterialized flap. Plast. Reconstr. Surg. 55:177, 1975.

39. McCraw, J., Dibbell, D., and Carraway, J.: Clinical definition of independent myocutaneous vascular territories. Plast. Reconstr. Surg., 60:710, 1977.

40. McCraw, J. B., Myers, B., and Shunklin, K. D.: The value of fluorescein in predicting the viability of arterialized flaps. Plast. Reconstr. Surg. 60:710, 1977.

41. McGregor, I. A., and Jackson, I. T.: The groin flap. Br. J. Plast. Surg. 25:3, 1972.

42. Nicholson, O. R., and Seddon, H. J.: Nerve repair in civil practice. Br. Med. J. 2:1065, 1957.

43. O'Brien, B. M.: Replantation surgery. Clin. Plast. Surg. 1:405, 1974.

44. O'Brien, B. M.: Replantation Surgery, Reconstructive Plastic Surgery. Philadelphia, W. B. Saunders Co., 1977, 3243.

45. Owens, N.: Compound neck pedicle designed for

repair of massive facial defects. Plast. Reconstr. Surg. *15*:369, 1955.

46. Peacock, E. A.: Dynamic splinting for the prevention and correction of hand deformities. J. Bone Joint Surg. *34A*:789, 1952.

47. Peacock, E. E., and Van Winkle, W. W., Jr.: Surgery and Biology of Wound Repair. Philadelphia, W. B. Saunders, Co., 1976.

48. Potenza, A. D.: Tendon healing within the flexor digital sheath in the dog. J. Bone Joint Surg. *44A*:49, 1962.

49. Press, E.: Wringer washing machine injuries. Am. J. Public Health *54*:812, 1964.

50. Roberts, G.R.: Impaling and transfixion injuries to the limbs. Br. J. Surg. *51*:135, 1964.

51. Rozner, L.: Anatomical and physiological factors in below-knee wounds. Lancet *1*:1362, 1965.

52. Sakellarides, H.: A follow-up study of 172 peripheral nerve injuries in the upper extremity in civilians. J. Bone Joint Surg. *44A*:410, 1962.

53. Seddon, H. J.: Three types of nerve injury. Brain *66*:238, 1943.

54. Seddon, H. J., Medawar, P. B., and Smith, H.: Rate of regeneration of peripheral nerves in man. J. Physiol. *102*:191, 1943.

55. Sherman, R. T., and Parrish, R. A.: Management of shotgun injuries; a review of 152 cases. J. Trauma *3*:76, 1963.

56. Smith, J. W.: Microsurgery of peripheral nerves. Plast. Reconstr. Surg. *33*:317, 1964.

57. Smith, J. W.: Blood supply of tendons. Am. J. Surg. *109*:272, 1965.

58. Stromberg, W. B.: Injury of the median and ulnar nerve. J. Bone Joint Surg. *43A*:717, 1961.

59. Sunderland, S.: The intraneural topography of the radial, median, and ulnar nerves. Brain *68*:243, 1946.

60. Tackett, A. D., and Sale, W. G.: Vascular injuries of the lower extremity. Am. Surg. *43*:488, 1977.

61. Thorraldsson, S. E., and Grabb, W. C.: Intravenous fluorescein test as a measure of skin flap viability. Plast. Reconstr. Surg. *53*:576, 1974.

62. Trueta, J.: Treatment of War Wounds and Fractures. London, Hamish Hamilton, 1939.

63. Vasconez, L. O., Bostwick, J., and McCraw, J.: Coverage of exposed bone by muscle transposition and skin grafting. Plast. Reconstr. Surg. *53*:526, 1974.

64. Wagle, M. B.: Gas gangrene — conservative management. Br. J. Plast. Surg. *16*:391, 1963.

65. Weber, E. H.: Cutaneous sensation. *In* Schafer, E. A. (ed.): Textbook of Physiology. New York, The Macmillan Co., 1900, 928.

66. Webster, G. V., Peterson, R. A., and Stein, H. L.: Dermal overgrafting of the leg. J. Bone Joint Surg. *40A*:796, 1958.

67. Weiland, A. J., et al.: Replantation of digits and hands: Analysis of surgical techniques and functional results in 71 patients with 86 replantations. J. Hand Surg. *2*:1, 1977.

68. Williams, G. R.: Replantation of the extremities. *In* Sabiston, D.C. (ed.): Textbook of Surgery. Philadelphia, W. B. Saunders Co., 1977.

69. Woodhall, B., and Beebe, G. W.: Peripheral Nerve Regeneration. Washington, D.C., V.A. Medical Monograph, 1956.

70. Young, J. Z.: The functional repair of nervous tissue. Physiol. Rev. *2*:318, 1942.

71. Young, J. Z., and Medawar, P. B.: Fibrin suture of peripheral nerves. Lancet *2*:126, 1940.

General

Cannon, B., et al.: Reconstructive Surgery of the Lower Extremity. In Converse, J. M., (ed): Reconstructive Plastic Surgery. Philadelphia, W. B. Saunders Co. 1977.

Committee on Trauma, American College of Surgeons: Early Care of Acute Soft Tissue Injuries. Philadelphia, W. B. Saunders Co., 1961.

Ellis, M.: The Casualty Officer's Handbook. London, Butterworth & Co., Ltd., 1962.

Flint, T., Jr.: Emergency Treatment and Management. Philadelphia, W. B. Saunders Co., 1975.

Kirkaldy-Willis, W. H., and Wood, A. M.: Treatment of Trauma. Baltimore, The Williams & Wilkins Co., 1962.

Schrire, T.: Emergencies. Springfield, Ill., Charles C Thomas, 1962.

CHAPTER 18

INJURIES OF THE HAND

Raymond M. Curtis, M.D.

Michael E. Jabaley, M.D.

James J. Ryan, M.D.

The strength and flexibility of the human hand are unequaled by any other part of the body. The hand is also an organ of expression, exposing the secrets of the heart and soul. This fact, coupled with concern regarding economic loss and inability to contribute to society, readily explains the psychological disturbances associated with crippling hand injuries.

Bunnell's[16] dictum that the *early* treatment of the acutely injured hand determines whether the hand is "doomed to disability" or "will regain usable function" cannot be overemphasized.

BASIC PRINCIPLES

A procedure of management so formalized that it may be followed by the emergency department nurse as well as the intern, resident or staff doctor should be available in the emergency department of every hospital. The following is suggested as an optimal routine.

History. Information pertinent to the injury must be as detailed as possible. Specific attention should be paid to the time of occurrence, the mechanism of injury and the position of the hand when injured. The degree of contamination should be determined as well as the nature of first aid administered.

Assessment of the Injury. Evaluation of total hand function is imperative. The examination must include a careful search

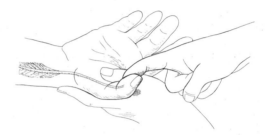

Figure 18–1. *Testing for the function of the flexor pollicis longus to the terminal phalanx of the thumb.*

for vascular injury, evaluation of flexor and extensor tendon function (Figs. 18–1, 18–2 and 18–3), an appraisal of sensation (Fig. 18–4), an assessment of all the small muscle functions of the hand (Figs. 18–5 and 18–6) and a roentgenogram if bone injury is suspected.

Initial Wound Management. The wound is covered with a small sterile gauze dressing, following which the in-

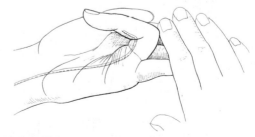

Figure 18–2. *Testing for the function of the flexor superficialis in ring finger by blocking the action of the flexor profundus tendon by holding the middle and ring fingers in extension.*

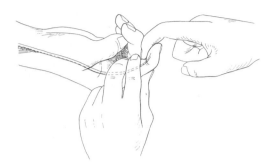

Figure 18-3. *Method of holding finger to block flexion of the proximal interphalangeal joint so as to test for flexor profundus function in the terminal phalanx.*

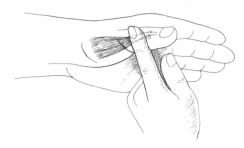

Figure 18-5. *Method of testing for function of the short abductor muscle of the thumb that is innervated by the median nerve.*

jured extremity is shaved properly and cleansed thoroughly with soap and water. This cleansing must be done carefully so that none of the solution enters the wound. The wound is irrigated with copious quantities of normal saline solution or, preferably, a buffered electrolyte solution such as Tis-u-sol,* since experimental work has demonstrated that "normal" saline alters wound pH. Following completion of irrigation, the wound is again covered with a sterile dressing, and the hand and forearm are prepared with an antiseptic solution and placed on a sterile arm board for examination.

Definitive Treatment. Suturing of hand lacerations in the emergency department is permissible only if the examiner can be certain that there has been no tendon or nerve damage. The repair of injury

---

*Travenol Laboratories, Inc. Morton Grove, Illinois.

to deep structures demands the following conditions:[21]

1. A well-equipped operating room.
2. Adequate hand instruments.
3. Capable assistants.
4. Complete anesthesia.
5. A realization of the importance of the procedure.
6. A bloodless operating field provided by a pneumatic tourniquet.
7. Meticulous atraumatic surgical technique.

It is both impossible and dangerous to explore a hand and perform the necessary repair without the aid of a bloodless operative field provided by a tourniquet. Even in those instances in which suturing of a minor laceration is accomplished under local anesthesia in the emergency department, the patient will tolerate a tourniquet for 25 to 30 minutes. The bloodless field allows visualization of the depth of the

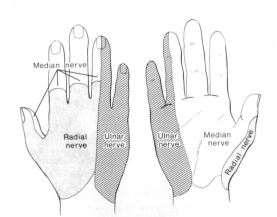

Figure 18-4. *Sensory distribution of median, ulnar and radial nerves to hand.*

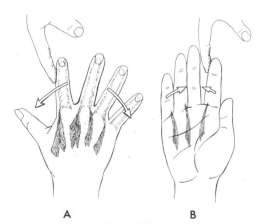

Figure 18-6. *Method of testing for function of the dorsal interossei (A) and the palmar interossei (B), which are innervated by the ulnar nerve.*

wound, and injuries not suspected clinically may be detected.

General anesthesia is employed uniformly when there are no contraindications so that unlimited operative time with complete tolerance of the tourniquet is provided. Recent experiences with bupivacaine hydrochloride (Marcaine) suggest that this drug will also provide satisfactory anesthesia for extended periods of time. Local anesthesia may be used for less severe injuries.

LOCAL ANESTHESIA. Lidocaine (Xylocaine), 1 per cent, locally infiltrated into the wound is adequate for small lacerations. Epinephrine must not be used with the local anesthetic for fear of producing digital artery spasm and thrombosis. Adequate preoperative sedation of the patient and supplementation with intravenous Demerol, if necessary, greatly facilitate the use of local and nerve block anesthesia.

NERVE BLOCK ANESTHESIA. Block of the median nerve at the wrist, the ulnar nerve at the elbow and the radial sensory nerve in the distal third of the forearm can be used for local procedures on the hand. The patient will not tolerate a tourniquet for more than 30 to 45 minutes.

AXILLARY BLOCK ANESTHESIA. It is well to supplement the axillary block with local infiltration of lidocaine in a circular fashion about the upper arm in order to increase tourniquet tolerance time. The use of bupivacaine hydrochloride (Marcaine) has expanded greatly the indications for axillary blocks.

BRACHIAL PLEXUS BLOCK ANESTHESIA. Brachial plexus block with lidocaine, 2 per cent, with epinephrine 1:1000,000, provides excellent anesthesia for hand surgery. It is particularly valuable for a patient who is not a suitable candidate for general anesthesia because of the recent intake of food or suspected injuries to other organ systems.

The special arm board first described by Boyes[5] (Fig. 18–7)[20] allows the operator to sit in the oval area and rest his elbows on the table for much of this work. This is of particular value for the more meticulous type of work and eliminates much of the fatigue associated with this finely detailed

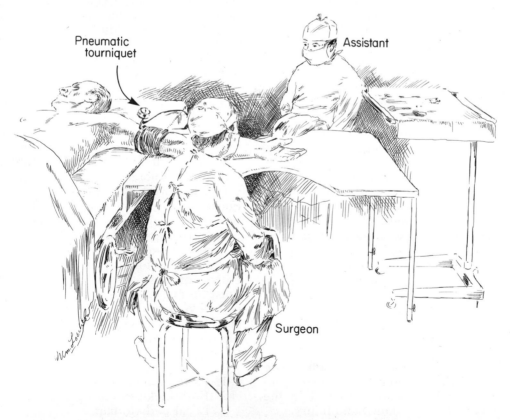

Figure 18–7. *Special Boyes arm board for hand surgery.*

surgery. An inflatable pneumatic tourniquet with an accurate manometer provides a bloodless field. Elevation of the arm for 5 minutes followed by inflation of the cuff will prevent bleeding during preparation of the extremity with antiseptic solution. Following the application of sterile drapes, the tourniquet is released, the extremity is wrapped firmly with a sterile Ace bandage from the fingertips to within 1 inch of the tourniquet to completely empty the extremity of blood, and the tourniquet is reinflated. A pressure of 300 mm. of mercury is utilized in adults. Children under 12 years of age require 260 mm. pressure; 150 mm. pressure provides adequate ischemia in infants.

The tourniquet may remain inflated for one and a half hours.[11] If the operation has not been completed at the end of this period, a light pressure dressing is applied to the wound and the tourniquet is released for 15 minutes. The tourniquet is reinflated after the arm has once more been wrapped with an elastic bandage. If the wound is infected, the extremity is emptied of blood by means of elevation rather than use of an elastic bandage.

In many civilian hospitals a busy operative schedule may impose a delay of several hours in the definitive treatment of an acute hand injury. In these circumstances, a sterile dressing is applied to the forearm and hand after initial wound management in the emergency department, and this dressing remains in place until the patient reaches the operating room. Administration of antibiotics is initiated preoperatively.

A patient who has been actively immunized against tetanus should have a booster dose of tetanus toxoid. Those who have not received prior immunization may need active immunization with initial dose of tetanus toxoid continued at weekly intervals until complete. Rarely, there may be an indication for hyperimmune human tetanus antiserum.

SKIN

The provision of adequate soft tissue coverage will determine, in many instances, the final result achieved in the management of a serious hand injury.

Primary closure can be secured at the time of initial management in the majority of acute injuries by strict observation of the surgical principles of thorough wound cleansing and debridement and by careful selection of the method of closure best suited to the situation. Delayed primary closure[31] is preferred for wounds that are severely contused or heavily contaminated or that must be treated after an unduly long interval following injury. Such wounds are thoroughly cleansed, surgically debrided and irrigated with copious quantities of a buffered electrolyte solution. The hand is dressed with a single layer of fine mesh gauze, padding and a plaster splint and elevated continuously until the patient is returned to the operating room for wound closure. This should ordinarily be accomplished in 3 to 5 days in order to avoid the development of granulation tissue and excessive deep scar and to permit active and passive motion of the joints and tendons.

There is no excess tissue on the hand. For this reason, closure of areas of skin loss simply by undermining and suturing the wound margins is doomed to failure. Tissue of questionable viability is far better excised primarily than allowed to become necrotic and secondarily infected. Accurate determination of viability is a decision of major importance. Observation of the return of circulation to the questionable tissue following release of the tourniquet can be of considerable value in making this judgment. Circulation within the skin margin may be assessed by small incisions into the dermis after the tourniquet has been deflated for 10 to 15 minutes. Intravenous fluorescein sodium (Fluorescite), followed by study of the tissue in question under Wood's light to determine presence or absence of fluorescence, can predict tissue survival.

Simultaneous repair of deep structures and provision for adequate soft tissue coverage comprise optimal management. It must be emphasized that the type of skin coverage provided is determined by the specific wound situation. The following plastic procedures are useful in providing the necessary coverage:

1. Partial-thickness skin grafts.
2. Full-thickness skin graft.
3. Local pedicle flap.
4. Distant pedicle flap.

Partial-Thickness Skin Graft

The decision to use a partial-thickness skin graft is based on the characteristics of the bed on which the graft is to be placed. In general, exposed tendons and compound fractures require pedicle flap coverage. An excellent clinical result can be obtained with a partial-thickness graft if the paratenon and epitenon overlying the extensor tendons are intact (Fig. 18–8). A partial-thickness skin graft may provide suitable coverage for the palm if the flexor tendons are within their sheaths. Pedicle flap coverage is required if the tendon sheaths have been denuded and the flexor tendons lie exposed in the wound. The partial-thickness graft is useful for the coverage of minor fingertip avulsions in which a good bed of subcutaneous tissue remains (Fig. 18–9). An alternative method for securing grafts employs steri-strips instead of sutures and allows the graft to conform better to the convex surface of the fingertip. Contraction of the graft with time will advance the normal skin of the finger distally so that at the end of a year there will be little evidence of the original injury and good sensation will be present over the tip of the finger.

In specific instances, the partial-thickness graft may be utilized to secure early temporary wound closure with the realization that pedicle flap replacement of the skin graft at a later date will be necessary to allow further reconstructive procedures. The approach is particularly suitable for battle casualties.

A thick graft, approximately 0.018 in., provides good permanent skin coverage. The graft is obtained with the Reese Dermatome. Perfect hemostasis, adequate pressure and strict immobilization are essential for a proper "take" of the graft. One should select a donor site that is hidden or will accommodate a cosmetically acceptable scar. This is especially true in female patients and members of races with pigmented skin.

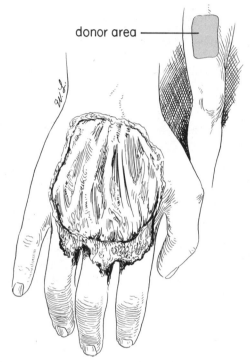

donor area

Figure 18–8. *Extensive avulsion of dorsum of hand and use of thigh as donor area for dermatome skin graft.*

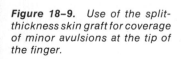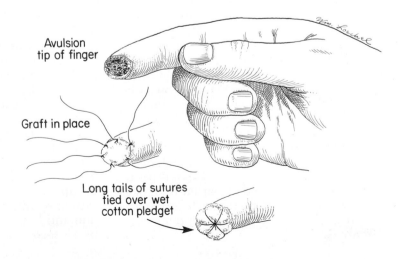

Avulsion tip of finger

Graft in place

Figure 18–9. *Use of the split-thickness skin graft for coverage of minor avulsions at the tip of the finger.*

Long tails of sutures tied over wet cotton pledget

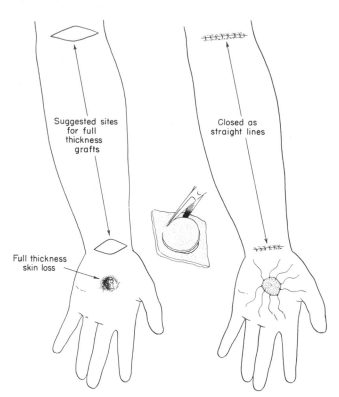

Suggested sites
for full
thickness
grafts

Closed as
straight lines

Full thickness
skin loss

Figure 18–10. The use of the full-thickness skin graft for replacement of skin loss. Note how sutures are left long to be tied over pressure dressing on graft and how graft is patterned to fit the defect perfectly.

Full-Thickness Skin Graft

Full-thickness grafts are valuable for the repair of small defects, particularly in those instances in which it is important that there be no subsequent shrinkage of the graft (Fig. 18–10). Full-thickness grafts are preferred by some for fingertip avulsion.

The antecubital fossa and the flexion crease of the wrist are preferred donor areas since closure of the defect is accomplished more easily than in the central, volar aspect of the forearm. A perfect pattern of the defect should be outlined on the donor area of the full-thickness graft to ensure suturing the graft into position with no more than normal skin tension (Fig. 18–10). All subcutaneous fat is removed from the graft either at the time of excision or by stretching the graft over the operator's finger and trimming away the fat with fine scissors. Full-thickness grafts demand meticulous attention to every detail if survival is to be achieved. A partial-thickness graft is preferred if there exists any question regarding the suitability of the recipient areas.

The skin avulsed by a severe injury may occasionally be defatted and replaced as a full-thickness graft. Severely contused skin is not suitable for this purpose.

Pedicle Flaps

Blood-bearing skin and subcutaneous tissue often are needed to provide cover for exposed tendon and bone. The surgeon dealing with acute hand injuries must be in a position to apply such coverage at the time of primary treatment or soon thereafter.

Local Flaps. ROTATION FLAP. A local rotation flap is particularly suitable for wounds on the dorsum of the hand and can be raised from the dorsal or lateral aspects of the fingers as well. Skin flaps are difficult to rotate on the palm because of the fascial attachments to the underlying structures.

CROSS-FINGER FLAP. The cross-finger flap is indicated in the management of fingertip injuries in which the loss of both skin and subcutaneous tissue exposes tendon and bone. A satisfactory result cannot be expected with a partial-thickness skin

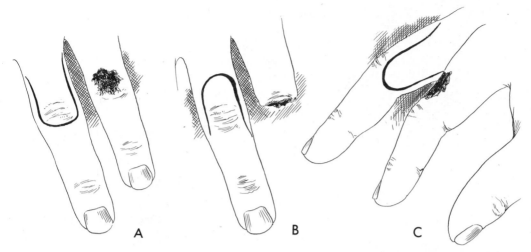

Figure 18–11. *An illustration of the fact that pedicle flap may be based distally, proximally or laterally.*

graft applied over a denuded flexor tendon. The cross-finger flap is of particular value for surfacing defects on the flexor surface of the finger and the fingertip.

Utilization of pedicle flap tissue from an adjacent finger offers many advantages. Vascular complications within the flap are unusual because of the abundant circulation. Only two adjacent fingers need be divided safely under local anesthesia 10 to 14 days postoperatively. The functional and cosmetic result is superior, and the recovery of sensation is frequently faster than with other methods. The major disadvantage consists of imposing scarring and possible stiffness on a normal finger.

The cross-finger flap may be based distally, proximally or laterally depending upon how it can best be rotated to fill the defect (Fig. 18–11). The flap should always be designed larger than the defect. The incision for creation of the laterally based flap should be carried to the mid-axial position to minimize the danger of residual scarring and stiffness (Fig. 18–12). As the dissection reaches the lateral margin of the finger, it is necessary to separate a layer of oblique fascia (Cleland's ligament) joining the skin on the lateral aspect of the finger to the extensor mechanism and phalangeal periosteum.[22] Release of these fascial bands adds approximately 0.25 in. to the

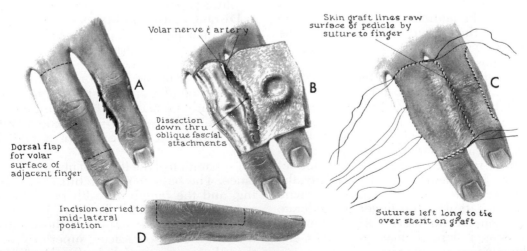

Figure 18–12. *Technique of preparation of cross-finger pedicle flap for large volar defect and partial thickness graft to donor area. (From Curtis, R. M.: Ann. Surg. 145:650, 1957.)*

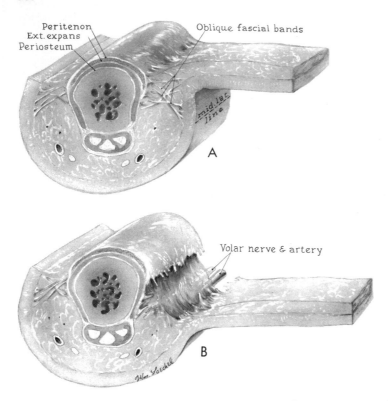

Peritenon
Ext. expans
Periosteum

Oblique fascial bands

mid. lat. line

A

Volar nerve & artery

B

Figure 18–13. A, *Cross section of finger through proximal phalanx, showing oblique fascial bands that fit skin to extensor tendon mechanisms and periosteum of phalanges. B. Release of skin obtained by dividing the oblique fascial fibers. (From Curtis, R. M.: Ann. Surg. 145:650, 1957.)*

length of the flap (Fig. 18–13). The flap is handled with meticulous atraumatic technique and sutured with fine nylon. The donor area is covered with a partial-thickness graft 0.015 to 0.018 in. in thickness. Care is taken to line the raw area of the pedicle flap completely with the skin graft (Fig. 18–12). A stent dressing is tied over the graft, and wet cotton is packed lightly between the two fingers. Care is taken not to jeopardize the circulation of the flap. The pedicle is divided in 10 to 14 days, and the margin of the pedicle on the donor finger is trimmed to lie in the mid-lateral position.

Cross-finger flaps may be required in late reconstructive procedures. Resurfacing of the volar aspect of a finger may be necessary prior to tendon grafting, and this is best accomplished with a cross-finger flap. In dealing with a severe flexion contracture requiring tenolysis, excision of tendon sheath and volar capsulectomy, the best results are obtained by Kirschner wire immobilization of the finger in moderate extension and immediate application of a cross-finger flap, if inadequate skin and subcutaneous tissue exist.

THENAR FLAP. The thenar flap[3] is of value in severe avulsions or amputations of the fingertips. The flap is elevated well posterior from the thenar area to avoid hyperflexion of the proximal interphalangeal joint; considerable care must be taken in resurfacing the donor site to prevent persistent discomfort in the resultant scar. Permanent stiffness of the proximal interphalangeal joint may follow immobilization of longer than 10 to 14 days, especially in older patients.

Distant Flaps. ABDOMINAL FLAP. An abdominal pedicle flap, elevated and sutured to the defect primarily, frequently is the procedure of choice for coverage of a large defect of the hand or forearm (Fig. 18–14). Complex and severely contaminated wounds are managed best by either immediate or delayed partial-thickness grafting or delayed application of a pedicle flap.

Preparation of the flap is of utmost importance. The base should be broad and flaring, and the length-to-width ratio should not exceed 2:1. The flap may be based above or below the umbilicus; those above the umbilicus are pedicled superiorly, and those below are pedicled inferiorly. Flaps, particularly if tubed, are raised in a plane

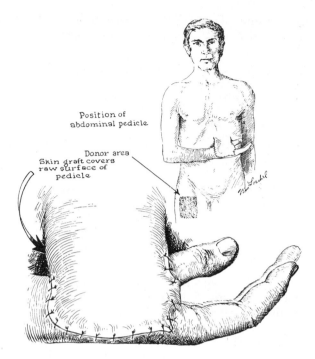

Figure 18–14. *Use of abdominal pedicle flap for coverage of extensive defect of wrist and hand. Note that abdominal donor site is covered primarily with dermatome skin graft. This graft also lines the raw surface of the pedicle.*

parallel to the rib over the anteriolateral aspect of the chest and abdomen, since thoracic vessels descend slightly obliquely. The flap should be precisely designed[37] by a pattern of the wound and elevated at a level to include a minumum amount of fat. This technique reduces the amount of "parasitic fat" that detracts from the blood supply and frequently makes unnecessary subsequent defatting procedures. A flap delay procedure may be utilized if a healed wound is being resurfaced; the flap is outlined as described, incised to the appropriate level and then the wound edges resutured. The flap is elevated and transferred to the defect 2 weeks later. Abdominal flaps may be partially defatted, if necessary, at the time of application. An open pedicle flap is never used on the hand because of the inevitable secondary infection and excessive scarring at the attachment of the pedicle. All pedicles are closed either by grafting of the raw surface or by tubing the base of the pedicle.

CROSS-ARM FLAP. The cross-arm flap is limited in the amount of tissue available but offers the advantages of being less bulky than an abdominal flap. The decision to employ a cross-arm flap, as opposed to an abdominal or infraclavicular flap, is based on its suitability in terms of thickness and availability.

TENDONS

Principles of Tendon Repair

The achievement of satisfactory results following tendon repair is dependent upon an understanding of the physiology of tendon healing. The experimental work of Skoog and Person,[60] Potenza,[53] and other investigators has demonstrated the peritenon to be the main source of the vascular bud that grows into the area of tendon injury.

Potenza[53] found in an experimental study of the healing process in the canine flexor digital tendons that the vascular bud was the source of fibroblasts from which collagen bundles develop. Fibroblastic activity was demonstrable within 10 days after injury. Initially, the collagen fibers are oriented in a plane perpendicular to the long axis of the tendon; they are realigned in the direction of the tendon fibers by approximately the 112th day.[53]

Tensile strenth studies indicate the juncture to be weakest on the third day following repair, conincident with maximal edema of the tendon ends. The degree of healing at the anastomosis will allow some active motion at 3 weeks, but it may be 6 weeks before the tendon can be considered strong.

Tendon repair demands sharp and meticulous dissection with a minimum of surgical trauma. The following principles of strictly atraumatic technique must be observed:

1. The tendon is handled when possible with the wet, gloved finger.

2. Traumatized tendon ends are removed sharply.

3. Stainless steel suture material on atraumatic needles is used.

4. The operative field is kept moist by frequent irrigation with a buffered electrolyte solution.

5. Sharp dissection is utilized exclusively; identification of dissection planes is enhanced by using a two- to three-power magnifying loupe.

6. Blood supply is preserved, and hematoma is prevented.

The tendon suture or juncture should be placed in tissue that has not been traumatized by the original injury or surgery. Severe, crushing or mangling injuries may contraindicate primary tendon repair. All scar must be removed at the time of secondary repair in order that the sutured tendon ends will lie in good tissue.

The character of the wound, the mechanism of injury, the degree of contamination and the elapsed time between injury and definitive treatment determine whether primary or delayed tendon repair is performed. A maximum elapsed time limit of 6 hours, during which definitive treatment may be undertaken, is generally satisfactory. The time limit may be extended when dealing with sharply incised wounds that have been cleansed and dressed with 1 hour of injury. When these requirements cannot be met, it is better judgment to defer tendon repair for 2 to 4 days. In crushing or mangling injuries in which there has been gross contamination, the tendon repair may be deferred for 4 to 6 weeks or until the wound is soft and pliable. Boyes[5] has stated: "It is difficult to prove that primary repair is superior to that done later, all other factors being equal. Unless the wound can be treated, unless healing can be obtained by primary intension, reactionless in type, the tendon and nerve repair probably should be delayed. We must approach the fundamental problem by graded steps and stages."

Suture materials should be inert, as fine as possible and swaged on atraumatic needles — stainless steel is preferred, but other synthetics such as Mersilene or Pro-

lene are also used. 4–0 or 5–0 size is used in the flexor tendon and 4–0 is used with the pull-out wire technique. The tendon being sutured should not be handled with forceps but rather with the moistened, gloved hand or with a transfixion needle. Utilizing the method of Bunnell, the tendon end that is held with clamp or forceps is trimmed away after the suture is inserted. Potenza[53] emphasizes that an adhesion is produced at each point of trauma. The Bunnell figure-of-eight buried suture (Fig. 18–15B) or the Bunnell pull-out wire technique (Fig. 18–15A) may be utilized. The latter is preferable for suturing of the flexor tendon to the terminal phalanx and for the repair of extensor tendon injuries on the dorsum of the hand. Interrupted sutures, 5–0 or 6–0 have been recommended for tendon repair by Verdan[67] and Mason[44] and are the method of choice for repairing extensor tendons

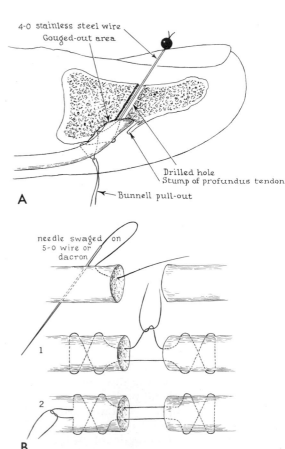

Figure 18–15. *The technique of tendon repair. A, Bunnell pull-out technique using 4–0 or No. 34 wire. B(2), Bunnell figure-of-eight tendon suture using 5–0 wire or Dacron. B(1), Technique modified to allow knot to be tied within the anastomosis.*

over the metacarpophalangeal and interphalangeal joints since wire sutures in
these locations irritate the skin and may
require removal.

Flexor Tendon Injuries

**Distal Third of the Forearm and
Wrist.** The flexor profundus tendons, the
flexor carpi radialis and the flexor carpi
ulnaris are repaired with a figure-of-eight
5–0 wire suture. A fold of synovium is interposed between the flexor profundus and
superficialis tendons are repaired with interrupted sutures of 6–0 wire in order to
produce a minimum of scarring between
the superficialis and profundus tendons.
Verdan[67] and other investigators have suggested not repairing the flexor superficialis
tendons at this level; certainly repair is not
recommended in the badly contused or
contaminated wound, but one should strive
for the ideal and repair all injured structures when possible.

Carpal Canal. Lacerations through the
transverse carpal ligament usually produce
extensive damage. Division of all the flexor
tendons and the median nerve is not uncommon. Adequate exploration and repair
demands excellent exposure, which usually requires extension of the wound into the
forearm and palm (Fig. 18–11B). The flexor
profundus tendons to the fingers and the
long thumb flexor are repaired with figure-
of-eight 5–0 wire sutures. Repair of the
flexor superficialis tendons should not be
performed if the flexor profundus tendons
are intact. Opinion differs as to whether the
flexor superficialis tendons should be re-

paired in the presence of divided flexor
profundus tendons. Repair of the flexor superficialis tendons, if undertaken, should
be accomplished with interrupted sutures
of 6–0 wire or 6–0 Ethiflex.

**Long Thumb Flexor in the Thenar
Area.** Testing sensation and opposition
and abduction is essential since lacerations
in the thenar area frequently divide the
volar digital nerves to the thumb and the
motor branch of the median nerve. Primary
repair of the tendon injury is accomplished
if not contraindicated by wound considerations. Retraction of the proximal tendon
above the wrist and difficulty in exposing
the point of tendon injury are the major
problems. The transverse carpal ligament
may be divided and the area of division
exposed after identification of the median
nerve (Figs. 18–16B and 18–17B), or a mid-
lateral thumb incision carried across the
palm, allowing retraction of the superficial
head of the short thumb flexor, may be
utilized (Fig. 18–17A). The latter incision
is used for secondary tendon repair and
tendon grafting in the thumb and, in most
instances, eliminates the need for dividing
the transverse carpal ligament. The tendon
is repaired with a figure-of-eight suture of
5–0 wire. An alternative technique is to use
a 4–0 pull-out wire suture placed proximal
to the laceration and several 6–0 wire sutures to approximate the tendon ends.

**Long Thumb Flexor within the Flexor
Tendon Sheath.** The results of primary
repair of the long thumb flexor within the
tendon sheath warrant this procedure. The
repair is accomplished with interrupted
fine wire sutures, and that portion of the

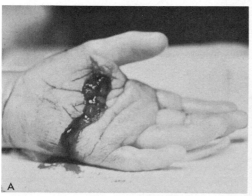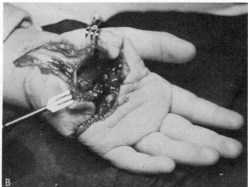

Figure 18–16. *A, Photograph illustrates laceration of palm of the hand. B, Method of extending the laceration proximally with division of transverse carpal ligament in order to expose the divided flexor tendons and the median nerve.*

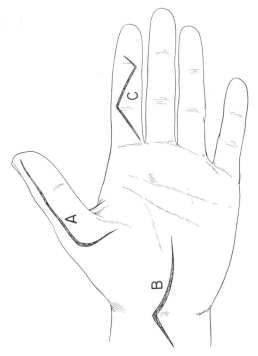

Figure 18–17. *A, Diagram illustrates incision for exposure of the flexor pollicis longus tendon within the thumb. B, Incision for exposure of flexor tendons and median nerve within carpal canal. C, Bruner zigzag incision for exposure of flexor tendons within the finger.*

sheath overlying the juncture is excised. A pulley mechanism must be retained either over the proximal phalanx or over the metacarpophalangeal joint. The tendon ad-

vancement technique is the procedure of choice for lacerations near the insertion of the long thumb flexor and yields good results if no more than 10 to 15 mm. shortening of the tendon is required.

Flexor Superficialis Tendon Alone. Careful exploration is required to rule out injury to the profundus tendon. The flexor superficialis tendon is not repaired except in certain skilled artisans who require function of both the superficialis and profundus tendons. The best functional result is achieved by carefully controlled early motion. If one elects to repair the flexor digitorum superficialis, he must be reasonably certain that he will not compromise the function of the flexor profundus in the process.

Flexor Profundus Alone. Primary repair of flexor profundus tendon lacerations yields good results in the presence of an intact flexor superficialis tendon, provided the wound is ideal. The Bruner zigzag incision[12] (Fig. 18–17C) may be used as an alternative to the standard midaxial approach in order to incorporate the wound into the incision. The advancement technique (Fig. 18–18), using the Bunnell pullout wire to anchor the tendon to the terminal phalanx, gives better results than tendon anastomosis but may be employed only if the distal stump of the profundus is short, i.e., 15 mm. in the index finger, and 10 mm. in the middle, ring and little fingers. Slight active motion may be initiated as

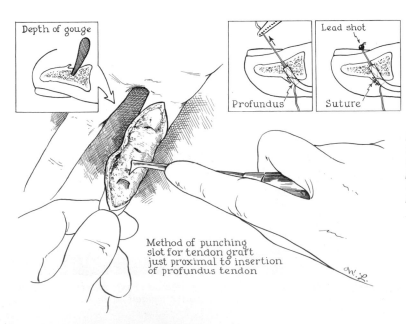

Figure 18–18. *Diagram illustrates Bunnell pull-out wire suture for advancement of flexor profundus tendon or for attaching a tendon graft to the terminal phalanx.*

early as 12 days following tendon advancement. Excision of an intact flexor superficialis tendon is never done under any circumstances. Secondary tendon grafting is the procedure of choice when the wound is less than ideal if a good passive range of motion persists in the distal interphalangeal joint.

Flexor Profundus and Flexor Superficialis Tendons within the · Flexor Tendon Sheath of the Finger.   The area of the flexor tendon sheath of the finger called "no man's land" by Bunnell,[42] the critical zone by Littler[42] and "the area of the expert" by Verdan,[67] represents the most difficult area in which to achieve a satisfactory end result following the division of both tendons. Primary repair may be attempted with reasonable anticipation of success in children under the age of 12. At the other end of the chronological spectrum, Boyes reports results with tendon grafting in patients over 50 years to be no better than with primary repair.[9] Thus, the area of contention involves the group between children and those over 50. Two schools of thought exist regarding definitive treatment of these patients: whether to perform primary repair or close the wound and tendon graft the profundus in 4 to 6 weeks. All authorities agree that simple wound closure is the treatment of choice when dealing with a less than ideal wound.

The best results of primary repair have been reported by Verdan[67] and Kleinert.[38] Both emphasize that the technique should be performed only by the skilled hand surgeon, under ideal circumstances, and with meticulous technique. Kleinert[38] excises only enough sheath to permit the anastomosis to glide freely (Fig. 18–19) and performs the suture with a modified Bunnell criss-cross combined with a running 6–0 or 7– Dexon, Ticron or monofilament nylon to the tendon edges. When circumstances preclude primary repair in an otherwise ideal situation, Madsen[43] has recommended wound cleansing and dressing, followed by delayed primary repair within a period of 7 days, provided the wound remains clean without drainage or infection.

Wakefield[68] doubts that conditions are ever ideal for primary repair in "no man's land," except possibly in children 4 to 6 years old, and states: "Some surgeons are endeavoring to perfect a technique which

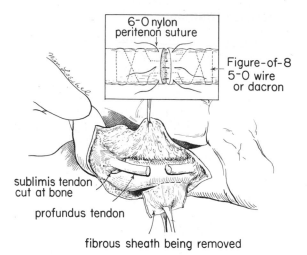

Figure 18–19.   *Method for primary repair of the flexor profundus tendon. Modified after techniques of Verdan and Kleinert.*

will permit successful primary repair within 'No man's Land.' Although prospects seem to offer some promise, the method is not of general application. Tendon grafting in this situation gives vastly superior results in most surgeon's hands." Verdan[67] reports that 50 per cent of his primary repairs and approximately 50 per cent of his tendon grafts in "no man's land" flex to within 3 cm. of the distal palmar crease; one third of the primarily repaired tendons required tenolysis. Boyes[8] reported the results of primary repair in a selected series of ideal injuries in 12 patients. Forty-three per cent of these flexed to within 4.0 cm. of the distal palmar crease; whereas, in a group of patients with secondary tendon grafts done under ideal conditions, all flexed to within 2.5 cm. of the distal palmar crease.[10] Dupont and Crikelair[26] reviewed the repairs done by resident surgeons on the Surgical Service at their hospital: of 33 primary repairs in "no man's land," three patients obtained a good result; of 23 tendon grafts, 21 patients obtained a good result. Van't Hof and Heiple[66] reviewed the current literature on this subject and reported that, of primarily repaired tendons, 38 per cent flexed to 2.5 cm. of the palm and 57 per cent flexed to within 4.0 of the distal palmar crease. Lister et al.,[41] achieved an excellent or good result in 75 percent of primary repairs in "no man's land" in 28 patients (flexion to within 1.5 cm. distal palmar crease and not more than 30° lack of extension).

Tendon Grafting

The major criterion determining the suitable time for tendon grafting is the softness and pliability of the wound. With proper wound care, the tissues may be satisfactory within the 4 to 6 weeks of the initial injury. On the other hand, massage, passive stretching and soaking of the hand may be required for a significantly longer period of time before the tissues become soft and pliable.

The sources of a tendon graft are listed preferentially as follows:

1. Palmaris longus.
2. Plantaris.
3. Extensor digitorum communis of index.
4. Extensor indicis proprius.
5. Common extensors of the second, third and fourth toes.

The palmaris longus is absent in 14 per cent and the plantaris in 7 per cent of the population. Considerable dissection is required in removing the common toe extensors, particularly if a long graft is needed. The common toe extensors fuse at the ankle, and sharp dissection is necessary to isolate a single tendon. The muscle belly of the extensor indicis proprius frequently extends to the wrist. For these reasons, the common extensor of the index finger is preferred in the absence of a palmaris longus. The extensor digitorum communis of the index finger is readily available; it provides a long graft; and no disability results from its sacrifice since the extensor indicis proprius provides full extension of the index finger. Sharp dissection is required to section the juncture tendinum.

A midaxial incision on the radial side of the index finger or on the ulnar aspect of the middle, ring and little fingers together with a separate incision in the palm are utilized for tendon grafting. If the original wound lends itself to a zigzag incision, this approach may be used instead. An associated digital nerve injury may determine whether the radial or ulnar aspect of the finger is explored. Better exposure is achieved by a continuous incision along the mid-lateral line of the finger and across the palm if the laceration is in the region of the metacarpophalangeal joint or the base of the proximal phalanx. In this area, sharp

dissection is required to excise the tendon sheath and remove the stumps of the divided tendons. Adequate removal of scar is essential to a good result. In some instances, scarring may be so severe that the surgeon must content himself with excision of the fibro-osseous canal, all the flexor tendon remnants and no reconstruction. In such instances, 4 to 6 months are allowed for complete healing, following which the flexor profundus tendon and new pulleys are provided by tendon grafts. An alternative approach to the badly scarred finger involves the insertion of a silastic tendon prosthesis at the time of scar and tendon excision.[30] The formation of a synovium-lined sheath about the prosthesis greatly simplifies the second stage of the reconstruction and appears to improve the functional result.

The flexor superficialis tendon stump is not removed if it has healed smoothly, as is so often the case with division of the tendon immediately proximal to the vincula. The flexor superficialis tendon must be excised to within a few millimeters of its insertion in the presence of dense scar for it may be limiting flexion of the proximal interphalangeal joint.

The amount of tendon sheath excised is determined by the degree of scarring within the sheath. In those instances in which the flexor superficialis tendon is intact and the graft is being inserted for flexor profundus action, the sheath usually is beautifully intact, and only that amount necessary to allow removal of the distal flexor profundus stump and exposure of the proximal stump for anastomosis need be resected. The sheath is subjected to minimal surgical trauma by passing the tendon graft blindly with a small probe or ureteral catheter. The sheath must be reduced to a two-pulley system, one at the base of the proximal phalanx and one over the middle phalanx, when dealing with a severely scarred or completely collapsed sheath.

Passive excursion of the flexor profundus tendon is tested prior to performing the proximal anastomosis. A passive excursion of 35 mm. in the adult with the tourniquet elevated (measured by grasping the relaxed proximal cut tendon end and stretching distally, the wrist in neutral position) is equivalent to an active excursion of 55 to 60 mm. with the normal range (demonstrated by repair under local anesthesia; tendon stretched to maximum length with the wrist in neutral position; patient asked to flex the finger).[24]

The proximal anastomosis is performed with a figure-of-eight suture of 4–0 or 5–0 wire. The figure-of-eight suture technique allows the anastomosis to lie at the point of origin of the lumbrical muscle from the profundus tendon and to recede proximally into an area not traumatized by dissection. The lumbrical muscle is excised if badly scarred. The graft is passed through an area of normal synovial tissue within the carpal canal and the anastomosis performed proximal to the wrist if a good range of passive motion cannot be obtained by moderate dissection in the proximal palm.

The proper tension for the tendon graft is determined by placing the palm flat on the table with the wrist in neutral position and the fingers extended, stretching the graft distally as tautly as possible, and marking the point on the graft corresponding to the insertion of the flexor profundus tendon into the distal phalanx. If 35 mm. of passive excursion have been demonstrated in the profundus muscle-tendon unit, the graft tension is adjusted so that the finger rests in a normal position of function. With less than 35 mm. of passive excursion, the graft tension is increased correspondingly so that the finger rests in more than normal flexion; in this instance, complete extension may not be obtained.

The distal anastomosis of the tendon graft is performed by anchoring the graft to a slot in the terminal phalanx beneath the stump of the flexor profundus tendon with a figure-of-eight pull-out suture of 4–0 wire (Fig. 18–18). A sharpened dental root extractor provides an excellent instrument for creating the slot in the terminal phalanx. Injury to the volar plate of the distal interphalangeal joint in dissecting up the stump of the flexor profundus tendon must be avoided to prevent adherence of the graft at this point, with subsequent lack of flexion of the distal phalanx. A single knot is tied over the button on the terminal phalanx and the position of the finger tested before excising any excess graft. The stump of the flexor profundus is sutured to the graft with interrupted sutures of 6–0 Mersilene. The pull-out wire is brought out through a single skin opening near the tendon insertion. This distal position of the pull-out wire minimizes irritation and

allows for better motion of the graft within the sheath than if the wire lies along the graft and exits over the middle phalanx.

Flexor tendon repairs and tendon grafts are immobilized with the wrist and fingers in slight flexion for 3 weeks. The hand is examined frequently to be certain that adjacent fingers are not becoming stiff. Slight passive extension of the proximal interphalangeal joint of the injured finger with the metacarpophalangeal joint held in flexion can be performed at the end of the second week. Protected active motion within the splint is begun at 2½ weeks, and graded active motion without the splint is allowed at 3 weeks. The suture is removed at the fourth week.

The minimum age at which tendon grafting may be performed successfuly is debatable. A minimum age of 5 years has been suggested by some; however, it must be realized that a finger lacking flexor tendon function does not grow normally, and operation at a younger age may be desirable. The senior author has performed tendon grafting successfully in a 13-month-old child.

Pulvertaft[54] reports a successful case of tendon grafting performed 17 years following the initial injury. In long-standing cases it may be necessary to use an adjacent flexor superficialis as the motor. The flexor profundus motor may be used if the tendon has been adherent within the finger and acting as a flexor of the metacarpophalangeal joint. In such instances, the tendon sheath must be reduced to a two-pulley system because of the absence of synovium within the sheath.

Extensor Tendon Injuries

The Bunnell pull-out wire technique, augmented by a few interrupted 6–0 sutures at the anastomosis, is the method of choice for the repair of extensor tendon injuries on the dorsum of the hand. Repair of the extensor mechanism over the metacarpophalangeal or interphalangeal joints is accomplished with 6–0 silk or Mersilene to avoid possible skin irritation by wire sutures. Splinting protects the sutured tendon.

Extensor tendon injuries distal to the wrist are immobilized for 3 weeks, with the wrist and metacarpophalangeal joints in moderate extension and the proximal in-

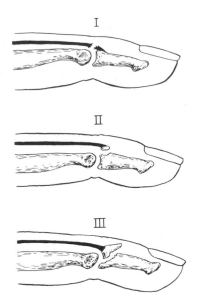

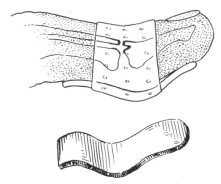

Figure 18–21. *Mallet finger with rupture of extensor tendon treated on a biconcave aluminum splint with a Band-Aid immobilizing only the distal interphalangeal joint. (Redrawn after Milford, L.: Campbell's Operative Orthopaedics. 4th ed. St. Louis, The C. V. Mosby Co., 1963.)*

Figure 18–20. *The three types of closed injury to the extensor tendon and its insertion to the terminal phalanx that produces the mallet finger deformity.*

terphalangeal joints in slight flexion. Extension of the wrist is maintained for four weeks following repair of the wrist extensors.

Mallet Finger. Mallet finger is produced by three types of closed injury (Fig. 18–20) in addition to open laceration of the extensor tendon inserting at the base of the terminal phalanx. Lacerations should be repaired by suturing of the tendon and immobilization of the distal interphalangeal joint in extension, either by splinting or Kirschner wire fixation.

1. Rupture of the extensor tendon or laceration of the distal interphalangeal joint.
2. Avulsion of a small fragment of bone with the extensor tendon.
3. Avulsion of a large segment of the articular surface with the extensor tendon.

Rupture of the extensor tendon (Type I) only and avulsion of a small fragment of bone with the extensor tendon (Type II) are treated by aluminum splint immobilization of the distal interphalangeal joint in slight hyperextension for 6 to 8 weeks (Milford[46]) (Fig. 18–21). The proximal interphalangeal joint is not immobilized. Patients lacking extension at the distal interphalangeal joint after a 2- to 4-week period of improper splinting usually will achieve a good result

following 8 weeks of splinting with progressively increased hyperextension of the distal interphalangeal joint. Some patients will respond to this course of treatment as long as 3 months after injury, provided slight active extension of the distal interphalangeal joint can be demonstrated prior to splinting.

Avulsion of a large segment of the articular surface (Type III) is managed by open reduction and Kirschner wire fixation (Fig. 18–22).

Tenolysis. Tenolysis is a very useful and rewarding procedure for dealing with tendon injuries in which a good functional result has not been achieved following primary repair, physiotherapy, dynamic splinting and active usage.

The procedure demands meticulous removal of all scar tissue and precise hemostasis. Active and passive motion is initiated within 72 hours postoperatively and

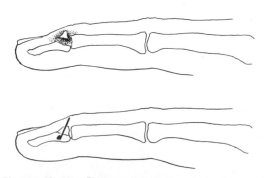

Figure 18–22. *Diagram illustrates reduction and Kirschner wire fixation of a large bone fragment avulsed from the base of the distal phalanx.*

consists of placing the finger through a full range of motion once daily. The finger is splinted between these brief periods of exercise in order to prevent a recurrence of adhesions secondary to the reaction produced by this tendon moving through a fresh wound. Rubber band traction may be utilized to stretch a finger into extension following tenolysis; the traction is removed and the finger placed actively and passively through a full range of motion once daily. Active exercise is gradually increased.

PERIPHERAL NERVES

Primary repair of peripheral nerve injuries is preferred to secondary repair when there is a clean, sharp laceration (Onné).[51] Lack of retraction of the nerve and the absence of a neuroma proximally and a glioma distally significantly reduce the amount of gap to be overcome. Secondary nerve suture is reserved for crushing and mangling injuries and situations in which a skilled surgeon is not available to perform the neurorrhaphy. If primary repair cannot be accomplished, the nerve is united with a single suture in the epineurium to prevent retraction. Repair should be performed as soon as the wound will allow — if at all possible, no later than 6 months after injury.[15] Considerable care must be observed in serially sectioning the nerve proximally and distally until an area of minimal intraneural scarring is encountered, and equal care must be observed in properly aligning the fascicles at the time of suturing. Sunderland[63] has pointed out that the fascicular pattern is constant for only 5 mm. in the median nerve. Onné[51] noted no difference in the results when comparing primary repair with secondary suture performed within 6 months of the injury. Seddon[58] strongly advocated secondary suture on the basis of electively choosing the incision for exposure, ease of determining the amount of damaged nerve and ease of suturing provided by the thickened nerve sheath. Certainly this is the procedure of choice in treating battle casualties, but most civilian injuries can be repaired primarily.

A gap of 2.5 to 4.0 cm. in the median and ulnar nerves at the wrist can be overcome simply by immobilizing the wrist in flexion. A gap of 10 cm. in the ulnar nerve can be overcome by mobilization of the motor branches and transplantation of the nerve anterior to the elbow joint. A gap of 7.5 cm. in the median nerve can be overcome by mobilization of the motor branches and transplantation of the nerve anterior to the pronator teres; flexion of the elbow will relax the tension on the suture line at the wrist. A nerve graft must be employed if the gap is greater than 10 cm. in the ulnar nerve or 7.5 cm. in the median nerve. Zachary[71] has emphasized that a successful outcome is unlikely following resection of a 5 cm. segment of nerve. The superior results reported by Millesi[47] will undoubtedly encourage surgeons to graft nerve gaps of smaller distances than these figures. The critical aspects of his technique are high magnification, topographical mapping of the nerve ends, resection of the epineurium, a minimum of fine sutures carefully placed and the absolute absence of tension. The suture material utilized for neurorrhaphy must be as fine and unreactive as possible. Most specialists now recommend size 9–0 or 10–0 nylon for epineural and interfascicular suturing. Precise placement of such material requires good quality magnifying loupes at the very least. Many authors advocate the operating microscope.

The suture material utilized for neurorrhaphy must be as fine and unreactive as possible. The technical difficulties encountered in using very fine wire lead most specialists to recommend nylon or silk, sizes 6–0 or 7–0. The sutures are placed only in the nerve sheath (Fig. 18–23).

The wrist is splinted in flexion for a minimum of 4 weeks following nerve repair. Abnormal tension on the suture line during

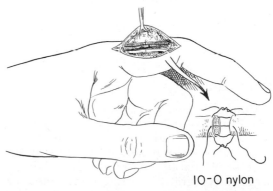

10-0 nylon

Figure 18–23. Drawing illustrates technique of peripheral nerve repair using epineurial suture.

the subsequent 4-week period is prevented by weekly application of a new dorsal plaster splint, and the amount of extension at the wrist is progressively increased until full extension is attained.

Repair of the digital nerve is mandatory and, if possible, should be accomplished primarily. Secondary suture of digital nerves divided in the palm frequently is impossible because of retraction of the nerve ends and the resection imposed by the neuroma and glioma. Nerve grafts are frequently necessary at this level. Repair of digital nerve injuries as far distally as the distal interphalangeal joint is possible.

Nicholson and Seddon[49] reviewed 305 nerve repairs in 277 patients in civilian practice. When the injury was at the wrist level, two out of three sutures of the median nerve were followed by useful motor recovery and four out of five times there was a good sensory recovery. The results of ulnar nerve suture at the wrist were slightly better, with four out of five making useful sensory and motor recovery; in one case out of three some degree of lateral movement of the fingers was regained.

The causes for failure to achieve a satisfactory result following nerve repair may be summarized as follows:

1. Excessive elapsed time between injury and repair. (Zachary and Holmes[72] reported 15 months to be the maximum interval compatible with a satisfactory result.)

2. Excessive nerve gap to be overcome. (Zachary[71] reported that a gap of more than 7 cm. yields a poor result.)

3. Excessive mobilization of the nerve being repaired. (Nicholson and Seddon[49] indicated that local mobilization with flexion of the wrist and elbow yields better results than transposition.)

4. Failure to adequately resect the neuroma and glioma.

5. Failure to properly align the motor and sensory fibers.

6. Postoperative suture line separation.

Nerve Grafts

Bunnell[16] described successful digital nerve grafts, and Bunnell and Boyes extended the technique to larger nerves.[17] They also demonstrated experimentally that small cable grafts survive whereas large nerve grafts, the size of the median

and ulnar nerves, undergo fibrosis before the growing axons reach the distal anastomosis. A nerve graft for the digital nerve can be obtained from the sural nerve or the lateral antebrachial cutaneous nerve. The sural nerve can provide multiple strands or nerve graft to allow for grafting larger nerves such as the median, ulnar or radial. Seddon[59] reported a 50 per cent success rate (69 per cent, if the partial successes are counted) in a series of 107 nerve grafts. The successful results compared favorably with the best results following direct suture; the partially successful results provided return of useful sensory and motor function; and the failures exhibited no functional benefit from the procedure. Millesi[47] reported his series of repair in 33 median and 32 ulnar nerves in 1972 using his technique for bridging the gap with multiple strands of sural nerve. His results indicate better quality of sensory and motor return in a greater number of patients than has heretofore been reported for any other method.

Nerve Compression Syndromes

Compression of peripheral nerves, whether acute or chronic, may result in pain, numbness and motor weakness. Failure to recognize and treat such compression may lead to swelling, stiffness and even causalgia. The most common site of compression of the median nerve is in the carpal canal, where it may produce the carpal tunnel syndrome. Carpal tunnel syndrome can result from fractures, sprains, burns, crush injuries and lacerations around the wrist. Treatment consists of incision of the transverse carpal ligament. Internal neurolysis of the median nerve should also be performed if there is evidence of thickening and scarring of the epineurium. On rare occasions, the median nerve may also be compressed by the pronator teres muscle.

The ulnar nerve may also be compressed and may produce similar symptoms. The most common sites are at the wrist (in Guyon's canal) and at the elbow. Decompression, sometimes combined with neurolysis, is usually sufficient treatment, although translocation is sometimes employed at the elbow.

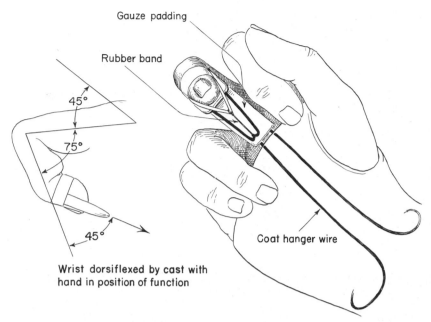

Gauze padding

Rubber band

45°

75°

45°

Wrist dorsiflexed by cast with
hand in position of function

Coat hanger wire

Figure 18–24. Drawing illustrates technique of using rubber band traction for fracture of phalanges and metacarpals. Insert shows angles which metacarpophalangeal and interphalangeal joints should assume during
traction. Note that coat hanger wire is molded to fit finger. The traction should immobilize only and not distract
the fracture site.

BONES AND JOINTS

Principles of Fracture Management

The optimal treatment of fractures involving the metacarpals and phalanges
achieves correct alignment, allows early
movement and prevents joint stiffness and
adherence of tendons. Correct alignment
usually may be achieved only at the time of
the initial manipulation. Closed manipulation, whenever possible, is preferable to
open reduction. The reduction is maintained by a molded plaster splint, the hand
splint suggested by Bohler[4] (Fig. 18–24) or,
if necessary, by traction or Kirschner wire
fixation. A Kirschner wire may be inserted
percutaneously under direct vision or at the
time of open reduction.

Malalignment produces malfunction.
Rotation at the fracture site in the metacarpal or phalanx may cause scissoring of the
fingers and malposition of a fractured phalanx is a frequent cause of adherent flexor
and extensor tendons. Pre- and post-
reduction radiographs are essential but do
not replace functional evaluation. Rotation
at the fracture site may not be detected on
the x-rays but becomes immediately appar-

ent on the basis of scissoring of the flexed
fingers.

The wrist and fingers are splinted in the
position of function. Motion, if only once
daily, is initiated in the fractured finger as
soon as possible.

Metacarpal. SIMPLE FRACTURE WITH-
OUT DISPLACEMENT. In the absence of
instability at the fracture site, treatment
consists of a volar plaster splint to the level
of the metacarpophalangeal joint. Active
motion of the fingers is allowed, but activity
is limited until the pain and swelling have
disappeared.

BASE OF THE THUMB METACARPAL
(BENNETT'S FRACTURE). Closed reduction is obtained by forcing the thumb metacarpal into opposition and abduction. It is
rarely possible to maintain the reduction
with the thumb in this position. James[33]
transfixes the thumb and index metacarpals
with a Kirschner wire, maintaining the reduction by thumb opposition (Fig. 18–25).
Traction has been suggested by others.
Open reduction with Kirschner wire fixation is indicated if reduction and fixation
cannot be achieved by closed manipulation
(Fig. 18–25). The recently introduced small
fragment instruments and appliances have

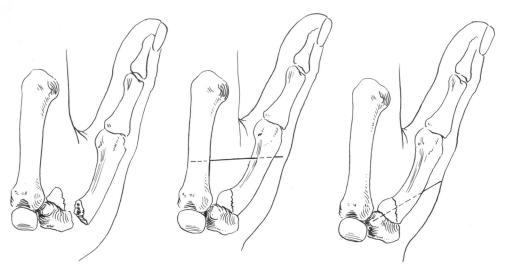

Figure 18–25. *Alternate techniques of immobilization of Bennett's fracture of first metacarpal. Kirschner wire fixation can be used with closed reduction or open reduction.*

been especially effective in treating metacarpal fractures.

OBLIQUE FRACTURES OF THE SHAFT. Closed reduction is preferred. Immobili-

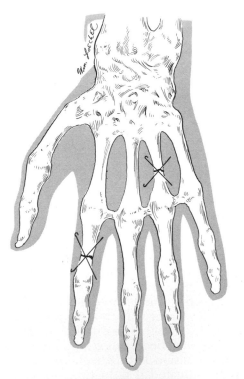

Figure 18–26. *Drawing illustrates use of fine Kirschner wires for immobilization of fracture of phalanx and metacarpal. If possible, wires should be inserted so as to allow joint motion while fracture is being immobilized. Criss-cross technique is also useful in metacarpal fracture.*

zation is by means of a plaster splint to the palm if the fracture is stable and without rotation or by Kirschner wire fixation (Fig. 18–26). Instability, rotatory deformity or inability to maintain length requires correction by closed or open reduction.

TRANSVERSE FRACTURE OF THE SHAFT. Closed reduction and immobilization occasionally may be accomplished. Open reduction and Kirschner wire fixation are frequently required as a result of the instability of the fracture. In testing the functional result following reduction, it is important to recall that all fingers point to the tubercle of the scaphoid when forced into full flexion at the metacarpophalangeal and proximal interphalangeal joints (Fig. 18–27). Axial rotation also is evaluated by examining the plane of the fingernails.

FRACTURE OF THE HEAD. Fractures of the distal metacarpal near the head usually are impacted. Volar angulation of as much as 30 degrees at the fracture site in the fourth and fifth metacarpals is compatible with an excellent functional result because of the mobility of these metacarpals, and treatment consists of immobilization in a volar plaster splint to prevent excessive use of the hand until the pain and swelling have disappeared. Lack of full flexion at the fourth and fifth metacarpophalangeal joints indicates excessive angulation at the fracture site and requires closed or open reduction. The index and middle fingers tolerate less angulation at the fracture site and require open reduction with Kirschner wire

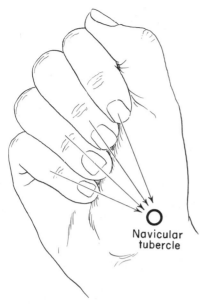

Figure 18–27. *Diagram illustrates that when fingers are fully flexed at metacarpophalangeal and proximal interphalangeal joints all fingers point to tubercle of navicular. Axial rotation at fracture site is detected by the horizontal plane of fingernail.*

a dorsal concavity resulting from angulation at the fracture site (Fig. 18–29). The adequacy of closed reduction is evaluated on the basis of active extension of the fingers: failure of full extension at the proximal interphalangeal joint indicates an unsatisfactory reduction. Open reduction with Kirschner wire fixation usually is required and is accomplished through a dorsal incision with splitting of the extensor tendon in the midline. A slight amount of dorsal concavity as a result of improper reduction prevents full extension because of a tendon imbalance in the extensor mechanism. Fractures through this cancellous area usually heal within 3 to 4 weeks.

SHAFT. A linear fracture may be treated by taping the injured finger to an adjacent finger. Open reduction is required for spiral fractures with rotation and for transverse fractures with displacement at the fracture site. Open reduction and internal fixation with Kirschner wires is accomplished through a dorsal incision and exposure of the fracture site by splitting the extensor tendon in the midline. Early motion in flexion and extension is allowed. Healing may be complete within 5 to 7 weeks.

DISTAL. Open reduction is necessary to properly position the fracture fragments when there has been a fracture of one or

fixation if proper alignment cannot be achieved by closed manipulation (Fig. 18–28).

Proximal Phalanx. BASE. The proximal third of the proximal phalanx frequently is the site of a compression fracture, with

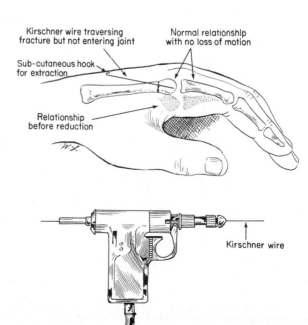

Figure 18–28. *Drawing illustrates method of inserting Kirschner wires for fixation of fracture of head of 1st metacarpal. Note use of electric motor to facilitate insertion of fine wire.*

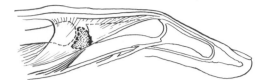

Figure 18–29. *Deformity with impacted fracture of base of proximal phalanx. Dorsal concavity produces imbalance preventing full active extension at proximal interphalangeal joint.*

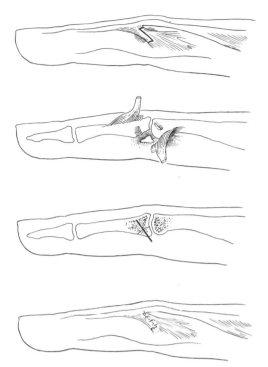

Figure 18–31. *Diagram illustrates technique of step cutting the retinacular ligament and removal of the lateral capsular ligament for exposure of the proximal interphalangeal joint and fracture fragment, with Kirschner wire fixation of fracture.*

both condyles (Fig. 18–30). Open reduction is accomplished through a mid-lateral incision with division of the retinacular ligament. Exposure of the lateral aspect of the joint and condyle is accomplished by removal of a portion of the capsular ligament (Fig. 18–31). Anchoring of the fracture fragment with Kirschner wire is performed under direct visualization of the joint surface. Repair of the collateral ligament may not be possible, but the retinacular ligament is always repaired.

Middle Phalanx. BASE. Subluxation of the proximal interphalangeal joint and injury to the lateral and volar capsules usually occur with fractures of the base of the middle phalanx. The capsular injury produces considerable swelling of the proximal interphalangeal joint. Severe disability due to joint stiffness results from improper treatment. Closed manipulation is attempted by placing the proximal in-

terphalangeal joint in 70 to 80 degrees of flexion. The traction technique described by Robertson et al.[56] is the method of choice for treating markedly comminuted fractures (Fig. 18–32). Open reduction is ac-

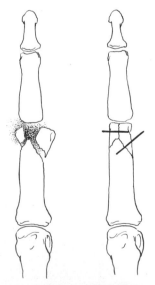

Figure 18–30. *Kirschner wire fixation following open reduction of T-type fracture of the condyles of the proximal phalanx.*

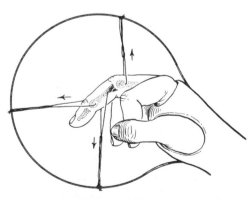

Figure 18–32. *Method of Robertson, Cawley and Faris for treatment of acute fracture-dislocation of the proximal interphalangeal joint, with traction from Kirschner wire in proximal and middle phalanges. (Curtis, R. M.: Joints of the hand. In Flynn, J. E. (ed.): Hand Surgery. © 1966, The Williams & Wilkins Co., Baltimore.)*

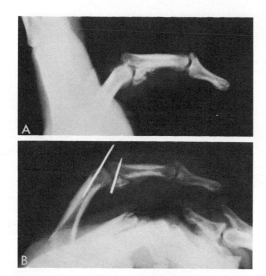

Figure 18-33. *A, Fracture-dislocation of proximal interphalangeal joint. B, Open reduction and Kirschner wire fixation of fracture with temporary Kirschner wire to prevent recurrence of subluxation. (Curtis, R. M.: Joints of the hand. In Flynn, J. E. (ed.): Hand Surgery. © 1966, The Williams & Wilkins Co., Baltimore.)*

complished through a midlateral incision, with division of the retinacular ligament and resection of the lateral capsular ligament to gain exposure of the proximal interphalangeal joint (Fig. 18–31). The reduction is maintained by Kirschner wire fixation (Fig. 18–33); lateral stability of the joint is provided by repair of the retinacular ligament. An additional Kirschner wire may be utilized to hold the proximal interphalangeal joint in slight flexion for 4 to 6 days (Fig. 18–26). Protected active motion is initiated within 5 to 7 days. Chronic fracture-dislocations in this area require capsulectomy to achieve reduction of the fragment and flexion of the proximal interphalangeal joint.[25]

SHAFT. Open reduction and Kirschner wire fixation (Fig. 18–26) are frequently required because of the severe displacement produced by the pull of the flexor superficialis on the proximal fragment. Linear, nondisplaced fractures and fractures proximal to the insertion of the flexor superficialis may be treated simply by using an adjacent finger as a splint.

DISTAL. The fracture usually is T-type with separation of one or both condyles from the middle phalanx. Open reduction with Kirschner wire fixation is accomplished through either a midlateral or dor-

sal incision. The Kirschner wire should be inserted in a manner that will permit early motion.

Distal Phalanx. BASE. Fractures producing large fragments involving a third or a half of the articular surface demand open reduction and Kirschner wire fixation (Fig. 18–22). Avulsion of a bone fragment volarly with the flexor profundus tendon requires immediate surgery consisting of fixation of the fragment with a Bunnell pull-out suture of 4–0 wire. T-type fractures of the base of the distal phalanx are managed by closed or open reduction; proper alignment of the articular surface is essential to a satisfactory result.

SHAFT AND TUFT. Fractures in this area are treated by means of simple splinting of the distal interphalangeal joint for 3 to 4 weeks. Radiographical evaluation frequently suggests nonunion although clinically the fracture is stable.

Dislocation

Carpometacarpal Joints. Closed manipulation rarely is successful in treating this severly disabling injury. Inadequate reduction of the metacarpal bases as seen on a lateral x-ray is indication for immediate open reduction with Kirschner wire fixation. Severe muscle and tendon imbalance with inability to flex the metacarpophalangeal joint follows improper treatment (Fig. 18–34).

Metacarpophalangeal Joint. FINGERS. Closed reduction should be attempted but infrequently is prevented by interposition of either joint capsule, natatory ligament or tendon (Kaplan[36]). Open reduction is indicated if there is any question as to whether a satisfactory reduction has been achieved.

THUMB. Closed manipulation should be attempted but should be followed by open management if the reduction is not entirely satisfactory. Exposure of the joint through a dorsal incision is accomplished by splitting the extensor tendon and retracting the extensor pollicis brevis. The reduction may be maintained with Kirschner wire fixation, if necessary.

Rupture of the ulnar collateral ligament of the metacarpophalangeal joint of the thumb may produce ulnar instability (gamekeeper's thumb) and requires open reduction (Stener[61]).

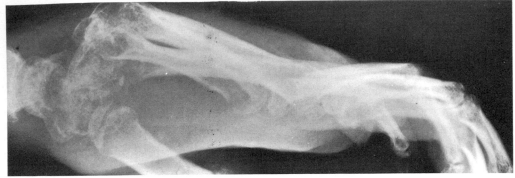

Figure 18–34. *Carpometacarpal dislocation. Radiograph shows bases of middle, ring and little finger meta-carpals dislocated on the carpus. Muscle and tendon imbalance produce hyperextension of proximal phalanx on metacarpal head and flexion at proximal interphalangeal joints. (Curtis, R. M.: Joints of the hand. In Flynn, J. E. (ed.): Hand Surgery. © 1966, The Williams & Wilkins Co., Baltimore.)*

Sprain

Finger sprains represent partial tears of the capsular ligament secondary to overangulation of the joint. Early treatment consists of splinting the finger in the position of function for 3 weeks; the patient removes the splint once daily after the first week and performs slight, active extension and flexion. Aspiration of the joint for hemarthrosis may be indicated early. Injuries seen late exhibit stiffness secondary to thickening of the colateral ligament; pain may be a prominent complaint. Relief of pain in chronic cases may be provided by the injection into the joint of 2 ml. of triamcinolone acetonide (Kenalog*).

*E. R. Squibb & Sons, Inc. New York, N.Y.

AMPUTATIONS

The two major problems encountered in dealing with amputations are adequate closure of the stump and management of the volar digital nerves. Closure of the amputation stump may be accomplished by a variety of procedures (Figs. 18–35 and 18–36).

1. Primary closure with or without resection of bone.
2. A combination of volar and dorsal flaps created by midlateral incisions.
3. A lateral or dorsal flap rotation with skin grafting of the donor area (Fig. 18–36).
4. A local or distant pedicle flap.
5. Combination of two triangular flaps

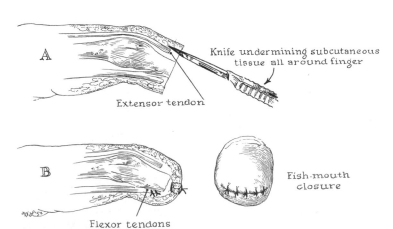

Knife undermining subcutaneous tissue all around finger

Extensor tendon

Flexor tendons sutured to sheath

Fish-mouth closure

Figure 18–35. *Closure amputation of finger by freeing dorsal and volar skin flaps. Lacerated flexor superficialis tendon sutured to tendon sheath.*

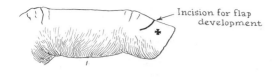

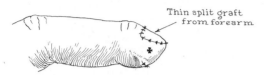

Figure 18-36. *Local rotation flap from dorsum of finger for closure of amputation.*

raised laterally from either side of the finger (Kutler method)[28] or a single volar flap on a subcutaneous pedicle.[2]

Partial thickness skin grafts do not provide adequate coverage over bone. Pedicle flaps from adjacent fingers are preferred to thick abdominal flaps. Divided volar digital nerves are placed in a drill hole in the phalanx to reduce the risk of disability from neuroma formation. Simple resection of the nerve, allowing the nerve end to retract proximally is frequently successful but may lead to compression of the neuroma between bone and objects coming in contact with the hand.

Thumb. Preservation of maximal length by all reconstructive techniques available is mandatory in most cases.

Fingers. Decisions regarding treatment must be based on considerations of the occupation and specific needs of the individual. The choice is between primary closure following resection of bone and complex reconstructive technique must be made carefully in every patient. Useful function may be retained if proper coverage can be provided with traumatic amputations through the terminal phalanx distal to the flexor and extensor tendon insertions. Amputations through the middle phalanx are best managed by shortening the phalanx and closing the wound with available skin. Care in handling the profundus tendon is necessary to avoid paradoxical extension of the proximal interphalangeal joint due to the "lumbrical plus" syndrome.[52] Maximal length is preserved with amputations through the proximal phalanx, particularly in the little finger. Retention of the proximal phalanx of the

index finger may prove a hindrance and require subsequent resection through the metacarpal.

REPLANTATION OF HANDS AND DIGITS

Jacobson and Suarez[32] introduced microvascular surgery by demonstrating the value of the operating microscope in 1960 as an aid in the repair of small blood vessels. They also developed instruments and suture materials. Further improvements in the instrumentation and suture materials were developed by Salmon and Assimacopoulos[57] and Buncke and Schulz.[13, 14] The successful anastomosis of vessels with a diameter of only 1 ml. became possible. Surgeons now had the tools for digital replantation.

The first successful complete survival of an amputated human index finger was achieved in January 1966, at the No. 6 People's Hospital of Shanghai in the People's Republic of China.[1] Komatsu and Tamai[40] reported the first successful replantation of a completely amputated thumb in 1968. Thereafter, Kleinert[39] in 1968, and O'Brien[50] in 1972 and others as well reported successful replantation of hands and digits.

Treatment of the Amputated Hands and Digits

Thumb and multiple amputations as well as wrist and transmetacarpal amputations should be replanted. With a single index finger amputation, replantation is usually not indicated. Amputated isolated digits should be replanted only under unusual circumstances such as for occupational or anesthetic reasons.

It has been demonstrated that if the totally amputated part is properly cooled, a successful result may be achieved even when 12 or more hours have elapsed before circulation is re-established in a digit and possibly longer for a hand.[69] Since the patient may be transported some distance to the replantation team and may have sustained considerable blood loss, his condition should be evaluated carefully. He should be resuscitated if necessary before transfer for surgery.

The wound should be flushed, prefera-

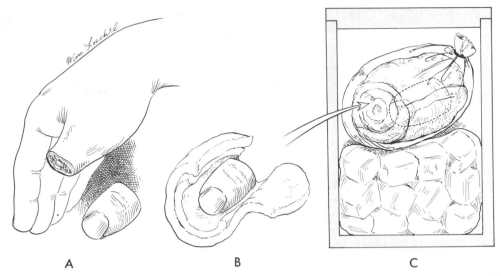

Figure 18–37. *Method of emergency care of totally amputated thumb or fingers. A, Thumb and hand. B, The amputated thumb wrapped in sterile gauze. C, Plastic bag containing amputated thumb placed in styrofoam container on top of separate plastic bag of ice cubes.*

bly with Ringer's lactated solution. Do not apply antiseptic solutions to the wound. Apply a sterile dressing, wrap the hand in soft gauze for pressure and elevate. The amputated part should be flushed, preferably with Ringer's lactated solution. Do not scrub or apply antiseptic solutions to the amputated part. Wrap the part in dry sterile gauze or towel, depending on the size, and place in a plastic bag. The part is then placed in a container, preferably styrofoam, and cooled by separate plastic bags containing ice (Fig. 18–37).

Surgical Technique. The surgical technique now employed is done by two teams when possible; while one team prepares the stump the other team prepares the amputated part. Following debridement, some bone shortening may be necessary so as to allow good vessel anastomosis without tension. When there is bone stabilization the arterial repair is carried out using 10–0 nylon with the microscope. The digital nerves are repaired with 10–0 nylon and the flexor tendons with 4–0 Prolene or Mersilene. Two dorsal veins are repaired for each artery and the extensor tendon is repaired. The skin is loosely approximated and a bulky dressing applied. Vein grafts can be used when necessary for the arterial or venous anastomoses.

The success rate in replantation varies as to whether the part is sharply amputated or severed by a crushing blow. The present survival rate for digits or hands ranges from 76 to 90 per cent.[64, 65, 69] Useful function with recovery of sensibility has been achieved in replanted hands and digits.

Contraindications for replantation may be severe crushing injuries, avulsion injuries, digits with multiple level lacerations, severe contamination and improper care of the amputated part.

Treatment of the Partially Amputated Digits and Hands

The revascularization of a partially amputated finger or thumb is of equal importance for, without one good digital vessel, survival is not likely and nor will there be good sensory recovery after digital nerve repair.

For partial amputation, flush with Ringer's lactated solution. Place the part in a functional position, apply a dry sterile dressing, soft gauze bandage and splint. Apply coolant bags to the outside of the dressing (Fig. 18–38).

Surgical Techniques. Using the microscope, the digital arteries are repaired with 10–0 nylon and the flexor and extensor tendons with 4–0 or 5–0 Prolene or Mersilene. If the dorsal veins are interrupted, at least two of these should be repaired using 10–0 nylon. Vein grafts are frequently indicated for repair of the arteries or veins in the partial amputation since the anastomosis must be achieved without tension between the ends of undamaged vessels.

INFECTION

Chemotherapy and an appreciation of the importance of hand infections have contributed equally to a decreased incidence and improved management. An attitude of complacency can lead only to disaster in the form of life-threatening systemic infection and permanent crippling of the hand.

Principles of Management

All hand infections of more than minor proportions require hospitalization. The most common organisms are staphylococcus, streptococcus, gram-negative and combination staphylococcus and gram-negative organisms. Antibiotic coverage with a bactericidal drug should be instituted at once on their presumed presence and adjusted when cultures and sensitivities become available.[29] Heat in the form of continuous warm, moist dressings (used with care so as not to produce a burn), elevation and immobilization by plaster splint in the position of function are essential. Sedation is frequently necessary in that most serious hand infections are excruciatingly painful. Seriously ill patients require bedrest and parenteral fluid therapy.

The choice between conservative and surgical management demands exceedingly fine judgment. Space infections and localized soft tissue infections require immediate drainage. Premature surgical treatment is to be strictly avoided in the process of cellulitis and progressing lymphangitis. Therapy must be aggressive, whether conservative or surgical.

Operative management of hand infections demands adherence to the same principles employed in elective hand surgery. Virtually all hand infections require general or brachial block anesthesia for adequate drainage. Local infiltration anesthesia is hazardous, and digital gangrene is produced readily by finger block anesthesia. A bloodless field is essential. Incisions and dissection must be anatomically accurate so that important structures are not damaged and uninvolved areas are not contaminated. If there is a wound of entry, it should be explored and drained first before proceeding to other areas. The dictum "go where the pus is," is appropriate. Through-and-through drainage is to be avoided. Drains, when utilized, are either soft rubber or grease gauze wicks. Proper postoperative management is of utmost importance and consists of sterile dressing technique, continuous moist dressings and physiotherapy as early as possible to prevent joint stiffness. Frequent examination during the postoperative period is essential. The persistence of pain and tenderness is most often due to undrained infection, and a second exploration may be indicated. When doubt exists as to the presence of pus, exploration is advised, especially in children. A negative exploration is much preferred to an overlooked infection. Lastly, the surgeon who overrelies on antibiotics courts disaster; the ideal treatment of closed space infection is still surgical incision and dependent drainage.

Anatomy

Hand infections may be classified into those involving primarily soft tissue and those involving the various potential spaces within the hand. A sound knowledge of anatomy is essential to proper diagnosis and treatment.

Tendon Sheaths. The tendon sheaths of the thumb and little finger extend from the terminal phalanx to a point 2 to 3 cm. proximal to the proximal flexion crease of the wrist. A septum occasionally separates the proximal and distal halves of the sheaths. The proximal halves of the thumb and little finger sheaths are referred to as the radial and ulnar bursae, respectively. The radial and ulnar bursae communicate proximal to the transverse carpal ligament. The tendon sheaths of the index, middle and ring fingers extend from the terminal phalanges to a line joining the radial extremity of the proximal palmar crease with the ulnar extremity of the distal palmar crease. The proximal extremity of the index finger sheath overlies the thenar space. The proximal extremities of the middle and ring finger sheaths overlie the mid-palmar space. The tendon sheaths of the index, middle and ring fingers rarely communicate with the ulnar bursa.

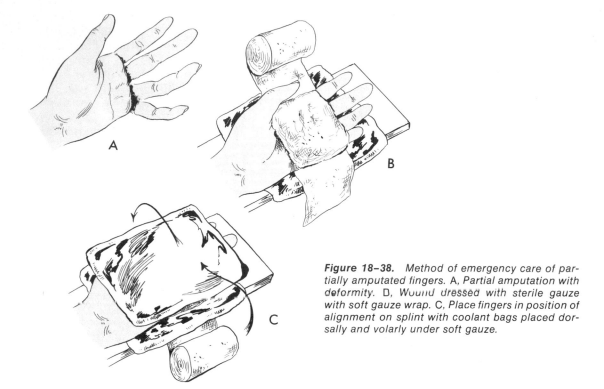

Figure 18–38. *Method of emergency care of partially amputated fingers. A, Partial amputation with deformity. B, Wound dressed with sterile gauze with soft gauze wrap. C, Place fingers in position of alignment on splint with coolant bags placed dorsally and volarly under soft gauze.*

Thenar Space. The thenar space is separated from the mid-palmar space by a fibrous septum extending from the palmar aponeurosis to the third metacarpal (Fig. 18–39). The thenar space extends from the third metacarpal to the thenar eminence and from the transverse carpal ligament to within 1 cm. of the proximal flexion crease of the index finger. It lies between the flexor tendons and lumbrical muscle of the index finger and the adductor pollicis and extends radially between the deep aspect of the adductor pollicis and the palmar aspect of the first dorsal interosseous muscle.

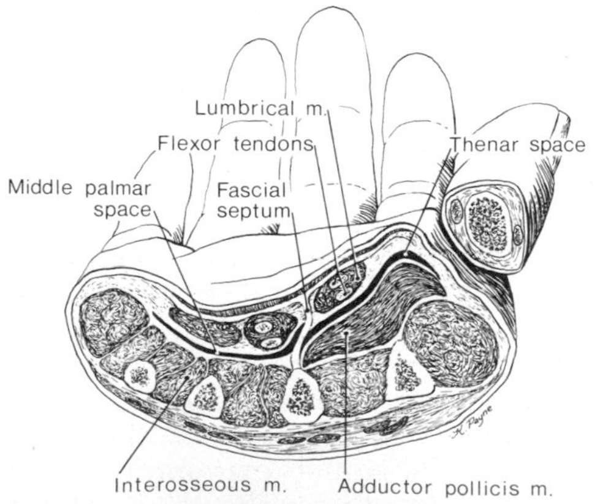

Mid-palmar Space. The mid-palmar space (Fig. 18–40) extends from the third metacarpal to the hypothenar eminence; it reaches slightly more proximally than the thenar space. The roof of the mid-palmar space is formed by the sheaths of the lubrical muscles to the middle, ring and little fingers.

Parona's Space. Parona's space is a potential space lying between the flexor pollicis longus and the flexor digitorum profundus tendons and the pronator quadratus muscle.

It must be emphasized that infections confined initially to a given space may subsequently involve adjacent spaces. The firm attachment of the palmar aponeurosis to the thenar and hypothenar muscles prevents the formation of a space in which pus may accumulate. The dorsal subaponeurotic space is not often infected because of the barrier provided by the metacarpals and interosseous muscles.

Figure 18–39. *The mid-palmar space and the thenar space and related anatomical structures in cross section of hand approximately 3 cm. proximal to the metacarpophalangeal joints.*

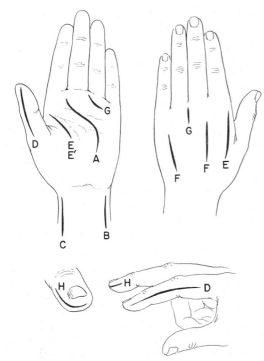

Figure 18–40. Indication of sites for incisions for drainage. A, For midpalmar space and palmar portion ulnar bursae. B, For ulnar bursae above wrist. C, For radial bursae above wrist. D, For tenosynovitis of flexor tendon. E, For thenar space abscess. E', For palmar portion radial bursae. F, For subaponeurotic space. G, For collar button abscess palm and dorsum of hand. H, For felon. (Redrawn from Boyes, J. H.: Bunnell's Surgery of the Hand. 4th ed. Philadelphia, J. B. Lippincott Co., 1964.)

Lymphatic Drainage. The lymphatics of the fingers, web areas, distal palm, and thenar and hypothenar eminences drain to the lymphatic lakes within the loose areolar tissue on the dorsum of the hand; the lymphatic trunks from the dorsum accompany the cephalic and basilic veins. The cephalic vein lymphatics drain directly into the nodes of the deltopectoral triangle, whereas the lymphatics accompanying the basilic vein pass through the epitrochlear and axillary nodes. The lymphatics of the central and proximal palm accompany the superficial and deep venous arches to the lymphatics associated with the radial and ulnar arteries. Tremendous edema of the dorsum of the hand is commonly associated with hand infection and, too frequently, is interpreted as localized infection in this area.

Soft Tissue Infections

Folliculitis. A low-grade infection involving the hair follicles occurs most commonly on the dorsum of the proximal phalanx. The process usually clears rapidly with placing the hand at rest and employing continuous warm soaks.

Furuncle. Subcutaneous abscesses usually occur on the dorsum of the proximal phalanx. General or proximal nerve block anesthesia is required for adequate drainage.

Carbuncle. Carbuncles are relatively uncommon but may occasionally be seen on the ulnar aspect of the dorsum of the hand. General or proximal nerve block anesthesia is required for adequate drainage; a linear rather than cruciate incision is utilized.

Collar Button Abscess (Web Space Infection). The thickness of the palmar skin permits formation of a localized abscess immediately beneath the cuticular layer (subcuticular abscess). A collar button abscess has perforated the dermis to form a deeper abscess or, in the palmar web area, has perforated the palmar aponeurosis to reach the dorsum of the web. Web space infections may extend proximally within the lumbrical sheaths to enter the thenar or mid-palmar spaces.

Paronychia (Run Around). Localized infection between the nail and the cuticle constitutes a paronychia. Pain is a prominent symptom; the cuticle appears erythematous and tense. Early cases are treated simply by elevation of the cuticle; incisions proximally on the dorsum are not necessary. When the nail has become undermined, it acts as a foreign body, and the proximal third of the nail must be excised. Chronic cases exhibit exuberant granulation tissue beneath the cuticle; the granulation tissue and the proximal nail must be removed.

Felon. The multiple fibrous septa attaching the skin to the terminal phalanx form expansionless closed spaces. Infection and only slight swelling within these closed spaces readily produce thrombosis of the terminal branches of the digital arteries with resultant necrosis of the tuft of the terminal phalanx. Severe pain is an outstanding feature of a felon. The distal phalanx is tense, ischemic, hard and exquisitely tender. Drainage is accomplished through a midlateral incision paralleling the volar surface of the distal phalanx (Fig. 18–40H). The knife must extend to, but not through, the skin of the opposite side of the finger and must divide all the fibrous septa. The so-called "fish mouth" incision is to be avoided. Persistent drainage and the presence of exuberant granulation tissue within the incision or a sinus tract indicate osteomyelitis of the terminal phalanx. The bone is not attached surgically; adequate drainage is provided and sequestration allowed.

Human Bite. Wounds produced by human teeth contain virulent anaerobic organisms and spirochetes as well as streptococci and staphylococci and can result in truly devastating hand infections. The wound usually overlies a metacarpophalangeal joint, and there is injury of the extensor tendon mechanism and direct contamination of the joint. Extension of infection to the palm occurs via the lumbrical sheaths. The wound is sometimes sustained with fist clenched; later, when the hand opens, the tissues slide back and seal the wound. Under no circumstances are wounds secondary to human bites sutured. Treatment consists of thorough cleansing, irrigation, debridement, adequate drainage, antibiotic therapy, splinting and elevation. Bone sequestration is allowed to separate spontaneously. Reconstructive procedures are deferred until wound healing is complete and the tissues are soft and pliable.

Herpetic Whitlow. Infection of the subcuticular layer of the skin by herpes simplex virus begins as an area of irritation and shortly becomes intensely painful.[62] Deep vesicles appear and spread. This may be resistant to all forms of treatment. Sudden improvement usually occurs within about 10 days. The herpetic lesion may become secondarily infected with staphylococci and need drainage.

Unusual Infections

Mycobacterium Marinum. Human infections with *Mycobacterium marinum* are becoming more common. Infection in man usually follows an injury or abrasion sustained while in an environment contaminated with the organism, such as tropical fish aquariums, swimming pools, ponds and brackish water. To identify the organism the laboratory worker needs pertinent information on the location of the lesion and the history of exposure; for example, injury sustained while working in aquarium, or swimming in contaminated water, or from barnacles or fish fins.

It is essential to culture specifically for mycobacteria. This includes standard cultures at 37° C as well as special cultures at 31° C, to detect *Mycobacterium marinum*, which generally will not grow at the higher temperature. Recommended drug regimen is isoniazid with ethambutol, rifampin, or both.[27]

Animal Bites. Infection due to *Pasteurella multocida* from cat or dog bites is more common than realized.[19] Soon after the bite, the area becomes painful, red and swollen, with an ascending lymphangitis and lymphadenopathy. An abscess may develop. When cultures are sent to the bacteriology laboratory, special note should be made about the possibility of such infection since these organisms may be interpreted as other gram-negative bacteria. Penicillin is the antibiotic of choice.

Symbiotic Infection. The combination of microaerophilic nonhemolytic streptococcus and hemolytic *Staphylococcus aureus* produces a lesion destructive to the skin and subcutaneous tissue.[20] The lesion usually is painful and tender. The gross appearance is quite characteristic. There is an outer zone of erythema, a sharply defined purple middle zone, and an inner zone of gangrenous skin. A portion of the overlying area of the gangrenous skin may have a vesicle on the surface.

Treatment is surgical debridement of the necrotic tissue (plus antibiotics that are effective against the causative organisms) as demonstrated by sensitivity tests. Since this may extend to involve the fascia of the hand and forearm, it has been described by Wilson[70] as "necrotizing fasciitis."

Space Infections

Tendon Sheath. Suppurative tenosynovitis usually is secondary to a puncture wound over the volar aspect of the distal interphalangeal or proximal interphalangeal joints. Rapid extension of infection within the closed space provided by the tendon sheath leads to early necrosis of the flexor tendon secondary to pressure obstruction of the vincula and may produce systemic symptoms out of proportion to the wound. Severe pain is the outstanding symptom. The diagnosis is established readily on the basis of Kanavel's[34] four cardinal points:

1. The finger is held in flexion.
2. There is uniform swelling over the entire course of the tendon sheath, as opposed to the localized swelling seen with soft tissue infection.
3. There is discrete tenderness over the entire course of the sheath.
4. Passive extension of the finger produces intense pain.

Treatment must be prompt and efficient and consists of early, adequate drainage of the tendon sheath. Delayed treatment results in destruction and loss of function of the flexor tendons; the entire hand may be incapacitated by exudate. Drainage is accomplished through an incision extending from the base of the distal phalanx to the proximal flexion crease of the digit or through a zigzag incision. Finger incisions are placed on the ulnar aspect of the index finger and the radial aspect of the little finger. The sheath is opened throughout its length. The proximal cul-de-sac of the sheath is drained through a transverse incision in the palm immediately distal to the proximal palmar crease. Incisions utilized for draining the tendon sheath of the thumb must extend no farther than the midpoint of the first metacarpal in order to avoid injury to the motor branch of the median nerve. Anatomical landmarks may be entirely absent as a result of swelling, and if care is not taken the incision may be found to lie in the volar midline following resolution of the edema. The dorsal ends of the finger flexion creases provide the most accurate guides to placement of the incision (Fig. 18–40D).

Radial Bursa. Extension of infection to the radial bursa is manifested by tenderness from the distal phalanx of the thumb to above the carpal ligament. Draining is accomplished through an incision paralleling the thenar eminence and extending from the proximal flexion crease of the thumb to within 2 cm. of the transverse carpal ligament. It must be emphasized that the sensory rami of the median nerve, as well as the motor branch, cross the tendon sheath.

Ulnar Bursa. The earliest sign of infection within the ulnar bursa is an area of maximal tenderness at the point at which the distal palmar crease crosses the hypothenar eminence. Drainage is accomplished through an incision paralleling the hypothenar eminence and extending from the proximal palmar crease to the transverse carpal ligament (Fig. 18–40A).

Adequate drainage of the proximal extremities of the radial and ulnar bursae requires an incision in the mid-ulnar line of the wrist immediately proximal to the transverse carpal ligament (Fig. 18–40B). The radial and ulnar bursae almost always communicate, and an infection in one is followed by infection in the other. A "horseshoe abscess" involves the tendon sheaths of the thumb and little finger together with the radial and ulnar bursae.

Parona's Space. Infection within Parona's space is secondary to infection of the radial or ulnar bursae or to infection within the mid-palmar space. The diagnosis is based on localized swelling and tenderness on the volar aspect of the wrist immediately proximal to the transverse carpal ligament. Drainage is accomplished through an incision in the mid-ulnar line of the wrist (Fig. 18–40B).

Thenar Space. Thenar space infections are secondary to direct puncture wounds or suppurative tenosynovitis of the index finger. The typical appearance of the hand consists of massive swelling of the soft tissues between the thumb and index metacarpals, with the thumb pushed away from the hand. Tenderness is maximal in the first interosseous space. Drainage is accomplished through an incision on the dorsal aspect of the thumb-index web paralleling the web margin and extending between the heads of the thumb and index metacarpals (Fig. 18–40E and E').

Mid-Palmar Space. Infections within the mid-palmar space are secondary to direct puncture wounds or suppurative tenosynovitis of the middle or ring fingers. Severe pain and marked systemic toxicity are characteristic. The normal palmar concavity is lost, and the palm is flat and extremely tense. Tenderness is maximal in the center of the palm. Drainage is accomplished through a transverse incision immediately proximal to the distal palmar crease (Fig. 18–40A).

CHEMICAL INJURIES

Injection Injuries

A variety of devices in modern America are capable of injecting foreign and frequently caustic substances such as plastic and paint into the hand at pressures varying from 1000 to 15,000 lbs./sq. in.[45] Popularly known as "grease gun" or "paint gun" injuries, they may appear deceptively innocuous initially but rapidly progress to ischemia and gangrene if unrecognized and untreated. The clues to diagnosis are the history, a small puncture wound and mild discomfort that rapidly changes to exquisite pain. Initial redness about the wound becomes ashen gray, hard and tender. Treatment is wide surgical incision and exploration of all suspicious areas. Involved tissue must be debrided, removing as much of the offending agent as possible and employing open treatment. The postoperative course is often indolent and further debridement may be necessary. Many such cases eventually result in amputation.

Drug-Related Injuries

In the current epidemic of drug addiction, injection injuries of the hands and arms are seen with increasing frequency. These problems have a wide spectrum of presentation and pathophysiology, and range from the most common, a painful nodule at the site of injection, to the rare and often tragic intra-arterial drug injection.[55]

The most frequently seen presenting problem is a painful nodule occurring at the site of a subcutaneous injection. These nodules are chemically induced fat necrosis of the subcutaneous tissues with attendant low-grade inflammation and fibrosis. They can be difficult to distinguish from low-grade intercurrent infection but on culture seldom grow virulent organisms and frequently resolve with local measures. The second most common problem is that of acute infection and abscess forma-

tion about an injection site. The most frequently cultured organisms are gram-positive but in addition there may be gram-negative organisms and antibiotic coverage should be for both. It must be borne in mind that in the course of treatment the acutely injured hand of the addict often does not respond in the usual way to therapeutic measures; indeed, the retrograde spread of lymphangiectic infection is seen. The third most common presenting problem is chronic nonpitting swelling of the hands and digits, most often confined to the nondominant hand. It is most often seen in long-term addicts and accompanies long-standing subcutaneous injection. Study of the pathogenesis of this chronic swelling has demonstrated associated lymphatic obstruction.[48] Skin biopsy reveals dense dermal fibrosis and marked collagen tissue deposition subcutaneously. It is of interest to note that heroin is frequently cut with quinine, and this substance has been used experimentally to produce lymphatic obstruction in experimental lymphedema. Chronic nonhealing cutaneous ulcerations are the fourth common presenting problem, arising from cutaneous necrosis over a site of abscess formation or subcutaneous fat necrosis and sepsis. These are characteristically punched out, indurated ulcerations with pale chronic granulations; they respond slowly to local measures. A less common but most tragic complication of drug injection is the gangrene and tissue loss attending intra-arterial injection.

Gangrene of the extremity following intra-arterial drug injection has been frequently reported and is the subject of several experimental studies. A clear antecedent to this gangrene is intra-arterial thrombosis. The importance of the factors leading to this intra-arterial clotting is less clear. The factors implicated have been vascular spasm, intimal injury with vasculitis and subsequent thrombosis and drug-blood interaction with immediate intravascular cellular agglutination and clotting. The pathophysiology would appear to vary with whether the injected drug is a parenteral preparation or an oral medication in an nonphysiological suspension.

Thiopental, which gave rise to the initial iatrogenic injuries, has been most thoroughly studied. Vascular spasm does not seem to be a major component with this parenteral preparation, but the evolution of intimal damage and vasculitis with subsequent thrombosis is the major focus of injury. In experimental studies therapeutic measures that have reduced the amount of gangrene following intra-arterial thiopental injection in animals are: (1) sympathectomy preceding the injection and (2) heparinization. The intra-arterial administration of Procaine as well as other antispasmotic agents has been without definite benefit. Intra-arterial dexamethasone was the most effective agent in ameliorating gangrene following intra-arterial Hydroxyzine injection. Clinical reports have recommended some additional measures. Brachial plexus block is favored over stellate ganglion block as it provides analgesia as well as sympathetic blockade. A continuous brachial plexus block with indwelling catheter has proved useful in heparinized patients.

When the injected drug is a nonphysiological suspension of an oral medication, the injury and subsequent evolution of gangrene may be much more rapid and severe. The large amount of insoluble particulate matter injected results in rapid agglutination of cells intravascularly with diffuse embolization and subsequent thrombosis. The rapidity of onset of this effect would make the measures directed against the evolution of vasculitis, as in parenteral agents, less effective. This has been the clinical experience. Once thrombosis is established, an entirely different therapeutic regimen, centered about clot lysis, would seem indicated. The reports of restoration of circulation with this regimen following intra-arterial thrombosis of varying causes within the hand are most encouraging and certainly this modality deserves a primary place in care once thrombosis is established.[35] Fasciotomy has seemed to have been of benefit in limiting the adverse effects of the attendant massive edema on the intact circulation. We strongly recommend this mode of therapy.

An awareness of the altered pathophysiology of acute infections in the chronically injured hands of addicts is helpful. Dorsal swelling may not subside and often limitation of hand motion has preceded the acute episode and has not resulted from it.

These patients' indifference to their injuries is often monumental. Their self-destructive tendencies causing unreliability, uncooperativeness and unwillingness to return for follow-up visits greatly compound the difficulty of treatment for the hand surgeon.

REFERENCES

1. American Replantation Mission to China: Replantation surgery in China. Plast. Reconstr. Surg. 52:476, 1973.
2. Atasoy, E., Ioakimidis, E., Kasdan, M. L., Kutz, J. E., and Kleinert, H. E.: Reconstruction of the amputated fingertip with a triangular volar flap. J. Bone Joint Surg. 52A:921, 1970.
3. Beasley, R. W.: Reconstruction of amputated fingertips. Plast. Reconstr. Surg. 44:349, 1969.
4. Bohler, L.: Treatment of Fractures. 4th ed. Baltimore, William Wood & Co., 1935.
5. Boyes, J. H.: A philosophy of care of the injured hand. Bull. Am. Coll. Surg. 50:341, 1965.
6. Boyes, J. H: Bunnell's Surgery of the Hand. 4th ed. Philadelphia, J. B. Lippincott Co., 1964.
7. Boyes, J. H.: Demonstration of Arm Board for Hand Surgery. American Academy of Orthopaedic Surgeons, 1950.
8. Boyes, J. H.: Discussion of paper by Van't Hof, A., and Heiple, K. G.: Flexor tendon injuries. J. Bone Joint Surg. 40A:262, 1958.
9. Boyes, J. H.: In Cramer, L. M., and Chase, Robert A. (eds.): Symposium on the Hand. St. Louis, C. V. Mosby Co., 1971, p. 191.
10. Boyes, J. H.: Evaluation of digital flexor tendon grafts. Am. J. Surg. 89:1116, 1955.
11. Bruner, J. M.: Safety factors in the use of the pneumatic tourniquet for hemostasis in surgery of the hand. J. Bone Joint Surg. 33:221, 1951.
12. Bruner, J. M.: The zig-zag volar-digital incision for flexor-tendon surgery. Plast. Reconst. Surg. 40:571, 1967.
13. Buncke, H. J., Jr., and Schulz, W. P.: Experimental digital amputation and reimplantation. Plast. Reconstr. Surg. 36:62, 1965.
14. Buncke, H. J., Jr., and Schulz, W. P.: Total ear replantation in the rabbit utilizing microminiature vascular anastomosis. Br. J. Plast. Surg. 19:332, 1966.
15. Bunnell, S.: Surgery of nerves of the hand. Surg. Gynec. Obstet. 44:145, 1927.
16. Bunnell, S.: The early treatment of hand injuries. J. Bone Joint Surg. 33:807, 1951.
17. Bunnell, S., and Boyes, J. H.: Nerve grafts. Am. J. Surg. 44:64, 1939.
18. Burkhalter, W. E., Butler, B., Metz, W., and Omer, G.: Experiences with delayed primary closure of war wounds of the hand in Viet Nam. J. Bone Joint Surg. 50A:945, 1968.
19. Byrne, J. J., Boyd, T. F., and Daly, A. K.: Pasteurella infection from cat bites. Surg. Gynecol. Obstet. 103:56, 1956.
20. Byrne, J. J.: The Hand. Springfield, Charles C Thomas, 1959, p. 70.
21. Curtis, R. M.: Reconstruction of the acutely injured hand. Maryland Med. J. 5:675, 1956.

22. Curtis, R. M.: Cross-finger pedicle flap in hand surgery. Ann. Surg. 145:650, 1957.
23. Curtis, R. M.: Joints of the hand. In Flynn, J. E. (ed.): Hand Surgery. Baltimore, The Williams & Wilkins Co., 1966.
24. Curtis, R. M.: Lecture, Repair of Flexor Tendon Injuries. Emory University Hospital, April 1, 1966.
25. Curtis, R. M.: Capsulectomy of the interphalangeal joints of the fingers. J. Bone Joint Surg. 36A:1219, 1954.
26. Dupont, C. G., and Crikelair, G. F.: A review of 135 cases of tendon lacerations in the hand and wrist. J. Bone Joint Surg. 42A:913, 1960.
27. Gunther, S. F., Elliott, R. C., Brand, R. L., and Adams, J. P.: Experience with a typical mycobacterial infection in the deep structures of the hand. J. Hand Surg. 2:90, 1977.
28. Fisher, R. H.: The Kutler method of repair of finger tip amputations. Proceedings Am. Soc. Surg. Hand. J. Bone Joint Surg. 48:606, 1966.
29. Friedberg, A., and Waddell, J. P.: Proceedings of the American Society for Surgery of the Hand. J. Bone Joint Surg. 54A:896, 1972.
30. Hunter, J. M., and Salisbury, R. E.: Flexor-tendon reconstruction in severely damaged hand. J. Bone Joint Surg. 53A:829, 1971.
31. Jabaley, M. E., and Peterson, H. D.: Early treatment of war wounds of the hand and forearm in Vietnam. Ann. Surg. 177:167, 1973.
32. Jacobson, J. H., and Suarez, E. L.: Microsurgery in anastomosis of small vessels. Surg. Forum 11:243, 1960.
33. James, J. I. P.: Fractures of the phalanges and metacarpals. Proceedings of meeting British Hand Club for Surgery of the Hand, May 14, 1965.
34. Kanavel, A. C.: Infections of the Hand. (7th Ed.). Philadelphia, Lea & Febiger, 1939.
35. Kartchner, M. M., and Wilcox, W. C.: Thrombolysis of palmar and digital arterial thrombosis by intra-arterial thrombolysin. J. Hand Surg. 1:67, 1976.
36. Kaplan, E. B.: Dorsal dislocation of the metacarpophalangeal joint of the index finger. J. Bone Joint Surg. 41A:1081, 1959.
37. Kelleher, J. C., Sullivan, J. G., Baibak, G. J., and Dean, R. K.: The Distant Pedicle Flap in Surgery of the Hand. Orth. Clin. N. Am. 1:227, 1970.
38. Kleinert, H. E., Kutz, J. E., Ashbell, T. S., et al: Primary repair of lacerated flexor tendons in "no man's land." Proceedings, Am. Soc. Surg. Hand. J. Bone Joint Surg. 49A:577, 1967.
39. Kleinert, H. E., Serafin, D., Kutz, J. E., et al: Replantation amputated digits and hands. Orthop. Clin. North Am. 4:957, 1973.
40. Komatsu, S., and Tamai, S.: Successful replantation of a completely cut-off thumb. Plast. Reconstr. Surg. 42:374, 1968.
41. Lister, G. D., Kleinert, H. E., Kutz, J. E., and Atasoy, E.: Primary flexor tendon repair followed by immediate controlled mobilization. J. Hand Surg. 2:441, 1977.
42. Littler, J. W.: The severed flexor tendon. Surg. Clin. N. Am. 39:435, 1959.
43. Madsen, E.: Delayed primary suture of flexor tendons cut in the digital sheath. J. Bone Joint Surg. 52B:264, 1970.
44. Mason, M. L.: Fifty years of progress in hand surgery. Surg. Gynec. Obstet. (Int. Abst. Surg.) 101(6):541, 1955.
45. Meagher, S. W.: Special Wounds. In Flynn, J. E. (ed.): Hand Surgery. Baltimore, The Williams & Wilkins Co., 1966.
46. Milford, L.: The hand. In Crenshaw, A. H. (ed.): Campbell's Operative Orthopedics. (4th Ed.). St. Louis, C. V. Mosby Co., 1963, vol. 1.
47. Millesi, H., Meissl, G., and Berger, A.: The interfascicular nerve-grafting of the median and ulnar nerves. J. Bone Joint Surg. 54A:727, 1972.
48. Neviaser, R. J., Butterfield, W. C., and Wieche, D. R.: The puffy hand of drug addiction. J. Bone Joint Surg. 54A:629, 1972.
49. Nicholson, O. R., and Seddon, H. J.: Nerve repair in civil practice. Br. Med. J. 2:1065, 1957.
50. O'Brien, B. M., and Miller, G. D. H.: Digital reattachment and revascularization. J. Bone Joint Surg. 55A:714, 1973.
51. Onné, L.: Recovery of sensibility and sudomotor activity in the hand after nerve suture. Acta Chir. Scand. (Suppl. 300), 1962.
52. Parkes, A.: The "lumbrical plus" finger. Hand 2:164, 1970.
53. Potenza, A. D.: Tendon healing within the flexor digital sheath in the dog. J. Bone Joint Surg. 44A:49, 1962.
54. Pulvertaft, R. G.: Tendon grafts for flexor tendon injuries in fingers and thumb; study of technique and results. J. Bone Joint Surg. 38B:175, 1956.
55. Ryan, J. J., Hoopes, J. E., and Jabaley, M. E.: Drug injection injuries of the hands and forearms in addicts. Plast. Reconstr. Surg. 53:445, 1974.
56. Robertson, R. C., Cawley, J. J., Jr., and Faris, A. M.: Treatment of fracture, dislocation of the interphalangeal joints of the hand. J. Bone Joint Surg. 28:68, 1946.
57. Salmon, P. A., and Assimacopoulos, C. A.: Microsurgery: Review of the literature and description of a modified technique. Minn. Med. 47:679, 1964.
58. Seddon, H. J. (ed.): Peripheral Nerve Injuries. Medical Research Council Special Series No. 282. London, Her Majesty's Stationery Office, 1954.
59. Seddon, H. J.: Nerve grafting. J. Bone Joint Surg. 45B:447, 1963.
60. Skoog, T., and Persson, B. H.: An experimental study of the early healing of tendons. Plast. Reconstr. Surg. 13:384, 1954.
61. Stener, B.: Displacement of the ruptured ulnar collateral ligament of the metacarpophalangeal joint of the thumb. A clinical anatomical study. J. Bone Joint Surg. 44B:869, 1962.
62. Stern, H., Elek, S. D., Millar, D. M., and Anderson, H. F.: Herpetic whitlow. Lancet 2:871, 1959.
63. Sunderland, S.: The intraneural topography of the radial, median, and ulnar nerves. Brain 68:243, 1945.
64. Tamai, S., Tasumi, Y., Shimizu, T., Hari, Y.,

Okuda, H., Takita, T., Sakamoto, H., and Fukui, A.: Traumatic amputation digits: The fate of remaining blood. J. Hand Surg. 2:13, 1977.

65. Urbaniak, J. R.: Digital replantation. Letter to the editor. J. Hand Surg. 2:82, 1977.

66. Van't Hof, A., and Heiple, K. G.: Flexor tendon injuries of the fingers and thumb. J. Bone Joint Surg. 40A:256, 1958.

67. Verdan, C.: Practical considerations for primary and secondary repair in flexor tendon injuries. Surg. Clin. N. Am. 44:951, 1964.

68. Wakefield, A. R.: Management of flexor tendon injuries. Surg. Clin. N. Am. 40:267, 1960.

69. Weiland, A. J., Villarreal-Rios, A., Kleinert, H. E., Kutz, J. E., Atasoy, E., and Lister, G.: Re-
plantation of digits and hands: Analysis of surgical techniques and functional results in 71 patients with 86 replantations. J. Hand Surg. 2:1, 1977.

70. Wilson, B.: Necrotizing fasciitis. Am. Surg. 18:416, 1952.

71. Zachary, R. B.: Results of nerve suture in peripheral nerve injuries. In Seddon, H. J. (ed.): Peripheral Nerve Injuries. Medical Research Council Special Report Series No. 282, London, Her Majesty's Stationery Office, 1954, pp. 354–388.

72. Zachary, R. B., and Holmes, W.: Primary suture of nerves. Surg. Gynecol. Obstet. 82:622, 1946.

CHAPTER 19

PERIPHERAL VASCULAR INJURIES

Robert B. Rutherford, M.D.
Glenn L. Kelly, M.D.

The first crude vascular repair was performed by Hallowell over 2 centuries ago,[30] and the basic suture techniques as we know them today, including the use of autografts and homografts, were well worked out by the end of the first decade of this century and summarized in the classic works of Carrel[3] and Guthrie.[10] By 1910, over 100 lateral repairs and 46 end-to-end anastomoses or segmental vein grafts had been performed clinically.[24] The stage was set for the application of these techniques to vascular injuries by the outbreak of World War I, and yet it was not until the Korean conflict was well under way over 35 years later that this came to pass. The development and use of high-velocity missiles and high explosives during World War I, the treatment priorities imposed by mass casualty situations, and the inordinately long evacuation times from embattled trench to operating theatre combined to perpetuate a discouragingly high failure rate and established the attitude that there was no place for primary vascular repair in military surgery. The emphasis shifted to the management of the delayed complications of vascular injury, arteriovenous fistulas and false aneurysms. Even under the more optimal conditions of civilian practice, treatment rarely went much beyond hemostasis, and not only was the injured artery ligated at the expense of patency but so was the accompanying vein. For inexplicable reasons, this attitude was perpetuated through World War II, as indicated by DeBakey and Simeone's review,[5] which revealed that direct repair was attempted in only slightly over 3 per cent of 2471 arterial injuries with end-to-end anastomosis being performed in only eight instances. The overall amputation rate was 49 per cent.

The Korean War shared a period of very rapid advancement with cardiovascular surgery when bold innovative approaches seemed commonplace. Rapid evacuation, ample blood replacement, antibiotics, new vascular instruments and a more stable fighting front with trained surgeons at forward (M.A.S.H.) hospitals set the stage for a complete reversal of the previously conservative military approach to vascular injuries. Immediate repair was attempted in 88 per cent of arterial injuries.[12] In these cases, the amputation rate was only 13 per cent compared to 51 per cent for those in whom ligation of the injured vessel was carried out. The present-day (aggressive) approach to vascular injuries can be said to stem from this experience, although important additional refinements have been added by subsequent experiences in civilian practice and in the Vietnam conflict, as will be brought out later. However, it should be realized that today's relatively optimistic outlook toward peripheral vascular injuries is not due solely to adopting

596

a policy of immediate operative repair. Rapid transportation, availability of blood and antibiotics, abandonment of mass tourniquet techniques, a better appreciation of the true nature of certain forms of arterial injury (high-velocity and blunt trauma), the increased use of arteriography, recognition of the importance of fracture stabilization, thorough debridement (including the traumatized arterial segment), fasciotomy, repair of concomitant venous injuries and the success of vein grafts in bridging major vascular defects in the face of major contamination and tissue destruction, heparin anticoagulation, Fogarty balloon catheters, use of antiplatelet drugs, Doppler flow detectors and improved suture material and instruments all have contributed greatly to this advance.

ARTERIAL INJURIES

A wide spectrum of arterial injuries may be encountered, depending on the mechanism of injury. Examples of these are shown in Figure 19–1. Penetrating wounds may take the form of a small puncture, a lateral or through-and-through (knife) laceration or a gaping (low-velocity) bullet hole. An artery will be cleanly transected if directly hit by a high-

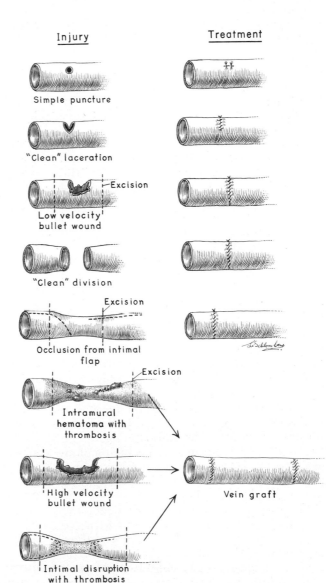

Figure 19–1. *Common forms of arterial injury with the likely method of repair.*

Injury   Treatment

Simple puncture

"Clean" laceration

Low velocity bullet wound — Excision

"Clean" division

Occlusion from intimal flap — Excision

Intramural hematoma with thrombosis — Excision

High velocity bullet wound — Vein graft

Intimal disruption with thrombosis

velocity bullet or, on a near miss, it may be literally torn apart by the explosive energy released in the temporary cavity that develops in the bullet's wake.[1] Blunt trauma may result in contusion and segmental spasm of the artery or, more commonly, its occlusion by intramural hematoma and segmental thrombosis, flap-like intimal tear or circumferential intimal disruption. Arteriovenous fistula and false aneurysm are the most common late complications.

In the majority of instances, the arterial injury is not an isolated consideration. Associated injuries to the accompanying vein and nerves, concomitant fractures or dislocations, varying degrees of muscle and other soft tissue destruction and contamination of the wound with bacteria and foreign material frequently compound the problem. Other factors that play a role in the end result are the level of injury, the collateral circulation and, occasionally in civilian practice, underlying occlusive arterial disease. A good example of the significance of the level of injury is the popliteal artery, which may be injured by displaced fractures above or below the knee joint or dislocation of the joint itself in addition to penetrating trauma. It is the only major artery traversing this section of the lower extremity and most of its collaterals (the geniculate arteries) depart from it over a relatively short segment so that they may be involved primarily by the injury itself or secondarily by a relatively short segmental occlusion of the popliteal artery. The high amputation rate associated with ligation of an injured popliteal artery was documented early by Makins.[22] Even more recently, popliteal artery repair carried an amputation rate of 32 per cent in the Vietnam War experience, almost twice that of the next most serious site of peripheral arterial injury, the common femoral.[27] It should be understood that higher amputation rates are to be expected in the natural course of an acute traumatic occlusion than with acute thrombotic occlusion of an already arteriosclerotic vessel, in which there has been time for the development of collateral channels.

Iatrogenic arterial injuries are becoming legion with the advent of newer invasive procedures, including diagnostic and therapeutic arteriography, cardiac catheterization, arterial blood gas sampling and pressure monitoring and intra-aortic balloon pumping. Even use of the Fogarty embolectomy catheter has produced untoward effects by elevating some distant intimal plaque, or more commonly, by rupturing the artery during overinflation of the balloon.[9] Delay in diagnosis and surgical treatment of these injuries is often great, probably owing to the physician's natural reluctance to concede his ill fortune. Often a second opinion by another consultant can help overcome this inertia. The inpatient setting should not offer false security but rather should provide an opportunity for careful observation with frequent examinations, noninvasive testing or even arteriography.

DIAGNOSIS

The possibility of an arterial injury should be entertained whenever a penetrating wound is found along the course of a major vessel, particularly if there is excessive bleeding from the wound or a rapidly expanding hematoma. However, if the artery has been completely severed and its ends have contracted and become occluded by thrombus, the wound itself may not arouse suspicion. Nonpenetrating injuries are a less obvious and therefore more treacherous cause of arterial injury. The existence of a displaced fracture, dislocation or extensive soft tissue injury in particular should lead to the consideration of concomitant arterial injury. This is particularly true with injuries about the knee and elbow and fractures of the first rib, which have an increased association with subclavian artery injury.[29] Of course, the state of the extremity distal to the wound usually reflects the presence of ischemia. Pallor or mottled cyanosis may be apparent. Palpation reveals coolness and absent or diminished pulses. Occasionally, however distal pulses may be intact due to large collateral channels, thus disguising the presence of acute arterial injury. In 271 civilian arterial injuries reported by Shires et al.,[32] distal pulsations were palpable in 69 and were normal in 40. In a later review,[26] the incidence of normal distal pulses in association with arterial injuries was approximately 10 per cent. Capillary filling should be noted, not only as an aid to diagnosis, but as an indication of viability, to help establish priority of treatment when other significant injuries are present. Decreased sensation and motor strength are common early results of peripheral nerve ischemia owing to the high oxygen demands of this tissue. However, careful neurological examination must be made to differentiate ischemic neuropathy from associated direct nerve damage.

Difficulty may arise in examining extremities in the presence of shock. This may not only mask the aforementioned signs but, in association with subclinical degrees of arteriosclerosis, may lead to confusing differences between compared extremities. In a similar regard, it may be difficult to decide in older patients if absent peripheral pulsations are due to the extremity injury or to pre-existing disease. A history of claudication or the presence of trophic skin changes or absent hair growth on the foot being examined should be sought to clarify this situation. Repeated examinations of the extremity for evidences of arterial injury are important in detecting delayed occlusion, the pulsating hematoma of a false aneurysm or the bruit of an arteriovenous fistula.

Doppler flow studies are of positive but limited assistance in diagnosing extremity arterial injuries. Although gaping avulsion injuries or severe fractures occasionally may interfere, usually a standard blood pressure cuff can be applied to the forearm or ankle and arterial pressures measured. Flow sounds can be evaluated without use of the cuff if its application is impossible. A decrease in velocity and absence of normal biphasic arterial flow sounds coupled with significantly decreased ankle or wrist pressures are strongly suggestive of proximal arterial injury but may also reflect compression, spasm or pre-existing occlusive disease. Similarly, a totally normal Doppler examination suggests arterial integrity but cannot completely rule out a tangential or nonoccluded arterial injury. Perhaps of most importance is its use in predicting viability of an extremity. If flow is reduced but audible at the wrist or ankle, especially in conjunction with a wrist or ankle pressure of greater than 30 mm. Hg, then the current viability of that extremity is probably guaranteed. This information may be useful in establishing priorities for multiple organ repairs or if evacuation to a more sophisticated facility is contemplated. Repeated sequential Doppler examinations should be done in this setting to detect any deterioration of flow due to propagation of arterial thrombus, tissue swelling or concomitant venous thrombosis. These techniques are also useful to monitor patients with severe extremity fractures before, during and after orthopedic repair. Alterations from the normal arterial signals would warrant arteriography. Furthermore, venous flow may be assessed for evidence of occlusion or pulsatile sounds suggesting that an arteriovenous fistula may be present.

Finally, the value of arteriography in evaluating arterial injuries cannot be overemphasized.[33] It is particularly useful in dissociating arterial spasm from actual occlusion, in providing earlier diagnosis in cases in which clinical evidence is not decisive (as following blunt trauma), in identifying the level of occlusion for more precise exploration (especially in the case of multiple penetrating injuries, multiple fractures or the elderly patient), in assessing the condition of collateral circulation and in detecting incomplete occlusions, false aneurysms and arteriovenous fistulas. When an extremity is markedly swollen from extensive crush injury to soft and bony tissue, physical examination is usually more difficult. Tense subcutaneous and muscle compartments alone may obliterate normal pulses and capillary filling and produce ischemic neuropathy. Only arteriography can delineate the state of the arterial system in these cases. It is unnecessary only in penetrating wounds in which the existence and location of the arterial injury are obvious.

Preoperative venography has little to recommend its use. If arterial exploration is planned, the vein will be visually inspected. Furthermore, radiographical extravasation from the low pressure venous system is not likely when adjacent hematoma and swelling are present and only occlusion could be determined. Occlusion can more easily be detected by Doppler examination if it exists at the popliteal level or more proximally.

TREATMENT

Once an arterial injury has been diagnosed, its relative priority in the overall management of the injuries to the patient must be established. Such a decision depends greatly upon the significance of the associated injuries as well as the immediate threat presented by the arterial injury itself. Although it is axiomatic that repair should be performed as soon as possible, it is equally true that once the possibility of exsanguinating hemorrhage has been recognized and dealt with, there may be no immediate threat of loss of life or limb from this injury, and trauma to other vital areas may deserve first or at least concomitant attention.

Nevertheless, the consequence of delay in restoring arterial circulation to the extremity must be taken into account in making such decisions. Although it is recognized that the often quoted 6- to 12-hour "golden period" is only relative, the results of treatments do correlate well with this concept. Edwards and Lyons[6] noted that gangrene was rare following successful repairs undertaken within 6 hours of injury but occurred in over 50 per cent beyond 12 hours. In Jahnke's experience[13] with 77 consecutive arterial repairs during the Korean conflict, no amputations were required when the delay was 12 hours or less but were required in 29 per cent after this lapse of time. Makin et al.,[21] reporting results with arterial injuries associated with fractures or dislocation, found the late amputation rate to be 16 per cent when delay was less than 12 hours and 80 per cent beyond that, with the remaining 20 per cent of the patients suffering permanent disability.

The degree of urgency for repair is often decided by the apparent viability of the skin. However, it should be recognized that outward appearances may be deceiving because muscle and especially nerves are much less tolerant of prolonged ischemia than is skin. The work of Malan and Tattoni[23] indicates that myelin degeneration and axon retraction begin after 4 to 6 hours of ischemia and that discoid degeneration with progressive loss of contractility may affect 90 per cent of the muscle fibers by 12 hours, beyond which time only partial recovery is possible. Failure to recognize this may lead to serious late disability from nerve deficits or ischemic muscle contractures. Areas of skin anesthesia and digital paralysis or foot drop should be considered *late* warning signs of serious limb ischemia. In this regard, Lavenson et al.[19] have shown a good correlation between viability and audible flow through nonpalpable distal vessels, e.g., the posterior tibial artery at the ankle, using an ultrasound flow detector.

In addition, before electing not to repair immediately a peripheral arterial injury in which there is no threat to viability of the extremity, consideration must be given to the possible dire consequences that distal propagation of thrombus with occlusion of additional collaterals might bring to the marginally viable extremity. If there is good reason to favor delayed reconstruction, one must still continue close observation and be prepared to reverse this decision at the first sign of deterioration. At the other extreme is a controversial thesis proposed by Brisbin[2] that noncritical arterial combat injuries be ligated rather than repaired when optimal conditions are not present. Such opinion was fostered by postoperative disruption of five superficial femoral repairs and one popliteal artery repair performed at forward hospitals in Vietnam. It was emphasized that, particularly in the young, it is ordinarily not essential to limb survival to repair the brachial artery between the profunda and elbow collaterals, the ulnar or radial artery alone at any level, the profunda femoris artery, the superficial femoral artery proximal to the geniculate collaterals and the anterior tibial, posterior tibial or perineal artery alone at any level. By the same token, vascular repair in the face of serious neuromuscular or skeletal injuries that preclude the return of useful limb function must be avoided. However, in a more favorable environment and particularly when not restricted by priorities dictated by other injuries, it is probably wise to at least explore all potential injuries to "name" vessels regardless of how inconsequential the injuries may seem, for even if viability is not at issue, late aneurysms and arteriovenous fistulas may be avoided and those successfully repaired may serve an unexpected later purpose.

The most pressing indication for treatment following arterial injury is, of course, exsanguinating hemorrhage. This should be controlled initially with direct application of pressure over the site of injury or the course of the artery proximal to this.

The use of a tourniquet is condemned except under the most extreme circumstances since this technique occludes collateral circulation as well as the injured vessel. In addition, improper application of the tourniquet frequently succeeds only in stemming venous outflow. In large wounds over superficial arteries, hemostasis may be achieved by direct clamping. However, blind clamping into the depths of a bleeding wound only allows additional blood loss at a time when it can be least well tolerated. Unless vascular clamps are available, the artery injury may be compounded by this practice, necessitating a more extensive debridement and possibly the need for a graft.

Once control of hemorrhage has been established, it should be maintained until circulating blood volume has been restored and additional blood is on hand to support definitive exploration. Tetanus prophylaxis should be administered and, in most cases, broad spectrum antibiotic coverage should be provided for the indications of shock, tissue ischemia or gross contamination.

The actual technique of surgical exploration and repair of arterial injuries must be individualized, but certain principles should be considered. Ordinarily, general anesthesia can be used, but such considerations as an associated head injury, alcoholic intoxication or the desire to continue observation for suspected thoracic or abdominal trauma may dictate the use of regional anesthesia. Many surgeons actually prefer the latter because of the theoretical benefit of vasodilatation, and continuous epidural anesthesia is gaining popularity for elective vascular procedures in the lower extremity. The entire extremity and adjacent areas of the trunk as well as the area over the upper saphenous vein in an uninvolved extremity should be prepared and draped. Provision should *always* be made for intraoperative arteriography where available.

One of the first steps should be to gain proximal control of the injured artery. Occasionally it is easiest to use a small, separate incision to tape and occlude the artery proximally. This provides a relatively bloodless field for exploring the injured vessel. Usually it is expeditious to explore directly through a penetrating tract or over an area of blunt injury. The missile entry site can be excised with the same incision. Extremity incisions should be oriented longitudinally with the patient in the supine position. This is of critical importance when surgical wounds need to be lengthened for increased exposure or if a bypass is necessitated. These incisions will generally correspond to those used for elective exposure of this part of the arterial tree.

Although it is not necessary in early operations on simple peripheral arterial injuries, consideration should be given in other cases, as soon as hemostasis has been established, to inserting a temporary arterial shunt, using a length of thromboresistant plastic tubing to bridge the defect. This technique, as recommended by Eger et al.,[7] provides several advantages: early restoration of flow and prevention of further ischemia during the course of the operation; the ability to perfuse the distal vascular bed with heparin solutions (under pressure if necessary to overcome high critical closing pressures); allowance of more accurate debridement of nonviable tissues, repair of damaged veins *before* arterial repair and fixation of concomitant fractures prior to the vascular repair as well as the performance of most of the vascular reconstruction without interruption of flow. An important additional technical suggestion, to be carried out prior to use of this technique and again just prior to the completion of the final anastomosis, is the removal of thrombus from the distal arterial tree using Fogarty balloon catheters. The presence of back bleeding cannot be considered reliable evidence of distal patency. Only intraoperative arteriography can reliably provide evidence of distal patency and should be used whenever normal distal pulses are not completely restored. Systemic heparinization is not without its dangers in the face of other injuries or prior to wound debridement. In such cases, brief intermittent release of the controlling clamps, with or without installation of a small dose of heparin (30 mg.) or a heparin-Ringer's lactated solution into the distal artery, may provide a reasonable alternative. Of course, this so-called "distal" or "regional" heparinization is only possible while circulatory interruption is maintained. In less complicated situations, systemic heparinization (1 mg./kg. every 2 to 3 hours) may be carried out as in elective arterial surgery.

Accurate assessment of the true nature and extent of the arterial injury is of utmost importance. One common mistake is to assume that an intact but narrowed arterial segment represents spasm alone when, in fact, mechanical obstruction exists from intimal disruption or dissection or from intramural hematoma and segmental thrombosis. In general, it is wiser to assume that arterial spasm is associated with some significant intramural injury and to open the vessel than to persist with external efforts to relieve it or to close the wound with the expectation that the "spasm" will eventually abate.

However, if either exploration or a good arteriogram has ruled out mechanical intraluminal problems, a number of maneuvers may be attempted to relieve the arterial spasm (Fig. 19–2). Segmental periarterial neurectomy, by excision of the adventitial layer, is worthwhile. In addition to this, the topical application of warm saline solutions of Xylocaine, sodium nitrite, papaverine or Priscoline has been recommended, either by infiltration of the arterial wall or application of a gauze sponge soaked in these solutions. Howev-

er, neither of these is as effective as mechanical dilation in overcoming simple segmental spasm. If the vessel has been opened, this may be achieved by spreading a clamp within the lumen of the segment or drawing an inflated balloon catheter through it. In the closed vessel, injection of saline into the lumen of the segment isolated between two vascular clamps may achieve the same effect. Although secondary diffuse spasm may respond to regional sympathetic block or intra-arterial injections of vasodilators, the segmental spasm more frequently encountered in arterial injuries appears to result from local, myogenic reflexes that are usually refractory to these latter measures. Finally, if all local measures fail to relieve segmental spasm, it is usually wiser to resect the involved segment and replace it with a vein graft. Careful examination of such segments will usually reveal evidences of more extensive intramural damage than suspected.

Another common mistake is to underestimate the *extent* of the injury to the arterial wall beyond the gross limits of the penetrating wound itself. This has proved particularly important in Vietnam, where high-velocity missile wounds are common. In such situations, histological studies

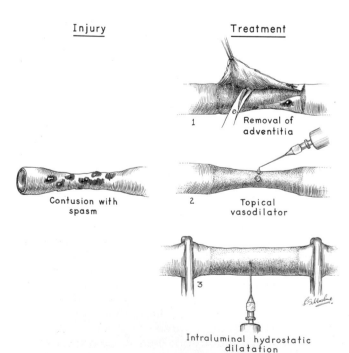

Injury   Treatment

1   Removal of adventitia

Contusion with spasm

2   Topical vasodilator

3

Intraluminal hydrostatic dilatation

Figure 19–2. *Local measures commonly used to relieve segmental arterial spasm.*

have shown microscopic damage for more than a centimeter beyond the limits of grossly visible injury. However, Rich[28] no longer recommends the arbitrary resection of 2- to 3-cm. margins, the policy that was initially suggested following these studies.

The method of reconstruction will depend on the extent of injury to the arterial wall. Figure 19–1 illustrates the usual repairs employed for the most common forms of arterial injury. Basically, they include reapproximation of cleanly incised wounds, wedge excision of small penetrating wounds with primary closure or saphenous vein patch graft, and segmental excision with reanastomosis or interposition of a hydrostatically dilated reversed segment of saphenous vein. The actual suture techniques have not changed greatly from the principles layed down by Carrel in 1907.[3] The adventitia should be cleared from the margins of repair. The suture should traverse the full thickness of the arterial wall; repeated inspection is necessary to ensure inclusion of the intima. The size of the suture material, its pattern of placement and the choice of interrupted or continuous technique must be individualized. In general, finer interrupted technique is used in smaller arteries, and simple through-and-through sutures are preferred to everting mattress sutures. The newer synthetic suture materials are preferable to silk.

End-to-end anastomosis may be possible after mobilization of the proximal and distal ends of the artery, but suture line tension and narrowing must be carefully avoided. To this end, the use of autogenous vein for patch or circumferential grafting has been invaluable. The preference for an autogenous vein over a prosthetic graft is particularly valid for peripheral arteries and in the presence of gross contamination or significant tissue damage. An acceptable alternative to use of the saphenous vein that is still preferable to the use of a prosthesis in this situation is provided by the cephalic or even the basilic veins in the arm. If the physician is already operating inside the abdomen, the hypogastric artery may be sacrificed if it is essential to replace a segment of iliac artery with autologous vessel of similar diameter, especially in the face of widespread contamination. One can expect in the adult to be able to harvest a length of hypogastric artery measuring 4 to 5 cm. with an average diameter of 7 to 8 mm.[34] Any injury that is extensive enough to warrant the use of a graft is likely to be associated with injury to the accompanying vein or to require prolonged immobilization. To avoid an additional threat to the venous system in such an injured extremity, it is recommended that the saphenous vein graft be obtained from the uninvolved side whenever possible. Otherwise, the technique of saphenous vein grafting does not differ from that normally employed. The segment must be reversed to maintain normal orientation to flow. This is preferable to leaving it in its original orientation to the extremity and avulsing or excising its valves. Its lumen should be distended to physiological pressure with heparinized Ringer's lactated solution, and, ideally, its distended diameter should be almost equal to or slightly exceed that of the artery it is to replace. Repair of small, noncritical arteries is certainly not obligatory, especially in the face of other more serious injuries. However, tandem injuries to radial-ulnar or tibial-peroneal arteries may necessitate intervention to preserve limb viability. Also, the amputation rate following brachial artery occlusion of up to 4 per cent[20] and possible subsequent arm claudication make brachial artery repair almost mandatory. Techniques of repair are essentially the same as for larger vessels but should include the use of fine (6–0 or 7–0) interrupted monofilament (polypropylene) sutures placed with the aid of optical magnification. Postoperative antiplatelet medication (ASA gr. 10 by mouth or rectum b.i.d. for 2 weeks) probably aids in maintaining patency.[15]

Following arterial repair, pulses should be palpable at a distal position in the extremity (usually the wrist or ankle), which have been included in the sterile field for this very purpose. If pulses are not easily felt, the surgeon should not assume that this is due to reversible spasm but should perform an intraoperative arteriogram. This can be done easily by rapidly injecting 15–25 ml. of contrast material through an 18-gauge needle connected to a syringe by a short segment of sterile IV tubing. Momentary bulldog occlusion of the artery just proximal to the injection site can help avoid washout of the contrast agent and provide high-quality films. The x-ray cassette can be wrapped in a sterile Mayo stand cover and placed under the free-draped extremity. Defects in the arterial profile must be assumed to be thrombi and further efforts must be made to retrieve them.

There are frequently other problems requiring attention, although the repair of the arterial injury usually takes precedence. One common exception to this involves the management of concomitant fractures, the stable reduction of which must be coordinated with the arterial repair. In such a circumstance, certain questions arise, the answers to which determine the sequence to be followed. How will reduction and stabilization best be achieved? How urgent is restoration of flow? Will subsequent reduction and stabilization of the fracture imperil the repaired artery or be interfered with by it? Will the final position of fixation cause tension on or kink the repaired vessel? Will skeletal shortening accompanying the reduction influence the length of the arterial segment of interposed graft to be anastomosed? Ordinarily, in civilian practice, the repair can follow reduction and fixation of the fracture and, in instances in which there is urgency to restore flow, a temporary internal shunt may be employed as suggested previously. The Vietnam experience has shown, however, that rigid adherence to this preferred sequence is not necessary and individualization should be allowed. In fact, the current trend is toward vascular repair first with *external* fixation being carefully applied at the end of the procedure to avoid introducing foreign material into the wound. The Hoffmann or Vidal-Adrey device[14] is a helpful adjunct that allows skeletal pins, placed at a distance from the injury, to be externally stabilized by a metal frame. The risk of osteomyelitis secondary to internal fixation can thereby be eliminated. The extremity subsequently can be dressed without plaster, which facilitates wound care and examination of pulses and tissue viability. An alternative method is to incorporate the Steinman pins into a cast, which is immediately bivalved to avoid constriction.

Concomitant injuries to the accompanying nerves and veins are frequent, and their management in this setting bears comment. Distal motor and sensory function will have been assessed prior to operation, but the weakness and numbness that accompany ischemia may be misleading. Delayed repair of injuries to peripheral nerves is the usual rule in complicated, high-velocity or seriously contaminated wounds, but even in these situations, the operator can facilitate the subsequent repair by carefully assessing the appearance of the nerves at time of exploration and tagging their ends in line with the perineural vessels for future orientation. Although there is still considerable disagreement over immediate versus delayed (3 weeks to 3 months) repair, most investigators now recommend concomitant nerve repair under less complicated circumstances than those just described, provided a surgeon experienced with these injuries is available. The decision to repair concomitant venous injuries will be dealt with later in this chapter, but in general is recommended.

Thorough irrigation and debridement of damaged muscles and other soft tissues should follow the principles outlined in the previous chapter. Skin coverage can normally be achieved by mobilization of surrounding skin, but if a flap is necessary, the defect it produces can be filled by a split-thickness graft. It is undesirable to have a repaired artery covered only by skin, not only because it will be exposed if the skin closure breaks down, but because it will be more susceptible to trauma in the future. In addition, delayed skin closure may be dictated by the degree of contamination of the wound. This goal cannot always be easily achieved because of injury to surrounding muscle, but a muscle flap can usually be mobilized to cover the site of repair. In the femoral triangle, for example, the sartorius is usually available and can be used in the manner employed in radical groin dissections.

When there has been early and adequate repair of a discrete arterial injury, little more need be done to achieve excellent results. In other instances, ancillary measures bear consideration, particularly fasciotomy. The rationale for fasciotomy is that ischemia, particularly if associated with some degree of venous obstruction, will lead to swelling of muscles within the fascial compartments of the calf or forearm with eventual impairment of capillary flow to the muscles and, finally, necrosis and fibrosis. Although it has been debated that swelling alone cannot be responsible for this consequence (since the extravascular pressure it creates can hardly exceed the intravascular pressure that generates it), those who have seen the tense, pale muscle expand through fasciotomy incisions and become pink again think that this argument is academic and cite venous gangrene of distended, obstructed gut and swollen pedicle flaps as a precedent.

Patman and Shires[25] have advocated fasciotomy under the following circumstances: undue delay, prolonged shock, extensive soft tissue damage, damage to venae comitantes and preoperative swelling of the limb. Their low amputation rate (3.8 per cent) has been partly attributed by them to the liberal use of these criteria. Theoretically, most vascular surgeons support the use of fasciotomy in most of these circumstances but, in practice, few employ it quite so liberally for "prophylactic" in-

dications. The proponents of prophylactic fasciotomy argue that it can be carried out through small skin incisions with little additional time and risk and that it is only effective if carried out early, before irreversible changes in the muscle have taken place. More objective methods that measure the pressure within the fascial compartments have been devised and are advocated by some authors.[36] Perhaps the best of these devices employs a porous wick that is placed percutaneously into the muscle compartment and resists occlusion by adjacent tissue. Compartment pressure that approaches the arterial diastolic pressure should prompt fasciotomy. However, the results of these pressure-measuring techniques have been difficult to reproduce, leading most trauma surgeons to abandon their use in favor of the clinical indicators already mentioned.

The standard fasciotomy (Fig. 19–3) calls for three small vertical linear skin incisions in the mid-calf over each of the anteror, lateral and posterior muscle com-

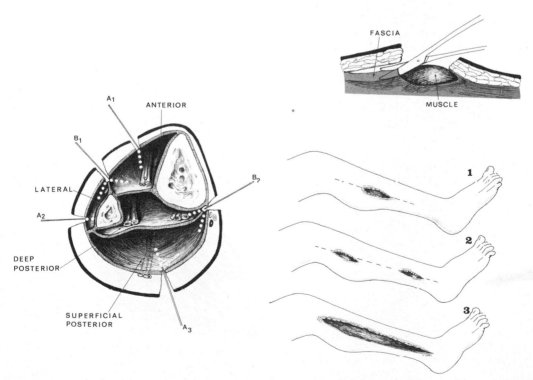

Figure 19–3. *The "standard" fasciotomy approach involving three linear incisions (A$_1$, A$_2$ and A$_3$) through the outer fascia of the anterior, lateral and superficial posterior muscle compartments of the calf. This may be accomplished by one or two short skin incisions (1 and 2) through which the scissors may be passed and slid along the cut edge of the fascia (insert) or by a long incision (3) which may be loosely closed or left open for secondary closure or grafting. This approach does not decompress the deep posterior compartment. All four compartments can be opened through two incisions (B$_1$ and B$_2$) but full-length incisions (3) must be made.*

partments. Through these the overlying fascia can be slit for most of its length by sliding the cutting edges of the partly opened scissors against the superior and inferior ends of the fascial defect. Skin closure may defeat the purpose of fasciotomy and may not even be possible without undue tension once the swollen muscle compartment expands. Some believe that the fasciotomy skin incision should be as long as the fascial incision, but most feel that should be done only if, after fascial incision, the skin can be seen to be providing a constricting effect. In order to decompress the fourth or deep posterior compartment, the posteromedial calf incision must be deepened to allow the surgeon to incise the fascia overlying the deep plantar flexor muscles. This is essential in the markedly swollen or contused extremity. Finally, four compartment decompression can also be achieved by the more radical fibulectomy-fasciotomy, as originally advocated by Kelly.[17] This procedure employs removal of the middle three fifths of the fibula through a single lateral calf inci-

sion (Fig. 19–4). Although removal of this portion of the fibula causes little or no functional disability, it leaves a major open wound to contend with. For this reason, most surgeons reserve this fibulectomy-fasciotomy for the more advanced situations and use the standard approach in early or prophylactic situations.

Fasciotomy of the hand, foot and even individual digits is occasionally necessary when those parts are tense and interfering with adequate perfusion. Classic incisions to avoid weight-bearing surfaces and later contracture are recommended. Sympathectomy is another adjuvant measure, but one of debatable effectiveness. Although the relief of arterial spasm is its usual justification, local rather than peripheral nervous factors appear to be more important in the spasm associated with direct arterial trauma,[18] and the local measures outlined previously seem to be more effective than sympathetic blockade. However, sympathectomy has been shown to acutely increase resting nutrient flow to muscle, skin and bone, particularly in the more distal

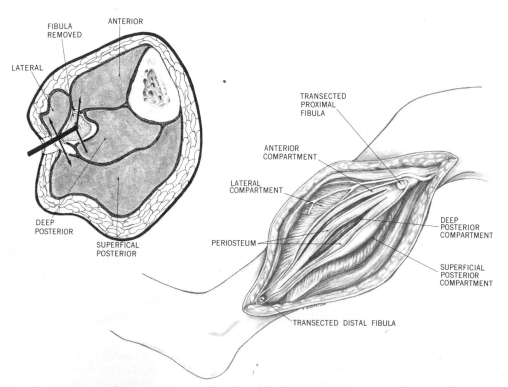

Figure 19–4. The "radical" fasciotomy of fibulectomy fasciotomy in which all four muscle compartments of the calf are exposed, incised and decompressed through the bed of a subperiosteal fibulectomy.

part of the extremity.[30] This occurs even in the face of proximal arterial occlusion, but the flow increases are not as great as flow-meter studies would suggest since much of the increase in flow passes through opened arteriovenous shunts and does not nourish the tissues. Nevertheless, this non-nutrient flow may help in keeping grafts patent during the early days. Nonetheless, it is the authors' opinion that it will rarely spell the difference between success or failure in arterial injury repair, and obviously it will not cover up for technical inadequacies. During that short initial postoperative period when sympathetic denervation may be useful, intermittent lidocaine infusion through an indwelling epidural catheter can usually achieve this effect and an additional operative procedure can be avoided.

The previously discussed, and other, measures are commonly resorted to when satisfactory return of circulation has not been achieved or when the level of circulation initially achieved by surgery deteriorates. Before attributing this state of affairs to arterial spasm or compartmental swelling, technical failure at the site of repair must be ruled out by arteriography or re-exploration. The latter possibility is particularly likely whenever there is an abrupt deterioration in the peripheral pulses, skin temperature or capillary filling. This underscores the importance of frequent monitoring of the state of the circulation of the injured limb in the early postoperative period. Doppler flow sounds and limb pressure determinations help to reflect normal restored flow and significant alterations in these parameters can provide early warning of arterial reocclusion. Routine intraoperative arteriography after the reconstruction has been completed and before closure will do much to uncover these problems before they become manifest, and provides welcome assurance to the surgeon during those early hand-wringing hours that nothing important has been overlooked in providing the best possible chance for restoration of limb viability and function.

VENOUS INJURIES

Venous injuries of significance may be isolated but more commonly occur in association with injury to the accompanying artery. They will be discovered if sought at the time of arterial exploration, but even a major deep venous occlusion will frequently be missed if it is an independent injury. It should be suspected whenever early swelling or cyanosis occurs distal to the injury.

Simple, clean lacerations of major veins should be repaired primarily after removal of secondary thrombus formation. Repair of more extensive injury rarely results in permanent patency and is more likely to lead to thromboembolic complications. However, in the Vietnam experience, in which repair of the concomitant venous injury has been accomplished in approximately one third of the cases, the threat of pulmonary embolism did not become manifest. Even though it is realized that eventual thrombosis of the venous repair is likely to occur in the majority of cases, repair of major venous injuries is currently being advised because it is believed that the success of the arterial repair is jeopardized when major venous outflow obstruction exists, and if this can be avoided by even a few days of patency of the venous reconstruction, it will be worthwhile. This is dramatically evident in the superior results obtained with popliteal artery repair when concomitant popliteal vein injuries were repaired rather than ligated.[35] Fortunately, the situation in which the injury is severe enough to involve the major venous collaterals and dictate repair of the major vein also favors the patency of the repair because of the high rate of obligatory flow that must pass through the anastomosis. If the vein is not the major portal of venous return or is too badly damaged to repair, double ligation is recommended with the proximal ligature placed just distal to the next large tributary whenever feasible. Significant disability following such ligation is usually temporary if a careful postoperative regimen, similar to that employed following thrombophlebitis, is adhered to and additional venous thrombosis avoided. However, unlike the postphlebitic limb in which recannulization with valvular incompetence occurs and leads to permanent disability, elastic support and intermittent elevation may not be necessary indefinitely following uncomplicated ligation, and the tendency to dependent edema often subsides with the development of adequate collateral tributaries. The use of postoperative heparin may increase the likelihood of permanent patency following vein repair. A regimen of low-dose (5,000 units every 8 hours) heparin for the first 48 hours followed by full-dose heparin for 10 days has been suggested by one author.[16]

Amputation

Amputation may be indicated from the outset if the damage to the tissues of the extremity, and particularly the nerves, is so extensive that successful vascular repair and reconstruction of the remaining structures would not provide a useful appendage. In marginal cases, this decision requires experienced judgment and, unless the situation is clearly hopeless, it is better to proceed with reconstruction. Amputation may be necessary later if the arterial reconstruction fails and the causes of this failure cannot be overcome. Unless the threat of systemic toxic effects from crushed, infected or gangrenous tissues becomes manifest, delayed amputation is preferred if for no other reason than that its unquestionable need will become clearly apparent to and better accepted by the patient. Even in this situation, the so-called "debridement amputation" has great merit as a preliminary procedure to control infection and allow the definitive amputation to be carried out with a higher degree of success in primary healing. Furthermore, the additional time allows for the development of collateral circulation and potentially a lower level of amputation. Immediate fitting of prostheses is important in the elderly to avoid unretrievable loss of walking skills and in the young for morale purposes. The details of definitive amputations are beyond the scope of this chapter.

LATE SEQUELAE AND RESULTS

The results of failure to achieve adequate arterial repair have already been mentioned. The degree of success achieved may not be apparent until the adequacy of circulation has been tested by normal use. Even then, the late results of arterial repair, particularly when grafts are used, may be hard to document and evaluate since these procedures are ordinarily performed for occlusive arterial disease of later life. Whether the repaired vessels of younger patients will be the site of predilection for arteriosclerosis and other degenerative changes will only be answered in time, but these considerations do not invalidate the procedures presently employed.

The most common late sequelae of arterial injury are false aneurysms and arteriovenous fistulas. The impression that these are delayed complications of arterial injuries is probably not justified. Rather it is their recognition that is delayed, a carry-over from the time when wounds not presenting an immediate threat to limb survival were not explored. Early exploration and definitive treatment of suspected arterial injuries, as practiced in the past 15 years, should continue to reduce the incidence of these sequelae.

The early recognition of an arteriovenous fistula usually depends upon the auscultation of a bruit in the region of a recent penetrating wound. Pulsatile arterial sounds heard by the Doppler apparatus with the probe placed over the effluent vein is also diagnostic. Later, attention may be attracted by symptoms of decreased arterial circulation distal to the fistula, increased venous collaterals and, eventually, even varicosities in the vicinity of the fistula or, finally (in large, proximal fistulas), the signs and symptoms of high-output cardiac failure. The hemodynamic alterations associated with arteriovenous fistulas and their therapeutic implications have been thoroughly documented by the work of Holman[11] and Elkin.[8]

In general, an arteriovenous fistula should either be attacked early when it is little more than a poorly organized communicating hematoma and before major venous collaterals have had time to develop, or operated on 6 weeks to 3 months later when the acute inflammatory reaction has subsided. When done within the first day or so, fistulas are technically not much more difficult than any other acute arterial injury. The procedure of choice is repair of both artery and vein or at least repair of the artery and double ligation of the vein. If for some reason both artery and vein have to be sacrificed, the rationale for quadruple ligation (artery and vein proximal and distal to the fistula) as well worked out by Holman[11] should be heeded.

Traumatic false aneurysms are usually

allowed to develop because the possible significance of an innocuous-appearing wound over the course of a major artery is not considered. One should be particularly suspicious of excessive bleeding or hematoma formation following such wounds. The expansile or pulsatile nature of such hematomas may not be apparent until later. The same preference for early operation that has been expressed in regard to arteriovenous fistulas applies to false aneurysm. At the time of operation, proximal and distal control of the involved vessel is necessary before approaching the aneurysm itself. It is frequently necessary to use a partial or circumferential graft to repair the vessel after excision of the aneurysm, although success has been reported in the use of endaneurysmorrhaphy, in which the communication is closed through the opened aneurysmal sac.

REFERENCES

1. Amato, J. J., Rich, N. M., Billy, L. J., Grubner, R. P., and Lawson, N. S.: High-velocity arterial injury. J. Trauma 11:412, 1971.
2. Brisbin, R. L., Geib, P. O., and Eiseman, B.: Secondary disruption of vascular repair following war wounds. Arch. Surg. 99:787, 1969.
3. Carrel, A.: The surgery of blood vessels. Johns Hopkins Bull. 18:18, 1907.
4. Carrel, A.: Heterotransplantation of blood vessels preserved in cold storage. J. Exp. Med. 9:226, 1907.
5. DeBakey, M. E., and Simeone, F. A.: Battle injuries of the arteries in World War II. Ann. Surg. 123:534, 1946.
6. Edwards, W. S., and Lyons, C.: Traumatic arterial spasm and thrombosis. Ann. Surg. 140:318, 1954.
7. Eger, M., Gokman, L., Goldstein, A., and Hirsch, M.: The use of a temporary shunt in the managment of arterial vascular injuries. Surg. Gynecol. Obstet. 13:67, 1971.
8. Elkin, D. C.: The treatment of aneurysms and arteriovenous fistulas. Bull. N. Y. Acad. Med. 22:81, 1946.
9. Foster, J. H., et al.: Arterial injuries secondary to the use of the Fogarty catheter. Ann. Surg. 171:971, 1970.
10. Guthrie, G. C.: Heterotransplantation of blood vessels. Am. J. Physiol. 19:482, 1907.
11. Holman, E.: Arteriovenous aneurysm. Abnormal Communication Between the Arterial and Venous Circulations. New York, The MacMillan Co., 1937.
12. Hughes, C. W.: Arterial repair during the Korean War. Ann. Surg. 147:555, 1958.
13. Jahnke, E. J., Jr., and Seeley, S. F.: Acute vascular injuries in the Korean War: An analysis of 77 consecutive cases. Ann. Surg. 138:158, 1953.
14. Karlström, G., and Olerud, S.: Percutaneous pin fixation of open tibial fractures. J. Bone Joint Surg. 57A:915, 1975.
15. Kelly, G. L., and Eiseman, B.: Management of small arterial injuries. J. Trauma 16:681, 1976.
16. Kelly, G. L., and Eiseman, B.: Civilian vascular injuries. J. Trauma 15:507, 1975.
17. Kelly, R. P., and Whitesides, T. E., Jr.: Transfibular route for fasciotomy of the leg. J. Bone Joint Surg. 49A:1022, 1967.
18. Kinmouth, J. B.: The physiology and relief of traumatic arterial spasm. Br. Med. J. 47:59, 1952.
19. Lavenson, G. S., Rich, N. M., and Baugh, J. H.: Value of ultrasonic flow detector in the management of peripheral vascular disease. Am. J. Surg. 120:522, 1970.
20. Machleder, H. I., Sweeney, J. P., and Barker, W. F.: Pulseless arm after brachial artery catheterization. Lancet 1:407, 1972.
21. Makin, G. A., Howard, J. M., and Green, R. L.: Arterial injuries complicating fractures or dislocations: The necessity for a more aggressive approach. Surgery 59:203, 1966.
22. Makins, G. W.: Gunshot Injuries to the Blood Vessels. Bristol, England, John Wright & Sons, Ltd., 1919.
23. Malan, E., and Tattoni, G.: Physio- and anatopathology of acute ischemia of the extremities. J. Cardiovasc. Surg. 4:2, 1963.
24. Nolan, B.: Vascular injuries. J. R. Coll. Surg. 13:72, 1968.
25. Patman, R. D., Poulos, E., and Shires, G. T.: The management of civilian arterial injuries. Surg. Gynecol. Obstet. 118:725, 1964.
26. Perry, M. O., Thal, E. R., and Shires, G. T.: Management of arterial injuries. Ann. Surg. 173:403, 1971.
27. Rich, N. R., et al.: Popliteal artery injuries in Vietnam. Am. J. Surg. 118:531, 1969.
28. Rich, N. R.: Vascular trauma in Vietnam. J. Cardiovasc. Surg. 11:368, 1970.
29. Richardson, J. D., McElvein, R. B., and Trinkle, J. K.: First rib fracture: A hallmark of severe trauma. Ann. Surg. 181:251, 1975.
30. Rutherford, R. B., and Valenta, J.: Extremity blood flow and distribution. The effects of arterial occlusion, sympathectomy and exercise. Surgery 69:322, 1971.
31. Schumacker, H. B, Jr.: Arterial suture techniques and grafts: Past, present and future. Surgery 66:419, 1969.
32. Shires, G. T., and Patman, R. D.: Vascular Injuries in the Care of the Trauma Patient. New York, McGraw-Hill Book Co., Inc., 1966.
33. Sinkler, W. H., and Spencer, A. D.: The value of peripheral arteriography in assessing acute vascular injuries. Arch. Surg. 80:300, 1960.
34. Stoney, R. J.: The arterial autograft. In Rutherford, R. B. (ed.): Vascular Surgery. Philadelphia, W. B. Saunders, 1977, p. 363.
35. Sullivan, W. G., et al.: Early influence of popliteal vein repair in the treatment of popliteal vessel injuries. Am. J. Surg. 122:528, 1971.
36. Whitesides, T. E., et al.: A simple method for tissue pressure determination. Arch. Surg. 110:1311, 1975.

CHAPTER 20

INITIAL MANAGEMENT OF FRACTURES AND JOINT INJURIES: THORACIC AND LUMBAR SPINE, PELVIS AND HIP

James L. Hughes, M.D.

The physician in the emergency department setting, by his expertise in the diagnosis and initial management of an injured patient, can play a major role in how rapidly the patient may return to normal activity. Many long-term problems can be prevented by the appropriate initial management. This chapter will be limited to the general principles of initial diagnosis and treatment so as to guide a house officer or generalist prior to a consultation with the appropriate specialist. When applicable, an outline of definitive care will be given.

Each physician responsible for the initial care of an accident victim must recognize that each injury requires a rapid diagnosis coupled with steps to prevent deterioration. Nowhere is this more applicable than in fractures of the spine and the pelvis. It must be remembered that these fractures are frequently associated with other injuries. It is good practice to alert the patient and his family, if possible, that other injuries may remain undisclosed for several days while attention is directed toward obvious life-threatening problems.

THORACOLUMBAR SPINE

Spinal injuries range from a paravertebral muscle contusion with little or no effect on the patient, to a dislocation of the thoracolumbar vertebrae with paraplegia. In all cases of trauma, damage to the spine must be considered and ruled out by appropriate examinations. It is estimated that approximately 7000 new cases of permanent injury to the spinal cord occur each year. Improper care in the emergency department may contribute to permanent damage, and it is this fact that governs the protocol for emergency care.

Evidence of Injury. Every accident victim should be quickly examined for weakness or paralysis, sensory impairment and pain or tenderness along the spine. A thorough neurological examination should not be done at the time the patient is first seen but should be performed later when all parameters are stable. Until confirmation of stability is made via specific examinations, all spinal injuries are to be considered unstable.

Initial treatment should actually begin at the scene of the accident by a well-trained ambulance crew. If the patient arrives in the emergency department in a position other than a prone or supine one, this change of position should be accomplished immediately. An emergency stretcher, such as that manufactured by the Stryker Corp., is useful in maintaining the proper position. Upon arrival into the emergency department, all clothing is removed without altering the position of the patient. If a neurological deficit is present, great care is taken to prevent the patient from lying on any objects that may begin pressure necrosis of the skin (decubitus ulcer).

Documentation should be made immediately as to the adequacy of the airway, the presence or absence of shock and the level of consciousness. Neurological injuries may cause a distortion of physical findings. Injuries to the abdomen may be masked by spinal cord injury. Loss of the normal pain sensation may cause a ruptured viscus to go unrecognized. With flaccid paralysis the abdomen may remain soft when the presence of blood, intestinal contents or urine in the peritoneal cavity would normally cause board-like rigidity. The opposite may also occur, in that with partial cord transection, rigidity of the abdomen may occur when no intraabdominal pathology is present.

Spinal shock is a state that may immediately follow spinal trauma in which the cord is transected. Transection may occur either as a result of a complete laceration of the cord or by temporary loss of the blood supply, a physiological transection. In spinal shock all muscles below the level of the lesion are completely paralyzed, tone is lost and reflexes are initially abolished. When the lesion is above the thoracolumbar area, there is a temporary drop in blood pressure due to peripheral pooling of blood. In spinal shock the decrease in blood pressure is usually not accompanied by tachycardia. When one finds tachycardia and a falling hematocrit, attention should be turned toward the extremities, chest or abdomen in an attempt to find a source for hemorrhage.

A careful examination should be made of the lower extremities. In paraplegia the normal "pain signal" will be absent and a fracture or major vascular injury may be easily overlooked. A thorough manual examination should be made of all major joints and long bones, and the distal pulses checked.

Approximately 30 per cent of patients having thoracic or lumbar spine injuries have concomitant lesions, with the majority being craniocerebral in nature. A comatose or stuporous patient presents a difficult evaluation problem. Attention should be paid to any movement the patient makes in order to analyze the presence or absence of muscular activity. Only in profound coma will the normal withdrawal to painful stimulus be absent, provided the cord is intact. Usually, if one foot is raised and dropped directly over the other, the descending heel will not strike the resting foot unless paralysis is present in the falling limb. Care must be taken to control the comatose patient on the stretcher. Straps over the lower extremities should be separated from the skin by soft pliable material.

Preliminary Management. An adequate airway is the first priority. The standard procedures for maintaining an adequate airway have been covered elsewhere and may be applied here.

Circulatory support is next in order and this is accomplished by an intravenous infusion through a number 18 needle. When the IV is being started, blood should be drawn for type and cross-match, hematocrit, white blood count and differential and electrolytes.

Attention should be paid next to the urinary tract. A No. 14 or 16 French foley catheter should be utilized under strict aseptic technique. The amount of urine obtained should be carefully recorded. The catheter should then be placed to straight drainage.

Definitive Diagnosis and Management. Once emergency care has been rendered and the patient's condition is stable and under control, a careful and thorough examination can be undertaken.

If the patient is conscious, a history should be obtained as to how the injury occurred and, if paraplegia is present, whether the onset was acute or gradual. In addition to this brief but important history, the patient should be asked to pinpoint any area of pain or tenderness. Directions should be given to move the lower extremities and the presence or absence of movement recorded.

A detailed neurological examination should now be undertaken covering every dermatome of the trunk and lower extremity. It is helpful to have a chart, showing the dermatome distribution, on the wall in the emergency department. Movement, sensation, tone and reflex changes should be recorded. This initial record is critical, for without an accurate and thorough recording of this examination, future changes in the neurological picture cannot be appreciated. Table 20–1 shows the common findings in injuries to the thoracic and lumbar vertebrae with cord damage.

An examination of the back should next be undertaken without moving the patient. If the patient is supine, the examining hand may be slipped gently beneath the patient. Prominence of spinous processes, local tenderness, palpable or visible deformities and the presence of muscle spasm help to delineate the area of injury. Abrasions should be noted about the abdomen, for this may lead one to suspect a seatbelt injury.

If a thorough physical examination of the extremities, abdomen, chest and head was not accomplished initially, it should now be done.

Special Diagnostic Procedures. After the probable level of injury is determined, AP and lateral radiographs are made without moving the patient. This study should include at least four vertebral bodies above and below the suspected level of injury. These roentgenograms are examined for the contour and alignment of the vertebral bodies and the presence or absence of bone fragments protruding into the spinal canal. The most common area of injury in which the cord is damaged is at the junction of the mobile lumbar spine and the less mobile thoracic spine. Special attention should be paid to this area, looking for a slice fragment of the upper border of the body of the lower vertebrae (Fig. 20–2B and C). This represents the most unstable of all the injuries to the thoracolumbar spine. It must be kept in mind that all fractures of the spine will appear stable in the supine or prone position. If any questions arise as to the presence or absence of stability after the initial x-rays, tomograms should be taken.

Spinal taps should not be done as a routine procedure on these patients. This procedure should only be done in conjunction with a myelogram. There is a great difference of opinion as to when these procedures should be carried out. Consideration should be given to doing them if one suspects a block in a fracture dislocation or if protrusion into the cord by a fragment of bone or an intervertebral disc is suspected. Normal manometric studies in the spinal tap are more significant than an abnormal study, for tears in the dura or cord edema may prevent a rise in pressure on jugular compression.

Early Definitive Therapy. Open injuries of the vertebral column and spinal cord are extremely rare. When these are present, surgical repair is carried out as in

---

TABLE 20–1. Typical Findings with Injury to the Thoracic or Lumbar Spinal Cord

1. INJURY OF T1 TO T12

   a. Paraplegia.
   b. Initial absent deep tendon reflexes in lower extremities, absent cremasteric and plantar reflexes; upper abdominal reflexes may be preserved in low thoracic lesions.
   c. Anesthesia below the dermatome level on the trunk corresponding with level of cord damage.
   d. Bladder and bowel retention; priapism in male.

2. INJURY OF L1 TO L5

   a. Partial flaccid paraplegia, the extent depending on which roots of the cauda equina are involved.
   b. Above L2 knee and ankle jerks and plantar reflexes are absent; cremasteric reflexes present. Below L2 knee jerks are present.
   c. Anesthesia of perineum, sacral area and lower extremities may be spotty and asymmetrical.
   d. Bladder and bowel retention at least temporarily but perhaps with some retention of sensation.

any other soft tissue injury. A laminectomy is indicated if there is a persistent spinal fluid leak, indicating a laceration of the dura either by bone or a foreign body. All tears of the dura should be closed, utilizing fascial graft if necessary. Antibiotic coverage intravenously is indicated in conjunction with copious and frequent irrigation during surgery in an attempt to prevent meningitis. Many of these injuries will be secondary to a puncture wound with the point of entry away from the midline.

Types of Injury

Paravertebral Muscle Tear. A paravertebral muscle tear will reveal acute spasm and a list toward the injured area. X-ray examination will be within normal limits save perhaps for a scoliosis secondary to muscle spasm. Treatment is directed toward ablation of pain by the appropriate analgesics, bed rest and warm compresses.

Intervertebral Disc Injury. Protrusion of an intervertebral disc may be diagnosed by the history and physical findings that include a positive straight-leg-raising test in association with reflex and sensory changes. Positive identification is made by a myelogram. Conservative care of an acute disc should be undertaken initially just as was recommended for the paravertebral muscle tear.

Wedge or Compression Fractures. Wedge or compression fractures (Fig. 20–1A) are the most common fractures of the thoracic-lumbar spine in persons under 50 years of age. These occur most commonly as a result of a fall from a height in which the patient lands on his feet, transmitting acute flexion forces to the spine. The injury may well be coupled with a fracture of the os calcis. Occasionally, falling objects may strike the patient's shoulder, causing acute flexion of the spine and a compression fracture of the thoracic spine. In persons over 50 certain pathological conditions such as multiple myeloma, metastatic tumors or osteoporosis may predispose the patient to a fracture of the vertebral bodies with a minimum of external force. Occasionally, coughing, sneezing or just getting out of a chair may be the only history obtained.

X-rays will show a diminution in the anterior height of the vertebral body. This

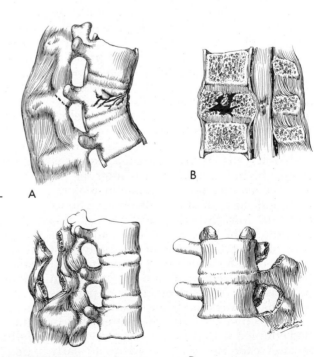

Figure 20–1. *Stable thoracolumbar spine fractures.*

diminution in height may be from 10 to 90 per cent of the vertebral body. Neurological deficit rarely occurs with this fracture, for the posterior elements remain intact.

Early treatment in the younger age group can be outlined as follows. The patient must at all times remain supine, having been given enough sedation to overcome the severe discomfort. It must be kept in mind that adynamic ileus may occur secondary to the paravertebral hematoma accompanying this fracture. If ileus occurs, IV fluids along with a nasogastric tube must be utilized. If the collapse of the vertebral body is over 30 per cent of the total height of the body, the patient should be carefully placed with his head at the foot of a hospital bed in order that the knee-gatch can be utilized to obtain hyperextension of the fractured area. A hinged fracture board is placed between the mattress and springs. The knee-gatch is then gradually elevated at approximately one turn of the crank per hour until it is believed that sufficient extension has been accomplished to reduce the fracture. This method should produce some reduction by tension on the anterior longitudinal ligament. A lateral x-ray should be taken to confirm the amount of reduction obtained. When the patient's spine stabilizes, he should be transferred to a Goldthwait frame for application of a hyperextension plaster jacket. Care must be taken in applying this plaster jacket to obtain pressure over three important bony prominences: the upper sternum and anterior chest, the iliac crests and the spine directly overlying the level of the fractured vertebra. Care must be taken to cover the iliac crest, rib margins, pubic and upper sternum with felt pads. Hyperextension exercises should be initiated very early after the injury, for maintenance of an adequate paravertebral musculature is of prime importance in lowering the morbidity of this fracture. If the collapse is less than 30 per cent of the total height of the body, rest followed by hyperextension exercises will be sufficient treatment for a good result. In persons over 50 years of age or in persons who have sustained minimum trauma, complete bed rest with the patient flat in bed coupled with the early use of hyperextension exercises will be adequate early treatment. Early ambulation of the patient

can be accomplished by the use of the Taylor back brace. Appropriate attention should be paid to any pre-existing pathology that predisposed to the fracture.

"Burst" Fracture. "Burst" fractures (Fig. 20–1B) are similar to compression injuries except that in this instance the line of force is almost perpendicular to the vertebral column. As the forces are transmitted down the column, the affected vertebral body appears to explode. Owing to the projection of fragments posteriorly, there may occasionally be a neurological deficit. This deficit is usually transitory in nature but if not, a myelogram should be done. If a block is demonstrated, appropriate surgical decompression should be accomplished.

If decompression is not necessary, treatment consists of bed rest in neutral position. The hyperextended position should be avoided. When the patient stabilizes, a plaster jacket should be applied in neutral position, or an appropriate spinal brace may be used. Owing to the multiplicity of fragments coupled with intact ligamentous structures surrounding these fragments, the fracture will heal very rapidly.

Transverse Process Fractures. Transverse process fractures (Fig. 20–1D) occur occasionally in the lumbar spine as an avulsion injury secondary to violent, sudden muscle contraction. The injury may also occur from a direct blow or may frequently accompany substantial intra-abdominal or retroperitoneal trauma. Radiographical evidence of this fracture may be obtained on the AP view. The jagged line found at the fracture, along with the findings of tenderness and spasm, will differentiate this entity from a congenital separation. Treatment for this fracture should be directed toward making the patient comfortable. Bed rest for several days along with the appropriate analgesic is all that is necessary. Care should be taken to explain to the patient that he has no chance for neurological damage. Avoidance of overtreatment is strongly encouraged.

Spinous Process Fractures. The spinous processes (Fig. 20–1C) may be fractured by direct trauma, as with an object falling from a height and striking the patient's flexed spine, or indirect trauma, such as the violent muscle pull associated with "clay-shoveler's" fracture. This latter fracture occurs primarily at the T1 level. Diagnosis is made on physical examination and by lateral x-ray. No attempt at reduction should be undertaken and the patient should be treated symptomatically. No neurological deficit is found with this injury.

Unstable Fractures. All patients with acute traumatic injury to the spine should be treated as though the injury is unstable until proved otherwise. Any degree of malalignment, however small, in either AP or lateral view of the spine should make the physician suspect instability. A "slice wedge" fracture of the upper part of the lower vertebra, when seen on both the AP and lateral x-rays, is indicative of a fracture-dislocation and denotes a very unstable situation (Fig. 20–2B and C). Almost all of the fractures that are unstable will be found in the T2, L1 area. Even with severe trauma the thoracic spine remains stable owing to the rib attachments. L1, L2, and L3 are most commonly involved in seatbelt injuries (Fig. 20–3A and B). Almost all of these fractures have either

a complete or partial neurological deficit. Regardless of whether the neurological deficit is partial or complete, extreme caution must be maintained in the movement and care of these patients, for there may be the possibility of some neurological return. Any motor power or sensation present below the level of cord damage indicates a partial lesion of the cord. Total loss of sensation below the cord lesion is an indication of cord transection, especially if reflexes controlled by the segments below the lesion are present. Holdsworth believes that if complete loss of motor power and sensation persist longer than 24 hours, irreparable damage to the cord is certain.[1]

Fractures of the posterior elements (Fig. 20–2A) may occur as a result of direct trauma or from hyperextension. These are rare injuries but may be associated with injury to the spinal cord and should be considered unstable.

When the diagnosis of instability is made, appropriate nursing care is begun in order to prevent decubitus ulcers. Circoelectric beds should not be used in pa-

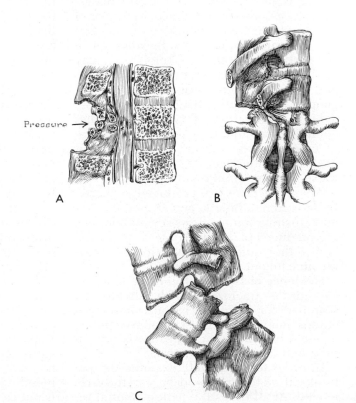

Figure 20–2. Unstable thoracolumbar spine fractures.

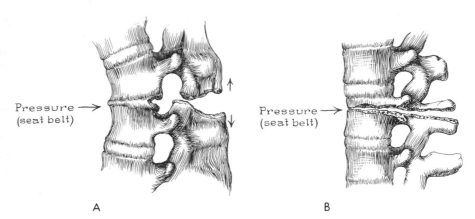

Figure 20–3. *Unstable thoracolumbar spine fractures.*

tients with a neurological deficit. These beds may cause serious ulceration, especially in the lower extremities. An orthopedist and neurosurgeon should be consulted in order that a decision for definitive therapy may be made.

FRACTURES OF THE PELVIS

The pelvic ring is composed of the ilium, ischium, pubic and sacral bones, providing multiple functions. A number of early and late complications are associated with fractures of the pelvis. Because one of the early complications, hemorrhage, may lead to death, it is important to consider and diagnose fractures of the pelvis early. In all types of pelvic fractures, there is an average blood loss of two units. Other complications found in a high percentage of cases include rupture of the bladder, urethra or intestine. Any combination of these may be found in any patient.

These fractures are produced primarily by falls from a height, automobile crashes and crushing trauma. Less severe fractures are produced in the elderly by a simple fall and in the young by an avulsion of a muscle attachment.

Evidence of Injury. Evidence of a pelvic girdle fracture, which should be searched for in any accident victim, includes mobility of the symphysis pubis, lower limb paresis or hypesthesia, hematuria and perineal ecchymosis.

In order to adequately examine the patient, all clothing should be carefully removed. At all times the patient should re-main in a supine position on a stretcher. Examination of the pelvic ring may be carried out in the following manner. The examining hands should be placed on the anterior-superior iliac spines and outward pressure gently applied. If the ring is broken, there will be an opening of the fracture and the patient will experience discomfort. Pressure over the symphysis pubis will demonstrate tenderness in a fracture of the pubic rami. Leg length discrepancy can be noted visually and documented by measuring the distance from the anterior-superior iliac spines to the medial malleoli. Attention should be directed toward the perineum, for swelling or discoloration in this area may indicate extravasation of urine or blood. Prior to any treatment of the fractures it is necessary that the patient's condition be stable. The blood pressure is monitored and recorded every 5 minutes or more frequently if shock is present. A No. 18 needle or larger is utilized for transmission of IV fluids. A blood sample is sent promptly for typing and cross-matching; a minimum of five units of whole blood is set up. The monitoring of central venous pressure, urine output and hematocrit is a useful guide to fluid replacement. The presence of profound shock may necessitate utilizing a plasma expander such as dextran. If blood replacement is not keeping up with the loss, consideration is given to an abdominal exploration to look for a tear of the iliolumbar or internal pudendal arteries or the iliac veins. If a retroperitoneal hematoma is found it should not be opened, for more bleeding will occur, and this complication is not easily controlled. Ligation of the internal iliac artery is not helpful because of the rich collateral circulation. No manipulation of the fracture should occur prior to control of the bleeding, for this will only increase the blood loss. The degree of blood loss is proportional to the number of fractures of the pelvis. Bleeding from the fracture sites can be controlled by reduction and stabilization of the fractures.

Injury to the genitourinary tract, especially to the bladder, may complicate even the most minor injury to the pelvis. The integrity of the urinary tract should be confirmed in every patient with pelvic injury regardless of how insignificant the injury may appear. A distended bladder is extremely vulnerable to any trauma about the pelvis. The bladder rupture may produce intraperitoneal extravasation of urine, resulting in acute peritonitis, or more commonly the rupture may be extraperitoneal, thus permitting urine to escape into the regional tissue spaces. Urethral injuries occur primarily in the male, usually in association with fractures involving the pubic rami and symphysis. The urethra is usually torn at the apex of the prostate and in most cases the tear is complete. If a urethral tear is present, the prostate may be freely moveable or not felt at all on rectal examination. Bleeding from the urethral meatus should alert one to a probable urethral tear. The diagnosis of a tear is confirmed by retrograde urethrogram. Urine is then obtained and examined for blood. Hematuria is not by itself significant, for this may occur simply from contusion to the bladder. Tears of the bladder are confirmed by the injection of radiopaque contrast material into the catheter followed by a roentgenogram. Extravasation of the contrast material may be noted, or the bladder may simply be pushed aside by a pelvic hematoma. An intravenous pyelogram may reveal a lacera-

tion of the renal parenchyma. In profound shock this latter study is not indicated, as the kidneys will not visualize.

Actual laceration or entrapment of the bowel may occur in the more severe fractures. Other known associated injuries include laceration of the vagina, rectum and diaphragm.[2]

Diagnostic Confirmation. An anterior-posterior x-ray of the pelvis is sufficient to permit classification of a fracture into the stable (Fig. 20–4) or unstable (Fig. 20–5) variety. Occasionally, a lateral x-ray is indicated to document displacement of a sacral fracture.

Specific Fractures. The pelvic skeleton is anchorage for powerful locomotor muscles. In youth sudden contraction of a muscle against resistance, such as in a hurdler or sprinter, may avulse the anterior superior iliac spine or the ischial tuberosity (Fig. 20–4). In the ischial tuberosity avulsion by the hamstring muscles, the buttock is found to be tender, swollen, and painful. The thigh cannot be flexed and the knee extended without pain in the buttock area. Maximum displacement occurs at the time of injury and does not usually exceed 2 cm. Bed rest and control of pain should be provided until ambulation with crutches is tolerated. Operative repair is contraindicated.

Avulsion of the anterior iliac spine occurs as a result of a sudden pull from either the sartorius or rectus femoris. Displacement is usually limited to 3 cm. or less by the surrounding fascial connections. Treatment consists of bed rest with the thighs flexed for 1 or 2 weeks in conjunction with mild analgesics. Operative treatment is not indicated.

A shear fracture of the ilium occurs almost exclusively in a motorcyclist who, at the point of impact, is thrown forward,

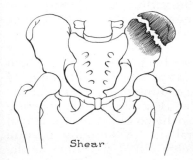
Shear

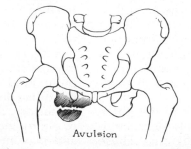
Avulsion

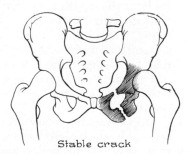
Stable crack

Figure 20–4. Stable pelvic fractures.

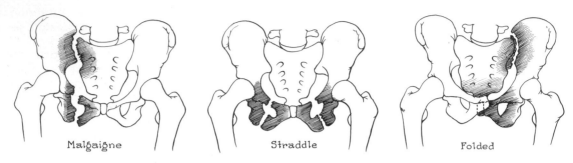

Figure 20–5. *Unstable pelvic fractures.*

catching his iliac crest on the handlebar. Occasionally, this fracture will be associated with an open abdominal wound with or without rupture of a viscus. Attention is directed toward surgical cleansing of the wound followed by the appropriate repair of the viscus if necessary. The shattered ilium is treated as follows. If there is no other pathology present, bed rest followed by gradual ambulation will give an excellent result. If an open wound complicates the fracture, the broken fragments may be removed, reduced or left undisturbed as the local circumstances dictate.

Isolated fractures of the pubic rami in which the ring of the pelvis is not significantly altered may be treated symptomatically by early ambulation if no other injuries are present (Fig. 20–4). With fractures about the obturator ring the patient may be more comfortable on bed rest for a few days with a pillow beneath the knees. Before releasing these patients from the emergency department, one must make sure that the patient is in stable condition, has a patent urinary tract and a normal abdominal examination. Even the most benign-appearing injury may produce pathology in the systems just mentioned.

Stable fractures of the pelvic ring also include diastasis of the symphysis in association with "spraining" of the sacroiliac joints. Depending on the severity of the separation, treatment may range from bed rest for several days to application of a pelvic band to provide support and relief of pain. Surgery is not indicated as early treatment.

Stress fractures may occur in the pubic rami as a result of excessive physical activity in an otherwise sedate individual. These should not be confused with bone tumors

that may arise in this area. Treatment is rendered only as symptoms dictate.

Fractures involving the sacrum are difficult to diagnose by x-ray and are usually found when the patient continues to complain of discomfort or when sacral nerve hypesthesia is seen in the perineal or posterior femoral cutaneous nerve areas. If displacement is noted, an attempt should be made to reduce the fracture by placement of the finger into the rectum and gentle manipulation of the fracture. Follow-up treatment consists of bed rest until the patient can ambulate normally.

Unstable fractures in which there are breaks in the anterior-posterior segments of the pelvic ring are treated only after the patient's condition is stabilized, for these are the fractures in which blood loss may lead to severe shock and death. In addition the bladder, bowel or urethra may be involved.

"Straddle" injuries (Fig. 20–5) occur as a result of direct trauma to the pubis or perineum, producing grossly unstable fractures limited to the anterior segment of the pelvic girdle. Rupture of the urethra is common with this injury. After treatment of associated injuries, the patient should be treated in a semi-sitting position in an effort to neutralize the various muscle pulls in the fracture fragments. A supine position may produce gross displacement of the fragments.

A Malgaigne fracture is one in which fracture lines are present through one set of pubic rami and through the region of the sacroiliac joint (Fig. 20–5). The fracture posteriorly may be on either the ipsilateral or contralateral side of the pubic fracture and may involve either the ilium or the lateral mass of the sacrum. On physical examination the affected lower extremity lies in external rotation and appears shortened. A palpable, tender hematoma is noted frequently over the separated fracture anteriorly. Shock and urinary extravasation are frequently found. Reduction should be accomplished as soon as possible, for no other special care can be undertaken until this is done. Small separations are reduced simply by placing the patient in a lateral position with the normal side up and allowing the body weight to reduce the two pelvic fragments. Reduction is maintained by a canvas sling placed beneath the buttocks with weight and pulley systems attached to the sling elevating the pelvis until it is barely touching the bed. Buck's traction (Fig. 20–6) should be applied to the affected lower extremity in order to prevent cephalad displacement of the unstable fragment. This traction should be maintained until fibrous union occurs after several weeks. After stability is obtained, a plaster spica can be used in place of the suspension hammock.

In the case of an "infolding" or "telescoping" fracture of the pelvis (Fig. 20–5), the hip on the affected side is flexed and inwardly rotated in association with eleva-

tion of the thigh and buttock from the examining table. Urethral or bladder injuries occur as a result of overlapping of the pubes. The displaced pelvic bone may be either anterior or posterior to its mate. Reduction is relatively easy if the displacement is anterior, for simple pressure on the iliac crests with the patient supine will usually reduce the dislocation. If reduction is not accomplished easily or if the dislocation is posterior, it is necessary to place the uninvolved lower extremity in flexion, lateral rotation and abduction, and have an assistant hold this position while the affected extremity is likewise flexed, internally rotated and hyperabducted. The fracture dislocation will then be stable when reduced and the patient can be nursed while supine. A suspension hammock is not necessary in this injury. Bed rest is utilized for 6 to 8 weeks with the affected lower extremity held in Buck's traction to prevent proximal migration of the unstable pelvic segment.

Crush injuries in children usually show multiple fractures of the "immature" pelvic bones with no joint disruption. Healing occurs rapidly as displacement of the fractures is not marked. When the integrity of

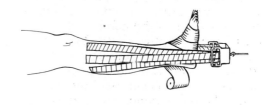

Figure 20–6. *Buck's traction.*

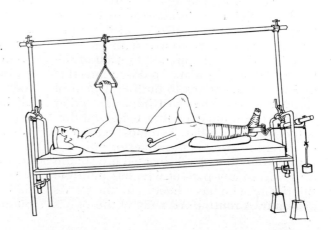

the abdominal contents is confirmed, the child may be treated on bed rest in a supine position until healing occurs.

FRACTURES OF THE ACETABULUM AND DISLOCATIONS OF THE HIP

A normal hip maintains stability by the proper relationship of the femoral head to the acetabulum, the muscular framework surrounding the hip joint and the hip capsule reinforced by accessory ligaments. When the thigh is flexed and abducted, a powerful force along the longitudinal axis of the limb forces the femoral head through the capsule posteriorly. This occurs most often in automobile accidents when the knee strikes the dash, and is described as a "dashboard" dislocation. If the force along the longitudinal axis of the femur is applied with the thigh crossed and abducted, there results a classical posterior dislocation. With less abduction of the thigh a dislocation of the proximal femur occurs in association with a fracture of the acetabular rim. If the thigh is abducted, either a simple fracture of the acetabulum with or without a central protrusion of the head or a fracture of the femoral neck occurs. In any dislocation of the hip or fracture of the acetabulum, the knee on the ipsilateral side should be investigated by physical examination and x-ray because a great percentage will demonstrate fractures of the patella.

Acetabular Fractures. In describing fractures of the acetabulum, it is useful to divide the acetabulum into three components.[3] The ischium comprises the posterior pillar; the pubic ramus, the anterior pillar; and the ilium, the superior pillar. While a central fracture dislocation of the hip into the acetabulum may disrupt all three pillars, one should try to ascertain on x-ray exactly what has happened to each of the three individual pillars. In doing this, it is possible many times to outline a plan of reconstruction. The most important pillar of the acetabulum in relation to hip stability is the posterior pillar. The most important to weight-bearing is the superior pillar.

Consideration of a dislocated hip should be given to any patient who has multiple injuries or who has a fracture of the pelvis or femur. A routine AP x-ray of the pelvis may show one of the femoral heads to be smaller or larger than the opposite side and would lead one to suspect a dislocation. A stereoscopic AP or a tube lateral x-ray will confirm the dislocation. Other x-rays should be taken on any fracture of the acetabulum, or if there has been a dislocation. If a dislocation is present, these x-rays are taken only after reduction is accomplished. The first x-ray should be taken with the patient tilted 45 degrees on his sound side and the x-ray tube placed directly over the injured acetabulum. By this method the posterior acetabular rim will be shown in detail. By tilting the patient 45 degrees with the injured side down and the x-ray tube directly over the injured side, an excellent view of the anterior acetabular rim may be obtained.

An acetabular fracture with central dislocation of the hip occurs as a result of a blow to the knee with the extremity in abduction or as a result of a direct blow on the greater trochanter. The latter mechanism occurs most frequently when a pedestrian is struck by a car. This is a severe injury and attention must be given initially to replacement of the blood volume. Blood loss may be massive with this fracture and steps should be taken to ensure that adequate blood is available for replacement. At least five units of blood should set up for replacement as necessary. The abdominal viscera and the gastrointestinal tract should be considered and their integrity proved. Shortening of the involved extremity may be present with this injury; otherwise a normal attitude exists. Any attempt to move the extremity will be extremely painful.

When the patient's condition is stabilized, traction is applied in the lateral and longitudinal directions under general anesthesia. One person stands along the injured side and applies traction with a sheet placed on the inner aspect of the proximal thigh. When another person applies longitudinal traction, the resultant force should reduce the dislocation. After this is accomplished, x-rays should be taken, and if the superior weight-bearing portion of the acetabulum is intact, the extremity may be treated with skeletal traction through a distal femoral pin and balanced suspension for several weeks with 25 to 30 pounds initially, with later reduction to 10 to 15 pounds. Other techniques for reduction have been used, such as placing a large wood screw or crossed Steinman pins in the greater trochanter for lateral traction; however, this is to be discouraged as initial management. On rare occasions it may be necessary to open the hip in order to re-establish a satisfactory weight-bearing surface.

Anterior Dislocation of the Hip. Anterior dislocation of the hip occurs most commonly as a result of a fall from a height with the blow being administered on the posterior aspect of an abducted, externally rotated thigh. The deformity of the leg is diagnostic (Fig. 20–7) and consists of a flexed, abducted, externally rotated extremity that may appear longer than the uninjured limb. The femoral head usually comes to rest in the obturator foramen.

Reduction is usually accomplished rather easily, often without anesthesia, by applying traction to the hip in the direction of the deformity. After the musculature surrounding the hip has been relaxed, the ex-

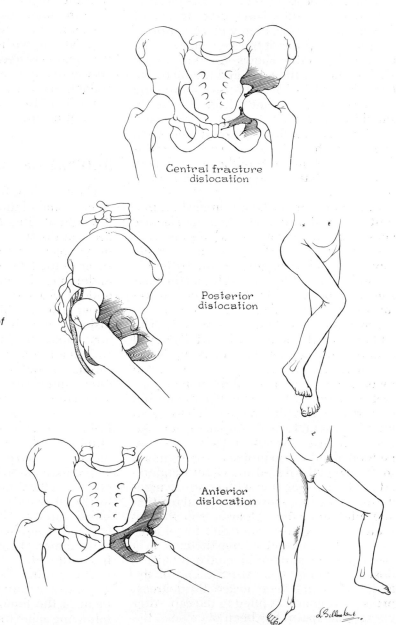

Figure 20–7. Basic types of hip dislocation.

Central fracture
dislocation

Posterior
dislocation

Anterior
dislocation

tremity is gently internally rotated and abducted. Post-reduction films are then made to determine reduction and also to check for any loose fragments of bone that may be in the joint. If loose fragments are found, they should be removed through an anterior approach to the hip. If no fragments are found, Buck's traction, using 5 to 7 lbs., is then applied to the injured extremity. Bed rest in a semiflexed position is maintained until soft tissue healing is present in about 3 weeks.

Posterior Dislocation. This is the most common dislocation and is often associated with injury to the sciatic nerve. It may or may not be in association with a fracture of the posterior pillar of the acetabulum. The typical deformity shows the hip to be slightly flexed, abducted and internally rotated (Fig. 20–7). There is also a shortening of the involved extremity. This dislocation should be considered an emergency, and manipulative reduction takes precedence over most other injuries. The late complication of aseptic necrosis of the femoral head is directly related to how long the head was dislocated.

Reduction cannot be accomplished in a posterior dislocation without satisfactory anesthesia. Several methods have been advocated for relocation of the hip. In Bigelow's circumduction method the patient is anesthetized on the x-ray table and the physician accomplishing the reduction removes his shoes and takes a position standing over the patient on the x-ray table. The adducted thigh and leg each are fully flexed over the abdomen. As traction is applied to the thigh, lateral circumduction followed by external rotation and abduction may effect reduction. This maneuver should not be carried out with force, especially in an elderly patient, for a fracture of the femoral neck may ensue. Another effective and safe method of reduction utilizes strong traction in the axis of the flexed and slightly abducted thigh in association with gentle maneuvering of the thigh toward external rotation and mild abduction. Stemson's method of reduction is an excellent one for elderly people. The patient is anesthetized in a prone position and the affected extremity is flexed at 90 degrees over the end of the table. With the knee flexed 90 degrees, pressure is gently applied to the calf. After the muscle spasm has been overcome, the hip will easily reduce. This method takes longer than the previously described procedures but it is probably the safest.

After reduction another series of x-rays should be obtained in order to check the reduction as well as the integrity of the acetabulum. If there has been an associated posterior pillar fracture with this dislocation, an x-ray utilizing the technique previously described will show whether or not this fragment has been reduced. Indications for opening a posterior dislocation include posterior instability of the hip, significant displacement of the acetabular fracture fragment, loose bone fragments in the joint and persistent or increasing signs of sciatic nerve injury. At all times, both pre- and post-reduction, the status of the sciatic nerve should be ascertained. After reduction is accomplished, Buck's traction, using 5 to 7 lbs., is applied with the hip in a neutral position.

INJURIES OF THE HIP

The hip joint, functioning as the cornerstone of ambulation, is subjected to trauma throughout life. Most injuries, however, occur at the two extremes of life, either in the young prior to the closure of the epiphysis or in the later years when the bone has undergone degenerative changes. In the middle years of life when the proximal femur is strong, the most common injury is dislocation of the femoral head. In any injury about the hip, efficient and precise early management is essential, for complications of delayed management are frequent and severe.

In children, owing to the presence of epiphyses, various injuries may occur. Prior to closure of the proximal femoral epiphysis, the femoral head and the femoral neck have separate blood supplies. The blood supply to the femoral head enters via the femoral neck; thus any injury to the neck may cause disruption of the blood supply. This is the reason for the frequent complication of aseptic necrosis of the femoral head after an injury to the hip in childhood.

The capital femoral epiphysis is the major site of injury in childhood. Displacement of the femoral epiphysis may occur following acute trauma as an "acute" slip or it may gradually slip over a period of several months. The slip takes place through the zone of hypertrophied cartilage, occurring more commonly in boys between the ages of 10 and 16. The body habitus of these youngsters is either of the obese "Fröhlich" type or of the rapidly growing "beanpole" type.

In an acute slip there is usually a history of a severe injury coupled with acute pain. On entrance into the emergency department the child will appear to be in severe pain and the lower involved extremity will be shortened and externally rotated. Any movement of the involved lower extremity will precipitate increased pain in the hip. A gradual slip will not be associated with any history of acute trauma, and the patient usually complains of pain in the knee region, fatigue and a limp. Physical examination here reveals a limitation of internal rotation. If the slip is quite severe when the leg is brought into flexion, the limb will rotate externally and move into abduction.

If one suspects an acute slip the involved extremity should be immobilized in a Thomas splint prior to any radiographical examination. Immobilization will reduce pain and minimize any damage that may occur to the remaining vascular attachment. X-rays taken by the AP and tube lateral techniques will reveal the true pathology. In an acute slip there will be a fracture through the epiphyseal line with the head lying inferior and posterior to the neck. There will be no evidence of new bone formation. If a gradual slip has occurred, there will be widening of the femoral neck and a tilting posteriorly and inferiorly of the femoral head. This tilting may be minimum or severe. It must be remembered that an acute slip may occur superimposed upon a chronic slip.

A patient with chronic slip should be placed on bed rest or on non-weight-bearing with crutches until a decision can be made by the appropriate specialist as to the type of treatment needed. An acute slip, however, should be treated as a fracture, with all the general principles of immobilization followed. Buck's traction should be utilized with 5 pounds and plans outlined for early reduction. This reduction may be closed or open. A gentle closed reduction may be attempted under an image intensifier, taking care not to injury any remaining blood supply. If this is accomplished easily, a spica cast may be applied. Open reduction is recommended by many authors utilizing atraumatic surgical technique with internal fixation being accomplished at the time of surgery.

Fractures of the hip in children are the result of severe trauma. These are uncommon injuries and are associated with a very high incidence of complications. The classification most commonly used divides the type of fractures into transepiphyseal, transcervical, cervical trochanteric (base of neck) and intertrochanteric fractures of the hip.[4] The most common fracture in a child is the base of neck type.

Because of the severe trauma that is necessary to produce these fractures, the child must be examined carefully for other injuries. The most common complicating injury found on examination will be that of cerebral trauma. A consideration of the battered child syndrome should be entertained if no significant history of trauma is present or if no underlying disease such as osteogenesis imperfecta is present.

Examination of the involved extremity will usually reveal the limb to be shortened and externally rotated. Rarely, the limb may be normal in appearance if the fracture is impacted. When one suspects a fracture about the hip, a Thomas splint should be applied immediately. Only after this is accomplished should an AP and tube lateral x-ray be taken. A frog leg lateral should not be taken as this may further injure the blood supply of the hip.

After documentation of the type of fracture present, several avenues of therapy are open to the physician, depending on his skill and experience. Gentle, closed reduction coupled with a spica cast may be utilized, or open reduction attempted with atraumatic surgical technique and internal fixation by several pins. A nail should not be used in these fractures. Neither of these two methods of treatment has yet proved superior to the other. The complication of aseptic necrosis remains quite high in either treatment. It is very important, however, to carry out one or the other method of initial management early, if possible within the first 6 to 8 hours after injury, for in this manner the high complication rate may be reduced.

Occasionally, the lesser trochanter is avulsed by the iliopsoas, or the greater trochanter by the abductor muscles. These avulsion injuries do not require operation and may be treated by non-weight-bearing with crutches for several weeks or until the pain subsides.

Fractures of the femoral neck (intracapsular) and of the trochanteric region (extracapsular) of the femur are primarily injuries of the elderly. Eighty per cent of these fractures occur in people over 60 years of age. Because of osteoporosis, a longer life expectancy and a natural tendency toward coxa vara, women with this injury outnumber men about 3 or 4 to 1. The mortality rate of 15 to 35 per cent is a result not of the fractures themselves but of their complications. Pneumonia, pulmonary embolism and cardiovascular complications are responsible for the high death rate.

The mechanism of injury responsible for these fractures is usually a fall onto the injured side. Occasionally, however, the patient will actually fracture the bone before the fall as a result of a misstep or a twisting motion.

The chief complaint on admission is usually severe pain in the hip area with radiation into the knee. The injured extremity will usually appear to be shortened and externally rotated. These two findings are not always present, for the fracture may be impacted.

Roentgenograms in two planes are necessary to confirm and identify the type of fracture. In addition to an AP x-ray of the hip, a tube lateral should be taken. A frog leg lateral should never be taken of the hip in the emergency department setting.

Throughout all examinations the injured extremity should not be moved about. As soon as possible, Buck's traction with a pillow under the knee should be applied.

In considering future management of these patients, several considerations are in order. As detailed a history as possible is obtained from the patient or the patient's family in an effort to determine the status of the patient's ambulation prior to the injury. A patient who was bedridden or confined to a wheelchair, or one in whom there was a history of previous malignant disease or other major medical problems, may best be treated by conservative means. If none of these factors is present, then the treatment

of choice is operative intervention. After an EKG, chest x-ray and other studies appropriate to a geriatric work-up are obtained, the patient should be scheduled in preparation for early operation. Usually the patient is in the best physiological condition at the time of the accident, and any lengthy delay will predispose the patient to thrombophlebitis, cystitis, decubitus ulcers or pneumonia. Delays in operation are only justified in an attempt to correct diabetic acidosis, cardiac failure and arrhythmia, acute myocardial infarction, cerebral hemorrhage, or dehydration secondary to the fracture occurring over 24 hours prior to the admission of the patient to the hospital. Treatment of any of these problems should be accomplished in association with an internist in an attempt to prepare the patient for early surgery. By operating early and mobilizing the patient quickly after surgery, postoperative complications of surgery in the elderly are diminished.

Intracapsular fractures can be classified according to the angle of inclination of the fracture as described by Pauwel. Type I fractures show an angulation of 30 degrees to the horizontal, type II 50 degrees and type III 70 degrees (Fig. 20–8). Because these fractures are intracapsular, they are not associated with significant hemorrhage.

A type I intracapsular fracture occurs most commonly from a fall causing a direct blow on the involved hip. These fractures may be considered stable if there is no posterior tilt on the tube lateral x-ray, the head on the AP x-ray is in slight valgus and on physical examination the involved leg can be moved slowly without pain. If these factors are all present, the patient may be treated on bed rest with Buck's traction for several weeks followed by non-weight-bearing ambulation until healing takes place. If there is any question of instability, then the fracture may be fixed in situ by use of three Knowles pins.

Treatment of the unstable types II and III is best accomplished either by open reduction and internal fixation or by replacement of the head with an endoprosthesis. The use of an endoprosthetic replacement in fresh fractures should be considered in any patient over 70 years of age if his general condition would not permit possible secondary surgery if the nailing of

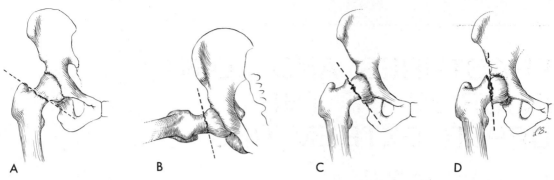

Figure 20–8. *Femoral neck fractures.*

the femoral head failed; if Parkinson's disease, spastic hemiplegia or severe arthritis of the hip is present; or if the patient is subject to pathological fractures. If the patient comes in late with a displaced fracture of the femoral neck, he should be considered for primary prosthetic replacement.

In the operative treatment of these fractures, great care must be taken to achieve adequate reduction, proper fixation of the fragments and atraumatic handling of all tissues.

Intertrochanteric fractures of the hip occur outside the hip capsule and therefore have an adequate blood supply, which allows for satisfactory union if the fracture is properly immobilized. Closed methods may be accomplished by means of traction and plaster immobilization, but the associated mortality rate is quite high. The type I or nondisplaced intertrochanteric fracture can be treated by a nail and plate, thus enabling the patient to resume early non-weight-bearing ambulation. If the patient's general condition does not permit surgery, he may be managed on bed rest with frequent careful turning. The healing time is shorter for this than for any other hip fracture.

In a type II intertrochanteric fracture there will be some displacement, but an intact medial calcar will allow good surgical results. These fractures are reduced at operation on the fracture table under biplane x-ray control, and then internally fixed by use of a nail and side plate.

In a type III intertrochanteric fracture there is comminution of the medial calcar, which predisposes to instability and late varus deformity. These fractures are treated by medialization of the femur and implantation of the medial femoral calcar into the distal intramedullary cavity in association with internal fixation by a nail and side plate. Prior to transferring the patient from the operating table, biplane x-rays should be taken. Technical errors include too long or too short a nail, too long or too short a plate, or an inadequate reduction of the fracture. Postoperatively, the patient is gotten out of bed and transferred to a chair within 24 hours after the operation. It is not necessary after an adequate reduction and internal fixation to immobilize these patients for any period of time in bed or in a cast. Metastatic disease causing a fracture of the femoral neck is best treated by an endoprosthesis. If the bone destruction results in an extracapsular fracture, internal fixation may be accomplished by a nail and plate enabling the patient to be nursed in a more comfortable manner.

REFERENCES

1. Holdsworth, F. W.: Early orthopaedic treatment of patients with spinal injury. *In* Spinal Injuries, Proceedings of a Symposium (P. Harris, ed.) London, Morrison & Gibb, Ltd., 1963, pp. 93–100.
2. McLaughlin, H. L.: Trauma. Philadelphia, W. B. Saunders Company, 1959.
3. Müller, M. E., Alligower, M., and Willenegger, H.: Manual of Internal Fixation. New York, Springer-Verlag, 1970.
4. American College of Surgeons: Fractures and dislocations of the lower extremity. *In* Early Care of the Injured Patient. Philadelphia, W. B. Saunders Company, 1972, pp. 263–276.

CHAPTER 21

FRACTURES AND JOINT INJURIES OF THE UPPER EXTREMITIES

Paul R. Manske, M.D.

INTRODUCTION

Since the skeletal framework of the upper extremity lies superficially within the soft tissues, it is relatively easy to visualize and palpate the osseous structures and be suspicious of most fractures and dislocations. In addition to bone and joint injuries, upper extremity trauma can result in injuries to important vascular, neural and other soft tissue structures. Therefore, the examining physician must question and evaluate the injured patient concerning pain, abnormal sensation and the ability to move the upper extremity.

All suspected skeletal injuries should be properly splinted before the injured patient is moved to a location where the injury can be further evaluated and treated. Failure to do so may result in (1) increased pain and discomfort for the patient, (2) increased swelling and edema of the entire injured extremity and (3) possible additional damage to vital soft tissue structures.

Suspected injuries of the upper arm and forearm can be immobilized with standard wooden or pneumatic air splints. When injuries of the elbow are suspected, the extremity should be splinted in the position of injury rather than changing the position to conform to the shape of the available splint. Injuries of the shoulder girdle can be supported with a sling or immobilized

against the thorax with a sling and swathe, i.e., sling held in place with an elastic or gauze bandage.

Peripheral Neurovascular Injuries

It is most important to examine all patients with upper extremity trauma for peripheral neurovascular injuries. Any abnormality should be noted and carefully recorded. Not only is this of utmost importance in the subsequent evaluation and treatment of the patient, it is of value in avoiding medicolegal problems. Such an evaluation can be performed quickly and without significant loss of time in treating the patient.

The brachial, radial and ulnar arteries lie superficially beneath the skin at the antecubital fossa and on the volar surface of the wrist. They are easily palpated. If the distal arteries cannot be palpated the physician may be forced to rely on less exacting parameters such as capillary filling of the nail bed, skin color and skin temperature. If vascular injury is suspected, further evaluation with a Doppler recorder, strain gauge plethysmograph or arteriography by a surgeon trained in vascular surgery is necessary.

Although specific skeletal injuries are more frequently associated with particular nerve injuries, it is appropriate to note the motor and sensory functions of all major peripheral nerves with any upper extremity trauma. Since patients may be reluctant or unable to move the traumatized extremity because of the pain associated with fractures or dislocation, the physician must either palpate the involved muscle to assess the motor function or he can rely entirely on the sensory examination. Table 21–1 is a helpful guide for a cursory examination of the major peripheral nerves of the upper extremity.

Although peripheral nerve injuries must be noted, they do not constitute medical emergencies. If the nerve deficit is secondary to a neuropraxia lesion, the function will return spontaneously. Unless a nerve is thought to be severed, it does not require immediate treatment. Delayed repair of peripheral nerve lacerations (particularly if due to a gunshot wound) is preferred by some surgeons.

SHOULDER GIRDLE

Sternoclavicular Joint Dislocation

This injury results either from a blow to the shoulder or a direct force to the medial end of the clavicle. Most dislocations are anterior beneath the skin, but the medial clavicle can also dislocate posteriorly. These retrosternal (posterior) dislocations may compress and partially obstruct major thoracic vascular structures or the trachea and produce life-threatening problems.

Anterior dislocations are easily diagnosed since the medial end of the clavicle is palpable just beneath the skin and is quite prominent compared to the opposite side. Retrosternal dislocations produce a depression in the sternoclavicular joint region that might not be noted clinically because of the soft tissue swelling. Standard x-rays of the sternum and clavicle may not define the dislocation, and special oblique or tomographic views comparing the affected joint with the opposite side are often necessary.

The anterior dislocation is usually easily reduced by applying lateral traction to the abducted arm and direct pressure to the medial end of the clavicle. However, the dislocation tends to recur when the traction and pressure are released. A reverse figure-of-eight bandage may maintain the reduced position. If the anterior disloca-

tion does recur, it is best to accept the deformity rather than to perform an open reduction using internal fixation with metal pins. These pins have a propensity to migrate to the structures within the thoracic cavity and convert a simple deformity into a life-threatening problem.

Posterior dislocations can be reduced by pushing the shoulder posteriorly while the patient is lying on his back with a folded sheet placed between his scapulae. If this fails, the medial end of the clavicle can be grasped with a towel clip and elevated back into place, using appropriate anesthesia in the operating room. The medial clavicle is usually stable and the patient can be treated in the standard figure-of-eight dressing for 6 weeks (Fig. 21–1).

Clavicle Fractures

Clavicle fractures (Fig. 21–2) are frequently seen in children and teenagers. Since the clavicle is the osseous link between the upper extremity and the trunk, it is subject to severe compressive and torsional forces with any trauma to the arm. The clavicle can also be fractured by direct blows to the superior aspect of the chest. The fracture fragments frequently displace and override at the fracture site because of muscle pull and the weight of the extremity (Fig. 21–3).

This fracture is easily diagnosed by pain, swelling and deformity at the site of the injury. Rarely there may be associated injuries of the great vessels, brachial plexus or lungs, which lie posterior and just beneath the mid-portion of the clavicle.

All clavicle fractures should be held in a figure-of-eight bandage (Fig. 21–1). This

TABLE 21–1. Guide for Examination of Major Peripheral Nerves of the Upper Extremity

NERVE	MOTOR FUNCTION	SENSORY AREA
Axillary	Shoulder abduction (deltoid muscle)	3 cm. diameter area at insertion of deltoid muscle
Radial	Wrist and finger extension	Dorsal web space between thumb and index finger
Median	Thumb abduction and opposition	Volar tip of thumb, index and middle finger
Ulnar	Radial abduction of index finger	Volar tip, small finger

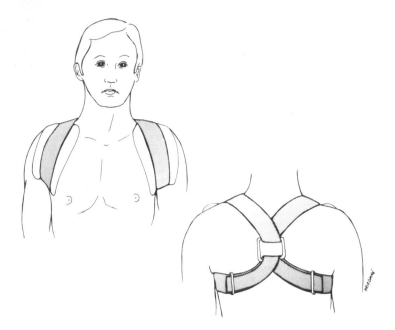

Figure 21-1. *Figure-of-eight dressing holding shoulders back. It is frequently used to treat posterior dislocations of the clavicle and fractures of the clavicle.*

type of immobilization will restore general alignment to the fracture. These fractures usually heal with proper immobilization, and operation is rarely indicated.

The straps should be adjusted to pull on the lateral ends of the clavicle rather than at the fracture site. Since all figure-of-eight bandages tend to loosen, the straps should be tightened daily, especially in the first week after application. In heavily muscled individuals, partial venous obstruction and edema of the extremities can result if the straps are too tight. This problem can usually be treated by requiring the patient to lie supine with a small towel rolled between the scapulae at frequent intervals during the day. The fractures are immobilized for 3 weeks in children and for 6 weeks or more in adults.

A mass of callus forms at the fracture site and the physician is well advised to forewarn the patient of this large subcutaneous lump. The mass usually regresses even if it does not completely resolve. Although women may object to the lump, it is usually preferable to a surgical scar.

Acromioclavicular Joint Injury and Dislocation

Injury to the acromioclavicular ligaments usually is the result of a direct fall or blow on the point of the shoulder. If the

force is minimal, the injury is limited to these ligaments and there is no loss of shoulder girdle stability. However, with greater force the coracoclavicular ligaments also may be torn and the clavicle displaces superiorly as the weight of the

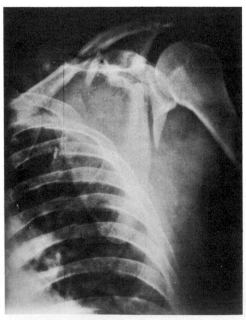

Figure 21-2. *Fractures of both the clavicle and scapula.*

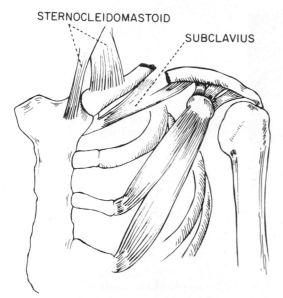

Figure 21-3. Clavicle fracture displaced by attached musculature.

upper extremity pulls the acromion inferiorly (Fig. 21–4).

The upward displacement of the clavicle is usually apparent on physical examination. However, x-ray confirmation is essential since some patients have swelling of the soft tissue surrounding the acromioclavicular joint because of the trauma to the shoulder (Fig. 21–5). Anteriorposterior x-rays of both shoulders should be obtained with the patient holding about 10 pounds of weight in each hand to accentuate the deformity of the dislocated clavicle.

Injury to the acromioclavicular ligaments alone can be treated with a sling until the soreness resolves since the shoulder girdle is structurally stable. However, if the acromioclavicular joint is dislocated secondary to associated coracoclavicular ligament tear, strapping and bandaging are usually ineffective in holding the dislocation reduced. In order to adequately reduce and hold the dislocation, the integrity of coracoclavicular ligaments must be restored operatively using screws, wires, Mersilene tape, and so forth. Although some patients prefer the deformity to an operative procedure, the shoulder is usually weak and painful and the deformity is cosmetically displeasing.

Scapular Fracture

The scapula is infrequently fractured; most fractures are undisplaced. It is necessary to make the patient as comfortable as possible until the bone has healed. Relief of pain can usually be accomplished with a simple sling or by immobilizing the arm in a stockinette Velpeau bandage. Because of potential problems of painful "frozen" shoulder, it is wise to initiate daily active range of motion exercises at 7 to 10 days after injury.

Shoulder Dislocation

Dislocation of the glenohumeral joint occurs more frequently than at any other joint of the body. The predilection for this injury at the shoulder joint is due to many

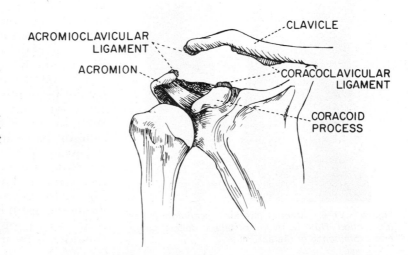

Figure 21-4. Acromioclavicular joint dislocation with associated coracoclavicular ligament disruption.

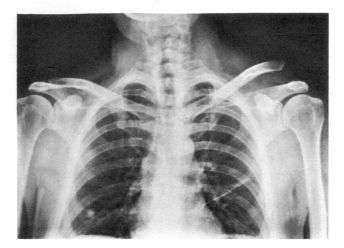

Figure 21–5. Left acromiocla-vicular joint dislocation.

factors, including the relative instability of the articulating osseous structures, the relatively loose and weak ligamentous supporting structures, the extensive range of motion of the joint and the torsional forces

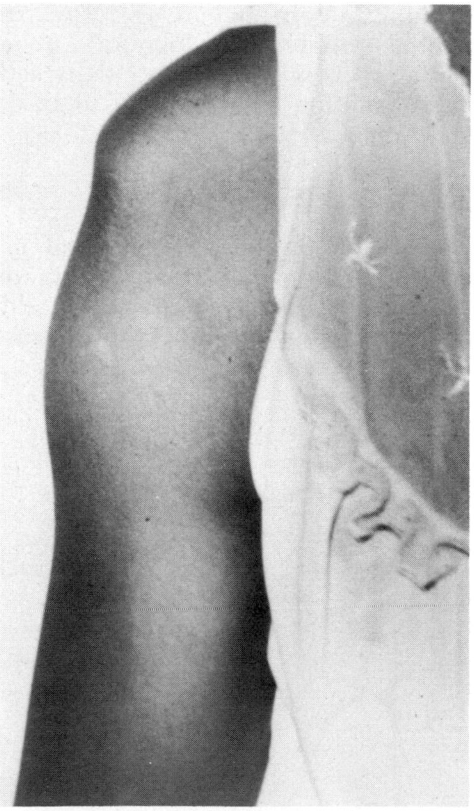

Figure 21–6. Anterior-inferior scapulohumeral dislocation. Note flattening of lateral deltoid bulge and prominence of the acromion.

that can be applied through the long lever of the extended arm. Although the head can dislocate in any direction, it most frequently displaces anteriorly beneath the coracoid process. The dislocation occurs as the arm is abducted and externally rotated. The head passes through a tear in the anterior-inferior portion of the capsule.

The patient experiences immediate pain and is reticent to move his extremity, which is displaced forward and externally rotated at the shoulder. Although there is a prominence anteriorly where the head lies in the subcoracoid region, the lateral aspect of the shoulder is flattened (Fig. 21–6). If proper facilities are readily available, it is best to obtain an x-ray of the shoulder before attempting reduction. However, it is not wise to delay an attempted reduction since this delay often leads to increased pain, increased muscle spasm and increased difficulty in obtaining reduction.

It is important to assess the axillary, radial, median and ulnar nerve function since one or all of these may be injured with this dislocation. If a nerve injury is noted prior to attempted reduction, the manipulation cannot be implicated as the causative factor. Fortunately, nerve deficits usually resolve by 6 to 8 weeks and nerve exploration or reconstructive surgery is rarely necessary. With certain nerve injuries it is necessary to apply a splint temporarily; e.g., wrist cock-up splint for radial nerve injury, to prevent joint contracture until the nerve again begins to function.

Reduction of a dislocated shoulder should only be attempted by a physician or a paramedical person familiar with the nature of the injury since serious secondary complications can be produced by improper techniques. The simplest way to obtain reduction is to apply forward traction to the affected arm while the patient relaxes. This is most easily accomplished by placing the patient prone on a table with the arm hanging forward over the side (Stimson method). Traction may be applied manually or by suspending weights from the wrist or hand.

Another relatively simple maneuver is the Kocher method. With counter traction applied against the thoracic cage by an assistant using a sheet, (1) distal traction is applied to the extremity with the elbow flexed, (2) the arm is externally rotated and abducted and (3) as the humeral head slips into the glenoid, the arm is internally rotated and adducted.

If these methods fail, it is imperative that x-rays of the shoulder be obtained since there may be an associated fracture complicating the dislocation. Occasionally it is necessary to perform the reduction under general anesthesia.

After the shoulder is reduced, it must be immobilized in adduction and internal rotation continuously for a minimum of 3 weeks while the torn structures of the anterior shoulder capsule heal. This immobilization is most comfortably accomplished using a Velpeau stockinette bandage (Fig. 21–7). The incidence of recurrence of the anterior dislocation is related to the age of the patient (higher incidence with younger patients), degree of causative force (higher incidence with minimal force) and time of immobilization (higher incidence if less than 3 weeks). Even though it is apparent that the physician can

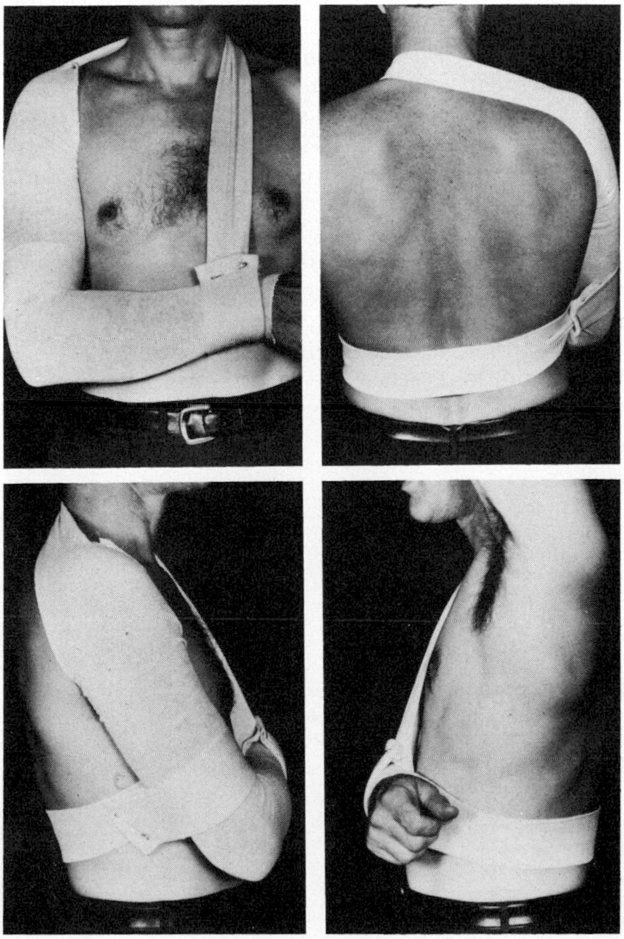

Figure 21–7. Stockinette velpeau dressing for lightweight immobilization of the shoulder. A long piece of stockinette tubing is slit in two places to allow insertion of the arm and emergence of the hand. The two ends are pinned or tied around the limb after encircling the neck and waist.

only influence the time of immobilization, he is obliged to impress this fact on the patient.

Rotator Cuff Ruptures

The rotator cuff is composed of the common tendon of four muscles that insert into the humeral head (supraspinatus, infraspinatus, teres minor, subscapularis). The tendinous fibers of the cuff demonstrate attritional changes associated with age. When the tendon fibers are further stressed by a fall, a direct blow or even minor trauma to the shoulder, they can lose their integrity and a rupture can occur. Consequently, this injury is usually observed in older patients. Ruptures can involve the entire cuff but more frequently are confined to a single tendon unit. (The supraspinatus is the most frequently injured.)

The function of the rotator cuff is to stabilize the humeral head in the glenoid and produce the initial 40 degrees of shoulder abduction. In the case of small tears (confined to a minimal portion of the tendon), the cuff can continue to function even though movement of the shoulder is painful. However, with massive tears of an extensive portion of tendon, the cuff fails to function and the patient is unable to initiate shoulder abduction. One can test for an extensive tear by passively abducting the shoulder and asking the patient to gradually lower his arm. If the arm suddenly drops at approximately 40-degree abduction, one must be suspicious of a massive tear. The diagnosis of a small or an extensive tear in the rotator cuff can be made by shoulder arthrography (Fig. 21–8).

Undoubtedly, many small tears of the rotator cuff heal and corrective surgery is not required. However, if a large tear is suspected, the advantages of early surgery are apparent in terms of improved shoulder function and the avoidance of a long period of painful watching and waiting.

HUMERUS

Fractures of the Proximal Humerus

Fractures of the proximal humerus at the level of the surgical neck can be treated initially with the limb in a sling or a stockinette Velpeau for 7 to 10 days, followed by institution of range of motion exercises. Displaced fractures of the tuberosity require open reduction and internal fixation since the tendons of the rotator cuff insert at that level.

Interarticular and comminuted fractures of the proximal humerus are difficult to treat by open reduction and internal fixation. Even if the surgeon is talented and fortunate enough to align the fragments with internal fixation, the resultant motion of the shoulder is often poor. Many surgeons prefer to treat these intra-articular proximal humerus fractures with a sling and swathe or a stockinette Velpeau for 7 to 10 days and then institute range of motion exercises. Even though the x-rays show poor reduction of the fragments, the

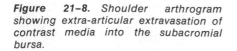
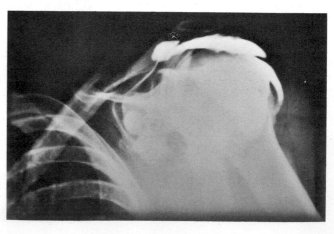

Figure 21–8. Shoulder arthrogram showing extra-articular extravasation of contrast media into the subacromial bursa.

patients frequently obtain reasonably good shoulder motion and adequate function. In markedly interarticular comminuted fractures of the proximal humerus, a humeral head prosthesis is recommended.

It is important to note that much of the post-traumatic shoulder pain is secondary to capsular adhesions. Therefore, it is important to begin range of motion exercises early no matter whether operative or nonoperative methods are used.

Fractures of the Shaft of the Humerus

Fractures of the shaft of the humerus are usually obvious by the total instability of the upper arm. The fracture deformity is visible and palpable when the limb is lifted. Since the radial nerve spirals around the posterior to lateral aspect of the humerus at the junction of the middle and distal thirds, injury of this nerve is not uncommon. Consequently, particular attention should be given to radial nerve function in the routine evaluation of peripheral neurovascular function.

Most radial nerve injuries are neuropraxia lesions and will resolve within 6 to 12 weeks. Electromyography at approximately 6-week intervals will assist the physician in determining whether nerve recovery is progressing. If nerve function fails to return, the nerve should be surgically exposed since it may be encased in fracture callus or caught in the fracture site.

The fracture may be temporarily splinted with padded wooden splints placed medially and laterally or the arm held against the chest wall with a sling and swathe until appropriate x-rays are obtained. If the patient is unable or unwilling to abduct the arm to obtain a lateral view x-ray, a transthoracic lateral x-ray should be obtained.

Humeral shaft fractures are frequently treated and held with a form of ambulatory traction known as a "hanging cast" (Fig. 21–9). An above-elbow circumferential cast is applied with the elbow flexed. The forearm is supported with a collar and cuff sling. By adjusting the position of the cuff, angulation at the fracture site can be corrected. It is important that the proximal margins of the cast are either above or

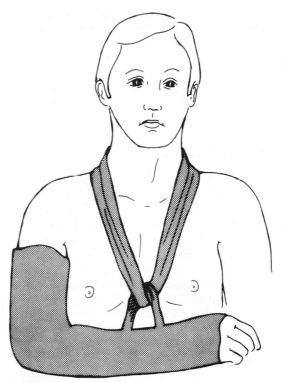

Figure 21–9.   *Hanging cast. A plaster of Paris long arm cast is suspended by a stockinette collar around the neck. This method of ambulatory traction allows the weight of the forearm and the cast to reduce the humerus fracture. Proper alignment of the fracture can be obtained by appropriate placement of the stockinette collar and loop on the cast.*

below the fracture site but not directly at it. Since the weight of the cast aligns the fracture fragments by gravity traction, it is necessary that the patient never be completely recumbent, even when sleeping at night.

Some physicians prefer to immobilize the fracture with "sugar tong" splints. A long plaster splint is placed longitudinally along the medial aspect of the upper arm, wrapped around the flexed elbow, and then along the lateral aspect of the arm to the shoulder. It is molded in place with a gauze roll when the plaster is still wet. Occasionally a shoulder spica with the arm in abduction and forward flexion is necessary to properly align the fracture.

Open reduction and internal fixation with an intramedullary rod or a compression plate are necessary when adequate reduction cannot be obtained or the fracture fails to unite by the nonoperative technique. Internal fixation is also indicated when the radial nerve is exposed prior to fracture healing. No matter which technique is used to obtain reduction of the fracture, it is important to begin pendulum range of motion exercises to the shoulder at approximately 2 weeks to avoid stiffness of that joint caused by prolonged immobilization.

INJURIES TO THE ELBOW

Trauma to the elbow can produce a variety of fractures and dislocations. Consequently, x-rays are extremely important to accurately diagnose the injury. In moving the patient to an x-ray facility, it is important to splint the injured elbow properly to avoid additional osseous and soft tissue damage. In general, one should not attempt to straighten the elbow in applying the splint, but to immobilize the extremity in the position of the deformity. The splint should be modified to fit the deformity rather than the deformity distorted to conform to the splint (Fig. 21–10). This can be accomplished by placing padded wooden splints medially and laterally rather than using the commercially available posterior aluminum splint (which places the elbow at 90-degree flexion) or the inflatable air splint (which extends the elbow).

Since there is a limited amount of soft tissue covering the osseous structures in the region of the elbow, the integrity of the three peripheral nerves (median, radial and ulnar) and the brachial artery may be jeopardized by the initial injury or by subsequent edema and hematoma formation. Therefore, it is imperative to determine the neurovascular status in the initial evaluation of all elbow injuries and to note any

change during the period immediately after treatment.

Fractures of the Distal Humerus

Nondisplaced fractures of the distal humerus of adults can be immobilized in a long arm splint for about 3 to 4 weeks. Gentle range of motion exercises are begun at approximately 2 weeks after injury by removing the splint once a day.

In general, anatomical alignment of displaced fractures by open or closed methods is desired. However, if there is marked comminution of the fragments, it is often wise to accept the deformity, treat the fracture with a posterior splint and institute range of motion exercises at approximately 2 weeks. Alternatively, adequate alignment can often be obtained with a pin through the olecranon (Fig. 21–11), known as Dunlop's traction.

If the fracture consists of a displaced single fragment, e.g., fracture line through the capitulum or trochlea, one should strive for anatomical reduction, usually requiring open reduction and internal fixation. However, it is not necessary to perform open reduction of epicondylar fractures since the articular surface is not involved.

Among the most serious and common injuries in children is the supercondylar fracture. Even when the fracture is not displaced, the potential obstruction of the arterial circulation by soft tissue edema and fracture hematoma makes this a serious injury. It is imperative that the distal radial pulse be monitored at hourly intervals by attentive parents or properly trained hospital personnel. In most cases, the physician should hospitalize children with this

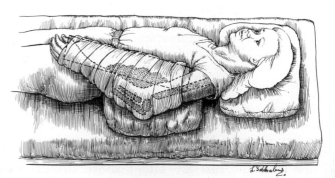

Figure 21–10. *The injured elbow should be splinted to maintain the existing position. It should not be flexed or extended. A wood splint, properly wrapped to the limb with knitted gauze, is therefore preferable to an air splint.*

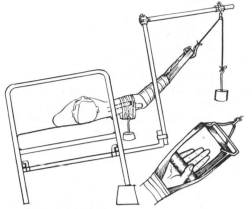

Figure 21–11. Dunlop's traction. (Schmeisser, G., Jr.: A Clinical Manual of Orthopedic Traction Techniques. Philadelphia, W. B. Saunders Co., 1963.)

injury in order to properly follow the vascular patency.

Supercondylar fractures in children frequently displace posteriorly (Fig. 21–12). In reducing this fracture, the physician must be certain to correct rotational, as well as the lateral, medial and posterior angulation deformities. This can usually be accomplished by manipulative reduction with the elbow flexed. If attempts at manipulative reduction fail, Dunlop's traction is a safe and frequently successful method.

When the fracture will not stay in the reduced position, a percutaneous Kirschner pin can be used to maintain alignment. Although infrequently necessary, one should not hesitate to perform open reduction and internal fixation to obtain adequate alignment.

Following reduction, the elbow is immobilized in at least 90-degree flexion with a long arm plaster cast or splint. Attention must be given to the radial pulse in the post-treatment period.

Volkmann's ischemia, secondary to pressure and swelling within the fascial envelope surrounding the elbow, is a devastating but preventable complication of elbow fractures in children. Impending ischemia is noted initially by increased pain, decrease in pulse volume and altered sensation of the digits. If ischemia is suspected, the physician should immediately attempt to relieve the vascular compression by splitting or removing the immobilizing plaster cast and elevating the extremity. At times, the pressure must be relieved by extending the elbow to a less acute angle. If these measures fail, a fasciotomy of the elbow and volar forearm compartment should be performed to reduce the pressure and restore circulation.

Olecranon Fractures

Displaced fractures of the olecranon are interarticular fractures and require open reduction and internal fixation. These cannot be reduced and held by closed methods. The length of immobilization in a posterior plaster splint depends on the type of internal fixation used.

Radial Head Fractures

Fractures of the radial head and neck in adults are frequently undisplaced and can be treated in a posterior splint for 3 to 4 weeks. In order to avoid stiffness of the elbow, the splint should be removed once a day and gentle range of motion exercises begun at 2 weeks. If more than 30 per cent of the articular surface is destroyed or if the fracture is angled more than 20–30 degrees, surgical excision of the head is indicated. Some surgeons prefer to place a silastic radial head implant, but this treat-

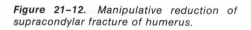

Figure 21–12. Manipulative reduction of supracondylar fracture of humerus.

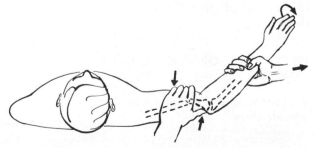

ment is not universally accepted. The radial head should never be excised in children following fracture since the epiphyseal growth plate is involved and the forearm will be shortened and deformed on the radial side.

Dislocated Elbow

In an elbow dislocation, the olecranon is usually displaced posteriorly to the distal humerus. These dislocations are quite easy to reduce with forward traction on the forearm if there are no associated fractures. Post-reduction x-rays are essential to determine the radius-capitellum and the ulna-trochlea relationship on both anterior-posterior and lateral x-ray views. The fracture should be held for 3 weeks at 90-degree flexion in a plaster cast or splint, and daily range of motion exercises begun at 2 weeks by removing the splint once a day.

Subluxation of the Radial Head in Children

"Nursemaid's elbow" or subluxation of the radial head usually follows forcible traction on the extended forearm of young children. The child complains of pain in the elbow, holds the forearm pronated and refuses to use the arm. Flexion-extension is uninhibited. X-rays are negative and the diagnosis must be made based on the clinical examination.

The subluxation is treated by manipulative reduction. The physician grasps the elbow with one hand, the thumb in position to apply pressure to the radial head. The elbow is extended by holding the wrist with the other hand. The forearm is forcibly supinated as pressure is applied to the radial head. Only slight force is necessary and no anesthesia is required. The child has a sudden pang of discomfort, but the pain is immediately relieved. The forearm is held in a flexion sling for several days.

FRACTURES OF THE FOREARM BONES

Fractures of the Midshaft of Radius and/or Ulna

Fractures of either the radius or ulna can occur in adults and children as a result of direct trauma to the forearm. Because of the muscle forces pulling on the proximal and distal fracture fragments, fractures are frequently displaced. Since forearm supination and pronation require proper maintenance of the interosseous space, anatomical reduction of the fracture(s) is necessary in order to restore proper function of the forearm. In adults, anatomical reduction of displaced fractures of the radius or ulna is difficult to obtain by closed methods. Consequently, open reduction and internal fixation must be performed using intramedullary rods or compression plates, and the extremity immobilized in a long arm cast for 6 weeks. Nondisplaced fractures are treated with long arm casts and immobilization.

Anatomical reduction of radius and ulna fractures of children is not essential since the healing callus will remodel as the child grows. These fractures will heal adequately as long as manipulative reduction can restore end-to-end apposition of the fracture fragments. The fracture is immobilized in a long arm cast from 4 to 6 weeks with the forearm in neutral pronation-supination position.

Monteggia Fractures

This fracture consists of a mid-shaft fracture of the ulna associated with radiocapitellum dislocation. This injury can be produced by a direct blow or a severe pronation force to the forearm. Manipulative reduction should be attempted by first reducing the ulna shaft fracture using longitudinal traction and then pressing the radial head to its normal position. The forearm is immobilized in supination with the elbow flexed about 45 degrees. If postmanipulation x-rays do not show anatomical reduction, the fracture must be operatively reduced and held with internal fixation and then the radial head reduced. At times the annular ligament must be repaired or a fascial graft sutured about the radial neck in order to stabilize the dislocation.

Fracture of the Distal Radius

The most common adult fracture is the dorsally displaced distal radius fracture described by Abraham Colles (Fig. 21–13). This is one of several fractures that can occur by a fall on the outstretched arm.

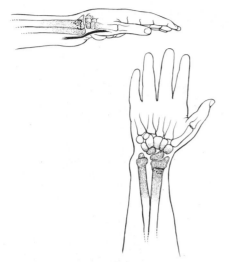

Figure 21-13. Colles' fracture.

X-rays show dorsal angulation of the distal fragment resulting in relative shortening of the radius in relation to the ulna. It is necessary to correct the deformity and restore the length for proper forearm and wrist function.

Manipulative reduction is frequently successful in aligning the fracture using local or regional anesthesia. A long arm cast is applied with the wrist in ulnar deviation and slight flexion and the forearm in a neutral or slightly pronated position.

When the Colles fracture is comminuted on the dorsal aspect of the radius, the fragments can "settle" and the deformity can recur even though they had been anatomically reduced initially. This can be prevented by frequent postoperative x-rays and reapplication of a snug-fitting cast as the swelling and edema subside. Alternatively, the fracture fragments can be held in place with percutaneous Kirschner wires placed at the time of initial reduction.

In the post-reduction period, the extremity should be elevated above the level of the heart until the swelling subsides.

Obviously a sling places the injured extremity in a dependent position and fails to provide sufficient elevation in the early treatment period.

The median nerve can be compressed by swelling and fracture hematoma at the level of the wrist and is noted by decreased sensation of the thumb, index and long-finger tips. If symptoms of median nerve compression develop, the cast and padding should be split, even if this results in loss of fracture position. It is important to evaluate the patient for excess swelling and signs of median nerve compression at 24 and 72 hours after application of the cast.

This chapter has outlined the basic principles and concepts regarding treatment of fractures and joint injuries of the upper extremity. The reader is encouraged to consult the following excellent references for a more extensive review of the subject.

REFERENCES

1. Bateman, J. E.: The Shoulder and Neck. Philadelphia, W. B. Saunders Co. 1972.
2. Conwell, H. E., and Reynolds, F. C.: Management of Fractures, Dislocations and Sprains. Chapters 11–15, 7th Edition. St. Louis, C. V. Mosby Co., 1961.
3. Crenshaw, A. H.: Cambell's Operative Orthopaedics. Chapters 5–8, 5th Edition. St. Louis, C. V. Mosby Co., 1971.
4. DePalma, A. F.: The Management of Fractures and Dislocations. 2nd Edition. Philadelphia, W. B. Saunders Co., 1970, pp. 486–930.
5. Rockwood, C. A., and Green, D. P.: Fractures. Chapters 8–11. Philadelphia, J. B. Lippincott Co., 1975.
6. Schmeisser, G.: A Clinical Manual of Orthopedic Traction Techniques. Philadelphia, W. B. Saunders Co., 1973.
7. Smith, F. M.: Surgery of the Elbow. 2nd Edition. Philadelphia, W. B. Saunders Co., 1972.
8. Wilson, J. N.: Watson-Jones — Fractures and Joint Injuries. Chapters 18–21, 5th Edition. New York, Churchill-Livingstone, 1974.
9. Tachdjian, M. O.: Pediatric Orthopaedics. Philadelphia, W. B. Saunders Co., 1972, pp. 1532–1651.

CHAPTER 22

INJURIES OF THE LOWER EXTREMITIES

Perry Schoenecker, M.D.

Jordan Ginsburg, M.D.

The general condition of the patient either from disease or associated trauma dictates priorities in management of trauma. In the critically injured patient, the immediate problem is one of resuscitation and maintenance of vital functions. Once this is accomplished, all major extremity bones and joints should be systematically evaluated for the extent of both open and closed injuries. Management of lower extremity and musculoskeletal injuries should not be sequestered from the total care of the patient. A methodical evaluation of all extremities in both the conscious and the unconscious patient is critical for the detection and successful management of unsuspected as well as obvious injuries. The basic clinical examination must determine possible fractures and joint dislocations and the extent of associated soft tissue injury. Neurovascular integrity of the extremities must be documented prior to instituting care of even the simplest fractures and dislocations. Radiological evaluation of all suspected areas of injury is also critical in the acute assessment of the traumatized patient. Proper radiological evaluation includes x-rays of one joint above and below all suspected areas of trauma (Fig. 22–1).

Open injuries demand immediate definitive care of the wound. Sterile dressings should be applied and proper splinting of the extremities is mandatory to minimize further soft tissue trauma. Antibiotics and tetanus immunization are started at this time. After the patient's general condition has stabilized, a working diagnosis of the extent of extremity trauma will have been realized and a plan of general acute management should be formulated.

Definitive treatment of closed fractures not associated with circulatory impairment can be delayed while life-threatening injuries are being treated. All fractures should, however, receive immediate treatment sufficient to control deformity and minimize further tissue damage. Definitive care of the closed fractures may then be performed when the patient's general condition has stabilized.

As acute resuscitation and evaluation is accomplished, each physician who manages trauma must determine if he and other members of the staff can provide definitive care for all the patient's problems at that institution; if not, then the patient's condition should be stabilized and he should be transferred to the nearest facility so prepared.

The goal of the physician in the treatment of fractures is to restore the injured part or parts to normal function at the earliest possible time with the least risk to the patient. Open fractures should be converted to closed fractures as early as possible, again with the least risk to the patient.[32] Treatment of an open fracture,

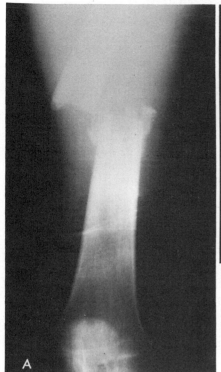
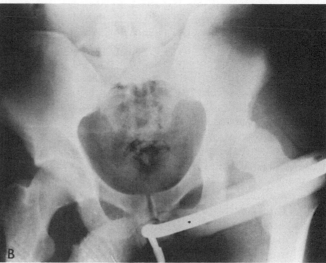

Figure 22–1. Traumatic hip joint dislocation with ipsilateral femoral shaft fracture. A, Anteroposterior view of left femoral mid-shaft fracture; note the adducted attitude of the proximal fragment. B, Anteroposterior view of pelvis of same patient with unsuspected posterior dislocation of left hip.

therefore, is treatment of the wound. It matters not how well the fracture may be reduced and maintained if the wound becomes infected. With an infected fracture, the result at best is destruction of bone, loss of position and delayed or non-union of the fracture; at worst, it is loss of limb or life.

The factors that determine success or failure of wound treatment have been outlined by Reynolds: (1) the virulence of the organism contaminating the wound, (2) the number of organisms, (3) the length of time the organisms remain in the wound, (4) the health of the tissue contaminated and (5) the resistance of the host. The physician has no control over the concentration of virulence of the organisms that contaminate the wound at the time of injury. He can minimize further contamination by immediate application of a sterile dressing and protection of the wound while the extremity is being prepared for wound surgery. Organisms initially contaminating a wound exponentially grow in number with time, so that early debridement minimizes contaminating organism concentration. With the possible exception of small puncture wounds and wounds caused by low-velocity missiles, all open fractures and/or dislocations must have a formal debridement. There is no substitution for good wound surgery, for it is this treatment that reduces the number of organisms, shortens the time they remain in the wound and is a vital factor in determining the viability of the contaminated tissue. The fifth factor, the resistance of the host, is augmented by appropriate blood replacement, antibiotic administration and nutrition.

The operation described is that of a thorough debridement of the entire wound similar to that described by Hugo of Lucca circa 1200 A.D. The initial preparation consists of copious lavage and concomitant appropriate mechanical scrubbing of the wound edges to remove the gross contamination of particles of clothing, road gravel and dirt. Following this, a skin-preparing solution of choice is applied and routine draping is performed. The wound is then irrigated copiously from within out. Debridement in the lower extremity is best done without a tourniquet. This makes it easier to determine the viability of tissue. In certain instances it may be advisable to use a tourniquet to prevent excessive blood loss, but if used, complete hemostasis must be accomplished at the end of the procedure after the tourniquet is deflated and before a final dressing is applied. The margins of the skin and all devitalized soft tissue structures are excised; the wound may be extended until the most inaccessible recess is thoroughly opened and in clear view and all foreign substances within the wound are meticulously removed. After thorough exposure, the wound is again copiously irrigated with Ringer's solution and finally an antibiotic irrigating solution to further deplete bacterial contamination.

After the soft tissues are thoroughly debrided, attention should be turned to the bone: small pieces of bone completely detached from soft tissue should be removed. However, large detached fragments, even if contaminated, are best cleaned and replaced in most instances. Care should be taken to minimize further iatrogenic devitalization of bone by the unnecessary denuding of its soft tissues.

Damaged major vessels should be repaired by a surgeon capable of this. Techniques of vessel repair have been im-

proved considerably since World War II, as has the prognosis from such an injury.[39] Successful surgical repair is now possible of arteries associated with fractures as distal as the wrist and ankle. Concomitant with reconstitution of circulation to an ischemic extremity is mandatory, adequate compartmental decompression distal to the site of repair.[12, 39]

When arterial repair has been accomplished, the addition of internal fixation of the fracture remains controversial. Connolly et al.[9, 10] showed that this is not always necessary and that the decision to use internal fixation should depend on local factors such as bone fragments and tissue loss. They felt that the key to extremity viability was in minimizing the delay before revascularization, the status of collateral channels, the development of infection and degree of soft tissue damage (Fig. 22–2). The repaired vessel should be covered by soft tissue if possible; the remainder of the wound may be packed open.

Primary nerve repair is not advisable when extensive soft tissue trauma has oc-

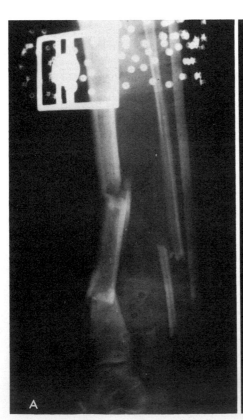
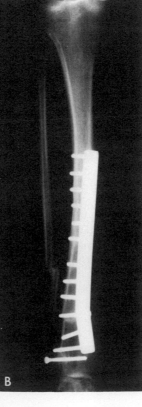

Figure 22–2. *Tibia-fibula fractures with laceration of posterior and anterior tibial vessels. A, Segmental distal tibia-fibula fractures. B, Healed fractures 8 months after operation for repair of vascular injury and concomitant plate fixation of tibia.*

curred, particularly when one is unsure of the extent of nerve damage.[37] Nerve repair may be performed at a later date but within a time reference such that healing of the nerve repair coincides with healing of the fracture. This minimizes prolonged immobilization of joints. Major tendons may be repaired in clean wounds; however, for the most part, soft tissue structures are best treated by delayed primary repair, when one is sure about the absence of wound infection.

Adequate immobilization of the bone fragments is often problematic. To protect the soft tissues, the fracture must be appropriately immobilized (Fig. 22–3). In most situations this can be accomplished by traction, external plaster fixation or pins above and below the fracture site incorporated into plaster or an external fixation frame.[5, 18, 26] The latter is applicable when there is extensive soft tissue loss associated with a very unstable fracture, such as of both bones of the leg (Fig. 22–4). In this situation, secondary procedures, perhaps several, will be required to close the wound and stability of the fracture facili-

tates wound management. If internal fixation is selected, an intramedullary rod should be employed if possible.[26]

Open wounds are routinely left open and closed at a later time. Loosely packed fine mesh gauze has proven to be a satisfactory agent for an open wound dressing; it affords excellent wound drainage with minimal skin maceration. It is far safer to pack all wounds open. They may then be closed by delayed suture or appropriate skin grafts or flaps, or allowed to heal by secondary intention. Once the wound is closed and healed without infection, internal fixation may be used if indicated.

FRACTURES OF THE FEMUR

Closed fractures of the shaft of the femur are common injuries secondary to trauma. They are often seen in young children subjected to torsional force or a direct blow. These are often isolated injuries and may be treated definitively as soon as a full medical assessment is performed. The treatment of choice in patients up to age 10

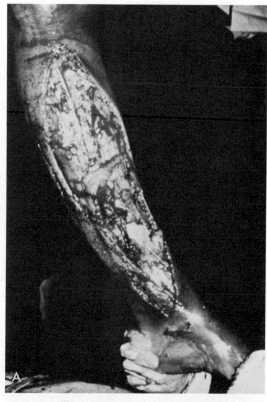

Figure 22–3. Unstable open mid-shaft tibial fracture. A, Extensive soft tissue damage.

Illustration continued on following page.

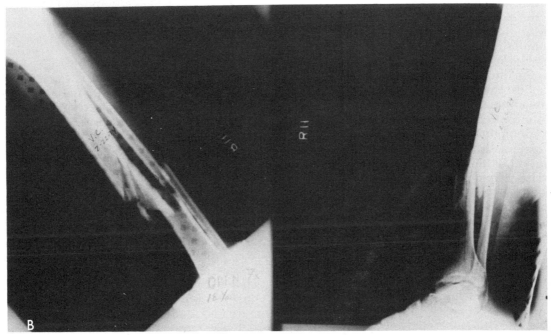

Figure 22–3 Continued. B, *Comminuted mid-shaft tibial fracture.*

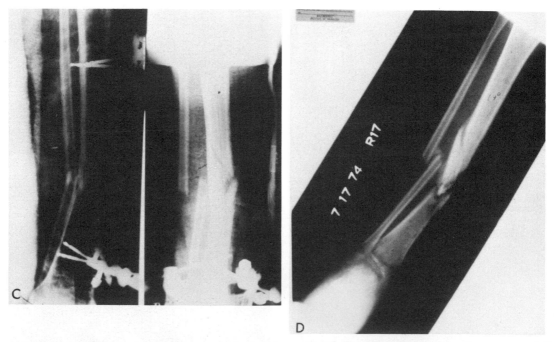

Figure 22–3 Continued. C, *Fracture immobilized in Roger-Anderson device for total wound management.* D, *Soft tissues healed after multiple surgical procedures and delayed osseous union.*

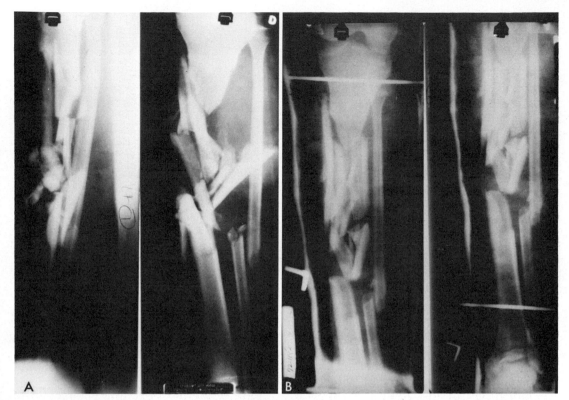

Figure 22-4. *Unstable open tibial fracture. A. Extensively comminuted tibial fracture. B. Immobilization of fracture with cross pins incorporated into a plaster cast.*

or 11 is Russell's skin traction.[33] If the patient is heavy and requires more than 5 lbs. of skin traction, a threaded pin may be placed in the proximal tibia, taking care to avoid the open epiphysis of the tibial tubercle.

Traction is then maintained until the fracture is minimally painful and clinically "sticky" with x-ray evidence of early callus formation. At this point a spica cast is applied and the patient can be treated at home. Recently there have been reports of excellent results of immediate spica application in children up to 10 years of age.[17] Optimal position is side-by-side apposition with 1 cm. of overriding and no angulation. End-to-end apposition in children may result in overgrowth and lengthened extremity. More than 1 cm. of overriding results in a shortened extremity.[3]

Fractures of the shaft of the femur in adults are often associated with major local soft tissue trauma as well as injuries to other organ systems. Treatment must be directed toward the patient as a whole rather than focusing on fracture manage-

ment. Special attention must be paid to head, chest and abdominal trauma. Attention to the basics of trauma managment, including establishing an airway, controlling hemorrhage and treating shock, is mandatory. It should be remembered that in a closed femoral shaft fracture it is reasonable to assume that one to two units of blood may be sequestered in the leg. The vascular status of the extremity must also be determined as this is far more critical to the immediate fate of the leg than is the fracture itself. Early treatment of a femoral shaft fracture in the emergency department should be oriented toward stabilizing the bone and protecting the soft tissues rather than toward definitive reduction. Open wounds should be dressed without attempts at closure. When the patient's general condition allows, the wound should be explored, debrided, irrigated and packed open in the operating suite.

Once the patient's condition is stabilized, definitive treatment is possible. The classical mode of therapy is skeletal traction with balanced suspension (Fig. 22–5). This is done with a threaded pin through

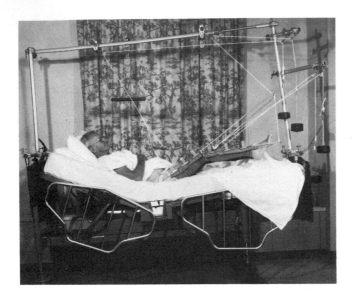

Figure 22–5. An adult patient in balanced suspension and skeletal traction. This is a common method of management for fractures of the shaft of the femur.

the tibia. Traction is maintained until the fracture is "sticky" and then a spica cast is applied. If adequate alignment can be maintained, this is effective therapy with a minimal rate of non-union or infection. Complications in the adult can produce high hospital cost, increased morbidity from thromboembolic phenomena, decreased range of motion especially at the knee joint, problems with skin care and a lengthy rehabilitation period.

Open reduction of femoral shaft fractures has gained in popularity in the past 30 years. This is because of the significant advantages of shortened hospital stay, early ambulation and early joint motion. Either intramedullary rods or plates and screws have been used successfully. The selection of fractures for internal fixation is important since each of these devices has its limitations. Rods are useful only for fractures in the area of the isthumus, while plates are difficult to apply to a high fracture or at the point of maximal femoral bowing. Comminuted fractures are not amenable to either form of open treatment. The disadvantages of open reduction and internal fixation are an increased infection rate, increased non-union rate and morbidity of a major surgical procedure. These disadvantages are magnified in the presence of an open fracture. In recent years there has been a resurgence in some centers of closed reduction and intramedullary nailing utilizing special equipment and intraoperative fluoroscopy.[26]

This is certainly attractive in relation to decreasing the chance of devascularizing fracture fragments during operative exposure but this technique is not widely available.

One of the most exciting changes in femoral shaft fracture management was originally reported by Smith in 1855.[38] This is the concept of functional bracing. This utilized the precept of applying external support while allowing function. Several studies have shown that with weight-bearing in a cast brace there is maintenance of adequate alignment as well as early fracture healing with the advantage that joint motion is maintained and muscle wasting minimized.[6, 24, 25] This method is recommended for both open and closed fractures (Fig. 22–6). Initial skeletal traction is utilized until the fracture is "sticky" and soft tissue swelling has resolved. The cast-brace technique facilitates early rehabilitation while minimizing the chances of infection, non-union or joint stiffness. This is a time-consuming and somewhat demanding technique that does not lend itself well to all fractures, especially those with high shaft involvement. Sometimes the multiplicity of injuries dictates open reduction to facilitate general patient care and free the patient of traction apparatus. Often open reduction with internal fixation makes ipsilateral fractures of other bones easier to manage.

Supracondylar fractures, especially those with intra-articular extension, are

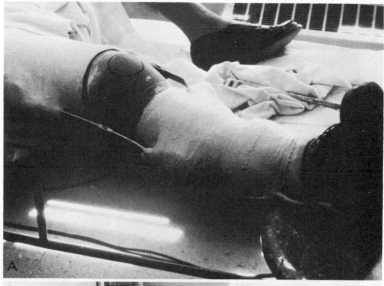

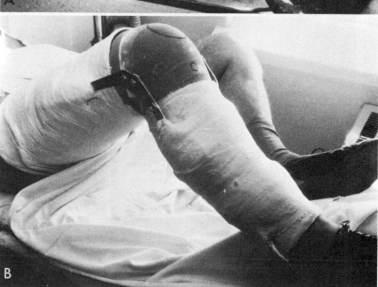

Figure 22–6. Cast brace. A and B, Femoral fracture immobilized in a cast brace 6 weeks after the fracture; an active range of knee motion exercises are prescribed to facilitate rehabilitation.

difficult to treat. Skeletal traction, occasionally in conjunction with manipulation, is often adequate to align these injuries. Treatment is then completed with either a spica or cast-brace. Often when the condyles are disrupted it is not possible to obtain joint congruity by closed means, and to minimize later degenerative changes this alignment is necessary. This may be done by open reduction and internal fixation. Webb bolts, Knowles pins or a blade plate apparatus have all been used with some success (Fig. 22–7). The problems of infection, non-union and residual loss of motion of the knee are unfortunately all too common.

INJURIES TO THE KNEE JOINT

Injuries to the knee joint are quite common, especially from athletic trauma. In these cases, the fact of injury is obvious, but the challenge lies in definitive diagnosis and treatment. The trauma surgeon must not neglect the knee injury in the patient who has suffered vehicular trauma with multisystem involvement. If the diagnosis of ligament injury is missed, the opportunity for early repair and the expectation of a satisfactory result may be irretrievably lost. Without a systematic examination it is quite easy to overlook an

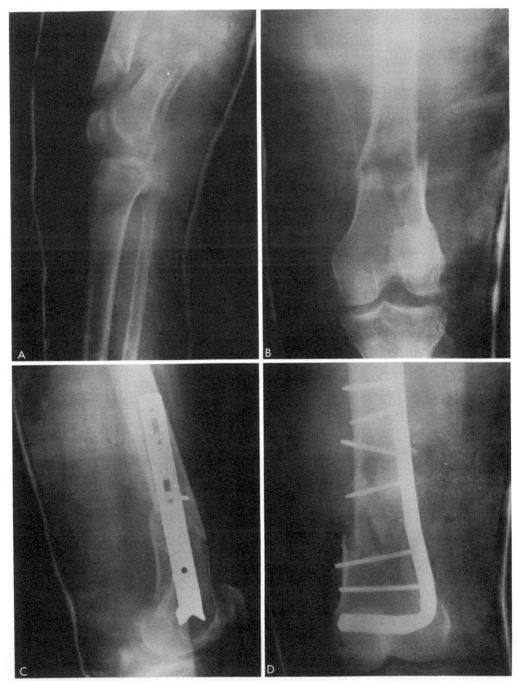

Figure 22–7. *Anteroposterior (A) and lateral (B) views of the left knee in a 65-year-old woman, showing a markedly displaced intracondylar and supracondylar fracture of the left femur. This patient had comparable injury of the right femur as well as rib fractures that resulted in a bilateral flail chest. Closed manipulation and traction failed to achieve a satisfactory reduction of these fractures. C and D, Open reduction and internal fixation were required but could not be done for approximately 1 month, which was the amount of time required for stabilization of the thoracic injuries.*

unstable knee in a comatose patient or one with abdominal trauma and shock.

The correct diagnosis of knee ligament injuries precludes a basic knowledge of knee anatomy.[4] The medial collateral ligament originates near the adductor tubercle. The deep portion inserts just below the tibial plateau while the superficial portion inserts farther distal under the pes anserinus. The posterior medial corner of the knee is stabilized by the capsule, semimembranosis tendon and the posterior oblique ligament. The lateral aspect is stabilized by the iliotibial tract, which inserts on the tibia at Gerde's tubercle. The lateral collateral ligament and the biceps femoris attach to the fibular head and the arcuate ligament and popliteus tendon reinforce the posterior lateral knee. The musculature about the knee can contribute greatly to stability, especially during a static examination, and for this reason it is essential to get patient cooperation for an adequate examination. It may be necessary to aspirate large effusions prior to stress testing.

The aim in the treatment of knee injuries is to establish an accurate diagnosis as soon as possible. It is a great help to know the status of the knee prior to injury but this is only available in organized athletics with preseason physical examinations. In the absence of prior injury, however, the opposite extremity can serve as a control. History is often quite helpful in making the diagnosis. With a serious ligament injury the patient-athlete may not have been able to continue activity due to pain or instability. With a meniscal injury or mild knee sprain, pain may initially be mild and the athlete may continue playing until pain and swelling increase. The occurrence of an audible or palpable "pop" in conjunction with a noncontact hyperextension injury is good evidence for an anterior cruciate ligament rupture.[14] The presence of an almost immediate large effusion is also suggestive of cruciate injury.

A careful physical examination is important in assessing ligamentous structures. The prime stabilizers to abduction stress are the medial collateral ligament, the posterior medial capsule and its reinforcements, and the anterior cruciate.[40] If the knee opens to abduction stress, especially in full extension, some or all of these struc-tures are injured. If the knee opens to adduction stress, injury to the iliotibial tract, lateral collateral ligament, biceps tendon and anterior cruciate may be suspected. There are several types of rotatory instability that have been described but a full discussion of these is beyond the scope of this chapter. Abduction stress with a torsional component may damage the cruciate ligaments as well as either meniscus. A positive posterior drawer sign indicates damage to the posterior cruciate ligament. This is rarely an isolated injury and is often associated with capsular, meniscal and extensive ligamentous damage. Hyperextension or a positive anterior drawer sign is often present in anterior cruciate injuries but occasionally cannot be elicited initially even with proven cruciate avulsions.

X-rays are not usually helpful in assessing damage. Stress x-rays will confirm instability but rarely add anything that is not clinically suspected. Occasionally a ligament will be avulsed with a fleck of bone that serves as a radiopaque marker. This most commonly comes off the fibular head or tibial spines (Fig. 22–8). One must

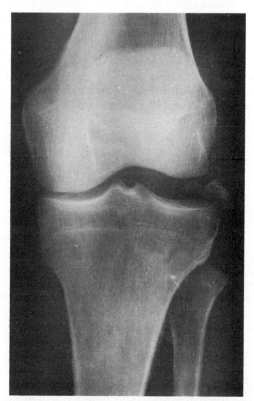

Figure 22–8. *Avulsion of the lateral collateral ligament and biceps tendon with a portion of the upper fibula. (Courtesy of Dr. Bernard Rineberg.)*

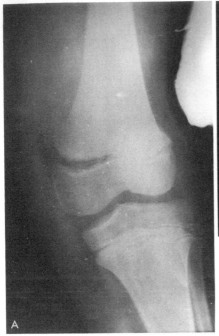
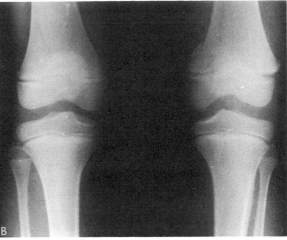

Figure 22–9. A, *Anteroposterior view of right knee with epiphyseal injury.* B, *Anteroposterior view of right knee. Epiphyseal injury simulating tibial collateral ligament rupture.*

always be sure that the instability one feels in a child is not due to an epiphyseal fracture. For these reasons in all cases plain films should be obtained (Fig. 22–9).

Once the anatomical location of injury is ascertained, it is imperative to assess its severity and initiate treatment. With gross instability the chances are nil that the ends of the ligament will anatomically approximate and heal and therefore surgical repair is indicated.[28] With partial injuries when the bulk of the ligament is contiguous, nonoperative measures have a good chance of success. In cases when there is indecision as to whether an injury should be operatively or nonoperatively treated, the conservative course is to surgically approach the knee and be certain that the ligament ends are in apposition.[11] The best surgical results come with surgery in the first 2 to 3 days because tissue planes and anatomic structures become very difficult to delineate as time goes by. By all means repair should never be delayed more than 10 days if possible.

It is our feeling that cruciate ligaments should be repaired whenever possible. The best results come when the ligament is avulsed from bone rather than torn at its mid-portion. There is considerable in-

terest in the recent orthopedic literature in primary reconstruction for irreparable cruciate injuries and this should certainly be considered in the knee with cruciate instability.[22]

Ligamentous injuries that are treated nonoperatively have often been treated with plaster immobilization. The quadriceps atrophy resulting from such immobilization prolongs morbidity and rehabilitation. Recovery time from this injury is appreciably shortened without adverse results if treatment consists of early range of motion and quadriceps exercises. As range of motion and muscle function improve and swelling decreases, weight-bearing as well as a progressive resistance program can be initiated. This has consistently given good functional results with minimal muscle atrophy and little residual loss of motion. Postoperatively, patients who are reliable and have good muscle control can be treated in much the same manner after 3 to 4 weeks of casting. It is possible in extremely reliable patients with excellent muscular control to have even less immobilization.[11, 14]

Meniscal injuries are more common than ligamentous tears. These are generally the result of rotational injuries with the medial side affected more often than the lateral. The menisci have a weight-bearing and shock absorbing function and their removal does not leave a normal knee joint.[19] The chance that degenerative changes will take place in a knee after meniscectomy is indeed higher than in an intact knee. Nonetheless, in a knee with a torn meniscus, we believe that meniscectomy is indicated. The rationale for meniscectomy lies with the immediate symptoms coupled with the mechanical wear pattern on the articular surfaces of the involved compartment. It seems reasonable to us to preserve a rim of normal meniscus at its capsular attachment when possible, as in a bucket handle tear, in order to attempt to preserve some meniscal function. We think that there is no place for immobilization just after meniscectomy; we institute immediate non-weight-bearing exercises and progress as just outlined for ligament injuries.

The diagnosis of a torn meniscus has classically rested on the physical examination and history. Recurrent effusion, locking, joint line pain and a positive McMurray click are indicative of meniscal tear. Double-contrast arthrography and the advent of arthroscopy have helped considerably in curtailing the incidence of negative arthrotomies. We cannot condemn strongly enough the practice of removing a meniscus that appears normal merely because an arthrotomy was performed.

Injuries to the patellar tendon or quadriceps tendon are not uncommon. The mechanism of injury is generally a severe, sudden quadriceps contraction against a fixed lower extremity. The physical findings include pain, swelling, a soft tissue defect and loss of active knee extension power. The treatment for this is surgical repair and cylinder cast application for 4 to 6 weeks.

More common than patellar mechanism injuries are fractures of the patella caused by direct trauma. Nondisplaced fractures may be treated simply with immobilization. Displaced fractures must be treated surgically or loss of extensor power results. If the patella is to be salvaged, the fragments must be anatomically aligned or else degenerative changes of the patellofemoral joint are inevitable. In a severely comminuted displaced fracture a patellectomy and repair of the tendon may be performed. Some patellar function may be preserved if a major fragment (one third or greater) can be salvaged and the patellar tendon sutured to this.

Acute patellar dislocations are a controversial problem. Whereas the disability from recurrent dislocations is well recognized and is a definite surgical problem, there is considerable difference of opinion regarding acute dislocations. These dislocations are almost always lateral and occur with the knee in flexion. Reduction is often spontaneous and usually can be affected by slowly extending the knee and applying pressure to the lateral aspect of the patella. The classical treatment is immobilization in a cylinder cast for 6 weeks.

There are certain conditions that predispose to dislocations of the patella. Abnormally lateral insertion of the patellar tendon, shallow femoral grooves and hypoplastic vastus medialis musculature all contribute to this problem. Most procedures to correct recurrent dislocations are combinations of medial reefings, lateral releases and realignment of the patellar tendon attachment. There is good rationale for surgery after an initial dislocation in those individuals with predisposing anatomical factors. Initial surgical intervention may be indicated in the high-performance athlete with an acute dislocation.[29]

FRACTURES OF THE TIBIA

The crest of the tibia is subcutaneous in its entire length and fractures of the shaft of the tibia may penetrate this thin tissue. Any suspected fracture of the leg should be immediately splinted, immobilizing the knee and the ankle. Proper initial treatment of a closed fracture will prevent it from becoming an open fracture due to skin necrosis and slough. Initial treatment of an open fracture should be with a dressing over the wound and an adequate splint; no attempt should be made to push an exposed piece of bone back under the skin, and no real attempt should be made at reduction unless there is a grotesque deformity of the leg with vascular embarrassment.

Fractures of the proximal tibia often result from a varus or valgus stress applied on the knee joint or axial impaction. Fractures in the proximal one third of the tibia unite readily; however, these fractures are often intra-articular and disrupt the articular surfaces of either the medial or lateral tibial plateau, resulting in various degrees of traumatic arthritis. Nondisplaced fractures of the proximal end of the tibia involving the articular surface can be managed by splinting the extremity. Traumatic effusions should be aspirated. Once the acute symptoms have subsided, usually in 1 or 2 weeks, the patient can be started on non-weight-bearing range of motion exercises. Weight-bearing can begin as soon as radiological evidence of union occurs. Displaced or depressed fractures are managed by either traction and early motion with cast brace protection or open reduction and reassembly of the fracture fragments.[16, 31] If this latter course is chosen, the depressed fragments are elevated and held in position with supplemental bone grafts and fixed internally with either Webb bolts or Knowles pins (Fig. 22–10). Fixation should be secure enough to allow early active motion before fracture healing has occurred. In any fracture involving the tibial articular surfaces, early motion in the post-injury period is essential to restoring knee function and augmenting articular cartilage nutrition. This can be accomplished with Apley's traction and/or cast-brace protection.[16, 31] Prolonged immobilization of these fractures until union occurs

carries a high risk of significant joint stiffness and permanent loss of motion.

Fractures of the shaft of the tibia may occur from a direct force, a torsional force or a penetrating injury. If the fibula remains intact, the fracture may be stable and can be managed by a cast and early weight-bearing.[27] Isolated fractures of the tibia are rarely significantly displaced, although occasionally the fracture will be angulated toward the fibula. Closed reduction, plaster immobilization and early weight-bearing is the treatment of choice for this injury. Fractures of both bones of the leg are all potentially serious unstable injuries. Spiral fractures of the tibia and fibula occur secondary to torsional forces; these fractures occur with the least amount of energy absorption and usually can be managed with closed techniques (Fig. 22–11). All adult patients with this injury should be hospitalized for a 24- to 28-hour period of observation for possible neurovascular compromise. Ambulatory care is then possible with appropriate plaster cast techniques and weight-bearing as indicated. Comminuted and segmental fractures of the leg are grossly unstable fractures (Fig. 22–4). These injuries occur with maximal energy absorption and often are open, comminuted fractures. Again for the closed injury, closed treatment is indicated. Plaster casts with possible pins above and below the fracture site to properly

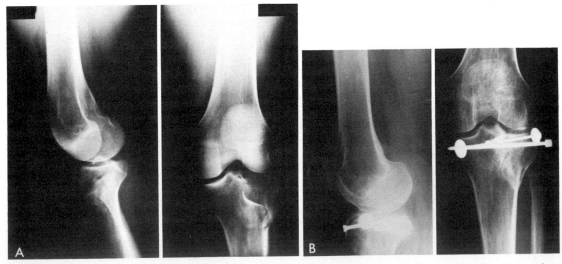

Figure 22–10. *Tibial plateau fracture. A, Depressed lateral plateau fracture. B, Six months after open reduction, internal fixation and bone graft.*

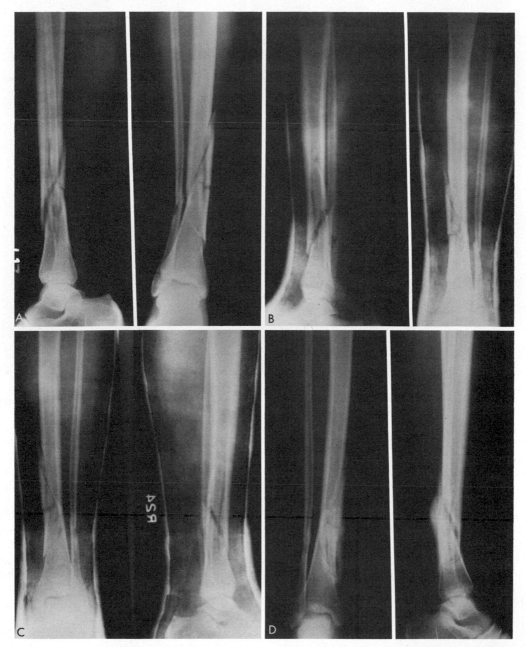

Figure 22–11.   *A closed fracture of the shaft of the tibia and fibula in a 19-year-old college girl, sustained in a twisting injury while ice skating. A, X-rays of the leg on admission to the hospital. A spiral comminuted fracture is apparent, with lateral angulation of the distal fragment. B, The patient was hospitalized for a week, and under general anesthesia the fracture was manipulated. Appearance of the limb immediately after manipulation and application of a long leg patellar tendon-bearing cast. The angular deformity has been corrected and the alignment restored. C, After application of the cast weight-bearing was allowed. Appearance of the limb after weight-bearing for 4 days. Some minimal posterior angulation of the fracture fragments is apparent, but otherwise there is no change in position. D, Three months after injury. The fracture is united. The position is unchanged since weight-bearing began.*

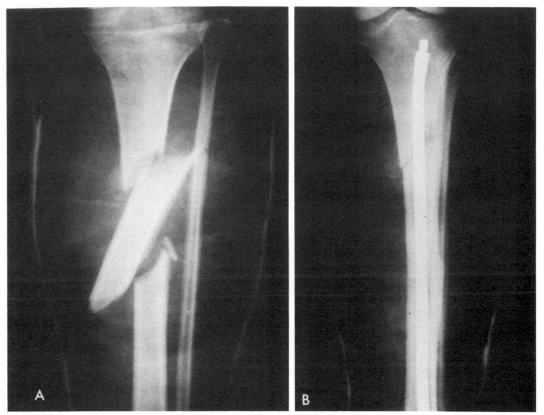

Figure 22–12. *Tibial fracture in patient with multiple traumatic injuries, including peroneal nerve palsy. A, Unreducible, segmental tibial fracture. B, Eight months after intramedullary nailing of same fracture; fracture has united.*

control the fracture are used. Judicious weight-bearing at a later date with properly applied long leg or short leg patellar tendon-bearing casts are employed. Careful observation of the fracture site with serial x-rays for the development of unacceptable angulation is necessary.[5, 35]

Open fractures of the tibia should be debrided in the operating room under anesthesia. The fracture is reduced and a cast applied. At an appropriate later time the cast and dressings are removed, the wound inspected and possibly closed or covered with a skin graft or muscle pedicle flap.[13] Often such closure is impossible; in such cases, the wound should be allowed to heal by secondary intention. When care of the wound has been realized, the fracture is managed with an appropriate plaster cast utilizing pins above and below the fracture to achieve stability of the osseous fragments (Figs. 22–3, 22–4). These pins can be secured by a plaster cast or an external fixation frame.[8, 26]

Internal fixation is indicated in open tibial fractures only if associated injuries are present that will necessitate repeated handling of the patient.[26] It is often difficult to maintain tibial fracture alignment in a recumbent patient with associated injuries. However, one must consider that open reduction and internal fixation of a tibial shaft fracture is a particularly hazardous procedure with associated risks of infection and non-union. We prefer to internally fix the tibia with an intramedullary nail.[21, 26] Once the nail has been inserted and the fracture reduced, weight-bearing can begin in a long leg cast as the patient's condition permits (Fig. 22–12). There are even fewer indications for internal plate fixation of an open tibial fracture; the catastrophic risks of infection and non-union are inherently high with such an operation (Fig. 22–13).[7]

FRACTURES INVOLVING THE ANKLE JOINT

The types of fractures and ligamentous injuries about the ankle joint are deter-

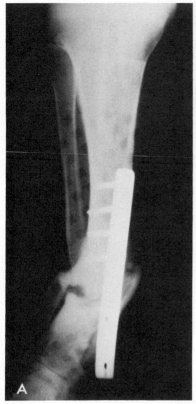
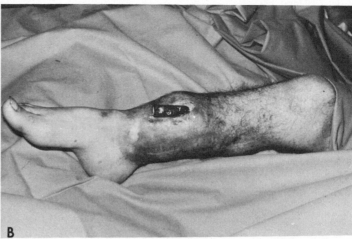

Figure 22–13.   *Open tibial fracture treated acutely with plate fixation. A, Radiographical evidence of screw-plate fixation failure and non-union 2 years following initial treatment. B, Clinical appearance of same infected extremity. Draining non-union was treated at this time with open amputation.*

mined by the mechanism of the injury: inversion of the foot in relation to the tibia, eversion of the foot, rotation of the foot about the distal tibia, forceful plantar of the foot, a direct blow or a combination of these.[23, 30] The magnitude and direction of the forces applied are also important factors: a twisting injury in an athletic activity will produce injuries quite different from those sustained in a high-speed vehicular accident. In his clinical examination and review of ankle x-rays, the examiner must understand the basic mechanisms of ankle injury. This will allow him to make a meaningful, correct assessment of the extent of damage. In evaluating the fracture roentgenograms, the surgeon must first decide whether the fracture is stable or unstable. In general, closed stable fractures and ligamentous injuries are adequately treated by external means: splint or cast. Unstable fractures are made stable by open reduction and adequate internal fixation of fracture fragments and suture of ligaments followed by short-term external plaster support.

The emergency room evaluation and initial splintage of the unstable fracture-dislocation of the ankle or foot or both

often leaves much to be desired. Too often, a grossly dislocated foot is unwisely left unattended and cutaneous elements are haphazardly treated, often leading to undue ischemia and skin loss (Fig. 22–14). It behooves the responsible physician to align the foot with the ankle as soon as the clinical and x-ray evaluations are complete. An adequate, comfortable splint from toe to groin then should be applied, allowing for intermittent determination of the neurovascular integrity of the foot. In closed injuries, such treatment will minimize the morbidity of pain, swelling and loss of viable skin until definitive treatment is begun at an appropriate time. Open fractures or fracture-dislocations about the ankle constitute surgical emergencies and these wounds must be treated as previously recommended.

Ankle sprains, laterally and medially, are a common traumatic affliction of the foot-ankle junction. A careful assessment of the extent of swelling, tenderness and instability must be made. Again ankle x-rays are an essential part of the emergency department evaluation. We have not routinely relied on stress ankle views in assessing instability. The less severe grade I

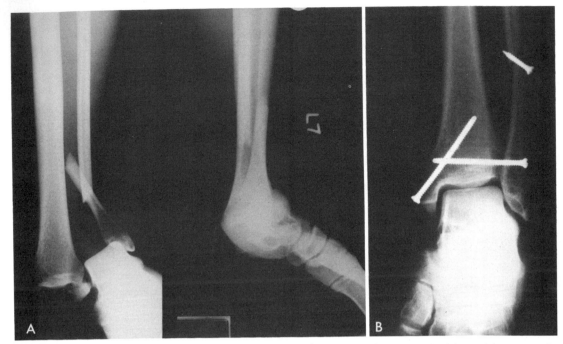

Figure 22–14. *Dislocation of foot on ankle. A, Radiograph shows grossly dislocated foot with osseous impingement of soft tissues medially. B, Radiograph following open reduction and internal fixation.*

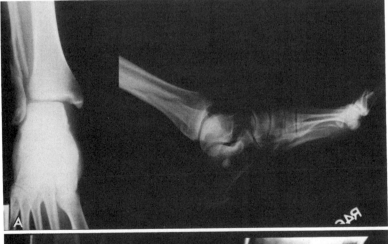

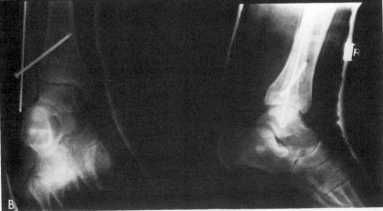

Figure 22–15. *Bimalleolar ankle fracture. A, Initial views showing distal fibular fracture proximal to the syndesmosis and medial mortise spread. B, Postoperative x-rays; mortise is reduced with suture of the deltoid ligament medially and internal fixation laterally.*

and II injuries are managed with soft dressings and crutches. We strongly feel that the more severe grade III injuries are best treated with soft or hard casts and non-weight-bearing in the acute stages of the injury.[8] Associated small avulsion fractures of the tarsal bones do not alter our management plans. We have not noted significant late disability with this regimen, providing that a strengthening rehabilitation program for the foot and ankle is incorporated into the treatment.

Innocent-appearing lateral malleolar fractures, usually the result of a fall and twisting injury, may also involve injury to the medial side of the ankle. An AP lateral and internal rotation x-ray of the ankle is necessary to assess the integrity of the ankle mortise. The articular cartilage space between medial and lateral malleoli and the talus should be equal to the space between the dome of the talus and the distal tibial articular surface (plafond) on the x-ray, and, if any widening is not immediately apparent but suspected, x-rays of the normal ankle should be taken for comparison. If the medial or lateral space is widened (Fig. 22–15), a disruption of the

normal anatomy of the ankle joint has occurred that must be appropriately treated to restore ankle function. If closed manipulation of the lateral malleolar fragment does not succeed in restoring the normal medial and lateral ankle articular space, then soft tissue may be trapped in the medial space and must be removed by operation and direct suture of the deltoid ligament. Often in such an injury the lateral malleolus requires open reduction and internal stabilization (Fig. 22–16).

Bimalleolar fractures may be reduced closed and maintained in anatomical position by plaster cast if the medial malleolar fragment is distal to the tibial plafond. With fractures at the level of the plafond or proximal to it, loss of reduction is common (Fig. 22–17) and elective open reduction and internal fixation is recommended. Plaster immobilization is used postoperatively for 4 to 10 weeks, varying with the security of internal fixation. Fractures of the lateral malleolus proximal to the joint line may also coincide with disruption of the distal tibial fibular ligament and subsequent widening of the ankle mortise. Operative reduction of the syndesmosis

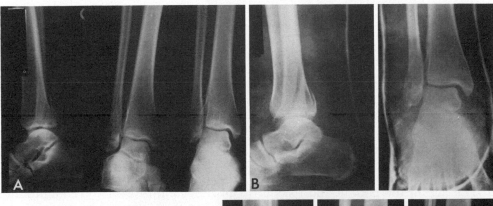

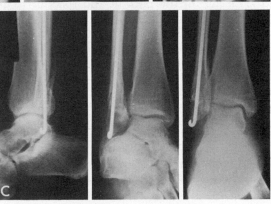

Figure 22–16. *Eversion injury: fracture of the lateral malleolus with deltoid ligament tear. A, Closed reduction attempted. B, Persistent widening of the talomedial malleolar joint space indicating entrapped deltoid ligament. C, Open reduction: ligament disengaged and repaired and fibula fixed with Rush rod.*

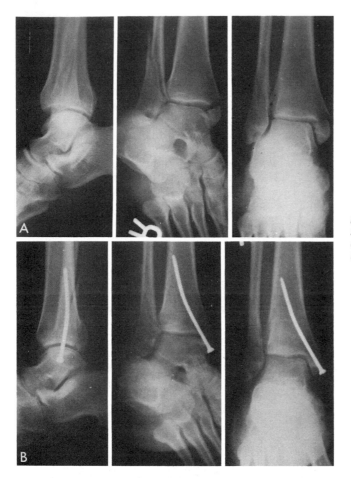

Figure 22–17.   *Bimalleolar fracture–inversion injury. A, Initial injury with minimal displacement. B, Two months after injury union of fracture fragments is evident.*

diastasis and fixation by a screw or bolt across the tibia and fibula is usually necessary (Fig. 22–15).

Trimalleolar fractures and fracture-dislocations are produced by severe trauma to the ankle joint. The size of the posterior malleolar fragment, medial malleolar fragment and any evidence of disruption of the tibial fibular ligament must all be evaluated. The age of the patient and risks of operative intervention versus morbidity from prolonged closed plaster treatment must be considered in selecting the appropriate management plan. If the posterior malleolus (posterior articular surface of the tibia) involves more than a fourth of the joint surface, then open reduction and internal fixation of this fragment is mandatory to restore the major weight-bearing surface of the ankle (Fig. 22–18).

In falls from a height, not only may the ankle mortise be disrupted but the distal tibia may be severely fractured as well

(Fig. 22–19). Closed manipulation under anesthesia is first attempted, and if the ankle mortise and alignment of the knee and ankle can be satisfactorily restored, open reduction may not be necessary. Open reduction may be advisable if a fairly large fragment is present, in which case screw fixation and attempt at restoration of the anatomical surface are indicated. If extensive compression and comminution are present, reduction may prove to be extremely difficult technically. The patient must be advised preoperatively that traumatic arthritis is a common accompaniment of any extensive injury around a joint and that future procedures in the form of arthrodesis for pain relief may be necessary.

Open fracture dislocations may be evaluated at surgery and internally stabilized only if necessary to protect the neurovascular supply to the foot. The chances of chronic osteomyelitis can be minimized

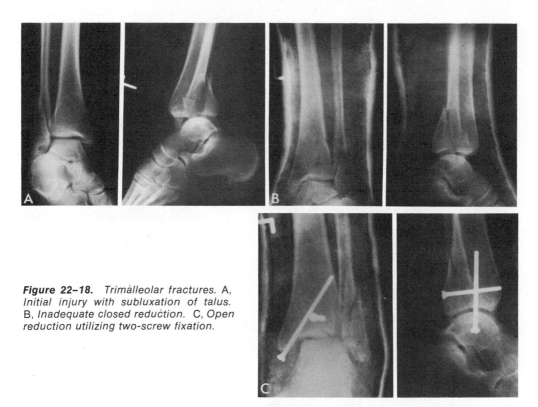

Figure 22–18. Trimalleolar fractures. A, Initial injury with subluxation of talus. B, Inadequate closed reduction. C, Open reduction utilizing two-screw fixation.

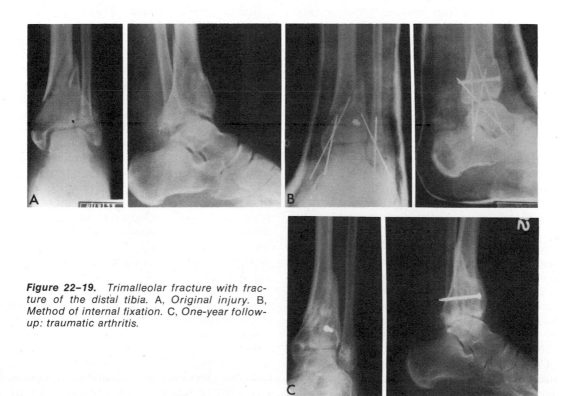

Figure 22–19. Trimalleolar fracture with fracture of the distal tibia. A, Original injury. B, Method of internal fixation. C, One-year follow-up: traumatic arthritis.

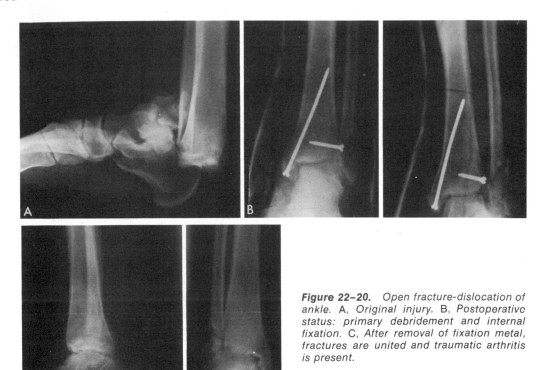

Figure 22–20. *Open fracture-dislocation of ankle. A, Original injury. B, Postoperative status: primary debridement and internal fixation. C, After removal of fixation metal, fractures are united and traumatic arthritis is present.*

only by meticulous wound toilet, gentle manipulation of tissues and adequate immobilization. Even then, the complication rate is high (Fig. 22–20).

FRACTURES AND DISLOCATIONS OF THE FOOT

Injuries to the foot vary in severity from minor inversion sprain to severe multilative partial amputations. The management of the severe injury begins in the emergency department with a gross assessment of the neurovascular status, skin integrity and tendon. Radiological examination completes the initial assessment of injury and further defines the mode of appropriate treatment. Swelling is a common sequel of any major trauma to the foot and most often presents dorsally. A good deal of the lymphatic and venous drainage of the foot and toes occurs across the dorsum of the foot; this drainage can be compromised by soft tissue and laceration injuries with or without fracture and dislocations of the underlying osseous structures.

Initial management of any significant foot injury is with a bulky splinting, soft dressing and elevation of the limb. Closed reduction of specific closed fracture or dislocations can be accomplished in the emergency department by qualified personnel. Occasionally such a reduction will be necessary as an emergency procedure to prevent sloughing of skin secondary to bony displacement. This is often seen in dislocations of the subtalar joint. However, many fractures and dislocations of the foot are not readily reducible without the benefits of anesthesia. Closed or possible open reduction with adequate anesthesia is often the only reasonable plan of management for these injuries.

Any significant open injury of the foot obligates appropriate, definitive treatment in the setting of an operating room. Meticulous debridement of open fractures and fracture-dislocation injuries is a necessity. Internal fixation is often done with Kirschner wires used as temporary holding devices. Soft tissues are best closed in a delayed fashion to minimize infection. Again attention must be directed to minimizing the postoperative swelling and

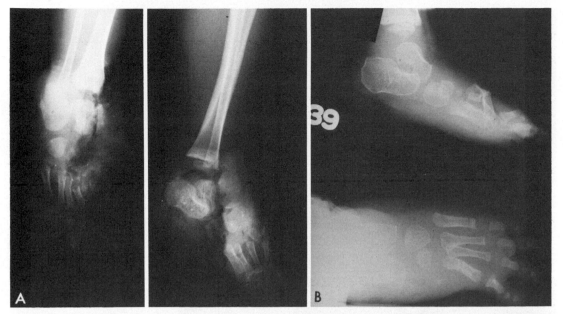

Figure 22–21.   *Severe foot and ankle laceration and partial amputation in a 2-year-old boy who fell off the seat of a riding lawn mower onto the rotating blade. A, Initial x-ray. B, Radiograph 1 year after injury following multiple surgical procedures. Tibial-epiphyseal plate is open, and foot is plantigrade with active motion and protective sensation.*

pain with appropriate bulky soft dressings and extremity elevation.

Severe lacerations of the foot are frequently seen as a result of lawn mower accidents. All too often these injuries occur in the growing youngster and are potentially mutilative (Fig. 22–21). These wounds are always grossly contaminated. Proper examination and determination of viability of tissues can be best performed in the operating room. Meticulous, thorough debridement of necrotic tissue and foreign matter is mandatory to minimize the ensuing infection. Repeated debridements are often indicated and at times a surprisingly functional, albeit cosmetically unappealing, foot can be salvaged. At times, the normal anatomy is so extensively disrupted that initial open definitive amputation is indicated.

Major injuries to the talus, calcaneus, navicular and tarsometatarsal joints are common. Fractures of the talus often occur following foot impaction against the floorboard of a rapidly decelerating automobile or airplane. These fractures are often nondisplaced and can be treated with appropriate plaster immobilization. Displaced fractures of the talus are severe injuries often necessitating a closed or possible open reduction with adequate anesthesia (Fig. 22–22). Avascular necrosis and

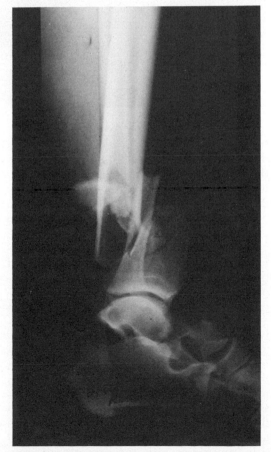

Figure 22–22.   *Displaced fracture of the talus and ipsilateral distal tibial fracture.*

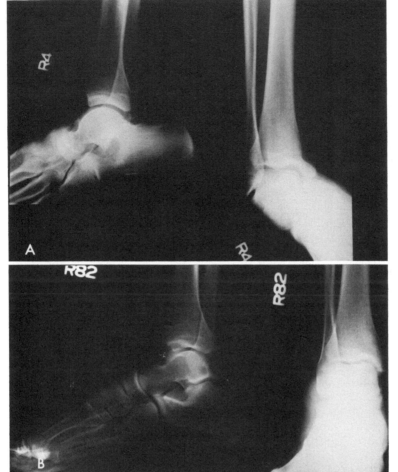

Figure 22–23. *Subtalar dislocation.* A, *Radiograph showing medial dislocation of foot with tenting of skin on lateral aspect of the foot.* B, *Post-reduction x-rays showing anatomical restoration of articulation of talus and calcaneus with general anesthesia.*

traumatic arthritis often result from such a disabling injury.[15] Subtalar joint dislocations are often recognized by the characteristic deformation of the foot (Fig. 22–23). Such an injury must be treated as an emergency to prevent sloughing of skin under displaced tarsal bones. Definitive anatomical reduction can then be performed in the operating suite. Fractures of the calcaneous generally require only appropriate soft-dressing splinting in the emergency setting. The examiner must be aware that lumbar spine injuries frequently occur in association with this injury. Regardless of the method of treatment the prognosis with and without reduction from this potentially crippling injury is often poor because of ensuing traumatic arthrosis of the subtalar joint. Fractures through the body of the navicular may involve the talonavicular joint and displacement of this injury generally requires closed, pos-

sibly open, reduction with adequate anesthesia at an appropriate time.

Fracture dislocation at the tarsometatarsal joint occurs secondary to severe twisting injuries about the foot. The anatomy of the joint must be precisely restored for a good long-term outcome.[2] This injury is best treated at the emergency department with an appropriate soft-tissue splinting dressing. Definitive care with adequate anesthesia is performed in the operating room. Open reduction and internal fixation of this injury is often necessary (Fig. 22–24).

Trauma to the digits of the foot is associated with severe pain. This is particularly true in closed injuries to the great toe. After appropriate x-rays have been taken, sterile decompression of subungual hematomas may be indicated. However, the treating physician must realize that he may be opening a previously closed fracture.

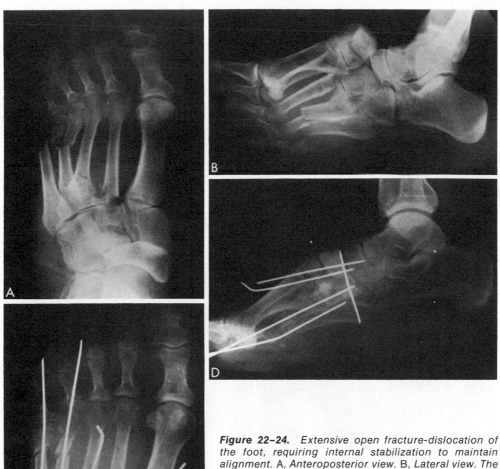

Figure 22–24. *Extensive open fracture-dislocation of the foot, requiring internal stabilization to maintain alignment. A, Anteroposterior view. B, Lateral view. The midfoot dislocation is apparent on this view. C, Anteroposterior view after reduction. D, Lateral view after reduction.*

Open fractures of the toes must be treated with the same meticulous wound care as open fractures elsewhere. Facilities in the emergency department are often inadequate for the proper irrigation and debridement of severe toe injuries. For the less severely injured digits, appropriate dressings and splinting to an adjacent intact digit will usually suffice.

FRACTURES IN CHILDREN

The general principles discussed for fracture management are applicable for children. Most fractures in children are closed fractures, and, whenever possible, are best handled by closed methods. With certain notable exceptions, internal fixations is to be avoided. The x-ray diagnosis of fractures in infants and children is frequently difficult because large portions of the ends of growing bones are composed of cartilage and cannot be visualized on routine x-ray examination. Adequate x-ray evaluation of these secondary epiphyseal growth centers and radiolucent epiphyseal growth lines is possible only with awareness of the chronological appearance of these structures and comparing x-rays of the injured and uninjured extremity.

Treatment should be directed at achieving the best possible alignment and in most cases this can be achieved by closed means. Gross angulation, however, should never be accepted. Rotational deformities must always be corrected at the time of initial treatment. A certain amount of persistent angulation at the fracture site may be acceptable and may be compatible with

a perfectly satisfactory end result, depending on the location of the fracture as related to growth centers and the amount of growth potential present.

The amount of residual angulation that can be accepted and the degree of remodeling that can be expected are dependent on several factors: (1) the age of the child,

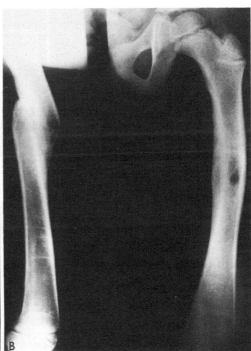

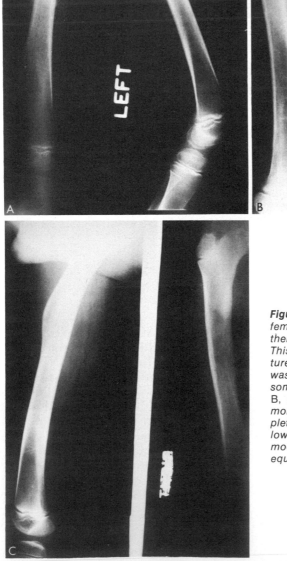

Figure 22–25. A, *Fracture of the shaft of the femur, treated in skeletal traction for 3 weeks, then immobilized in a hip spica for 11 weeks. This x-ray shows the appearance of the fracture when the cast was removed. The fracture was allowed to heal in bayonet apposition with some overriding and slight lateral angulation. B, Follow-up x-rays of case shown in A 4 months after cast removal. Healing is complete and remodeling is progressing. C, Follow-up x-rays 12 months after injury. Remodeling is nearly complete and leg length is equal.*

(2) the location of the fracture with relationship to the end of the bone and (3) the severity of the angulation. In a very young child or infant with a fracture close to the epiphysis, more residual angulation may be accepted. Conversely, in an older patient with a fracture near the middle of the long bone, an accurate reduction is demanded. The greatest degree of angular deformity can be accepted when the apex of the deformity is in the direction of motion of neighboring hinge joints. Lateral angulation, on the other hand, is more likely to persist to some extent, and rotational deformities will not be corrected by the growth and remodeling process.

End-on reduction of fractures in long bones of children is of little importance. These fractures may be allowed to unite with bayonet apposition in most patients, with an excellent prognosis. Indeed, bayonet apposition with some degree of overriding is desireable in fractures of the long bones to compensate for the acceleration of longitudinal growth resulting from the injury. Fractures of long bones resulting in overgrowth and leg length inequality for whatever reason result in a permanent difference in leg length for which there is no spontaneous compensation.

As a general rule, an excellent result may be obtained by traction or closed reduction and plaster immobilization. Certain fractures of long bones (e.g., the shaft of the femur) are best treated by Russell's skin traction or skeletal traction followed by plaster immobilization (Fig. 22–25). Bryant's traction should not be used except occasionally in infants because of the possibility of vascular damage[20] (Fig. 22–26). Except for specific instances, open reduction and the use of metallic fixation devices are never justified.[3]

Trauma about the ankle and knee in children often results in a fracture involving the open epiphyseal growth line. These injuries are quite common and because of the involvement of the epiphyseal plate, may cause premature closure of the involved growth plate resulting in inequality in leg lengths or angular deformities. These injuries usually are the result of a

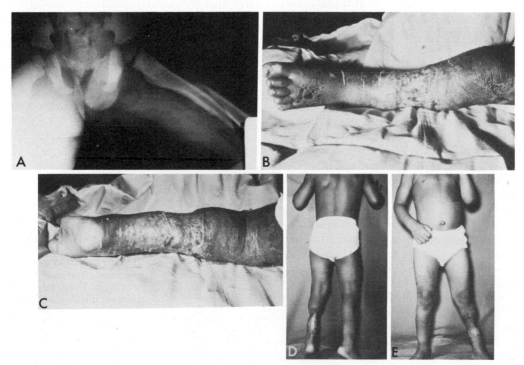

Figure 22–26. A, *Fracture of the shaft of the femur in a 2-year-old child. Treated initially in Bryant's traction. This x-ray shows the spiral fracture in good position and alignment. This fracture ultimately healed with a good result on the right. B and C, Front and back views of the injured leg. The patient developed a Volkmann's ischemic contracture with skin slough from the Bryant's traction. D and E, Front and back views of the final result of the injury shown in A. This required a skin graft and resulted in loss of all the muscles in the left leg below the knee. Lengthening of the Achilles tendon and triple arthrodesis were done later.*

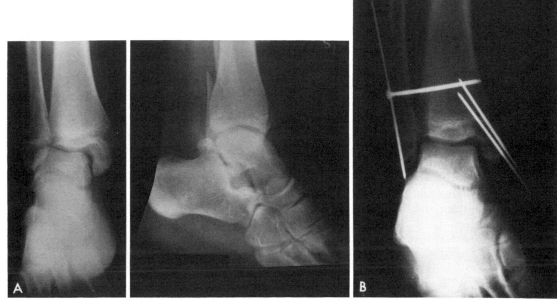

Figure 22–27. *Epiphyseal injury about the ankle. A, Salter type IV fracture of the distal fibula and tibia. B, Intraoperative x-rays; smooth pin was removed at 4 weeks and syndesmosis screw at 8 weeks after injury.*

shearing force applied across the epiphyseal plate with disruption of the plate and displacement of the epiphysis. These epiphyseal injuries have been classified in severity and in regard to prognosis by Aitken[1] and by Salter and Harris.[34]

Such classifications are helpful to the surgeon by providing some indication of the ultimate prognosis and also some indication as to the best method of treatment. Injuries involving a shearing force with displacement of the epiphysis with or without a fragment of metaphysis can usually be managed by closed reduction and plaster immobilization. These injuries are at the end of the long bones where the effects of future growth and remodeling will be the greatest, and providing that reasonable alignment can be obtained, anatomic reduction is not always necessary. Occasionally, these injuries, particularly those involving the distal femoral and distal tibial epiphyses, may be sufficiently unstable that some form of temporary internal fixation is necessary until healing provides stability. This fixation should always be minimal and should be removed as early as possible. The more severe types, in which a vertical fracture line runs through the epiphysis and frequently the articular surface of the joint, demand accurate reduction and maintenance of reduction and frequently require surgical treatment (Fig. 22–27). Since it is not always possible to be certain as to the degree of damage to the epiphyseal plate, regardless of the x-ray appearance of the injury, the prognosis must always be guarded and the parent must always be alerted to the possibility of growth disturbance in the future.

REFERENCES

1. Aitken, A. P.: Fractures of the epiphyses. Clin. Orthop. *41*:19, 1965.
2. Aitken, A. P., and Poulson, D.: Dislocations of the tarsometatarsal joint. J. Bone Joint Surg. *45A*:246, 1963.
3. Blount, W. P.: Fractures in Children. Baltimore, The Williams & Wilkins Company, 1955.
4. Brantigan, O. C., and Voshell, A. P.: The mechanics of the ligaments and menisci of the knee joint. J. Bone Joint Surg. *23*:44, 1941.
5. Brown, P. W., and Urban, J. G.: Early weight-bearing treatment of open fractures of the tibia. J. Bone Joint Surg. *51A*:59, 1969.
6. Brown, P. E., and Preston, E. T.: Ambulatory treatment of femoral shaft fractures with a cast-brace. J. Trauma *15*:860, 1975.
7. Cahill, B.: AO plating of tibia fractures. A.A.O.S. Instructional Course Lectures, Snowmass, Colorado, 1976.
8. Chapman, M. W.: Sprains of the ankle. A.A.O.S. Instructional Course Lectures. St. Louis, The C. V. Mosby Co., 1975, pp. 294–308.

9. Connolly, J. F., and Brooks, A. L.: Vascular problems in Orthopedics. A.A.O.S. Instructional Course Lectures. St. Louis, C. V. Mosby Co., 1973, pp. 12–17.
10. Connolly, J. F., Whittaker, D., and Williams, E.: Femoral and tibial fractures combined with injuries to the femoral or popliteal artery; a review of the literature and analysis of 14 cases. J. Bone Joint Surg. 53A:56, 1971.
11. Ellsasser, J. C., Reynolds, F. C., and Omohundio, J. R.: The non-operative treatment of collateral ligament injuries of the knee in professional football players. J. Bone Joint Surg. 56A:1185, 1974.
12. Geoffrey, W., Sheridan, M. D., and Frederick III, A. M.: Fasciotomy in the treatment of the acute compartment syndrome. J. Bone Joint Surg. 58A:112, 1976.
13. Ger, R.: Muscle transposition for treatment and prevention of chronic post-traumatic osteomyelitis of the tibia. J. Bone Joint Surg. 59A:784, 1977.
14. Ginsburg, J. M., and Ellsasser, J. C.: Problem areas in diagnosis and treatment of knee ligament injuries. Clin. Orthop. 132:201, 1978.
15. Hawkins, L.: Fractures of the neck of the talus. J. Bone Joint Surg. 52A:991, 1970.
16. Hohl, M.: Tibial condylar fractures. J. Bone Joint Surg. 49A:1455, 1967.
17. Irani, R. N., Nicholson, J. T., and Chung, S. M. K.: Long term results in the treatment of femoral shaft fractures in young children by immediate spica immobilization. J. Bone Joint Surg. 58A:945, 1976.
18. Karlstrom, G., and Olerud, S.: Percutaneous pin fixation of open tibial fractures. J. Bone Joint Surg. 57A:915, 1975.
19. Krause, W. R., Pope, M. H., Johnson, R. J., and Wilder, D. G.: Mechanized changes in the knee after meniscectomy. J. Bone Joint Surg. 58A:599, 1976.
20. Lansche, W. E., and Stamp, W. G.: Management of complications of femoral shaft fracture in children. South Med. J. 56:101, 1963.
21. Lottes, J. O.: Medullary nailing of infected fractures of the tibia. J. Bone Joint Surg. 45A:1548, 1963.
22. Marshall, J. L., and Rubin, R. M.: Knee ligament injuries — a diagnostic and therapeutic approach. Orthop. Clin. North Am. 8:641, 1977.
23. McDade, W. C.: Treatment of ankle fractures. A.A.O.S. Instructional Course Lectures. St. Louis, The C. V. Mosby Co., 1975, pp. 251–293.
24. Moll, J. F.: The cast-brace walking treatment of open and closed femoral fractures. South. Med. J. 66:345, 1973.
25. Mooney, V., Nichek, V. V., and Harvey, P. J.: Cast-brace treatment for fractures of the distal part of the femur. J. Bone Joint Surg. 52A:1563, 1970.
26. Mueller, K. H.: Intramedullary nailing of long-bone fractures — current concepts. A.A.O.S. Instructional Course Lectures. St. Louis, The C. V. Mosby Co., 1973, pp. 159–217.
27. Nicoll, E. A.: Fractures of the tibial shaft. J. Bone Joint Surg. 46B:373, 1964.
28. O'Donoghue, D. M.: Surgical treatment of fresh injuries to the major ligaments of the knee. J. Bone Joint Surg. 32A:721, 1950.
29. O'Donoghue, D. M.: Treatment of Injuries to Athletes. 2nd Edition. Philadelphia, W. B. Saunders Company, 1970.
30. Quigley, T. B.: Analysis and treatment of ankle injuries produced by rotatory, abduction and adduction forces. A.A.O.S. Instructional Course Lectures. St. Louis, The C. V. Mosby Co., 1970, pp. 172–182.
31. Roberts, J. M.: Fractures of the condyles of the tibia. J. Bone Joint Surg. 50A:1505, 1968.
32. Rosenthal, R. E., MacPhail, J. A., and Oritz, J. E.: Non-union in open tibial fractures. J. Bone Joint Surg. 59A:244, 1977.
33. Russell, R. H.: Fracture of the femur: A clinical study. Br. J. Surg. 11:491, 1924.
34. Salter, R. B., and Harris, W. B.: Injuries involving the epiphyseal plate. J. Bone Joint Surg. 45A:587, 1963.
35. Sarmiento, A.: A functional below-the-knee cast for tibial fractures. J. Bone Joint Surg. 49A:855, 1967.
36. Schoenecker, P. L., Manske, P. R., and Sertl, G. O.: Traumatic hip dislocation with ipsilateral fractures. Clin. Orthop., 130:233, 1978.
37. Simmons, J. C. H.: Peripheral nerve injuries. In Crenshaw, A. H. (ed.): Campbell's Operative Orthopaedics. St. Louis, The C. V. Mosby Co., 1971, pp. 1754–1756.
38. Smith, H. H.: On the treatment of ununited fracture by means of artificial limbs, which combine the principle of pressure and motion at the seat of fracture, and lead to the formation of an unsheathing callus. Am. J. Med. Sci. 29:102, 1855.
39. Spencer, F. C.: Peripheral arterial disease. In Schwartz, S., et al. (eds.): Principles of Surgery. McGraw-Hill Book Co., New York, 1969, pp. 735–739.
40. Warren, L. F., Marshall, J. L., and Girgis, F.: The prime static stabilizer of the medial side of the knee. J. Bone Joint Surg. 56A:665, 1974.

CHAPTER 23

CARE OF THE THERMALLY INJURED PATIENT

Martin C. Robson, M.D.
Thomas J. Krizek, M.D.
Robert C. Wray, Jr., M.D.

Thermal destruction of the skin produces local and systemic alterations so severe and so diverse that burn injury forms the prototype for the study of all major trauma. The initial and continued systemic hemodynamic, metabolic and nutritional changes and an altered host defense mechanism against infection are merely a reflection of the profound changes in the local wound. The management of the systemic changes is the means of sustaining the patient; the therapeutic imperative, however, is closure of the wound. No matter how elegant the treatment, ultimate survival, convalescence and functional recovery can occur only when the local wound is healed. An understanding of burn injury must begin and end with the burn wound.

Success in treatment is not necessarily reflected in survival statistics. Hideous deformity, limiting contractures and scarred personalities may all reflect well in data that report only mortality. Functional rehabilitation and social acceptance should constitute our measure of success. Our challenge is not how well we treat burns but how well we treat burned patients.

ANATOMY AND FUNCTION OF THE SKIN

The skin is by size and weight one of the largest organs in the body, being second only to muscle. It is also a vital organ; loss of a substantial area is, if unreplaced by the patient's own skin, incompatible with life. So too, invasive bacterial infection, limited to the skin and subcutaneous tissue, may be lethal without visceral spread. Despite wrinkles, we are not possessed of any excess skin. Moreover, it has only limited powers of regeneration and lacks much of the functional reserve characteristic of visceral organs.

Skin has the obvious functions of protection from the environment, sensibility and heat regulation. It is also that portion of ourselves that we present to the world and may, therefore, be a source of visual beauty. If scarred, it is a physical and potential social handicap.

Skin Area

The skin of an adult has a surface ranging from 1.5 to 1.9 square meters (average 1.7 sq. m.). More exact calculations can be obtained from the formula:[202]

$$\text{Area of skin sq. cm.} = \text{height in cm.}^{0.725} \times \text{weight in kg.}^{0.425} \times 71.84$$

In actual weight the skin represents from 14 to 17 per cent of our total body weight. For practical purposes, however, and in particular for assessing thermal injury, it is customary to think in terms of percentage of total surface area and the functional significance of the area, rather than the actual area or weight.

Anatomy

An understanding of functional disturbances and reparative processes of the skin requires consideration of its anatomy (Fig. 23–1). The skin is a two-layered covering resting on a subcutaneous padding of fat. The outer, highly cellular epidermal layer measures 0.06 to 0.8 mm. in thickness and is in contact with the dermis by way of multiple irregular, interpapillary ridges and grooves, often inappropriately called rete pegs (in three dimension they are ridges and grooves, not pegs). These ridges result in increased surface contact between the two layers; they provide much of the resistance of normal skin to tangential stress. The innermost layer of the epidermis is the basal or germinal layer (stratum germinativum) containing the cells destined for keratin production

(95 per cent of total cells) and melanocytes (5 per cent of total). This layer is the total epidermal contact with a neurovascular supply. Injury through this layer may spare sufficient keratin-producing cells to allow regeneration; melanocytes, however, are of neural origin and do not regenerate. This anatomical fact accounts for the depigmented appearance of scars.

Cells generated from this layer are gradually extruded toward the surface, forming first the prickle-layer (stratum spinosum), characterized by prominent, interlocking cell wall projections that further aid the skin's ability to withstand shearing forces. The next layer of evolution is the granular layer (stratum granulosa), which merges imperceptibly with the clear zone (stratum lucidum). These layers have a high, transferable water content (70 per cent), which is intimately concerned with water retention and heat regulation. These cells finally die and form the outer, nonliving, waterproof, fibrous protein that is keratin

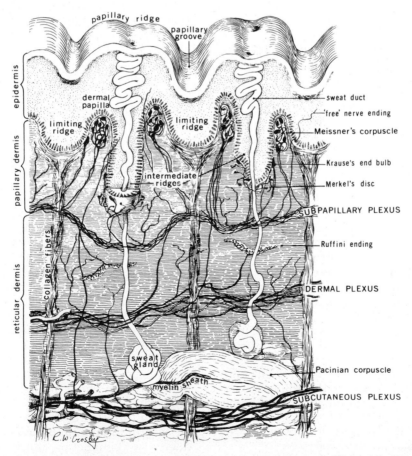

Figure 23–1. *Normal cross-sectional anatomy of the skin. (Courtesy Michael E. Jobalay.)*

(stratum corneum). Keratin contains only 15 per cent water, which when increased by immersion causes softening and "wrinkles," whereas decreased water content results in calluses.

The underlying dermis is 20 to 30 times thicker and contains the nervous, vascular, lymphatic and supporting structures for the epidermis as well as harboring the epidermal appendages. Dermal fibrocytes produce the fibrous proteins, collagen and elastin and give skin its strength. Mastocytes (mast cells) containing histamine and heparin also probably produce the mucopolysaccharides of hyaluronic and chondroitin sulfuric acid that form the interfibrillary matrix of the dermis. Histiocytes or tissue macrophages are distributed around blood vessels and hair follicles. The appendages of the skin include hair follicles and their associated sebaceous glands, the eccrine sweat glands that enter through interpapillary ridges, and the apocrine glands located in the axillary and inguinal regions.

Functions

Sensibility. There are three plexuses of nerves supplying sensibility to the skin. They are the subpapillary, the intradermal and the subcutaneous plexuses, which roughly correspond to the vascular plexuses. Branches of these plexuses go to the dermal papillae of the papillary dermis, where the greatest concentration of receptors are located. The receptors are of three types: mechanoreceptors, thermoreceptors and nociceptors; each of these is differentially sensitive to certain types of incident energy. Some nerve endings are capped with specialized endings such as Meissner's corpuscles or pacinian corpuscles, which filter out certain types of energy and enhance others. Each ending or set of endings connects to an identifiable area of the sensory cortex and each can elicit only one type of sensation. It is important to view these endings not as isolated entities but rather as points in a complicated matrix whose impulses are amplified or damped until they reach the cortex and are interpreted with other input. The cortex then responds with a symptom complex that is identifiable with burns of varying depths.

Heat Regulation. Body heat is generated by the metabolic oxidative processes and is added to by the environment from conduction (the transfer of heat from one molecule to another), convection (transfer of heat through a moving liquid or gas) and radiation (via electromagnetic waves).

To maintain thermal equilibrium, heat is dissipated by evaporation, conduction, radiation, convection and, in trifling amounts, via excreta. To be lost, internal heat must be brought to the surface. There is a rich dermal network that sends branches outward to form a subpapillary plexus. Characterized by multiple arteriovenous shunts, this vascular bed, if need be, can accept up to one sixth or one fifth of the cardiac output. Thus, in addition to its obvious nutritional function for the skin, it has great capacity for delivering blood for heat dissipation. Normally, man loses 70 per cent of the body heat load via conduction, 25 per cent by evaporation and the rest by convection or radiation.

Heat moves by molecular conduction and is dependent upon the specific conductivity of the tissues, with the physiological gradient (hotter to cooler) being toward the surface. The heat exchange is accomplished by thermal gradients obeying physical laws and varying not only with body temperature but also with ambient air temperature and moisture. When the air temperature exceeds the body temperature, the gradient is reversed and heat can be dissipated from the body only by evaporation.

Sweating will occur at 37°C air temperature at 0 per cent humidity. When the air is saturated and has a temperature exceeding body temperature, heat cannot be lost and fever will result (heat stroke). The eccrine sweat glands are capable of excreting 10 liters per day. Since water vapor molecules have a higher kinetic energy than molecules in water, thermal energy is required to convert sweat to water vapor. Five hundred and eighty calories of energy are required to convert one liter of water to vapor at 37°C. This energy is provided by the oxidative processes and normally accounts for 20 to 30 per cent of our total metabolic heat production.

Thermal equilibrium is, therefore, primarily a problem of delivery to the vascular system (dilatation or constriction), conductivity, convection and radiant loss supplemented, when necessary, by evaporative loss and the expenditure of energy.

Protection. The continuity of the skin and an intact sensibility are the major factors in protection. In addition to being an obvious barrier against mechanical and chemical trauma, it protects against thermal injury by heat dissipation and against cold injury by heat conservation. It is nearly waterproof, so that immersion in water does not cause swelling of tissues. Perhaps of major importance is the barrier it presents to bacterial invasion. The skin is never sterile, nor can it be easily sterilized. It is colonized by two major groups of organisms, its resident flora and a transient flora (Table 23–1). The bacteria are not normally recoverable from the surface or from the sweat glands, but rather are harbored in the hair follicles, particularly near the orifices of the sebaceous glands. The quantitative distribution of bacteria is related to the distribution of hair, and in levels ranging from 5 to 865,000 aerobic bacteria and 50 to 200,000 anaerobic bacteria per sq. cm.[230]

The skin exists in a nicely balanced state with its resident flora but actively resists the presence of its transient flora. The exposure to streptococci, staphylococci and enteric bacteria is frequent, and random cultures may recover any of these on occasion. The antibacterial qualities of the skin are related to active and passive activities. The secretion of sebaceous glands, sebum, contains high levels of fatty acids, particularly oleic acid. In addition to lubricating the skin surface, sebum actively destroys streptococci and, less effectively, staphylococci.[117] However, any break in the skin or any inflammation results in serum accumulation, which inactivates sebum and in this situation streptococci may colonize rapidly.[248] Staphylococci are also susceptible to desiccation on the normally dry skin surface; the application of a wet dressing with an impervious outer layer will both remove sebum and provide moisture, and staphylococcal furunculosis may rapidly appear. The enteric bacteria are not affected by sebum but are readily killed by desiccation on dry skin. The presence of moisture or maceration can result in colonization of enteric bacteria. Pseudomonas, particularly, is susceptible to desiccation and can be recovered from only 5 to 10 per cent of random skin cultures. Since bacteria tend to colonize in hair follicles, random skin swabs may often be sterile, and special techniques are necessary to accurately identify the bacteria.

Regeneration. The often presented concepts of wound healing are not totally applicable to thermal injury. The cleanly incised, coapted wound heals by a lag or inflammatory stage followed by the laying down of new collagen, realignment of fibers and the return of structural integrity. Implicit though not stated in this description is an intact epithelial covering. The understanding of healing in burns requires some conceptual alterations since burns constitute horizontally as well as vertically directed wounds. Loss of epidermal continuity requires ingrowth of new epidermis from the margin, or re-epithelialization from remaining epidermal elements. For practical purposes, this means regrowth from remaining basal cells or hair follicle epithelium since the glands contribute very little. Until epidermal continuity is

TABLE 23–1. Bacteriology of Normal Skin

I. RESIDENT FLORA
  A. Aerobic gram-positive cocci
    1. *Micrococcus luteus*
    2. *Staphylococcus epidermidis*
  B. Coryneform group
    1. *Corynebacterium xerosis*
    2. Lipophilic diphtheroids
  C. Fungi
    1. *Pityrosporum ovale*
    2. *Pityrosporum orbiculare*
  D. Anaerobic bacteria
    1. *Propionibacterium acnes*

II. TRANSIENT FLORA
  A. Aerobic gram-positive cocci
    1. *Staphylococcus aureus*
    2. *Streptococcus pyogenes*
    3. *Streptococcus faecalis*
  B. Aerobic gram-positive rods
    1. *Corynebacterium pyogenes*
    2. Mycobacterium spp.
    3. Bacillus spp.
  C. Fungi
    1. *Candida albicans*
    2. Other candidas
    3. Dermatophytes
    4. Phycomycetes
  D. Enteric bacteria
    1. *Pseudomonas aeruginosa*
    2. *Escherichia coli*
    3. *Enterobacter aerogenes-Klebsiella pneumoniae*
    4. *Proteus mirabilis*
  E. Anaerobic bacteria
    1. *Peptostreptococcus constellatus*

re-established by this regeneration or marginal ingrowth (or artificially, by applying a graft), there will be no healing. There will be little progress beyond the lag or inflammatory stage, characterized grossly and histologically by granulation tissue. Perhaps the greatest single advance in burn therapy is the realization and acceptance of the fact that a wound lacking epidermal covering cannot heal.

MECHANISMS OF THERMAL INJURY

At an internal temperature of 37°C we are only 6°C below our thermal death point (43 to 44°C for visceral cells). Our ability to rapidly dissipate heat is related to blood supply, thermal conductivity and evaporative water loss from the skin. The amount of external heat energy delivered to the skin is related to the intensity of the heat and the time of exposure. The skin can maximally dissipate heat at the rate of 0.04 cal./sec./sq. cm.; however, since a flash exposure may deliver 30 cal./sec./sq. cm., the ability to dissipate this falls short by a factor of almost 1000.

Experimentally, the time of exposure and intensity of the heat are easily measured and controlled. Although the response of the skin follows the same basic laws of physical energy, it is also subject to great biological variability. The water content of the skin, its varying thickness within a given area, pigmentation, the presence of hair, oil and dirt, as well as the rapid changes in peripheral circulation, all influence the tissue response to heat. These variations occur not only among species but also within very limited areas of the skin itself. The uniform application of heat to the surface does not result in a biologically uniform injury.

Within the limits of biological variability, skin will tolerate temperatures up to 40°C if the time of exposure is short. Thereafter, increased temperatures result in a logarithmic increase in tissue damage irrespective of time of exposure; fleeting exposure to 70°C will produce epidermal necrosis (Fig. 23–2). The rate of damage at 60 to 65°C is 10 million times greater than it is at 45°C.[107]

Short of incineration, thermal injury will destroy cells by interference with necessary biological function. The mechanics of injury are the result of denaturation of cell protein, interference with cell metabolism and secondary interference with vascular supply.

LOCAL RESPONSE TO THERMAL INJURY

The body reacts to thermal injury with a series of responses that are not unique for burns; rather, it is the intensity and magnitude of the responses that differentiate the burn injury. The severity of the injury is related to both depth and spatial distribution. The alterations result from the initial injury and, more significantly, the subsequent loss of skin function.

Although totally interrelated, the local reaction to burning may be artificially divided into: (1) the response of the thermally injured cell, (2) the local vascular response to injury, (3) local response related to depth of injury and (4) burn wound sepsis.

Response of the Thermally Injured Cell

The depth of thermal injury is determined by the combination of the burning agent, temperature, time of exposure and the series of events set in motion by the injury. There is a direct, vertical decrease in the severity of injury from the surface to the depth of the wound. Some cells are immediately destroyed, some are irrevocably injured, and some cells although injured are capable of surviving under suitable conditions. The vertical decrease is also reflected in a decrease concentrically in all directions from the central point of injury. Three concentric zones of a significant thermal injury have been described relating to the intensity of the thermal stimulus[127] (Fig. 23–2B). The outermost zone, the zone of hyperemia, is the area of the burn least affected and is usually healed by the seventh day. The innermost zone, the zone of coagulation, is irreversibly damaged from the outset and therefore its fate is determined at the time of injury. Between these two zones lies the zone of stasis. This represents an area of intermediate injury that initially resembles the zone of hyperemia but by the end

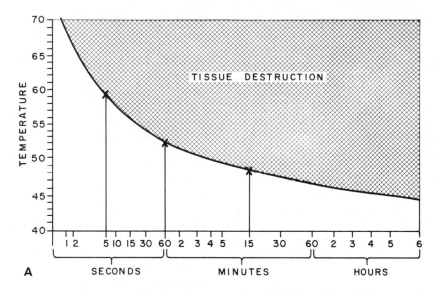

THREE ZONES WITHIN A MAJOR BURN

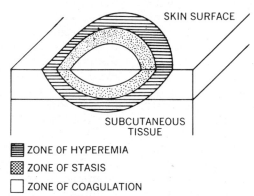

ZONE OF HYPEREMIA
ZONE OF STASIS
B ZONE OF COAGULATION

Figure 23–2. A, *Tissue destruction as a function of time and temperature (in degrees Centigrade). Exposure of the skin to 70° C. for one second results in damage. At lesser temperatures, increasing length of exposure is necessary, such as that at 45° C. exposure for six hours is required to cause damage. (Based on data of Moritz and Henrique.*[149]*) B, Diagram conceptually describing burn wound as concentric areas of decreasing damage.*

of 24 to 48 hours develops changes that eventually make it indistinguishable from the zone of coagulation.

The earliest cytological evidence of injury is a redistribution of the fluid and solid components of the cell nuclei. Imbibition of fluid results in nuclear swelling, membrane rupture and pyknosis. Cell cytoplasm first becomes granular and finally homogeneously coagulated. Progressive denaturation of cell protein occurs as temperatures rise. These latter changes in the thermally injured cell are theoretically reversible since protein is constantly being denatured by the body and being replaced. Only at temperatures in excess of 45°C does this denaturation exceed the re-

parative ability of the cell.[198] Therefore, reducing the temperature should reduce the denaturation of protein. Indeed, experimentally this has proved to be the case.

Cells are also injured and destroyed by interference with vital metabolic processes. Thermolabile enzyme systems are blocked at approximately the same temperatures that effect protein denaturation.[55] The metabolic response of an individual cell is quite variable, even within a homogeneous cell population. A decrease in enzyme activity below 50 per cent of normal results in cell death, whereas lesser degrees of injury may be reflected in altered survival.

The specialized functions of the various types of cells composing the skin are affected differently. In deeper injuries the dermal collagen and elastic fibers show coagulation and dissolution. Hair follicles show pyknosis of nuclei and rupture of the follicle from basal cell attachments. Lysis of epithelium of the sebaceous and sudoriferous glands may occur.

The response to thermal injury on the cellular level is neither uniform nor static. Much of the result will be determined by the vascular supply and the local environment of the wound. Additional heat, mechanical or chemical trauma or bacterial invasion will further destroy the injured cell that had a potential for survival.

Local Vascular Response to Injury

The local vascular response can be divided into immediate and delayed fluid and cellular phases. This is the normal inflammatory response and in mild thermal injuries (51 to 60°C for 20 seconds) is indistinguishable from that following mechanical trauma.[209] Longer or more severe exposure brings about more characteristic changes due to the heat itself.

Fluid Response. The cardinal feature of thermal injury is accumulation of fluid within the injured area. This fluid and electrolyte shift within the wound is related to the type and magnitude of injury. There is an immediate and reversible vascular response to burning. It is characterized by spasm of venules and dilatation of capillaries. An initial arterial and arteriolar vasoconstriction is followed by vasodilatation.[175] Capillaries and venules in the burned area become immediately permeable to plasma proteins of a molecular weight of 125,000 or below.[190] This capillary permeability occurs throughout the vascular tree in patients with greater than 30 per cent body burns. This type of response is transient, reversible and stimulated experimentally by histamine, serotonin and other vasoactive substances such as certain of the prostaglandins. It may be prevented experimentally by antihistamines and delayed by previous serotonin depletion.

The initial response is followed in 1 to 6 hours by a delayed response.[15] This delayed response appears indistinguishable from the response to injection of bacteria.

It may be initiated by histamine or the complement cascade but is probably sustained by slower-acting vasoactive substances in the kinin system[7] or the prostaglandin family.[132] It appears to develop at the capillary rather than the venule level. The greatest loss of both plasma and fluid occurs in the first 12 hours post-burn. During this period, leukocytes, platelets and red cells marginate on the vessel wall and plugging of the capillaries takes place. This results in egress of fluid from the capillaries and edema formation.[79]

Fluid and electrolyte changes occur in the thermally injured tissue by other mechanisms than capillary permeability. If capillary permeability alone accounted for fluid accumulation, externally applied pressure in excess of hydrostatic pressure could prevent it. This is not the case. In fact, fluid will accumulate in uninjured tissue around the site of pressure in almost equal amounts. Nor does it explain loss of fluid into areas of the body not involved by burns. Experimentally, burned tissue, even if immediately transplanted and devoid of a direct vascular supply, accumulates fluid far in excess of unburned, transplanted tissue.[205]

Normal protein (macromolecules) of the skin has an adsorption coefficient for water and electrolytes that may be very high. For comparison, the adsorption coefficient for a simple system such as water-charcoal is 37,000 atmospheres. These normal coefficients may be disturbed by burning and cause cellular tissue swelling irrespective of vascularity, and would theoretically occur at pressures far in excess of hydrostatic pressure. It would also tend to explain the more marked fluid and electrolyte accumulations in cell populations of injured and recovering cells, as opposed to areas where all cells are dead.[92]

This fluid and electrolyte shift is related to the type of injury. Thermal injury breaks down cell membrane, and potassium is released into the extracellular space. The concentration gradient between arteries and veins in the burned area may reach 0.72 mEq. per liter within a few hours.[192] Fox demonstrated that after a severe flash burn with immediate death of cells, the water, sodium and potassium content was less than in normal skin, although the underlying muscles showed increased water and sodium concentration.[92] In contrast, a low-intensity scald burn with severe injury to cells but less immediate cell necrosis results in increased water (three times greater than flash burn), sodium and potassium in both the burned tissue and the underlying muscle. This sequestering of fluid has been shown to be due to an uptake of water and sodium by injured collagen.[185, 205] In addition, an abnormality of the sodium pump exists with the intracellular sodium content increasing and a potassium efflux.[59]

The fluid-electrolyte-protein loss described is obligatory. It enters a "functional third space" and represents an overall hemodynamic deficit. Those vascular alterations are an integral part of the response to burning. In milder injury, the response may be limited to subpapillary vessels; whereas, in full-thickness skin destruction the vascular response will occur in the subcutaneous tissue and at the margins of the wound.

Cellular Response. The cellular response is characterized by neutrophil emigration from vessels to the tissues. This begins on a small scale immediately but progresses to a peak over 5 to 6 hours. The stimulus for emigration is not known, although it is probably related to a decreased expulsion force between the endothelial cell and the leukocyte. It is an integral part of the basic inflammatory response to any injury and may be stimulated by any substance that increases vascular permeability.

Once the neutrophil emerges through the permeable capillary membrane, it is attracted by chemotaxis to the site of injury. Chemotaxis does not necessarily proceed normally in the burned patient. When an impairment exists it appears to be due to a primary transient defect in polymorphonuclear leukocytes and not to a chemotactic inhibitor in the serum.[86] Once the neutrophil reaches the site of injury phagocytosis of the bacteria that have broached the burned portal of entry occurs. Phagocytosis proceeds normally in burned patients, but once phagocytized the bacterial intracellular kill ratio is decreased.[4]

Monocytes enter the injured area with the neutrophils, although in much smaller numbers. Because of their longer life span, they predominate in the wound after the first few days. These monocytes evolve into tissue macrophages and are effective against the remaining bacteria.

Red blood cells are affected in proportion to the severity of the vascular injury in the burn area. Loss of red cells into the tissue is not a part of the burn injury. However, a variable number of red cells in the area of the injury will be destroyed immediately and others will die prematurely. Decrease in blood flow, agglutination, sludging and eventual thrombosis will add to red cell loss.[137] Platelets are removed from the circulatory system in a similar fashion and an initial thrombocytopenia develops.

Although the cellular losses are an integral part of the early response to burning, the functionally important response is the noncellular fluid and electrolyte loss.

Local Response Related to Depth of Injury. The ultimate significance of depth of injury is not what has been lost but rather the functional capacity of that which remains — whether there is adequate capacity in the injured skin to withstand bacterial invasion and to provide regeneration. Although clues to depth may be obtained by clinical observation, the true extent of injury is usually determined only in retrospect. Although, in any given area, the depth will vary tremendously, it is conceptually easier to view burns as a uniform injury.

Superficial Burn. FIRST DEGREE. In low-intensity–prolonged exposure injury or high-intensity flash exposure the damage is superficial (Fig. 23–3). The local response is characterized by erythema due to the vascular response in subpapillary vessels. Edema will occur in basal layers, irritating naked nerve endings at this level and causing discomfort, although clinical swelling and blistering are not seen. Denaturation of the outer nonliving keratin layer does occur, accompanied by some cellular destruction, often delayed, in the underlying stratum granulosa. Premature cell death may result in desquamation at this level, which is noted as "peeling" a few days after the burn. Other than discomfort, there is no clinical significance to injury at this level. All germinal cells of the basal layer survive. Healing occurs by evolution of cells to the surface and is not accompanied by scarring or discoloration.

Partial-Thickness Burn. SUPERFICIAL, SECOND DEGREE — A. As intensity of

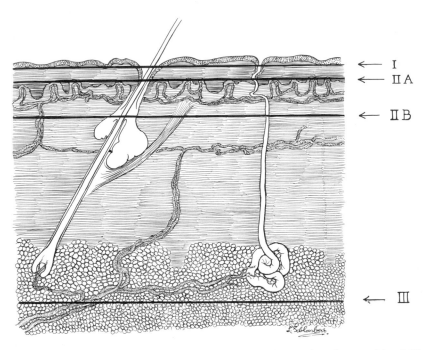

Figure 23–3. *Depth of injury from burns. I, Superficial burn, involves only subcorneal level. IIA, Partial thickness — superficial: involves some but not all the basal layer. Healing should occur spontaneously but perhaps with some depigmentation due to loss of melanocytes. IIB, Partial thickness — deep: loss of basal layer is complete. Only potential for spontaneous healing lies in the viable epidermal elements present in the skin appendages. III, Full thickness: by definition, all epidermal elements have been destroyed and spontaneous healing is impossible other than from the margins of the wound.*

heat or time of exposure is increased, there is increased tissue destruction. Since any injury short of full-thickness loss is "partial thickness," this injury requires further subdivision. Included in superficial partial thickness is any injury that does not totally destroy the basal layer. This injury is clinically and histologically characterized by fluid accumulation. Erythema is seen but the distinguishing finding is blistering. When the edema of burning is close to the surface, it is easily visible. The same vascular response occurs with edema formation either at the dermal-epidermal junction or within the epidermis itself. Cells of stratum granulosa are destroyed and, together with the stratum corneum, form the covering of the blister. Intercellular processes of "prickle cells" dissolve; edematous separation and often destruction of these cells are seen. Marked dilatation of the subpapillary plexus occurs, but the structural integrity of the dermis remains intact. Basal cells may be destroyed in part and nerve endings at this level irritated.

Intact blisters maintain a sterile, waterproof covering of the wound, and healing occurs by continued growth of the remaining basal cells. Removal or breaking of blisters results in a weeping wound and loss of "membrane-barrier" of the skin. Stripping this layer of epidermis results in an increase in evaporative water loss, attended by the necessary metabolic expenditure of thermal injury.[83] Loss of the blister also exposes naked nerve fibers and increases discomfort. Once the blister is broken, the edema fluid forms a coagulum or "crust," under which healing will also usually proceed uneventfully.

Blistering is not a phenomenon limited to superficial burns but can also be seen in full-thickness loss when the intensity of the heat is sufficient to cause "steam" within the epidermis. In these cases, it appears promptly in conjunction with the fluid phase of the injury (first 8 hours). The appearance of blisters after this time is suggestive of bacterial invasion and should be investigated in this light.

Since basal cells are not destroyed in quantity, regeneration is usually prompt and complete without scarring. Temporary discoloration may occur, and some permanent changes toward a lighter color may be related to loss of melanocytes. The cellular barrier to bacterial invasion is generally intact at this level, although the presence of plasma inactivates the antistreptococcal potency of sebum and streptococcal invasion may be a danger.

DEEP, SECOND DEGREE — B. This level of injury is characterized by disruption of epidermal continuity and loss of much of the basal cell layer, but with survival of viable epidermal elements in hair follicles and glands.

The major histological changes occur in the subpapillary plexus. The initial fluid and cellular phases of vascular response occur with edema accumulation at the dermal-epidermal junction. Coagulation necrosis of epidermal cells occurs as vascular injury progresses to vascular blockage, thrombosis and dissolution of endothelial cells. An inflammatory leukocyte response beneath the basal layer occurs.

There may be blistering in this injury but more often there is the development of dry coagulum of plasma and necrotic cells — an eschar. Fluid loss is quantitatively similar to weeping or blistered superficial wounds but is deceptively hidden beneath the coagulum. Since naked nerve endings in the basal layer are destroyed, the wound is not responsive to pinprick, although pressure sensation remains intact. The membrane barrier to water is lost and evaporation through coagulum is 15 to 20 times that of normal skin.[46] This wound is clinically indistinguishable from full-thickness loss.

The cellular barrier to bacterial invasion is also lost, and wound sepsis is the major clinical determinant of healing of this wound.

Injury at this level, if not further traumatized or subjected to bacterial invasion, has the potential for spontaneous regeneration. Undamaged epithelial cells in hair follicles and the margins of the wound will proliferate and resurface the wound. If the eschar is removed prematurely, the clinical appearance will be that of a granulating wound with multiple punctate epithelial islands. These will progressively enlarge and coalesce to form a new surface. When coverage is complete, underlying collagen fibers degenerate. New collagen is laid down and remodeling will occur over a period of time. The new epithelium is thin

and lacks sebaceous secretions to lubricate the surface, sensation is diminished and since most melanocytes are destroyed, it will be lighter than surrounding tissue. Failure to redevelop interpapillary ridges results in prolonged susceptibility to even minor, tangentially directed stress forces.[140]

Full-Thickness Burn. THIRD DEGREE. As the depth of injury increases in more severe trauma, all epidermal elements and dermal supporting structures are destroyed. Whereas the more superficial injuries are characterized by increased vascularity, this is an avascular injury. The fluid and cellular response to injury occurs at the margins, in normal viable tissue and in the depths of the subcutaneous tissue. Coagulation necrosis of cells, thrombosis of vessels, accumulation of fluid and cellular infiltrate in the margins of the wound characterize the injury. Fluid accumulation is related to the initial intensity of the heat. It is as great as in superficial injuries or injuries from lower-intensity exposure, in which cell death is more gradual.

Clinically characterized by the same eschar as deep partial-thickness burns, third-degree burns are also insensitive to pinprick. The leathery eschar also permits evaporative water loss to an excess degree and forms no functional barrier to bacterial invasion.

This injury cannot heal itself. There will be a natural progression of increased marginal and subcutaneous inflammatory response, development of granulation tissue and autolysis at the junction of viable and nonviable tissue with eventual slough of eschar. Resurfacing can occur only from the margins of the wound or by application of skin graft.

FOURTH DEGREE. Occasional severe incineration injuries occur in which the depth of injury extends through the subcutaneous tissue to involve fascia, muscle, periosteum or bone. The natural history of the wound is not dissimilar to other full-thickness injury, except for the individual problems of skin coverage that they present. Extensive destruction of muscle will also impose a myoglobin load on the renal tubules.

The burn wound, therefore, represents an injury of mixed severity and depth. The vascular and cellular response is more representative of the nonspecific inflammatory response than unique to thermal injury. The natural history of the wound is related to the amount of cellular destruction and the capacity for regeneration. These concepts, however, are presented as though they occur in the germ-free patient. Such is not the case and, clinically, the major determinant in the healing of burns and the survival of patients relates to the altered functional capacity of the skin to resist bacterial invasion.

Burn-Wound Sepsis

The local cutaneous defense against bacterial invasion is a function of an intact membrane barrier, antibacterial substances in sebum, desiccation on dry skin and a natural competition with the normal flora of the skin. Each of these is altered following thermal trauma. Contributing to the altered local defense mechanisms are modifications in systemic response such as hypovolemia and an altered immune mechanism.

Bacteria of the resident flora of the skin are resistant to heat injury in approximately the same proportions as are the skin cells. Those on the surface are heat-killed as are the surface cells, and initial swab cultures are usually sterile.[308] The bacteria in the hair follicles and glands, however, survive and quantitative counts of *biopsy* specimens show the same 10^3 bacteria per gram of tissue as found in the tissue prior to burning.[16] These organisms, *Staph. epidermidis* et al., we would now classify as "amphibionts." Not normally prime invaders, they do indeed have the potential for becoming the infecting organisms.

The initial danger to the burned patient is most often the *beta-hemolytic Streptococcus*, the most common of the transient flora, present in most patients. The rich vascularity of the inflammatory phase of early injury, the edema and the neutralization of the bacteriocidal defense mechanisms of sebum all render the burn particularly prone to streptococcal invasion. Historically, the recognition of "burn shock" and its management in the early 1940's resuscitated patients only to have them succumb to streptococcal invasion in the first few days after burning. The introduction of penicillin provided both effective treatment and prophylaxis against streptococcal burn sepsis. Although strep-

tococci remain exquisitely sensitive to penicillin and its use in the early phases of burn care remains appropriate today, it proved to be no panacea.[16]

With shock controlled and streptococcal sepsis prevented, the 1950's recorded only prolonged rather than increased survival. Opportunistic, ubiquitous, penicillin-resistant *Staphylococcus aureus* replaced streptococci as the offender.[239] Unchecked by competition with normal skin flora and flourishing in the warm, moist environment of the fresh burn wound staphylococci were able to colonize the wound. A quantitative increase in staphylococci resulted in microabscesses in and around hair follicles, then showering of bacteria into the blood stream, resulting in secondary abscesses. The aerobic nature of the staphylococci and their dependence on a good blood supply made the development of penicillinase-resistant antibiotics both timely and effective. Their apparent disappearance has been deceptive and a 900 per cent increase in *Staphylococcus aureus* septicemia between 1968 and 1970 was noted at the U.S. Army Institute of Surgical Research.[57] This increase appears to have continued over recent years.

The control of staphylococci did not produce a "germ-free" patient. Indeed, the first of the true "amphibiont" organisms, *Pseudomonas aeruginosa*, appeared as a major threat in the 1960's. The "amphibionts" are those organisms previously classified as "nonpathogens," which under conditions of altered host resistance and disturbed bacterial ecology can become predominant in a wound and reach sufficient quantitative levels to be truly pathogenic. Previously thought to be a harmless saprophyte, pseudomonas was encountered in only 8 per cent of burned patients in 1948; by the early 1960's it was encountered in 70 per cent of burned patients within one week after burning and was the leading cause of death.[165]

Indigenous to man, pseudomonas can be identified in 15 to 20 per cent of random nasopharyngeal and stool cultures. It is now ubiquitous in most hospitals; isolation has been ineffective prophylaxis. In mixed full- and partial-thickness injury, early pseudomonas colonization occurs within the lumen of hair follicles and glands; in full-thickness wounds it may not gain access until the eschar cracks.[222] Lodgement and quantitative growth to levels not exceeding 10^5 bacteria per gram, as determined by biopsy techniques, are compatible with survival and healing of deep dermal elements in partial-thickness injury. If the count exceeds 10^5 bacteria per gram, the bacteria spread from the hair follicles and colonize along the dermalsubcutaneous interface.[293-295, 301] Perivascular growth is accompanied by thrombosis of vessels and necrosis of any remaining dermal elements, converting partial-thickness burns to full-thickness loss. Levels of growth in excess of 10^5 bacteria per gram of tissue constitute "burn-wound sepsis," and levels of 10^8 to 10^9 bacteria per gram may be associated with lethal burns.[223] Since the process occurs in a subeschar plane, surface swabs may be deceptive. So too, lethal burn-wound sepsis may occur with no spread of viable organisms into the blood stream and without secondary visceral lodgement; negative blood cultures provide no security.[196]

The vascular changes of full-thickness burns with local occlusion of small vessels isolate the wound from many normal host defense mechanisms. So too, they prevent the adequate delivery of potent systemic antibiotics to the foci of bacterial growth. The use of topical antibacterial agents applied directly to the wound has been both rational and effective. Quantitative bacterial cultures of biopsy specimens have been a useful guide to management. Wound biopsy for culture and microscopic examination is very important. The mere presence of bacteria is not so critical as the quantitative level of bacterial growth.

Evidence suggests that pseudomonas burn sepsis has yielded to a variety of topical antibacterial agents and techniques. The repetition of history suggests, however, that this is leading to the emergence of the opportunistic growth of new and different "amphibiont" organisms. Prominent among these is Candida. Mycotic infection from *Candida Albicans* was not recognized in one series in the period from 1953–1959, appeared in 24 cases in the next 8-year period, and in the 3 years 1967–1970 there were 50 cases of candida septicemia identified.[63] Candida, although part of the normal bowel flora, is clearly a secondary invader. Predisposition is provided by decreased host resistance seen in the chronic burn patient, and potentiated by the dis-

turbance in the bacterial ecology resulting from antibiotic therapy. Long-standing indwelling catheters may provide a portal of entry, but more often it is the bowel. Candida septicemia is heralded by hypothermia, leukopenia, agitation and later vasculitis with purpura. There are no specific features to distinguish it from bacterial infection. Its presence in the gut, burn wound, or even the blood stream can be misinterpreted as "harmless" contamination. The finding of candida in the urine, however, particularly in the noncatheterized patient, is ominous and should be considered an indication for antifungal therapy.[155, 174, 214]

In addition to candida, mycotic burn-wound sepsis has been associated with Phycomycetes and the Aspergillus species. Infection with these species is identified by a change in the clinical appearance of the wound, development of purplish or black spots, ulceration of the burn wound, unexplained fever or unusual tenderness. Biopsy and histological identification are mandatory. Cultures are positive in only 30 per cent of histologically proved cases and follow only after a 3-to-5 day lag for growth on culture media.[38] Pathologically, all produce fat necrosis, ischemia of underlying muscle, vascular invasion and systemic dissemination. Of 30 cases reported in one series, 22 were of the Phycomycetes class (two were Rhizopus and the remainder probably Mucor) and the other eight from Aspergillus.[38]

Among the bacterial species emerging as threats to the burned patient, most prominent are the gram-negative bacteria, particularly the Enterobacteriaceae family.[62] Among these are *Serratia marcescens*, the Klebsiella-Enterobacter group, Erwinia species and, of particular note, the Providencia species. Providencia species, formerly known as *Proteus inconstans*, are gram-negative rods that fall into the general category of paracolon bacteria. *Providencia stuartii* has been identified with increasing frequency in the burn population, and in 1970 at the U.S. Army Institute of Surgical Research, it supplanted Pseudomonas as the predominant fatal blood stream pathogen.[57] Whereas staphylococcal septicemias were identified more frequently in 1970, only 37.2 per cent of patients affected died. The mortality with Providencia or pseudomonas bacteremia was 70 to 75 per cent.

During the 4-year period 1967–1970, there was a 700 per cent increase in the rate of recovery of Providencia from sputum cultures and a 61.8 per cent mortality rate in those patients with positive cultures.[57] Of particular concern was the observation that only 12 per cent of isolates were sensitive to antibiotics at the usual therapeutic blood levels achieved. An epidemic of totally antibiotic-resistant providencia has been reported by Zawacki.[314] Rather than invasive burn sepsis as such, much of the mortality seems to be associated with pulmonary complications.

Reports of viral burn sepsis have been frightening. One report of six cases of herpesvirus infection included two fatalities.[71] Also cytomegalic virus (CMV) has been reported in the burn patient with disseminated cytomegalic inclusion disease.[162]

Finally, not peculiar to burn wounds but common to all ischemic injuries with large masses of devitalized tissue, is clostridial infection.

Clostridium welchii and others of this group (*Cl. septique* and *Cl. novyi*) can manifest themselves in burn injury as either a crepitant cellulitis or a more lethal myositis. The cellulitis form spreads rapidly along fascial planes, does not involve muscle and is clinically manifest by a sudden increase in pain prior to appearance of swelling, erythema or crepitus. Slough of overlying skin may occur and is associated with variable systemic toxicity. Clostridial myositis is a more highly lethal infectious gangrene of the underlying muscle. It also tends to appear early (24 to 48 hours after injury) and is ushered in with sudden increase in pain, pallor, listlessness and, eventually, circulatory collapse. Crepitation may be a late finding. Overlying normal skin may develop a dusky appearance and, later, vesicles; drainage of the area is productive of a foul-smelling brown discharge.

Tetanus may occur from any wound, even if apparently insignificant. Proper tetanus prophylaxis is mandatory.

SYSTEMIC RESPONSE TO THERMAL INJURY

The function of all organ systems will eventually be altered due to the effects of a major burn. Some of the changes are in response to the stress of injury; some are related to burning itself; most, however, are due to the altered functional capacity of the skin. Although interrelated and interdependent, the systemic response is presented by organ systems and functions rather than in a chronological fashion.

Hemodynamics. Hemodynamic instability ("burn shock") was for centuries the major cause of death in burned patients. Buhl in 1855 noted that burn patients looked like those dying from cholera and reported their need for fluid. Yet as late as 1943, fully 50 to 75 per cent of burn deaths occurred in the first 48 hours from shock.[15] Blalock in 1930 observed that burn fluid was qualitatively similar to plasma and quantitatively sufficient to cause shock.[29]

Fully 60 per cent of the extracellular fluid volume may be lost in a major burn. Most of the loss occurs within the first 8 to 12 hours, but fluid loss continues for at least 48 hours after injury.[21] Patients may easily gain 10 per cent of their body weight during the course of replacement. This massive fluid loss is a combination of loss through the wound and a translocation into a "functional third space" that is lost to the circulating blood volume.

Added to this volume loss into the burn is an obligatory loss by respiration and urine, plus a suddenly increased evaporation from the burn surface. Loss of the stratum corneum increases the evaporative water loss 10 to 70 times over the loss from intact skin. Roe and Kinney have demonstrated that there may be a loss of 6 to 8 liters of fluid per day by evaporation alone.[250] Blood flow is further reduced by rising hematocrit, increased viscosity and sludging of cellular elements.

Compensation for these hemodynamic changes occurs at the expense of adequate perfusion. Hypovolemia results in splanchnic vasoconstriction, decreased renal, hepatic and intestinal perfusion, and subsequent compromised function of these organs.

Cardiac Function. Cardiac alterations originally thought to be in response to hemodynamic changes are now known to precede them. A precipitous drop in cardiac output occurs before any significant change in blood volume.[68] This may amount to as much as a 50 per cent decrease. This initial decrease suggests that there is a direct myocardial depressant factor active after thermal injury. As blood volume and plasma fall, the cardiac output decreases further and may reach a low of 20 per cent of normal.[190] Experimentally in lethal burns, the cardiac output continues to decrease until death occurs. However, in surviving animals the cardiac output returns toward normal — reaching preburn levels by 36 hours. Plasma volume, however, does not return as rapidly — again suggesting a direct myocardial effect. Evidence for this myocardial depressant factor has been accumulated from cross-perfusion studies between burned and unburned animals.

Pulmonary edema is difficult to produce in a patient with a normal heart. However, in the elderly or in a patient with previous cardiopulmonary embarrassment, fluid overload may become a problem. This becomes increasingly important because of the increase in pulmonary blood volume and pulmonary vascular resistance that has been demonstrated in the immediate postburn period.[50]

Renal Function. Renal function is altered in the burned patient as a direct effect of the stress of injury and secondarily as the result of the loss of extracellular fluid volume.

In response to the stress of trauma itself the posterior pituitary releases antidiuretic hormone (ADH) and maximum reabsorption of water occurs. So, too, aldosterone is released from the adrenal cortex and maximum sodium reabsorption results. In the untreated burn under the ADH-aldosterone influence, the kidney will excrete only an amount of urine necessary to handle the normal solute load, represented largely by urea. The result is oliguria (15 to 25 ml./hr.), increased urine concentration and decreased urine sodium concentration.[311]

Early destruction of red cells may present free hemoglobin in the urine. This situation may result in tubular necrosis only if accompanied by prolonged renal ischemia.

As volume loss is replaced in kind, renal blood flow is re-established. This results in an increased glomerular filtration rate and increased urine volume. Normally in this situation the urine volume reflects solute load and glomerular filtration rate, and changes are not the result of fluctuating ADH levels. The ADH response to stress will continue for variable periods of time,

and the high urine specific gravity continues. This cannot be lowered by hydration, and a large free-water load will cause water intoxication without changing the urine concentration. An osmotic diuretic such as mannitol will increase urine volume as a result of the increased solute load.

Renal function, therefore, is altered in the burn patient in a manner similar to that in any injured patient. Decreased renal function is almost inevitably a result of inadequate fluid and electrolyte replacement. Sodium and chloride are lost into the injured tissue in the same proportion as their plasma levels. As isotonic depletion results and, unless adversely influenced by treatment, alterations in serum concentration are not seen.

Respiratory Function. The response of the respiratory system to thermal injury may be violent and may of itself prove lethal. It is not, however, due to "burning." Moritz et al. demonstrated that application of a blow torch at 350°C through an endotracheal tube caused minimal injury beyond the carina.[199] The pulmonary tree is thus protected by the cooling produced by rapid vaporization. Only the inhalation of live steam results in true "burning" of the trachea or bronchi.

Edema of the epiglottis and larynx with burns of the face may endanger the upper airway. More commonly, particularly in burns sustained in close spaces, inhalation of products of incomplete combustion (including carbon monoxide, sulfides, acrolein, aldehydes, acid anhydrides, or even phosgenes) may lead to chemical pulmonary irritation, edema and pneumonitis. The pathological changes include congestion and edema of the respiratory tree, particularly small bronchi, with denudation of respiratory mucosa and obstruction from the denuded epithelial cells. Alveoli similarly may be filled with edema fluid and cellular debris. Scattered atelectasis and emphysema are early signs followed by evidence of bacterial invasion, septic microemboli and focal or diffuse bronchopneumonia.

Pulmonary function studies show that minute ventilation increases in the postburn period. This increase peaks at about 5 days and appears to be related to the size of the burn more than to any other measurable parameter. Oxygen consumption has shown a similar rise after thermal injury. Vital capacity may show a decrease up to 35 per cent of the predicted normal. Hypoxemia has been demonstrated in the initial period but usually returns to normal during the first week if severe inhalation injury has not accompanied the burn. The blood gas changes seen following the thermal injury are not dissimilar to those following other major nonthermal injury.[235] Most of these changes are due to impairment of diffusion and uneven distribution of alveolar gas and blood.[78] This may be due to the immediate increase in pulmonary extravascular water, which appears to be universal and not necessarily in association with toxic inhalation.[197]

Metabolic and Nutritional Response. The metabolic rate of a patient with a major burn is greatly accelerated. Oxygen consumption is increased and nitrogen losses are magnified. Urinary excretion of nitrogen (normally 10 to 15 gm. per day) may increase to 30 gm. per day in the first week post-injury. The water-holding lipid in skin is destroyed by the burn so that up to four times the normal amount of water vapor is transmitted by burned skin.[130] Since it requires 580 kcal. per liter to convert water to vapor, the loss of 5 liters per day would result in an expenditure of 2880 kcal. per day just for the increased evaporative loss.

The increased evaporative water loss (and accompanying heat loss) results in cooling of the body. This produces shivering and a further increase in the metabolic rate (30 to 300 per cent). Increasing the environmental temperature in which a burned patient is maintained has been shown to decrease his catabolism. The critical temperature appears to be about 34°C.[14] A decrease in urinary excretion of nitrogen has been found in burns of 10 to 50 per cent treated in environments of 32°C compared to those treated at 22°C.

Zawacki et al. have questioned the causal relationship between evaporative water loss and hypermetabolism.[315] They showed that reducing evaporation from the burned surface by application of an impermeable membrane did not reduce the metabolic rate. Recently, data have appeared showing a very close correlation between energy production during the hypermetabolic response and urinary catecholamine secretion.[309] The hypermetabolic response can be blocked by the administration of alpha- and beta-adrenergic blocking agents.

Nitrogen loss occurs into the burn wound itself in addition to the urinary losses. These losses are proportional to the size and depth of the burn and have been calculated by Nylen and Wallenius to reach levels of 2 to 3 gm. for each per cent body burn per day.[218] The amount of nitrogen per square meter that is necessary for equilibrium varies with the phase of wound recovery after burning.[281] Prolonged protein depletion is associated with lowered serum proteins, weight loss (up to a pound a day), decreased muscle tone, poor appetite, decreased pain threshold, depression, poor resistance to infection and possibly delayed wound healing.[31] Granulation tissue may enter a chronic phase in which the pink color is lost and it becomes pale, gray, fibrotic and accepts grafts poorly.

Protein anabolism and catabolism during the hypermetabolic period following extensive thermal trauma are regulated by both glucagon and insulin. Glucagon results in increased glucose production, decreased concentration of glucogenic amino acids and normal or slightly elevated levels of the branched chain amino acids. Insulin, conversely, inhibits gluconeogenesis and increases amino acid uptake by muscles. Glucagon: insulin ratios have been shown to be markedly decreased in patients with prolonged catabolism following thermal trauma.[58]

Profound intracellular cation alterations occur during hypermetabolic states such as occur after burning. Intracellular sodium concentration remains elevated for 30 to 40 days. This increase appears related to the patient's energy balance and will occur if the hypermetabolic burn patient has a daily intake of less than 1000 calories for more than 8 to 9 days.[58] However, with an intake of greater than 5000 kcal./day, the intracellular sodium concentration increase can be reversed within 72 hours.

Vitamin metabolism has been poorly studied. Vitamin C is obviously necessary for collagen formation and maintenance. Recently the role of vitamin A in collagen has been demonstrated.[77] B-complex vitamins are assumed to be necessary in normal doses. There is some evidence to suggest that alpha-tocopherol (vitamin E) may be useful in wound healing.[118]

Trace metals may become depleted in major burns. Zinc deficiency has been found to cause indolent-chronic wounds with minimal epithelialization and poor skin-graft acceptance.[154] Cohen has demonstrated decreased taste acuity with low zinc levels.[45] This contributes to further lack of appetite, thus deterring correction of the zinc deficiency by dietary means. These changes can be reversed with zinc administration.

Blood Elements. Progressive anemia occurs during the first week post-injury. Whereas previously this had been attributed to direct thermal damage to the erythrocyte itself and sequestration in the burn wound, newer findings suggest that an extrinsic mechanism produces the observed reduction in red cell survival.[24] Red blood cells from nonburned patients have decreased survival when injected into burned patients. Conversely, red cells from burned patients survive normally in nonburned patients. Sheldon has also demonstrated that the anemic hypoxia stimulus to erythropoietin production is removed in the burned patient because of increased production of 2,3-diphosphoglycerate by the erythrocytes.[267]

Platelet changes after thermal injury are biphasic. Immediately post-burn a thrombocytopenia exists.[119] This is accompanied by a decrease in fibrinogen levels and a brief episode of diffuse intravascular coagulation.[80] By 24 to 36 hours, the platelet count and fibrinogen levels rise and remain elevated for up to 3 weeks.

Liver Function. Liver function is measurably altered following thermal injury, but frank liver necrosis is unusual. Changes are probably due more to altered circulation and hypoxia in the early stages; later alterations may be the result of toxic waste products. Liver biopsies have shown early cloudy swelling and evidence of glycosis at 3 hours post-burn. Later changes may include some hepatocellular necrosis, vacuolization and fatty degeneration. After 4 weeks, reparative proliferation may still be present. Necropsy specimens show congestion, periportal necrosis or other changes indicating shock or sepsis.[25] Almost all liver function tests are abnormal at some time after a severe burn.[284]

Neuroendocrine Response. Epinephrine and norepinephrine release are increased greatly by all forms of trauma, including burns, as quantitatively reflected in urinary excretion. The amount of epinephrine excreted seems to parallel the size of the injury; norepinephrine responds out of proportion to other types of trauma, and levels may be seen comparable to those observed with pheochromocytomas.[105]

Although the resynthesis of both hormones is quite rapid, fatal burns may be accompanied by evidence of severe depletion. Such sympathetic depletion has been noted in up to 70 per cent of lethal burns. Although not the cause of death, this depletion may help to explain its mechanism.

Adrenal Cortical Response. Studies of the adrenal cortical response have revealed initially high and sustained levels of plasma 17-hydroxycorticosteroids, which return to normal with healing. Higher levels develop in patients with infected burns. Patients with burns of less than 40 per cent respond adequately and continuously to stress; it is doubtful that any burn ever becomes depleted of its adrenal steroids.[15]

The increased secretion of aldosterone seen in response to injury is principally due to the renin-angiotensin stimulus. However, its secretion is enhanced in situations that result in a falling serum sodium and rising potassium such as seen with burns. The effect of the aldosterone is to conserve the sodium as a compensatory mechanism for combating hypovolemia.[122]

Gastrointestinal Tract Function. The initial response to thermal trauma is similar to the response to any major trauma. As a result of severe splanchnic vasoconstriction, an early and sustained reflex ileus may occur. Acute gastric dilatation may occur early and be accompanied by abdominal distention, regurgitation and possible aspiration.

Although gastroduodenal mucosal ulceration is frequently seen following burns, it does not appear to be due to gastric hyperacidity. O'Neill has shown that Pavlov and Heidenhain pouches in dogs do not secrete increased levels of acid following burning.[220] When hyperacidity does occur, it appears to be related to hypercarbia and not to the thermal injury per se.[221] The amount of gastric mucus is decreased, and it may be this lack of protection to normal or even decreased amounts of acid that is responsible for mucosal ulceration. Although true gastric hyperacidity does not appear to be the cause of gastroduodenal mucosal ulceration in the burned patient, there does appear to be a correlation between the condition of the mucosa as observed by endoscopy and the basal acid output. Patients with acute gastroduodenal injury, present within 72 hours post-burn, tend to have higher basal acid outputs than do patients without gastrointestinal injury.[259] In these patients, gastrin levels were not increased and there was no correlation between serum gastrin levels and gastric acid secretion.[259]

Immune Response. The systemic immune response is altered by thermal injury. The presence or absence of a "burn toxin" has not been completely defined in humans. However, immunity relative to bacterial invasion has both theoretical and practical importance. Munster has documented that most mechanisms active in normal host defenses are affected in patients with severe burns.[209]

Thus burn patients appear more susceptible to infection than do unburned patients and experimental thermal injury increases susceptibility to bacterial infections in animals; these infections become refractory to treatment with antibiotics.[106] The role of the host's humoral and cellular immunological defense mechanisms has recently been appreciated.[8, 211]

Impaired cellular immunity in the burned patient is suggested by lymphocytopenia, delayed rejection of allografts, and anergy to delayed hypersensitivity antigens. Meakins et al. have related the incidence of septic complications and death to the response of five common antigens: mumps, PPD, candidin, trichophytin, and streptokinase-streptodornase.[180]

Humoral defects also have been demonstrated. Depression of the immunoglobulins, specifically IgG, has been shown post-burn and this did not appear to be entirely due to capillary permeability.[212] Complement titer decreases immediately after injury and may be due to protein leakage. However, its subsequent rise appears to be inversely correlated with burn severity, suggesting the presence of an inhibitor in the more severe burn.[64] An immunosuppressive peptide has been isolated from burn patients' serum that may explain some of the immunodepression seen with thermal trauma.[49] This may be responsible for the lymphocyte hypoactivity.

Other changes in host defense mechanisms, although not entirely immune in nature, affect the ability of the burned patient to withstand bacterial invasion.[254] Most important is the loss of integrity of defenses at the portal of entry because of the obvious mechanical injury to the skin. The inflammatory reaction is less than optimal because of venular stasis, microthrombosis and impaired margination of the leukocytes. Alexander has shown that neutrophil phagocytosis progresses normally but the intracellular killing is decreased.[4] He has related this to decreased levels of three hydrolases within the neutrophil (beta glucuronidase, lysozyme and acid phosphatase). For phagocytosis and intracellular killing to take place, leukocytes must be present at the necessary site and opsonins must be at the proper level to facilitate the phagocytosis. Fikrig et al. have demonstrated impaired chemotaxis secondary to a primary transient defect in polymorphonuclear leukocytes that might delay the neutrophil migration.[86] The presence of contamination in the burn injury can consume the opsonic proteins so as to lower their level below that necessary for optimal function.[6] Phagocytosis within the reticuloendothelial system is impaired. Together with the immunological deficiencies, these responses result in an overall deficit in host defense mechanisms.

How the evidence of a "burn toxin" fits into the specific immune defects noted is not understood. The relationship of this large molecular weight toxin to the smaller molecular weight inhibitor or supressor seen in serum is likewise not understood. Evidence appears to be overwhelming that defense mechanisms are less able to respond in the burned patient compared to the nonburned patient. The reason for this has yet to be explained. Recently, the role of malnutrition as an explanation for the immune defects has been raised.[312] If this is documented in humans, then the resistance of the burn patient might well be enhanced by total prevention of protein malnutrition.

Although survival chances after burning appear to be related to the area and depth of the body surface involved, the mortality is not a direct function of the per cent of body burn. Instead, a plot of mortality versus per cent of burn yields a sigmoid-shaped curve characteristic of a dose-mortality plot for a drug or toxic substance.[204]

Early reports on burn toxins, antitoxins, and convalescent burn sera have proved not to be due to any generalized toxic product but instead related to bacteria and their products. Sera and vaccines have been developed in several centers specifically to supplement the immune mechanisms against *Pseudomonas aeruginosa*. This is not to be construed as evidence for a generalized "burn toxin."

Isolation of a lipid-protein complex from thermally treated mouse skin fulfills criteria postulated for a true "burn toxin."[9] This substance is lethal when injected into recipient mice. The same physicochemical and biological activity was obtained for this complex when germ-free donor and recipient animals were used, thus eliminating the bacterial role previously confusing the issue. Also the toxic effect was demonstrated in genetically identical animals, proving that immunological incompatibility was not responsible for the toxicity. Preliminary animal data show that antitoxic serum can be produced to this substance that markedly increases survival.

Skeletal Changes. Localized as well as generalized skeletal abnormalities accompany burns and are not usually reflected in altered urine or blood biochemical changes.

Bone may be involved directly in deep thermal injury causing necrosis of periosteum and outer cortex.[17] Also it may be involved with either local or generalized osteoporosis related to local disease or immobilization. Periosteal new bone growth is not uncommon in children, particularly near areas of open granulation tissue. Recent reports of heterotopic calcification around joints following burns have appeared.[210] Articular destruction with fibrosis and even bony ankylosis can appear in children. These changes do not necessarily occur near areas involved in the burn wound; other changes are more directly related to exposure from burning or to sepsis.[81]

PSYCHIATRIC IMPLICATIONS

Patients adjust to the burn situation in a manner reflecting their total personality adjustment prior to injury.[161] Pain, helplessness, change in appearance and potential deformity all tend to bring about a situational depression aggravated by some very real financial and social adjustments. Sleeplessness, restlessness, loss of libido, or a sensation of being "closed in," and increasing acuity to lesser degrees of discomfort are normal in the burned patient. It is tempting to attribute all such personal changes to "psychological factors"; however, psychoses are rare unless the patient was previously psychotic. Such manifestations are more often toxic in origin.

Evidence of delirium should be a danger signal. Alterations in perception are manifest as hallucinations; disturbed interpretation results in illusions and delusions. There may be altered activity patterns with overtalkativeness, tremors, restlessness, laughing and crying. Moods may suddenly swing from euphoria to fear and temper tantrums. More progressive disturbances occur in the form of disorientation, diminished sensibility and coma.

The most common causes of these toxic psychotic symptoms in the burned patient are shock, hypoxia, altered water load (water excess and hypotonicity), electrolyte disturbances and sepsis. Later in the burn course there may occur vitamin deficiencies and protein and glucose intoxication from forced feedings. Excessive alcohol intake, epilepsy and drug addiction may all have preceded the burning and may result in withdrawal symptoms.

Drugs must be prescribed cautiously; narcotics and barbiturates may easily become necessary to the patient. Many of the phenothiazine tranquilizers will cause toxic symptoms, including twitching, nystagmus and other extrapyramidal signs.

The presence of wound sepsis and fever results in a wide variety of toxic manifestations including restlessness, decreased emotional control, inability to concentrate and vivid dreams. These may precede, accompany or follow an acute febrile episode and, in children, may be accompanied by convulsions and postictal depression.

Toxic psychotic disturbance in burns is rare after the first week except with sepsis. Multiple dressing changes and persistent, chronic pain tend to produce a very real situation disturbance characterized by detachment despondency, crying and lack of patient cooperation.

CLINICAL AND THERAPEUTIC IMPLICATIONS

Etiology and Incidence

Each year between 2,000,000 and 3,000,000 people in the United States are burned seriously enough to require medical attention. The 12,000 deaths per year reflect the tragic mortality. The 120,000 hospitalized patients with total or partial disability and problems in rehabilitation reflect the tremendous cost in time, money and suffering. Almost 50 per cent of major burns occur during growing and formative years (under age 20) and 30 per cent occur in children under 10 years of age.[30] People over the age of 65 years (9 per cent of the population) experience 28 per cent of the deaths from fire and explosion.[16]

In general, for children up to the age of 3 years, scalds are the most common form of burns. From 3 to 15 years, flame burns from ignition of clothing are most common. For those over the age of 60 years, smoking in bed and house fires predominate. Hot bath water (above 115° F.) is a serious cause of burns in young children, the disabled and the aged. Fully 80 per cent of burn accidents occur within the home.

Mortality

Meaningful data are extremely difficult to acquire. A great many burned patients die before reaching a hospital. Many patients with minor burns never seek professional care. Inclusion of either group would obviously influence the statistics. Thorough probit analyses of burn mortality are available and demonstrate that the most important criteria influencing survival are the size of the burn and the age of the patients (Fig. 23–4A).[39, 171, 241]

There have been two distinct trends in the last 30 years. The incidence of death in the early period from shock has almost disappeared. This has been reflected more in prolonged rather than increased survival. Secondly, with prolonged survival, sepsis has become a major cause of death, particularly burn-wound sepsis.[298] In recent years, however, respiratory complications have caused more deaths than burn-wound sepsis.[276]

In the first 24 hours following burn injury, the major causes of death are incineration and respiratory failure. From 2 to 21 days post-burn, infection is the major cause of death. Included with infection beyond 3 weeks are stress ulcers and from 10 to 12 weeks, hepatitis.[303] Except in hospitals particularly interested in burn care, autopsies tend to be cursory, and unless there is some striking finding such as a perforated ulcer, the death is attributed solely to "burns."

EVALUATION OF THE BURNED PATIENT

History. A careful history is as important in caring for the burned patient as in any other patient. Often done hurriedly, it should nevertheless be thorough and include the circumstances of the injury.

Pre-existing cardiovascular, renal, respiratory or metabolic diseases will complicate care and increase mortality. Epilepsy and alcohol or drug intoxication tend to predispose patients to burns, and the subsequent withdrawal symptoms or convulsions complicate treatment. Specific inquiries regarding previous tetanus immunization and drug allergies should be made.

Careful questioning of the patient as well as the firemen, police or ambulance emergency medical technicians who bring the patient to the hospital must ascertain the circumstances of the burning. A history of the burns being sustained in confined areas, accompanied by considerable smoke inhalation, will alert the physician to possible respiratory damage better than x-ray or physical findings. Evidence of suicide attempt and, in children, the battered child syndrome will indicate problems in later social adjustment.

Extent of Injury. The ultimate determinant in burn injury is the volume of tissue destroyed. Although it is difficult to determine depth, the extent of the burn can be assessed by careful observation and is important from a therapeutic, statistical and prognostic point of view. It is customary to record burns in terms of per cent of body surface area. Original estimates of surface area by location were introduced by Berkow[26] and have since been modified by Lund and Browder to make them applic-

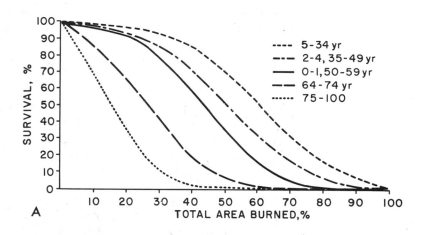

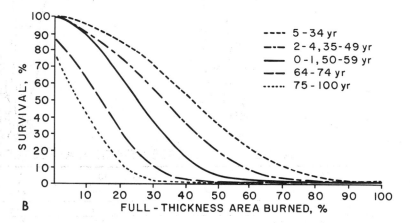

Figure 23–4. A, *Probit survival curves as a function of total percentage of body surface burned and age. (Modified from Feller et al.[84]). B, Probit survival curves as a function of percentage of full-thickness burn and age. (Modified from Feller et al.[84]) C, Probit survival curves showing tolerance to burns for males and females. (Modified from Feller et al.[84])*

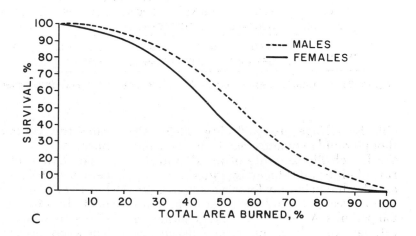

BURN SHEET

NAME _____ AGE_____ NUMBER_____

BURN RECORD.   AGES 7 TO ADULT.   DATE OF OBSERVATION _____

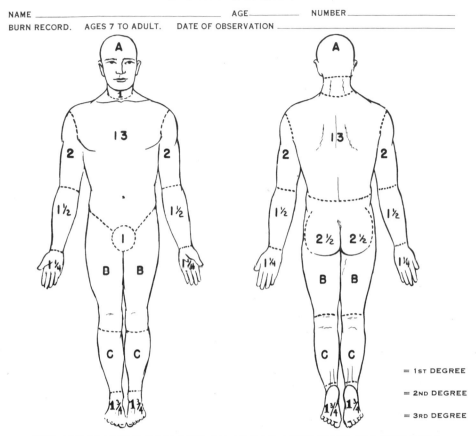

	= 1ST DEGREE
	= 2ND DEGREE
	= 3RD DEGREE

RELATIVE PERCENTAGES OF AREAS AFFECTED BY GROWTH

AREA	AGE 10	15	ADULT
A $^1/_2$ OF HEAD	$5^1/_2$	$4^1/_2$	$3^1/_2$
B $^1/_2$ OF ONE THIGH	$4^1/_4$	$4^1/_2$	$4^3/_4$
C $^1/_2$ OF ONE LEG	3	$3^1/_4$	$3^1/_2$

% BURN BY AREAS

PROBABLE { HEAD_____ NECK_____ BODY_____ UP. ARM_____ FOREARM_____ HANDS _____

3RD° BURN { GENITALS_____ BUTTOCKS_____ THIGHS_____ LEGS_____ FEET _____

TOTAL BURN { HEAD_____ NECK_____ BODY_____ UP. ARM_____ FOREARM_____ HANDS _____

{ GENITALS_____ BUTTOCKS_____ THIGHS_____ LEGS_____ FEET _____

Figure 23–5. *Chart for estimating body surface area in burned adults based on Lund-Browder figures.*[125]

able for all age groups[170] (Fig. 23–5). Although rapid estimates may be made using the Lynch-Blocker rule of fives[30] and the rule of nines introduced by Pulaski,[242] they are of value primarily for triage; more accurate assessment should be made on individual patients. A more direct and quantitative estimate of volume of burned tissue has been introduced by Klein et al.[136] Hydroxyproline, a degradation product of collagen, is serially measured in urine; the level indi-

cates the volume of tissue destroyed by burn.

The extent of the burns in terms of per cent of surface is meaningless in discussing burns of special areas including the face, neck, hands, feet and genitalia as it is in burns in young children and the elderly. These are all serious burns.

Burn injuries can be divided into categories. A major burn is considered to be partial-thickness burns of greater than 25 per cent body surface area (20 per cent in children); all full-thickness burns 10 per cent body surface area or greater; all burns involving hands, face, eyes, ears, feet and perineum; all burns with concomitant inhalation injury; electrical injuries; those associated with fractures or other major trauma and those in all poor-risk patients. Moderate burn injuries include partial-thickness burns of 15–25 per cent body surface area (10–20 per cent in children) with less than 10 per cent full-thickness burns that do not include the special areas and exclude electrical injury, inhalation injury, other trauma and poor-risk patients. Patients in both these categories probably require care in the hospital setting. The remaining burn injuries are categorized as minor and the patients can often be treated on an outpatient basis. An intelligent and dependable patient or family is a prerequisite for successful outpatient care.

Depth of Injury. As emphasized before, the biological response to thermal injury is exceedingly variable within even a limited area. Superficial burns can be ascertained from the history and the appearance of erythema without blistering, and the patient can be dismissed from the office or emergency department with topical analgesics and the reassurance that healing will occur inevitably and without noticeable sequelae.

A careful history will also prove valuable in assessing deeper burns. Flash and flame burns are all at least partial-thickness and often full-thickness injuries. Scald burns in adults tend to be superficial partial thickness but they may well be full thickness in children and in the elderly.

Attempts at differentiation on clinical grounds are also misleading. Sensation is deceptive since even full-thickness burns have pressure sensation. Pinprick is more accurate, but even here partial-thickness burns may be anesthetized by loss of naked nerve fibers in the basal layer.

Blistering is characteristic of superficial burns but may also occur with very deep burns from steam accumulation in the epidermis or, later, from infection. The appearance of a tough, leathery, anesthetic eschar is seen in full-thickness injury but also is seen frequently in deep partial-thickness injury as well.

Although many elaborate tests have been proposed for differentiating depth of burn, none has been reliable. All studies assume that (a) the injury is uniform, at least within a given area, (b) that the depth of the injury remains the same and (c) that if we knew the depth exactly, we would somehow change our treatment. However, the injury is not uniform, nor is it static. Infection or further trauma may well convert superficial injury to full-thickness loss. So, too, deep burns thought to be full-thickness injury may later re-epithelialize from viable epidermal islands if infection is prevented. The important triage concept is to differentiate the patients with deep burns from those with superficial burns who may be treated as outpatients. Further classification into numerical "degrees" is difficult, often incorrect, and does not materially affect the course of treatment.

Hemodynamic Evaluation. The hemodynamic response is a direct systemic manifestation of the type of injury and magnitude of tissue destruction in the local burn wound. Attention to the burn wound should not take precedence over the life-saving hemodynamic support of the burned patient any more than this phase of treatment should assume exclusive importance in burn care. The various new topical agents introduced in burn therapy result in profound fluid and electrolyte alterations in addition to changes imposed by the wound itself. Proper patient care demands that the burn wound, the accompanying systemic changes and the alterations produced by treatment be conceptually viewed as a dynamic interrelated process, not as isolated phenomena.

TREATMENT

Immediate Care. The burned patient demands the same thorough attention to cardiorespiratory function, hemorrhage and associated injuries as any other emergency trauma victim. Immediate treatment of his impending shock is begun by introducing a large-bore needle or catheter into the central venous system, preferably through unburned skin. Antibiotic ointment and a sterile dressing should be placed around the site of catheter entry. If an intraluminal catheter is used, suppurative thrombophlebitis must be watched for throughout the treatment period.[240] Blood is drawn for typing, complete blood count, serum electrolytes, glucose and urea nitrogen. Arterial blood gases are obtained if there is any evidence of smoke inhalation or pulmonary dysfunction. An infusion of buffered electrolyte solution is begun at a brisk rate. A urinary catheter is inserted, attached to a closed drainage system. Tetanus immunization should be provided as recommended by the American College of Surgeons Committee on Trauma.

Respiratory distress must be evaluated early. If present when the patient is first seen, it is more likely to be due to an unyielding eschar about the thorax than to inhalation injury. This causes restriction of rib motion and thoracic excursion with resultant impaired ventilatory function and CO_2 accumulation. Early and adequate chest escharotomy is indicated as an emergency procedure. An encircling eschar may cause vascular embarrassment to the extremities. This must be relieved either by a surgical escharotomy or by enzymatic decompression.[145]

Initial Volume Replacement. The weight of the patient, the type of burn wound (scald versus flame) and the extent of the initial injury in per cent of body area provide the initial guide to thinking. Rigid applications of formulas ignore the variability of patients. The greatest loss of plasma and fluid occurs during the first 12 hours after burning and then continues much more slowly for another 12 hours. Replacement therefore must be most rapid immediately and then can be slowed to correspond with the rate of loss.

Formulas have been advanced to predict the amount and type of fluid correction needed. Originally replacing suspected plasma loss with plasma to maintain a normal hematocrit, they have evolved into a volume/weight scale in relation to the percentage of body surface burn. A realization of the need for crystalloid replacement as well as plasma has resulted in the change in proportion and type of fluid used in resuscitation. Critical analysis of the various popular formulas reveals that the total volume replacement recommended varies only 2 per cent over 48 hours and the total milliequivalents of sodium vary only 6 per cent during the same period.[188]

The problem with formulas, besides their inherent rigidity, is that their adequacy of fluid replacement has been measured by survival alone. This has led to erroneous conclusions since it can be demonstrated that survival is compatible with a cardiac output as low as 25 per cent of normal and a plasma or blood volume deficit of 30 to 50 per cent.[190]

Simultaneous measurements of cardiac output, plasma volume and extracellular fluid have shown that plasma volume replacement during the first 24 hours postburn is dependent only upon the rate of fluid replacement.[238] The type of fluid, whether colloid or crystalloid electrolyte solution, does not matter. Sodium ion seems to be most important in the replacement. Therefore, a sodium-containing electrolyte solution is now recommended as the sole replacement for the first 24 hours. The obligatory loss of fluid from the vascular compartment has been shown to remain uncompensated until the replacement rate of administration exceeds 4.4 milliliters per kilogram of body weight per hour.[190] Above this rate plasma volume is not only maintained but actually expanded. Extracellular fluid volume replacement requires 3 to 4 ml. per kg. per cent body burn. Therefore, it can be predicted that this volume of fluid will be required and the rate of administration will have to exceed 4.4 ml./kg./hr. The rate will have to be greatest during the first few hours after injury.

Because of the capillary permeability occurring after thermal injury, colloid administration is of no benefit in the immediate post-burn period. Osmotic pressure cannot be built up over a freely permeable membrane; Starling's law is negated. Edema fluid will not be pulled back into the vascular compartment; rather, the colloid will leak into the extravascular spaces.

Some proponents of electrolyte-containing fluids only for resuscitation have suggested the use of hypertonic sodium-containing fluids to decrease the amount of fluid given. It is known that 0.52 mEq. of sodium/kg./per cent body burn is required for adequate resuscitation. A mixture containing 300 mEq. sodium, 200 mEq. lactate and 100 mEq. chloride per liter has been recommended as an alternative to more isotonic solutions.[184] The advantages of a hypertonic sodium-containing fluid are that cumulative sodium loads equal hypotonic resuscitation solutions but that total infusion volume is only one half to two thirds that required when using hypotonic solutions.[268] The decreased fluid volume results in decreased edema. Since edema significantly reduces dermal perfusion by the microcirculation and wound oxygen tension, a decrease in edema should ultimately benefit the burn wound. However, measurements of cardiac output during resuscitation with hypertonic solution reveal that it remains up to 40 per cent less than cardiac output seen with isotonic replacement. Extracellular fluid volume replacement occurs at the expense of intracellular volume loss. Even so, a persistent deficit in extracellular fluid volume has been documented.

Just as it has been demonstrated that a sodium-containing electrolyte solution alone should be given during the first 24 hours and that colloid is of no demonstrable benefit, the reverse is true during the next 24 hours.[190] Capillary integrity returns and Starling's law appears to be restored. Colloid is now effective in maintaining plasma volume, and further administration of sodium tends to aggravate the edema. Therefore, the only non-colloid required during this period is that to cover insensible obligatory losses.

MONITORING REPLACEMENT. In monitoring the adequacy of fluid and electrolyte replacement, one must assess the patient carefully by clinical observation, vital signs, hematocrit, serum electrolytes and urine output. The adequacy of fluid and electrolyte replacement is determined neither by ability to fulfill a previously outlined formula nor by any single clinical or laboratory finding. However, a urine output of 30 to 50 ml./hr. in the adult or 1.2 ml./kg./hr. in the child is the best single guide to adequacy of fluid replacement. If the urine output decreases, the rate of intravenous fluid administration must be increased.

The patient should remain alert; evidence of confusion may suggest hypoxia, fluid deficit or improper drug administration. Blood pressure and pulse rate are of value, but insufficient alone; arterial pressure remains compensated until late in shock and a tachycardia of 100 to 120 per minute may be quite compatible with adequate replacement.

The hematocrit will gradually rise in the first 24 hours to levels of 55 to 60 per cent,

even in the presence of adequate fluid replacement and excellent clinical response. Attempts to lower it may lead to dangerous over-replacement of fluid. Moreover, there is no information to suggest that the implied dangers of a high hematocrit have any correlation in fact.

Central venous pressure has been of debatable use in burns. Reports of its lack of value in the acute stage suggest that reliance on CVP readings may be dangerous.[261] If urine output is maintained, there is far greater tendency to give too much rather than too little fluid. The central venous pressure frequently does not reflect this overload. As shown by Achauer et al., with a falling cardiac output, the left ventricle can become transiently overloaded and go in and out of failure for brief periods.[2] This results in a left atrial pressure exceeding 25 mm. Hg, thus causing pulmonary transudation. This increase in interstitial water in the lung can occur without causing gross change in the right atrial pressure that would be reflected in CVP readings. A more reliable guide in the acute post-burn period would be pulmonary artery pressure. However, even measurements with a Swan-Ganz catheter have shown the pressure to remain low during early resuscitation; attempts to raise pulmonary capillary wedge pressure to "normal" are fraught with danger.[116]

After stabilization of the capillary membrane and the return to normal of cardiac output, central venous pressure monitoring may be indicated in patients with inhalation injury and in children or elderly patients with pre-existent cardiopulmonary disease.

Treatment of an isotonic fluid loss with balanced electrolyte solution should maintain normal serum electrolyte values. Hypernatremia and hyperchloremia may result from either administration of excess saline or lack of water; hyponatremia and hypochloremia can occur only with the administration of excess water relative to electrolytes. Treatment of hyponatremia with hypertonic saline solution will expand the entire extracellular fluid to isotonicity but may overload the patient. Such a situation is best treated by restriction of water or by administration of a solute diuretic (mannitol 50 gm. as a 10 per cent solution in saline infused over a few hours). All fluid replacement in the early burn stage is administered intravenously. Attempts at oral replacement in other than the most minor burns are discouraged by evidence of gastric dilatation and ileus.

Renal Failure. In the burn patient acute renal failure can occur only after prolonged and profound shock from unrecognized or untreated hypovolemia. The patient seen for the first time a few hours after burning who has oliguria and perhaps hemoglobinuria should not be assumed to have renal failure. To assume this diagnosis and to delay needed volume replacement will only insure the accuracy of the diagnosis. Acute renal failure is properly diagnosed by exclusion and with great reluctance.

In the initial evaluation it should be assumed that oliguria reflects the presence of hypovolemia. Ten to 15 gm. of mannitol should be infused rapidly in order to provide an osmotic load that will insure urine output if the mannitol can be filtered and the tubules are intact. However, osmotic diuresis will result in obligatory increase in urine volume even at the expense of dehydrating a hypovolemic patient, so volume replacement must begin rapidly. After an initial load of balanced salt solution (4.4 ml./kg./hr.) in an hour, plasma may have some particular value. By virtue of the large molecular protein components, it remains in the vascular compartment for slightly longer periods than do crystalloids. The adequacy of volume replacement is assessed only on the basis of therapeutic results, namely, the appearance of adequate urine output. There is little guide to overload during this test. Central venous pressure may reflect only the rapidity of the fluid administration if elevated and not the increased interstitial lung water if normal or depressed.[2] Pulmonary artery pressure monitoring may be useful in this situation. Only the absence of urine output and an elevated pulmonary pressure suggest acute renal failure.

Later Fluid Changes. Major loss after the initial sequestration (48 hours postburn) is from evaporative water loss from the wounds. These losses are not entirely free of electrolytes, and the administration of large amounts of free water may induce hyponatremia. Measurement of the serum sodium should guide therapy. Urine output is not an accurate guide to the patient's

state of hydration after the initial 48- to 72-hour post-burn period.

Use of Blood and Blood Products. BLOOD. The initial hematocrit readings deceptively understate the amount of red cell loss that occurs, both at the time of injury and with delayed hemolysis (up to 40 per cent of the total red cell mass).[208] As the hematocrit falls, the need for blood transfusion becomes obvious (fourth to seventh day). Multiple transfusions to maintain a hematocrit between 35 and 40 per cent are indicated. Approximately 1 ml. of blood for each per cent of body area burned is needed daily. The advisability of blood administration in the first 48 hours is open to considerable doubt; however, the maintenance of a hematocrit near normal in the later stages is accepted as beneficial.

PLASMA. The use of plasma or other colloids was discussed under initial volume replacement. Its use should be in the form of stored plasma, Plasmanate, or albumin to reduce the dangers of serum hepatitis. Plasma has been documented to have value in children, but perhaps on an immunological rather than a hemodynamic basis.[176, 177]

GAMMA GLOBULIN. Gamma globulin has been suggested in children in a dose of 1 ml. per kg. of body weight on the first, third and fifth post-burn days.[52, 133] Its value has not been totally documented.

HYPERIMMUNE AND CONVALESCENT SERUM. Definite benefit from hyperimmune and convalescent serum has not been adequately demonstrated in humans. Passive immunization has been shown by Jones in animals.[131] However, he warns that immunization by antiserum causes risk of allergic reactions and occasionally anaphylactic shock. The benefits of any antibacterial resistance may be overshadowed by these hazards.

VACCINES. Vaccination against *Pseudomonas aeruginosa* has been used to decrease the incidence of pseudomonas sepsis.[5, 228] When used, it must be a polyvalent variety made from numerous strains of Pseudomonas. Regardless of the number of strains used to develop the vaccine, new strains of *Pseudomonas aeruginosa* continue to emerge, limiting its usefulness.

Zellner and Metzger recently reported on a test group of 239 patients.[316] Using active immunization with a polyvalent vaccine, they made the following observations:

1. No relationship existed between the onset of infection and active immunization.
2. No relationship existed between the extent of the burn and the increase of the agglutination titer.
3. There was no relationship between the age of the patient and the increase in antibody titer.
4. No connection between positive blood cultures in vaccinated and nonvaccinated patients was observed.
5. No connection was seen between the antibody titer and the presence of a positive blood culture.
6. Even nonvaccinated patients showed an antibody reaction of sufficient strength to combat infection.

They concluded that active immunization is not a very effective means of combating septicemia. This may be due to the fact that a toxin exists that leads to immunosuppression and a definite reduction in antibody production in the patient. Therefore, vaccination still is not used in most burn centers. However, the further development of immunotherapy may be the most important means to decrease mortality from burns.

Respiratory System. Pulmonary dysfunction after burns may be divided into four general categories: that caused by restrictive unyielding eschar; that due to inhalation of smoke; those complications secondary to burn injury such as pneumonitis, pulmonary edema and thromboembolism; and multiple physiological alterations best classified as progressive pulmonary insufficiency. Patients with a history of flash burns or being burned indoors and having burns of the face (especially if deep) have a much increased incidence of pulmonary dysfunction. A combination of these factors resulted in 88 per cent chance of respiratory problems. Respiratory problems have been reported to eventually occur in 67 per cent of all patients with greater than 40 per cent burns.[225, 226, 227]

Both the patient's history and physical examination are helpful in raising the suspicion of significant smoke inhalation. While obtaining a history, it is important to note if the burn occurred in closed quarters and if so what materials were burning and how long the patient was exposed to the noxious fumes. It is also important to determine any first aid treatment the patient received prior to arrival, such as use of an oxygen mask. Physical findings that should raise one's index of suspicion are conjunctivitis, burned nasal vibrissae, carbon deposits in the oral cavity and carbonaceous sputum.

However, the most sensitive indicator is blood gas determinations with carboxyhemoglobin measurement. Although carbon monoxide per se is not detrimental, its presence suggests that other more noxic gases have also been inhaled. [133]Xenon lung scans permit the early diagnosis of inhalation injury by identifying impaired ventilatory removal of radioactive gas.[207]

The initial treatment for smoke inhalation is humidification of inspired air with a high oxygen content and careful tracheobronchial toilet.

The treatment is directed to improve the alveolar ventilation and increase the alveolar oxygen tension so that by mass action the oxygen will displace the carbon monoxide on the hemoglobin molecule.[317] For patients with moderately severe inhalation demonstrated by bronchospasm and wheezing, bronchodilators and mucolytic agents are helpful. Diagnostic bronchoscopy to assess the degree of damage and remove carbonaceous sputum plugs is of documented value. However, routine repeated bronchoscopy has not been shown to be significantly useful.

If hypoxemia with a decrease in arterial oxygen tension below 60 mm. Hg develops or an increase of carbon dioxide tension above 55 mm. Hg despite the use of an oxygen mask, intubation and respirator support are indicated. If a concentration of oxygen in the inspired air of greater than 50 per cent is required to keep the arterial oxygen tension above 75 mm. Hg, positive end-expiratory pressure (PEEP) of up to 15 cm. of water may be useful. Tracheostomy should be avoided unless absolutely necessary. Antibiotic coverage is no substitute for good technique, and antibiotics should only be employed in response to specific cultured bacteria. Steroids appear to have no beneficial effect upon acute pulmonary dysfunction due to inhalation and may actually be detrimental.[206, 307]

Bronchopneumonia and pulmonary edema tend to occur later in the burn course. Often this is in the perioperative period. Fluid replacement must be meticulously monitored intraoperatively and careful tracheopulmonary toilet is essential in the postoperative period. Unexpected pulmonary edema of pneumonia may be a manifestation of systemic extension of burn wound sepsis. Pulmonary embolism is rare in the uncomplicated burn course. When it occurs, it is usually associated with cannula-induced thrombophlebitis of large veins.

Pruitt has described the syndrome of progressive pulmonary insufficiency in patients with thermal injury.[236] This complex includes pulmonary capillary permeability resulting in interstitial and alveolar accumulation of fluid, protein, fibrin and cellular elements of the blood. This in turn may alter pulmonary vascular flow, ventilation dynamics and diffusion characteristics. Many insults to the lung may lead to this syndrome in the burn patient, including prolonged hypotension; fluid overload; myocardial infarction; bacterial, viral or fungal sepsis; smoke inhalation; fat embolism; aspiration; or disseminated intravascular coagulopathy. If the process worsens, increased airway resistance develops, with a decreased lung compliance and increased right-to-left shunting of blood in the lungs. Treatment is based on improving ventilation and correcting the underlying triggering disease mechanism. Intubation, respiratory support with PEEP, and consideration of myocardial support are helpful in limiting the progressive pulmonary insufficiency.

Metabolic and Nutritional Needs. Negative nitrogen balance and increased metabolic needs begin abruptly and continue progressively until the wound is closed. Protein loss into the wound, loss of muscle from disuse and increased metabolic rate from evaporative water loss are all aggravated by poor oral intake. In addition, alterations in hormonal relationships occur with increased secretion of catabolic hormones such as glucocorticoids, catecholamines and glucagon and impaired secretion of the anabolic hormone insulin.[270] Soroff and his associates have calculated the nitrogen requirements necessary to overcome this negative nitrogen balance to be at least 20 gm. nitrogen/m² body surface/day during the first month post-burn, and 13 to 16 gm. nitrogen/m²/day during the second post-

burn month. Not until wound closure has been achieved does the requirement fall to the normal 3 to 4 gm. nitrogen/m²/day.[210]

Arguments are occasionally raised that malnutrition does not reduce the rate of wound healing or increase the incidence of infection. Vast clinical experience, however, has demonstrated the increased morbidity in the nutritionally depleted burn patient. Recovery of intestinal motility allows oral intake usually by the fifth post-burn day. As lack of appetite is typical in the post-burn patient, attention should be directed toward attractively presented and tastefully prepared foods. Total caloric needs are about 60 cal./kg. per day in the average adult.[203]

Vitamin needs are not defined but a regimen probably should include 1 gm. of ascorbic acid, 50 mg. of thiamine, 50 mg. of riboflavin and 500 mg. of nicotinamide as well as twice the usual amounts of vitamins A and D daily.

Tube feedings may occasionally be required. Diarrhea may develop during tube feedings and is usually due to inadequate water intake. This can be controlled with bulk laxatives such as Metamucil in the dosage of 7 gm. per liter of liquid formula.[96] Solutions containing up to 1.5 cal./ml. with an osmolar concentration of not more than 600 appear to be well tolerated. If oral or tube feedings are not tolerated, intravenous hyperalimentation can be used. Up to 5000 calories per day can be provided by vein with resultant positive nitrogen balance, weight gain and even normal growth in children.[310]

Pseudodiabetes. Total parenteral nutrition can be associated with significant and life-threatening complications. Sepsis (especially due to candida), hyperglycemia, hyperosmolar coma and central vein thrombosis have all been related to hypertonic dextrose infusions. The recent introduction of a soybean oil emulsion (Intralipid) that is isotonic yet contains 1.1 kcal./ml. allows infusions through peripheral veins.[224] This appears to be much safer in the burned patient. A syndrome of hyperglycemia, glycosuria without acetonuria, acute dehydration, shock, coma and renal failure was described originally by Evans and Butterfield and has been called burn-stress pseudodiabetes.[82] Hyperglycemia resulting from the stress of trauma is well known and includes a diabetic-type glucose tolerance curve and decreased sensitivity to insulin. Arney et al. studied two cases carefully and noted that hyperglycemia followed high carbohydrate, high caloric forced feedings.[11] They also noted a high urine specific gravity and intense solute diuresis with subsequent dehydration and a rising BUN, hematocrit, serum sodium and serum chloride accompanied by a brisk urine flow. The severe hyperglycemia probably reflects an inability to utilize large amounts of glucose.[258] These patients had intakes of four to five times normal amounts of glucose. Experience with intravenous hyperalimentation suggests that a tolerance to these extreme solute loads can be developed and that insulin needs will be decreased.

Gastrointestinal System. Due to loss of peristalsis, initial therapy of most major burns should include nasogastric intubation for 24 to 48 hours. No oral feeding should be given until evidence of active peristalsis is present.

CURLING'S ULCERS. Curling's ulcers develop clinical significance in 12 to 25 per cent of patients with major burns.[111, 195] However, if superficial mucosal ulcerations are routinely looked for via endoscopy, 86 per cent of patients with large burns will develop gastric ulcerations.[60] In the study of Czaja et al.,[60] 74 per cent of these had ulcerations within 72 hours postburn. The exact mechanism is unknown, but the ulcers are not accompanied by hyperacidity. The incidence of ulcers increases with increasing burn size and are more common in patients who develop sepsis. The ulcers may be gastric or duodenal, and 15 per cent of the patients will have both gastric and duodenal ulcers. Duodenal ulcers are twice as frequent in children as in adults.[266] Bleeding is the usual manifestation and may be very brisk. Perforation occasionally occurs and is an indication for surgery. In a controlled study, neutralization of gastric acid and maintenance of the gastric pH above 7.0 has been shown to protect against these clinically significant complications.[179] Indications for surgery in a patient with bleeding are shock unresponsive to blood replacement and loss of 2500 ml. of blood over a 12-hour period in an adult (or a proportional amount in a child). Patients surviving such a major bleeding episode and not operated upon have a 30 per cent

chance of having a subsequent hemorrhage.[237] The incision may on occasion necessarily be made directly through eschar. Most authors feel that the ulcer-bearing portion of the gastrointestinal tract should be removed; subtotal gastrectomy alone or combined with a vagectomy, are equally successful. In children under age 15, vagectomy, over-sewing of the ulcer and an adequate drainage procedure have resulted in increased survival.[71] The incision should undergo delayed closure.

SUPERIOR MESENTERIC ARTERY SYNDROME. Compression of the distal duodenum at the level of the superior mesenteric artery may result in partial or complete duodenal obstruction. Reckler et al. have reported 19 cases of such obstruction.[247] This obstruction causes problems in the burned patient both because of the intestinal obstruction complications and the interference with alimentation at the time of increased metabolic needs. Post-feeding fullness, bile-stained vomitus or excessive nasogastric drainage suggests the need for barium studies. The diagnosis can best be made by cinefluorography. The syndrome may require operative intervention by means of a duodenojejunostomy but conservative means should be tried. These include feeding in the prone or the lateral decubitus position, attempting to pass a long intestinal tube beyond the obstruction for feeding and/or intravenous hyperalimentation. In a recent series of 37 patients with this syndrome, conservative measures were successful in 24.

COLONIC ULCERATIONS. Lower gastrointestinal bleeding can also occur in the patient with a major burn. This is usually due to ulcerations of the mucosa and muscularis mucosa. Colonoscopy has proved an aid in identifying the source of bleeding. Authors reporting one series have raised the possibility that these ulcers are secondary to yeast or sepsis.[243]

ACALCULOUS CHOLECYSTITIS. Biliary stasis leading to cholecystitis must be considered in the patient with right upper quadrant pain, unexplained vomiting or fever of unknown origin. The diseased gallbladder can perforate with very few symptoms if systemic sepsis occurs in a patient with undiagnosed acalculous cholecystitis. The treatment for this complication is cholecystectomy when feasible or temporary cholecystotomy if necessary. Kirksey et al.

reported nine patients with this complication while reviewing 1291 burn patients.[135]

Fever. Because of the inability of the burned patient to regulate temperature in the area of his burn, small environmental changes in the wound may be reflected in markedly fluctuating body temperature recordings. The appearance of sustained fever, however, demands systematic evaluation of the patient. Investigation should begin and end with the burn wound. Dressings clogged with coagulum or wet dressings that have dried out may prevent heat exchange, and a dressing change itself may eliminate the fever. The development of wound sepsis may independently increase the metabolic rate and, unaccompanied by heat loss, result in increased body temperature.

Smears of the wound drainage should be stained and cultures performed. The smear is vital for identification of clostridia. Biopsy of the wound can be obtained for microbiological and histological examination. Although complete examination of this tissue will require 36 to 48 hours, a 10-minute slide test can be performed to accurately predict whether greater than 10^5 organisms per gram of tissue are present.[115] Histological examination is important to determine the depth of invasion of the bacteria.[217] The pulmonary status of the patient must be carefully evaluated by sputum smear and culture as well as by chest x-ray. The urinary tract, especially if an indwelling catheter is being used, is a common site of infection. Cellulitis or phlebitis secondary to the use of an intravenous catheter is a possibility. Repeated blood cultures may be necessary to identify causative organisms. A helpful guide during the fever investigation is the level of the patient's blood glucose. Blood glucose levels of over 130 mg. per cent are statistically associated with septicemias from gram-positive organisms, whereas the presence of a blood glucose of less than 110 mg. per cent suggests gram-negative organism septicemia.[147, 253]

The patient's state of hydration should be carefully reconsidered and electrolytes checked, since either dehydration or salt excess may produce fever. Many drugs may also cause fever as a result of allergic reactions (e.g., penicillin) or as a side effect (e.g., atropine and derivatives).

Systemic Antibiotics in Burns

Although there is ample evidence that systemic antibiotics fail to reduce the incidence of burn-wound sepsis, this does not mean that they are totally ineffective.[187] There is, for instance, documentation that streptococcal infection, a major threat in the early post-burn period, can be prevented by prophylactic administration of penicillin. Although topical antibacterials may be antistreptococcal, most burned patients should receive intravenous penicillin in dosages of 1 to 5 million units every 6 hours. This is particularly true in patients who are not getting topical antibacterial treatment. It should be continued through the edema phase of 48 to 72 hours and then stopped to reduce chances of emergence of resistant organisms.[10] Since the goal of therapy is specifically antistreptococcal, the alternate choices in the patient allergic to penicillin are lincomycin or erythromycin rather than broad spectrum coverage.

Beyond the first few days no systemic antibiotics are used without specific indications and documentation of burn sepsis on quantitative cultures of the wound or blood stream isolates. Although staphylococci were not a major problem of the last decade, increased identification of staphylococcus bacteremias has been noted in the last few years.[57] Quantitative cultures of staphylococci exceeding 10^5 bacteria per gram of burn-wound tissue or positive blood cultures require systemic penicillinase-resistant antibiotics and possible alteration in the topical antibacterial regimen.

The key to pseudomonas burn sepsis is clearly prophylaxis with topical antibacterial agents. Identification of greater than 10^5 pseudomonas per gram of burn tissue demands intensive local wound care and probable change of topical agents. Although lethal pseudomonas burn-wound sepsis may indeed occur without visceral spread, systemic coverage with gentamicin, tobramycin, or carbenicillin is indicated when quantitative levels exceed 10^5 bacteria per gram or positive blood cultures are obtained.

The plethora of strains of Pseudomonas has resulted in an increasing incidence of resistance to systemic antibiotics. The other gram-negative infections, particularly *Providencia stuartii,* have been disturbingly resistant to all antibiotics.[314] So too, futile efforts to provide the patient with a broad spectrum of "blanket" prophylactic coverage only seems to predispose to their emergence. This is particularly true of the mycotic infections. In a survey of 233 patients with candidiasis, only 8 had not been on systemic antibiotics and 140 had been receiving multiple drugs.[174] Since the source of infection is usually the bowel, oral Mycostatin is administered. When candida invasion of the blood stream occurs as diagnosed by blood culture, urine culture and retinopathy, amphotericin B or other antifungal drugs are indicated. Systemic antibiotics also should be discontinued in an effort to allow the normal bacterial flora to return.

If total antibacterial control is to be attempted, the aggressive approach of Collentine[47] and Waisbren[300] is perhaps most reasonable. Meticulous wound care and topically applied antibiotics (neomycin, polymyxin B and nystatin) are supplemented by massive amounts of penicillin, methicillin, polymyxin and chloramphenicol. Results are comparable to those obtained with topical antibacterial agents in other institutions. The use of such an antibacterial "potpourri," however, is not without hazard and demands vigilance to potential toxicity and exquisite supervision of management.

As with antibiotics in any other phase of surgical practice, the agent must be chosen with precision and administered at a time, by a route and in a dosage most likely for it to be effective.

Pain. All burns are initially painful. The amount of discomfort thereafter is related to the depth and area of the burn, the method of treatment and the individual response of the patient himself.

All analgesics administered in the acute period should be given intravenously and in small amounts. Morphine 4 mg. or meperidine (Demerol) 20 mg. may be given initially and repeated as needed to insure comfort. Other routes of administration are contraindicated because of the dangers of delayed absorption. Long-term analgesia in a chronically painful injury is a difficult problem, and every effort should be made to avoid making the patient drug-dependent.

Aspirin has a lytic effect on gastric and duodenal mucus; repeated and prolonged administration should be avoided, particularly in this already ulcerogenic situation. Large amounts of tranquilizers may cause hepatotoxicity and may produce neurological aberrations. A mild antidepressant such as Elavil may be of value.

Dressing changes should be accomplished without the necessity of general anesthesia whenever possible; moderate amounts of appropriately timed analgesia will usually be sufficient. Ketamine has been of particular value in children both for dressing changes and grafting procedures.

Hypnosis may be of value in long-term management, particularly during manipulation of the wounds. Constant reassurance, full explanation of procedures and conversational diversion are forms of hypnosis used by all surgeons when the services of trained hypnotherapists are not available.

LOCAL CARE OF THE BURN WOUND

The principles of local care must be directed to:

1. *Primum non nocere* ("First, do no harm").

2. Prevent infection and allow survival of all remaining viable tissue.

3. Obtain the best functional and aesthetically attractive coverage as quickly as feasible.

Superficial Burn. FIRST DEGREE. Clinically, superficial burns are usually due to minimal exposure to flash, contact or scalding. There is evidence to suggest that immediate cooling by immersion in ice water for 15 to 20 minutes will diminish the amount of edema and subsequent discomfort. Since discomfort is aggravated by air currents over the injured area, application of any ointment or cream will reduce discomfort. Application of thick layers of gauze saturated in oil-based materials or use of any impermeable materials will prevent proper drainage of sebaceous glands, lead to maceration and may result in staphylococcal furunculosis. Thin layers of water-soluble creams, which may be readily washed off, are probably best. Healing without scarring will occur in 3 to 7 days, perhaps accompanied by "peeling."

Partial-Thickness Burns. SUPERFICIAL, SECOND DEGREE. Unless complicated by infection or treatment, this injury also heals spontaneously and promptly, with minimal discoloration. Blistering is usually present and if left intact will provide a barrier to infection and allow prompt healing. In practice, however, the patient rarely finds it possible to keep a blister intact. Once broken, serum and desquamated cells form a crust that is more susceptible to bacterial invasion, particularly streptococcus. Except in the palm of the hand, where a very tough blister is often present, blisters are best trimmed away and the wound gently cleansed with bland soap and dressed. Dressings should be inspected frequently and changed promptly when dirty, dislodged or saturated with exudate. Healing should occur in 7 to 14 days. Temporary biologic dressings that do not allow vascular ingrowth can be utilized in uniform superficial partial-thickness wounds. For this purpose porcine xenografts and amniotic membranes are better than human allograft skin since they can be used to prevent vascularization. If amniotic membranes are used, the amnion (shiny) side is placed against the wound surface because the chorion side will, indeed, allow vascular ingrowth.[255] A dressing with many of the same properties as a biologic dressing is Hydron, a two-component dressing made of polyhydroxyethylmethacrylate and polyethylene glycol. Sprayed on the burn wound, it prevents desiccation and exogenous contamination and allows epithelialization.[216] The key in using biologic dressings or Hydron is to apply them only to uniformly superficial wounds. Since the pathogenesis of burning rarely results in a uniform wound, they probably have little role. In the non-uniform wound containing even punctate areas of deeper injury, coverage with these dressings risks formation of abscesses and conversion of the entire wound.

Any superficial burn of this type in excess of 15 per cent in adults, any in areas of special importance (face, hands, etc.), or any occurring in geographical areas in which dependable follow-up care is not possible should be treated initially in the hospital. These burns are usually of major significance only if neglected.

Deeper Burns. PARTIAL THICKNESS, DEEP; SECOND DEGREE — B; AND FULL THICKNESS, THIRD DEGREE. It has been repeatedly emphasized that differentiation into degrees is artificial since the initial treatment of these burns is similar whether or not they are full thickness. Except for limited area injuries in highly intelligent, dependable people, all patients burned to this degree should be cared for in a hospital.

The initial care of these injuries is directed to removing dirt, debris, charred clothing and any grease or ointment applied as an emergency measure on the scene.

A decision must then be made as to the best form of local care. The choices available include: (1) occlusive dressing technique, (2) exposure, (3) semi-open, including topical therapy, and (4) excision.

Occlusive Dressings ("Closed")

Choice of the occlusive dressing technique should be based on definite indications and must be done properly if it is to be effective. The reason for an occlusive dressing is not to reduce edema; nothing short of the pressure that will result in ischemic necrosis will affect the fluid accumulation. Rather, the functions of a proper dressing are (1) to protect the wound from further mechanical or bacterial contamination, (2) to absorb any external drainage and (3) to immobilize the injured part. The classic indication is the burned extremity. Burns of the trunk, face and perineum lend themselves poorly to this technique.

To accomplish these purposes, the dressings should be carefully constructed from a variety of materials and thoughtfully applied. The inner layer, in contact with the wound, should be fine-meshed gauze, either plain or impregnated. The purpose of impregnating gauze is not to prevent sticking to the wound since macerating amounts of impregnate are necessary to accomplish this; rather, it provides a coating to the fibers and therefore promotes drainage through to absorptive layers. Plain gauze tends to entrap the drainage and form a coagulum at the innermost layer. Commercially impregnated gauze must be "wrung out" since its heavy impregnation tends to prevent drainage and to macerate tissue.

The rest of the dressing consists of bulky, absorptive materials; however, cotton-containing gauze should not be applied next to a weeping wound, since later removal is difficult. The dressing is completed by the application of firm, even compression using roller bandage or Kling. Kerlix does not provide firm or regular compression, being much too distensible. The use of Ace or elastic bandages is mentioned only to be condemned. An even, controllable amount of compression is not possible and dangerously constrictive dressings may result as the wound swells with fluid. The dressing is completed only by positioning and immobilizing in the appropriate position, which often requires the use of plaster splints. The functional position of the burn differs from the position of function often described. Except for the hand, all burns involving the flexor aspects of extremities or neck should be splinted in full extension.

Dressing should be changed when necessary, a nonspecific recommendation, but based on the variability of wounds. Actively weeping wounds may require changes 2 or 3 times per day; dry wounds may not require altering the dressing for 4 to 5 days. Evidence of odor, pain and unexplained fever are absolute indications for prompt inspection of the wound.

Exposure Method ("Open")

Exposure therapy was reintroduced by Wallace in 1949 in an attempt to reverse the practice of applying noxious compounds, such as tannic and picric acids, to the burn wound.[302] The basis for this form of therapy is the formation of a coagulum of protein and debris on the surface of the wound (an eschar), which will theoretically protect against mechanical and bacterial trauma. It sustains the principle that we should actively "do no harm," but it violates another well-known principle of surgery — that an open wound should be covered with a sterile dressing or skin. The classical indications have included burns of the perineum, the face and those limited to one aspect of the trunk.

If such a method is chosen, the room is prepared and reverse isolation techniques (gowns, masks and gloves when touching the patient) should be instituted. Clean sheets (not necessarily sterile) are placed under and cradled over (not touching) the patient. Adequate environmental heat can be provided by infrared lamps or by the Apollo heat shield. In 24 to 48 hours burned tissue and coagulum will form a thick, leathery surface, a process that may be hastened by use of fans. In superficial burns, a spontaneous regeneration of epithelium will occur beneath the crust or eschar, which will then separate in 14 to 21 days, a process that is unfavorably altered by mechanical trauma or bacterial invasion. In full-thickness injuries, the eschar will also separate in 14 to 21 days, leaving a granulating bed suitable for the application of grafts.

The objections to this form of therapy are numerous and valid. It is not a particularly good mechanical barrier and this function is lost when the eschar cracks. Nor is it a barrier to the increased heat and the water lost by evaporation; Cohen noted evaporation to occur at a rate 10 to 12 times that of normal skin through even the toughest, driest eschar.[46] It also seems to have little value in preventing bacterial proliferation. The bacteria are either beneath it from the beginning, arrive endogenously through the blood stream, are autogenously deposited by the patient or enter exogenously by a break in technique. Whatever the source, the natural history of exposure therapy is all too often burn-wound sepsis.

Semi-open (Topical Therapy)

Somewhere between the occlusive dressing technique and exposure are a variety of techniques that include continuous wet dressings (0.5 per cent silver nitrate) and topical antibacterials. Since the realization that the prevention of infection involves the maintenance of an equilibrium between ever-present bacteria and the factors of host resistance, the early care of the burn wound has been aimed toward preventing the numerical proliferation of bacteria.[254] As the bacteria that reside deep in the dermal appendanges proliferate to numbers greater than 10^5 organisms per gram of tissue, they begin to migrate through the tissue, surround and occlude blood vessels and cause thrombosis.[293-295] This thrombosis in the vessels in the wound, causing an avascular type of burn wound sepsis, necessitated the use of topical antibacterial agents. A brief review of these agents and methods of their use follows.

Silver Nitrate. The continuous wet dressing technique employing 0.5 per cent silver nitrate, evolved from Moyer's efforts to develop a method of burn care that would simultaneously reduce the nutritional and metabolic deficit related to evaporative water loss and control burn-wound sepsis.[203] In the 0.5 per cent concentration, silver nitrate does not seem to injure regenerating epithelium in the burn wound, yet is effectively bacteriostatic against *Staphylococcus aureus, Escherichia coli* and *Pseudomonas aeruginosa.*[33, 187]

The patient to be treated is carefully cleansed of debris and particularly of any previously applied ointment, which will prevent diffusion. The wounds are covered with multilayered coarse-mesh dressings saturated with the solution. These are held in place with a nonelastic dressing, and the complex is covered with dry sheeting to prevent evaporation and cooling. The dressings are kept wet with 0.5 per cent silver nitrate solution and are completely changed every 12 hours.

Like any agent, silver nitrate has both advantages and disadvantages. Benefits include the rather nondiscriminating bacteriostatic properties of the free silver ion, which gives broad spectrum protection to the fresh burn wound. Silver nitrate also reduces nutritional and metabolic losses by decreasing evaporative water loss. These losses are further diminished by the dry sheeting over the dressing.[203] There are both bacterial and metabolic disadvantages associated with the use of this agent. The Klebsiella of the Enterobacteriaceae group and Providencia species are not as susceptible as other bacteria.[33] *Enterobacter cloacae* can convert the nitrate to nitrite, causing methemoglobinemia.[296]

Metabolically, the use of silver nitrate is not without hazard and should be approached with great care. Silver nitrate in 0.5 per cent solution contains 29.4 mEq/l. and is thus hypotonic. The permeable nature of the burn wound requires prompt equilibration, and sodium, chloride and other ions are drawn into the dressings as deposits of silver chloride, carbonate and proteinate are formed. Such osmolar dilution can rapidly produce severe electrolyte deficits and cause hyponatremia and hypochloremia. Potassium is also lost but the gradient (5 mEq./l. in serum to 0 in dressing) is less. Careful salt replacement, initially intravenously and later orally, is necessary. Careful monitoring of serum electrolytes is vital and should be done initially every 3 to 4 hours in children and every 12 hours in adults and continued until oral supplements are being tolerated well and serum electrolytes are stable. If the wet dressings are allowed to dry or if the dressings are covered by an impervious material, hyperpyrexia develops. Again, this is extremely dangerous in children.

The silver ion precipitates on the surface and therefore penetrates eschar poorly. A singular limitation observed in the experimental animal[138, 141, 142] and confirmed clinically is its relative ineffectiveness in established infection;[183] to be most valuable it must be begun immediately as the definitive form of treatment.[232, 249]

Problems in the quality of wound healing with silver nitrate have been described. Deep partial-thickness burns tend to heal with hypertrophic scars, particularly in flexor areas and the hands; resurfacing with split grafts is an integral part of the rehabilitation. The surface of these spontaneously healed wounds tends to be thin and susceptible to minor abrasive trauma (Fig. 23–6). So too, erysipelatous-type inflammatory reactions seem to develop in apparently healed tissue.[203] Care must be taken to avoid applications of cocoa butter or other emollients that definitely aggravate these complications.

Sulfamylon (Mafenide Acetate). Mafenide acetate is available in both a 10 per cent water soluble cream and a 5 per cent solution. Mendelsohn and Lindsey suggested its use in burns.[181] After prolonged experimental trial,[164] using the excellent Walker burn-wound model, Lindberg and Moncrief introduced it for clinical trial in 1963.

The cream is applied as a thin layer to the burn surface twice daily after the wound has been cleansed of debris and the wound is allowed to remain exposed to the air. If the drug is accidentally removed by the patient while turning in bed, it is promptly reapplied. The 5 per cent solution is applied in a saturated gauze dressing and changed every 8 hours.[274] It is effective at

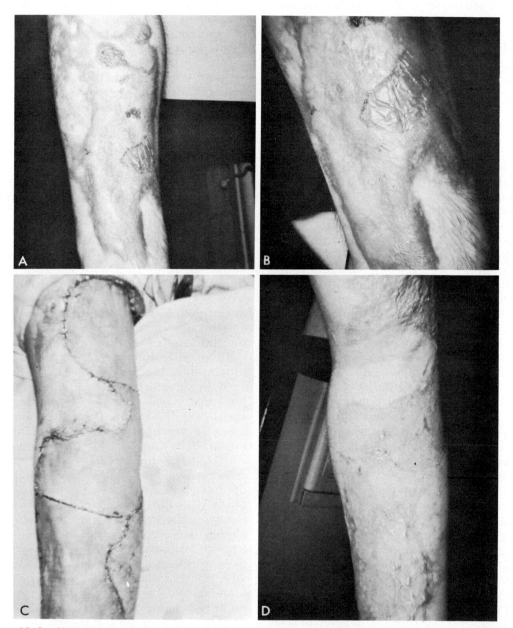

Figure 23–6. *Hypertrophic scarring. A, Deep partial-thickness burn of right forearm healed spontaneously with 0.5 per cent silver nitrate therapy. Photographs at four months indicate hypertrophic scarring and blistering. B, Close-up of A. Epithelium very susceptible to minor abrasive trauma, tending to be "wiped-off." C, Entire area excised and split-thickness grafts applied. D, Result two months later.*

penetrating the eschar and appears to be especially effective after the eschar has been removed from the granulating bed.[108] Among the major advantages of Sulfamylon are its ability to control pseudomonas burn wound sepsis, its ease of application and the lack of a need for dressings. It has several major disadvantages. It is metabolized by monamine oxidase to p-sulfamoylbenzoic acid, a carbonic anhydrase inhibitor.[33] Therefore, it has a tendency to produce a state of metabolic acidosis in the patient. In the normal burn patient a mild respiratory alkalosis exists, so an imbalance does not occur. If an inhalation injury with its attendant respiratory acidosis is present, the combination with metabolic acidosis from this agent could prove fatal. Early deaths, unrelated to burn wound sepsis, have been seen in the burn course with the use of Sulfamylon. These seem to be due to respiratory difficulties related to pulmonary edema.[219] This complication is not seen when the agent is first applied later in the burn course.

Mafenide acetate causes pain when applied to superficial partial-thickness burns with intact free nerve endings. This is not a true disadvantage because the agent was not designed for use in minor burns and its use is not painful on large full-thickness injuries. The necessity that it remain exposed for antibacterial potency can be a relative disadvantage when a dressing such as a splint is required for a severely burned hand. The 5 per cent aqueous solution can be used in a wet dressing covered by the splint.

Sulfamylon effectively penetrates intact eschar and experimentally and clinically reduces the flora to less than 10^4 bacteria per gram, a level compatible with survival of epithelial islands and "take" of skin.[109, 166, 193]

Experience with this agent has been wide and acceptable.[178, 191, 234, 271] Significant reduction in mortality, particularly in burns ranging from 40 to 60 per cent of body surface area, can be achieved. Boswick reports a reduction of mortality of burns in the 30 to 50 per cent body surface area from 70 to 34 per cent with mafenide (from 49 to 32 per cent in all burns).[32] Clearly, Sulfamylon remains the agent against which any new agent must be measured.

Gentamicin. Gentamicin sulfate (Garamycin) is a broad-spectrum antibiotic structurally similar to neomycin and kanamycin, with an unusual bacteriocidal potency against *Pseudomonas aeruginosa*.[27, 288] Clinical application has been best in the 0.1 per cent cream form (the ointment penetrates eschar poorly), applied either by semi-open or occlusive dressing technique. Dressing changes are variously recommended from twice a day to twice a week.[285] Although the drug is absorbed, the amounts rarely reach 10 per cent of toxic levels.[286] In the presence of sepsis, it should be supplemented by systemic antibiotic therapy.[289]

Disadvantages outweigh any benefits of this drug. Gentamicin sulfate is an excellent systemic antibiotic and use of the same drug topically decreases the effectiveness of the systemic preparation. The major disadvantage is the reported rapid emergence of resistant strains of *Pseudomonas aeruginosa*.[287] The strains have been shown to demonstrate a cross-resistance to silver sulfadiazine, rendering both agents ineffective.[114] Potential ototoxicity and nephrotoxicity can be associated with its continued absorption. For these reasons, gentamicin sulfate is not really recommended for routine use in major thermal injuries.

Silver Sulfadiazine. The best of silver nitrate, the silver ion, has been compounded with sulfadiazine as a 1 per cent cream for use as a topical antibacterial agent.[91, 95, 282] The binding with silver apparently prevents inactivation of the sulfonamide by altered pH or para-amino benzoic acid.[23] The release of the sulfa is apparently slow and systemic toxicity has not been a problem. The silver apparently binds with the DNA of the bacteria, thus releasing the sulfadiazine.[95] Its use has included semi-open and closed dressing techniques, usually with a once or twice daily application. Its use is not associated with unusual discomfort and local skin allergies have been surprisingly few. The eschars become soft and a thick creamy discharge is seen on the wound; however, this represents drug, some leukocytes and amorphous protein material, but not necessarily bacteria. Bacterial control is measured by quantitative cultures rather than by observing the deceptive purulent-appearing wound.

Serial biopsy cultures in one large series confirm its wide antibacterial spectrum.[23] *Pseudomonas aeruginosa* organisms were the most common isolate followed by *Enterobacter aerogenes. E. coli,* Proteus, Serratia and Candida were seen less frequently. The organisms that have not been effectively covered by this agent are *Staphylococcus aureus* and some strains of Klebsiella.[23, 219]

Reports of reduced mortality have been encouraging, and comparative studies indicate that its effectiveness is comparable to Sulfamylon but without the side effects.[90, 94, 95] During the past 3 years, this agent has become the most frequently used topical antibacterial for thermal burns. A disadvantage may be a reported associated granulocyte depression.[44, 299] To date this has seemed to be reversible and in the only controlled study available it has been questioned that the leukopenia was indeed secondary to the drug.[134]

Betadine Ointment. Betadine (povidone iodine) is an antibacterial agent of documented value in skin preps and surgical scrubs. Its effective ingredient is iodine; however, its use on intact skin has not been accompanied by a high incidence of allergenicity or toxic side effects. Betadine is effective in dilutions of 1:400 or even greater against most common burn pathogens as well as fungi and viruses. Its use in burns includes the aerosal spray and the solution full-strength as a wet dressing. Most interest has been in 10 per cent Betadine ointment.[100, 157] It should be applied at least every 6 hours and may be used either semi-open or in dressings. It shares with Sulfamylon a discomfort to the patient with application. Skin sensitivity and systemic side effects have not been recorded.

Experimental and clinical data suggest that like silver nitrate it is not effective against established burn sepsis, and to be effective, it should be used early as prophylaxis. Its efficacy in the management of major burns has not been well documented. Pietsch and Meakins suggested that Betadine be limited to burns of less than 20 per cent body surface since they found that iodine absorption leads to metabolic acidosis and renal failure when treating patients with large burns.[229]

Newer Topical Agents

Silver Lactate. Silver lactate is a silver-lacto-allantoin complex prepared in a hydrophylic ointment. It is easily applied and can be applied in a dressing or as a butter. Early studies suggested that it may be of use in the burned patient.[51, 121, 143]

Silver Nitrate Cream. A water-soluble cream incorporating silver nitrate has been investigated experimentally and clinically. Its advantages are its neatness of application and the absence of hypotonicity seen in the 0.5 per cent solution. Its ability to penetrate eschar is not proven.[73]

Cerium Nitrate. Cerium salts are toxic to both bacteria and fungi and show almost no absorption through the burn wound. Therefore, cerium nitrate has recently been tested clinically and found to be effective in decreasing surface bacteria in the burn wound.[186] Used alone it appeared to be most effective against the *Pseudomonas aeruginosa.* Combined with silver sulfadiazine it appears to provide a broad spectrum of protection against both gram-positive and gram-negative organisms.[93] Larger trials are under way. However, the combination cerium nitrate-silver sulfadiazine may actually be antagonistic and less effective than silver sulfadiazine alone.[113]

Zinc sulfadiazine and silver-zinc allantoin are two additional agents being evaluated in experimental and clinical trials.

Any agent, to be suitable for application to a burn wound, should ideally not produce pain when applied and be innocuous to the viable cells of the wound or to the patient if (and when) absorbed, nonallergic and most importantly, bactericidal. It would be nice if it were simple to apply and cheap, and even more salutary if it would both allow drainage and prevent evaporative water-heat loss. No agent yet available fulfills all these criteria. The history of topical therapy has been the introduction of new agents, attended by initial success and abandonment when they have become obviously toxic, ineffective or both. The introduction of any new agent or form of treatment is enthusiastically received by physicians and hospital personnel, who, in their curiosity, render meticulous and diligent patient care that this agent might be properly evaluated. One must be careful lest the apparent benefit be the result of this new interest in the burned patient rather than the agent or the form of therapy. There is also a tendency to evaluate results uncritically in comparison to what was accomplished in the years prior to the introduction of the new treatment, ignoring other factors, including a changing bacterial ecology, which would influence results.

Topical antibacterial efficacy can best be monitored by quantitative and qualitative analyses of burn wound tissue biopsies. Until recently, no in vitro tests were available to help one choose the most effective antibacterial agent for a given patient. Reports by Nathan and his co-workers have demonstrated an effective method of testing the burn wound bacteria against the various topical agents that are available.[215] The test bacteria are spread over an agar plate and the topical antibacterial agents are placed into wells in the agar. Zones of inhibition predict an agent's effectiveness. As these methods improve and more comparative data emerge, one will be able to more objectively choose the proper antibacterial agent for the patient. As the data are developed and new agents are discovered, however, the bacteria will continue to change so that at no time will the mythical "antibacterial of choice" be available for treatment of the burn patient.

PRIMARY EXCISION AND GRAFTING

The burned patient is never in better shape to tolerate an operation than moments after he has been burned. His course thereafter is downhill until the wound is closed.

Many studies have been undertaken to test the feasibility of early full-thickness excision of major burns.[18, 53, 173] Although burns of less than 10 per cent of body surface area can be readily excised and skin grafted, attempts at removing larger areas have been attended by excessive blood loss.[48] Most studies have failed to document a reduced mortality from such an approach.[173, 291] However, new grafting techniques, the availability of biologic dressings for temporary wound coverage, and hypotensive anesthesia have stimulated new interest in this approach.

Law and MacMillan have recently performed 52 excisional procedures on 35 patients with a mean body surface area of 35 per cent full-thickness burn, usually at about the tenth post-burn day.[156] Coverage was obtained with meshed skin grafts expanded from 3:1 to 6:1 in large areas. Blood loss in such massive excisions can be minimized by use of a CO_2 laser[85, 283] or the plasma scalpel or by the use of controlled hypotensive anesthesia. Burke has totally revolutionized the concept of full-thickness burn excision. In children with less than 35 per cent body surface area burns, he promptly excises the full-thickness eschar and replaces it by autograft skin.[40] In patients with larger than 35 per cent body surface area full-thickness burns he excises the wound and closure is obtained with matched and typed allograft from parental donors and "take" maintained with Imuran immunosuppression. As donor sites heal they are used again until all allograft has been replaced. Nineteen children with total burn size of over 80 per cent body surface area and with a full-thickness component of over 70 per cent body surface area treated with temporary skin transplantation and immunosuppression have been reported.[41, 42]

An alternative to full-thickness eschar excision has recently become quite popular. Based on the concentric wound concepts elucidated by Jackson, an intradermal or tangential excision can be performed. Janzekovic has pioneered this treatment and reported on 4370 patients treated by tangential excision and grafting performed 3 to 5 days post-burn.[128] She lists several advantages to this type of partial-thickness wound excision: (1) by excision of deep dermal surfaces, healthy tissue is not sacrificed and potentially damaged tissue that would have died if left to spontaneous demarcation is saved; (2) by autografting the excised areas, the biological properties of the skin are saved and contractures are prevented in the grafted areas; (3) when areas are too large to be autografted or very superficial, allografts can be applied to the dermal areas to eliminate infection and allow spontaneous epithelialization. Although proponents to this type of early excision have stated that it decreases length of hospital stay and is more cost effective than conventional treatment, controlled studies have not corroborated this.[280] Disadvantages to this technique include destruction of viable epidermal elements in partial-thickness areas, bleeding and the opening of portals of infection in the presence of sepsis. Also, the graft take on the tangentially debrided dermis has been reported to be less than optimal.[120]

SKIN GRAFTING

Over 100 years ago, George David Pollock performed the first skin graft on a burned patient and speculated that employing grafts early would promote healing and reduce contractures.[97] A century later, wound closure remains the therapeutic imperative. Large areas of the body should be covered as the first priority in efforts to reduce the size of the wound. Second priority is given to areas of great functional importance, particularly the hand and flexion areas.

The preservation of epidermal islands by prevention of burn-wound sepsis may result in spontaneous healing in many deep burns. However, the process is often prolonged and depleting to the physical and emotional resources of the patient. So too, the quality of healing from these wounds is often disappointing with unstable epithelium, hypertrophic scarring and contractures.

Preparation of the Wound

Historically, eschar separation occurred predictably between the tenth and fourteenth post-burn days. Clearly, much of this pattern was due to bacterial growth and autolysis of necrotic tissue and even destruction of remaining viable dermal tissue in deep burns. Successful control of burn wound sepsis by topical antibacterial agents has been attended by prolonged adherence of eschar, delay in preparing of the wound for grafting and even retardation of normal wound healing. Preparation of the wound requires persistence in mechanical debridement and perhaps enzyme therapy.

Mechanical Methods

Physical removal of necrotic debris may take the form of early, total excision of the burn, intradermal or tangential debridement or, more commonly, daily surgical cleansing of loosening eschar. This tedious approach is accompanied by minimal blood loss and discomfort and may be performed by paramedical personnel.

The frequent changing of dressings and the use of tub baths are additional mechanical methods of removing necrotic debris. The use of tub baths has additional salutary effects of providing patient comfort and an opportunity to maintain muscle tone and joint motion by subaqua exercises. Previous drug applications are washed away, debris is softened and loosened, and this presents an appropriate time for trimming away eschar prior to reapplying topical antibacterials. Prolonged immersion in hypotonic bath water will tend to leach out electrolytes from the wound, and salt should be added to the water if prolonged tubbing is employed. It is recognized that anything added to the immersate may also be absorbed, interdicting the use of pHisoHex or other hexachlorophene compounds in the tank.

Enzymes

Enzymes of many types have been introduced to dissolve the necrotic tissue. Each new agent has been later abandoned as uncontrollable, ineffective or potentially dangerous by allowing bacterial proliferation. A newer agent, Travase, is currently gaining popularity.[99, 277] A product of *Bacillus subtilis*, the enzyme works only in a moist environment and is inactivated by any of the free silver- or iodine-containing topical antibacterials (although apparently compatible with silver sulfadiazine and Sulfamylon). Applied every 6 to 8 hours in a moist dressing, it will dissolve eschar within hours and often debride a wound completely within 2 to 3 days. However, it will often expose the subcutaneous fat layer, which it will not debride, and which forms granulation tissue slowly and presents a difficult bed for skin grafting. More importantly, unless combined with continued antibacterial therapy, its use may dispose the wound to rapid bacterial proliferation. Hummel and co-workers reported sepsis in patients enzymatically debrided with Travase when concomitant topical antibacterials were not used.[123]

TEMPORARY WOUND COVERAGE

In a 50 per cent full-thickness burn in an adult, the amount of skin necessary to obtain coverage has been estimated at 6000 square centimeters. Such large amounts of donor areas are not readily available. Temporary biologic dressings applied to the burn wound render it less painful, reduce fluid and protein loss, and will preserve bacteriological control of the wound while donor sites re-epithelialize prior to re-use.

Allografts

The first allograft on a burn patient was performed by Pollock on the same patient who received the first autograft with his own arm used as a donor.[97] Until Brown demonstrated that postmortem allografts could be used,[36, 126] the necessity of using live donors limited the use of the technique. Although the depressed immune response of the burned patient leads to prolonged survival of allografts, permanent take has been realized only in identical twins. Burke has prolonged allograft survival in selected patients with immunosuppressives,[40-42] and recent work suggests that temporary storage of allograft in tissue culture reduces the antigenicity of the skin and may lead to indefinite and perhaps permanent survival when transplanted. Such a breakthrough, if confirmed, could lead to fulfillment of the burn surgeon's dream, an inexhaustible and readily available bank of skin.

At the present time, allografts are customarily used only as a temporary cover.[112, 172, 269, 272, 273, 313] Harvested within 6 to 12 hours after death, allograft may be stored up to 2 weeks at 4° C. Applied to a bacteriologically receptive wound, the allograft will clearly establish a vascular connection with the bed and truly "take." A bacterial flora containing more than 10^5 organisms per gram of tissue will usually prevent take and under such circumstances the allograft should be changed every 24 to 48 hours until take occurs. Such frequent changes will, of themselves, reduce the bacterial counts. Successful take of the allografts documents potential receptiveness of the bed to autografts. The allografts should be changed every 48 hours lest complete vascularization make later removal difficult and attended by profuse bleeding. Allowing the graft to reject merely reproduces the necrotic surface that was presented by the burn eschar itself.

In practice, allografts are not readily available in the general hospital and re-quire that a surgical team be kept on hand ready to procure the grafts if a suitable cadaver donor becomes available.

Xenografts

To substitute for the scarce allograft supply, a variety of xenograft tissues have been employed. Canine xenografts seemed to provide adequate temporary coverage but are tedious to obtain and not aesthetically pleasing.[290] Because of certain structural similarity to human skin, porcine xenografts have become popular and most successfully distributed commercially.[34]

Porcine xenografts are provided fresh, frozen and in a lyophilized form. Sterility is maintained by irradiation or by antibiotics. Their size is limited by the dermatome used to obtain the tissue, but they are aesthetically acceptable and easy to use, albeit quite expensive. As with allografts, porcine xenografts should be changed every 48 hours. There is controversy regarding take, and although vascular continuity has been occasionally seen on histological sections, injection of India ink fails to penetrate the graft. The biological adherence by fibrin clot, however, may be more important to effectiveness than actual take.

Xenografts reduce evaporative water loss, reduce exudation of protein from the wound and promote patient comfort.[246] They are neither experimentally nor clinically as effective as allografts in reducing or maintaining a low bacterial wound flora. A recent use of porcine xenograft has been as a dressing after being meshed and expanded at 1.5:1 or 3:1. This allows topical antibacterials to be used with the porcine skin. Early reports of this technique demonstrate its usefulness.[278]

Amniotic Membranes

Introduced by Sabella in 1912 as a cover for burn wounds,[262] amniotic membranes have found minimal favor in reported trials.[61, 67, 69] The histological similarity to skin and a presumed immunological immaturity led to hopes of permanent take and coverage. Although vascularization clearly occurs, autolysis and rejection are inevitable as with any allograft tissue.[70] The realization that temporary biologic dressings should be changed frequently has led to a rebirth of interest in fetal membranes.

Fresh amniotic membranes are obtained from sero-negative mothers with no history of endometritis or premature rupture of the membranes. The membranes are aseptically passed through four rinses of saline, one of 0.025 per cent hypochlorite and an additional four rinses of saline prior to storage at 4° C. Cultures confirm sterility prior to application and storage time up to 6 weeks has been reported. The membranes are applied with the amnion side up and the chorion in contact with full-thickness wounds and are changed every 48 hours until the time of autografting.

In vitro experiments demonstrate no inherent bacteriocidal substance in amnion.[256] However, applied as a membrane to infected burns and other open wounds in the experimental animals, it was superior to both allograft and xenograft skin and the equal of the animal's own skin in reducing the bacterial flora of their monocontaminated wounds. In a series of clinical cases that now exceeds 1000, amniotic membranes provided bacteriological control that was the equivalent of allograft and superior to xenograft.[256] They are readily available, and come in large sizes and at no cost to the patient.

Other Covers

No synthetic skin substitute has proved the equal of the biological adherence achieved with biologic dressings. Although many materials will reduce water loss and protein exudation, none totally provides bacterial protection and all tend to allow bacterial proliferation and potential wound sepsis at the interface with the wound. However, experimental and clinical studies continue and a synthetic substitute may soon be found that meets all of the requirements of a biological dressing.

Predicting Skin Graft Survival

There are certain conditions that must prevail to insure the successful application of a skin graft to an open wound. They are unchanged since George Lawson enumerated them in 1871:[158]

1. That the new skin should be applied to a healthy granulating surface.
2. That skin *only* should be transplanted, and special care should be taken that there is no fat adherent to it.

3. That the portions of skin be accurately and firmly applied to the granulating surface.
4. That the new skin be kept in its new position without interrruption.

However, each surgeon tends to apply his own criteria to a wound, which are largely subjective and in reported series have resulted in a failure rate as high as 21 per cent.[168]

More objective data may be obtained by serial quantitative cultures of biopsy specimens of the open wound.[15, 252] It has been observed that a graft take of 94 per cent was achieved in wounds containing 10^5 or fewer bacteria per gram of tissue.[146] When the bacterial counts exceeded 10^5 bacteria per gram, the survival rate for grafts fell to 19 per cent. It has also been observed that when allografts are applied an apparent take is associated with take of subsequently applied autografts.

In a series of 30 patients these two test methods were compared.[257] Allografts were changed until a take was observed; an average of 3.7 applications was necessary before this occurred. Simultaneous quantitative cultures of biopsy specimens indicated that such allograft take was associated in all cases with a bacterial flora of 10^5 or fewer organisms per gram. In 77 of 81 failures of allograft take, a bacterial flora exceeding 10^5 organisms per gram was identified. Successful autografting proceeded in 29 of 30 cases as predicted by these two tests.

TECHNIQUES OF SKIN GRAFTING

Donor Sites

In extreme situations, any and all available skin can be and has been used as a donor site, including the scalp and soles of the feet. However, when lesser amounts of skin are needed, consideration should be given to the long-term results; an unsightly donor site may later be of more concern to the patient than the original injury. Although no area of the body is immune to exposure, the buttocks and lower abdomen should be used first, particularly in young girls. The thighs provide more accessible donor sites, but are more visible postoperatively and the skin is less thick. Donor sites should be dressed with an impregnated fine-mesh gauze or a biologic dressing, and spontaneous re-epithelialization will occur in 10 to 14 days. If thin grafts are used and the donor site heals kindly, the donor sites may be re-used every 2 to 3 weeks.

Obtaining a Graft

It is rarely possible to cover more than 20 to 30 per cent of the body area at one time. In general, it is best to cover the anterior or posterior trunk at separate times. Grafts may be obtained with a freehand knife or any of the standard dermatomes. The Reese dermatome takes an even graft and is very useful on irregular surfaces, but it has the disadvantage of the necessity for changing the dermatome tape after each drum of skin. The Padgett dermatome also requires reapplication of tape after each drum of skin. The infant Padgett dermatome is of great value in children and in all patients for inaccessible areas. Reese or Padgett dermatomes are particularly useful in obtaining a large uniform sheet to cover the hands or an aesthetically important unit of the face. The Brown air-driven or electric-driven dermatomes have great value in burns, particularly for obtaining long sheets of skin quickly and easily. However,

Brown dermatomes require a flat surface (which may be obtained by ballooning the skin with saline injections) and produce a graft of irregular thickness.

Due to variations in skin thickness, a graft of 0.010 inch thick may produce a thin split graft when taken from the back, but may result in full-thickness loss when taken from the medial aspect of the thigh. In general, grafts should be 0.008 inch to 0.010 inch thick in children and 0.012 to 0.014 inch thick in adults. Where insufficient donor skin is available, thin grafts are used as the take is more predictable and donor sites may be re-used quickly. In areas of great functional stress, such as the hand, a thicker graft is probably preferable. Full-thickness grafts require an ideal recipient site and have little place in the treatment of acute burns. Pinch grafts offer no advantage and produce full-thickness loss at the donor sites.

"Postage-stamp" grafts are of value if it is necessary to cover large areas with small amounts of skin; these grafts will also allow drainage in contaminated areas. The graft is cut into sections, laid raw side up on wet fine-mesh gauze and implanted as a unit. The raw areas between the small grafts

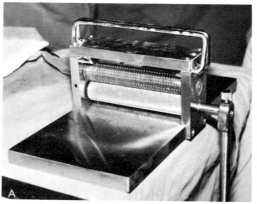
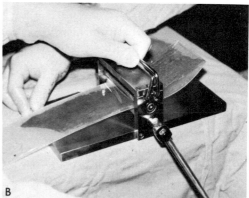
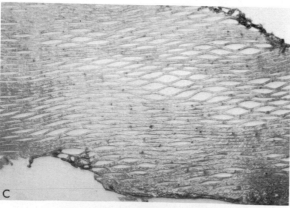

Figure 23–7. *Tanner-Vanderput mesh graft. A, Zimmer Dermatome. B. Split-thickness graft is placed against backing and run through "mesh grafter." C, Multiple linear perforations enable the graft to be expanded to three times its original width. Intervening areas spontaneously re-epithelialize.*

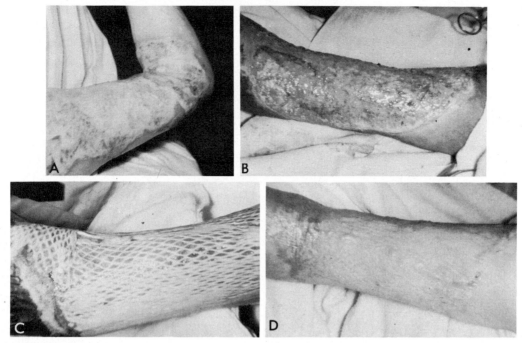

Figure 23–8. *Use of mesh graft. A, Full-thickness burn, upper extremity. B, After treatment with 0.5 per cent silver nitrate, a clean granulating bed is present. C, Mesh graft applied and silver nitrate occlusive dressings continued. D, Result at two months shows complete re-epithelialization with minimal cosmetic deformity and good functional skin.*

rapidly re-epithelialize from the graft margins. A more elegant modification is the Tanner mesh graft (Figs. 23–7 and 23–8), which produces multiple slices in the graft, allowing it to be opened to 3 to 9 times its original size. The interspersed raw areas heal by marginal ingrowth from the many edges of the graft. Mesh grafts should not be used on the face, hands, feet or flexor aspects of the body. When large sheets of skin are laid on the trunk, neither sutures nor dressings will be required. Dressings are useful on the extremities for compression and immobilization, but open grafting is suitable if skeletal traction is used to elevate the limb and allow circumferential grafting. It should be re-emphasized that any open area not covered with graft can only heal by scar.

Special Groups of Patients

Children. The tragedy of the burned child is that the injury was usually preventable. Children are the innocent victims of their own curiosity and ignorance and carelessness and lack of supervision on the part of their guardians. A small but significant number represent the effects of deliberate injury — "the battered child." Fully 70 per cent of burns occur in the home and more than 50 per cent occur in the formative years of life. Thermal burns are the number-one cause of fatal accidents in the preschool child.[1] Mortality figures do not cover the social significance of the burn-scarred child.

The etiology of these injuries is about equally divided between scalds and flash burns. The thinner skin of the child predisposes him to full-thickness loss from hot liquids. The overturning of coffee pots and other containers on the stove results in a high incidence of burns of the face, neck, shoulders and arms. The curious child is also highly subject to burns of the palm of the hand. Hot bath water can produce full-thickness loss in areas difficult to treat, including the soles of feet and the perineum.

Children are not small adults, and their initial and continued therapy should be appropriately altered. Special charts should be consulted to determine the size of the burn (Fig. 23–9), which is usually overestimated, whereas depth is usually underestimated. There is an even greater danger of fluid overload in children than in adults, and fluids should be administered

BURN SHEET

NAME _____   AGE_____   NUMBER_____

BURN RECORD.   AGES — BIRTH — 7 ½   DATE OF OBSERVATION _____

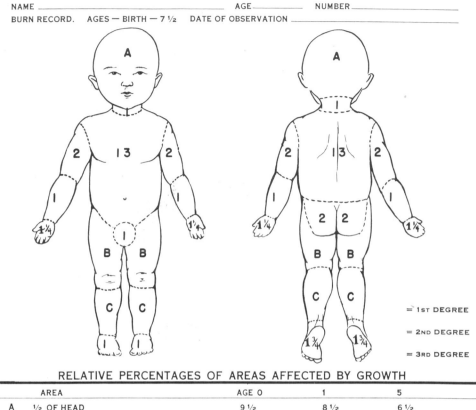

		= 1ST DEGREE
		= 2ND DEGREE
		= 3RD DEGREE

RELATIVE PERCENTAGES OF AREAS AFFECTED BY GROWTH

	AREA	AGE 0	1	5
A	½ OF HEAD	9 ½	8 ½	6 ½
B	½ OF ONE THIGH	2 ¾	3 ¼	4
C	½ OF ONE LEG	2 ½	2 ½	2 ¾

% BURN BY AREAS

PROBABLE 3RD° BURN	HEAD_____ NECK_____ BODY_____ UP. ARM_____ FOREARM_____ HANDS_____ GENITALS_____ BUTTOCKS_____ THIGHS_____ LEGS_____ FEET_____
TOTAL BURN	HEAD_____ NECK_____ BODY_____ UP. ARM_____ FOREARM_____ HANDS_____ GENITALS_____ BUTTOCKS_____ THIGHS_____ LEGS_____ FEET_____

SUM OF ALL AREAS _____   PROBABLY 3RD° _____   TOTAL BURN _____

Figure 23–9. Chart useful in estimating body surface area in burned children, based on Lund-Browder figures.[125]

with the same caution. The use of large amounts of colloid has demonstrated value in children if not in adults and may be more important immunologically than hemodynamically. The same interdiction against early oral replacement applies in children; gastric dilatation may be even more common. Indwelling catheters for urine measurement are used reluctantly in small children, but the need exceeds the dangers. Tracheostomy, a management problem in the young, is only rarely indicated.

Orthopedic complications are more com-

mon in children, and ankylosis may occur in joints remote from the burn. The local response of children to thermal injury and their reactions to burn-wound sepsis and appropriate local therapy are no different from those of adults. Current experience would suggest the use of some form of topical therapy.

Hospitalization is often prolonged and the diversionary value of "play ladies" and the facilities for continued schooling in the hospital are important. Early psychiatric and social consultation and support for the family will do much to relieve some of the anxiety and profound guilt the parents experience following the burning of a child. Prophylactic measures devoted to safety education of the parents concerning flammability of clothing and thermostatic control on hot water fixtures are all steps in the proper direction.

The Elderly. The elderly patient faces a dismal prognosis, far out of proportion to other age groups. The attenuation of the skin, diminished reflexes and the lack of agility which attend the aging process render this group prone to thermal injury. Scald burns have the same propensity for full-thickness loss as those in infants and similarly may be sustained in the bathtub.

Associated cardiovascular, renal pulmonary and metabolic derangements in this age group render resuscitation difficult. The principles are the same, but the execution must necessarily be altered, depending on the circumstances. The tendency to overload the circulation is perhaps the most common early mistake.

Local burn-wound care is similar to other groups. Thin skin makes split grafts difficult to obtain. Healing is slow and even minor injury or infection in the donor site will result in full-thickness loss. The ultimate goals of treatment must be altered. The healed wound is vital, even to the extent of accepting some functional limitation. Prolonged bed rest presents problems of its own, and efforts at continued ambulation or wheelchair use are attempted even during the course of treatment of the semiacute burn.

Others. Other frequently encountered groups of patients present unique problems. The obese patient is a particularly poor surgical risk for many reasons, including pulmonary problems and the difficult mechanical task of postoperative mobilizaton. The burn wound itself tends to be different, often demonstrating exceedingly slow separation of eschar and a tendency to develop a thin, collagenous film over the fatty wound rather than healthy granulation tissue. This results in poor graft take and prolonged disability. The application of a dry dressing to this wound, normally a poor surgical maneuver, may result in irritation and stimulation of granulation tissue.

The alcoholic, the drug addict, the epileptic and the suicide-prone all tend to be subject to thermal injury and present both therapeutic and social problems of rehabilitation.

Burns in Special Areas

Burns in areas of significant functional or aesthetic importance often require reconstruction. However, the prompt recognition of the unique problems of these areas, accompanied by aggressive attention to small detail, may prevent many of the deformities that are so resistant to later reconstruction. Consideration of these areas must begin immediately; a delay of a few days while efforts are directed toward the more dramatic systemic alterations may result in irreparable damage. The responsibility rests with the physician initially in charge of the patient, not with the reconstructive surgeon, who may not be consulted until some days, weeks or months later.

Hands. The hands represent to most patients the key to functional rehabilitation. The goals of treatment are preservation of a functional range of motion and adequate resurfacing as the prime area of skin grafting.

Initial care is directed to evaluation of the vascular status. Circumferential burns either of the hand or more proximally in the forearm or arm can result in ischemia, as an obligatory fluid accumulation occurs beneath an often unyielding eschar. Doppler ultrasound is a useful method of serially evaluating the adequacy of vascular perfusion. Decompression of the eschar should be done at first suggestion of vascular compromise. It is of particular importance to decompress the intrinsic musculature of the hands as well. Decompression can be performed using enzymatic debriding agents or by a classical escharotomy. In a large clinical series the nonsurgical decompression has proved to be rapid, safe and effective.[145] It preserves vascularity, minimizes the need for surgical intervention to re-establish circulation and enables the patient to maintain an effective range of motion.

The hand should be splinted in a position of advantage from which motion can be most easily regained and that most completely neutralizes the forces tending to produce deformity. The wrist should be extended just beyond neutral, thumb abducted and the metacarpophalangeal joints placed in complete flexion to avoid shortening of the collateral ligaments. The interphalangeal joints should be placed in a position near full extension. Since no position is functional if the fingers can't move, it is imperative that early and persistent efforts be made to maintain a full active and passive range of motion. Elevation helps reduce the contribution of gravity to edema formation. Topical antibacterials are equally indicated to prevent burn-wound sepsis.

Most burns of the hands occur on the dorsum as the hands are thrown up to protect the face against flashes of flames. So too, most burns are superficial and will be sufficiently healed within 2 weeks that topical medications may be discontinued. All burns that heal spontaneously within two weeks will be accompanied by acceptable skin cover and a good functional result. Another small group of patients have burns limited to the hand, whose depth is obviously deep as a result of contact with hot objects. In this group of patients, primary excision of the entire burn wound is indicated, with either immediate or delayed (24–48 hours) application of skin grafts.

A disturbing group of patients fail to have spontaneous healing within 2 weeks. The depth of their wounds may have been initially unclear or systemic problems may have prevented definitive early surgery.

There exists great confusion as to how to best manage these hands. Krizek et al. have recommended total excision of these wounds if they have not healed within 2 weeks.[144] They rightfully point out that this treatment can be considered a delayed primary excision since topical antibacterials have maintained bacteriological control. The biology of wound healing makes excision of the entire wound reasonable and appropriate. Others have recommended early tangential excision and grafting between the third and fifth day post-burn. Labanter states that conservatism without surgery results in good functional results.[149] Recently, a randomized series of deep dermal hand burns that had remained unhealed for 14 days has been reported.[76] After a 3-year follow-up, no differences were found between hands treated by delayed primary excision and grafting and those treated without grafting. It appeared that range of motion exercises, accurate splinting and controlled pressure on the healed wound allowed optimal healing and prevented stiffness and contractures in both groups.

When grafting is required in the burned hand, sheets of skin should be employed (Fig. 23–10). Adequate skin should be dressed into web spaces and adequate attention paid to abduction of the fingers as part of the physiotherapy. Burn syndactyly is a common complication requiring later Z-plasty release or further grafting. Post-

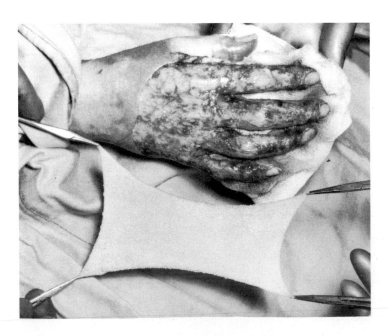

Figure 23–10. *Primary excision and grafting of a full-thickness dorsal burn of the hand. A definite effort is made to preserve the venous network. (Courtesy of John E. Hoopes, M.D.)*

operative splinting is also in the position of advantage and early motion is paramount.

Early and successful treatment of the burned hand has functional and psychological importance; a useful hand gives the patient needed reassurance of recovery and allows him to participate in his own care.

Face. Fortunately, the nature of burning and the vascularity of the facial skin usually prevent full-thickness loss. However, explosions, flash burns and scalds in children may indeed result in significant skin loss. The initial wound is often covered with grease, oil, dirt and other debris, which should be meticulously removed. Burned hair should be shaved (except the eyebrows). Blisters tend to break early and are best opened surgically and the devitalized epithelium meticulously trimmed away. The wound should then be gently cleansed with a bland soap and choice of treatment made.

These initial maneuvers require considerable intellectual discipline since they are to be done at a time when all efforts are normally expended in resuscitation. Immediate care, however, is the most appropriate; it is the least uncomfortable and avoids the development of a thick, dirty coagulum, which is present the next morning.

Vigorous scrubbing is to be avoided since it may destroy injured cells. Bacterial wound sepsis will be a determinant in conversion to full-thickness skin loss, as in other areas of the body. The use of silver nitrate is technically unsatisfactory, but the other topical antibacterials are suitable.

Eyes. The eyes are usually protected in other than chemical burns, but often at the expense of the eyelids. Burns of the eyelids are often full thickness and will result in ectropion and corneal ulcers unless grafts are applied. Initial therapy includes liberal irrigation of eyes, the use of scleral lenses and the consideration of tarsorrhaphy. Early skin grafting must remain a major priority. Contracture, even to separating a healed tarsorrhaphy, will occur unless sufficient skin is applied.

Ears. The ears are particularly exposed to thermal injury. The skin is thin and its loss results in perichondritis and avascular dissolution of cartilage. Such a complica-

tion presents an exceedingly difficult reconstructive problem since surrounding tissue is usually injured as well.

Particularly gratifying results may be obtained with the application of topical creams to the ear. Sulfamylon seems to be extremely well suited because of its ability to penetrate through the eschar to provide antibacterial protection to the cartilage. Bacterial invasion is resisted, and skin may well be salvaged.

Neck. The neck is an area of priority because of its propensity to early and severe flexion deformity. Such contracture is not only disabling but it renders anesthesia for any other procedure difficult and dangerous. The neck should be splinted in full extension and skin grafts applied early and in sufficient quantity to prevent this deformity. Postoperative splinting is also of value and may reduce the contraction of split-thickness grafts applied in this area.

Feet. Burns of the feet can cause special problems because of the propensity for edema when the burned foot is in the dependent position. The increased edema renders the burn wound more susceptible to streptococcal invasion.[248] Burns of the feet need elevation and the patient requires a specific systemic streptococcocidal antibiotic such as penicillin. The decreased temperature of pedal skin slows the healing time of the burned foot. Grafting of the deep dermal burn is often indicated to hasten recovery.

Team Care

One of the great advances in burn care has been the team concept of management. In addition to surgical and nursing care, the physical and occupational therapists, nutritionists, mental health specialists, social workers and basic scientists have assumed a proper role in the early and continued management of the patient.

It may not be as important that all patients be localized in a special area ("burn unit") as that they be cared for by a single team of interested trained personnel. Distribution of patients in several areas of the hospital is not as convenient as in a unit but may have the psychological advantage of allowing recovering patients to mingle with other than burned patients. An as yet unresolved danger of the "unit" concentrating all patients with major open wounds in a single area is the constant possibility of cross-contamination.

QUALITY OF HEALING AND REHABILITATION

The criterion of success is how well we treat burned patients.

Prevention of invasive burn-wound sepsis sustains lives. It also preserves epidermal elements in deep partial-thickness injuries. Such wounds reepithelialize from the follicles and glands, usually over prolonged periods of time. Such healing is attended by problems.[140] Pruritus is frequent and persistent for many months. Lack of adequate skin oils to lubricate the surface and regenerating sensory fibers contribute to this irritating problem. Spontaneously healed burns also are covered by a thin, fragile epithelium that tends to crack and be easily abraded by minor tangential stress. In important functional areas, resurfacing may be required. So too, spontaneously healed deep burns are prone to infection. Lacking the protective antibacterial qualities of the sebaceous glands, these wounds are susceptible to streptococcal infection and may require long-term prophylaxis with penicillin.

The normal biology of normal healing includes contraction. The duration and intensity of the inflammatory stage of healing, prior to coverage, will help determine the amount of scar and the amount of contraction. Myofibroblasts with contractile function are found in granulating wounds secondary to thermal injury. Larson believes there is a centripetal force due to these contractile cells.[153] Skin grafts applied to granulating beds retard but do not prevent such contraction. If sufficient, the clinical correlate of contraction, which is contracture, will develop.

Prevention of contracture is both more desirable and more effective than correction of deformity. The principles include splinting at all times in the optimal position to avoid contracture. The position of comfort is the position of contracture. The burn wound will shrink until it meets an opposing force.[152]

Prolonged pressure of healing tissue seems to reduce hypertrophic scarring, increase pliability and preserve contouring. This technique appears not only to arrest or suppress the production of additional hypertrophic tissue but also appears to enhance the natural remodeling process that normally occurs long after the initial injury. These changes have been elegantly documented using scanning electron microscopy.[20] Adequate resurfacing of areas that have been lost to burn injury and cannot be retrieved by splinting and pressure is the sine qua non. Finally, the greatest enemy and ally of the reconstructive surgeon is time; an enemy because all patients are desirous of early definitive correction of scarring and deformity, and an ally since time will mature scar and reduce disfigurement.

Marjolin's Ulcers

Originally noted by Celsus and accurately described by Marjolin in 1828, these ulcers are carcinomas arising in scars, particularly burn areas.

An estimated 2 per cent of all squamous cell carcinomas arise in old burn scars;[297] the incidence of burn scars becoming malignant is unknown. The presumed cause is persistent stimulation to marginal epithelialization for repeated growth and repair in irritated areas. Scar tissue is particularly liable to trauma since it is raised, tense, relatively avascular and unable to glide over underlying tissue.[13] Glover and Kiehn have failed to identify carcinoma developing in skin areas properly grafted.[101]

The age of the scar is more important than the age of the patient, with a median time interval of about 35 years, although acute carcinomas have been noted as early as 2 to 12 months post-burning. Marjolin's ulcers have a prevalence for the lower extremities and scalp and have a high incidence of regional metastasis (35 per cent) when first seen. Although the true incidence is unknown, the major hospitals treating burns report a frequency of about one new case a year.[12, 13]

It is readily apparent from the reported cases that the neglected burn scar is the one prone to carcinoma. Evidence of skin breakdown or constant irritation makes proper skin coverage imperative.

ELECTRICAL INJURIES

Robert C. Wray, Jr.

ELECTRICAL BURNS

Electricity causes 1300 deaths annually in the United States. Lightning accounts for one fourth of this number. The remainder are accidents from defective electrical equipment, momentary carelessness on part of the workers on high-tension lines and the curious child exploring electric outlets and wires. Although the number of deaths is great, serious and disabling injuries are more frequent.

EFFECTS OF ELECTRICITY

The most important factors in determining the extent of injury are intensity of current and duration of contact. Resistance at points of contact, efficiency of grounding and the pathway of current through the body also affect the severity of the injury. Low-voltage direct current is less dangerous than alternating current. In general, the higher the voltage and the longer the contact, the more severe the injury. Skin resistance is increased by thick skin and oil or grease and is decreased by thin skin and moisture. The larger the area of grounding, the greater the current flow. The current probably follows a direct line between the points of grounding. If the pathway of the current includes the heart or brain, cardiac or respiratory arrest is much more likely than if the path involves only the limbs.[37] Ineffective cardiac action may be due to asystole or fibrillation.

Three typical types of skin damage may result from electrical injury: (1) contact burns (entry and exit wounds), (2) arc burns and (3) thermal burns from ignition of clothing.

Local Tissue Effects

It is unclear whether the local tissue effects of electricity are due to the heat generated or cellular damage from electricity itself. The contact lesions (entry and exit) are quite characteristic and almost always consist of three concentric areas: (1) a charred black center, (2) a middle zone of gray-white coagulation necrosis, and (3) an outer bright red zone of partial coagulation. The area of coagulation may increase over a period of several days following the injury; this is thought to be due to progressive vascular thrombosis.

The second type of injury is from the arc burn. This burn is produced by current passing external to the body from the contact (entry) point to the exit point or ground. Burning from this source is usually not too extensive. It most commonly develops only when the entry and exit wounds are in close physical proximity. With extremely high voltages (50,000–100,000) arcing may produce extensive body burns. The third type of injury following electrical injury is a flame burn from ignition of clothing. The treatment of this is essentially as outlined previously for flame burns.

Blood Vessel Reactions

Intravascular thrombosis often leads to extensive ischemic destruction of tissue surrounding the initial injury. Furthermore, the extensive destruction of arteries may lead to secondary hemorrhage hours or days after the initial accident. Electrical injury is said to result in friability of the vessels, making control of hemorrhage difficult or impossible.

Experimental arterial lesions were produced in dogs by using 110- and 220-volt alternating and direct currents.[129] Lesions resulted only when the vessel was occluded and the circulation was stopped. From this observation it was concluded that the destructive effect of electricity on the vascular wall resulted from overheating. During free circulation heat was dissipated by the flow of blood and damage to the vascular wall was prevented. The arterial lesions that were produced in this experimental model were similar to those observed clinically. The involved wall was grossly thin and friable. The media was most strikingly involved, with marked destruction of the individual muscle cells. The internal elastic lamina was in time disrupted. In the most extensive injury, the endothelial cells were swollen and destroyed. Thrombosis was not a feature of these acute, sharply localized, experimental lesions, but widespread thrombosis is frequently observed clinically.

In another experimental study it was found that deep muscle injury occurred in dogs only if 500 or more volts were used.[124] The same authors conducted a more extensive study on rats, and the effects of 250 volts were studied. Skin resistance partially protected against electrical injury; the degree of muscle damage was much more severe if the contacts were placed directly on the muscle instead of on the skin. The limb involved with the experimental injury seemed to act as a volume conductor. Thus if the limb was of smaller diameter (distally), the severity of the injury was much greater than if the electrodes were placed more proximally. Theoretically, current conduction varies in the different tissues, but the temperatures obtained in the bone and muscle were the same after a few minutes. Arterial injury in the rats developed immediately with the passage of the current; there was no evidence of delayed or progressive vascular occlusion. This experimental finding is in contrast to the progressive occlusion when repetitive arteriograms are done in humans.[125]

Bone Destruction

Extensive destruction of bone is common in very high voltage electrical injuries. Grossly, the bone is avascular and appears whitened. Histological section shows the cells to be swollen and destroyed. Following very high voltage injuries, about 15 per cent of the patients develop bone sequestra.[22] The gradual sequestration and discharge of devitalized areas of bone results in prolonged delay in healing.

Nervous System Injury

In addition to the fairly common respiratory paralysis, other temporary paralyses may occur (particularly in the lower limbs). Ill-defined pain syndromes are often observed in addition to serious and persistent headache. Although these sequelae may subside spontaneously over the course of days, permanent residual disability has been reported.[275] Hemiplegia, aphasia, cerebellar dysfunction and epilepsy have all been reported following electrical injuries. Physiological spinal cord transection developed in 25 per cent of patients with high-voltage (> 5000 volts) electrical injury.[22] Similarly, late evidence of localized neurological injury may be reflected by the appearance of Parkinsonism and a variety of cranial nerve defects including auditory and vestibular dysfunction, facial paresis and optic atrophy. One third of patients with high-voltage injury involving the limbs developed sympathetic dystrophy.[22] A few instances of mononeuritis, with permanent loss of function of one or more peripheral nerves, have been observed. Among the more common sequelae of electrical injury is the occurrence of post-traumatic psychoneurosis, which may be prolonged and disabling.

Eye Injuries

The occurrence of cataracts following electrical injuries is of particular importance since their appearance may develop many months after the initial injury. Cataracts developed in 25 per cent of patients with high-voltage (> 5000 volts) injuries.[3] Cataracts usually follow accidents in which electrical contact was made near the eyes and may be unilateral or bilateral. In the majority of cases, the first changes appear in the anterior capsule as punctate opacities and vacuoles; this may proceed to complete opacification of the lens. Although electrical cataracts are relatively rare, patients with evidence of electrical contact near the eyes should be followed by an ophthalmologist.

Renal Dysfunction

Abnormalities of the urine sediment are commonly observed in electrothermal injuries. The problem of anuria following these accidents has been emphasized. Taylor and his co-workers[292] noted seven instances of prolonged renal complications in a consecutive series of seven patients with 22 electrical injuries treated at the Brooke Army Medical Center. Six of these seven patients expired and at autopsy acute tubular necrosis was observed in each. Shock undoubtedly plays a significant role in the production of this lesion. Fischer[87] has emphasized the importance of myoglobinuria and hemoglobinuria in predisposing the kidney to acute failure following electrical injuries. Significant hemoglobinemia may be observed following electrical accidents as a result of electrothermal injury and lysis of red cells. Similarly, the release of myoglobin from destroyed muscle may further increase the levels of circulating chromoprotein. Most authorities agree that precipitation of myoglobin and hemoglobin in the renal tubules, if not the cause of, is certainly contributory to the development of acute renal failure.[43]

Gastrointestinal Tract Abnormalities

Nausea, vomiting and prolonged paralytic ileus are as common following electrothermal injuries as they are after thermal burns and other major trauma. Although the ileus is usually brief, other gastrointestinal tract problems are more severe. In one study[22] about 15 per cent of the patients developed massive hemorrhage from gastric or duodenal ulcers. Pancreatic necrosis as well as necrosis and perforation of the gallbladder and intestine has been observed following electrical injuries.[19] The etiology of these intra-abdominal lesions is uncertain; however, diffuse vascular injury seems the most likely cause. In one study about 15 per cent of the patients developed cholelithiasis 3 months to 3 years after their injury.[22]

Fluid and Electrolyte Disturbances

The coexistence of electrical and thermal injuries is relatively common when clothing is ignited by arcing in high-tension injuries. Fluid loss in most of these patients is proportional to the area of the thermal burn. However, in severe electrical injuries with death of large volumes of muscle, extremely large fluid loss may occur.[263] Significant blood loss may occur as a consequence of vascular injury or from associated fractures and chest and abdominal trauma. Shock must not be accepted as a manifestation of the uncomplicated electrical injury; the possibility of associated hemorrhage or perforation of an intra-abdominal viscus must always be considered.

Associated Injuries

The violent, tetanic muscular contraction that results from contact (particularly with alternating-current sources) may result in a variety of fractures and dislocations. However, in a recent study,[22] falls resulting from electrical contact caused the only fractures noted. Fractures were found in about 10 per cent of the patients.

TREATMENT

Resuscitation

Immediate first aid involves mouth-to-mouth respiration and external cardiac massage if cardiorespiratory arrest has occurred. Prolonged respiratory support may be required as coma is occasionally observed following electrical injury. The associated injuries just mentioned must be treated. Continuous nasogastric suction for 24 to 48 hours is required following major electrical injuries. The fluid and electrolyte requirements are usually due to any associated thermal injury, but in massive electrical injuries large volumes of fluid must be administered. No formula is available for calculating the requirement, but sufficient lactated Ringer's solution to produce an adequate urine output is recommended. Due to the possibility of renal failure from precipitation of myoglobin and hemoglobin, urine output should be 40 to 50 per ml. per hour. Alkalinization of the urine with intravenous sodium bicarbonate is probably helpful, although its value is not proven. If urine output decreases despite apparently adequate volume loading solute diuresis with mannitol is indicated.

Antimicrobial Treatment

The most frequent cause of death following electrical injury is the same as that following thermal injury, systemic infection. In one recent series,[22] 7 per cent of the deaths were due to sepsis. In another series,[194] approximately one third of the patients developed sepsis sometime during their hospitalization. Sepsis can arise from necrotic muscle mass, bacterial invasion in the associated thermal burn or from perforations of the gastrointestinal tract. The topical antibacterials recommended for thermal burns (silver sulfadiazine, silver nitrate, Sulfamylon) may all be used for electrical injuries. Sulfamylon is of documented value because of its ability to penetrate eschar into underlying tissue. The overall mortality for isolated thermal burns and electrical injuries is about the same (15 per cent).[194]

Surgical Treatment

The cornerstone for surgical treatment is early escharotomy and fasciotomy. Fasciotomy will almost always be needed after high-voltage electrical injuries. It is now clear that the escharotomies and fasciotomies should usually begin at the most distal portion of the limb that is injured. Thus, mid-lateral escharotomies in the fingers and toes and decompression of the dorsal intrinsic muscles in the hand are necessary to maintain or salvage maximum function of the hand.

Both primary excision and watchful waiting have their place in the management of electrical burn wounds.[251] The proper choice is determined by the nature and location of the initial wound. The progressive necrosis that occurs with electrical injuries often leads to underestimation of the severity in the early stages. Difficulty with early excision lies in determining the depth of injury. Attempts at early primary closure may fail as a result of extension of the necrosis. On the other hand, the irretrievably damaged limb may serve as a source for the absorption of substances that destroy the kidneys and provide a culture medium for bacteria. In massive injury, early open amputation may be life-saving. Injuries involving the volar surface of the forearm and the hand are among the most challenging. Although the tendon and nerve may not be involved in the primary wound, they may be jeopardized when subsequently exposed by tissue slough. Early excision and closure by pedicle flap have been used to prevent secondary involvement, but loss of the tendon still occurs in the majority of cases.

Several recent studies have defined the commonness of amputation following high-tension (greater than 1000 volt) electrical injuries. In cases in which the limb is one of the points of entry or exit, about 70 per cent of the limbs will require major amputation.[169, 244] When the limb is ischemic on presentation, the rate of major amputation probably will be even higher. When the limb is not ischemic, about 40 per cent of the patients will still have residual dysfunction or will require minor amputations.[169] When the entry and exit points are not considered, about 50 per cent of the patients will require a "usually major" amputation of the upper or lower limb.[110, 194, 266] From 30 to 50 per cent of the remaining patients have residual dysfunction or require minor amputation.

It is generally agreed that the conservative approach is preferred in children with electrical burns about the mouth.[231] Delayed reconstruction appears to provide the most satisfactory results. Similarly, delayed debridement seems most satisfactory in electrical burns of the head. Large areas of the calvarium may be exposed and devitalized bone should be allowed to sequestrate spontaneously before a program of reconstruction is begun.

CHEMICAL BURNS

Robert C. Wray, Jr.

Most chemical burns are due to contact with acid or alkali. The most important step in the care of these burns is the removal of the noxious agent. Copious irriga- tion with water is the best initial treatment for all chemical burns.[35] If the patient has come into contact with hydrofluoric acid of greater than 20 per cent concentration, subcutaneous injection of a 10 per cent solution of calcium gluconate (about 0.5 ml./cm.² of burn) is the second step in treatment.[65] (Newer information[139] has suggested that intra-arterial perfusion of 4 per cent calcium gluconate is more effective than subcutaneous 10 per cent calcium gluconate. Excellent results were obtained with the intra-arterial route in experimental animals and patients.) The second step in the treatment of white phosphorus burns is irrigation with 1 per cent copper sulfate; re-irrigation with water and de-bridement of the particles should follow.[56] Other acid and alkali burns require only water irrigation for about 24 hours. Tissue repair cannot proceed until the agent has been inactivated by combination with tissues, neutralization or disposal. Following initial management, the basic principles utilized in thermal injury are applicable. Early excision and grafting usually cannot be employed because of uncertainty regarding the depth of injury. Definitive wound closure awaits the appearance of healthy granulation tissue.

COLD INJURY

Robert C. Wray, Jr.

CLINICAL FEATURES

The impression that trench foot and frostbite are distinct clinical entities has caused considerable confusion. Although the thermal conditions that lead to trench foot or frostbite may be quite different in degree, the common factor is cold.

TRENCH FOOT

Trench foot develops slowly over a period of hours or days due to exposure to moisture and cold (at temperatures usually above freezing). The extremity first becomes anesthetic; pain is noted only during extremes of motion and during weight-bearing. Considerable swelling later develops and the skin appears white and cold. As the lesion progresses, blisters filled with serous or serosanguineous fluid appear; eventually, the overlying skin desiccates and becomes gangrenous. The limb is never actually frozen.

In the late stage, the skin overlying the digits or indeed the whole lower limb may appear nonviable. It is difficult to estimate the depth of injury since the nonviable skin may separate, leaving pink, newly formed underlying skin or granulation tissue. If there is more severe damage, the deeper tissues are involved. These extensive injuries ultimately become shrunken and there is a sharp line of demarcation between the viable and nonviable parts.

FROSTBITE

Frostbite occurs rapidly and as a consequence of exposure to extreme cold; in the past this was frequently due to exposure at high altitudes while flying. The skin becomes blanched, and a stinging sensation is noted. The involved part becomes numb and a sensation of clumsiness is often reported. The member is firm to the touch and is, in fact, frozen. However, swelling is not an early manifestation. Thawing is attended by severe, dull, aching pains; the limb rapidly becomes hyperemic and swelling and blister formation are soon observed. Vesicles are filled with straw-colored or blood-tinged fluid. In time, the involved areas of skin become black and firm, producing the appearance of gangrene. Again, it is impossible to determine the depth of injury since the blackened skin may peel off, revealing healthy granulation tissue or newly formed skin. In the most severe injuries, however, gangrene may involve the entire substance of the extremity.

The frequency of frostbite in civilian practice depends primarily upon the latitude of the hospital. In Helsinki, Finland (latitude about 60° N) 110 patients were treated for frostbite at a single hospital within 2 years[148]; at Barnes and Allied Hospitals in St. Louis, Missouri (latitude approximately 38° N), we see about 10 patients every 2 years. In the study from Finland almost all of the patients had been drinking heavily before their injury. Both trench foot and true frostbite were present in the patients; this duality exists in the usual nonmilitary practice. The other potential victims are hunters, mountain climbers and explorers.

PREDISPOSING FACTORS TO INJURY

The most important environmental factors that influence the effects of cold are humidity and wind. Increase in the humidity or wind velocity increases the rate of heat loss from tissues. Anything that decreases local tissue perfusion (e.g., atherosclerosis, arteritides, constriction due to tight clothing, etc.) will increase the susceptibility of tissue to cold injury. Smoking and alcohol intake both increase the severity of cold injury. The elimination of drunkenness would prevent the vast majority of cold injuries in civilians.

PATHOPHYSIOLOGY OF COLD INJURY

The application of cold produces an immediate and marked arteriolar vasoconstriction.[162] Profound tissue anoxia results from the disturbance of blood flow that accompanies arteriolar vasoconstriction and the derangement in oxygen transport that is produced by the influence of cold upon the dissociation of oxyhemoglobin.

With thawing, the arterioles reopen and blood flow returns to the involved vascular bed, changing the white frozen appearance to that of hyperemia. This "flare" is soon accompanied by swelling, which results from the loss of intravascular fluid into the interstitial spaces as edema. Lewis[162, 163] related the occurrence of this wheal and flare response to the local release of a tissue substance (possibly histamine). After mild cold injury, this may be the only consequence; with more severe degrees of injury, however, an additional sequence is observed. Coincident to the development of interstitial edema, blood flow again slows and the dilated vessels become engorged with masses of erythrocytes.[150] For an undetermined period of time, these masses of erythrocytes can be broken up by gentle manipulation and

only later are true occlusive thrombi formed. The importance of thrombotic arterial occlusions in cold injury seems often to have been overlooked.[98, 245]

Weatherley-White and his co-workers[306] reported the results of an instructive experiment that defines the importance of the vascular lesions in the pathogenesis of cold injury. Injury was produced in one rabbit ear by its immersion in a mixture of solid carbon dioxide and ethanol. A circular full-thickness skin graft was then removed from both ears and each graft was reimplanted on the opposite ear — frozen skin on the normal ear and normal skin on the frozen ear. Uniformly, the frozen skin survived when transplanted to the normal ear, whereas normal skin necrosed on the frozen ear. However, the ability of various tissues to withstand cold injury is inversely proportional to their water content. The most easily injured tissues are vessels, followed by muscle, nerve, skin, dense connective tissue and bone. Thus, cell death is usually produced by direct impairment of cellular metabolism but tissue loss in the clinical circumstances appears to be more dependent upon the status of the local circulation following cold exposure. The anatomy of the vascular lesions apparently determines the eventual extent of tissue necrosis.

Since the extent of ischemic tissue loss following cold injury seems ultimately related directly to vascular occlusion, arteriography should afford a useful means of evaluating the extent of these injuries. Although Leriche and Kinlin[159] published in 1940 the results of Thorotrast arteriography in extremities injured by cold, there seems to have been little subsequent interest in their observations.

TREATMENT

Local Therapy

Since cold exerts its influence from exposure of the body surface and human tissues are imperfect thermal conductors, the extent of injury diminishes from the surface toward the deeper tissue levels. The superficial layers of skin are most strikingly involved; therefore, it is difficult to assess the eventual extent of tissue loss from the early appearance of the part. Consequently, it is expedient to avoid premature excision of apparently nonviable extremities after cold injury. A few days' to weeks' delay will allow a clear demarcation between viable and nonviable tissues and obviate the risk of removing salvageable and potentially useful tissue.

Rapid warming of the injured area is the most important step in treatment.[182, 304] The frozen extremity is placed in water having a temperature of 40 to 44° C. Rewarming for 20 to 30 minutes is usually sufficient. Dry heat should never be used and the application of blankets alone results in slow warming. The injured area should be cleansed carefully, and if injury involves the lower limbs, the toes should be separated by gauze. The area is then allowed exposure to air as bacterial proliferation in the tissue is not a common problem. Tetanus prophylaxis is given. Prophylactic antibiotics are usually administered, although proof for their effectiveness is lacking. Early amputation is indicated only in the face of uncontrolled or gas-producing sepsis. As a clear line of demarcation between viable and nonviable tissues becomes apparent, surgical debridement is undertaken. The normal vascularity of tissues immediately proximal to those destroyed provides the opportunity for a variety of reconstructive procedures. Useful limbs can, as a rule, be salvaged. In planning these procedures as well as in evaluating the eventual extent of tissue loss, arteriography may have considerable value.

The unpredictability of the eventual extent of tissue loss makes evaluation of the measures that have been proposed to diminish the tissue loss difficult.

Sympathectomy

Enthusiastic reports from Europe concerning the results of sympathetic block and of sympathectomy in the treatment of cold injuries during World War II were soon followed by reports of similar experiences in this country. Controversy continues about the precise role of sympathectomy in the acute lesion. This is based partly on the lack of an adequate means of assessing the results of treatment and partly on a lack of general agreement concerning the rationale of sympathectomy in the treatment of cold injury. It seems significant, however, that the precise role remains poorly defined more than 25 years after Ducuing[74] reported the results of sympathetic nerve interruption in some 300 patients.

It has been suggested that the vascular stasis that is observed after cold injury reflects the presence of arterial vasospasm. It has also been suggested that arteriovenous shunting may reduce effective tissue perfusion after cold injury. In support of this latter suggestion, it has been observed that the venous oxygen content is increased during recovery from cold injury. Fontaine and his co-workers[89] observed a rapid rise in the venous oxygen content during cooling of the canine limb. This rise in venous oxygen content, to a level nearly equal to arterial blood, apparently reflects the diminished metabolism of the limb occasioned by cooling as well as the influence of cold upon the oxygen dissociation curve of hemoglobin. With warming, the venous oxygen difference never returned to the control level. In the absence of direct measurements of blood flow in the limb or of a quantitative measure of tissue damage in the limb, these data cannot be conclusively interpreted to support the suggestion that arteriovenous shunts are opened by cold injury.

If an influence of the sympathetic nervous system is primarily concerned in the pathophysiology of cold injury, it seems reasonable that early sympathectomy should protect against tissue loss. On the contrary, experimental evidence indicates that sympathectomy performed within the first few hours of injury increased the edema formation and accelerated the pathological process of tissue destruction.[104, 305] It is difficult, therefore, to assign the sympathetic nervous system a primary role in the production of cold injury. It has been demonstrated in an experimental cold injury involved in the rabbit ear, however, that sympathectomy performed 24 to 48 hours after thawing hastens the resolution of edema and reduces the extent of tissue loss.[104] These experimental findings coincide with the clinical observation of the many proponents of sympathectomy.[102, 103, 264] The apparent beneficial effects of sympathectomy seem to reflect an increase in collateral circulation in the injured limb. The prominent element of arterial occlusion in relationship to cold injury has been emphasized. Sympathectomy apparently effects an increase in collateral circulation about these vascular occlusions.

In summary, sympathectomy 36 to 72 hours after injury is recommended only in those patients who may be anticipated to have a significant loss of a portion of the limb.

Anticoagulants

It has been noted that vessels shortly after thawing are dilated and filled with clumps of erythrocytes. In this early stage there is no evidence that thrombosis has occurred, since the erythrocyte clumps can easily be dislodged by gentle manipulation. The mechanism that leads to clumping is not known, but it may reflect the presence of a cold-induced increase in blood viscosity. This possibility suggests that low-molecular-weight dextran might be useful in the early treatment of cold injury. No controlled clinical study of the influence of this substance on the natural history of cold injury has been reported. Experimentally, however, treatment with low-molecular-weight dextran in doses of one gm./kg./day has been demonstrated to protect against tissue loss in rabbits.[305] Therefore, 1,000 ml. of 6 per cent dextran should be given on the day of injury and 500 ml. of the same solution every day for 5 days.

It is generally agreed that thrombi eventually form in the dilated, erythrocyte-filled vessels, possibly as late as 72 hours after thawing. This observation led to the suggestion that heparin might be useful in treatment of cold injury. The early favorable clinical experimental results were reported by Lange and his co-workers.[151] Subsequent workers,[54, 265] however, have been unable to substantiate these findings, and at the present time there is no evidence that heparin alters the natural history of the disease. Due to the aforementioned and the dangers of the use of heparin, I do not recommend the administration of heparin in the treatment of cold injury.

Intra-arterial reserpine has been used for the treatment of frostbite, and in experimental animals some benefit can be shown. Slow rewarming was compared with slow rewarming combined with intravenous dextran, intra-arterial tolazoline, intra-arterial reserpine and various combinations of the drugs. All of the drug treatments were superior to simple slow rewarming. The combination of intra-arterial tolazoline and reserpine with or without dextran was the most effective regimen. However, rapid rewarming was as effective as any drug treatment.[279] Only five patients have been reported to be treated with intra-arterial reserpine.[233] Three of these patients were treated within 2 weeks of their injuries. Angiography before injection of reserpine was followed by angiography after injection of reserpine. Reserpine seemed to be effective in relieving vascular spasm. Treatment did not seem to affect the progression of cutaneous gangrene. Reserpine relieved pain and paresthesias in two patients treated late after their cold injuries. Oral reserpine has not been shown to be effective in the treatment of cold injury.

LATE SEQUELAE

A particularly informative study of the late sequelae to cold injury was reported by Blair et al.,[28] who observed a group of 100 veterans of the Korean conflict 4 years after their injuries. They found that the late symptoms, in order of decreasing frequency, included excessive sweating, pain, coldness, numbness, abnormal skin color and pain and stiffness of the joints. In addition, frequent asymptomatic abnormalities of the nails, including ridging and inward curving of the edges, were observed.

It is likely that hyperhidrosis is both a cause and result of cold injury. Hyperhidrosis suggests the presence of an abnormality involving the sympathetic nervous system induced by cold injury and, indeed, hyperhidrosis is abolished by appropriate sympathetic denervation. Sensitivity to cold and the predisposition to recurrent cold injury are, in some respects, analogous to the consideration of hyperhidrosis. Blanching and pain upon subsequent cold exposure may be quite troublesome and at times so dramatic as to suggest a diagnosis of Raynaud's phenomenon. These symptoms are commonly dramatically relieved by sympathetic interruption. It seems quite unjustified, however, to imply that hyperhidrosis or cold sensitivity is necessarily the manifestation of an abnormality of the sympathetic nervous system or of an abnormal vascular response to sympathetic vasoconstrictor impulses. Hyperhidrosis and cold sensitivity may both precede and follow cold injury.

The late abnormalities of change in skin color, including depigmentation in the black and an appearance resembling erythrocyanosis in the white patient, are most likely the result of ischemia. Similarly, the abnormalities of the nails are comparable to those seen with ischemia, regardless of its cause. Neither of these abnormalities usually requires specific treatment.

Late symptoms of joint stiffness and pain on motion are relatively common and undoubtedly are often related to overlying scars and to mechanical problems occasioned by the variety of amputations required. Blair and his co-workers,[28] however, frequently observed "punched-out" defects in the subchondral bone of the involved limbs. These localized areas of bone resorption generally appear within 5 to 10 months after injury and may heal spontaneously. Vascular occlusion was felt to represent the most likely cause of these lesions. These bone changes, in close proximity to joint surfaces, help explain the joint symptoms.

The effects of frostbite on the growing hand have been recently re-emphasized.[72] All seventeen patients (26 hands) had premature closure of at least one epiphysis. The extent of premature closure was correlated with the severity of the frostbite but closure occurred with only partial-thickness injury. In the fingers, premature closure was more frequent from a distal to proximal direction (that is, the distal interphalangeal joint more frequently than the proximal interphalangeal joint and the proximal interphalangeal joint more frequently than the metacarpophalangeal joint). The thumb was less often involved than the fingers. In 2 per cent of the patients partial epiphyseal closure caused angular deformities.

REFERENCES

1. Abramson, D. J.: The care of severely burned children. Surg. Gynecol. Obstet. *122*:855, 1966.
2. Achauer, B. M., Allyn, P. A., Furnas, D. W., and Bartlett, R. H.: Pulmonary complications of burns: The major threat to the burn patient. Ann. Surg. *177*:311, 1973.
3. Adam, A. L., and Klein, M.: Electrical cataract: Notes on a case and a review of the literature. Br. J. Ophthalmol. *29*:169, 1945.
4. Alexander, J. W.: Serum and leukocyte lysosomal enzymes. Derangements following severe thermal injury. Arch. Surg. *95*:482, 1965.
5. Alexander, J. W., Fisher, M. W., and MacMillan, B. G.: Immunological control of *Pseudomonas* infection in burn patients: A clinical evaluation. Arch. Surg. *102*:31, 1971.
6. Alexander, J. W., McClellan, M. A., Ogle, C. K., and Ogle, J. D.: Consumptive opsoninopathy: Possible pathogenesis in lethal and opportunistic infections. Ann. Surg. *184*:672, 1976.
7. Alexander, J. W., and Meakins, J. L.: Natural defense mechanisms in clinical sepsis. J. Surg. Res. *11*:148, 1971.
8. Alexander, J. W., and Moncrief, J. A.: Immunologic phenomena in burn injuries. J.A.M.A. *199*:105, 1967.
9. Allgöwer, M., Cueni, L. B., Stadtler K., et al.: Burn toxin in mouse skin. J. Trauma *13*:95, 1973.
10. Altemeier, W. A., MacMillan, B. G., and Hill, E. O.: The rationale of specific antibiotic therapy in the management of major burns. Surgery *52*:240, 1962.
11. Arney, G. K., Pearson, E., and Sutherland, A. B.: Burn stress pseudodiabetes. Ann. Surg. *152*:77, 1960.
12. Arons, M. S., Lynch, J. B., Lewis, S. R., and Blocker, T. G., Jr.: Scar tissue carcinoma. Part I. A clinical study with special reference to burn scar carcinoma. Ann. Surg. *161*:170, 1965.
13. Arons, M. S., Rodin, A. E., Lynch, J. B., Lewis, S. R., and Blocker, T. G., Jr.: Scar tissue carcinoma. II. An experimental study with special reference to burn scar carcinomas. Ann. Surg. *163*:445, 1966.
14. Arthurson, G.: Evaporation and fluid replacement: Research in burns. *In* Matter, P., et al. (eds.): Transactions of the Third International Congress on Research in Burns. Berne, Hans Huber Publishers, 1971, p. 520.
15. Artz, C. P.: Understanding thermal burns and principles of management. *In* Davis, J. H. (ed.): Current Concepts in Surgery. New York, McGraw-Hill Book Co., 1965.
16. Artz, C. P., and Moncrief, J. A.: The Treatment of Burns. Philadelphia, W. B. Saunders Co., 1969.
17. Asch, M. J., Curreri, P. W., and Pruitt, B. A., Jr.: Thermal injury involving bone: Report of 32 cases. J. Trauma *12*:135, 1972.
18. Backdahl, M., Liljedahl, S. O., and Troel, L.: Excision of deep burns. Acta Chir. Scand. *123*:351, 1962.
19. Baldwin, W. M., and Dondate, M.: High frequency current burns in rats. Proc. Soc. Exper. Biol. Med. *27*:65, 1929.
20. Bauer, P. S., Larson, D. L., Stacey, T. R., Barratt, G. F., and Dobrkovsky, M.: Ultrastructural

analysis of pressure treated human hypertrophic scars. J. Trauma 16:958, 1976.

21. Baxter, C. R.: Burns. In Shires, G. T. (ed.): Care of the Trauma Patient. New York, McGraw-Hill Book Co., 1966.

22. Baxter, C. R.: Present concepts in the management of major electrical injury. Surg. Clin. North Am. 50:1401, 1970.

23. Baxter, C. R.: Topical use of 1.0% silver sulfadiazine. In Polk, H. C. and Stone, H. H. (eds.): Contemporary Burn Management. Boston, Little, Brown, 1971, pp. 217–225.

24. Baxter, C. R., Loebl, E. C., and Curreri, P. W.: Mechanism of erythrocyte destruction in the early post-burn period. Presented, fifth annual meeting of The American Burn Assocaton. Dallas, Texas, April 7, 1973.

25. Benain, F., Pattin, M., and Rappaport, M.: Puncture biopsies of the liver in critical burns. In Artz, C. P. (ed.): Research in Burns. Philadelphia, F. A. Davis Co., 1962, pp. 185–193.

26. Berkow, S. A.: A method for estimating the extensiveness of lesions (burns and scalds), based on surface area proportions. Arch. Surg. 8:138, 1924.

27. Black, J., Calesnick, B., Williams, D., and Weinstein, M. J.: Pharmacology of Gentamicin, a new broad-spectrum antibiotic. Antibiot. Chemother. 138–147, 1963.

28. Blair, J. R., Schatzki, R., and Orr, N. D.: Sequelae to cold injury in one hundred patients: Follow-up study four years after occurrence of cold injury. J.A.M.A. 163:1203, 1957.

29. Blalock, A.: Experimental shock. VII. The importance of the local loss of fluid in the production of the low blood pressure after burns. Arch. Surg. 22:610, 1931.

30. Blocker, T. G., Jr.: Burns. In Converse, J. M. (ed.): Reconstructive Plastic Surgery. Philadelphia, W. B. Saunders Co., 1964.

31. Blocker, T. G., Lewis, S. R., Kirby, E. J.: Levin, W. C., Perry, J. H., and Blocker, V.: The problem of protein disequilibrium following severe thermal trauma. In Artz, C. P. (ed.): Research in Burns. Philadelphia, F. A. Davis Co., 1962, pp. 121–124.

32. Boswick, J. A., Jr.: Topical therapy of the burn wound with mafenide acetate. In Polk, H. C., and Stone, H. H. (eds.): Contemporary Burn Management. Boston, Little, Brown, 1971, pp. 193–202.

33. Brentano, L., Moyer, C. A., Grovens, D. L., and Monafo, W. W.: Bacteriology of large human burns treated with silver nitrate. Arch. Surg. 93:456, 1966.

34. Bromberg, B. E., and Song, I. C.: Homografts and heterografts as skin substitutes. Am. J. Surg. 112:28, 1966.

35. Bromberg, B. E., Song, I. C., and Walden, R. H.: Hydrotherapy of chemical burns. Plast. Reconstr. Surg. 35:85, 1965.

36. Brown, J. B., Fryer, M. P., Randall, P., and Lu, M.: Postmortem homografts as "biological dressings" for extensive burns and denuded areas. Ann. Surg. 138:618, 1953.

37. Brown, K. L., and Moritz, A. R.: Electrical injuries. J. Trauma 4:608, 1964.

38. Bruch, H. M., Nash, G., Foley, F. D., and Pruitt, B. A.: Opportunistic fungal infection of the burn wound with Phycomycetes and Aspergillus. Arch. Surg. 102:476, 1971.

39. Bull, J. P., and Squire, J. R.: A study of mortality in a burns unit: Standards for the evaluation of alternative methods of treatment. Ann. Surg. 130:160, 1949.

40. Burke, J. F., Bondoc, C. C., and Quinby, W. C.: Primary burn excision and prompt grafting for the treatment of thermal burns in children. J. Trauma 14:389, 1974.

41. Burke, J. F., May, J. W., Albright, N., Quinby, W. C., and Russell, P. S.: Temporary skin transplantation and immunosuppression for extensive burns. N. Engl. J. Med. 290:269, 1974.

42. Burke, J. F., Quinby, W. C., Bondoc, C. C., Cosimi, A. B., Russelel, P. S., and Szyfelbein, S. K.: Immunosuppression and temporary skin transplantation in the treatment of massive third degree burns. Ann. Surg. 182:183, 1975.

43. Bywaters, E. G. L.: Ischemic muscle necrosis; crushing injury, traumatic edema, crush syndrome, traumatic anuria, compression syndrome; type of injury seen in air raid casualties following burial beneath debris. J.A.M.A. 124:1103, 1944.

44. Chan, C. K., Jarret, F., and Moylan, J. A.: Acute leukopenia as an allergic reaction to silver sulfadiazine in burn patients. J. Trauma 16:395, 1976.

45. Cohen, I. K., Schecter, P. J., and Henkins, R. I.: Decreased taste acuity and zinc loss following thermal injury. Presentation, American Society of Plastic Surgeons, Las Vegas, September 1972.

46. Cohen, S.: An investigation and fractional assessment of the evaporative water loss through normal skin and burn eschars using a microhydrometer. Plast. Reconstr. Surg. 37:475, 1966.

47. Collentine, G. E., Waisbren, B. A., and Mellender, J. W.: Treatment of burns with intensive antibiotic therapy and exposure. J.A.M.A. 200:939, 1967.

48. Conizaro, P. C., Sawyer, R. B., and Switzer, W. E.: Blood loss during excision of third degree burns. Arch. Surg. 88:800, 1964.

49. Constantian, M. B.: Association of sepsis with an immunosuppressive polypeptide in the serum of burn patients. Ann. Surg. 188:209, 1978.

50. Cook, W. A., Baxter, C. R., and Ferrell, J. M., Jr.: Pulmonary circulation after dermal burns. Vasc. Surg. 2:1, 1968.

51. Cossman, D. V., and Krizek, T. J.: Effect of silver lactate and silver sulfadiazine on experimental burn wound sepsis. Surg. Forum 22:495, 1971.

52. Craig, R. D. P.: Immunotherapy for severe burns in children. Plast. Reconstr. Surg. 35:263, 1965.

53. Cramer, L. M., McCormack, R. M., and Carroll, D. B.: Progressive partial excision and early grafting in lethal burns. Plast. Reconstr. Surg. 30:595, 1962.

54. Crismon, J. M.: Science in World War II. Advances in Military Medicine. Boston, Little, Brown, 1948, p. 176.

55. Cruickshank, G. N. D., and Hershey, F. B.: The effect of heat on the metabolism of guinea pigs' ear skin. Ann. Surg. *151*:419, 1960.

56. Curreri, P. W., Asch, M. J. and Pruitt, B. A.: The treatment of chemical burns; specialized diagnostic, therapeutic and prognostic considerations. J. Trauma *10*:634, 1970.

57. Curreri, P. W., Bruck, H. M., Lindberg, R. B., Mason, A. D., Jr., and Pruitt, B. A.: *Providencia stuartii* sepsis: A new challenge in the treatment of thermal injury. Ann. Surg. *177*:133, 1973.

58. Curreri, P. W.: Metabolic and nutritional aspects of thermal injury. Burns *2*:16, 1976.

59. Curreri, P. W., Wilmore, D. W., Mason, A. D., Jr., et al.: Intracellular cation alterations following major trauma: Effect of supranormal caloric intake. J. Trauma *11*:390, 1971.

60. Czaja, A. J., McAlhany, J. C., and Pruitt, B. A.: Acute gastroduodenal disease after thermal injury. N. Engl. J. Med. *291*:925, 1974.

61. Dahinterova, J., and Dobrkovsky, M.: Treatment of the burned surface by amnion and chorion grafts. Sborn. Ved. Prac. Lek. Fak. Karlov. Univ. (Suppl.) *11*:513, 1968.

62. Davis, B., Lilly, H. A., and Lowbury, E. J. L.: Gram-negative bacilli in burns. J. Clin. Pathol. *22*:634, 1969.

63. Dennis, D. L., and Peterson, C. G.: Candida and other fungi. *In* Polk, H. C., and Stone, H. H. (eds.): Contemporary Burn Management. Boston, Little, Brown, 1971, pp. 329–338.

64. Dhennin, C., Pinon, G., and Greco, J. M.: Alterations of complement system following thermal injury: Use in estimation of vital prognosis. J. Trauma *18*:129, 1978.

65. Dibbell, D., Iverson, R. E., Jones, W., Laub, D. R., and Madison, M.: Hydrofluoric acid burns of the hand. J. Bone Joint Surg. *52A*:931, 1970.

66. Dimick, A. R.: Experience with the use of proteolytic enzyme (Travase) in burn patients. J. Trauma *17*:948, 1977.

67. Dino, B. R., Eufemio, G. G., and DeVilla, M. S.: Human amnion: The establishment of an amnion bank and its practical applications in surgery. J. Phillip Med. Assoc. *42*:357, 1966.

68. Dodson, E. L., and Warner, G. E. Early circulatory disturbances following experimental thermal trauma. Circ. Res. *5*:69, 1957.

69. Douglas, B.: Homografts of fetal membranes as a covering for large wounds — especially those from burns. J. Tenn. Med. Assoc. *45*:230, 1952.

70. Douglas, B., Conway, H., Stark, R. B., Jesslin, D. and Nieto-Cano, G.: The fate of homologous and heterologous chorionic transplants as observed by the transparent tissue chamber technique in the mouse. Plast. Reconstr. Surg. *13*:125, 1954.

71. Dorr, L. D., Asch, M. J., and Zawacki, B. E.: Re-evaluation of surgical therapy of Curling's ulcer in children: Report of five patients with four survivors. Presented, fifth annual meeting of the American Burn Association, Dallas, Texas, April 6, 1973.

72. Dowdle, J. A., Leven, J. H., House, J. H., and Thompson, W. W.: Frostbite: Effect on the juvenile hand. J. Hand Surg. (in press)

73. Dressler, D. P., and Skornick, W. A.: The laboratory evaluation of topical silver nitrate in experimental burn wound sepsis. J. Trauma *12*:791, 1972.

74. Ducuing, J., D'Harcourt, J., Folch, A., and Bofill, J.: Les troubles trophiques des produits par de froid sec en pathologie de guerre. J. Chir. *55*:385, 1940.

75. Eade, G. G.: The relationship between granulation tissue, bacteria, and skin grafts in burned patients. Plast. Reconstr. Surg. *22*:42, 1958.

76. Edstrom, L. E., Robson, M. C., Macchiaverna, J. R., and Scala, A. D.: Prospective randomized treatments for burned hands: Nonoperative vs. operative. Preliminary report. Scand. J. Plast. Reconstr. Surg. (in press)

77. Ehrlich, H. P., Tarver, H., and Hunt, T. K.: Effects of vitamin A and glucocorticoids upon inflammation and collagen synthesis. Ann. Surg. *177*:222, 1973.

78. Epstein, B. S., Hardy, D. L., Harrison, H. N., Teplitz, G., Villareal, Y., and Mason, A. D.: Hypoxemia in the burned patient. A clinical-pathologic study. Ann. Surg. *158*:924, 1963.

79. Eriksson, E., and Robson, M. C.: New pathophysiologic mechanism explaining postburn edema. Burns *4*:153, 1978.

80. Eurenius, K., McManus, W. F., McEuen, D. D., et al.: Coagulation dynamics after thermal injury. Presented, fifth annual meeting of The American Burn Association, Dallas, Texas, April 7, 1973.

81. Evans, E. B., and Blumel, J.: Bone and joint changes following burns. *In* Artz, C. P. (ed.): Research in Burns. Philadelphia, F. A. Davis Co., 1962, pp. 26–32.

82. Evans, E. I., and Butterfield, W. J. H.: The stress response in the severely burned patient. Ann. Surg. *134*:588, 1951.

83. Fallon, R. H., and Moyer, C. A.: Rates of insensible perspiration through normal, burned, tape-stripped and epidermally denuded living human skin. Ann. Surg. *158*:915, 1963.

84. Feller, I., Flora, J. D., and Bawol, R.: Baseline results of therapy for burned patients. J.A.M.A. *236*:1943, 1976.

85. Fidler, J. P., MacMillan, B. G., Law, E. J., et al.: CO_2 laser excision of acute burns with immediate autografting. Presented, fifth annual meeting of The American Burn Association, Dallas, Texas, April 1973.

86. Fikrig, S. M., Karl, S. G., and Suntharalingma, K.: Neutrophil chemotaxis in patients with burns. Ann. Surg. *186*:746, 1977.

87. Fischer, H.: Pathological effects and sequelae of electrical accidents. J. Occupat. Med. *7*:564, 1965.

88. Foley, F. D., Greenawald, K. A., Nash, G., and Pruitt, B. A., Jr.: Herpesvirus infection in burned patients. N. Engl. J. Med. *282*:652, 1970.

89. Fontaine, R., Klein, M., Bollack, C., Kuhlman, N., and Sapicas, I.: Clinical and experimental contribution to the study of frostbite. J. Cardiovasc. Surg. 2:449, 1961.

90. Fox, C. L., Jr.: Clinical experience with silver sulfadiazine: a new topical agent for control of pseudomonas infection in burns. J. Trauma. 9:377, 1969.

91. Fox, C. L., Jr.: Silver sulfadiazine — a new topical therapy for *Pseudomonas* in burns. Arch. Surg. 96:184, 1968.

92. Fox, C. L., and Lasker, S. E.: Response to fluid therapy and tissue electrolyte changes in scalded and flash burned monkeys. Surg. Gynecol. Obstet. 112:274, 1961.

93. Fox, C. L., Monafo, W. W., Ayvazian, V. H., Skinner, A. M., Modak, S., Sanford, J., and Condict, C.: Topical chemotherapy for burns using cerium salts and silver sulfadiazine. Surg. Gynecol. Obstet. 144:668, 1977.

94. Fox, C. L., Jr., Rappole, B. W., and Stanford, W.: Control of *Pseudomonas* infection in burns by silver sulfadiazine. Surg. Gynecol. Obstet. 128:1021, 1969.

95. Fox, C. L., Jr., Sampath, A. C., and Stanford, J. W.: Virulence of *Pseudomonas* infection in burned rats and mice: comparative efficacy of silver sulfadiazine and mafenide. Arch. Surg. 101:508, 1970.

96. Frank, H., and Green, L.: Successful use of a bulk laxative to control the diarrhea of tube feeding. Presented, fifth International Congress on Burn Injuries, Stockholm, Sweden, June 20, 1978.

97. Freshwater, M. F., and Krizek, T. J.: Skin grafting of burns: A centennial. J. Trauma 11:862, 1971.

98. Friedman, N. B.: The pathology of trench foot. Am. J. Pathol., 21:387, 1945.

99. Garrett, T. A.: *Bacillus subtilis* protease: A new topical agent for debridement. Clin. Med. 76:11, 1969.

100. Georgiade, N. G., and Harris, W. A.: Open and closed treatment of burns with Povidone-iodine. *In* Polk, H. C., and Ehrenkranz, N. J. (eds.): Medical and Surgical Antisepsis with Betadine Microbicides. Purdue Frederick and Co., 1972.

101. Glover, D. M., and Kiehn, C. L.: Marjolin's ulcer; a preventable threat to function and life. Am. J. Surg. 78:722, 1949.

102. Golding, M. R., deJong, P., Sawyer, P. N., Nehigar, G. R., and Wesolowski, S. A.: Protection from early and late sequelae of frostbite by regional sympathectomy. Mechanism of "cold sensitivity" following frostbite. Surgery 53:303, 1963.

103. Golding, M. R., Martinez, A., deJong, P., et al.: The role of sympathectomy in frostbite with a review of 68 cases. Surgery 57:774,1965.

104. Golding, M. R., Mendoza, M. F., Hennigar, G. R., Fries, C. C., and Wesolowski, S. A: On settling the controversy on the benefit of sympathectomy for frostbite. Surgery 56:221, 1964.

105. Goodall, McC., and Moncrief, J. A.: Sympathetic nerve depletion after severe thermal injury. Ann. Surg., 162:893, 1965.

106. Hakim, A. A.: An immunodepressive factor from serum of thermally traumatized patients. J. Trauma 17:908, 1977.

107. Hardy, J. D.: Summary: Physiology. *In* Artz, C. P. (ed.): Research in Burns. Philadelphia, F. A. Davis Co., 1962, pp. 385–392.

108. Harrison, H. N., Bales, H. W., and Jacoby, F.: The absorption of Sulfamylon acetate from 5 percent aqueous solution. J. Trauma 12:994, 1972.

109. Harrison, H. N., Bales, H., and Jacoby, F.: The behavior of mafenide acetate as a basis for its clinical use. Arch. Surg. 103:449, 1971.

110. Hartford, C. E., and Ziffren, S. E.: Electrical injury. J. Trauma 11:331, 1971.

111. Haynes, B. W.: Current problems in burns. Arch. Surg. 103:454, 1971.

112. Haynes, B. W., Jr.: Skin homografts — a lifesaving measure in severely burned children. J. Trauma 3:217, 1963.

113. Heggers, J. P., Ko, F., and Robson, M. C.: Cerium nitrate/silver sulfadiazine: Synergism or antagonism as determined by minimum inhibitory concentration. Burns (in press)

114. Heggers, J. P., and Robson, M. C.: The emergence of silver sulfadiazine resistant *Pseudomonas aeruginosa*. Burns 5:184, 1978.

115. Heggers, J. P., Robson, M. C., and Ristroph, J. D.: A rapid method of performing quantitative wound cultures. Milit. Med. 134:666, 1969.

116. Heinrich, J. J., Fichandler, B. C., Barash, P. G., and Koss, N.: The Swan-Ganz catheter: Useful or not? Presented, Ninth annual meeting of The American Burn Association, Anaheim, California, April 1, 1977.

117. Hellat, A.: Studies on the self-disinfecting power of the skin. Ann. Med. Exper. Biol. Fenniae 26:1, 1948.

118. Hellstrom, J. G.: Vitamin E — A general review of the literature with assessment of its role in the healing of burns and wounds. Med. Serv. J. Canada 17:238, 1961.

119. Hergt, K.: Blood levels of thrombocytes in burned patients: Observations on their behavior in relation to the clinical condition of the patient. J. Trauma 12:599, 1972.

120. Hiebert, J. M., Golden, G. T., Edgerton, M. T., Rodeheaver, G. T., and Edlich, R. F.: Graft take: Tangential vs. full excision. Presented, Ninth annual meeting of The American Burn Association, Anaheim, California, April 1, 1977.

121. Hoopes, J. E., Butcher, H. R., Margraf, H. W., et al.: Silver lactate burn cream. Surgery 70:29, 1971.

122. Hume, D. M.: Endocrine and metabolic responses to injury. *In* Schwartz, S. I. (ed.): Principles of Surgery. New York, McGraw-Hill Book Co., 1969, p. 17.

123. Hummel, R. P., Kautz, P. D., MacMillan, B. G., and Altemeier, W. A.: The continuing problem of sepsis following enzymatic debridement of burns. J. Trauma 14:572, 1974.

124. Hunt, J. L., Mason, A. D., Masterson, T. S., and Pruitt, B. A.: The pathophysiology of acute electric injuries. J. Trauma 16:335, 1976.

125. Hunt, J. L., McManus, W. F., Haney, W. P., and

Pruitt, B. A.: Vascular lesions in acute electric injuries. J. Trauma 14:461, 1974.

126. Ivanova, S. S.: The transplantation of skin from dead body to granulating surface. Ann. Surg. 12:354, 1890.

127. Jackson, D. McG.: The diagnosis of the depth of burning. Br. J. Surg. 40:588, 1953.

128. Janzekovic, Z.: The burn wound from the surgical point of view. J. Trauma 15:42, 1975.

129. Jaffe, R. J., Willis, D., and Backem, A.: The effect of electric currents on the arteries. Arch. Pathol. 7:244, 1929.

130. Jelenko, C. III, and Ginsburg, J. M.: Water-holding lipid and water transmission through homeothermic and poikilothermic skins. Proc. Soc. Exp. Biol. Med. 136:1059, 1971.

131. Jones, R. J.: Passive immunization against gram-negative bacilli in burns. Br. J. Exp. Pathol., 51:53, 1970.

132. Kaly, G., and Weiner, R.: Prostaglandin E: A potential mediator of the inflammatory response. Ann. N.Y. Acad.Sci. 180:338, 1971.

133. Kefalides, N. A., Arana, J. A., Bazan, A., and Stastny, P.: Clinical evaluation of antibiotics and gamma globulin in septicemias following burns. In Artz, C. P. (ed.): Research in Burns. Philadelphia, F. A. Davis Co., 1962, pp. 219–228.

134. Kiker, R. G., Carvajal, H. F., Mlcak, R. P., and Larson, D. L.: A controlled study on the effects of silver sulfadiazine on the white blood cell counts in burned children. J. Trauma 17:835, 1977.

135. Kirksey, T. D., Moncrief, J. A., Pruitt, B. A., and O'Neill, J. A.: Gastrointestinal complications in burns. Am. J. Surg. 116:627, 1968.

136. Klein, L., Curtiss, P. H., and Davis, J. H.: Collagen breakdown in thermal burns. Surg. Forum 13:459, 1962.

137. Knisley, M. H.: Post burn pathologic circulatory physiology. In Artz, C. P. (ed.): Research in Burns, Philadelphia, F. A. Davis Co., 1962, pp. 51–57.

138. Koehnlein, H. E., and Lemperle, G.: Experimental studies on local treatment of pseudomonas-infected burn wounds. Plast. Reconstr. Surg. 45:558, 1970.

139. Koehnlein, H. E., Achinger, R., and Seitz, H. D.: A new method of treatment in hydrofluoric acid burns of the hand. Presented, annual meeting of The American Society of Plastic and Reconstructive Surgeons, November 1978.

140. Krizek, T. J.: Topical therapy of burns — Problems in wound healing. J. Trauma 8:276, 1968.

141. Krizek, T. J., and Davis, J. H.: Experimental Pseudomonas burn sepsis — evaluation of topical therapy. J. Trauma 7:433, 1967.

142. Krizek, T. J., Davis, J. H., DesPrez, J. D., and Kiehn, C. L.: Topical therapy of burns —experimental evaluation. Plast. Reconstr. Surg. 39:248, 1967.

143. Krizek, T. J., and Cossman, D. V.: Experimental burn wound sepsis: Variations in response to topical agents. J. Trauma 12:553, 1972.

144. Krizek, T. J., Flagg, S. V., Wolfort, F. G., and Jabaley, M. E.: Delayed primary excision and skin grafting of the burned hand. Plast. Reconstr. Surg. 51:524, 1973.

145. Krizek, T. J., Robson, M. C., Koss, N., Heinrich, J. J., and Fichandler, B. C.: Emergency non-surgical escharotomy in the burned extremity. Ortho. Rev. 4:53, 1975.

146. Krizek, T. J., Robson, M. C., and Kho, E.: Bacteria growth and skin graft survival. Surg. Forum 18:518, 1967.

147. Kucan, J., Heggers, J. P., and Robson, M. C.: Blood glucose level as an aid in diagnosis of septicemia. Burns (in press)

148. Kyaosola, K.: Clinical experiences in the management of cold injuries: A study of 110 cases. J. Trauma 14:32, 1974.

149. Labanter, H., Kaplan, I., and Shairtt, C.: Burns of the dorsum of the hand: Conservative treatment with intensive physiotherapy versus tangential excision and grafting. Br. J. Plast. Surg. 29:352, 1976.

150. Lange, K., and Boyd, L. J.: The functional pathology of frostbite and the prevention of gangrene in experimental animals and humans. Science 102:151, 1945.

151. Lange, K., and Loewe, L.: Subcutaneous heparin in the Pitkin menstruum for the treatment of experimental human frostbite. Surg. Gynecol. Obstet. 82:256, 1946.

152. Larson, D. L., Abston, S., Evans, E. B., and Linares, H. A.: Techniques for decreasing scar formation in the burned patient. J. Trauma 11:801, 1971.

153. Larson, D. L., Bauer, P., Linares, H. A., Willis, B., Abston, S., and Lewis, S. R.: Mechanisms of hypertrophic scar and contracture formation in burns. Burns 1:119, 1975.

154. Larson, D. L., Maxwell, R., Abston, S., and Dobrkovsky, M.: Zinc deficiency in burned children. Plast. Reconstr. Surg. 46:13, 1970.

155. Law, E. J., Kim, O. J., Stieritz, D. D., and Mac-Millan, B. G.: Experience with systemic candidiasis in the burned patient. J. Trauma 12:543, 1972.

156. Law, E. J., and MacMillan, B. G.: Excision of acute burns with immediate meshed autografting. Presented, fifth annual meeting of The American Burn Association, Dallas, Texas, April, 1973.

157. Law, E. J., and MacMillan, B. G.: Topical treatment of small burn wounds with Povidone-iodine. In Polk, H. C., and Ehrenkranz, N. J. (eds.): Medical and Surgical Antisepsis with Betadine Microbiocides. Purdue Frederick and Co., 1972.

158. Lawson, G.: On the transplantation of portions of skin for the closure of large granulating surfaces. Trans. Clin. Soc. London 4:49, 1871.

159. Leriche, R., and Kunlin, J.: Pathologic physiology and frostbite illness. Mem. Acad. Chir. 66:196, 1940.

160. Lescher, T. J., Sirinek, K. R., and Pruitt, B. A.: S.M.A. syndrome in thermally injured patients. Presented, 38th annual meeting of The American Association of the Surgery of Trauma, Lake Tahoe, Nevada, September 15, 1978.

161. Lewis, S. R., Goolishian, H. A., Wolf, C. W.,

Lynch, J. B., and Blocker, T. G.: Psychological studies in burn patients. Plast. Reconstr. Surg. *31*:323, 1963.

162. Lewis, T.: The Blood Vessels of the Human Skin and Their Responses. London, Shaw and Sons, Ltd., 1927, p. 51.

163. Lewis, T., and Love, W. S.: Observations upon the regulation of blood flow through the capillaries of the human skin. Heart *13*:1, 1926.

164. Lindberg, R. B., Brame, R. E., Moncrief, J. A., and Mason, A. D., Jr.: Prevention of invasive *Pseudomonas aeruginosa* infection in seeded burned rats by use of a topical Sulfamylon cream. Fed. Proc. *23*:388, 1964.

165. Lindberg, R. B., Moncrief, J. A., and Mason, A. D., Jr.: Control of experimental and clinical burn wound sepsis by topical application of Sulfamylon compounds. Ann. N.Y. Acad. Sci. *150*:950, 1968.

166. Lindberg, R. B., Moncrief, J. A., Switzer, W. E., Order, S. E., and Mills, W.: The successful control of burn wound sepsis. J. Trauma *6*:407, 1966.

167. Link, W. J., Zook, E. G., and Glover, J. L.: Plasma scalpel excision of burns. Plast. Reconstr. Surg. *55*:657, 1975.

168. Lowry, K. F., and Curtis, G. M.: Delayed suture in the management of wounds: Analysis of 721 traumatic wounds illustrating the influence of time interval in wound repair. Am. J. Surg. *80*:280, 1970.

169. Luce, E. A., Dowden, W. L., Su, C. T., and Hoopes, J. E.: High tension electrical injury of the upper extremity. Surg. Gynecol. Obstet. *147*:38, 1978.

170. Lund, C. C., and Browder, N. C.: The estimation of areas of burns. Surg. Gynecol. Obstet. 79:352, 1944.

171. Lynch, J. B.: Thermal burns. *In* Grabb, W. C., and Smith, J. C. (eds.): Plastic Surgery. Boston, Little, Brown, 1968.

172. MacMillan, B. G.: Homograft skin — a valuable adjunct to the treatment of thermal burns. J. Trauma 2:130, 1962.

173. MacMillan, B. G., and Altemeier, W. A.: Massive excision of the extensive burn. *In* Artz, C. P. (ed.): Research in Burns. Philadelphia, F. A. Davis Co., 1962.

174. MacMillan, B. G., Law, E. J., and Holder, I. A.: Experience with *Candida* infections in the burn patient. Arch. Surg. *104*:509, 1972.

175. Majno, G., and Palade, G. E.: Studies on inflammation. I. The effect of histamine and serotonin on vascular permeability: An electron microscopic study. J. Biophys. Biochem. Cytol. *11*:571, 1961.

176. Markley, K., Boconegra, M., Bazan, A., Temple, R., Chiaporri, M., Morales, G., and Carrion, A.: Clinical evaluation of saline solution therapy in burn shock. II. Comparison of plasma therapy with saline solution therapy. J.A.M.A., *170*:1633, 1959.

177. Markley, K., and Kefalides, N.: Further studies in the evaluation of saline solutions in the treatment of burn shock. *In* Artz, C. P. (ed.): Research in Burns. Philadelphia, F. A. Davis Co., 1962, pp. 81–88.

178. Mason, A. D., Jr., Pruitt, B. A., Jr., Lindberg, R.

B., et al.: Topical sulfamylon chemotherapy in the treatment of patients with extensive thermal burns. *In* Matter, P., Barclay, T. L., and Konicfova, Z. (eds.): Research in Burns: Transactions of Third International Congress of Research in Burns, Prague, September 20–25, 1970. Berne, Hans Huber Publishers, 1971, pp. 120–123.

179. McAlhany, J. C., Czaja, A. J., and Pruitt, B. A.: Antacid control of complications from acute gastroduodenal disease after burns. J. Trauma *16*:645, 1976.

180. Meakins, J. L., McLean, A. P. H., Kelly, R., Bubenik, K. O., Pietsch, J. B., and McLean, L. D.: Delayed hypersensitivity and neutrophil chemotaxis: Effect of trauma. J. Trauma *18*:240, 1978.

181. Mendelson, J. A., and Lindsey, D.: Sulfamylon (mafenide) and penicillin as expedient treatment of experimental massive open wounds with *C. perfringens* infection. J. Trauma *3*:239, 1962.

182. Merryman, H. T.: Tissue freezing and local cold injury. Physiol. Rev. 37:233, 1957.

183. Monafo, W. W.: The Treatment of Burns: Principles and Practice. St. Louis, Warren H. Greene, 1971.

184. Monafo, W. W.: Hypertonic balanced saline solutions in the treatment of burn shock. *In* Fox, C. L., and Nahas, G. G. (eds.): Body Fluid Replacement in the Surgical Patient, New York, Grune and Stratton, 1970, p. 237.

185. Monafo, W. W.: Hypertonic sodium solutions for the treatment of burn shock. *In* Polk, H. C., and Stone, H. H. (eds.): Contemporary Burn Management. Boston, Little, Brown, 1971, pp. 33–42.

186. Monafo, W. W., Tandon, S. N., Ayvazian, V. H., Tuchschmidt, J., Skinner, A. M., and Deitz, F.: Cerium nitrate: A new topical antiseptic for extensive burns. Surgery *80*:465, 1976.

187. Monasterio, F. O., Serrano, R. A., Barrera, G., Araico, J., Gutierrez-Bosque, R., Escobosa, J. E., and Barreto, F. R.: Comparative study in treatment of extensive burns with and without antibiotics. *In* Artz, C. P. (ed.): Research in Burns. Philadelphia, F. A. Davis Co., 1962, pp. 229–234.

188. Moncrief, J. A.: Editorial: Burn formulae. J. Trauma *12*:538, 1972.

189. Moncrief, J. A.: Effect of various fluid regimens and pharmacologic agents on the circulatory hemodynamics of the immediate postburn period. Ann. Surg. *164*:723, 1966.

190. Moncrief, J. A.: Medical progress — Burns. N. Engl. J. Med. *288*:444, 1973.

191. Moncrief, J. A.: The status of topical antibacterial therapy in the treatment of burns. Surgery *63*:862, 1968.

192. Moncrief, J. A.: Thermal and radiation injuries. *In* Zimmerman, L. M., and Levine, R. (eds.): Physiologic Principles of Surgery. Philadelphia, W. B. Saunders Co., 1964, pp. 62–85.

193. Moncrief, J. A., Lindberg, R. B., Switzer, W. E., et al.: Use of topical antibacterial therapy in the treatment of the burn wound. Arch. Surg. 92:558, 1966.

194. Moncrief, J. A., and Pruitt, B. A.: Electric injury. Postgrad. Med. 48:189, 1970.

195. Moncrief, J. A., Switzer, W. E., and Teplitz, C.: Curling's ulcer. J. Trauma 4:481, 1964.

196. Moncrief, J. A., and Teplitz, C.: Changing concepts in burn sepsis. J. Trauma 4:233, 1964.

197. Morgan, A., Knight, D., and O'Connor, N.: Lung water changes after thermal burns. Ann. Surg. 178:288, 1978.

198. Moritz, A. R., and Henrique, F. C., Jr.: Studies of thermal injury; the relative importance of time and surface temperature in the causation of cutaneous burns. Am. J. Pathol. 23:695, 1947.

199. Moritz, A. R., Henrique, F. C., Dutra, F. R., and Weisiger, J. R.: Studies of thermal injury. IV. An exploration of the casualty producing attributes of conflagrations; local and systemic effects of general cutaneous exposure to excessive circumambient air and circumradiant heat of varying duration and intensity. Arch. Pathol., 43:466, 1947.

200. Morris, A. H., and Spitzer, K. W.: Pulmonary pathophysiologic changes following thermal injury. U.S. Army Institute of Surgical Research. Annual Research Progress Report. Brooke Army Medical Center, Ft. Sam Houston, Texas, Section 52, 1, 1971.

201. Morris, P. J., Bondoc, C., and Burke, J. F.: The use of frequently changed skin allografts to promote healing in the non-healing infected ulcer. Surgery 60:13, 1966.

202. Moyer, C. A.: Burns. In Harkins, H., Moyer, C. A., Rhoads, J. E., and Allen, J. G. (eds.): Surgery, Principles and Practice. Philadelphia, J. B. Lippincott Co., 1961.

203. Moyer, C. A., Brentano, L., Grovens, D. L., Margraf, H. W., and Monafo, W. W.: Treatment of large human burns with 0.5 per cent silver nitrate. Arch. Surg. 90:812, 1965.

204. Moyer, C. A., and Butcher, H. R., Jr. (eds.): Burns, Shock and Plasma Volume Regulation. St. Louis, C. V. Mosby, 1967, p. 355.

205. Moyer, C. A., Margraf, H. W., and Monafo, W. W.: Burn shock and extravascular sodium deficiency — treatment with Ringer's solution with lactate. Arch. Surg. 90:799, 1965.

206. Moylan, J. S.: Inhalation injury — a major problem. Presented, Tenth annual meeting of The American Burn Association, Birmingham, Alabama, April 1, 1978.

207. Moylan, J. A., Wilmore, D. W., Mouton, D. E., and Pruitt, B. A.: Early diagnosis of inhalation injury using 133Xenon lung scan. Ann. Surg. 176:477, 1972.

208. Muir, F. K.: Red cell destruction in burns with particular reference to the shock period. Br. J. Plast. Surg. 14:273, 1961.

209. Munster, A. M.: Alterations of the host defense mechanisms in burns. Surg. Clin. N. Am. 50:1217, 1970.

210. Munster, A. M., Bruck, H. M., Johns, L. A., et al.: Heterotopic calcification following burns: A prospective study. J. Trauma 12:1071, 1972.

211. Munster, A. M., Eurenius, K., Katz, R. M., et al.: Cell-mediated immunity after thermal injury. Ann. Surg. 177:139, 1973.

212. Munster, A. M., Hoagland, C., and Pruitt, B. A.: The effect of thermal injury on serum immunoglobulins. Ann. Surg. 172:965, 1970.

213. Nash, G., Asch, M. J., Foley, F. D., and Pruitt, B. A., Jr.: Disseminated cytomegalic inclusion disease in a burned adult. J.A.M.A. 214:587, 1970.

214. Nash, G., Foley, F. D., and Pruitt, B. A.: Candida burn wound invasion: a cause of systemic candidiasis. Arch. Pathol. 90:75, 1970.

215. Nathan, P., Law, E. J., Murphy, D. F., and MacMillan, B. G.: A laboratory method for selection of topical antimicrobial agents to treat infected burns. Burns 4:177, 1978.

216. Nathan, P., Robb, E. C., Srirastava, R., and MacMillan, B. G.: A bacterial barrier for skin donor sites. Presented, Tenth annual meeting of The American Burn Association, Birmingham, Alabama, March 31, 1978.

217. Neal, G. D., Marvin, J., Lindholm, G. R., Barker, E. A. and Heimbach, D. M.: Burn wound biopsy: Comparison of new culture technique to quantitative cultures. Presented Tenth annual meeting of The American Burn Association, Birmingham, Alabama, March 30, 1978.

218. Nylen, B., and Wallenius, G.: The protein loss via exudation from burns and granulating wound surfaces. Acta Chir. Scand. 122:97, 1961.

219. Ollstein, R. N., Symonds, F. C., Cricklair, G. F., and Pelle, L.: Alternate care study of topical sulfamylon and silver sulfadiazine in burns. Plast. Reconstr. Surg. 48:311, 1974.

220. O'Neill, J. A., Jr.: The influence of thermal burns on gastric acid secretion. Surgery 67:267, 1970.

221. O'Neill, J. A., Jr., Pruitt, B. A., Jr., Monerret, J. A., et al.: Studies related to the pathogenesis of Curling's ulcer. J. Trauma 7:275, 1967.

222. Order, S. E., Mason, A. D., Jr., Walker, H. L., et al.: Vascular destructive effects of thermal injury and its relationship to burn wound sepsis. J. Trauma 5:62, 1965.

223. Order, S. E., and Moncrief, J. A.: The Burn Wound. Springfield, Ill., Charles C Thomas, 1965.

224. Paradis, C., Spanier, A. H., Calder, M., and Schizgal, H. M.: Total parenteral nutrition with lipid. Am. J. Surg. 135:164, 1978.

225. Phillips, A. W., and Cope, O.: Burn therapy. II. The revelation of respiratory tract as principal killer. Ann. Surg. 155:1, 1962.

226. Phillips, A. W., and Cope, A.: Burn Therapy, III. Beware the facial burn. Ann. Surg. 156:759, 1962.

227. Phillips, A. W., Tanner, J. W., and Cope, O.: Burn therapy. IV. Respiratory tract damage (an account of the clinical, x-ray and post mortem findings) and the meaning of restlessness. Ann. Surg. 158:799, 1963.

228. Pierson, C., and Feller, I.: A reduction of Pseudomonas septicemias in burned patients by the immune process. Surg. Clin. N. Am., 50:1377, 1970.

229. Pietsch, J., and Meakins, J. L.: Complications of povidone-iodine absorption in topically treated burn patients. Lancet 1:280, 1976.

230. Pillsbury, D. M., Shelley, W. B., and Kligman, A. M.: Dermatology. Philadelphia, W. B. Saunders Co., 1956.

231. Pitts, W., Pickrell, K., Quinn, G., et al.: Electrical burns of lips and mouth in infants and children. Plast. Reconstr. Surg. 44:471, 1969.

232. Polk, H. C., Monafo, W. W. Jr., and Moyer, C. A.: Human burn survival: study of the efficacy of 0.5% aqueous silver nitrate. Arch. Surg. 98:262, 1969.

233. Porter, J. M.: Intra-arterial sympathetic blockade in the treatment of clinical frostbite. Am. J. Surg. 132:625, 1976.

234. Pruitt, B. A., and Curreri, P. W.: The burn wound and its care. Arch. Surg. 103:461, 1971.

235. Pruitt, B. A., Jr., DiVincenti, F. C., Mason, A. D., Jr., et al.: The occurrence and significance of pneumonia and other pulmonary complications in burned patients: comparison of conventional and topical treatments. J. Trauma 10:519, 1970.

236. Pruitt, B. A., Erickson, D. R., and Morris, A.: Progressive pulmonary insufficiency and other pulmonary complications of thermal injury. J. Trauma 15:369, 1975.

237. Pruitt, B. A., Jr., Foley, F. D., and Moncrief, J. A.: Curling's ulcer: A clinical pathological study of 323 cases. Ann. Surg. 172:523, 1970.

238. Pruitt, B. A., Jr., Mason, A. D., Jr., and Moncrief, J. A.: Hemodynamic changes in the early postburn patient: The influence of fluid administration and of a vasodilator (Hydralazine). J. Trauma 11:36, 1971.

239. Pruitt, B. A., and Moncrief, J. A.: Current trends in burn research. J. Surg. Res. 7:280, 1967.

240. Pruitt, B. A., Stein, J. M., Foley, F. D., et al.: Intravenous therapy in burn patients: Suppurative thrombophlebitis and other life-threatening complications. Arch. Surg. 100:399, 1970.

241. Pruitt, B. A., Tumbusch, W. T., Mason, A. D., and Pearson, E.: Mortality in 1100 consecutive burns treated at burns unit. Ann. Surg. 159:393, 1964.

242. Pulaski, E. J., and Tennison, C. W.: Quoted in Artz, C. P., and Reiss, E. (eds.): The Treatment of Burns. Philadelphia, W. B. Saunders Co., 1957, p. 9.

243. Pulito, J., and Parshley, P. F.: Colonic bleeding with ulceration associated with severe burn wound injury. Presented, Eighth annual meeting of The American Burn Association, San Antonio, Texas, April 1, 1976.

244. Quinby, W. C., Burke, J. F., Trelstad, R. L., and Caulfield, J.: The use of microscopy as a guide to primary excision of high-tension electrical burns. J. Trauma 18:423, 1978.

245. Quintanilla, R., Krusen, F. H., and Essex, H. E.: Studies on frost-bite with special reference to treatment and the effect on minute blood vessels. Am. J. Physiol. 149:149, 1947.

246. Rappaport, I., Pepino, A. T., and Dietrick, W.: Early use of xenografts as a biologic dressing in burn trauma. Am. J. Surg. 120:144, 1970.

247. Reckler, J. M., Bruck, H. M., Munster, A. M., et al.: Superior mesenteric artery syndrome as a consequence of burn injury. J. Trauma 12:979, 1972.

248. Rickells, L. R., Squire, J. R., Topley, E., and Lilly, H. A.: Human skin lipids with particular reference to the self-sterilizing power of the skin. Clin. Sci. 10:89, 1951.

249. Richetts, C. R., Lowbury, E. J. L., Lawrence, J. C., et al.: Mechanism of prophylaxis by silver compounds against infection in burns. Br. Med. J. 1:444, 1970.

250. Roe, C. F., and Kinney, J. M.: The caloric equivalent of fever. II. Influence of major trauma. Ann. Surg. 161:140, 1965.

251. Robinson, N. W., Masters, F. W., and Forest, W. J.: Electrical burns: A review and analysis of 33 cases. Surgery 57:385, 1965.

252. Robson, M. C., and Heggers, J. P.: Bacterial quantification of open wounds. Milit. Med. 134:19, 1969.

253. Robson, M. C., and Heggers, J. P.: Variables in host resistance pertaining to septicemia. I. Blood glucose level. J. Am. Geriatr. Soc. 17:991, 1969.

254. Robson, M. C., Krizek, T. J., and Heggers, J. P.: Biology of surgical infection. Current Problems of Surgery, March 1973.

255. Robson, M. C., and Krizek, T. J.: Clinical experiences with amniotic membranes as a temporary biologic dressing. Conn. Med. 38:449, 1974.

256. Robson, M. C., and Krizek, T. J.: The effect of human amniotic membranes on the bacterial population of infected rat burns. Ann. Surg. 177:144, 1973.

257. Robson, M. C., and Krizek, T. J.: Predicting skin graft survival. J. Trauma 13:213, 1973.

258. Rosenberg, S. A., Brief, D. K., Kinsley, J. M., Herrera, M. G., Wilson, R. E., and Moore, F. D.: The syndrome of dehydration, coma and severe hyperglycemia without ketosis in patients convalescing from burns. N. Engl. J. Med. 222:931, 1965.

259. Rosenthal, A., Czaja, A. J., and Pruitt, B. A.: Gastrin levels and gastric acidity in the pathogenesis of acute gastroduodenal disease after burns. Surg. Gynecol. Obstet. 144:232, 1977.

260. Rouse, R., and Dimick, A. R.: The treatment of electrical injury compared to burn injury: A review of pathophysiology and comparison of patient management protocols. J. Trauma 18:43, 1978.

261. Rubin L. R., and Bongiovi, J., Jr.: Central venous pressure: Unreliable guide to fluid therapy in burns. Arch. Surg. 100:269, 1970.

262. Sabella, N.: Use of fetal membranes in skin-grafting. Med. Rec. N.Y. 83:478, 1913.

263. Sachatello, C. R., and Stephenson, S. E., Jr.: High voltage burns. Am. Surg. 31:807, 1965.

264. Schumacher, H. B, Jr., and Kilman, J. W.: Sympathectomy in the treatment of frostbite. Arch. Surg. 89:575, 1964.

265. Schumacher, H. B, White, B. H., Wrenn, E. L., Cordell, A. R., and Sanford, T. F.: Studies in

experimental frostbite — The effect of heparin in preventing gangrene. Surgery 22:900, 1947.

266. Sevitt, S.: Duodenal and gastric ulceration after burning. Br. J. Surg. 54:32, 1967.

267. Sheldon, G. F., Sanders, R., Fuchs, R., Garcia, J., and Schooley, J.: Metabolism, oxygen transport, and erythropoietin synthesis in the anemia of thermal injury. Am. J. Surg. 135:406, 1978.

268. Shimzaki, S., Yoshioka, T., Tanaka, N., Sugimoti, T., and Onji, Y.: Body fluid changes during hypertonic lactated saline solution therapy for burn shock. J. Trauma 17:38, 1977.

269. Shuck, J. M., Bedeau, G. W. and Thomas, P. R. S.: Homograft skin for the early management of difficult wounds. J. Trauma 12:215, 1972.

270. Shuck, J. M., Eaton, R. P., Shuck, L. W., Wachtel, T. L., and Schade, D. S.: Dynamics of insulin and glucagon secretions in severely burned patients. J. Trauma 17:706, 1977.

271. Shuck, J. M., and Moncrief, J. A.: The management of burns. Part I: General considerations and the Sulfamylon method. Curr. Prob. Surg. February 1969.

272. Shuck, J. M., Moncrief, J. A., and Monafo, W. W.: The management of burns. Curr. Probl. Surg. 38–41, 1969.

273. Shuck, J. M., Pruitt, B. A., Jr., and Moncrief, J. A.: Homograft skin for wound coverage: A study in versatility. Arch. Surg. 98:472, 1969.

274. Shuck, J. M., Thorne, L. W., and Cooper, C. G.: Mafenide acetate solution dressings: An adjunct in burn care. J. Trauma 15:595, 1975.

275. Silversides, J.: The neurological sequelae of electrical injury. Can. Med. Assoc. J. 91:195, 1964.

276. Silverstein, P., and Dressler, D. P.: Effect of current therapy on burn mortality. Ann. Surg. 171:124, 1970.

277. Silverstein, P., Helmkamp, G. M., Walker, H. L., and Pruitt, B. A., Jr.: Laboratory evaluation of enzymatic burn wound debridement in vitro and in vivo. Surg. Forum 23:31–33, 1972.

278. Silverstein, P., Peterson, K., and Sadler, R.: Meshed pigskin as an adjunct to burn wound therapy. Presented, Fifth International Congress on Burn Injuries, Stockholm, Sweden, June 20, 1978.

279. Snider, R. L.: Treatment of experimental frostbite with intra-arterial sympathetic blocking drugs. Surgery 77:557, 1975.

280. Sorensen, B.: Acute excision/exposure treatment of acute burn injuries. A randomized controlled clinical trial. Presented, Fifth International Congress on Burn Injuries, Stockholm, Sweden, June 20, 1978.

281. Soroff, H. S., Pearson, E., and Artz, C. P.: An estimation of the nitrogen requirements for equilibrium in burned patients. Surg. Gynecol. Obstet. 112:159, 1961.

282. Stanford, W., Rappole, B. W., and Fox, C. L., Jr.: Clinical experience with silver sulfadiazine, a new topical agent for control of *Pseudomonas* infection in burns. J. Trauma 9:377, 1969.

283. Stellar, S., Levine, N., Ger, R., and Levenson, S. M.: Laser excision of acute third-degree burns followed by immediate autograft replacement: An experimental study in the pig. J. Trauma 13:45, 1973.

284. Stenberg, T., and Hogeman, K. E.: Experimental and clinical investigations on liver function in burns. In Artz, C. P., (ed.): Research in Burns. Philadelphia, F. A. Davis Co., 1962, pp. 171–176.

285. Stone, H. H.: Review of pseudomonas sepsis in thermal burns. Verdoglobin determination and Gentamicin therapy. Ann. Surg. 163:297, 1966.

286. Stone, H. H.: Wound care with topical gentamicin. In Polk, H. C., and Stone, H. H. (eds.): Contemporary Burn Management. Boston, Little, Brown, 1971, pp. 203–216.

287. Stone, H. H., and Kolb, L. D.: The evolution and spread of gentamicin-resistant pseudomonads. J. Trauma 11:586, 1971.

288. Stone, H. H., Martin, J. D., Huger, W. E., and Kolb, L.: Gentamicin sulfate in the treatment of pseudomonas sepsis in burns. Surg. Gynecol. Obstet. 120:351, 1965.

289. Summerlin, W. T., and Artz, C. P.: Gentamicin sulfate therapy of experimentally induced pseudomonas septicemia. J. Trauma 6:233, 1966.

290. Switzer, W. E., Moncrief, J. A., Mills, W., Order, S. E., and Lindberg, R. B.: The use of canine heterografts in the thermal injury. J. Trauma 6:391, 1966.

291. Taylor, P. H., Moncrief, J. A., Pugsley, L. Q., Rose, L. R., and Swtizer, W. E.: The management of extensively burned patients by staged excision. Surg. Gynecol. Obstet. 115:347, 1962.

292. Taylor, P. H., Pugsley, L. Q., and Vogel, E. H., Jr.: The intriguing electrical burn: A review of thirty-one electrical burn cases. J. Trauma 2:309, 1962.

293. Teplitz, C.: Pathogenesis of pseudomonas vasculitis and septic lesions. Arch. Path. 80:297, 1965.

294. Teplitz, C., Davis, D., Mason, A. D., and Moncrief, J. A.: Pseudomonas burn wound sepsis. I. Pathogenesis of experimental pseudomonas burn wound sepsis. J. Surg. Res. 4:200, 1964.

295. Teplitz, C., Davis, D., Walker, H. L., Raulston, G. L., Mason, A. D., and Moncrief, J. A.: Pseudomonas burn wound sepsis. II. Hematogenous infection at the junction of the burn wound and the unburned hypodermis. J. Surg. Res. 4:217, 1964.

296. Ternberg, J. L., and Luce, E.: Methemoglobinemia: Complication of the silver nitrate treatment of burns. Surgery 63:328, 1968.

297. Treves, N., and Pack, G. T.: Development of cancer in burn scars. Surg. Gynecol. Obstet. 51:749, 1930.

298. Tumbusch, W. T., Vogel, E. H., Butkiewicz, J. V., Graber, C. D., Larson, D. L., and Mitchell, E. T.: Septicemia in burn injury. J. Trauma 1:22, 1961.

299. Valente, P., and Axelrod, J. L.: Acute leukopenia associated with silver sulfadiazine therapy. J. Trauma 18:146, 1978.

300. Waisbren, B. A.: Antibiotics in the treatment of burns. Surg. Clin. N. Am. 50:1311, 1970.

301. Walker, H. L., Mason, A. D., Jr., and Raulston, G. L.: Surface infection with *Pseudomonas aeruginosa*. Ann. Surg. 160:297, 1964.

302. Wallace, A. B.: Treatment of burns; a return to basic principles. Br. J. Plast. Surg. 2:232, 1949.

303. Wartman, W. B.: Mechanisms of death in severe burn injury: The need for planned autopsies. *In* Artz, C. P. (ed.): Research in Burns. Philadelphia, F. A. Davis Co., 1962, pp. 6–13.

304. Washburn, B.: Frost-bite — what it is — how to prevent it. Emergency treatment. N. Engl. J. Med. 266:974, 1962.

305. Weatherley-White, R. C. A., Paton, B. C., and Sjöstrom, B. L.: Experimental studies in cold injury. III. Observations on the treatment of frostbite. Plast. Reconstr. Surg. 36:10, 1965.

306. Weatherley-White, R. C. A., Sjöstrom, B. L., and Paton, B. C.: Experimental studies in cold injury: II. The pathogenesis of frostbite. J. Surg. Res. 4:17, 1964.

307. Welch, G. W., Lull, R. J., Petroff, P. A., Hander, E. W., McLeod, C. G., and Clayton, W. H.: The use of steroids in inhalation injury. Surg. Gynecol. Obstet. 145:539, 1977.

308. Wickman, K.: Studies on burns. XIV. Acta Chir. Scand. 140 (suppl.) 408, 1970.

309. Wilmore, D. W., Long, J. M., Mason, A. D., Skreen, R. W., and Pruitt, B. A.: Catecholamines: Mediator of the hypermetabolic response to thermal injury. Ann. Surg. 180:653, 1975.

310. Wilmore, D. W., Curreri, P. W., Spitzer, K. W., et al.: Supranormal dietary intake in thermally injured hypermetabolic patients. Surg. Gynecol. Obstet. 132:881, 1971.

311. Wright, H. K., Gann, D. S., and Drucker, W. R.: Current concept of therapy for derangements of extra-cellular fluid. *In* Davis, J. H. (ed.): Current Concepts in Surgery. New York, McGraw-Hill Book Co., 1965.

312. Wunder, J. A., Stinnett, J. D., and Alexander, J. W.: The effects of malnutrition on variables of host defense in the guinea pig. Surgery 84:542, 1978.

313. Zaroff, L. I., Mills, W., Jr., Duckett, J. W., et al.: Multiple uses of viable cutaneous homografts in the burned patient. Surgery 59:368, 1966.

314. Zawacki, B. E., and Pearson, H. E.: Epidemic nosocomial infection by antibiotic-proof Providencia: Its origin, course and relation to topical chemotherapy on a large burn ward. Presented, fifth annual meeting of the American Burn Association, Dallas, Texas, April 1973.

315. Zawacki, B. E., Spitzer, K., Mason, A. D., and Johns, L. A.: Does increased evaporative water loss cause hypermetabolism in burned patients? Ann. Surg. 171:236, 1970.

316. Zellner, P. R., and Metzger, E.: Active immunization in burns. Burns 2:54, 1976.

317. Zikria, B. A., Budd, D. C., Floch, F., and Ferrer, J. M.: What is clinical smoke poisoning? Ann. Surg. 181:151, 1975.

CHAPTER 24

TRAUMA AND THE CHILD

J. Alex Haller, Jr., M.D.
James L. Talbert, M.D.
Dennis W. Shermeta, M.D.

INTRODUCTION TO TRAUMA IN CHILDHOOD

Accidents are responsible for more than half of all deaths among school-age boys and nearly two fifths of those among school-age girls in the United States. The National Health Survey indicates that 18 million children in the age range from 6 to 16 years (40 per cent of the total population at these ages) suffer injuries requiring medical attention and at least 1 day of restricted activity each year.

At 1 year of age, when presumably an infant is most watched and protected against accidental injury, an accident is the most common cause of death. During this period asphyxiation from inhalation or ingestion of food or foreign objects represents 30 per cent of the total accidental death toll. Motor vehicle accidents are responsible for almost a fifth of all accidental deaths in this age group, a number that has been increasing over the last 15 years. Other types of mortal accidents in the infant age group are burns, drowning and falls; all of these are preventable through proper protection and supervision.

In 1973, 4300 or 31.9 per 100,000 children from age 1 to 4 died as the result of accidental injury. Accidents kill more children in this age group than the next seven causes combined! The death rate from all other causes decreased 30 per cent between 1963 and 1973, while accident mortality remains unchanged despite widespread accident prevention efforts directed at those caring for the preschool child.

Accidents in the school-age group cause more than half of all deaths in males and nearly two fifths of those in females in the United States. This high mortality rate has been virtually unchanged between 1963 and 1973. The hospital morbidity and the long-term sequelae of these injuries in children have even greater medical and social significance than simple death rates. It has been conservatively estimated that 50,000 children are permanently crippled by accidents every year and that another two million are incapacitated for many weeks and months. This creates an enormous rehabilitation problem, which will increase each year simply on the basis of the increase in numbers of this segment of our population. The impact on our health care system is incalculable.

No evaluation of the expense and grief to the individual family with a severely injured child can be truly meaningful. From an objective viewpoint, however, this carnage represents an inestimable loss in potential earning power that could be coldly calculated in dollars and cents.

GENERAL PRINCIPLES IN THE CARE OF THE INJURED CHILD

In the management of major trauma, the necessity for immediate, accurate evaluation of the extent of injury is not unique to the child. The margin for error in this age group is far less, however, and some aspects merit special emphasis.

The responses of young children to serious trauma are qualitatively as well as quantitatively different from those of adults. For example, abdominal distention and diaphragmatic elevation from post-traumatic ileus are greater threats to the limited chest volume of children than to adults. Any blood loss assumes dramatic importance with the tiny blood volume of a young child. Increased surface area in a child allows excessive and rapid heat loss, especially in situations of multiple injuries and prolonged exposure during emergency management. Transfusion of large quantities of cold blood and fluids may lead to further serious loss of body heat. Associated congenital defects are much more likely to complicate the management of serious injury in children, especially those related to congenital heart abnormalities. The characteristic lability of a young child in his reaction to stress demands the utmost vigilance in detecting subtle signs of inadequate response to ongoing treatment. Blunt trauma is responsible for probably 80 to 90 per cent of serious injuries in children. External evidence of internal injury may be misleading and result in serious delay in operative treatment. This is especially true of multiple injuries that involve the head, and head injuries are associated with multiple trauma in children in a much higher percentage than in adults. Associated with these head injuries is a much higher incidence of subdural hematoma in children. Head injuries greatly increase the difficulty of evaluating generalized trauma in children, for it is similar to blunt trauma in a drunken adult. A young child may be unable to express his pain and to localize his symptoms even when he is conscious; this fact places multiple trauma in childhood almost in the category of veterinary medicine. Finally, serious injuries in an immature child may have disastrous effects upon his emotional well-being at this impressionable age. The terror of separation from familiar faces is greatly magnified by the usual busy and impersonal environment of a major emergency department. Serious emotional aftereffects are not uncommon from even minor injuries that are treated under threatening circumstances by physicians who are not aware of this important additional insult to a child.[14]

Each patient deserves his physician's maximal kindness and compassion. Unfortunately, this truism meets its most stringent challenge in a busy emergency department. The few moments required to win the confidence and trust of a child, however, reward the doctor by facilitating his examination and by ensuring the validity of his observations. There are few more difficult tasks than attempting to evaluate the abdomen of an apprehensive, struggling child.

After major injuries have been excluded, sedation is an important and useful adjunct in the treatment of minor trauma in children. Pentobarbital in a dosage of 5 mg. per kg. of body weight or the popular "lytic cocktail" may be employed for this purpose. The standard lytic cocktail used on the Pediatric Surgical Service of The Johns Hopkins Hospital is composed of Demerol (2 mg. per kg.), Phenergan (2 mg. per kg.) and Thorazine (2 mg. per kg.). These drugs are administered intramuscularly, 45 to 60 minutes prior to painful procedures. This regimen should not be employed in infants less than 1 year of age. The total dosage of Phenergan and Thorazine should not exceed 50 mg. each, and the dosage of Demerol should not exceed 150 mg. It must be remembered that any contraindication to general anesthesia is equally applicable to heavy sedation. Standard formulas are useful only as baselines and must be adapted by the physician to the individual child and situation.

Both preoperative sedation and local anesthesia require a critical delay period before their maximal effect is realized. Haste may obviate any reward that might otherwise be expected.

Positioning and restraint of children is particularly important for minor surgical procedures. Details of the techniques of restraining children (Fig. 24–1) as well as other forms of specialized treatment are ably presented by Hughes in his book, *Pediatric Procedures*.[18]

Most techniques in management of local

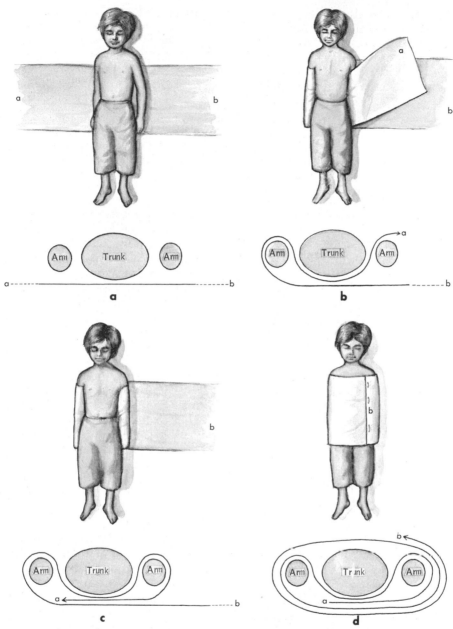

Figure 24–1. *A technique of body restraint for the infant and young child. (From Hughes, W. T., Jr.: Pediatric Procedure.)*

trauma and lacerations are no different in the child than in the adult. The physician should be encouraged, however, to use fine suture material in the younger patient, both for technical and cosmetic reasons.

Serious trauma in the young child presents the classic raison d'etre for a trauma unit directed by a general surgeon. In a few medical centers, new children's trauma units, distinct from but closely coordinated with adult trauma units, have been developed and offer innovative approaches to emergency care for this special group of patients. In such centers the children's trauma unit may be directed by a pediatric surgeon who is, in essence, a general surgeon for children. The need for command decisions cutting across specialty fields and the high incidence of injuries to multiple organ systems make the injured child a clear example of the need for a team approach to trauma.

The following cases illustrate the multiplicity of systems that may be involved in severe trauma and the importance of appointing a surgeon with a diversity of experience — in most instances a general surgeon — as the coordinator of patient care.

Case History No. 1.   K. B., JHH #111 65 97. A 4-year-old girl was brought to the emergency room in a semicomatose state shortly after being struck by an automobile. The remainder of the history was sketchy, but it was subsequently learned that the patient had been thrown into the air by the initial impact only to fall back onto the hood of the car, thereby suffering a second blow.

The vital signs on admission were surprisingly stable. Although she was semiconscious, the child's mental status appeared to stabilize under observation. In the course of the next hour a thorough evaluation, including multiple x-ray studies, revealed the following injuries:

1. Multiple fractures of the right pelvis.
2. Fractures of the left mandible.
3. Vaginal tear from a bone spicule of the pelvic fracture.
4. Contusion of the left cerebral hemisphere as manifested by decreased level of consciousness, right hemiparesis and clonus of the right leg.
5. Fracture of the right first rib.
6. Right pulmonary contusion.
7. Abrasion of right cornea.
8. Laceration of lip.
9. Multiple contusions and abrasions of the body.

Although mild hematuria was evident initially, an intravenous pyelogram failed to demonstrate any significant renal injury. The urethra and bladder were demonstrated to be intact on cystogram, although a larger right retroperitoneal hematoma from the pelvic fracture distorted the lateral bladder wall.

Despite some localization of cerebral signs, the absence of any significant deterioration combined with actual stabilization of the patient's condition appeared to allow further observation. The question of coexistent, unrecognized intra-abdominal trauma was another contraindication to immediate craniotomy. Accordingly, the patient was admitted to the Intensive Care Unit of The Children's Medical and Surgical Center where close monitoring of the vital signs, with fluid replacement, was undertaken. The pulmonary congestion secondary to the right lung contusion progressed, resulting in an acute episode of respiratory embarrassment. Tracheal intubation and positive pressure respiration were instituted. (We would now use continuous positive end-expiratory pressure breathing with a volume ventilator and with an end expiratory pressure of 5–10 cm. H_2O.)

The patient's general picture was one of gradual improvement. The positive pressure respirator was discontinued after 4 days because of clearing of the right lung. The level of consciousness also improved to the point that the patient responded to verbal stimuli by 12 days. A cerebral arteriogram obtained during this period confirmed the absence of a subdural hematoma. After 30 days the patient spoke her first words. In 6 months she had recovered completely from her injuries and had no evidence of either physical or mental retardation.

Although not used in this patient, one of the more important advances in the treatment of patients with head trauma is the placing of monitoring devices for the management of intracranial pressure. Whether an intraventricular catheter or a bolt-transducer is used, this monitoring technique is essential for the early detection and rapid treatment of increasing intracranial pressure. Accumulated experience with this monitoring procedure suggests that increasing intracranial pressure is not an irreversible complication of brain edema. Hypoventilation and noxious stimuli such as pain or endotracheal suctioning may also cause increases in intracranial pressure. Monitoring intracranial pressure permits rapid detection and treatment of these changes and may suggest a need for ventilatory support, narcotics or anesthesia. Furthermore, these devices help monitor the interaction of other therapeutic modalities on intracranial pressure, such as the use of positive airway pressure that may increase intracranial pressure by impeding venous return from the head. Finally, the use of these devices may become an integral part of the vigorous forms of therapy directed toward other causes of increased intracranial pressure, such as hypothermia and barbiturate poisoning.

It can be easily understood how associated serious injuries might escape detection in the natural concern that arises during treatment of any one of the many systems involved. Only with the appointment of a single coordinator of therapy can such errors of omission be minimized. Although some cases appear to involve only one specialty service, the importance of having all pediatric trauma patients seen by the general surgeon is again emphasized by the following example.

Case History No. 2. W. B., JHH #114 93 74. A 3-year-old boy was admitted to the accident room with a history of having been struck by an automobile. There was no suggestion that the patient had been crushed or run over. He had lost consciousness for several minutes, but his sensorium was relatively clear on admission. There was no subsequent deterioration in his mental state. Admission examination revealed a large contusion and smaller laceration of the left frontooccipital area of the skull. There were no localizing neurological signs. The remainder of the examination was within normal limits except for minimal contusions of the left flank. Specifically, there was no evidence of abdominal tenderness; bowel sounds were active.

The hematocrit was 34 per cent on admission, the white blood cell count was 22,000 and urinalysis revealed 25 to 30 red blood cells per high powered field. Skull x-rays demonstrated a large depressed skull fracture, but abdominal and chest x-rays were interpreted as normal. An intravenous pyelogram subsequently demonstrated good bilateral renal function.

Approximately one and a half hours following admission, at the termination of the work-up just outlined, the patient was first noted by the general surgical consultant to have developed left upper quadrant abdominal tenderness. The hematocrit was rechecked and remained 35 per cent. The central venous pressure was also stable. In view of the strong possibility of intra-abdominal injury and the necessity for elevation of the depressed skull fracture, simultaneous exploratory laparotomy and craniotomy were performed.

This decision was clearly justified by the physical signs of peritoneal irritation and was substantiated by the finding of a ruptured spleen at laparotomy. The postoperative course was uneventful, and the patient was discharged 13 days later.

The recognition of coexistent abdominal and cerebral trauma and the prompt institution of treatment avoided the confusion that inevitably results when a patient undergoing craniotomy for a head trauma develops hypotension at the time of surgery. Hidden bleeding from a ruptured spleen or other organ may pass unrecognized in these situations and may prove fatal. Screening of trauma cases by a pediatric surgeon helps to decrease the frequency of such problems. There can be no substitute for immediate total evaluation of the seriously injured patient. This fact is strongly underlined in the pediatric age group.

In this case, splenectomy and an open reduction of multiple skull fractures were performed; today in treating such an injury, attempts to repair and salvage the spleen would be the first course of action. Life-threatening, exsanguinating hemorrhage may result from lacerations of the spleen and therefore splenic injuries are a common cause for emergency laparotomy. In the past, little thought had been given to suturing the spleen or carrying out a partial resection under these circumstances because, until recently, removing the spleen was not recognized as carrying a hazard of overwhelming sepsis as a result of secondary immunological deficiency. The spleen is an important organ in the immunological defense mechanisms in children: It strains out all foreign matter, including bacteria, thus having an important sieve-like effect. In addition, it is the site of formation of specific antibodies that are necessary for defending against encapsulated gram-positive bacteria. It is this latter function, formation of specific opsonin-like antibodies, which is localized in early childhood to the spleen. Without a spleen a young child is exposed to the danger of overwhelming sepsis. As a result of this new understanding of splenic function, reasonably aggressive attempts should be made to preserve the spleen in children and probably also in adolescents.

Several approaches have been suggested to prevent unnecessary splenectomies.[8] These include radionuclide scans to visualize the spleen and document the presence or absence of rupture and arteriography to localize the sites of major bleeding. These specialized diagnostic modalities are indicated only in children who have no evidence of multiple systems injuries and who are hemodynamically stable. Following major blunt injuries, if no clear-cut clinical indications for abdominal exploration are present and if the peritoneal tap for blood is negative, then a child can be conservatively managed with the diagnostic studies just mentioned. Obviously, such children should be admitted to intensive care areas for observation during these procedures, and if their vital signs become unstable, rapid laparotomy is indicated.

If an exploratory operative procedure is indicated for blunt abdominal trauma and the spleen is found to be lacerated, attempts should be made to preserve the splenic tissue by suturing the laceration, by partial splenectomy and by preserving any accessory spleens that may be present. Mattress sutures supported by Teflon pledgets or small pieces of omentum often facilitate securing the soft splenic tissue. Autotransplantation of splenic tissue into muscle or retroperitoneal tissues may be feasible, but this is an experimental procedure at the present time. There is no good evidence that transplanted splenic tissue will be immunologically functional. All reasonable attempts should be made to preserve splenic tissue in children in order to decrease the chances of overwhelming postsplenectomy sepsis.

If it is necessary to remove the spleen to prevent exsanguinating hemorrhage or because the spleen has been completely transected from its vascular pedicle, the child should be placed on prophylactic antibiotics, preferably one of the penicillins, possibly for the rest of childhood. The recent introduction of polyvalent pneumococcal serum should also be added as a part of prophylaxis against overwhelming sepsis in a splenectomized child.

SPECIAL CONSIDERATIONS IN THE TREATMENT OF TRAUMA IN INFANTS

Size. The small size of the injured child is the single most influential factor differentiating his management from that of the adult. The margin for error is diminished correspondingly and may seem infinitesimal in the newborn and premature infant. Seemingly trivial details, which assume importance only in complicated cases of adult trauma, demand routine attention in the management of children.

The obvious discrepancies in physical size of adults and children are reflected in alteration of physiological function. The importance of a tiny blood volume is immediately apparent. In the newborn infant a single blood-soaked sponge may represent the difference between circulatory stability and shock.

Respiratory Reserve. From both an anatomical and physiological standpoint, the infant has a much lower respiratory reserve than the adult.[16] The vital capacity at 1 week of age is approximately 140 ml. and

the tidal volume is 15 ml. The trachea may be only 4 cm. in length and 6 mm. in diameter. These factors coupled with a weak thoracic musculature, flexible rib cage and narrow air passages all complicate the movement of tracheobronchial secretions.

Heat Loss. The increased surface area of the infant relative to his weight allows excessive heat loss under circumstances of debility. The thermal regulatory mechanism of children often is unable to meet the requirements of such situations, and great care must be taken to monitor and support the temperature of all infants. This inadequacy is magnified by the transfusion of large quantities of cold blood, a circumstance that may lead to rapid loss of body heat and even significant cardiac arrhythmias.

Fluid and Electrolyte Balance. Fluid and electrolyte balance presents an additional problem in these small patients. Although numerous formulas have been devised for the routine maintenance of fluid and electrolytes in children, they are usually inadequate in situations leading to rapid internal or external losses of fluids. The physiological maturity of the baby may play an important role in such circumstances. Renal immaturity in the newborn is reflected in decreased ability to concentrate and conserve fluid and electrolytes. There is a concomitant limitation in glomerular filtration rate. The combination of these two factors restricts the infant's ability to respond to conditions of stress and increased metabolic demand.

Drug Therapy. The general physiological immaturity of the infant also may exert its influence in other areas. Any physician caring for such patients must have a thorough knowledge of possible drug idiosyncrasies as well as proper dosages for this age group.

The necessity for adjusting medication dosages in infants to the variables of weight and surface area is immediately apparent. However, other factors such as alterations in rate of absorption and excretion, differences in distribution and, finally, variables in metabolism and detoxification are equally important in newborn and premature infants. it is recommended that any group caring for an injured child include a physician who is conversant with these problems.

Congenital Defects. Another potential

source of complications in the management of injured children is the coexistence of congenital anomalies. Cardiac defects are of particular significance. A unique example of a complicating anomaly was seen in a small child hospitalized for a supracondylar fracture of the elbow. There was no evidence of coexistent abdominal trauma. However, the child subsequently developed signs and symptoms of partial intestinal obstruction and was found to have a partial malrotation with volvulus of the small intestine.

Response to Trauma. Lability often is cited as the outstanding characteristic of the response of infants and children to trauma. *The smaller the size of the patient, the briefer the transition from health to illness and from illness to death.* The utmost vigilance is demanded in detecting the subtle signs that suggest alterations in the infant's condition. Fortunately, the elasticity of the healthy child's response seems boundless, allowing a rapid compensation for potential catastrophes if corrections can be instituted promptly.

SPECIAL TECHNIQUES IN THE MANAGEMENT OF TRAUMA IN CHILDHOOD

Fluid and Electrolyte Balance. As indicated, the single most difficult task in the management of a small infant or child may involve adequate fluid and electrolyte replacement. To the physician who infrequently handles children the maintenance of such a patient on prolonged parenteral replacement itself poses a formidable challenge. Knowledge of fluid and electrolyte therapy in infants and children has advanced tremendously in recent years, with an increased understanding of the physiological mechanisms that are involved.

Many formulas have been devised for the calculation of maintenance fluids in children, but the most rational ones appear to be those based on the rate of metabolic turnover. The use of this factor enables one to consolidate his thinking in terms of a single variable, that is, allows an integration of the basal requirements with the additional influences of activity and environmental temperature. With this approach, one is furnished simultaneously with the caloric requirements of his pa-

TABLE 24–1. Standard Basal Calories[°]

WEIGHT (kg.)	CALORIES/24 HOURS MALE AND FEMALE	
3		140
5		270
7		400
9		500
11		600
13		650
15		710
17		780
19		830
21		880
25	1020	960
29	1120	1040
33	1210	1120
37	1300	1190
41	1350	1260
45	1410	1320
49	1470	1380
53	1530	1440
57	1590	1500
61	1640	1560

Modified from Talbot.

Increments or decrements
1. Add or subtract 12 per cent of above for each degree C (8 per cent for each degree F.) above or below rectal temperature of 37.8° C (100° F.)
2. Add 0 to 30 per cent increments for activity.

[°]From Vaughn, V. C., III, McKay, R. J., and Behrman, R. E.: Nelson Textbook of Pediatrics. 1979.

tient. This figure becomes increasingly important in situations demanding long-term parenteral alimentation.

CALORIC REQUIREMENTS. Table 24–1 is a brief outline of basal caloric requirements in children varying in weight from 3 to 31 kg. The maintenance supply of water for the average patient varies from 110 to 120 ml. per 100 calories metabolized.[32] Thus, the maintenance fluid requirements of a child may be obtained easily by multiplying this last figure (110–120) by the calculated caloric requirement divided by 100 (the latter having been obtained by adjusting the standard basal caloric requirement [Table 24–1] to conditions of temperature and activity). The postoperative patient, of course, will have a tendency to retain water and certain electrolytes, and maintenance fluids should not exceed 80 to 90 ml. per 100 calories metabolized.

FLUID RETENTION. The tendency of pediatric patients to retain fluids postoperatively seems to vary directly with age. An infant, for instance, has a much briefer period of water retention postoperatively than an older child. There is also an individual variation in fluid and electrolyte excretion in children, especially during infancy. However, the average sodium requirement for parenteral fluid therapy is 2 to 4 mEq., and the potassium requirement is 2 to 3 mEq. for each 100 calories metabolized. A solution of 5 or 10 per cent glucose containing 30 mEq. of sodium and chloride and 20 mEq. of potassium per liter represents an adequate maintenance fluid that meets the usual requirements when administered intravenously at the rate of 110 to 120 ml. per 100 calories metabolized.

MASSIVE REPLACEMENT. The difficulties of fluid maintenance in infants and small children are compounded in situations demanding massive volume replacement. Little effort has been made to simplify this problem in the small patient, although great strides have been taken in monitoring similar shifts of fluids in adults. Fortunately, the elasticity of the child is such that he will often weather prolonged episodes of relative hyper- or hypovolemia without lasting damage. Even so, inaccuracies in replacement therapy may spell the difference in ultimate survival. In an effort to consolidate the various monitoring factors into a simplified, readily available scheme, the following approach has been adopted by the Pediatric Surgical Service of the Children's Medical and Surgical Center in The Johns Hopkins Hospital.

USE OF FLOW CHART. All patients admitted for major surgery or with severe trauma are monitored on a fluid and electrolyte flow chart with minimum 6-hour calculations of balance. Important features of this system include measurements of central venous pressure, total serum solids, hematocrit, urinary specific gravity and serum electrolytes, with precise calculations of all fluid intake and output. The patient's vital signs and clinical response remain the most important criteria of adequate return of homeostasis. Such signs may be misleading, however, under certain situations, and the addition of the supplemental information outlined previously allows a more controlled approach to patient management.

URINARY OUTPUT. Urinary output in the child is a sensitive index of volume expansion and renal perfusion, but here, again, one may be mislead. The newborn infant, for instance, may be limited in both his ability to increase volume and to concentrate urine.[24] As a result, urinary specific gravity in these patients may remain relatively low in the face of inadequate fluid intake. On the other hand, congestive failure may rapidly ensue from overhydration, since a diminished glomerular filtration rate limits the renal response in such situations. Older children present the same problems evident in the adult, in that the antidiuretic response of the immediate postoperative period may limit urinary output even with maximal hydration. Urinary output, then, is a valuable index of homeostasis only if intrinsic pitfalls are recognized.

CENTRAL VENOUS PRESSURE. The use of central venous pressure has found increasing advocates in recent years since its first application in the field of cardiac surgery.[3, 36] Again, this is not necessarily an absolute value. Rather, in the absence of a coexistent cardiorespiratory problem, this indicator provides an excellent index of functional intravascular volume. In essence, the central venous pressure is a direct reflection of the effective cardiac filling pressure. If there is decreased central venous pressure one may assume that additional fluids may be administered; whereas elevations of pressure, in the absence of local venous obstruction, indicate that the cardiac filling pressure is adequate for the state of cardiac function at that particular moment. In such circumstances other means of increasing cardiac output must be sought.

Introduction of Swan-Ganz right heart catheter allows continuous monitoring of right atrial pressure and mean pulmonary arterial pressure as well as pulmonary wedge pressure, which may be equated to left atrial pressure. Perfusion of the lung in children with blunt thoracic trauma may be of critical importance and percutaneous introduction of this catheter now provides such information with more reliability than the central venous pressure catheter.

In addition, the device's capability to monitor continuously cardiac output as a function of thermodilution is now currently employed in children undergoing massive transfusions and fluid shifts from multiple trauma. This technique of percutaneous introduction allows reproducible and accurate assessment of cardiac output.

One reason central venous pressure has not been applied so widely in the infant as

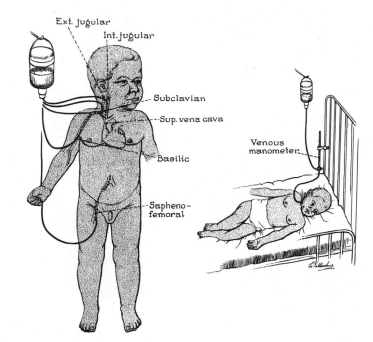

Figure 24–2. *Sites for central venous pressure monitoring in the infant. (From Talbert, J. L., and Haller, J. A., Jr.: Am. Surg. 32:767, 1966.)*

in the adult is the seeming sparsity of satisfactory sites through which central venous cannulation may be achieved.[30] Experience has indicated that catheterization of the inferior vena cava may be unfavorable in some children because of interference by abdominal pressure changes. Such situations may be particularly common in the infant and small child, in whom the changes in intra-abdominal pressure associated with distention, crying or breathing are much more pronounced than in adults. The sites for cannulation, therefore, are limited. Routes that have been chosen include the basilic vein in the antecubital fossa and the external and internal jugular veins in the neck (Fig. 24–2). In infancy, such cannulation usually necessitates a cutdown. The internal jugular particularly is a sizable vein in infancy and offers a readily accessible spot for introduction of a large-bore catheter *when other routes are inadequate*. Such cannulation conceivably may be performed percutaneously, but direct exposure appears surer and possibly safer (Fig. 24–3). Percutaneous puncture of the subclavian vein, however, via the subclavicular route offers an alternate route, although there is a definite hazard of producing pneumothorax with this method and it is chosen only when other sites seem poorer. Such a situation did arise in a severely burned 3-month-old infant whose

only area of uninvolved skin lay in the shoulder. Subclavian catheterization allowed fluid and antibiotic administration through this route for more than 4 weeks.

The importance of placing the monitoring catheter in a central position has been emphasized repeatedly. The effects of either venous spasm or valves interposed between the central and peripheral venous systems may lead to discrepancies if pressures are monitored peripherally.[36] When measured correctly, however, venous pressure provides an accurate guide to fluid volume, especially under conditions of massive replacement or hidden losses.

USE OF SERUM SOLIDS. The use of total serum solids as an indication of serum protein levels has become increasingly popular with the introduction of small, accurate refractometers (Fig. 24–3).[28] The measurements are particularly useful in situations associated with such massive fluid and concomitant protein losses as might occur in burns. The measurement has also been employed in monitoring major surgical and traumatic cases, however, and has been equally applicable in these instances. The losses incurred following major surgical dissections often consist primarily of protein rich fluid. Again, the measurement of total serum solids, coupled with simultaneous determinations of the hematocrit and venous pressure, allows considerable in-

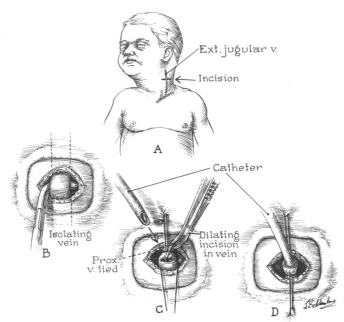

Figure 24-3. *Catheterization of the external jugular vein as performed in the infant (A and B). The vein is isolated with a small curved clamp through a short, transverse skin incision. (C) A 4-0 plain catgut ligature is tied about the cephalic end of the vein. A second ligature is placed distally, with traction exerted in opposite directions by clamping the ties to the adjacent drapes. A transverse incision is made in the anterior wall of the vein. This opening is then enlarged by inserting and spreading the tips of a small curved forceps. (D) While the vein lumen is exposed in this manner, a beveled cannula may be introduced with relative ease. When the catheter has been positioned at the level of the innominate vein or superior vena cava, the second ligature is secured. The use of fine, plain catgut avoids any necessity for subsequent removal of these ligatures. The skin incision is closed with a single vertical mattress suture of fine silk. This same suture may be tied about the cannula with a separate knot at a point 1.5 cm. from the skin. By dividing this distal knot, subsequent withdrawal of the catheter is possible and removal of the skin suture itself may be avoided. Finally the cannula should always be carefully taped to the skin of the neck as an additional safeguard against accidental dislodgment. (Talbert, J. L., and Haller, J. A., Jr.: Am. Surg. 32:767, 1966.)*

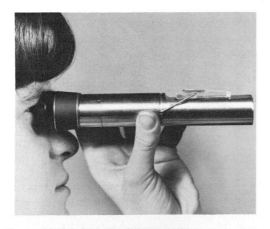

Figure 24-4. *A total solid meter. This visual refractometer provides accurate measurements (maximum error 0.1 per cent TS) of urinary specific gravity, total serum solids and total serum proteins when one drop of test solution is placed between the measuring prisms on top of the instrument. In general, the serum contained in two small microhematocrit tubes is sufficient for such determinations. (TS Meter Model 10400. American Optical Company, Instrument Division, Buffalo, New York.)*

sight as to whether the patient requires water, plasma or blood replacement at any particular moment.

ADDITIONAL PROBLEMS. A flow chart, as outlined previously, coupled with daily determinations of body weight gives a continuing picture of the patient's condition. These data on the state of hydration and intravascular volume are particularly valuable in situations in which one is uncertain whether the oliguria (or anuria) that so often follows severe trauma is a reflection of primary renal damage or of inadequate replacement. The flow chart also serves as a valuable indicator of unusual trends in therapy and may allow the physician to anticipate and avoid complications prior to their development. The danger of overhydration and excessive transfusion in small infants may thus be obviated. Since none of these observations requires elaborate equipment, they should be readily accessible to the physician and, when coupled with determinations of serum electrolytes, offer a precise guide to therapy.

An additional hazard of massive fluid replacement in infants and small children is encountered in the administration of cold blood or plasma. These solutions must be warmed prior to their administration, if by no other means than coiling plastic intravenous tubing in a container of warm water. The warming water should not be hotter than 43 to 46° C. Relatively inexpensive equipment is available that is designed specifically for this purpose. Large quantities of citrated blood may necessitate calcium replacement in small infants. This practice has been followed for many years in adults but is relatively unimportant in this group as compared to infants, whose calcium stores are more quickly expended and whose compensatory mechanisms are less able to respond to potential calcium depletion. A final complication of massive colloid replacement in children is the potentiation of the metabolic acidosis of shock by the infusion of stored blood or plasma. The seriousness of this problem is proportional to the size of the patient and the rapidity of replacement therapy. Administration of bicarbonate or TRIS buffer may be necessary in such circumstances.[18]

Another significant problem encountered in infants is the administration of small, precise quantities of parenteral fluids over prolonged periods. The use of a constant infusion pump such as the Holter Pump for this purpose has proved extremely useful (Fig. 24–5). Carefully measured volumes may be given at low flow rates with these units without fear of clotting in the intravenous tubing.

Although hypodermoclysis has proved helpful as a method of fluid administration in the past, the indications for its use on a trauma service are few indeed. Other routes of administration such as intraarterial, intraperitoneal or intraosseous infusions are not necessary. There is no situation in which the indications for these approaches would obviate the potential hazards of their use.

Airway Provision. The establishment of an adequate airway in a child may also present special problems. The older child should be managed as an adult. That is, when prolonged respiratory support is demanded, a tracheostomy should be performed, using an adapter tube for the res-

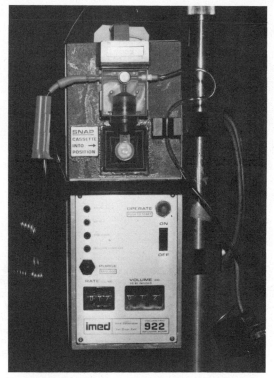

Figure 24–5. *IMED 922 infusion pump for constant intravenous infusion of hyperalimentation solutions as well as special medications.*

pirator. Tracheostomies in infants, however, are notorious for their accompanying complications. There are difficulties in the management of tiny tracheostomies and sometimes removal of the tube may be a problem. To obviate this problem some pediatric surgeons have resorted to prolonged use of endotracheal tubes. Many of these physicians have been enthusiastic about this technique, but we have found that it also creates difficulties, especially increased problems with tracheobronchial secretions and damage to delicate laryngeal tissues. The concomitant use of steroids may help to diminish any laryngeal edema resulting from prolonged irritation by such tubes but, in general, we have continued to utilize tracheostomies, attempting to remove them within 3 to 5 days to avoid the troublesome dependence on the tube that may develop and to decrease scarring and stricture of the tracheal wall.

Tracheostomy in infants and children should *not* be performed as is an adult tracheostomy (see Chapter 12). Three salient features of the operative technique of

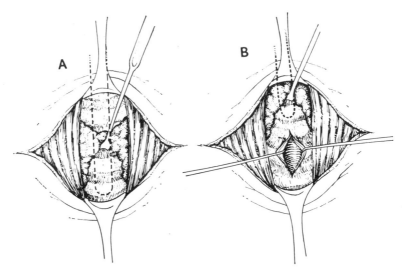

Figure 24–6. *Tracheostomy technique: A transverse skin incision has proved preferable for use of the Silastic tube which is equipped with an inferior "tracheostomy incision shield" that prevents angulation and erosion of the edge of the tube into the lower margin of the skin wound. The strap muscles are separated vertically by blunt dissection and the thyroid isthmus is reflected cephalad after division of the pretracheal fascia (A). The anterior tracheal wall is then incised vertically, dividing the second, third, fourth and, if needed, the fifth tracheal cartilages in the midline. No transverse counter incision is employed and no tracheal flap or window is ever removed in infants. The endotracheal tube is then withdrawn into the proximal tracheal, the tracheotomy margins are retracted laterally by small hooks, and an appropriate Silastic tube is inserted (B).*

tracheostomy in an infant need emphasizing:

1. Tracheostomy should never be attempted in a baby without first intubating the patient to ensure an adequate temporary airway.

2. No tracheal tissue should be excised. A vertical incision through two or three cartilages will provide a quite adequate opening, and the elastic tracheal rings will subsequently reconstitute the airway cylinder on tube removal. Traction on stay sutures on either side of the vertical incision can restore the airway and allow easy, controlled replacement of the tube, should it be inadvertently dislodged (Fig. 24–6). The adult technique of excising a window promotes tracheal instability in an infant, in view of the proportionately larger amount of the central part of the cartilaginous rings excised. The poorly supported trachea may collapse, and the soft tissues of the neck can fall into the lumen, narrowing it considerably during healing.

3. Finally, the infant's tracheostomy tube must be securely and snugly sutured or tied in position, since dislodgment occurs very easily, and reinsertion may be more difficult than in adults.

Proper nursing care is as critical to successful tracheostomy as the technical procedure itself. Several items deserve emphasis:

1. Because of his short neck, a baby must be positioned with his neck extended by a small roll under his shoulders, to prevent obstruction by his fat neck or chin.

2. Suctioning must be a sterile procedure using a fresh, sterile catheter and clean glove each time.

3. Adequate suctioning past the tip of the catheter is essential to prevent plugs. (Even the relatively inert Silastic tubes will plug at the tip if inadequately suctioned.) Adequate humidification is, of course, mandatory.

Failure to recognize significant anatomical difference between an infant's and an adult's tracheal anatomy has led to inappropriate miniaturization of adult metal tracheostomy tubes; these devices can prove unsatisfactory in size, length and configuration. Taking into account the narrow tracheal lumen of a child, the extreme flexibility of his cartilages and the increased activity and movement of his body, head and neck, a relatively larger tube lumen is required for an infant than an adult in order to achieve satisfactory air exchange and avoid additional airway resistance. Rigid tubes that cannot conform to the length and shape of the trachea can encourage mucosal ulceration and all its attendant morbidity, particularly if the constant movement of a mechanical ventilator is added.[34]

We have explored the use of flexible, synthetic tracheostomy tubes for our infants and children. We have been quite pleased with the basic tracheostomy tube designed by Aberdeen. Such tubes, constructed of very inert and well-tolerated silicone rubber, have been used in thousands of patients with no unusual complications, no permanent strictures and ready extubation in all babies who survived their original disease.[15, 34]

Attention to several factors is important:

1. The period of initial nasotracheal or orotracheal intubation before tracheostomy should be sufficiently brief to avoid subglottic inflammation and subsequent scarring and stenosis. Two to three days in older children and a week or more in small infants appears to be relatively innocuous.

2. Careful tracheostomy technique suited to children such as previously described can prevent scarring and narrowing at the tracheostomy site itself.

3. The use of flexible, inert tracheostomy tubes, such as the Silastic tubes (Aberdeen design), can help avoid inflammation and scarring of the distal trachea.

4. Finally, the tracheostomy tubes should be progessively diminished in caliber to the narrowest size over several days prior to extubation. The patient can become accustomed to breathing through the relatively wider trachea and pharynx, and the surgeon can observe how well the patient tolerates the normal ventilatory path. When this is accomplished, the small tube is simply removed with the child in a high humidity atmosphere.

Gastrointestinal Decompression. A final area demanding special consideration in children is that of gastrointestinal decompression following abdominal trauma and surgery. Nasogastric decompression of the stomach is an absolutely essential step prior to examining the traumatized child. Children who have been severely frightened will become aerophagic and the stomach will become grossly distended. An adequate abdominal examination, therefore, must begin with gastric decompression.[11] Not only can gastrointestinal decompression be achieved during the initial stages of convalescence but also early feeding may be administered through these tubes, thus conserving the strength of the patient during a critical phase of recovery. To avoid overdistention in infants during these initial feedings, a Y-tube arrangement has been employed that allows excessive pressure to be vented. In this way the frequent complications of regurgitation and aspiration of feedings in infants are avoided. A greater degree of freedom and mobility is also allowed the older child, resulting in a much happier convalescence. It should be emphasized, however, that a nasogastric tube satisfactory for short-term decompression in older children should be used when indicated.

Temperature Regulation. As mentioned previously, the thermal regulatory mechanism of pediatric patients often seems immature, and great care must be taken to monitor temperatures frequently and to provide some means of external warmth. Warming blankets can be employed for this purpose in older children. For infants, Isolettes are an ideal means of providing both warmth and moisture, and their use is encouraged in this age group. It should be emphasized, however, that all connections with intravenous tubes, drainage tubes and ancillary equipment should be arranged so that ready access to the Isolette is preserved. There is no more frustrating situation than that presented by a critically ill infant who requires instant attention but who is enclosed by a cage of tangled tubes and plastic walls.

Other facets of management in children are not unlike those employed for older patients. The use of extensive monitoring equipment, including electrocardiograms and pressure recorders, may become necessary and should be readily available. The radial artery at the wrist in older children and in infants is the most common site for positioning of catheters for monitoring arterial pressure.[10]

TRAUMA PECULIAR TO CHILDHOOD

Much of the trauma encountered in children is similar in both etiology and treatment to that seen in adults. Particular types, however, are distinguished by their predominance in infancy and childhood. Included in this latter group are neonatal trauma, the "battered child" syndrome and certain forms of home accidents.

Neonatal Trauma

Neonatal trauma constitutes an important percentage of birth mortality. Any practicing surgeon may be confronted with a seriously injured newborn and should be prepared to handle the varied aspects of such situations.

The most common area of traumatic birth injury in the neonate is the head. Superficial molding, erythema, abrasions, ecchymoses or even fat necrosis are not uncommon.[32] The caput succedaneum with passive edema of the presenting part is well recognized. Such injuries are usually of no consequence. A cephalohematoma with subperiosteal hemorrhage or actual skull fractures occasionally may be encountered. The neophyte may have difficulty in interpreting skull x-rays in these patients and, on palpation, may confuse suture lines with depressed fractures. Routine needle aspirations should be avoided and, in the absence of a depressed fracture or localizing neurological signs, close observation should be the only treatment necessary. The usual source of intracranial injury is the molding of the skull that occurs in the birth process rather than an actual impact force. Overriding of the sutures may lead to tearing of small veins and sinuses on the tentorium, producing subarachnoid or subdural bleeding.

Traumatic damage to the vertebrae and spinal cord may result from traction or forced movements of the neck during the delivery, producing compression or laceration of the vertebral arteries, tears in cervical joint capsules, dura or nerve roots, or compression of the spinal cord.[1] The premature infant is particularly susceptible to such damage. Injuries of this type may be more common than realized, since the signs are usually obscured by associated cerebral damage.

Peripheral nerve damage is another well recognized product of traumatic delivery, with a classic Erb-Duchenne paralysis (C5–6), Klumpke's paralysis (C7–8 and T1), phrenic nerve paralysis and facial nerve

paralysis the most common forms of this type of injury.

The skeletal injuries most commonly observed in newborns are clavicular fractures and fractures and dislocations of the extremities.[1] Of this group, clavicular fractures are most common and should always alert the physician to the possibility of an associated brachial plexus, pulmonary or phrenic nerve injury. A common manifestation of these last two complications is respiratory distress, induced either by pneumothorax or diaphragmatic paralysis.

Although figure-of-eight shoulder bandages are useful in treating clavicular fractures in older children, it may be extremely difficult, and probably unnecessary, to employ this technique in newborns. In tiny infants there is a tendency for such bandages to exert maximum pressure immediately over the fracture site rather than at an optimal point on the distal shoulder. Certainly, as emphasized previously, Velpeau dressings and arm slings are contraindicated for treatment of this problem in any age group. In the neonate the easiest, and safest, treatment is to avoid lifting the affected extremity. Maintaining the infant in the usual prone position achieves a result comparable to splinting with a figure-of-eight dressing and permits excellent healing.

Fractures and dislocations of the extremities are commonly associated with neurological and developmental anomalies such as meningomyelocele or arthrogryposis multiplex congenita. Detailed treatment of these fractures is outlined in the literature.

Respiratory embarrassment following delivery may result from injuries that compromise the nasal airway, from dislocations of the cricothyroid or cricoarytenoid articulations or pneumothorax.[15, 32] Dislocation of the cricothyroid or cricoarytenoid articulations may necessitate immediate tracheostomy. A tension pneumothorax may present a critical emergency necessitating immediate decompression by needle aspiration, with subsequent drainage for persistent leaks (Fig. 24–7). Minor degress of pneumothorax in infancy may be treated expectantly, since rapid absorption of air in the pleural or peritoneal cavities will occur within 24 to 48 hours, especially in the presence of high oxygen concentrations. There should be no hesitancy, however, in

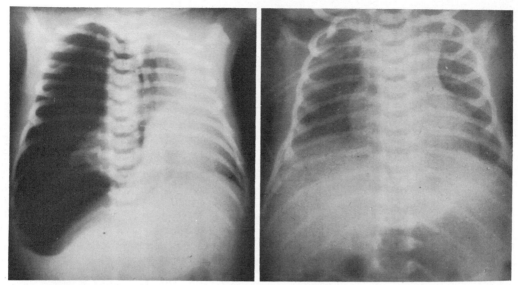

Figure 24–7. *Tension pneumothorax of the newborn relieved by tube drainage.*

inserting a small intercostal chest catheter attached to underwater seal drainage in those instances in which a continuing air leak is encountered (Fig. 24–8). Suction is rarely needed. In general, these tubes are best inserted laterally under direct vision, with care taken to prevent excessive medial protrusion into the mediastinum, either displacing the latter structure or preventing complete pulmonary expansion. A small removable stylet inserted through the catheter has been found to facilitate insertion of these tubes through lateral stab wounds. The use of a trocar is prohibitively dangerous in a small patient in whom deviations of a fraction of an inch may lead to major injuries.

Abdominal trauma is unusual in the neonate. Injury of the liver comprises the more frequent form. Adrenal hemorrhage has been attributed to trauma but it is questionable whether this is not a secondary rather than a primary condition.

Vascular injuries, especially those arising from blunt trauma, are rarely incurred in the pediatric age group. When they are present, however, they may compromise the future growth and function of the involved extremity. Early recognition and correction of vascular injuries are essential factors in assuring normal limbs.[36]

Battered Child Syndrome

Public Law 93-247, the Child Abuse Prevention and Treatment Act, is the latest in federal legislation designed to curb the increasing incidence of the "battered child syndrome." Such legislation has unfortunately awaited medical definition of what constitutes child abuse. Awareness of this clinical complex began in 1946 when Caffey* reported the association between subdural hematomas and fractures of the long bones in infants. In 1953, Silverman reported incidental findings of healed fractures in infants. It was his feeling that such injuries were secondary to trauma. In 1955, Wooley and Evans reached the conclusion that these fractures were not only traumatic but also were most often inflicted intentionally. Since this report, there have been many identical reports culminating in 1961 with Kempe's coining the phrase battered child syndrome. With the introduction of a precise permanent radiographic documentation of findings associated with the battered child syndrome, there ensued numerous epidemiological studies, investigations into etiology, methods of management, community wide programs and a large amount of social and legal work to determine the structure under which such cases should be managed. With the defining of the syndrome and the extensive publicity that it has received, reporting of the battered child syndrome in the literature has escalated from 7000 cases in 1967

---

*Caffey, J.: Multiple fractures in the long bones of infants suffering from chronic subdural hematoma. Am. J. Roentgenol. 56:167, 1946.

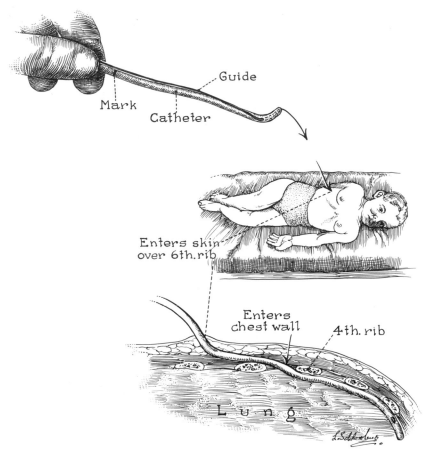

Figure 24–8.   *A technique for chest tube insertion in the infant. A short skin incision is made over the 6th rib in the midaxillary line following infiltration with 0.5 per cent procaine. A subcutaneous tract is then dissected bluntly with a small curved clamp over the superior margin of the 5th rib and through the intercostal muscles into the pleural cavity. A malleable probe is then inserted as a stylet into the proximal side-hole of a small French catheter (Nos. 10 to 12). The tip of the stylet is curved in order to facilitate introduction of the catheter through the skin incision and subcutaneous tract into the chest cavity. The catheter has been marked previously at the optimum depth of insertion in order to prevent excessive penetration into the thorax and possible injury to apical or mediastinal structures. The use of a stylet facilitates placement of the drainage tube in an optimum position along the lateral thoracic wall. Once positioning is achieved, the probe may easily be withdrawn. A lateral insertion site is preferable in infants, even in the treatment of pneumothorax. Introduction of a catheter through the second intercostal space anteriorly, as recommended in adults, is excessively difficult and hazardous in view of the limited pleural space and the close proximity of vital structures. In infants, direct insertion of the catheters into the chest, rather than tunneling through the subcutaneous tissues, as described, may result in a significant delay in healing of the tube tract.*

to 200,000 in 1974. Early identification of childhood battering is emphasized in the writing of Schmitt and Kempe in the most recent edition of the *Nelson Textbook of Pediatrics.* They state as follows:

> If the child who has been physically abused is returned to his parents without any intervention, 5 per cent are killed and 35 per cent are seriously reinjured.

Morse° has noted that injury from abuse is more common than appendicitis in children and that its mortality is many times higher. It is, therefore, imperative that pediatric surgeons develop diagnostic skills and a high index of suspicion, which will be equally applied in both appendicitis and battered child syndrome. In the past physicians have tended to transfer responsibility for follow-up supervisory care to the hospital social services department or community service agencies. Experience may indicate the need for continued medical involvement, with periodic examinations as prophylaxis against repeated injuries.

°Morse, T. S.: Child abuse: A neglected form of trauma. J. Trauma *15*:620, 1975.

Nearly two thirds of all recognized cases of battered child syndrome occur in youngsters in the first 2 years of life. The young nonverbal child, unable to escape and totally dependent upon those taking care of him, is at highest risk of injury and death.

The physical features most commonly associated with child abuse may usually be readily visible on the body surface. The hallmarks of this syndrome are abrasions, lacerations and ecchymoses that are incompatible with the level of the child's developmental age. They may be in groups, as burns, belt marks and lacerations of lip and gum; ears may be traumatized by twisting and the child may have unusual and unclean skin "rashes." The skeletal system may reveal tenderness, swelling or limitation of motion of an extremity; periosteal thickening of long bones; a variety of healing reactions of long bones in varying stages; and acute cephalohematomas. The abdomen may have both external signs of trauma as well as occult signs of peritoneal inflammation from ruptured organs following kicks or blows. We have personally seen complete transection of the lateral left lobe of the liver from a kick in the epigastrium; complete transection of the pancreas at the level of the spine; multiple small bowel perforations and hematomas; complete venous occlusion of the entire small bowel; rupture of the spleen, kidney and bladder from someone kneeling on the child's abdomen; and rupture of the gallbladder from a kick in the right upper quadrant.

These injuries are difficult to diagnose in the absence of a history of any trauma and are dependent upon an acutely high index of suspicion about an infant with external signs of trauma that might at first resemble a more routine case of sepsis. When presented with a child whose injuries seem most compatible with physical abuse, it is essential that the physician compile a careful history. Since parents, guardians or baby sitters tend to conceal the true mechanism of injury, it is important to question the possibility of recent "accidents." The physician must then ascertain whether the quoted circumstances of the "accident" are compatible with the location and extent of the injury sustained. If the child reportedly contributed to the "accident," it must be determined whether or not the personal involvement was compatible with the physical developmental age. If multiple injuries are present clinically or radiographically, the question of whether or not they are all compatible with the "accidental event" or whether they are of necessity separate events must be answered.

Statistically verified long-range permanent physical and emotional damage occurs in an alarmingly high percentage of the children we have seen. An appreciable number of these children appear retarded on subsequent psychological testing, but differentiation between innate genetic factors, emotionally based retardation and organic central nervous system damage is difficult.

The initial goal in the long-range treatment of the battered child syndrome is prophylaxis; that is, protection against the hostile environment. Identification of this adverse environment is based upon physician recognition with the first physical evidence of child abuse. Continued education and involvement of pediatricians, emergency room physicians and pediatric surgeons is the first step in achieving the goal.

An excellent example of the battered child syndrome is provided in the following case report:

Case History No. 4. W. B., JHH, 102 10 55. A 3-year-old white male child was admitted through the emergency room with complaints of "throwing up for 4 days." Except for previous admissions to The Johns Hopkins Hospital for repair of a cleft lip and palate, the child had remained asymptomatic until 3 days prior to admission. At that time he was noted to vomit on several occasions, the symptoms persisting with increasing frequency. The mother denied all knowledge of possible trauma until the patient was seen by a local physician, who inquired as to the etiology of numerous contusions over the abdomen and extremities.

The family and social history were pertinent, since the mother was divorced and the child had not been the product of the marriage.

On examination, the patient was obviously an acutely ill, dehydrated child with evidence of multiple areas of old bruising, particularly over the right abdomen (Fig. 24–9). Diminished bowel sounds were present, although there were no signs of peritoneal irritation. There was tenderness to direct palpation in the right lower quadrant of the abdomen, but no masses were evident. X-rays of the abdomen, chest and right arm revealed Colles' fracture of the right wrist and an adynamic ileus. The hematocrit was 30 per cent (the hematocrit on discharge 1

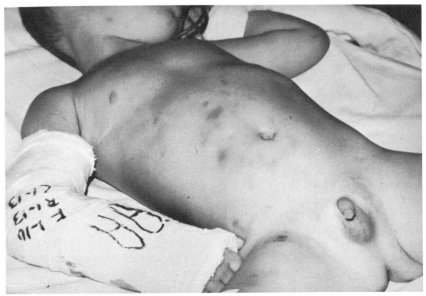

Figure 24–9. *The "battered child syndrome" as exemplified by abdominal ecchymoses and fracture of the right arm.*

month previously had been 34 per cent), the white blood count was 17,000, and the urinalysis revealed 4+ proteinuria and numerous red blood cells. Serum chemistries revealed a serum urea nitrogen of 75 mg. per cent; sodium, 127 mEq./l.; potassium, 7.2 mEq./l.; carbon dioxide, 18 mEq./l.; and amylase, 900 mg. per cent (reducing substance).

The clinical impression was one of generalized blunt trauma resulting in a fracture of the right wrist and right renal damage associated with retroperitoneal hematoma. An intravenous pyelogram confirmed the presence of a nonfunctioning kidney on the right. The blood pressure was noted to be normal on admission and remained so throughout the course of hospitalization.

The patient was admitted to the Intensive Care Unit of The Children's Medical and Surgical Center under the immediate supervision of the Pediatric General Surgical Service with consultant services supplied by Pediatrics, Orthopedics and Urology. Fluid and electrolyte replacement was instituted immediately and all chemistries, including the serum amylase, had returned to normal by the fourth hospital day. A gastrointestinal series demonstrated continuity of the intestinal tract. A retrograde pyelogram revealed evidence of dye extending out from the superior calyx into the renal parenchyma, suggesting a traumatic fracture. Renal scan showed no evidence of uptake of the radioactive material by the right kidney. Several repeat pyelograms during the subsequent months continued to reveal absence of function of the right kidney. The hematuria cleared during this

time, however. Since there was no evidence of developing hypertension or localized abdominal mischief, a conservative, watchful approach was directed toward the renal injury.

The social problem was quite involved and required a thorough evaluation of the home situation, both by the police and the social service division. The patient was finally discharged to the mother's care after she was cleared completely of any possible complicity in the child's injury. A third person was implicated by the investigation and was removed from all contact with the patient. Further steps in management have included efforts to improve the family's socioeconomic situation.

O'Neill and associates have presented an excellent review of the patterns of injury seen in battered children.[25] In their series of 110 battered children, the types of injuries in the order of frequency were soft tissue injuries, fractures and head injuries. Eight of the patients died from head injuries. Combined injuries were common. Evidence of chronic or prior injury was the rule.

Home Injuries

Any classification of injuries unique to childhood includes those occurring in the home. Such injuries may result from falls; from entanglements with various types of vehicles, including automobiles, wagons, bicycles, skateboards and skates; from body burns, either electrical or thermal; from ingestion of caustic substances and foreign bodies; or from so-called wringer injuries.

Body Burns. The treatment of body burns is particularly difficult in the infant and young child. This problem is reflected in the high mortality encountered in this age group. The body surface area of these patients is large in relation to their weight and differs in distribution from that observed in adults. As a result, standard charts that have been prepared for estimation of extent of burns in adults are useless when applied to infants or small children.[5]

Certain complications of burn therapy are encountered more frequently in children than adults. Airway obstruction due to laryngeal edema is a greater hazard because of the smaller structures. Alterations in metabolic response may also prove troublesome in these patients. Excessive sodium replacement is much more likely to occur in infants. Colloid loss in the adult may be balanced by normal physiological responses, whereas any serious burn in the young child usually will necessitate some form of extrinsic colloid replacement.[22] The introduction of topical therapy with either 0.5 per cent silver nitrate solution or Sulfamylon cream has proved both a tremendous boon and a potential hazard. Serious electrolyte dilution may develop within 6 hours in infants when Moyer's silver nitrate method of treatment is employed.[21] Severe hyperchloremic acidosis, particularly with a respiratory burn, may be a complication of Moncreif's method of Sulfamylon therapy.[20] Careful monitoring and electrolyte replacement are mandatory under these circumstances.

Although basic replacement formulas are useful in projecting fluid and colloid losses in burn patients, the addition of the monitoring routine outlined previously for management of other forms of surgical trauma may be particularly helpful in the infant or young child during the first 4 to 5 days of treatment. Other details of routine therapy are discussed in Chapter 23.

Ingestion of Caustic Materials. The accidental ingestion of strong acids or alkalies by children is largely limited to the preschool age group. This serious injury is a result of gross carelessness in leaving caustic substances within reach of 1- to 5-year-old children. The material most often swallowed is lye, either in crystalline form or as a liquid cleaner.[6] Strong solutions of ammonia may cause serious burns, but ammonia solutions have usually been diluted before use in the home. The ingestion of ammonia, therefore, is seldom a cause of significant esophageal burns. Concentrated acids are usually not found in the home and so are seldom swallowed by children.

Unlike the adult who swallows lye to commit suicide, the young child immediately tries to rectify his painful mistake by spitting and regurgitating any residual material. For this reason, gavage will not yield enough caustic solution in a child to make it worthwhile. In most lye ingestion suspects, only the mouth and pharynx will be burned but the minority with esophageal burns have a potentially grave injury.

Lye, which is practically pure sodium hydroxide, destroys tissue by producing a liquefaction necrosis.[4] This process results in deep penetration through the wall of the esophagus and may produce esophageal perforation. Acids, on the contrary, produce a coagulation necrosis that prevents deep penetration. Thus, the ingestion of acids usually does not result in serious injury.

The immediate problems are airway obstruction by epiglottal edema and esophageal perforation. Fortunately, both occur rarely. The most common complication is the dense scar tissue that circumferentially contricts the esophagus at the burn site and produces significant obstruction or total occlusion of the esophagus. Most of our intensive treatment is directed toward the prevention of this serious complication of caustic burns.

The first step in the examination of a child suspected of lye ingestion is a careful evaluation of the history. Usually the person who arrives with the child will bring the evidence and relate the exposure to the substance. If the material is a corrosive agent and the story of ingestion is plausible, an immediate examination of the mouth and pharynx is imperative. Often the lips and mucous membranes will be reddened and occasionally partially coagulated. Any evidence of pharyngeal edema or erythema raises the question of epiglottal edema and airway obstruction. This finding requires immediate hospitalization because the period of maximal edema and danger is between 6 and 24 hours.

All children with evidence of oral or pharyngeal burns must be assumed to have esophageal burns as well. It is our practice to esophagoscope all such children within 24 hours of the lye ingestion to document the presence or absence of the burn. There is no increased danger of instrumental perforation if the operator stops *when he sees the burn and does not attempt to visualize the extent of the burn.* Numerous authors, especially Kaplan and associates in this country and Palva in Finland, have pointed out that the best way to make a positive diagnosis of an esophageal burn is by immediate esophagoscopy.[19, 26] Certainly it is important to determine if a significant caustic burn has occurred before initiating any regimen of intensive therapy that will require close observation and expensive hospitalization.

High humidity and systemic steroids are the basic ingredients of treatment for airway edema. Prophylactic antibiotics, preferably penicillin or methicillin, are necessary only when a serious burn is suspected and esophageal perforation may be impending.

In most hospitals the time-honored treatment for prevention of esophageal stricture has been early and frequent dilatation of the acutely burned esophagus. This therapy was introduced by the Austrian Hans Salzer in 1920 and bears his name.[29] It is usually carried out blindly, using tapered bougies, and is then repeated once a day for several weeks, then every other day for 2 to 3 weeks and, finally, once a week for many months. Bougie dilatation alone has been reasonably effective in preventing complete stricture but has not prevented significant areas of serious stenosis in some patients.

Because of inherent difficulties with prolonged bougienage and many unsatisfactory long-term results, intensive short-term adrenal steroid therapy has been tried in many medical centers in an attempt to decrease the inflammatory reaction associated with the burn. The steroid therapy is entirely nonspecific and its use is based only on the antiphlogistic effect of these drugs. If the inflammatory response is largely prevented, the subsequent scar tissue will be much less extensive.

Based on these theoretical considerations, Haller and Bachman studied comparative effects of bougienage and steroid treatment in experimental caustic burns of the cat esophagus.[9] Their data strongly support the recent clinical experience that steroids are more effective than bougienage in preventing late stricture formation. Bougienage is currently being used in The Johns Hopkins Hospital only when a barium swallow shows evidence of beginning stenosis of the esophagus. Preliminary clinical experience would suggest that a steroid dosage of 1 to 2 mg. of prednisone per kg. of body weight per day in young children is adequate to control edema at the burn site.[13] The steroid is continued for a minimum of 3 weeks, at the end of which period a repeat esophagram is obtained. If there is no evidence of stricture formation at this time, the steroids are discontinued and the patient followed closely with repeat studies of the esophagus at 3-month intervals for a year. If, on the other hand, stricture formation is apparent at the completion of this initial treatment, the steroids are discontinued and a regimen of esophageal bougienage is instituted.

We have recently reviewed our long-term results with this type of treatment protocol for caustic burns of the esophagus. The conclusions of this study were as follows:

Two hundred eighty-five children with possible caustic burns of the esophagus were managed at 2 university hospitals using similar protocols. Of these, 235 (82 per cent) had immediate esophagoscopy and 69 (29 per cent) had demonstrated esophageal burns. They were treated with steroids and antibiotics. Eight (12 per cent) with proven burns developed strictures that responded to prolonged dilatations and none has required esophageal replacement. The remainder are free of swallowing symptoms. By contrast, eight patients from other hospitals who were not treated by this protocol were referred for esophageal replacement and prolonged dilatation.[11, 17] Our strong impression is that immediate steroid-antibiotic therapy greatly decreases the incidence of esophageal stricture but does not completely eliminate it. Those children who develop strictures on this treatment regimen seem to have milder esophageal scarring, which usually responds to dilatation rather than requiring esophageal replacement.[16]

Only more extensive experience will ultimately define the comparative roles of bougienage, steroids and antibiotics in the treatment of caustic burns of the esophagus. The need for good preventive therapy cannot be disputed, because a severe stricture of the esophagus is a major problem. Repeated dilatations with calibrated bougies may give adequate relief for the chronic stricture. If the stricture becomes too narrow and too dense, some type of resectional surgery becomes necessary. It is beyond the scope of this discussion to consider these operative procedures, but none is entirely satisfactory, for the esophagus is an organ that cannot be easily replaced.

Foreign Bodies. Young children test many small objects with their lips and mouth. This inquisitiveness explains most of the cases of aspiration and ingestion of foreign bodies. Aspiration, because it endangers the airway, usually presents a real emergency, but ingestion of a foreign body seldom requires immediate surgical intervention.

Aspiration probably occurs because a child becomes choked while attempting to swallow and, on vigorous inhalation, sucks the object into the larynx and trachea. The foreign body initiates a sudden spasm of coughing and wheezing, with varying degrees of cyanosis. Fortunately, most objects produce acute symptoms and proper treatment is instituted at once. Occasionally, smooth objects, especially food such as a peanut or bean, becomes lodged in a bronchus, with only transient acute symptoms. These children present later with recurrent pneumonia and lung abscesses due to bronchial obstruction.

Acute respiratory obstruction from a foreign body in a young child requires immediate bronchoscopy by the most skillful endoscopist available. Even diagnostic bronchoscopy in infants is a treacherous examination because of the small structures and tiny airway, but endoscopy to remove foreign bodies is more difficult. It is best done under very light anesthesia and requires great skill and experience.

Holinger has repeatedly emphasized that it is essential to use small caliber bronchoscopes to decrease instrumental trauma, and it is best to expose the larynx first with a small laryngoscope and then insert the bronchoscope under direct vision.[17] Aspirated foreign bodies are usually *not* radiopaque so that x-ray studies are not so helpful as in the diagnosis of objects in the esophagus or stomach.

Once the foreign body has been grasped and removed, the child should be kept in high humidity and given a brief course of steroid therapy for 3 to 5 days. Fortunately, after removal there are very few acute or chronic complications from an impacted foreign body.[17]

Swallowed objects may become lodged anywhere in the gastrointestinal tract, but unless it has sharp points any foreign body that passes the esophagus can be expected to pass out the rectum. The most frequent sites of lodgment in the esophagus are at the level of the cricopharyngeal muscle (beneath the clavicle) and at the esophagogastric junction, with the upper site being much more common. The initial symptoms of coughing, choking and gagging strongly suggest the presence of a foreign body, but if it becomes fixed in the esophagus, the symptoms may disappear and give a false sense of security. If the history and symptoms are suspicious, an x-ray examination, including a thin barium swallow, will usually confirm the diagnosis.

Coins and discs are most common, but any object or toy can be found in the esophagus. All sharp-pointed objects should be removed with reasonable speed, but esophagoscopy can be delayed for 12 to 24 hours if the object is smooth and there is no significant symptomatology. Often repeated attempts at swallowing will dislodge round foreign bodies, and they will pass on through the gastrointestinal tract. In a very young child general anesthesia, administered via an endotracheal tube, is desirable for the endoscopy, but older children tolerate the procedure quite well under moderate sedation and topical anesthesia.

The round or smooth foreign body that reaches the stomach can be followed expectantly without x-ray studies by carefully examining the stools until the object is passed. If the object is pointed or has sharp edges, such as an opened safety pin or a nail, a single abdominal x-ray should be taken 2 to 3 times a week to document its progressive passage. Operative intervention is indicated if the foreign body fails to move down the gastrointestinal tract. This lodgment implies penetration into the intestinal wall and may represent impending perforation.

The rectum and vagina occasionally harbor foreign bodies that have been inserted by the fingers of ever-inquisitive young children. Foreign bodies in the rectum are one of the commonest causes of rectal bleeding in childhood; the foreign body is always palpable on rectal examination. A remarkable assortment of small foreign bodies has been removed from the vaginas of little girls. A persistent vaginal discharge, especially if it is purulent, should prompt a thorough x-ray and/or digital examination. When the diagnosis is made, the treatment is simple removal.

Wringer Injuries. The wringer injury represents a particular type of crush injury that occurs almost exclusively in child-

hood. In spite of the introduction of spin dryers, an astounding number of the old wringer washers remain in use, judging by the persistent frequency with which this type of injury is encountered in an emergency department population. With the recognition of potential seriousness of such trauma the morbidity has diminished greatly. All children with wringer injuries extending above the mid-arm are immediately hospitalized. The extremity is wrapped in a bulky pressure dressing and suspended in an upright position for 24 hours, with close monitoring of sensation and circulation during this time (Fig. 24–10). The dressing is changed in 24 hours, and if any significant degree of swelling is evident, hospitalization is prolonged and treatment continued. If there is minimal swelling, the bulky dressing is reapplied and the patient discharged home with continuation of suspension of the extremity for 48 hours. Subsequent treatment in each case is adapted to individual evidence of ancillary damage such as skin loss or nerve paralysis.

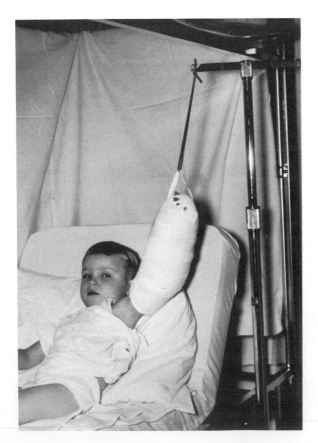

Figure 24–10. *A demonstration of the technique of treating "wringer injuries" of the arm with a bulky pressure dressing and suspension. Exposure of the finger tips allows hourly checks of sensation and circulation. Any evidence of impaired capillary filling or anesthesia may indicate compression of the nerves and vessels in the fascial compartment of the forearm by an expanding hematoma. The dressing should be removed immediately under such circumstances, and the arm should be carefully examined. Prompt performance of a fasciotomy may be necessary to prevent the progression of this process.*

Although this regimen probably represents overtreatment in the majority of cases, the infrequency of serious residual damage has led to its perpetuation. Under this program the only instances of persistent morbidity in recent years were those in which skin loss required grafting. There have been no cases in which increasing edema has led to impairment of blood supply to the distal extremity. Although fasciotomies have been recommended for patients with swelling and progressive vascular embarrassment, no such cases have been encountered since this treatment was instituted.

The "Accident-Prone" Child

Many children seem to suffer recurrent injuries and may be described as "accident prone."[33] At times, particularly in older children, such injuries appear to result from deliberate flirtation with danger. In younger children, the patient often appears to be a tense, high-strung individual who seems under pressure to be active — the type who must take a dare and who rushes headlong into situations without considering the risks. This behavior may be described as counterphobic, because a child attempts to cope with his unconsciously determined fear by exposing himself to the very danger of which he is afraid. Most of the resulting injuries are not unique and are handled in a standard way.

SUMMARY

Trauma in childhood is not fundamentally different from serious injuries at any age, but the potential earning power and social contributions make the injured child a trauma problem of special significance. The basic principles of rapid, careful evaluation and sequential correction of altered physiology are the backbone of successful therapy. The unique metabolic demands and miniature anatomic relationships of the infant or young child present the physician with a special challenge and great responsibility. However, the rewards are high; the younger the injured child, the greater is our total investment.

REFERENCES

1. Benson, C. D., Mustard, W. T., Ravitch, M. M., Snyder, W. H., Jr., and Welch, K. J.: Pediatrics Surgery. Chicago, Year Book Medical Publishers, Inc., 1962.
2. Benson, D. W.: Unpublished data.
3. Borrow, M., Aquilizan, L., Krausy, A., and Stefanides, A.: The use of central venous pressure as an accurate guide for body fluid replacement. Surg. Gynecol. Obstet. 120:545, 1965.
4. Bosher, L. H., Burford, T. H., and Ackerman, L.: Pathology of experimentally produced lye burns and strictures of the esophagus. J. Thoracic Surg. 21:483, 1951.
5. Conway, H.: Management of burns in children. Am. J. Surg. 107:537, 1964.
6. Crowe, J. T.: Poisoning due to lye. Am. J. Dis. Child. 68:9, 1944.
7. Done, A. K.: Developmental pharmacology. Clin. Pharmacol. Ther. 5:432, 1964.
8. Ein, S. H., Shandling, B., Simpson, J. S., and Stephens, C. A.: Non-operative management of traumatized spleen in children: How and Why. J. Pediatr. Surg. 13:117, 1978.
9. Haller, J. A., Jr., and Bachman, K.: The comparative effect of current therapy on experimental caustic burns of the esophagus. Pediatrics 34:236, 1964.
10. Haller, J. A., Jr.: Monitoring of arterial and central venous pressure in infants. Pediatr. Clin. N. Am. 16:637, 1969.
11. Haller, J. A., Jr., and Talbert, J. L.: Trauma workshop report: Trauma in children. J. Trauma 10:1052, 1970.
12. Haller, J. A., Jr., and Talbert, J. L.: Clinical evaluation of a new silastic tracheostomy tube for respiratory support of infants and younger children. Ann. Surg. 171:915, 1970.
13. Haller, J. A., Jr., and Andrews, H. G.: Pathophysiology and management of acute corrosive burns of the esophagus. Modern Treatment 7:1182, 1970.
14. Haller, J. A., Jr., Andrews, H. G., White, J. J., Tamer, M. A., and Cleveland, W. W.: Pathophysiology and management of acute corrosive burns of the esophagus: Results of treatment in 285 children. J. Pediatr. Surg. 6:578, 1971.
15. Haller, J. A., Jr., and Shermeta, D. W.: Acute thoracic injuries in children. Pediatr. Ann., 5:71, 1976.
16. Holder, T. M.: Problems peculiar to infants. In Gibbon, J. H., Jr. (ed.), Surgery of the Chest. Philadelphia, W. B. Saunders Co., 1962.
17. Holinger, P. H., and Johnston, K. C.: Foreign bodies in the air and food passages. Pediatr. Clin. N. Am. 1:827, 1954.
18. Hughes, W. T., Jr.: Pediatric Procedures. Philadelphia, W. B. Saunders Co., 1964.
19. Kaplan, J., Gandhi, K., Elsen, J., and Oppenheimer, P.: Early esophagoscopy for diagnosis of esophageal burns. Arch. Otolaryngol. 73:52, 1961.
20. Lindberg, R. B., Moncrief, J. A., Switzer, W. E., Order, S. E., and Mills, W.: The successful control of burn wound sepsis. J. Trauma 5:601, 1965.

21. Monafo, W. W., and Moyer, C. A.: Effectiveness of dilute aqueous silver nitrate in the treatment of major burns. Arch. Surg. *91*:200, 1965.

22. Moyer, C. A., Margraf, H. W., and Monafo, W. W., Jr.: Burn shock and extravascular sodium deficiency — treatment with Ringer's solution with lactate. Arch. Surg. *90*:799, 1965.

23. Nyhan, W. L., and Lampert, F.: Response of the fetus and newborn to drugs. Anesthesiology *26*:487, 1965.

24. Odell, G. B.: The magnitude of volume and solute disturbances in the neo-natal period associated with fasting and thirsting. J. Saint Barnabas Medical Center *2*:92, 1964.

25. O'Neill, J. A., Meacham, W. F., Griffin, P. O., and Sawyers, J. L.: Patterns of injury in the battered child syndrome. J. Trauma *13*:332, 1973.

26. Palva, T.: Corrosions of the esophagus. Acta Otolaryngol. Suppl. *158*:44, 1960.

27. Philippart, A. I.: Blunt abdominal trauma in childhood. Surg. Clin. N. Am. *57*:151, 1977.

28. Rubini, M. E., and Wolf, A. V.: Refractometric determination of total solids and water of serum and urine. J. Biol. Chem. *255*:869, 1957.

29. Salzer, H.: Early treatment of corrosive esophagitis. Wien. Klin. Wochenschr. *33*:307, 1920.

30. Talbert, J. L., and Haller, J. A., Jr.: The optimal site for central venous measurement in newborn infants: A critical comparison of superior versus inferior caval pressures with increasing abdominal distention. J. Surg. Res. *6*:168, 1966.

31. Thomas, D. V., Fletcher, G., Sunshine, P., Schafer, I. A., and Klaus, M. H.: Prolonged respirator use in pulmonary insufficiency of newborn. J.A.M.A. *193*:183, 1965.

32. Vaughan, V. C., III, McKay, R. J., and Behrman, R. E.: Nelson Textbook of Pediatrics. Philadelphia, W. B. Saunders Co., 1979.

33. Velcek, F. T., et al.: Traumatic death in urban children. J. Pediatr. Surg. *12*:375, 1977.

34. White, J. J., and Haller, J. A., Jr.: An improved technique for tracheostomy in infants and children. Resident Staff Physician, p. 11s, February 1972.

35. Whitehouse, W. M., et al.: Pediatric vascular trauma. Manifestation, management and sequelae of extremity arterial injury in patients undergoing surgical treatment. Arch. Surg. *111*:1269, 1976.

36. Wilson, J. N.: The management of acute circulatory failure. Surg. Clin. N. Am. *43*:469, 1963.

CHAPTER 25

WOUND SEPSIS: PREVENTION AND CONTROL

John F. Burke, M.D.
Conrado C. Bondoc, M.D.

GENERAL CONSIDERATIONS

The successful management of an injured patient rests on an accurate understanding of the physiological disturbances caused by trauma and their timely repair. Repair, in the medical sense, not only involves the restoration of anatomical continuity and alignment of soft tissue or fracture but, equally important, rests on the maintenance of this restoration and alignment while the processes of healing are carried out. Sepsis is the major stumbling block to this completion of accurate healing. Over the past 20 years, the considerable increase in physiological knowledge and its application to the traumatically injured patient have considerably improved his chance for immediate survival. Too often, however, the dramatic rescues of the emergency department and operating room are lost in the ensuing weeks on the hospital ward through bacterial infection. It is clear that the successful management of trauma depends not only on the early repair of physiological and anatomical defects but, equally important, on the prevention or successful treatment of a septic complication. In assessing the overall problems of sepsis in trauma, it appears that prevention is easier to accomplish and far more likely to lead to a satisfactory re-

sult than is the treatment of an infection that is established. This chapter is divided into two sections — the first and more important section deals with the problems and techniques useful in preventing infection, and the second section deals with the problems and techniques of treating established sepsis in traumatically injured patients.

PREVENTION OF SEPSIS

As already noted, it is almost always easier to prevent sepsis than it is to treat a bacterial lesion once it is established in the tissue. This concept is particularly important in the patient following trauma for tissue injury, and the surgical manipulations required for restoration of normal anatomy seriously decrease the patient's usual resistance to bacterial invasion, particularly in the localized area of trauma itself. Post-traumatic swelling, relative ischemia, areas of hematoma and direct soft tissue damage all combine with the systemic derangements of circulatory volume and cardiovascular instability to make the seriously injured patient an easy mark for bacterial invasion. This extensive defect in the patient's ability to defend himself against bacteria begins immediately after injury and is perhaps at its most serious immediately before resuscitation in the emergency department. With this in mind, it is obvious that if sepsis is to be avoided, preventive measures must begin as shortly after injury as possible (i.e., along with the life-saving measures instituted to establish an airway, halt blood loss or repair circulatory volume). In general, these preventive measures may be divided into several categories for the purpose of discussion. The categories are: (1) re-establishment of physiological stability, (2) prevention of further bacterial contamination of tissue, (3) elimination of the tissue bacterial contamination inflicted at the time of trauma, and (4) use of preventive antibiotics. Although these points are easiest to discuss separately, it is important to understand that they should not be carried out sequentially but simultaneously as early as possible in the post-injury period.

Establishment of Physiological Stability

In the overall treatment of the trauma patient, including those measures designed to prevent sepsis, the rapid and effective use of measures to bring the patient to the state of near normal physiology is perhaps the cornerstone on which all other measures must rest. The most extensive debridement, the most timely and accurate repair of vascular occlusion, or the most extensive use of antibiotics will accomplish little without the simultaneous resumption of normal physiological function. In addition to seriously compromising the function of the brain, heart and kidney, low cardiac output and systemic hypoperfusion produce other more subtle but nevertheless as potentially lethal effects. These effects are seen, in particular, on the bacterially contaminated, traumatic wound. It is widely recognized that immediate correction of circulatory failure is essential to prevent death from central nervous system or cardiac failure. It is not widely recognized that immediate correction of circulatory failure is an essential ingredient in the prevention of wound sepsis. The effects of hypotension on the ability to defend against bacterial invasion have been adequately documented.[1, 2] Therefore, both for the immediate

and the long-term well-being of injured patients, particularly those with open wounds or compound fractures, timely re-establishment of adequate circulation is indispensable. Unfortunately, the operational definition of "adequate circulation" is at times considered to be clinically achieved with the resumption of urine flow or the recording of a nearly normal central arterial pressure. It is important to realize that in this situation the peripheral muscle mass and skin may remain seriously underperfused. This defect in circulation in the area of a contaminated wound is a steppingstone for sepsis. It is not sufficient to prevent the patient's death from shock in the immediate post-injury period; the trauma surgeons must also prevent the development of sepsis in the area of the injury itself. Although sepsis may not be manifest for a few days or a week following trauma, the bacterial contamination causing suppuration occurs during or close to the time of injury, and prevention of infection is impossible without "adequate circulation" to the soft tissue injuries themselves. Restoration of circulation, therefore, includes not only the restoration of the central but also the restoration of the peripheral circulation, if wound infection is to be avoided. In this context, the peripheral hypoperfusion produced by vasoconstrictive agents provides a further reason to avoid their use in traumatic shock.

The exact method of repairing circulatory volume and achieving near normal peripheral as well as central circulation has been outlined in detail elsewhere in this book. It is, however, important to recognize that the physiological defects caused by red cell loss are, at this time, most effectively remedied by red cell replacement.

In addition to the problems of circulatory volume and level of vascular perfusion, there are further systemic abnormalities that must be corrected before physiological equilibrium and near normal antibacterial defenses can be expected. Normal respiratory function and adequate gas exchange are vital; acid-base equilibrium, electrolyte concentration and hydration are important areas to bring to balance. In addition, pre-existing disease states, such as diabetes, must be carefully controlled. It is well to remember that the patient's own bacterial defenses are the most important in preventing sepsis.

Prevention of Further Bacterial Contamination

Although for practical purposes bacterial contamination of a traumatically inflicted open wound occurs at the time of injury, further bacterial contamination continues until the wound is closed or otherwise protected through medical intervention. It is important to recognize that this further bacterial contamination of an open wound can be largely eliminated by the efficient use of dressings and sterile technique well known to all surgeons. In assessing the need to protect the wound from further contamination as early as possible following injury, it is particularly important to note that although the bacterial species likely to contaminate a wound at the time of injury may, on rare occasion, produce serious if not lethal infection, they are also likely to be sensitive to the available antibiotic agents. A conspicuous exception to this rule is the staphylococcus. In the past, most strains of *Staphylococcus aureus* acquired in the community were sensitive to penicillin. At this time, about 80 per cent of community-acquired staphylococci are resistant to penicillin so that a penicillinase-resistant penicillin such as oxacillin, nafcillin, cloxacillin or dicloxacillin should be used for IV or oral delivery. On the other hand, the bacterial species found in hospitals are perhaps, on the whole, more virulent; but, even more important, they are much more likely to be resistant to the antibiotic therapy. Therefore, infection generated by bacterial contamination of a traumatic wound in the factory, on the farm, or at the roadside almost always responds to active antibiotic therapy, but infection produced by hospital bacterial strains resulting from contamination in the hospital itself is likely to be antibiotic-resistant and difficult to treat successfully.

The preventive measures used to protect the patient from further contamination are simply those involved in accurate sterile techniques and the prevention of cross-infection. Unfortunately, many injured patients are thoroughly contaminated by hospital strains of bacteria in the emergency department because accurate attention to the details of sterile technique and prevention of cross-infection are temporarily pushed to the background by urgent measures that are required to deal with massive hemorrhage, respiratory insufficiency or cardiovascular collapse. Too often, intravenous catheters, tracheostomy tubes, Foley catheters, instruments and dressing sponges are contaminated in the hurry of emergency resuscitation of a seriously injured patient. Again, too often, the life saved by emergency resuscitation is lost later through the consequences during resuscitation of bacterial contamination that does not become manifest as sepsis for days or weeks later on the ward.

The wound does not provide the only portal of entry for bacterial invasion of the traumatically injured patient. The respiratory tract, the urinary tract and the blood stream, as well as the wound, are often infected, as just noted, by bacteria carried on catheters, tubes and instruments placed in the emergency situation without proper precautions for maintenance of sterility.

As in the restoration of normal physiology, the protection of the patient from further contamination must begin immediately on the patient's admission to the emergency department and continue unabated until the wound is closed and all catheters, tubes and drains have been removed.

Recently, a system of protective isolation has been developed for patients with large open wounds which cannot be rapidly closed.[3] This system of preventing bacterial cross-contamination of the patient on the hospital ward is called the bacteria controlled nursing unit (BCNU) and has been used extensively in the treatment of major burn injuries.

Elimination of Contaminating Bacteria and Devitalized Tissue

Ranking in importance close behind the establishment of near-normal physiology in preserving life and preventing wound infection are the measures that are taken to eliminate the bacteria, foreign bodies and devitalized tissue from the patient's wound when he is presented for medical care. These measures may be loosely collected under the title of "debridement." This is a simple and relatively clear-cut concept, but in clinical application it is likely to present considerable judgmental and technical difficulties. The maneuvers of debridement have their basis in experience gained in the First World War through the attempts by the French army surgeons to reduce the incidence of sepsis and gas gangrene in the wounded. In brief, debridement implies the removal of all foreign material, devitalized tissue and contaminating bacteria from a wound as early as possible following injury. Although the idea of removing dead tissue is simple enough, the actual problems faced in carrying out these concepts may be very difficult. The problems lie, on the one hand, in the difficulties of accurately differentiating tissue that has been injured and is destined to die from tissue that is injured but destined to recover, and, on the other hand, in the reluctance of the surgeon to sacrifice skin, muscle, bone or tendon (and along with it useful function) that he cannot be sure does not have the ability to recover. For these reasons, debridement is often incomplete, leaving devitalized tissue and bacteria in the wound and thereby producing the disasters of suppuration. Experience has therefore taught that following the debridement of a traumatic wound, unless the total removal of actual and potentially devitalized tissue can be ascertained with certainty, the wound must be left open to be closed after secondary debridement, if necessary, in 3 to 7 days. This technique is known as delayed primary or secondary closure.

Using the combination of early debridement, thorough irrigation with saline and delayed primary closure, both the risk of suppuration and of loss of function secondary to removal of potentially viable tissue can be held to a minimum. In the classic application of the principles of delayed primary closure, the edges of the wound are held apart by a thin layer of gauze covered by an occlusive dressing preventing further bacterial contamination. The wound is then splinted in a position of rest to prevent motion and strain. If pain, exudate, fever or other systemic reaction demands, the wound can be examined at any time without difficulty and further debridement can be carried out. If there is no sign of suppuration, the wound is prepared for closure, usually on the ward with supplemental local anesthesia. The gauze is removed, the wound edges examined, and, if necessary, further debridement is car-

ried out. If the wound edges are clean and beginning to granulate, the wound is closed by opposing the edges as in a primary closure. If suppuration is present, the gauze is replaced and a further delay is part of the treatment process.

The use of a thin layer of gauze between the wound edges in a delayed primary closure prevents pocketing of exudate and ensures drainage of purulent material if it occurs. It allows the wound to be examined on clinical demand without seriously interrupting the time schedule of healing. The amount of scar tissue, however, is increased if a foreign body such as gauze is allowed to remain in a wound a matter of days, and the loss of fluid, electrolyte and protein from large wounds is considerable. Recently, the use of split-thickness cadaver skin allografts or porcine xenografts has been substituted for a thin layer of gauze holding the wound apart.[4] The skin provides physiological closure of the wound edges while maintaining all of the advantages of delayed primary closure. Fluid, electrolyte and protein losses are reduced to zero, and scar tissue formation is not in excess of that seen in the usual primary healing. The technique of delayed primary closure and the use of split-thickness allografts as temporary primary closure are demonstrated in Figures 25–1 and 25–2.

Occasionally, soft tissue wounds, because of their size or because of the natural immobility of the skin, such as that found in the lower leg, may be impossible to close using the simple expedient of advancing the skin edge to repair the defect. Plastic surgical procedures, such as the swinging of a flap or the harvesting and transfer of a split-thickness autograft, may be required. In the emergency operative situation, these plastic surgical procedures further complicate the technical problems at hand and considerably prolong the operative procedure and the anesthesia time. Here again, the use of previously harvested, split-thickness skin allografts or xenografts, stored in the operating room, may be employed.[4] The cadaver skin allograft supplies all of the benefits of primary closure without the additional surgical problem or time required to harvest an autograft. This method has proved far superior to the use of gauze dressings in the management of wounds such as open fractures

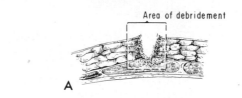

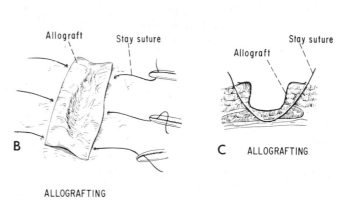

Figure 25–1. *Steps in technique of allografting followed by delayed closure showing (a) area to be debrided, (b) allograft placed as the usual split-thickness skin graft, and (c) relation of debrided area to allografted surface and stay suture tract.*

or open reduction of the lower third of the tibia and fibula, where soft tissue protection of the bony structures is largely absent if the leg skin cannot be primarily closed.

Along with the techniques of debridement, delayed primary closure and special wound management using skin allograft, it is essential to employ impeccable surgical technique. The use of foreign bodies should, in general, be avoided. Accurate hemostasis, general tissue management and precise use of sutures without tension, along with accurate anatomical reconstruction, will provide the optimal functional result with the least danger of wound sepsis.

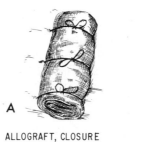

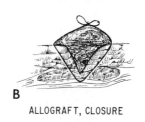

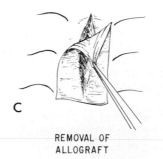

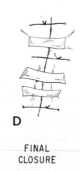

Figure 25–2. *Steps in the technique of allografting followed by delayed closure showing (a) and (b) stent holding allograft in place on debrided surface, (c) removal of allograft at time of definitive closure, and (d) appearance of wound following definitive closure.*

Preventive Antibiotics

The restoration of normal physiology and the preparation of the wound by removal of contaminating bacteria, foreign bodies and devitalized tissue, followed by a means of physiological closure, are the most important components of the therapeutic regimen leading to timely healing without suppuration. Unfortunately, it is not always possible to achieve these goals accurately, and in these clinical instances it is reasonable to consider supplementing the patient's sagging resistance to bacteria with antibiotic substances. In this instance, the term *preventive antibiotics* is used, for, to be effective, the antibiotics must be delivered before infection begins with the idea of preventing bacterial invasion, not with the idea of treating an already established lesion.

Over the past few years, considerable experimental and clinical evidence has been amassed, documenting the effectiveness of preventive antibiotics in both elective and emergency surgery.[5-8] This experience has demonstrated principles important to the prevention of sepsis in seriously injured patients. First, preventive antibiotics can markedly decrease the risk of postoperative sepsis if they are delivered at a time when they can supplement the activity of the tissue to prevent bacterial invasion. Second, use of preventive antibiotics is most effective when the antibiotic substance is in the tissue before the bacteria arrive and is progressively less effective over the next 4 hours.

Using these concepts as guidelines, it is clear that antibiotics must be delivered to the injured patient at risk as soon after injury as possible. In fact, if indicated, antibiotics should be given with the initial fluid requirement at the same time that shock or acidosis is being reversed. It is again pointed out that preventive measures designed to allow healing without sepsis, if they are to be effective, cannot wait until the more dramatic activities related to repair of shock or respiratory insufficiency are over. Antibacterial measures must be among the initial therapeutic measures in the resuscitation of a seriously injured patient.

The choice and dose level of antibiotic to be used cannot be easily categorized. Because of the danger of less than normal perfusion of traumatized areas, if renal function is intact, daily doses of antibiotic probably should range toward the upper end of the recommended dosage of the antibiotic chosen. The intravenous route of administration is perhaps the most useful because of the unreliability of the gastrointestinal tract and of intramuscular absorption in a patient with an unstable cardiovascular system. Further, it is urgently necessary to deliver antibiotic substance to the injured tissue as soon as possible. The choice of antibiotic must rest with the clinical judgment and experience of the surgeon. In general, a single antibiotic with low toxicity should be chosen. Multiple antibiotics should be used only in clinical situations in which risk of life-threatening infection is extensive. Oxacillin, cephalothin, ampicillin and tetracycline have been used with success. The combinations of kanamycin and oxacillin, or penicillin and tetracycline have also been used.

CONTROL OF WOUND INFECTIONS

The important first step in dealing with an established infection in a traumatic wound is establishing the diagnosis of infection itself. The earlier this can be accomplished on indirect clinical grounds, the less likely is the occurrence of generalized infection and the smaller the tissue damage secondary to local bacterial invasion. The final level of function of a joint or an extremity may well depend on the early recognition and prompt, effective treatment of developing infection in a traumatic wound. In small wounds, the diagnosis can easily be made by observing the cardinal signs of inflammation — pain, heat, redness and swelling. In large wounds complicating extensive trauma, which may extend into body cavities or deeply into the intramuscular spaces, the diagnosis of deep sepsis is far more difficult to make at an early time. The patient may complain of local pain, tightness or tenderness in the region of the wound, but these signs are not universally present. The systemic evidence of inflammation, consisting of spiking fevers, leukocytosis, malaise and, in extreme cases, shock, are those that must be carefully evaluated. Occasionally, a rapidly spreading cellulitis may be seen, often indicating a beta-hemolytic streptococcal infection, and, rarely, gas may be noted in the tissue, indicating infection caused by gas-forming organisms.

Once the diagnosis of infection is established, treatment must be begun immediately in order to confine the advance of the infection to as small an area of tissue as possible. The general principles of treatment of established infection in traumatic wounds are the same in small wounds treated as outpatient problems as they are for major life-threatening injuries. The principles are:

1. Establishing and maintaining drainage of loculated, purulent material.
2. Debridement of tissue devitalized by the septic process.
3. General systemic support of the patient, including antibiotics if bacterial invasion of the tissue surrounding the wound is present.

The exact technical method chosen for drainage and debridement, the need for systemic support and the decision to use or not to use antibiotics depends on the extent of the wound and its anatomical location. Wound infections involving abdominal or thoracic cavities or the brain cannot be handled in the same manner as sepsis following a compound fracture of the femur or sepsis in a small, soft tissue wound of the forearm. In all cases of sepsis requiring medical treatment, identification of bacteria should be carried out through cultures, and their antibiotic sensitivities should be determined. Although the treatment of wound infection in special areas of the body is detailed elsewhere in this volume, there are several general principles that are worth mentioning here. For practical purposes, the varying difficulty of bringing a post-traumatic wound infection under control is related directly to the possibility or impossibility of (1) establishing open, continuous drainage of the infection site, and (2) the possibility or impossibility of wide debridement of the bacterially involved tissue. In a soft tissue wound of an extremity, it is physiologically and functionally feasible to open an infected area wide for drainage and maintain this adequate drainage until in-

fection has been overcome by keeping the wound open. In the same wound, the sacrifice of skin, subcutaneous tissue and muscle is not limited by devastating loss of function. On the other hand, for physiological reasons, it is impossible to establish, much less maintain, wide-open drainage of an infection in the peritoneal or pleural cavities, and, for reasons of maintenance of function, it is impossible to debride wide areas of the brain in order to remove all bacteria-laden tissue. These special cases should be recognized and special methods of management employed.

Treatment of Specific Infection

Although the principles of treatment of bacterial infection in a traumatic wound are broadly similar no matter what species of bacteria is involved, there are important differences in the pathophysiological evolution of infection caused by certain bacteria; and, perhaps more important, the life-threatening alterations produced by specific bacteria are worth special note.

Beta-Hemolytic Streptococcus Infections. Infections caused by beta-hemolytic streptococcus are notable for their early onset, rapid invasion of tissue and frequent production of life-threatening blood stream invasion. These infections usually produce a rapidly evolving cellulitis, or lymphadenitis, at times called erysipelas, which may begin hours after the traumatic contamination of a wound and progress to fatal septicemia in a day or so. Fortunately, the beta-hemolytic streptococcus is exquisitely sensitive to antibiotic therapy, particularly to penicillin and, for practical purposes, does not develop resistance to the antibiotic. Because of the organism's sensitivity and inability to develop resistance, beta-hemolytic streptococcal infections are easily preventable by the early use of preventive antibiotics; or, if an infection develops, they are easily eliminated by the early use of therapeutic antibiotics. The danger in this infection lies in its ability to produce a rapidly evolving systemic infection, raising the possibility of extensive bacterial invasion before diagnosis and treatment are carried out.

Pseudomonas. Pseudomonas is often encountered as a mixed infection in burn or other extensive wounds when the patient is seriously ill and when large amounts of necrotic tissues are present. It is characterized by a musty, foul odor and often by the development of greenish discoloration of the surface of the wound. The wound may be rapidly invaded with a virulent strain, producing a severe invasive septicemia with a rapidly fatal course.

The treatment of pseudomonas infection rests on efforts to increase host resistance, particularly by improving nutritional status, along with adequate, early removal of necrotic tissues from the wound as well as by the use of both topical and systemic antibacterial agents. For topical use on the burn wound, Sulfamylon, Silvadene and 0.5 per cent $AgNO_3$ have been shown effective in preventing and controlling burn wound sepsis. Gentamycin and tobramycin with or without carbenicillin has proven effective for systemic use.

Meleney's Ulcer. Known as synergistic gangrene, this is a chronic progressive form of mixed infection caused by the combined presence of a microaerophilic nonhemolytic streptococcus and the aerobic hemolytic *Staphylococcus aureus*. It has an incubation period of 10 to 14 days and usually starts around wound edges as a wound complication.

The lesion begins as an area of pale red cellulitis with a purplish center, progressively turning gangrenous; finally, ulceration takes place. The ulcerated area becomes progressively larger and is characterized by its purplish, grayish, painful margins that extend peripherally. Treatment should include wide excision of gangrenous ulcerated margins and systemic antibiotics in the form of penicillin and/or erythromycin depending on bacterial sensitivity, and delayed primary closure.

Crepitant Cellulitis. This is another form of acute mixed infection, also known as necrotizing fasciitis. It usually develops as a complication following the contamination of wounds resulting from gastrointestinal perforations as in perforated colon carcinoma, perforated diverticulitis or ruptured perirectal abscess and from genitourinary discharges. The common etiological agents are bacteroids, anaerobic streptococcus and other coliform bacteria. Bacteroids produce thrombophlebitis and embolization of nutrient vessels, resulting in ischemic changes in the surrounding soft tissues. The lesion is characterized by severe acute necrotic changes in the areolar tissues along fascial planes (necrotizing fasciitis), resulting in progressive gangrenous changes to the overlying skin. Crepitation is also noted, which results from gas produced by the offending microorganisms in underlying tissues. Treatment should include wide excision and extensive decompression of all necrotic tissues with intensive systemic penicillin and clindamycin.

Human Bite. A human bite is the most dangerous bite produced by any mammalian species. The resulting infection is caused by synergistic action of anaerobic and aerobic bacteria, both gram-positive and gram-negative, including staphylococcus, streptococci, diphtheroids and spirochetes. These groups of bacteria cause severe destructive lesions of the skin, the underlying subcutaneous tissue, fascia, tendons and joints. This infection is characterized by high fever and chills and is marked by swelling and tenderness and a thick, foul-smelling purulent exudate originating from the underlying subcutaneous tissues. Wide excision of necrotic tissues, decompression, adequate immobilization, secondary closure and systemic antibiotic therapy are necessary. In this case, ampicillin is often the agent of choice.

Tetanus. Tetanus,[9] usually called lockjaw, is a clinical syndrome caused by a toxin produced by *Clostridium tetani*, a spore-forming, strictly anaerobic, gram-positive bacillus. The bacteria are found widely distributed in nature, being commonly found in the gastrointestinal tract of domestic animals and in soil. Unlike bacterial infections that produce clinical difficulties by direct invasion as well as by intoxication, the tetanus bacillus produces disease by elaborating a toxin that diffuses throughout the tissue. Severe or even lethal tetanus can be caused by minor bacterial growth with little inflammation in the most minor of wounds. Natural tissue resistance to the tetanus bacillus is high, so that under ordinary circumstances contamination of tissue with this bacillus or its spores does not result in bacterial growth or invasion. However, if devitalized tissue and/or foreign bodies are allowed to remain in a wound, anaerobic conditions may be produced and tetanus infection established. *Puncture wounds*[10] have particular importance in this context, for the depth of the wound and the narrowness of the opening to the surface can prevent efficient cleaning of the wound at initial treatment, and foreign bodies, such as dirt, rust, and bits of clothing, are not easily removed. In addition, purulent exudate resulting from inflammation in a puncture wound tends to pocket, for the external opening of the wound is soon sealed by a protein coagulum and a closed-space infection is produced. For this reason emergency treatment of puncture wounds should have special attention and for the most part the wounds should be opened wide in order to ensure adequate cleaning, debridement and drainage.

Tetanus is, perhaps, one of the easiest diseases to prevent, for active immunization using toxoid has proved to be effective in its prevention and the preventive effect is long-lasting. However, the civilian public health measures attempting to produce a uniformly immunized population have not been effective, and there are many patients who come to the emergency department following trauma who have not had adequate tetanus immunization. Although the clinical disease of tetanus is rare today, it is seen sporadically throughout the country so that its development must be considered and measures for its prevention routinely taken. Prophylaxis against tetanus is usually carried out using adsorbed tetanus toxoid in three subcutaneous doses of 0.5 ml. each. The second is given 4 to 6 weeks following the initial dosage, and the third is given 6 to 12 months following the second dose. This regimen produces effective, active immunization and a repeat booster dose of 0.5 ml. tetanus toxoid subcutaneously within the following 10 years produces a rapid rise in antitoxin titer. This response to a booster dose may occur for as long as 25 years after active immunization and in many patients may last throughout the lifetime.

For minor injuries treated early after they are incurred in a patient who has a clear history of tetanus immunization within the last 5 years, a booster dose is all that is required. In the immunized patient who has had a booster dose within the year, no specific antitetanus treatment is indicated. However, when the wound is more serious or more than 24 hours old, with extensive destruction of tissue and

contamination, 250 units of tetanus immune globulin (human) should be given. The use of penicillin or tetracycline should be considered. In the unimmunized patient, passive immunity can be established using human antitetanus globulin by intramuscular injection. The usual recommended dose is 250 units, although larger doses have occasionally been recommended. In addition to the administration of antibody for passive immunity, dosage for active immunity, according to the schedule in the previous paragraph, should be begun immediately.

The diagnosis of tetanus may be suspected in a patient who suffers insomnia, irritability, tremor, spasms and rigidity of muscles adjacent to a wound. The incubation period varies from 4 to 21 days, but is usually between 7 and 10 days. The severity of the clinical disease and the mortality rate are inversely proportional to the length of incubation. The shorter the incubation period, the more serious the disease.

The major objectives of treatment of tetanus are removal of the sources of tetanus toxin production and the neutralization of the circulating toxin already produced. The former is accomplished by thoroughly debriding any traumatic wound by wide excision. Anaerobic conditions must be prevented at all cost, and the wound, therefore, is usually left open following debridement. Circulating tetanus toxin is destroyed by administering 500 units of immune human globulin daily for about 10 days. Antibiotics, usually in the form of penicillin, cephalosporin or tetracycline,[11] are given to the patient in large doses in order to further prevent elaboration of the toxin by growth of the tetanus bacillus. Because the main symptoms are muscle spasms, sedation with valium and a quiet, dark environment are essential. In severely ill patients with pharyngeal spasm, tracheostomy should be performed and muscle relaxants used as necessary to ensure adequate respiration. Nutrition may be maintained with a nasogastric tube, and constant nursing care will be required.

Patients being treated for tetanus should receive immunization using tetanus toxoid. The clinical disease does not uniformly confer immunity.

Clostridial Infection (other than Tetanus). Infections with these organisms may cause two clinical forms of infection

A guide to prophylaxis against tetanus in wound management

1979 revision

Prepared by
The Committee on Trauma
of the American College of Surgeons

General principles

I. The attending physician must determine for each patient with a wound, individually, what is required for adequate prophylaxis against tetanus.

II. Regardless of the active immunization status of the patient, meticulous surgical care, including removal of all devitalized tissue and foreign bodies, should be provided immediately for all wounds. Such care is essential as part of the prophylaxis against tetanus.

III. Passive immunization with Tetanus Immune Globulin—Human (called human T.A.T.) must be considered individually for each patient. The characteristics of the wound, conditions under which it was incurred, its treatment, its age, and the previous active immunization status of the patient must be considered. It is not indicated, however, if the patient has ever received two or more injections of toxoid.[4]

IV. To every wounded patient, give a written record of the immunization provided, instructing him to carry the record at all times, and if indicated, to complete active immunization. For precise tetanus prophylaxis, an accurate and immediately available history regarding previous active immunization against tetanus is required.

V. Immunization in *adults* requires at least three injections of toxoid. A routine booster of adsorbed toxoid is indicated every ten years thereafter.[1] In *children* under seven, immunization requires four injections of diphtheria and tetanus toxoids combined with pertussis vaccine. A fifth dose may be administered at four to six years of age. Thereafter, a routine booster of tetanus and diphtheria toxoid is indicated at ten-year intervals.[2]

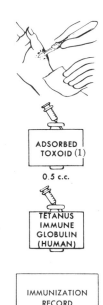

ADSORBED TOXOID (1)

0.5 c.c.

TETANUS IMMUNE GLOBULIN (HUMAN)

IMMUNIZATION RECORD

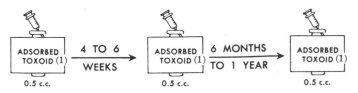

ADSORBED TOXOID (1)   4 TO 6 WEEKS   ADSORBED TOXOID (1)   6 MONTHS TO 1 YEAR   ADSORBED TOXOID (1)

0.5 c.c.   0.5 c.c.   0.5 c.c.

Figure 25–3.

Specific measures for patients with wounds

I. Previously immunized individuals

A. When the attending physician has determined that the patient has been previously fully immunized and the last dose of toxoid was given *within ten years:*

ADSORBED TOXOID (1)

0.5 c.c.

1. For nontetanus-prone wounds, no booster dose of toxoid is indicated;

2. For tetanus-prone wounds and if more than five years has elapsed since the last dose, give 0.5 cc adsorbed toxoid. If excessive prior toxoid injections have been given, this booster may be omitted.

B. When the patient has had two or more prior injections of toxoid and received the last dose *more than ten years previously,* give 0.5 cc adsorbed toxoid for both tetanus-prone and nontetanus-prone wounds. Passive immunization is not considered necessary.

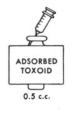

ADSORBED TOXOID

0.5 c.c.

II. Individuals NOT adequately immunized

A. When the patient has received only one or no prior injection of toxoid, or the immunization history is unknown:

1. For nontetanus-prone wounds:
   a. Give 0.5 cc adsorbed toxoid,[1]

2. For tetanus-prone wounds:
   a. Give 0.5 cc adsorbed toxoid,[1]
   b. Give 250 units (or more) of human T.A.T.,[3]
   c. Consider providing antibiotics, although the effectiveness of antibiotics for prophylaxis of tetanus remains unproved.

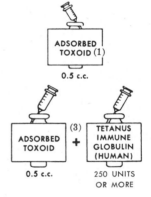

ADSORBED TOXOID (1)

0.5 c.c.

ADSORBED TOXOID + (3) TETANUS IMMUNE GLOBULIN (HUMAN)

0.5 c.c.   250 UNITS OR MORE

Footnotes

(1) The Public Health Service Advisory Committee on Immunization Practices in 1977 recommended DTP (diphtheria and tetanus toxoids combined with pertussis vaccine) for basic immunization in infants and children from two months through the sixth year of age, and Td (combined tetanus and diphtheria toxoids: adult type) for basic immunization of those over six years of age. For the latter group, Td toxoid was recommended for routine or wound boosters; but if there is any reason to suspect hypersensitivity to the diphtheria component, tetanus toxoid (T) should be substituted for Td.

(*Morbidity and Mortality Weekly Report, Vol. 26, No. 49, p 402, Dec 9, 1977, Center for Disease Control.*)

(2) Report of the Committee on Infectious Diseases, ed 18. Evanston, IL. American Academy of Pediatrics, 1977, p 2-11, 278-285.

(3) Use different syringes, needles, and sites of injection.

(4) Equine Tetanus Antitoxin: *Do not* administer equine T.A.T. except when human T.A.T. is not available, and only if the possibility of tetanus outweighs the danger of reaction to horse serum.

This guide from the Committee on Trauma of the American College of Surgeons is the work of an ad hoc subcommittee on prophylaxis against tetanus: Roger T. Sherman, MD, FACS, Tampa, Florida, Chairman; Wesley Furste, MD, FACS, Columbus, Ohio; and Richard Faust, MD, FACS, New Orleans, Louisiana.

Posters and reprints may be obtained from the Committee on Trauma, American College of Surgeons, 55 East Erie Street, Chicago, Illinois 60611.

Figure 25-3 Continued.

of surgical importance. Common species isolated from clostridial infections are *C. welchii*, *C. novyi* and *C. septicum*. *Clostridial cellulitis*, a septic process involving subcutaneous and areolar tissues, is characterized by rapidly spreading cellulitis along the fascial planes and is associated with crepitation, necrosis and sloughing of the overlying skin. The offending organism is usually *C. welchii*. There is marked swelling, edema and pain around the wound with a grayish-brown discharge from the wound. Treatment should include extensive wide excision, debridement and decompression and systemic penicillin or tetracycline.

Gas Gangrene (Clostridial Myositis). Gas gangrene[12] is a life-threatening infection involving destruction of muscle and must be clinically separated from gas-forming infections that do not carry the grim prognosis of clostridial myositis. Gas gangrene usually develops early after traumatic injury, often within 12 hours. It is characterized by extreme pain, rapid pulse, restlessness, a thin brownish discharge and a profound toxemia. There is swelling and edema of the affected tissue, crepitus may be present, and bubbles are occasionally seen in the discharging serosanguinous exudate.

For clinical success, treatment must be immediate and thorough. Early excision of the entire involved muscle mass should be carried out. If the wound is in an extremity, immediate amputation may be necessary. Antibiotics should be given by the intravenous route in large doses. Penicillin or, in the case of sensitivity to penicillin, tetracycline has proved effective. The use of gas gangrene antitoxin is not clearly established but, if used, it should be administered early and in doses consisting of 10,000 to 15,000 units per kilogram of body weight. Hyperbaric oxygen has been found to increase the effectiveness of surgical debridement and antibiotic therapy in certain cases of gas gangrene.[13]

REFERENCES

1. Miles, A. A., Miles, E. M., and Burke, J. F.: The value and duration of defense reactions of the skin to the primary lodgement of bacteria. Br. J. Exp. Pathol. 38:1, 1957.
2. Miles, A. A.: Nonspecific defense reactions in bacterial infections. Ann. N.Y. Acad. Sci. 66:356, 1956.
3. Burke, J. F., Quinby, W. C., Jr., Bondoc, C. C., Sheehy, E. M., and Moreno, H. C.: The contribution of a bacterially isolated environment to the prevention of infection in seriously burned patients. Ann. Surg. 186:377, 1977.
4. Burke, J. F., and Bondoc, C. C.: A method of secondary closure of heavily contaminated wounds providing "physiologic primary closure". J. Trauma 8:228, 1968.
5. Burke, J. F.: The effective period of preventive antibiotic action in experimental incisions and dermal lesions. Surgery 50:1, 161–168; 184–185, 1961.
6. Burke, J. F.: Preoperative antibiotics. Surg. Clin. N. Am. 43:665, 1963.
7. Burke, J. F.: The significance of time between injury and treatment. Conn. Med. 29:110, 1965.
8. Bernard, H. R., and Cole, W. R.: The prophylaxis of surgical infection: The effect of prophylactic antimicrobial drugs on the incidence of infection following potentially contaminated operations. Surgery 56:151, 1964.
9. Robles, N. L., et al.: Tetanus prophylaxis and therapy. Surg. Clin. N. Am. 48:799, 1968.
10. Committee on Trauma, American College of Surgeons: Prophylaxis against tetanus. *In* The Management of Fractures and Soft Tissue Injuries. 2nd Ed. Philadelphia, W. B. Saunders Co., 1965.
11. Goodman, L. S., and Gilman, A.: Pharmacological Basis of Therapeutics. 4th Ed. New York, Macmillan, 1970.
12. Altemeier, W. A., and Furste, W. L.: Collective review — gas gangrene. Surg. Gynecol. Obstet. 84:507, 1947.
13. Boerema, I.: An operating room with high atmospheric pressure. Surgery 49:291, 1961.

CHAPTER 26

EMERGENCY DEPARTMENT ORGANIZATION

Marla E. Salmon White, R.N., Sc.D.
Donald S. Gann, M.D.

INTRODUCTION

Several major components must be developed and integrated in order to effect an emergency department organization that can support quality patient care. In this chapter we discuss concepts underlying organization of *the physical plant, the patients, the resources and the management* of the emergency department, to provide a basis for examining and possibly improving the organization of specific emergency departments. We will not offer specific prescriptions for organization, since these must vary according to internal and external constraints of each facility.

Although there are other components, the interactions of the four just named primarily determine the function of an emergency department. Incorporation of each of these into an overall perspective allows one to examine and utilize his own setting to create improved emergency department organization, thus avoiding the "cookbook" attempt to emulate the "ideal." We believe that the only practical means for improvement of emergency department organization is building on what already exists. It is both unrealistic and wasteful to ignore the present in planning future emergency department improvements.

Others have described the relationships between organization of service and proc-

ess of care, including elaborate models to predict outcomes in relation to certain activities within organizations.[4] There is almost nothing in the literature describing these relationships within emergency departments, although problems stemming from faulty organization are usually apparent both to staff and to patients. If asked, staff members could easily enumerate reasons for suboptimal patient care, such as lack of space, staff and resources and unresponsive management. Therefore, in viewing one's own organization, it is important to ask those working in the emergency department for their views.

There are a number of historical reasons why emergency departments provide suboptimal care. Among these are a lack of adequate sources of primary and secondary care for large segments of the population, emphasis on inpatient care in institutional financial priorities and lack of recognition of emergency care as a unique service deserving some administrative self-determination. In addition, until recently, proponents of emergency care have been lacking among those physician-providers functioning in emergency departments. Few of these have made emergency care a priority professional commitment; most view it either as an interim or unfortunately necessary experience. As a result, the major advocates for improvement of emergency care have often been those with the least administrative voice — the nursing staff.

Recently, federal and private support of emergency medical systems and research efforts have provided the resources and knowledge necessary to begin improvement of emergency care. However, if issues concerning the organization of an emergency department are not resolved, improvement will not occur.

PHYSICAL PLANT

For purposes of this discussion, the physical plant is defined as the setting within which emergency care and supportive activities take place. It is essential that each emergency department define the patient care activities that will take place in terms of levels of care and of supportive activities. The most common supportive activities include registration and waiting, family counseling, patient counseling, administrative activities, teaching, staff resting and reading, research, laboratory and x-ray, examination and surgery. These vary according to the individual setting, but each will influence the allocation of space in the emergency department.

Certain concepts need to be understood in planning new construction, renovation or reorganization of the physical plant. With respect to immediate patient care one must consider several questions:

1. Accessibility. How easy is it for a patient and his family to come to the emergency department? How well identified is the location? How many physical barriers are there to entry? How much time is lost just "getting in?" The physical organization should minimize distance and barriers for the most severely ill or injured patients.

2. Observability. At what point are patients actually viewed by providers and how well is visual accessibility maintained throughout the care process? This is a critical factor for patients with major trauma or equally grave illnesses, whose conditions may change rapidly. The most advanced patient monitoring systems are not an adequate substitute for direct observation of the patient.

3. Privacy. Given visual accessibility, how much respect is demonstrated through the setting for the individual's need for privacy? In conditions of limited severity, this factor may supersede convenience for the staff.

4. Proximities. How close, temporally and spatially, to the patient are the people and diagnostic and therapeutic resources needed in care? One of the greatest pitfalls in adopting an architecturally "perfect" emergency department design is that the issue of the relationship of care and support activities may be neglected. Prior to adopting any floor plans, emergency department management should define carefully what needs to be located near to what.[8] Figure 26–1 illustrates a tool that can be utilized in defining proximities

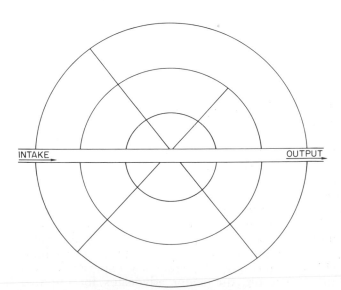

INTAKE   OUTPUT

Figure 26–1. Concentric circle model. Through use of this tool, it is possible to map out desired proximities, accesses and relative relationships among elements in emergency department structure for planning renovations or new construction, without constraints of floor plans. This permits an individualized approach to physical organization of an emergency department, rather than a "perfect emergency department" design approach. It also allows consideration of existing facilities in re-designing emergency departments.

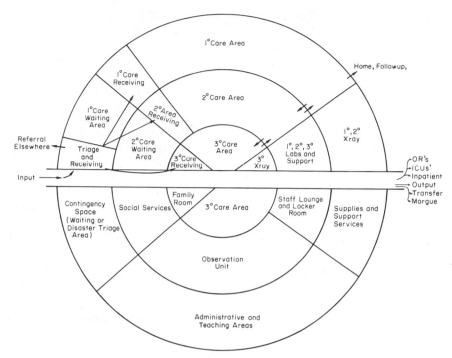

Figure 26–2.   *Sample emergency department proximity plan using concentric circle model.*

through locating activities in a compartmentalized concentric circle. The number of rings and compartments can be expanded according to the number of activities identified. The example in Figure 26–2 utilizes critical care as the center of all activity. This may vary among emergency departments, but is the mainstay of any emergency department oriented toward trauma care.

Separations should also be considered along with proximities. For example, it may be desirable to separate persons with minor complaints from those with severe injuries or to provide separate points of entry or egress for those with conditions of different levels of severity. In the figure, this can be accomplished by decreasing adjacencies.

5. Comfort. How attractive, quiet and accommodating to patients, friends or family members is the care setting?

6. Maintainability. How efficient and easily maintainable is the plant, so that provider time can be allotted to patient care rather than care of the "place"? Physical plants with multiple corridors, niches and "dust-catching" fixtures demand provider time.

By considering proximities and coupling these with optimal *accessibility, observa-*

bility, privacy, comfort, maintainability and *efficiency,* one produces the basis for realistic planning of the physical plant. At this point, one can plan in detail numbers and types of rooms and space and resources required. The result of this type of planning is an emergency department oriented to patient care rather than one into which patients must somehow be accommodated — that is, design should follow, not determine, function. The equipment and special facilities needed in a given emergency department will depend upon its patient load and selection. In terms of trauma care, the relation between function and facilities has been defined in detail by the Committee on Trauma of the American College of Surgeons.[3]

PATIENTS

The mix of patients, the plans for their care and the nature of the staff assigned to that care all have an impact on the organization of the emergency department. What happens to a patient during his stay in the department can be affected dramatically by what has transpired prior to his arrival and can in turn determine what will happen following this departure. Accordingly, three phases of patient care will be viewed organizationally:

1. The pre-emergency department phase
2. The emergency department phase
3. The post-emergency department phase.

The ability of the emergency department to direct the course of events during each of the three phases affects its organization and its response to patients during the emergency department phase.

The Pre-emergency Department Phase

How patients are managed prior to their arrival in the emergency department may determine the outcome of their care in the emergency department. This assumption has led to the development of emergency medical services systems (EMS) that utilize trained personnel (EMT's and paramedics) and sophisticated systems for communication and transportation and categorization of hospitals, and that attempt to optimize interaction among these components. Whereas there are controversies surrounding each of these elements, it has become clear that if emergency department representatives do not participate in discussions and decisions surrounding these aspects of EMS, their departments stand to suffer far-reaching consequences, to the ultimate detriment of patient care. For example, emergency department representatives who do not understand the role and potential value of skilled ambulance personnel may fail to utilize the observations of patients by these personnel or may ignore their ability to transmit vital information regarding a patient's history and status. This attitude, in turn, fails to reinforce and support the ambulance personnel in their roles. In addition, those in emergency departments need to inform those designing EMS systems about the resource potential of their institutions. Otherwise, a capable and appropriately equipped emergency department may be bypassed because patients are transported to an institution that *has* been involved in determining how the pre-emergency department care system is organized. (EMS as related to disaster situations is treated in

Chapter 27.) Although this does not suggest a logical method for design of EMS systems, it does indicate the political nature of the process. Without input, neither the interests of the emergency department nor the needs of patient care can be met. Emergency departments must be represented in planning efforts and must maintain continued communication and monitoring throughout the implementation of pre-emergency department care programs. Those representing emergency departments must be knowledgeable in relation to the care capacity, resources and growth potential of their departments and must have the requisite authority. Too often, commitments by institutions are empty because those making them have neither the information nor the authority to do so.

The Emergency Department Phase

This is the phase during which the patient is received, evaluated, treated and either released or admitted. Organization of the receipt stage of care should be designed to provide immediate assessment of all patients, whether arriving by ambulance, helicopter or private transportation. This requires trained personnel available at points of entry. The initial assessment should result in a matching of patients to resources in a fashion that best meets the patient's needs. Many emergency departments have instituted a triage process involving the nursing staff, whereby a nurse evaluates patients in terms of severity and nature of complaint in relation to services available in the emergency department or related referral services immediately available.[1] This nursing triage must be bypassed without delay or confusion in the case of severely injured or ill patients. Successful triage also requires that resources for care be carefully identified and that guidelines be established to describe criteria for patient referrals. It is vitally important that initial patient assessment be taken seriously and that those assessing the patient have the appropriate orientation and experience. This stage of care requires the exercise of the best judgment in the least amount of time and holds the gravest potential consequences. The more appropriate the initial determination of the nature of the problem and its severity, the more appropriate and timely the care for the patient will become. Physician back-up must be readily available for consultation when there is a question about the appropriate site for care. Under no circumstance should a nurse be given the option of referring a patient "to the street" without consultation and assessment by a physician.

The receipt phase should also include gathering of information about the patient for purposes of "registering," including names of family, addresses, demographic data and method of payment. Allowance should be made for patients who cannot register on arrival, with this to be handled at a later time by the patient, his friends or family. All patients should be registered for legal and informational reasons. Exceptions to this rule, even for friends of care providers, lead inevitably to legal and ethical dilemmas. Patient billing and considerations unrelated to patient care should be kept separate from appropriate documentation of the patient visit. This may be accomplished by use of special forms that permit retention of economic and other nonessential information at the registration/billing area.

Management of registration information that is not relevant to actual assessment should be done by the personnel not designated to carry out patient care. Confusion of these roles results in loss of vital information and time and contributes to neglect of patient care.

Following receiving of the patient, care should be provided in a timely and appropriate fashion. In the large emergency department, care has been segregated historically by service, e.g., medical, surgical, gynecological. Within each of these organizational areas, truly emergent patients usually are treated first and then others are addressed in a "first-come first-served" fashion. Thus, patients with problems of limited severity may experience very long delays. It seems desirable to consider the organization of care, separating patients into emergent, urgent and non-urgent categories. The development of specially trained emergency nurse practitioners[5] and emergency physicians[6] may facilitate this form of organization. Patients with non-urgent complaints can be cared for by mid-level health professionals in a designated area, thus decreasing waiting time for these patients and freeing physicians

for the care of the emergent and urgent patients. In addition to conservation of time and effort of physicians, improvement in staffing patterns for the nursing staff may be possible. Rather than assigning a predetermined number of personnel to each service area, whether needed or not, in this system there is greater ability to pool staff at the secondary or tertiary levels as needed, while continuing to provide care at the non-emergent level.

To minimize the number of staff assigned and thus cost, care in the emergency department should be organized to maximize utilization of each provider of care and at the same time to minimize patient waiting time. It is critical that staff nurses in emergency departments be equipped with the physical and psychosocial skills requisite for collaboration with physicians, social workers and others in initiating diagnostic procedures and patient therapy. Protocols for certain types of non-emergent patient conditions may be developed to allow the nurse, after initial assessment, to order diagnostic tests and x-rays. The patient's hospital records can also be ordered by the nurse at the time of assessment, if indicated. Social workers and other resource persons can also be mobilized by the nurse following assessment.

To minimize patient waiting time, laboratory and radiology resources must be highly responsive. Otherwise patients may wait hours for results of tests; this delays treatment and causes congestion in the care areas and poor patient management. In addition, a distinction must be made between results needed to make urgent decisions, such as those involving admission of emergency department cases, and results not needed until later.

It is essential that both nursing care and care involving physicians be documented and that these documents be easily accessible to all providers. Nursing documentation should include initial and periodic assessments and observations, medications, treatments and referrals. Special forms can be developed to provide a check-off format for critical care or long-term observations, in which much objective data are documented. Such a format should not preclude documentations of subjective impressions, however. The physician documentation should include history, physical tests, orders, diagnosis, treatment, referrals and disposition. All entries should indicate the time of observation or activity and should be signed by the provider.

Emergency department organization should involve the patient's family members and other support persons in the care process to the greatest extent feasible. Unfortunately, many emergency department staff members view such involvement as an inconvenience or disruption. Family and friends not only provide important information, e.g., medical and social histories and self-care skills, but also give the patient emotional support and comfort in a highly threatening and impersonal environment. Providers may be less effective at times in managing the patient's anxiety and fears than are relatives and friends. Some emergency departments utilize trained volunteers or provide patient advocates to assist in this process.[11] Such persons can help to identify patients' needs, provide communication between patients and families, intervene in crisis situations and answer questions about the care in the emergency department. However, advocates or volunteers should not be viewed as a remedy for provider negligence.

The Post-emergency Department Phase

The organization of care also needs to anticipate what happens after initial emergency care is completed. Historically, emergency departments have not ensured continuity of care for the patient. The most obvious result of this is the return of patients to emergency departments with exacerbated problems. This is costly in both financial and human terms.

If a patient is being admitted, providers need to inform the patient, and family if possible, of the reason for admission and of what to expect during the next phase of care. Family members should be directed to talk with persons who can counsel them about the financial and technical aspects of admission. Emergency admissions can be emotionally traumatic experiences for both patient and family. It is the responsibility of emergency department staff to minimize this trauma.

Patients who are not being admitted

should be interviewed prior to release (exit interview) to provide them with information on home care and schedules of return visits, and to explain the need for each. Both physicians and nurses should be involved in pre-discharge teaching. Physicians need to inform patients throughout the care process what is happening to them and why. This should terminate in a final discussion with the patient about his physical condition, his therapy and his follow-up care. Patients should be encouraged to ask questions and to demonstrate understanding. Nurses should utilize each patient care activity as an opportunity to teach the patient. Such teaching is highly meaningful and takes little time if done while procedures are being performed. Explaining to a patient during suturing why the wound has been thoroughly cleaned and draped helps to reinforce telling the patient of the need for keeping the wound clean later. An effective technique in the exit interview is to ask the patient to relate his knowledge of what happened to him during his visit and why, what medications he has been given, what they will do for him and what he should do in terms of his care following his visit. This allows the interviewer to correct misconceptions and to build on existing knowledge. After the interview, the patient and his family members should be able to demonstrate knowledge relating to the following:

1. Condition, diagnosis and prognosis.
2. Medications, directions for administration, indications and therapeutic and side effects.
3. Follow-up care: appointments; home activities, diet restrictions and resources available for carrying these out.
4. Signs of deterioration of the patient's condition and what to do if they appear.

Such information is crucial to post-emergency department care. The nurse needs to assess carefully the resources available to the patient and his ability to participate in his own care. Teaching a patient to soak a limb in warm water is a wasted experience if he has no hot water available, as is giving a patient who can't read a printed instruction sheet.

A follow-up mechanism should be part of the organization of care. This should be designed to serve two purposes: (1) to ensure adequacy of follow-up care, and (2) to provide feedback to providers. The system needs to relate to the needs of the patients. It can be a PRN approach, in which a provider requests that a follow-up person call or visit a patient about whom the provider has some specific concerns. Alternatively, there may be a continuous approach, carried out by defining the kind of follow-up needed by certain patients and by performing daily chart review. A nurse with a public health background can be very effective in this role. This person can review charts, make calls and visits and even mobilize community resources if appropriate.

Providers can benefit from follow-up information about the patient's condition, needs and impression of care. It is unfortunate that few providers in emergency departments ever know the consequences of their patient care. There is tremendous teaching and management value in this type of information. In its absence, there is no way a provider can judge the effectiveness of such care.

Emergency department organization also needs to plan for patients who die in the department. It is usually assumed (or hoped) that patients dying in the emergency department have no post-care needs. This results in family members receiving the "bad news," often in the waiting room, perhaps receiving a sedative and then being encouraged to leave the department as soon as possible. It should be the attitude of the department that the family be considered carefully both during and after the death of a patient. Ideally, families of critically ill patients should be given a private area in which to wait, with someone constantly available to them.[7] This person should be knowledgeable about the patient's care, be capable of providing information, support and crisis intervention, and be able to assist the family after the death of the patient. Every emergency department nurse needs to be prepared in this role and to view it as his or her responsibility. Medical social workers and trained clergy can also be helpful. Physicians also should be prepared to participate, and it is solely the physician's responsibility to inform the family of the death of the patient.

The family of the dead patient should be given the opportunity to see the patient in a secluded area, with a provider accompanying them, and should be allowed some time to begin the grief process before leaving. Emergency department personnel should arrange, if possible, for a friend or relative of the immediate family to accompany the family home when they are prepared to leave.

Emergency department personnel involved in the care of a dying patient require consideration as well. They should be given an opportunity to express their feelings and frustrations openly and to feel that this process is acceptable and supported. Some emergency departments provide counselors, psychiatric personnel or clergy members with whom staff can discuss their feelings. These people are most helpful and are most successful when administrative personnel recognize and support their functions.

RESOURCES

The ability of an organization to function depends largely upon the availability and deployment of resources. In planning organizational strategies, all potential resources should be identified and understood. Whereas financial resources are usually identified, numerous other resources that have equally significant impact on the ability of an emergency department to provide patient care may be overlooked. Among these are *human resources, continuing care resources* and *training and developmental resources.*

Financial resources are available to emergency departments through both internal and external sources of the institution. Income and allocated institutional support are the most common forms of emergency department support. Income is related to payment for services by the patient through whatever mechanism of payment is available to him (self-pay, third party, medical assistance or other federally supported programs). Who provides the service, how charges are generated and billing and collection procedures determine the extent of income. Emergency departments utilizing only house staff physicians are unable to bill for professional services, whereas those utilizing attending staff or full-time paid physicians have this

option. Some states are considering legislation that would enable non-physician
health practitioners to receive reimburse-
ment for professional services.

The system for generating charges is
critical. The decision of whether an emergency department charges an average visit
fee or bills only on the basis of procedures,
treatments and tests, or combines both,
should be made with a knowledge of the
ability to pay and care needs of the department population. If patients requiring the
most expensive care are not covered by
third-party payers and are not eligible for
other federal- and state-supported coverage, it may be necessary to generate an
average charge across the patient population in order to meet costs. To attempt to
avoid charging in this fashion, emergency
departments should attempt to enroll all
eligible patients in medical assistance or
other programs at the time of the patient's
visit. Social service referrals may be helpful in accomplishing this objective.

If the patient population is well insured,
charging for procedures and professional
fees, with a standard visit charge, is the
most desirable option. This method re-
coups actual costs of patient care. In order
to accomplish this, we must establish
mechanisms to provide accurate information about costs in terms of supplies,
overhead and provider time associated
with procedures and care for various
patient conditions.

The emergency department billing system should be organized to identify
charges both to the department and to patient or third-party payers. This process
should be completed as soon as possible
after the patient visit and each charge
should be defined in terms of patient care.
The system should also provide ongoing
information to management about the
types and frequency of procedures and patient care in the department.

Collection procedures should be designed to address three phases of collection: (1) at the time of the patient visit, (2)
after receipt of the bill, and (3) in the event
that payment is delinquent. The general
experience in collection suggests that the
collection of moneys from self-pay patients
is best accomplished immediately following the visit. Thus, a mechanism for collection should be developed at the time of
visit. The responsibilities for identifying

method of payment and instituting the collection procedure should not rest with the
provider, nor should the payment status of
the patient be a consideration in the care
he receives. Designated nonpatient care
personnel should be trained in financial
interviewing, counselling and collecting
procedures.

Allocated institutional support determines the extent to which the hospital supports the activities of the emergency department. In negotiating institutional
support, it is critical that the emergency
department director and administrator
have accurate knowledge of the actual
costs of operations and of the income generated. Trends and variations of visits,
costs and receipts are important. The administrator also must have a well-defined
operational plan that carefully projects directions and dimensions of growth as well
as related costs.

In negotiation of institutional support,
services provided by the emergency department to other areas of the institution
also should be considered. These include
processing of elective admissions; provision of examination areas, equipment, supplies and personnel for patients within the
hospital; laboratory or radiology services
or both; and float staffing. The related costs
need to be assessed and to be covered by
the institution. The financial picture for
emergency departments lacking this information will necessarily be poor and indicate an "in the red" operation, even in the
presence of sound fiscal management. Historically, this has been a major source of
institutional perspectives on the financial
viability of emergency departments.

Grants and traineeships also may be
found to help support some functions of
emergency departments. Emergency department administrators need to have a
sound, updated knowledge of federal,
state, local and private moneys available
for specific programs. Manpower-training
moneys and research and development
grants may be provided at federal and state
levels. Private foundation support may be
available for special programs related to
needs of the community.

Human resources must be identified and
deployed rationally within the emergency
department. Human resources should be
designated in terms of the work to be accomplished, rather than the organization

being built around the personnel within it. Activities must be defined and examined in terms of the category of personnel likely to be most effective and efficient in carrying out these activities. The process should begin when the expectations for provision of patient care are defined and when standards are set in relation to these. Examination of each phase of care should indicate type of personnel required. Then, information concerning frequency of conditions and hours to be worked by each provider allows inference of actual numbers of each category for staffing.[10] Indirect patient care activities such as patient registration, billing and administration must also be defined carefully in terms of work-related activities, their frequency and time required for their accomplishment.

Emergency departments should have contact with facilities that provide continuing and alternative care. In examining patient care needs, emergency department planners should have information about the continuing care needs of the patient population and about the extent to which outside resources can meet these needs. This information should be utilized in organizing emergency department follow-up approaches and actual follow-up care. A knowledge of alternative care sites is a requisite to responsible organization of the receiving phase of patient care. If alternative facilities are available and better able to meet patient needs, these should be incorporated into the triage process. Thus, "walk-in" clinics may, if available at appropriate hours, serve to alleviate overcrowding in the emergency department. Information about continuing and alternative care resources should include accurate assessment of the nature of services provided, eligible population and accessibility and availability of services. There should also be an appraisal of the acceptability of the services to the patient population.

DEFINING ADMINISTRATIVE STRUCTURE

Administrative History of Emergency Departments

Organizations exist to accomplish work. The degree to which work becomes "pro-

ductive" relates to the function of administration within the organization. Conceptually, administration is the system within an organization for initiating, facilitating, monitoring and controlling work. It is the means through which organizational direction is set, resources allocated and growth promoted. The ability of administration to carry out these functions is reflected in the effectiveness and efficiency of the organization in its work.

Historically, emergency departments have been subject to "default" management and administration. Because of their relatively low institutional status, emergency departments have been viewed as unpleasant administrative necessities requiring minimal administrative time, effort, resources and commitment. Emergency departments that have evolved as appendages of surgical services are examples of products of this attitude. Viewed often only as input mechanisms for inpatient surgical care, these departments had little support in the care of patients not requiring admission or not viewed as "surgical" patients. In the training situation, emergency departments evolved as teaching (by doing) sites for house staff, with little control or supervision of actual care. In both of these situations, administration has been generally removed, with primary interests lying in areas other than those of emergency medicine.

In many emergency departments, the only administrative staff having any working knowledge of the setting and any commitment to care provided there is the nursing staff, usually at the head nurse level. Often, this has resulted in adversary relationships between medical staff, who may be "passing through," and nursing staff, who feel some ownership for the department. When nursing staff is assigned on a PRN-float basis, even this bit of committed management is lost.

Other administrative arrangements for emergency departments have related to administration either provided by or coordinated with contracting physician groups. The success of this arrangement has depended greatly on the content of the contract and on the objectives of the parties participating in the agreement. If there is a commitment to emergency medicine as a discipline of value rather than as a concern for profit, there is some hope of producing effective patient care with this arrangement. If this commitment is lacking, however, the work of the emergency department and its organization will be geared to maximizing profit at the possible expense of safe and effective patient care.

The common grain seen in the administrative history of emergency departments is that there has been a lack of agreement about purposes, institutional commitment and support and administrative structures. The results are apparent today: emergency departments are often the stepchildren of hospitals.

Importance of the Organizational Mission

The administrative structure of an emergency department should be designed in relation to the organizational mission.[9] Too often, organizations adopt models for administrative structure that prove to be dysfunctional in relation to their purposes. The organization must carefully assess its reasons for existing and must list each in order of importance. Statements of organizational mission may seem simple and possibly unnecessary. However, this step in designing administrative structure is critical and should not be taken lightly. The definition of mission is the basis of understanding, necessary for those both within and outside the organization to relate productivity to its functions. Too often, people within organizations work at cross purposes with no real understanding of the direction of the organization. This leads to frustration, to wasted resources and to lack of growth. For example, settings in which generation of profit is the top organizational priority seldom share this priority with staff providing patient care. This places those attempting to maximize quality of care at odds with those attempting to minimize costs.

Following definition of mission, goals for each element of the organization should be established in relation to the mission.[2] If the mission of an emergency department is to provide care for major trauma, specific goals may include availability of staff and facilities, minimized waiting and transport time and isolation of these patients from non-critical patients. Similarly, if the mission of the organization includes providing ongoing nursing

care, specific goals may include increasing the professional-to-patient ratio or scheduling nursing staff according to patient load. The process of definition of mission and goals should involve those persons organizationally responsible and accountable for the work required for their accomplishment. The input of staff people at this stage is helpful both as a source of information and as a step in making possible more meaningful and less traumatic organizational changes.

The process of defining organizational mission, goals and then objectives should be viewed conceptually as movement from the ideal, overall direction of the organization to the specific, operationally defined and attainable work to be accomplished. Objectives should be the short-term expected accomplishments of the organization in relation to its goals and mission. To carry this a step further, objectives relating to providing major trauma care may include a staffing pattern for physicians to allow transfer from "intermediate" to "critical" care areas in order to supply vital support for a "peak load" of trauma without unnecessary use of assigned extra physicians. Similarly, if one goal is to schedule nurses according to patient load, objectives could include: (1) determine the numbers, types and care requirements of patients arriving during different work shifts in the department, to be accomplished every 6 weeks; and (2) evaluate the present numbers and types of staff and the shift distribution in relation to patient load, to be accomplished within 3 weeks following data gathering. Many other objectives could be established to relate to these examples. Each should define movement toward accomplishment of the goal.

Objectives and goals should be stated realistically on the basis of a knowledge of the constraints and enabling factors present both within and outside the organization. This requires a solid understanding of the work needed, resources of all types, the setting and the environment. Operationally attainable objectives and goals are those that are stated in terms of what it is that will be done, what resources are available and attainable to enable accomplishment, what constraints are present and how long it will take for the objectives and goals to be met. Sound objectives and goals also define means for determining whether or not they have been met, and thus provide a rational basis for evaluation.

Administrative Function

If an organization has carefully outlined its mission, goals and objectives, it has produced a set of documents that can serve as an administrative blueprint and as a basis upon which the administrative structure should be built. Earlier, administration was defined as the system through which work is initiated, facilitated, monitored and controlled. Given an understanding of the work to be done through the direction-setting phase of organizational development, which is the stating of mission, goals and objectives, these functions can be ascribed to roles and levels of administrative personnel in the production of an administrative structure.

If each goal and objective is defined in terms of how it is to be initiated, facilitated, monitored and controlled, the majority of the work of administration is described. The decisions then relate to how much of this work can best be done on an outgoing basis, at what level and by whom. Decisions about levels and numbers of people outline the administrative structural content and layers. Decisions about who administers, that is, who is responsible and accountable for administrative process, define lines of authority. These decisions should represent rational matching of preparation to function.

Administration itself needs to be viewed as a piece of work requiring expertise, technologies and abilities. Mere tenure in a staff position does not prepare one to move into an administrative role. Addi-

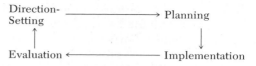

Figure 26–3. *Work process.*

tional training may do so. Conversely, it is important that those charged with administration of highly specialized areas such as emergency departments have appropriate practical knowledge and experience. Finally, the abilities to lead, to organize and to relate to others must be considered. It is unfortunate that few planners in health care settings demonstrate an operational understanding of the need for prepared administrative staff.

The work involved in any administrative function should be viewed in terms of ongoing process. Within this process are essentially four stages: *direction setting, planning, implementation* and *evaluation.* These stages represent elements of a cycle, as illustrated in Figure 26–3. The direction-setting phase of the organization has been covered earlier in this discussion. On the overall organizational level, this is followed by planning, implementation, evaluation and responsive iteration of the process. The actual length of the cycle is relative to the level within which the process takes place. Using a simplified organizational model, Figure 26–4 illustrates the relative time differences in relation to this cycle at various levels. This diagram illustrates the relation between the time required for completion of work cycles — the time between setting of direction and evaluation of product — and the level within the organizational hierarchy. Implicit in this is the scope of work. For the

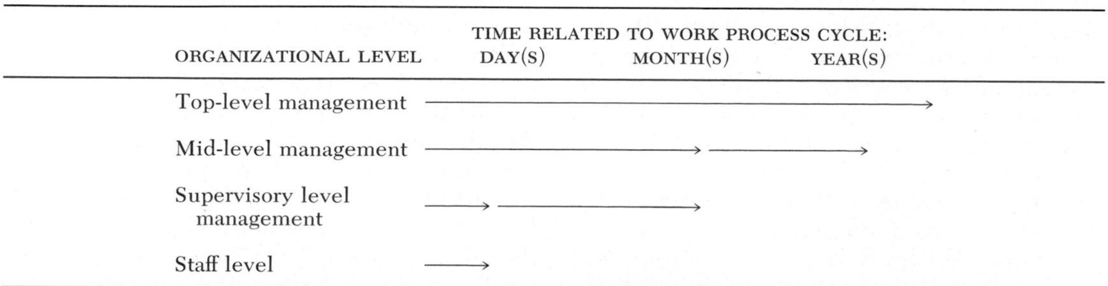

ORGANIZATIONAL LEVEL	TIME RELATED TO WORK PROCESS CYCLE:		
	DAY(S)	MONTH(S)	YEAR(S)
Top-level management	————————————————————→		
Mid-level management	———————————————→	————————→	
Supervisory level management	——→ ———————→		
Staff level	——→		

Time to complete cycle of work process for different levels in organization.

Figure 26–4. *Time to complete cycle of work process for different levels in organization.*

staff person, work is most often directed, planned, implemented and, perhaps, evaluated on a daily basis. The supervisor must orchestrate the duties of employees and see results of their work on a longer-term basis, relating not only to his own duties but also to those of his subordinates, peers and superiors. The mid-level manager has an even broader scope of work and thus requires greater time for that work to be brought to fruition. Finally, the work of the organization as a whole is brought together at the stage of the top-level manager or administrator, requiring even greater time.

In order to function productively, the staff person requires knowledge of the objectives, goals and mission of the organization and of the relationship of his duties to their realization. Otherwise, he cannot assess his worth to the organization. The converse process is a requisite to determining the success of the organization at all levels in meeting its mission, goals and objectives and revising these responsively. In the absence of an ongoing work cycle, administration and all other organizational work becomes reactive, stopgap activity lacking the means for optimal effectiveness, efficiency and meaning. Organizations that function in this fashion become institutional deficits and open themselves up to control by others within the institutional setting.

Each stage of the administrative process requires specific resources that will vary, depending upon the content of the work. The one common requirement at all stages of the process is information. Each administrative level needs ongoing, relevant and reliable information systems that provide the basis for direction setting, planning, implementation and evaluation. The content of these systems will vary according to the level of administration they serve. Each administrative level must identify indicators relating to productivity and means of evaluating progress toward meeting of the objectives, goals and mission of the organization. This information should be ongoing and regularly reviewed. Lack of readily accessible, reliable information is one of the most common administrative problems. Without this information, administrative decisions and actions are both irresponsible and unresponsive.

SUMMARY

The organization of emergency departments should reflect a rational process of matching resources to needs. Historically, emergency departments have been organized in a reactive fashion, lacking the direction setting, planning, implementation and evaluation necessary to productive, prospective organization.

Organization of the physical plant should be based on an understanding and application of concepts for optimal design, including observability, accessibility, privacy, efficiency, maintainability and proximities and must reflect the mission of that emergency department. The "model emergency room" floor plan adopted in planning emergency departments in some instances is responsive neither to the patient needs specific to that setting nor to the resources available for the meeting of those needs. The rational approach to facilities planning requires extensive knowledge of the setting, of the resources and of the constraints on the organization in meeting the needs of its patients.

Organization of patients must similarly reflect a rational matching of resources to needs. Phases of care before, during and after the patient's visit should be the basis upon which organization is built. This requires an understanding of optimal care and what is realistically attainable in the specific emergency department.

The organization of resources requires not only appropriate allocation of capital but also appropriate allocation of the broad range of human and developmental resources available to emergency departments. The basis for organizing, attaining and deploying resources in emergency departments must be a knowledge of what is needed, of what is available, of how to secure resources and of the most effective and efficient means for their utilization.

The actual administrative structure of the emergency department organization is key to the function of the other organizational components just discussed. It is through definition of the purpose or mission of the organization that its administrative structure is defined. This structure is the means through which the ongoing work process of direction setting, planning, implementation and evaluation is accomplished. The administrative work of initiating, facilitating, monitoring and controlling the functions of the organization can be accomplished best through a common understanding not only of the organization's mission but also of the specific goals and objectives required to fulfill that mission. Administrative roles and the preparation of those filling those roles are individually determined in relation to the content of the administrative work to be accomplished.

The underlying key to organization of emergency departments at any level is the knowledge of the mission of the organization. Without this requisite understanding any model organization of the physical plant, patient care, resources and administration is doomed to failure. The goals of the organization will be subordinated to individual goals. Ultimately, then, the emergency department must be organized around a set of missions that is responsive to the needs of the community to be served, that is coordinated to the purposes of other neighboring emergency departments, and that is a departmental reflection of the overall mission of the institution.

REFERENCES

1. Albin, S. L., et al.: Evaluation of emergency room triage performed by nurses. Am. J. Public Health 65:1063, 1975.

2. Charn, M. P.: Breaking through the tradition barrier: Managing integration in health care facilities. Health Care Management Review 1:56, 1976.

3. Committee on Trauma, American College of Surgeons: Optimal hospital resources for care of the seriously injured. Bulletin Am. Coll. Surg. 61:15, 1976.

4. Donabedian, A.: Promoting quality through evaluating the process of care. Med. Care 6:181, 1968.

5. Geolot, D., et al.: Emergency nurse practitioners: An answer to an emergency crisis in rural hospitals. J. Am. Coll. Emergency Physicians 6:355, 1977.

6. Jelenko, C., III, and Frey, C. F.: Emergency Medical Services, an Overview. Bowie, Md., R. J. Brady Co., 1976.

7. Kübler-Ross, E.: On Death and Dying. New York, Macmillan, 1969.

8. Rutherford, R. B.: Organization: Design, function and operation of outpatient clinics. In Hill, G. J. (ed.): Outpatient Surgery. Philadelphia, W. B. Saunders Co., 1973, p. 4.

9. Schaefer, M. J.: How should we organize? J. Nursing Administration 6:12, 1976.

10. Stevenson, J. S., et al.: A plan for nurse staffing in hospital emergency services. Monograph 20–1696. New York, National League for Nursing, 1978.

11. White, M. E. S.: Evaluation of the patient advocacy program at The Johns Hopkins Emergency Department. Doctoral dissertation, The Johns Hopkins University School of Hygiene and Public Health, Baltimore, 1977.

CHAPTER 27

MASS CASUALTY MANAGEMENT

Donald S. Gann, M.D.
Eugene L. Nagel, M.D.
John D. Stafford, M.D.
Frederick Walker, M.D.

A dictum in emergency care is that anything may happen, anywhere and at any time. Thus the *emergency care system* (EMS)* must be prepared to deal with any situation. Ideally, the regional EMS should be a realistically planned effort involving the hospital and fire, police and other community agencies aiding disaster victims.

When a sudden and unexpected occurrence overwhelms the initial response mechanisms of the EMS system, this is commonly termed a disaster. It should be clearly understood that the term is relative, since an absolute demand could be easily handled by one system but totally overwhelm another. For example, in an active war zone the EMS system may routinely care for hundreds of casualties per day, whereas several thousand would inundate its available resources. By contrast a small civilian hospital in an isolated rural setting might find two or three badly injured victims from an automobile wreck too much to manage in a timely and adequate manner.

A characteristic of the EMS is the mechanism by which sudden increasing demands on one local system are met by

shifting resources from less involved areas to the scene of the demand. A common term for the process by which resources are temporarily loaned to the system being taxed by emergency demands is "mutual aid." In this manner, peak emergency care demands are often met by use of shared facilities or temporarily borrowed resources from systems in neighboring areas. In most regional civilian EMS systems these mutual aid plans are triggered locally several times a year and therefore planning and operations are kept current through repeated use.

The plan for managing victims of disasters should be built around an existing EMS system. Since detection, notification and primary dispatch of rescue teams and on-site early care are all part of the EMS, it is the pre-hospital component of EMS that will commonly provide hospitals with their initial notification and assessment of the scope and nature of the disaster. This preliminary information, often sketchy and even inaccurate, furnishes the basis for initiating the hospital and medical components of the emergency care system.

Experience in handling large numbers of injured patients is relatively limited, and much of the accumulated experience has been military rather than civilian. In addition, there are virtually no controlled

---

*Abbreviation for Emergency Medical Services.

studies on the handling of mass casualties. Since the essence of the problem is too much work for too few people provided with inadequate facilities, it is unlikely that we will ever have much carefully controlled data on which to base our management of this type of problem. Naggan[2, 13] describes the experience of four wars and numerous mass casualty situations in determining mass casualty management. He states the principle that "evacuation is not urgent, only primary treatment and preparation for evacuation are urgent." Recognition of condition (primary assessment) is made more difficult in the mass casualty environment owing to many of the logistical and environmental components. The location and transportation of victims to a nearby casualty collection station will assist this process. This area (or areas) furnishes some degree of medical control and ancillary personnel can offer valuable assistance at this point.

Primary care consists mainly of basic life support (BLS) measures together with such advanced life support (ALS) measures as may be necessary. (These are usually devoted to airway and ventilation factors, control of hemorrhage, anti-shock treatment and preparation for transportation.) In the situation in which there are more casualties to be evacuated than transportation facilities can handle, an area should be designated where the less severely injured patients can wait. There is seldom need for medical personnel in the most forward areas, since rescue and ambulance personnel are trained to function in this environment.

PRINCIPLES OF DISASTER MANAGEMENT

Advance Planning

The most important and generally agreed-upon principle that has emerged from the experience of the medical profession in handling disasters is the need for realistic *advance planning*. In spite of the importance and wide acceptance of this principle, there has been less thoughtful planning for handling mass casualties than there should be. Shaftan[16] summarizes this well in stating that most descriptions of civilian disasters are concerned with implementation of hospital disaster plans and

casualty care after the patient reaches the hospital triage area. Little has been written on the coordinated rescue, resuscitation, transportation and management of the injured at the scene of the disaster. Much of what is written is not accurately descriptive of the actual events. Shaftan describes: "At the scene of the disaster the physicians found smoke, fire and confusion. Unauthorized requests for oxygen, morphine, demerol, plasma, blood, etc., as well as for ambulances and medical personnel, produced a veritable bedlam...."

In many cases central medical authority cannot be designated effectively in time for any important decisions to be made. Personnel arriving on the scene may find that decisions on access routes and casualty collection points and initial assessment of the situation have been made by police units whose arrival preceded theirs. Obviously, criteria for such decision making should have been discussed in planning sessions with representatives of all involved personnel (fire and police departments, medical planners and the support and mutual aid agencies commonly utilized, including nearby military resources). In many cases, an exercise can precede the development of an areawide plan to make it realistic and therefore worthwhile.

Opinion varies as to the effectiveness of medical treatment teams in the forward areas. Reports[4, 10] of the 1975 London underground disaster, in which a train ran into a wall in a blind tunnel, described setting up an efficient "stabilizing" medical post underground near the site. The area was a little-used and filthy underground platform that was plagued with heat, soot, bad air and insufficient lighting. Nevertheless, the volunteer doctor-nurse teams apparently were able to provide valuable initial treatment and to assist fire brigade, police and ambulance personnel effectively.

A differing opinion was offered by Rutherford,[15] centering on the experience of the Royal Victoria Hospital in Belfast in an area of civil unrest. Over a 3-year period this hospital received multiple casualties from bomb incidents on 48 occasions. There were 15 additional instances in which street rioting gave rise to a disaster situation. The large number of real experiences obviated the necessity for drills and circumvented the difficulty in creating realism in these exercises. Emphasis was on rapid movement of patients to the hospital with little or no resuscitation at the site. The evaluation process was not described, but Rutherford's conclusion was that urban bombing incidents can be handled adequately in this manner.

Disasters may range from episodes of violence in an urban setting, in which scope of the occurrence is relatively easy to define, to the large acts of nature with disruption of communication and transportation over wide geographical areas. In this case, true assessment of the scope of the disaster may take days or even weeks. Disasters may be natural (floods, earthquakes, windstorms, large fires, volcano eruptions) or man-made (transportation, explosion, fire, riot and civil unrest, war). (Effects of riots are discussed in a later section of this chapter.)

A large natural disaster may occur on a scale that defies any planned immediate response. The Bengal cyclone of November, 1970[12] is one such example. The storm struck on a broad front in a densely populated and impoverished area. The most severely affected area (2000 square miles) had an estimated population of 1.7 million. Overall mortality was estimated at 14 per cent with a range of 4.7 per cent in Amtali to 46 per cent in Tazumuddin. The overall mortality was estimated at 224,000. More than half of the deaths were of children under age 10, although this age group represented only a third of the pre-cyclone population. In this type of disaster survival is linked to ability to cling to such stable objects as trees and therefore the old, young, sick, malnourished and females in general were selectively lost to this storm. In disasters of this magnitude, a choice is often made between providing forward medical teams and providing food, clothing and shelter for the population remaining. In Bengal, water, field hospitals and preventive health measures were needed less urgently. However, World Health Organization and International Red Cross officials familiar with large-scale natural disasters tend to agree that the measure maximally associated with life-saving is in the provision of food, water and shelter. Immediate and definitive emergency medical measures are difficult to provide on the scale often needed, and in geographical areas with inadequate information, communication and transportation.

A somewhat differing opinion was voiced by Whittaker and colleagues[20] concerning the 1972 earthquake disaster in Nicaragua. Here an emergency tent hospital was erected and functioned as a triage and limited treatment facility for a period of 5 days. The plan was to classify victims according to severity of injury and refer the most severely injured to hospitals in nearby cities. The transportation facilities were good but communications were almost nonexistent. In addition, there were many patients with secondary injuries due to fires, transport accidents and criminal assaults. Since the geographical area of damage was relatively circumscribed, the utilization of the medical team and forward hospital was advantageous.

There are many proponents of planning and exercises designed to meet the needs of the hospital involved in a disaster. While the advantages of exercises should apply to a region, so many organizations would be involved in such an exercise that the undertaking would be difficult and expensive. Other problems with such exercises are the general lack of criteria as to what constitutes adequate response and/or behavior, and the lack of an adequate number of referees organized to evaluate results, with resultant inconclusive evaluation. Persons experienced in actual disasters tend to rely on established procedures, utilization of existing protocols and roles for personnel rather than on special plans that place people in unfamiliar roles to participate in unfamiliar procedures. Rutherford[15] suggests the use of normal routine rather than special documentation, labels, etc. He feels that a disaster is, among other things, a communication exercise and that confusion and error should be kept to a minimum. One way of accomplishing this end is to allow people to work in their usual area, using their normal routines. He says that experienced senior staff should be available to man the mobile teams, accident and emergency centers if they are to function effectively. In his view, the main use of the "medical team" is to assess the situation, advise the forward area teams if requested and advise the hospitals receiving the victims. Other investigators have organized and carried out elaborate exercises that, in their view, properly rehearse the planned activities that answer the disaster needs when they arise.[1, 5-9, 17, 18] Finally, persons with experience may extrapolate from one type of occurrence, say civil unrest, to include all manner of causes or to stress the hospital plan without attempts to integrate the hospital's function into the total EMS response to a disaster.[19]

It is obviously difficult to develop plans that will be suitable for the limitless type and magnitude of disasters that may occur. Some disasters cause a general disruption in a community and others are localized to a building or two. Some damage and disrupt the hospital itself, others do not. Some involve fire; some, collision; some, exposure to dangerous chemicals. There are certain features that are sufficiently common to enough different types and sizes of disasters to justify the effort involved in planning. By definition in mass casualty situations the demands always exceed the capacities of the personnel and facilities. The purpose of advanced planning is therefore to establish a system that will assure the optimal utilization of personnel and facilities for the particular situation.[3, 11]

Although the fundamental unit for handling the medical aspects of a disaster is the hospital, it should be but one part of mass casualty planning. The community at large and its various elements are vitally concerned in this planning and it is incumbent upon all medical personnel even remotely involved in mass casualty preparedness to thoroughly understand the EMS system of which they are a part.

It is estimated that in the average medium-sized city in the United States a disaster situation may occur only once in several years; thus the establishment of well-defined guidelines for caregivers is difficult. A further difficulty in establishing guidelines for civilian practice is accentuated by the fact that so much of past experience with mass casualties has been in a military setting. The problems involved in transferring lessons learned in military practice to civilian practice are obvious. As in all of medicine, we must be prepared to change our guidelines as new knowledge enables us to do so. The guidelines that are laid down today may become outmoded as a consequence of new concepts in casualty care. Nonetheless, at this time, certain principles in the handling of mass casualties seem to have emerged from our experience.

Casualty Predictability

As previously stated, the key to effective handling of disaster situations is realistic advance planning. A second principle of disaster preparedness is that, within broad limits, the number and type of casualties that will occur in various types of disasters may be predicted. For example, in a thermonuclear exposion one will probably see relatively few missile injuries in patients without hopeless radiation damage. Also, in most civilian disasters, as contrasted with military situations, a large percentage of the injured population will have multiple injuries. The estimation of the injuries likely to occur in various types of disasters has been reviewed.[21]

Use of Effective Maneuvers

A third principle is that certain maneuvers that are economical of personnel, facilities and time may produce a decrease in mortality, early morbidity and long-term functional loss. Such steps as provision of emergency ventilation, control of hemorrhage and other anti-shock measures can be carried out quickly by individuals with limited training and are an efficient use of resources in mass casualty circumstances. Conversely, more sophisticated techniques that require the prolonged services of highly trained individuals using complex equipment and many supplies, though extremely valuable in ordinary practice, may not be a wise investment of resources in handling large numbers of injured people in a brief period of time. Precisely how much of a shift must be made in the mass casualty situation from extensive procedures to simpler and more efficient ones will depend upon the circumstances of the particular situation.

Treatment Modifications

A corollary of this principle is that the way in which we handle specific types of injuries in ordinary practice must often be modified when we are dealing with casualties from a disaster.[21] This shift in thinking and action is extremely difficult for many physicians to make — a fact that should not be underestimated by those responsible for mass casualty management. Experience with civilian disasters has revealed that strong-willed physicians thoroughly familiar with their own particular specialty but unaware of the modifications that must be made in a mass casualty situation are likely to continue to utilize conventional techniques in such a situation unless there is forceful direction from those in charge.

Teamwork

This brings us to a fourth principle of mass casualty management: teamwork. In ordinary practice each physician is accustomed to working in a more or less independent capacity. The effective management of large numbers of casualties in a short time demands a totally different organizational structure. There must be someone in charge, in the person of the *disaster plan director*, who by experience and training is capable of giving orders, and others must be able and willing to follow directions. This individual should have control as close to absolute authority as is seen in medical practice. Although this is an environment that is quite different from that in which most physicians ordinarily function, repeated experience with civilian casualties has demonstrated conclusively that centralized authority is essential to optimal mass casualty management.

Philosophical Approach

Special attention should be given to the readjustment of thinking — literally of philosophy — that is necessary if the best possible results are to be obtained from the medical care of disaster victims. The physician is ordinarily committed to the highest quality of care for his individual patient. When a hospital is flooded with tremendous numbers of seriously injured individuals, an abrupt modification of this philosophy is essential. For example, certain individuals will arrive at the hospital in such condition that, under the disaster circumstances, there is no hope of salvaging them, though had they arrived in isolated circumstances, aggressive treatment might have permitted their survival. In the

disaster situation we have no reasonable choice but to regard these individuals as hopelessly injured and to turn the bulk of our efforts to those less seriously wounded.

The problems involved in this philosophical approach can run quite deep and deserve more discussion than can be devoted to them here. In most mass casualty situations decisions must be made regardng which patients should receive the attention of physicians. Difficult as the concept may be to entertain and to decide upon, those responsible for disaster planning in a community should give thought to the matter of whether usefulness to the community should be a criterion in selecting patients for the limited medical care that may be available. The handling of this problem in the event of a massive thermonuclear war or other major catastrophe could vitally affect the community in the months and years following the disaster. Though this idea may seem unattractive, it simply reflects the immense change in philosophy that is sometimes called for when we must shift from the ordinary practice of medicine to the care of casualties from a far-reaching disaster.

DISASTER PLANNING FOR THE HOSPITAL

Space Allocations

A key feature of the hospital management of disasters is the provision of separate space for triage, stabilization, major surgery, minor surgery and recovery. Special provision should be made for supplying space for waiting families of disaster victims, for the handling of the dead and for accommodation of representatives of communications media. The integration of these facilities, the provision of adequate resources and staff and the mobilization of a disaster plan require finely tuned coordination. Such coordination can be achieved only if the plan is exercised at regular intervals through disaster drills.

Surgery. In most hospitals, the major surgery area will be the main set of operating rooms in disasters. Ample numbers of surgical staff, anesthesia staff and nursing staff must be provided and a plan must be at hand for orderly addition of staff as needed. A minor surgery area (and possibly a special fracture area) should be provided so that patients need not remain for definitive care in the stabilization area and so that patients at the same time will not overload the major surgical area. The minor surgery area must be supervised by an experienced individual who can maintain a steady flow of patients. It is imperative to note that here, as elsewhere in the handling of disasters victims, it may be necessary to compromise the highest quality of care in the name of efficiency.

Recovery Area. Plans must provide for the easy evacuation of regular hospital patients from areas normally used for recovery or for intensive care to provide large open areas for recovering disaster victims. Intensive care unit personnel must constantly be aware of patients who could be moved out if a need should arise suddenly. It is particularly important that an appropriate individual have the authority to make decisions about patient moving and that a crisis of authority not be allowed to arise that would be superimposed on the crisis imposed by the disaster itself.

Also, the recovery area must be staffed by individuals with a high index of suspicion who are able not only to detect serious complications of therapy but who may also be able to detect injuries that have been overlooked in the initial evaluation and management procedures.

Family Waiting Area. Families of disaster victims must be provided with an area for waiting. If possible, this space should be adjacent to small rooms where conferences with physicians can be held, particulary in the event of death of a patient. Relatives and close friends may be needed to identify patients. The planning of the operation of this facility may cause it to serve to minimize anxiety, which if uncontrolled can lead to mass hysteria.

Morgue. In any major disaster, patients will inevitably die. Bodies must be stored in an orderly fashion that will permit their viewing for identification. Some plan should provide for a means of egress for families that have identified their dead so that they need not return to the area where other families are waiting.

Media Headquarters. Members of the press and other communications media must be kept informed; a room should be set aside for media representatives. Members of the hospital public relations department are probably best qualified to handle news dispatches and perhaps television coverage. Responsible medical personnel may communicate with members of the media at intervals. It is imperative, however, that members of the media not be allowed to roam through the hospital, since this will heighten both confusion and anxiety.

Logistics

The key feature in coordination of hospital disaster efforts is successful communication among those responsible for resources. In order to coordinate the various resources and facilities, an information system manned by trained personnel must provide the communications connection. A single individual should be in charge of coordinating disaster resources and facilities. That individual, the disaster plan director, or his alternate should be the only person who can activate a disaster plan. Such activation should result immediately in the gathering of key personnel in a disaster control center that will serve as the communication center while the plan is in effect and in the assigning of a reasonable number of personnel to the other key areas. Each member of the hospital staff should know his assignment in the event of a disaster. It is often desirable to have a disaster plan that enumerates two or more levels of disaster during which different numbers of staff will be called upon to serve. It is imperative that a distinction be made between disasters that occur inside the hospital and those that occur in the community, and to identify situations that require the mobilization of other types of medical personnel. The disaster control center should include representatives of the medical staff, nursing staff, administration, materials management, security, public affairs and support services. Specific communication support should be provided. The individuals in the control center must have the authority to call in staff from outside, to reallocate staff within the hospital and to allocate resources as indicated. They should have the knowledge to prevent forced inactivity of hospital disaster workers because of insufficient supplies as one example. They must be able to communicate effectively with external security officials and with the EMS coordinators should disturbances arise or should transient overloading occur.

Drills

As indicated earlier, the effective coordination of facilities, resources and manpower requires both planning and practice. It is commonplace that the requisite disaster drills are given little attention beyond that necessary to comply with external standards. Complex problems that may arise to challenge key coordinating staff in an actual disaster are not covered in many drills. This staff needs to meet periodically to consider such problems and to plan solutions to them that may be effective. Drills must focus on resource and staff allocation and reallocation as well as on the specifics of how to handle individual clinical problems. With the combination of planning and practice, however, the hospital itself may appropriately be regarded as a resource in the event of mass casualties.

Triage

The classification of patients into categories is critical in determining the success in handling a disaster. These categories may include patients who need immediate stabilization, those who can proceed to definitive care and those with relatively minor injuries. Physicians performing such triage must be experienced in the care of trauma patients and sensitive to unusual clinical problems. It is imperative that this task not be relegated to junior staff or house officers. The triage area must be capable of expansion to accommodate all patients that may be brought to a given hospital. Since triage is best performed at the entry point to the hospital, the emergency department should have been planned to serve this purpose. Ideally, the registration and waiting areas should be capable of conversion to triage.

The stabilization of patients who may be in shock or who have impending shock, airway problems or major hemorrhage should normally be carried out in the emergency department in an area immediately adjacent to the triage area. It is important that it be possible to open up relatively wide space for this purpose, so that patients will remain visible and not be sequestered in rooms. This area must be provided with equipment for fluid therapy, for airway maintenance and for stabilization of fractures. There must be easy egress from this area to areas for definitive care. The stabilization itself should not be used for definitive care. Patients should be sent to other areas for this purpose, even for relatively minor injuries.

The details of patient sorting will, of course, depend upon the particular circumstances. Patients arriving at the hospital may be classified into one of four major categories by the triage officer. These are:

I. Patients with minimal injuries who will do well on self-care or "buddy" care. Medicolegal responsibility makes it necessary not only to allow any patient to register if he desires but also to provide "medically trained" personnel to render care. This holds true for the disaster situation and may make the self-care or "buddy" system not feasible and force these patients to be grouped with Category II patients.

II. Patients whose injuries are less trivial and will require medical attention but are not of a serious nature; these patients will not require intensive care.

III. Patients whose injuries will require major medical attention. This group may be subdivided into the following:
    A. Require early operation
      1. Immediate
      2. After an interval
    B. Do not require operation or operation will be performed only later in their course.

IV. Patients who are either dead on arrival or so hopelessly wounded that under the circumstances of the disaster there is no reasonable chance of saving them.

In some disaster situations, the patient flow may be so great that initially triage should be made according to the most basic classifications, i.e., (A) those who will live no matter what, (B) those who will die no matter what and (C) those whose survival depends upon early critical care. It may be necessary to have "tiered" triage in which Category C patients are subdivided by another team according to whether or not there is need for surgery, and early operation or delayed operation.

The problem is compounded by the fact that the triage officer does not have everyone in front of him at once, making comparisons difficult. Two steps can be taken to minimize this disadvantage. One is good communication with EMS disaster field staff via the disaster plan director. A second is use of the "tiered" triage system in which the surgeon in charge of the operating room subdivides those patients referred to him into priorities of management. Considerable surgical sophistication is required in making the judgments that must be executed in the triage area. It is not simply a question of recognizing quickly the severity of various injuries and the urgency with which they must be tended to, though this is an important aspect. In addition, the triage officer must be familiar with the extent of the overall disaster because this will influence the categorization of patients. For example, in a limited disaster that will not tax resources extensively, few patients who arrive at the hospital alive will be placed in Category IV. On the other hand, in a major catastrophe that nearly wipes out an entire city, a triage officer who carelessly assigns patients to Category III who should be in Category IV will jeopardize many legitimate Category III patients. The triage officer knows the number and status of arriving casualties; the disaster plan director knows the conditions in the hospital. Each, then, has information that is essential for the decisions that the other must make; obviously, they should be in close communication.

In addition to sorting patients into categories, the triage officer may or may not be assigned two additional responsibilities. The first is the establishment of priorities among Category III patients. In other words, the triage officer may determine which patients most urgently need surgical attention, blood transfusions and other care. Except for those hospitals that are relatively small and have relatively limited staffs, it is probably not desirable for the triage officer to have responsibility for priority assignment on Category III patients. For the most part, it is better that the triage officer simply assign the patient to a category, send the patient on his way to the appropriate area and leave the determination of priority of management to those in the area to which the patient goes. The reasons for this are evident; the triage officer's judgement must be made hastily and on the basis of an exceedingly brief period of observation, while those in the area to which the patient goes will have a longer period of observation and perhaps better facilities with which to make a judgment.

The other responsibility sometimes assigned to triage officers is the institution of certain measures of immediate care such as the relief of airway obstruction and the control of hemorrhage. The ideal would be for those who are transporting patients to the hospital to institute these measures when they are called for; to some extent this ideal can be approached with proper planning on a community-wide basis.

If it is elected to assign to the triage officer the responsibility of priority of determination for Category III patients or the responsibility for execution of some immediate care measures, provisions must be made for this in the disaster planning by assigning to the triage officer adequate personnel for assistance in his work.

Patient Identification and Record-Keeping

Systems that serve to identify patients in a disaster situation should be different from the hospital routine in several respects. First, the identification number should be small. This saves transcription time and reduces chances of copying error. Most hospitals have "X" numbers for temporary identification. These are, however, 6- to 9-digit numbers. A system such as D1, D2, D3, would identify the disaster victim as being such. Later permanent hospital numbers could be assigned so that disaster numbers could be used again. Traditional wrist bands are often cut off in the era of arterial lines and use of the wrist for other purposes. Foot bracelets suffer the same fate; when saphaneous cutdowns are needed, the ID band gets cut off. We favor writing the number of the patient with marker that would wear off in 2 or 3 weeks; the bottom of the foot is an excellent location for this identification.

The use of pre-printed forms for x-ray, laboratory and especially blood bank would save both time and errors. Pre-printed checklist type of physical examination records are excellent in the disaster situation.

In many disaster situations, iatrogenic

disasters of an even greater magnitude may be precipitated by poor or inefficient identification systems.

Patient Care Categories

Patients in each category should be cared for in a separate location. The segregation of patients on this basis, which in ordinary hospital practice is called progressive patient care, is probably the most efficient means of handling large numbers of casualties in a brief period of time with limited resources. No triage officer is infallible and conditions may change after a patient is assigned to a category; consequently, someone should be given the authority to shift patients from one category to another after their initial assignment.

Category I — Minimal Care. Almost no medical personnel are necessary to handle patients in this category. Some responsible individual should be present in the area to be sure that order is maintained and if possible to supervise the administration of self-care and "buddy" care.

Category II — Light Medical Attention. Again, very little medical expertise needs to be expended. The principal duties to be carried out are perhaps the administration of tetanus shots, the application of light dressings and other chores that can safely be performed by medical students, nurses and paramedical personnel. The triage officer may assign a few individuals to this category in whom he suspects a more serious injury; consequently, some of these patients may require close observation.

Category III — Major Medical Attention. It is this category that will utilize most of the personnel, equipment and supplies. The specific organizational structure of Category III care is best determined by the individual hospital on the basis of its particular resources. The designation of a senior person to supervise this large portion of the mass casualty management is probably advisable in most hospitals. Patients with burns and other injuries that will not require initial operative care during the emergency situation (Category IIIB patients) can be attended by internists, pediatricians and other nonsurgical personnel, though it is desirable to have in the area in which these patients are being handled a member of the surgical staff who is familiar with the care of trauma patients. Many of the patients in this area will have blood volume problems that require attention.

Patients who require early operative treatment must, if priority has not already been determined by the triage officer, be sorted with respect to the urgency of operative intervention. The decision regarding the timing of operation will, of course, depend in large measure upon the nature and size of the disaster — several patients with moderately severe head injuries may require decompression quite early. On the other hand, in the event of a major catastrophe with hundreds of soft-tissue injuries to be cared for by a few surgeons, the talents of the neurosurgeon and his associates may be much better utilized in the performance of 30 or 40 wound debridements than in the performance of three or four cranial decompressions. This goes back to a principle outlined earlier, namely, that there are certain procedures that are rather simply performed but have a high yield in terms of reducing mortality and morbidity. In a major catastrophe it is wise for most medical attention to be directed at these. The disaster plan director should aid those attending Category III patients in making these decisions. He knows the scope of the overall size and nature of the disaster and the demands it is placing upon personnel, facilities and supplies.

It is probably desirable for a relatively high-ranking member of the surgical staff to serve as a deputy disaster plan director in charge of Category III patients. His major responsibility is to keep the workload reasonably well distributed among the personnel caring for these patients. These decisions will depend upon an assessment of the nature and extent of the disaster and upon his observation of conditions in his area.

The nonoperative care of patients in Category IIIA, both preoperative and postoperative, can be carried out by junior surgeons and by some nonsurgical physicians, though they should be supervised by one of the more senior surgical staff members.

Those with the greatest expertise and leadership ability should be utilized to fill the positions of disaster plan director, triage officer, deputy disaster plan directors and other "nonoperating" positions. In the latter stages of the mass casualty situations, as patients held for subsequent surgery come to the operating room, it may be possible to free individuals from these chores to head operating teams. When patients are assigned to operating teams with little training and experience, it is quite worthwhile for a senior member of the surgical staff to supervise the selection of operative procedures. The maximum use of an able and experienced surgeon can often be made by having him circulate among operating teams of less experienced surgeons, utilizing his judgment as to the procedures to be carried out by these less thoroughly trained individuals.

Other factors besides the availability and talent of surgeons will determine the type of surgical care that can be carried out in a disaster situation. As already suggested, the availability of anesthetists, anesthetic agents and oxygen may be limiting factors. It has been estimated that the average operating team in a disaster can handle about 15 cases every 24 hours. Naturally this figure will vary, depending upon the type of operative procedures that are carried out, but this does give a rough guide to the disaster plan director.

Category IV — Hopelessly Injured and D.O.A. The emotional difficulty involved in classifying these patients and the importance of assigning some patients who arrive at the hospital alive to this category have already been discussed. Without question, patients in Category IV should be made as comfortable as possible with the facilities at hand. A few nurses equipped with drugs can ordinarily do this. As the initial stages of a mass casualty situation pass, it may become evident that personnel, supplies and equipment will permit the care of additional patients in Category III and a physician may be assigned to screen surviving Category IV patients for transfer to Category III

FURTHER CONSIDERATIONS

The extent to which x-ray and laboratory facilities can be employed in managing patients in a mass casualty situation will depend upon the particular circumstances.

Both facilities are likely to reach use capacity quickly. Fortunately, few laboratory tests are ordinarily essential in handling the acutely traumatized patient. On the other hand, x-rays can be of immense help. Consequently, the senior radiologist on the hospital staff will have a critical responsibility in determining how the hospital's x-ray facilities are used.

In the confusion that goes with handling a disaster, it is essential that the hospital be adequately patrolled by authoritative individuals responsible for maintaining order and for directing ambulatory patients, relatives and friends, press and spectators to the appropriate locations. This function can be combined with a messenger function, and again hospital personnel displaced from their normal activities can be used.

It has already been mentioned that an area should be set aside for providing information to the relatives and close friends of patients. It is equally important that an experienced individual from the hospital staff be assigned the responsibility for handling this matter. This individual should be selected carefully and should be provided with the assistance and support necessary to carry out his job. A nonmedical person or a junior member of the medical staff can be assigned here if he can qualify. It is important in setting up a disaster plan that a means be provided whereby information can be easily relayed from treatment locations to the area in which families wait to receive information. In the disaster situation the possibilities for mass hysteria among the minimally injured and among relatives and friends of the seriously injured are very real. A little advance planning about the handling of these seemingly trivial problems can avert much serious trouble. Furthermore, it may be necessary to have friends and relatives identify seriously injured and deceased patients; this needs to be taken into account in setting up the disaster plan.

Much of what has been said about dealing with families also applies to relations with the news media. Here again the services of a tactful individual with sound judgment and some knowledge of the nature of the situation can avert much misunderstanding and confusion. A senior member of the hospital staff should be assigned this responsibility; many lay hospital directors are well suited to this job.

Throughout the emergency situation the disaster plan director must be fully cognizant of developments both outside and inside the hospital. He must know something of the continuing arrival of further casualties and he must know the status of his personnel and their supplies. Provisions should be made in disaster planning for such information to reach the disaster plan director. He cannot, however, hope to gain all the information he needs by remaining in one spot and having information brought to him. He must periodically tour the hospital and talk with his deputies and others who are involved in the care of patients and related activities.

AFTERMATH

Most mass casualty situations develop suddenly and without warning, but their effects go on for weeks, months and years. In this discussion we have been concerned with the early handling of the medical service aspects of a disaster. These aspects are the ones that require the greatest advanced planning because there is the least time to prepare for them. Subsequent events can be dealt with in a somewhat more orderly fashion.

In handling any mass casualty situation there is an initial flurry of exhausting activity that may last from a few hours to a few days. However, thought must be given to the "secondary" care of the casualties who survive and to the orderly return to normal hospital routine and normal community function. The amount of "secondary" care required of victims of a disaster will depend upon a number of factors. If the immediate situation has required that vast numbers of wounds be left open and a sizeable number of fractures left unreduced, then soon after the initial stage of disaster management will follow another period of high activity in caring for these injuries. Further rehabilitation may go on for months or years. The point to be emphasized here is that there is less need and less possibility for planning in this, though some attention needs to be directed to it in establishing a disaster plan.

SPECIAL CONSIDERATION: RIOTS

Because civil disturbances rank among the more probable mass casualty problems for urban hospitals and because they raise problems, particular attention should be directed in community and hospital planning to the handling of such disturbances. Unlike in most other mass casualty situations, injuries tend to occur in clusters over a period of several days. During this time the peak patient load is likely to be at night. Since the demands on hospital personnel are likely to occur somewhat erratically over a period of time, careful thought must be given by the disaster plan director to the optimal use of such personnel and to adequate rest for them.

The nature of the disturbance is likely to disrupt not only the transportation of casualties but also of personnel to and from the hospital. Ample provision must be made by the community to assure that both casualties and personnel will reach the hospital as expeditiously as possible. In addition, this is one type of disaster in which the security of the hospital itself is jeopardized. Community and hospital planning must provide protection for the hospital building and its occupants. A further complication is the presence in the hospital of large numbers of casualties who are likely also to be prisoners. Planning for this type of disaster must include some means of guarding such individuals.

By and large, the types of injuries seen do not differ greatly from those in other disaster situations. Usually, individuals exposed to the riot control gases, CN (including chemical Mace) and CS, require no special care other than removal to an area of clean air. Exposure to these agents initially leads to a burning sensation in the eyes with considerable lacrimation and usually some rhinorrhea; heavier exposure is likely to produce cough and a sensation of tightness in the chest; dense concentrations of the agents may cause nausea and vomiting. All of these symptoms also are ordinarily relieved upon removal to an uncontaminated atmosphere. Contact with the agents over a prolonged period, particularly in warm weather, may produce irritation of the skin. Since these "gases" are in actuality particulate solids in a finely divided state, heavy contamination of the body or clothing is best dealt with by removal of the clothing and washing the individual with water or a 5 per cent sodium bisulphite solution. If eye irritation is not relieved by removal of the individual to clean air, the eyes should also be washed out with water or physiological salt solution. As nearly as can be determined, these riot control agents produce no adverse effect on pre-existing respiratory, cardiac or other conditions.

CARE OF SPECIFIC DISORDERS

In the mass casualty situation, modifications must often be made in the handling of various types of injuries and disorders in order to achieve the maximum benefit for the greatest number of patients. These modifications do not come easily to some surgeons, but they are essential if the limited resources at hand are to be utilized effectively. Obviously, the ways in which ordinary care is altered for the disaster situation will depend upon the casualty load, the size of the hospital, the personnel present, the availability of supplies and equipment, whether there is damage to the hospital itself and a variety of other factors. A precise determination of these modifications must be made on the basis of the particular situation. Since in making these modifications various functions of the hospital must be coordinated, the ultimate responsibility for deciding how particular injuries are to be handled must rest with the disaster plan director. It is he who knows the casualty load, the availability of dressing materials, the extent of supply of oxygen and anesthetic gases, the fatigue factor in his personnel and other items that must enter into the decisions.

Because of the need for individualization to the specific circumstances of a particular disaster, it is not possible here to do any more than suggest some of the ways in which ordinary care may be modified in a disaster situation in an effort to obtain optimal utilization of resources. These suggestions are based upon military and civilian experience and emphasize the principle that certain simple maneuvers help in decreasing mortality and long-term functional loss. Only three specific areas will be discussed in detail: blood volume deficit, infection and burns.

Blood Volume Deficit

Blood volume deficit has been a major source of morbidity and mortality in past disasters. As in dealing with non-disaster patients, the first step in coping with massive acute blood loss is hemostasis. The application of a pressure dressing to an extremity or the clamping of a lacerated jugular vein can be carried out quickly; however, except in quite limited disasters, patients who are bleeding rapidly from intrathoracic or intra-abdominal injuries may have to be assigned to Category IV.

In disaster planning, the need for volume replacement in massive amounts must be taken into consideration. The stockpiling of materials to combat blood volume deficits in large numbers of patients is necessary. Certainly, 5 per cent plasma protein fraction and lactated Ringer's solution would be used extensively and should be in adequate supply. Some evidence suggests the crystalloid solution to be equally as satisfactory as the colloid in acute intravascular expansion.

Blood and blood components will be in great demand in most disasters. The use of Group "O" and type-specific blood may be necessary in the acute situation, but many patients will be adequately served by emergency and routine cross-matching. Coagulation factors, especially those found in fresh frozen plasma, will be needed. Each blood bank should develop guidelines for the rewarming and utilization of this vital component. A point to remember is that patients massively transfused with "O" red blood cells should receive AB plasma. The limited availability of this component makes use of "O" blood in mass casualty situations less satisfactory. It is a good idea for businesses and industries in which a mass casualty situation is possible to have all the employees blood typed. A list of this information would then be kept by both the company administration and the hospital most likely to receive the casualty victims. Many lives could possibly be saved by this simple preparation procedure.

A practice not needed in the usual administration of packed red cells is reconstitution. Urgent administration of packed cells will be both necessary and slow. The addition of 50 to 75 ml. of normal saline will cut administration time by one third to one half. This is best done under blood bank supervision but can also be done at the triage area.

The administration of intravenous fluids of any type requires certain supplies, and there is no value in having available solutions to combat blood volume deficits unless sufficient supplies of intravenous therapy equipment are also available.

In almost every major disaster that has occurred in the past, hypovolemia has been a major cause of death among patients who arrived at the hospital alive. Proper handling of the hypovolemia problem by advance planning and the execution of sound clinical judgment with regard to managing blood volume deficits in the disaster situation will be important determinants of the success of the medical operation in the disaster.

Infections

Wound infection has often been a major problem in mass casualty situations. Keystones in the management of infection once it has developed are adequate drainage and the administration of antibiotics. However, in a major catastrophe the available supply of antibiotics may be limited even a few days after the catastrophe when infection becomes a problem. This gives infection prophylaxis a high priority. However, infection prophylaxis is not easy in the disaster situation. On one hand, many wounds are deep and contain large amounts of devitalized tissue and foreign material, providing a superb medium, and on the other, it is quite difficult to maintain adequate sterility. Two measures that experience has shown are quite valuable in infection prophylaxis in mass casualty situations are the wide debridement of wounds and the postponement of wound closure.

Though one cannot say with finality that prophylactic antibiotics are not useful in preventing infection following trauma, the bulk of evidence available today suggests that they are not. Furthermore, the limited supply of antibiotics is a practical curb on their use for prophylactic purposes even if one concedes their value. Evidence suggests that when the risk of infection is high, the administration of antibiotics in massive dosage at the time of wounding and immediately thereafter may act as an effective prophylaxis against infection. If antibiotics are available in some quantity, patients who are otherwise salvageable and who arrive at the hospital soon after sustaining extensive wounds with much devitalized tissue, which cannot all be removed and in which there is heavy contamination, might profitably be treated by the administration of massive doses of antibiotics immediately upon arrival at the hospital and for a short period thereafter.

Burns

The number of burns occurring in a mass casualty situation will, of course, depend upon the nature of the disaster. The amount of care that can be rendered to burns will depend upon the number of burn and other victims and the status of facilities at the hospital. In limited disasters the majority of burns can be cared for quite adequately. However, in major catastrophes patients with burns over a certan percentage of body surface area are placed in Category IV if the maximum number of patients are to be salvaged.

The bulk of medical attention in major catastrophes will be directed toward those patients with 20 to 50 per cent body surface burns. Whatever the relative merits of open and closed dressings of burns in ordinary practice, there can be little doubt that in the mass casualty situation open treatment is generally preferable. Silver nitrate and Sulfamylon therapy may be used but both are responsible for major problems in metabolic derangements and in the case of silver nitrate, damage of the hospital equipment and facilities. Silver sulfadiazine will be the mainstay of most burn therapy. Also, the newer techniques of tangential excision and early grafting will not be feasible in the mass casualty situation.

Though the decisions regarding burn management in a mass casualty situation hinge on particular circumstances, some advance thought during the disaster planning stage concerning the techniques to be employed is valuable. If the disaster plan director knows at the time of arrival of the first burn victim what resources will be at his disposal for burn therapy and has an idea of the alternatives that will be available to him, much time can be saved at a period when time is at a premium.

CONCLUSION

Optimal medical care in disasters of all sizes and types is dependent upon realistic advance planning by the community and its hospitals. The type of catastrophe that will occur in a particular community cannot be anticipated, but planning can assure that when a disaster occurs, appropriate individuals will be in a position to deal effectively with the specific problems that arise. The fact that planning cannot be complete is no justification for the absence of preparation. The integration of hospital disaster planning to the regional EMS plan is essential for realistic preparedness in the event of a real disaster.

REFERENCES

1. Abelson, L., Star, L., and Goldner, A.: Twenty years of medical support in aircraft disasters at Kennedy Airport. Aerospace Medicine May 1973, p. 560.
2. Adler, Y., and Naggan, L.: Reanimation strategy and equipment at the front line. *In*: Proceedings of the 21st International Congress of Military Medicine and Pharmacy, Bucharest, May 1973, pp. 63–65.
3. Caro, D.: Major disasters. Lancet *11*:1309, 1974.
4. Ebel, P.: Medical teams to the rescue. Daily Telegraph March 6, 1975, p. 81.
5. Evans, D.: Simulated aircraft disaster instructional exercise at Baltimore-Washington International Airport. Aviation, Space and Environmental Medicine April 1976, p. 445.
6. Fisher, C.: Mobile triage team in a community disaster plan. J. Am. Col. Emergency Physicians 6:10, 1977.
7. Gierson, E., and Richman, L.: Valley triage: An approach to mass casualty care. J. Trauma *15*: 193, 1975.
8. Gill, W., Champion, H., Long, W., Stega, M., Nolan, J., Decker, R., Misinscky, M. and Cowley, R.: A clinical experience of major multiple trauma in Maryland. Md. State Med. J., January 1976, p. 55.
9. Hays, M., Stefanki, J., and Cheu, D.: Planning an airport disaster drill. Aviation, Space, and Environmental Medicine 47:556, 1976.
10. Lister, J.: Conflicting loyalties in a damaging dispute — an ancient rivalry. Disaster on the Tube. Medical Intelligence 292:1171, 1975.
11. Moles, T.: Planning for major disasters. Anesthesiology 49:643, 1977.
12. Mosley, W.: Bengal cyclone of November 1970: Logical approach to disaster assessment. Lancet *I*:1029, 1972.
13. Naggan, L.: Medical planning for disaster in Israel. Evaluation of the military surgical experience in the October 1973 War, and implications for the organization of the civilian disaster services. Injury 7:297, 1976.
14. Rutherford, W. H.: Surgery of violence. II. Disaster procedures. Br. Med. J. *1*(5955):443, 1975.
15. Rutherford, W. H.: Experience in the accident and emergency department of the Royal Victoria Hospital with patients from civil disturbances in Belfast 1969–1972 with a review of disasters in the United Kingdom 1951–1971. Injury *4*:189, 1972.
16. Shaftan, G.: Disaster and medical care. J. Trauma 2:111, 1962.
17. Star, L., Abelson, L., and Goldner, A.: Operation S.A.F.E. (simulated aircraft fire and emergency). Aerospace Medicine 45:888, 1974.
18. Theoret, J.: Exercise London: a disaster exercise involving numerous casualties. CMA J. *114*:697, 1976.
19. Walt, A., and Wilson, R.: Disaster planning: A modern reality. Preparation and planning for emergencies and trauma. Management of Trauma. Philadelphia, Lea & Febiger, 1975, pp. 13–24.
20. Whittaker, R. Fareed, S., Green, P., Barry, P., Borge, A., and Fletes-Barrios, R.: Earthquake disaster in Nicaragua: Reflections on the initial management of massive casualties. J. Trauma *14*:37, 1974.
21. Whyte, A.: Disaster wound treatment. Br. **Med. J.** 2:43, 1975.

CHAPTER 28

THE EPIDEMIOLOGY AND PREVENTION OF INJURIES

Susan P. Baker, M.P.H.
Park Elliott Dietz, M.D., M.P.H.

Each year 75 million Americans are injured severely enough to need medical attention. In 1977, 152,000 were fatally injured, including 20,000 victims of homicide and 27,000 suicides. Surgeons and others who treat these injured patients also have opportunities to decrease the extent of trauma in large groups of people whom they will never see. To do so most effectively requires awareness of the factors contributing to the frequency and severity of injuries.

In describing the epidemiology of major types of trauma, this chapter illustrates concepts applicable to the occurrence and prevention of all injuries. Some injuries, such as nonsurgical trauma (poisoning, drowning), are not specifically discussed, but the basic concepts are the same. The chapter emphasizes the role of the environment — everything that is external to the person, ranging from clothing to transportation systems. This emphasis is made because of the importance of the environment in determining the probability and nature of the injuries, as well as the many opportunities for making changes in the environment that will reduce injuries.

Preparation of this chapter was supported in part by the Insurance Institute for Highway Safety, Washington, D.C.: the Robert Wood Johnson Foundation, Princeton, N.J.; the Philadelphia Foundation; and the Maryland Medical-Legal Foundation. The opinions, conclusions and proposals in the text are those of the authors and do not necessarily represent the views of the sponsors.

RISK FACTORS AND HIGH-RISK GROUPS

Injuries, like diseases, do not occur at random. Certain population groups are at increased risk owing either to greater exposure to hazards, decreased ability to avoid hazards, decreased resistance to injury or less likelihood of a favorable outcome when injured. While the predominant population groups vary with type of injury, many important risk factors are common to a wide variety of injuries.

Age

For all injuries combined, population-based *death* rates are highest in the elderly: 164 per 100,000 for people age 75–84, compared with 86 per 100,000 for people age 15–24[102] (Fig. 28–1), who have a very high death rate as well as the highest injury rate. Age differences in *injury* rates reflect not only differences in activities, behavior and physical capabilities but also in injury thresholds. The complexities of age differences in fracture rates were described by Buhr and Cooke, who divided bones into three groups: (1) bones with high fracture rates in the young, such as the distal humerus and clavicle, that do not become osteoporotic in the elderly; (2) bones with high fracture rates in the wage-earning population, especially bones of the hands and feet; and (3) bones that fracture more readily in the elderly because

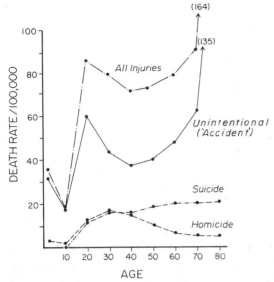

Figure 28–1. *Injury death rates by age, per 100,000 population in the United States, 1976. (From National Center for Health Statistics, U.S. Department of Health, Education and Welfare, 1978.)*

they tend to become excessively brittle and osteoporotic with age, especially in females — examples are the proximal femur, pelvis and proximal humerus.[15]

In *children under 5*, high injury rates reflect developmental patterns: the largest number of burn injuries in this age group occurs during the second year of life,[104] when ability to move and explore increases. Pedestrian injuries, on the other hand, become common around age 4, as parental supervision is decreasing. For the

under-5 age group, falls are the leading cause of nonfatal injuries, but the largest numbers of fatalities (Table 28–1) result from vehicle occupant injuries, housefires and drownings (about 750, 750, and 700 deaths, respectively), with pedestrian deaths a major problem in urban areas. For ages 0–4, firearms are almost as common a cause of death (80 per year) as poisoning by solids and liquids, but this fact is neither widely recognized nor reflected in preventive efforts. Between 1960 and 1976, the number of young children killed by firearms changed very little, but fatal poisonings dropped from 450 to 80[72] as lead-based paint was used less commonly and manufacturers modified the contents and packaging of medicines and other potentially poisonous agents.

Teenagers and young adults are exposed more than other age groups to such high-risk activities as contact sports, motorcycling, high-speed driving and hanggliding. They have especially high death rates from vehicle crashes, firearms and drowning. In the 15–24 year age group, about three fourths of all deaths result from injuries: 24,000 unintentional, 5000 homicidal, 5000 suicidal.

In the *working age* population, motor vehicle crashes cause almost half of all deaths from unintentional injuries. Nonfatal injuries among males, however, are incurred primarily at work. Even though occupational risks are low for females and white-collar workers, for the entire labor

TABLE 28–1.   Leading Categories of Unintentional° Injury Deaths, in Order of Frequency, for Selected Age Groups

AGE <5	15–24	75+	ALL AGES°
Mot. veh. occ.†	Mot. veh. occ.	Falls	Mot. veh. occ.
Housefires	Drowning	Mot. veh. occ.	Falls
Drowning	Poisoning	Pedestrian	Pedestrian
Pedestrian	Pedestrian	Suffocation°°	Drowning
Suffocation°°	Firearms	Housefires	Poisoning
Falls	Falls	Clothing ignition	Housefires

°If homicides and suicides were included, firearms (which cause about 30,000 deaths annually) would be the second leading category for all ages combined.

†Motor vehicle occupant.

°°Inhalation or ingestion of food, vomitus or other object causing obstruction or suffocation.

Data from the National Center for Health Statistics, U.S. Department of Health, Education, and Welfare (1976), unpublished.

force the National Health Survey shows injuries to be even more common at work than in the home: 120 versus 80 per thousand, respectively. Fatal job-related injuries are most numerous on the highway (about 4000 deaths annually) and among construction workers and farmers (2000 each). Even higher death rates per worker characterize other occupations such as fire-fighting and mining.[72]

Among the *elderly*, extremely high death rates (Fig. 28–1) reflect their generally poorer clinical course and susceptibility to complications following injury. Moderately severe trauma (that is, with an Injury Severity Score on the scale of Baker et al. of 10–19) is about nine times as likely to prove fatal to patients over 70 as to patients younger than 50.[4] While people 65 and older comprise only one tenth of the population, one fifth of all injury deaths occur in this group. For certain types of trauma — notably falls and burns — the incidence of nonfatal injury also increases markedly in the elderly,[29, 52] probably owing in large part to their decreased perception and slowed responses.

Sex

The risk of fatal injury is two and one half times as great for males as for females. Males have 50 per cent more nonfatal injuries and predominate especially with regard to injuries associated with transportation, recreation, work and assaults. Not only the number of injuries but also the proportion of very severe injuries is greater for males. For motor vehicle crashes, the ratio of deaths to injuries is much higher for males than females and is especially high for males age 15–24, as a result of more severe crashes in this group. Similarly for falls, males of all ages have a higher ratio of deaths to injuries.[52] (A ratio of deaths to injuries is similar to a case fatality rate but includes all injuries, not just hospital admissions.)

Sex differences in resistance to injury are most notable in postmenopausal women, as a result of the greater prevalence of osteoporosis in this group. Buhr and Cooke reported that the likelihood of fracture of the femoral neck was 30 times as great for men over 80 as under 40, and 300 times as great for women over 80 as under 40.[15]

Alcohol and Other Drugs

Alcohol is an important contributor to all types of injuries. The likelihood of its presence increases with the severity of injury and cannot be discounted even in young teenagers. More than half of fatally injured drivers and substantial proportions of adults injured in falls, fires or assaults are likely to have blood alcohol concentrations (BAC's) exceeding 100 mg. per 100 ml., which in most states is presumptive evidence of intoxication in a motor vehicle operator. One fourth of the patients admitted to one trauma unit had BAC's of at least 100 mg. per ml. and 42 per cent had measureable concentrations.[17] In a study of emergency department patients, alcohol was detected in 30 per cent of the patients injured on highways, 22 per cent injured at home, 16 per cent injured on the job, and 56 per cent injured in fights or assaults. BAC's above 50 mg./100 ml. predominated in the latter group and were least common in those injured on the job.[105] For "fall repeaters," i.e., people injured in two or more falls in a single year, hospital records suggested alcohol as a contributory factor in 23 per cent of the cases, compared to about 10 per cent of other fall patients; since the patients included children, these percentages underestimate the proportion of adults who had been drinking.[50]

Alcohol's causal role in injuries is shown by (1) the high BAC's commonly found in people who are most "responsible" or "at fault" in the events leading to injury (Fig. 28–2), (2) the rarity of high concentrations in comparable groups of people who are *not* injured and (3) the increase in frequency and severity of injury associated with increases in BAC.[6, 46, 54, 103] For many teenage and elderly drivers, alcohol increases the likelihood of vehicular crash involvement even at concentrations below 50 mg. per 100 ml. For ages 25–59, serious crashes generally involve extremely high concentrations, and the majority of fatally injured "at fault" drivers have BAC's of 150 mg. per 100 ml. or higher[6] (Fig. 28–2). While there are substantial differences between individuals, the average 155-pound person would reach a BAC of approximately 50 mg. per 100 ml. after consuming 5 ounces of 80-proof whiskey, or a BAC of 150 mg. per 100 ml. with 10 ounces, if drinking after a meal. A given amount of alcohol

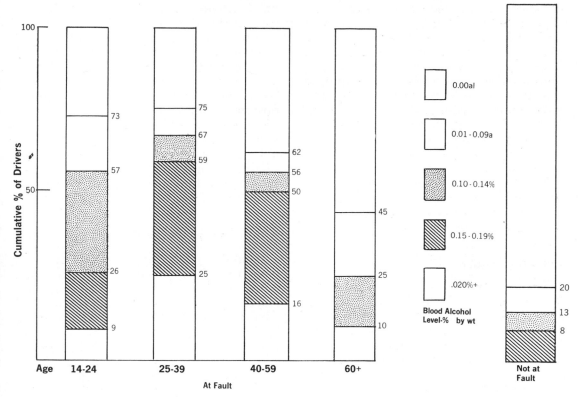

Figure 28–2. Blood alcohol concentrations in drivers killed in crashes in Baltimore. Left hand columns, drivers at fault, by age. Right hand, drivers not at fault, all ages combined. (From Baker, S. P., and Spitz, W. U.: J.A.M.A. 214:1079, 1970.)

will have less effect on a heavier person (because the alcohol consumed is distributed throughout the entire body) and greater effect if consumed on an empty stomach.

The prominent role of alcohol in relation to trauma is not limited to its adverse effect on perception, judgment and performance. Experiments indicate that a blow of specified force to the brain, spinal cord or precordium is more likely to produce severe impairment or death in animals pretreated with alcohol than in those without alcohol.[32, 65] Further deleterious effects of high BAC's on the trauma patient include problems in diagnosis and treatment of injury as well as the complication of delirium tremens (see Chapter 29). In some instances the ability to rule out or recognize alcohol intoxication can be vital to successful diagnosis and management; this can be achieved using portable breath-testing instruments or taking advantage of the close correlation between BAC and serum osmolality.[17]

To date, *drugs other than alcohol* have not been shown to play a causal role in a substantial proportion of injuries, although abuse of amphetamines, marijuana or other drugs can seriously impair performance. Multiple drug use, especially the combination of alcohol with one or more other drugs, creates additional problems. Some drugs in common use (benzodiazepines, barbiturates, phenothiazines, for example) have an additive or synergistic effect in combination with alcohol.[55, 71] While the roles of drugs other than alcohol are poorly understood in injury causation, their presence in the trauma patient is not uncommon and, especially if not recognized, may complicate the clinical course (see Chapter 29).

Socioeconomic Status

Socioeconomic status influences the incidence of homicide and extrafamilial assaultive injuries and of pedestrian and house fire fatalities, all of which are most common among the urban poor. While wealth places certain people at especially high risk of death — adults with private planes, for example, or children in neighborhoods with swimming pools — the burdens of injury nevertheless rest disproportionately on the poor. High-risk jobs, low-quality housing and use of more hazardous products such as space heaters tend to be concentrated among people of lower socioeconomic status. Tragic socioeconomic imbalances are reflected in high injury rates among blacks[7, 59] and in nonwhite death rates that are about six times the white rate for assaults and three times the white rate for burns.[52, 102]

Time and Place

Marked seasonal fluctuations characterize most injuries. Deaths from fires are more common in the winter months, those from drowning and motor vehicle crashes (especially motorcycles) in the summer. A November peak in unintentional shootings coincides with the beginning of hunting season. Variations with geography and population density are also pronounced: motor vehicle death rates are highest in sparsely settled areas, with the rates per 100 million vehicle miles ranging from two in New Jersey to six in Wyoming.[72]

Geographic and temporal factors influence not only the incidence of injuries but also the corresponding need for appropriately organized trauma services. The fact that the majority of serious crashes occur in rural areas creates problems in transportation and delays in definitive treatment of the injured. Similarly, serious injuries, especially those related to use of alcohol, are especially common at night and on weekends, when hospital staffing may be minimal. One study showed that 86 per cent of the patients who required hospitalization following highway crashes arrived at the hospital during the weekend, evening or nighttime shifts, and the more serious the injury, the greater the likelihood of arrival during these shifts.[5] Similar relationships have been observed for injuries from falls[50] and assaults.

Protecting High-Risk Groups

What do infants, teenagers and the aged have in common with one another and with self-employed laborers, impoverished ghetto dwellers and people with alcohol problems? Whether for maturational, economic, psychological or other reasons, members of most high-risk groups *tend to be harder to influence with approaches that require changes in individual behavior in order to prevent injury.* Seatbelt use laws in Ontario, for example, had little effect on teenagers (Fig. 28–3). In Miami, elderly pedestrians admonished by police for jaywalking did so again at their next opportunity.[45] Scofflaw drivers whose licenses are revoked are even more likely than the average licensed driver to be involved in fatal crashes.[58, 82] People who live in "firetrap" housing can least afford smoke detectors. And not only are young children hard to influence, but in-

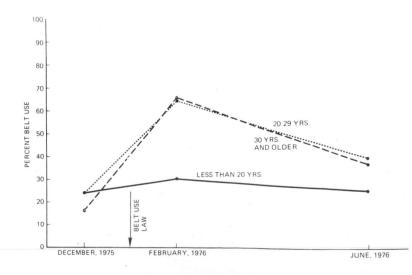

Figure 28–3. *Per cent driver and right front passenger shoulder belt use in equipped cars before and after mandatory belt use law went in force January 1, 1976 in Ontario, Canada, by estimated age. (From Insurance Institute for Highway Safety Status Report 11:10:2, 1976.)*

tensive efforts at a well-baby clinic had no effect on dangerous maternal behavior such as leaving knives and matches in reach of young children.[24]

The tendency to attribute injuries to "human error" has nourished false hopes that they can be prevented through education. Neither public education campaigns nor driver education programs have yet been shown by scientific evaluation to justify the veneration and large budgets accorded them. Many injuries (including highway injuries) result less from lack of knowledge than from failure to apply what is known. This is true not only of the individuals who may be affected (the student who knows he should wear a seatbelt, the mother who knows she should keep her child away from the stove) but it is also true of the decision-makers who determine the probability of injury for others (including manufacturers who know that their cars, stoves, etc., will be used by less-than-perfect people yet who fail to design products to minimize the likelihood of injury).

Because people whose behavior is especially hard to influence predominate among the injured, successful preventive approaches generally involve improved product designs and changes in the man-made environment that will protect *everyone*.[44, 107] Such automatic ("passive") protection, now taken for granted in insulated hand tools and household fuses, is gradually gaining acceptance in other realms because of its unmatched potential for preventing deaths and injuries. The following sections mention a variety of underexploited technological approaches to the prevention of injury, for their application is among the most promising challenges of modern science.

MOTOR VEHICLE CRASHES

In 1977, highway deaths numbered 47,000, occurred at a rate of 21 per 100,000 population and accounted for 90 per cent of all transportation fatalities (Fig. 28–4). Roughly one death in 40 in the United States involves a motor vehicle. The societal costs of highway injuries, exclusive of property damage, total about $18 billion annually. Underscoring the potential value of modifications to cars and other

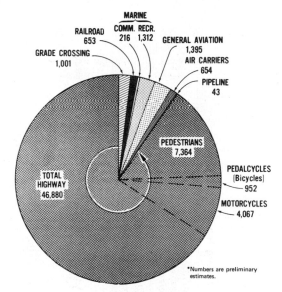

Figure 28–4. *Transportation fatalities in 1977. (From U.S. National Transportation Safety Board.)*

motor vehicles, about one in 25 is involved at some time in its "life" in a crash resulting in death or hospital admission. Although the discussion of transportation injuries focuses on highway crashes, the same principles apply to air, rail and water transport.[45]

Mechanical energy is the etiological agent for all fractures, concussions and lacerations, whether they result from crashes, falls, assaults or other events.[42] As with diseases, prevention is a matter of keeping the etiological agent from reaching a susceptible person in amounts or at rates that exceed injury thresholds. Regardless of age and other risk factors, the mechanisms of injury and the basic preventive strategies (Table 28–2) are the same for everyone.

Injury patterns have changed in response to vehicle improvements and use of protective equipment. In Queensland, Australia, for example, major head injuries as a proportion of all major injuries in highway fatalities dropped from 43 to 34 per cent in car passengers and from 53 to 30 per cent in motorcyclists in connection with laws requiring seatbelt use in automobiles and helmet use by motorcyclists. The proportion of head injuries did not

TABLE 28–2.   Examples of 10 Basic Strategies for Reducing Injuries and Deaths

STRATEGY	Injury to Motor Vehicle Occupants	EXAMPLES Injury to Football Players	Injury by Handguns
1. Preventing marshalling of potentially injurious agents or 2. Reducing their amounts	Alternative travel modes; reductions in speed limits and speed capabilities of cars	Fewer games; shorter quarters; speed restrictions in tackling drills	Reduced production of handguns, bullets
3. Preventing inappropriate release of agent	Vehicle and road designs that simplify driver's task	Playing surfaces that reduce likelihood of falls	Locking up guns; eliminating motive for shooting, e.g., no cash
4. Modifying release of agent	Use of seat belts to decelerate occupant with vehicle	Short cleats on shoes allowing foot to rotate rather than transmitting sudden force to knee	Single-shot guns requiring reloading between firings
5. Separating in time or space or 6. With physical barriers	Restricting transport of hazardous materials to certain times and places; highway medians	Limited-contact practice drills; placing fixed structures farther from field; face masks	Bulletproof vests; bulletproof glass
7. Modifying surfaces, basic structures	Airbags to spread forces over wide area of body; removing projections in car	Changing outside of helmets to reduce injuries to other players	Soft, doughnut-shaped bullets for target shooting (require less initial velocity, unlikely to penetrate humans)
8. Increasing resistance to injury	Therapy for osteoporosis	Musculoskeletal conditioning	
9. Emergency response or 10. Medical care and rehabilitation	Systems that route patients to appropriately trained physicians	Personnel trained to recognize serious injuries; physicians on call	Occupational rehabilitation for paraplegics

change in fatally injured pedestrians and bicyclists during the same period; bicyclists had the highest proportion of head injuries, and almost three fourths sustained skull fractures.[99]

Motor Vehicle Occupants

Motor vehicle occupant deaths — about 35,000 in 1977 — comprise the largest group of fatal injuries for all ages up to 75 (Table 28–1). Among the most important factors affecting the risk of occupant injury or death are amount of highway travel, road characteristics, speed, vehicle crashworthiness and restraint use.[43, 45] The correlation between *amount of travel* and exposure to risk of injury is obvious; less obvious, perhaps, is the possibility of reducing highway deaths by reducing the need to travel or substituting safer modes — trains or buses, for example, since their death rates per passenger mile are only a fraction of that for cars (Table 28–3).

Road characteristics influence the likelihood of crashes and often determine whether a crash will result in injury or death. The effect of better designed highways is reflected in lower death rates per vehicle mile (one third as high on interstates as on other roads) and per passenger mile (one sixth as high for intercity buses as for all buses combined).[72] Highway design features that reduce crashes include separating opposing streams of traffic, as with one-way streets or median dividers; eliminating intersections; improving illumination, signing and lines of sight; designing roadsides so straying cars can recover safely; removing roadside structures or using only structures that attenuate crash forces (breakaway light poles, for example, or barrels filled with energy-absorbing materials). A few physicians, notably Haddon and Waller,[56] have disputed the notion that people whose cars stray from the traffic lanes "get what they deserve," and have fought such practices as replacing demolished roadside poles with stronger structures that will survive a crash while ensuring more human damage. The sides of major highways, especially interstates, are beginning to reflect the more modern philosophy, but the 16,000 motor vehicle occupants killed annually in single-vehicle crashes illustrate the size of the remaining problem.

Speed is a major factor in crash causation because at higher speeds humans and vehicles are less able to respond in time to avoid a crash. Moreover, once a crash occurs, speed becomes an important determinant of the likelihood and severity of injury, since the energy dissipated in a crash increases with the square of the change in velocity (in a deceleration-to-zero velocity). Thus the forces on a properly restrained occupant in a forward crash at 70 mph may be roughly twice the forces at 50 mph. Stapp, who was experimentally decelerated from 632 mph to zero mph in 1.4 seconds without irreversible injury, proved that a properly restrained person can withstand extremely abrupt deceleration.[92] The 55 mph national speed limit reduced the speed of travel on roads with previously higher limits and was a major factor in the decreased death rate per 100 million vehicle miles — from 4.2 in 1973 to 3.5 in 1974 and subsequent years. The overall drop of some 10,000 deaths per year was partly due to other factors, but an estimated 5000 lives annually have been saved by the 55 mph limit. Perpetuation of the 55 mph limit and appropriate reductions in speed capabilities of vehicles would do much to prevent unnecessary death and injury.

Vehicle size has consistently been shown to correlate inversely with the likelihood of death or serious injury. Small cars are involved in more crashes per mile

TABLE 28–3. Death Rates per Person Mile of Travel for Users of Vehicles (United States, 1975–1977)*

TYPE OF TRAVEL	DEATHS/100 MILLION PERSON MILES
Motorcycle	17
General aviation	12
Automobile	1.4
Bus	0.15
Train	0.07
Scheduled plane	0.04

*From Haddon, W., Jr., and Baker, S. P.: Injury control. *In* Clark, D., and MacMahon, B. (eds.): Preventive Medicine, 2nd ed. Boston, Little, Brown & Co., in press.

and associated with more deaths and injuries per crash than larger cars. While it is true that the risk of injury to occupants of a vehicle decreases as the size of the other vehicle in a collision decreases, the problem would not be solved if all cars were small. This is because (1) 40 per cent of occupant deaths occur in single-vehicle crashes, in which the likelihood of death or severe injury increases as vehicle size decreases, (2) larger cars give better protection in crashes with trucks, which figure prominently in crashes fatal to car occupants and (3) when two cars of equal size collide, the probability of survival increases with vehicle size.[45]

Much can be done to vehicles of all sizes and types to improve the protection of their occupants by spreading out the decelerative forces in space or time. This can be achieved, for example, with vehicle front ends that optimally manage crash decelerations, energy-absorbing steering wheels and windshields and instrument panels that dissipate some of the energy by deforming* when struck by a head or knee; eliminating, rounding or sufficiently padding all surfaces that project into the occupant compartment; and by ensuring that occupants are neither thrown out of the compartment nor endangered by its collapse. States[93] and other physicians interested in auto racing safety have pushed manufacturers to extend to highway vehicles — through rollbars and other changes in vehicle design — the lessons learned in sports car racing, where it is not uncommon for drivers to escape injury in rollover crashes at 80–100 mph.

Since creation of the United States Department of Transportation's National Highway Traffic Safety Administration in 1966, first directed by Dr. William Haddon, Jr., federal safety standards for new motor vehicles have been developed to reduce the frequency of crashes, e.g., standards for brakes, and to make cars more crashworthy, e.g., standards for restraint systems, door locks and fuel systems. The standards were credited with saving some 25,000 lives by 1974.[45]

Restraint systems, such as seatbelts and airbags, allow occupants to decelerate with their vehicles rather than more abruptly when thrown against unyielding structures inside or outside the vehicles. Restraints also spread the decelerative forces over a wider area rather than focusing them on a small area of the body, as do mirrors, knobs and other objects with small radii of curvature. Use of the combined lap and shoulder belt reduces the likelihood of death or serious injury by about 60 per cent. In Australia, after seatbelt use was required by law, decreases of 21 to 25 per cent in occupant deaths were reported; spinal cord injuries also decreased.[45, 81] In the United States, although seatbelts have been standard equipment for more than a decade, only about 20 per cent of front seat occupants wear them. Usage increases somewhat with educational level, but the basic problem is not lack of information or conviction. (This can be demonstrated with a one-minute survey: ask any roomful of people how many believe that their chance of death or injury is less if they wear seatbelts. Many hands that go up will come down when you ask how many fastened their own seatbelts that morning.)

The ability of "passive" designs to automatically protect all occupants in a crash, without requiring the cooperation of the person who needs protection, has resulted in a federal requirement that by 1983 all new cars must automatically provide substantial crash protection to front seat passengers in frontal crashes, which produce the majority of severe or fatal injuries. Testimony from a number of physicians and medical organizations helped to prevent congressional override of this requirement; one surgeon pointed out that, in contrast to the relatively few instances in which his own efforts could spell the difference between life and death, the senators' decision could save thousands of lives every year.[31] The designs presently available to meet the federal requirement are the airbag and the passive seatbelt, which is automatically positioned diagonally across an occupant's torso when the door is closed and which has been shown to substantially reduce occupant deaths and injuries.[20, 45]

Airbag-equipped cars, which have been driven more than half a billion miles, have given good protection in crashes without

---

*The forces on a person in a crash, fall or other deceleration are inversely proportional to the stopping distance, which often is largely determined by the deformation or "yield" of the object struck.

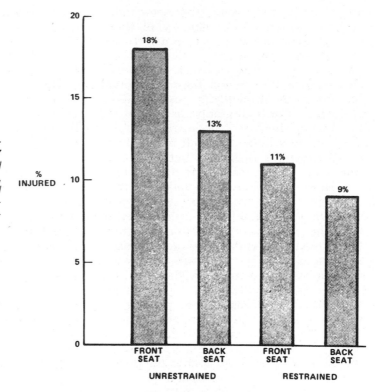

Figure 28–5. *Injury rates of passengers less than 15 years of age in 1967 and later model year crash-involved automobiles in North Carolina, 1973–1974, by seating location and restraint use. (From Insurance Institute for Highway Safety Status Report 11:8:1, 1976.)*

causing significant side effects such as damage from eyeglasses or cigarettes. Their record for preventing serious injury to the head, face, neck or internal organs is excellent.[45, 51]

Children are at special risk as occupants because they are even less likely than adults to be properly restrained; only 7 per cent wear seatbelts or ride in adequate infant and child seats. Few parents realize that in a crash they would be unable to hold a child in their arms and, if unrestrained themselves, could even crush the child. Placing children in the back seat reduces their risk of injury, but restraints give even better protection. The best protection for a child is to ride in the back, properly restrained[108] (Fig. 28–5). Although a federally approved infant or child restraint provides ideal protection for a young child, a child who is able to sit unsupported is far safer when protected with a lap belt than when held on a lap or riding unrestrained. Among the promising approaches to the problem is legislation requiring children to be restrained either with seat belts or in infant or child seats whenever they travel.

Recently it was discovered that infants less than six months old have very high occupant death rates: 9.1 per 100,000 population, decreasing to 4.8 for 1-year-olds and to 2.6 by age 6.[4] Physicians should therefore encourage parents to transport children safely, beginning with the trip home from the hospital. A hospital program designed to increase use of acceptable infant carriers achieved substantial improvement in usage rates when carriers were given to the mothers, but despite careful instructions three fourths of the infant carriers were not attached to the cars. The net effect of this program in terms of child protection was therefore minimal, showing the importance of evaluating the overall results of such efforts.[79]

Pedestrians

The 7400 pedestrian deaths annually — about 4 per 100,000 population — comprise one sixth of all highway fatalities. Two thirds occur in urban areas, accounting for more than half of the highway fatalities in large cities. Those killed tend to be the aged, the very young or people impaired by alcohol; these three groups account for three fourths of the pedestrian deaths in Baltimore. About two thirds of the injured children under 5 years of age

are struck when crossing between intersections, whereas the majority of those
over 65 are struck at intersections.[72] In the
first instance this suggests the prominent
effect of immaturity and lack of supervision and in the second both perceptual
limitations and difficulty in crossing quickly enough. For both groups, as well as for
the alcohol-impaired pedestrian,[46] solutions are less likely to result from educational programs than from better *separation* of pedestrians from moving
vehicles — that is, using spatial separation
(as in pedestrian malls and underpasses),
temporal separation (traffic lights timed to
favor the pedestrian) and physical barriers.
Other promising approaches include major
reductions in the use of private vehicles in
urban areas, elimination of high-hazard situations (as by having buses stop on the far
side of intersections, where pedestrians
are not likely to cross in front of the buses)
and better illumination. Such measures
would benefit *all* pedestrians, including
the high-risk groups. As of now, the pedestrian environment is designed primarily
for the mature, alert, sober and agile. Similarly, all would benefit from improvements
to vehicle exteriors: rounded contours,
"soft" front ends, appropriate bumper
heights and elimination of protrusions, all
of which are now featured in research safety vehicles.

Motorcycles, Mopeds and Bicycles

About 4000 motorcyclists and 1000 bicyclists were killed in 1977; the figure for
motorcyclists represented a 24 per cent increase over 1976, partially because of
widespread repeal of helmet laws. The
popularity of mopeds (motorized bicycles)
is too recent a phenomenon for separate
statistics to be readily available (they are
commonly classed with motorcycles), but
their numbers are rapidly increasing as
states liberalize their policies and allow
them on highways without requiring helmet use or, in many cases, licensure. European statistics indicate that death rates per
100,000 vehicles are roughly 170, 50 and 8
for motorcycles, mopeds and bicycles, respectively, with the differences being
partly due to differences in annual mileage
and type of usage. Death rates per million
miles have been estimated as being twice
as high for motorcycles as for bicycles.[78]

The median age is about 15 years for bicyclists killed in the United States and 23
years for motorcyclists. As in most other
types of highway deaths, alcohol is a major
factor in motorcycle fatalities.

The basic strategies are similar for protecting riders on all types of two-wheeled
vehicles.[27, 45] Collisions could be reduced
by such measures as reducing speed capabilities, separating cycles from cars and
trucks, improving visibility with lights and
reflectorized materials on cycles and riders
and improving operator competence and
road design. Injuries resulting from impact
with the cycle itself — especially injuries
to the trunk and legs — could be reduced
by widening and softening handlebars and
other structures at likely contact points as
well as by use of protective clothing.

Thus far, the most effective strategy for
reducing motorcyclist deaths has been the
required use of helmets (Fig. 28–6). Enact-
ment of such laws, in which surgeons often
played a leading role by testifying to the
efficacy of helmets, reduced deaths by
about 30 per cent.[80] The effectiveness of
the laws has been tragically demonstrated
in states that repealed laws once they were
no longer federally required. In Kansas,
repeal resulted in an increase in head injuries from 77 to 130 per 1000 crashes.[66]
When the law was repealed in Minnesota,
the number of deaths jumped from 57 in
1976 to 94 in 1977. Ironically, the repeals
have generally applied only to motorcyclists 18 or older, thus exempting from required helmet use those of the ages with
about 80 per cent of the fatalities. The
demonstrated success of helmet laws for
motorcyclists and the severity of head injuries in moped riders[61] and bicyclists[98]
point to the urgent need to increase helmet use among *all* cyclists.

FALLS

Falls injure 14 million Americans each
year. The 15,000 deaths annually (7 per
100,000 population) are surpassed only by
motor vehicle crashes and shootings. Fatal
falls occur most often in the home. They
are also a prominent cause of occupational
deaths, especially in construction work,
the occupation with the largest number of
work-related injury deaths.[72] Almost 60 per
cent of all fall deaths are of persons 75 or

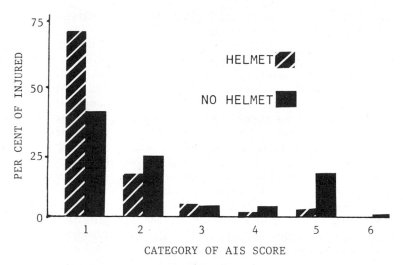

Figure 28–6. Distribution of severity of head injuries in motorcyclists in relation to helmet use. The most severe injuries (AIS grades 4–6) were most common among motorcyclists not wearing helmets. Kansas, 1975–76. (From: Lummis, M., and McSwain, N. E.: Proceedings of the 21st Conference of the American Association for Automotive Medicine, 1977.)

over, among whom falls are both the leading type of fatal injury and a major cause of morbidity and disability. Reflecting both the frequency and serious consequences of falls in the elderly, at one general hospital patients 60 and older accounted for 24 per cent of all fall injuries treated, 63 per cent of admissions for fall injuries, and 80 per cent of the related days of hospitalization. In a single year, treatment costs for the 1740 fall patients at this hospital (16 per cent of whom were admitted) totalled half a million dollars.[50]

Head injuries predominate as a cause of death in fatal falls except among the elderly, in whom death is most often associated with fractures and their sequelae. Fractures account for the majority of hospital admissions, and soft tissue injuries for the majority of emergency room visits for falls. Lacerations are the most common fall injury treated in the young, fractures in the elderly.[50]

The mechanisms and determinants of injury, as well as the injuries themselves, are the same for falls as for crashes. The forces increase with the square of the velocity at impact, which is largely determined by the height from which a person falls. The distance that people can fall must therefore be reduced in high-risk situations ranging from bridge construction, where lifelines can limit a worker's fall, to hospital beds, which should be appropriately low. One hospital found that about one patient out of 40 fell out of bed during the average stay of 20 days.[40]

Snyder and others have found that "vir-

tually any headfirst fall of greater than 10 feet onto a rigid surface may be expected to cause skull fracture or concussion" at any age.[89] Falls from heights are an important cause of death and severe injury among children in some cities. In New York City, following a campaign combining intensive public information efforts and provision of free window guards, deaths of young children resulting from falls from windows dropped sharply from 57 in 1973 to 37 in 1975. An important result of the New York City Health Department's campaign was a statute requiring landlords to install window guards in apartments where young children live.[91]

As in car crashes and the majority of sports injuries, the forces transmitted to a person who falls are inversely proportional to the stopping distance, which generally is determined by the combined deformation of the person, his clothing and the surface struck. DeHaven's 1942 study of survivors of falls from heights, which played an important role in the beginnings of crash injury research, showed that under the proper conditions the human body could withstand enormous forces. Illustrating the importance of increasing the stopping distance and spreading the decelerative forces was a female who fell 55 feet and landed at a speed of 37 mph on her side and back, depressing the earth to a depth of 4 inches. There was no loss of consciousness or other sign of injury.[22]

The effect of a smooth, soft landing surface is further illustrated by data from paratrooper training; the injury rate was 18 per 1000 landings on rough terrain, about three times the rate on sand dunes.[47] Failure to appropriately modify surfaces where falls are likely to occur results in injuries in playground falls onto unnecessarily hard surfaces and in thousands of injuries to elderly people who fall onto hard, unpadded floors in homes, hospitals, nursing homes and institutions. Protective apparel can ameliorate impact forces and should be considered for groups at high risk of fall injury: helmets for horseback riders and bicyclists, for example, and padded clothing for the elderly.

Man-made structures landed on by a falling person often determine the likelihood and severity of injury. Sharp edges and corners have become an accepted part of our environment even though they add unnecessarily to the likelihood of injury when anyone falls against them. In one study of falls, the object struck was identified in 388 instances; furniture caused the injury in half of these cases, with coffee tables predominating (85 of 193 cases).[50] The corners of tables, metal drawers and eye-level cupboards are common examples of the need to consider injury potential in the design of furniture and housing. Falls on stairs caused 10 per cent of all fall deaths in Sweden[97] and 37 per cent of the slips and falls of elderly people studied in England.[86] About three fourths occur when people are going *down*stairs. Sometimes ramps or elevators eliminate the need for steps, but wherever stairways are present, falls and associated injuries can be reduced by proper illumination, evenly spaced steps, handrails and adequate friction between shoes and stair covering.

The importance of fall injuries as a source of morbidity and mortality is not reflected in adequate scientific attention to their etiology and prevention. In a recent study of injuries in an occupational setting it was noted that a fall due to unsure footing was the most common injury-producing event; yet instead of pointing out the need to improve the footing and modify the surfaces against which employees fell, emphasis in the study was on preventing hurrying, risk-taking and negligence. The recent burgeoning of crash injury research is unlikely to spread to falls until attention is focused on the *injuries* and their prevention rather than on "accidents" and behavioral changes.

BURNS

Burns are the fourth leading cause of accidental death and a major source of morbidity, disability and disfigurement. An estimated 1.2 million burns each year are severe enough to require medical attention or limit activity. The incidence of new burns that require hospitalization is 26–28 per 100,000 population annually, based on estimates from national surveys of hospital discharges and an intensive survey in upstate New York.[29] Nationwide, this means some 60,000 new burn cases admitted to hospitals each year. The total number of admissions is about 25 per cent higher, since many patients require multiple admissions.

Although the etiology of burns is well understood, preventive efforts do not match our knowledge. Even in occupational settings, where control should be easiest, the hazards are such that almost half of all hospitalized burns among men ages 20–64 are incurred at work.[29]

Residential fires or conflagrations cause almost two thirds of the 6000 burn deaths annually in the United States. Because these deaths usually occur before the person can be hospitalized, they have often escaped the attention of physicians. Burns from house fires comprise about 5 per cent of hospital admissions for burn injuries and also have the highest case fatality rate among hospitalized burn patients: about 15 per cent compared to about 3 per cent for all other burns (Table 28–4). Table 28–5 shows a chain of common conditions that can result in a fatal house fire. Other conditions could be easily added to the diagram. The elimination or correction of any one of the contributing conditions might be sufficient to prevent this hypothetical fatality. The final condition listed ("only one means of egress from apartment") illustrates the need to improve building codes: two thirds of a group of 107 persons who died at the scene of fires in Baltimore had made unsuccessful attempts to escape from the building. Of the preventive approaches mentioned in Table 28–5, education has been the most commonly relied upon and the least effective. Few parents do not know that "you shouldn't leave matches within reach of young children" and that "every home should have a fire extinguisher," yet the knowledge often is not reflected in practice.

**TABLE 28–4.   Top 10 Hazards and Case Fatality Rates 1974–1975
Upstate New York Survey of Hospitalized° Burn Injuries**

HAZARDS	TOTAL PATIENTS No.	DIED No.	%
Hot liquids	1654	20	1.2
Clothing	583	62	10.6
Gasoline	367	10	2.7
Automotive	354	2	0.6
Chemicals	342	5	1.5
Cooking grease	305	1	0.3
Conflagrations	213	25	11.7
Stoves and ovens	192	5	2.6
Propane gas	78	1	1.3
Furnaces	68	0	0.0
Subtotal, top 10	4,156	131	3.2
Other	1,376	34	2.5
Not stated	259	11	4.2
Total	5,791	176	3.0

°Excludes DOA's (predominantly from house-fires).
From Feck, G. A., Baptiste, M. S., and Tate, C. L., Jr.: An Epidemiologic Study of Burn Injuries and Strategies for prevention. Albany, New York State Department of Health, 1977.

Housefires initiated by smoldering cigarettes cause an estimated 2000 deaths each year and even larger numbers of serious injuries. Most of these fires would not occur if cigarettes were to self-extinguish after not being puffed on for a few minutes. Some brands already have this property and the American Burn Association has proposed that all cigarettes be required to meet standards for self-extinguishment.

More than 40 per cent of burn injuries in patients requiring hospitalization are *scalds;* one fourth of these scalds occur in children under 5 years of age. Hot beverages, especially coffee, cause half of all scalds in young children.[29] Sorensen reported that in Copenhagen such scalds were commonly the result of tipped-over coffee filters, prompting the plastic surgeons to actively encourage the development and use of more stable coffee makers.[90]

Hot water is the leading cause of all scalds and of all hospital admissions for burns. Hot tap water, especially in bathtubs and showers, is the primary harmful agent.[29] In homes as well as hospitals and nursing facilities, water heating and delivery systems can and should be modified so that water either is not heated to a temper-

TABLE 28–5.   Fatal House Fire: A Chain of Contributing Conditions

CONTRIBUTING CONDITIONS (EXAMPLES)	PREVENTIVE APPROACHES
Cigarette lighter or matches easy for child to light	Product design
Cigarette lighter or matches left within reach of child	Parental education
Draperies easily ignited	Product design and material
Smoke detector not installed	Housing regulations; education
Fire extinguisher not available	Education
Paint, walls, other construction materials not flame retardant	Housing construction and materials
Only one means of egress from apartment	Housing design

ature likely to cause a second- or third-degree burn or is automatically shut off at shower and bathtub if it exceeds a certain temperature. Such simple precautions, incorporated into housing and equipment codes, could virtually eliminate this major cause of burn morbidity.

Clothing ignition leads to an estimated 6000 hospital admissions each year in the United States. In 1974, clothing ignition was cited on 445 death certificates — a 54 per cent reduction compared to 1968, when such information was first collected; the largest drop in deaths was for children under 15 years of age, who had a 79 per cent reduction. In Baltimore, the number of clothing ignition deaths for ages 0–14 decreased from an average of five per year prior to 1966 to zero for 1970–77; this drop preceded the flammability standard for children's sleepwear and appeared to be partly due to changes in clothing styles and fabrics. The flammability standard also appears to have had effect: one pediatric burn unit that averaged 12 admissions annually for sleepwear ignition prior to the standard had three such cases in 1975 and one in 1976.[68] Clothing burns of patients treated or admitted or both at Pittsburgh hospitals occurred at high rates in children, elderly females, working males and low-income groups. Compared with other burns, clothing-related burns were more likely to be full-thickness and to involve multiple parts of the body.[7]

The most common ignition sources reported by the New York State study were gasoline, stoves, smoking materials and matches. Recommended countermeasures include use of recently developed matches that create less heat and self-extinguish when dropped and close-fitting garments for high-risk groups, and greater use of fabrics that because of their basic composition, tight weave or smooth finish are less likely to ignite, melt, burn with intense heat and/or release toxic gases.[29] Although one chemical (TRIS) chosen by manufacturers to make certain materials flame retardant was subsequently banned because of possible carcinogenicity, the various ways to make fabrics flame retardant include treatment with other chemicals as well as modifying the basic material.

Electrical burns from appliances or extension cords (4000 per year)[21] occur at high rates in young children and can be

extremely disfiguring. Their prevention is both important and feasible. Efforts at a pediatric clinic succeeded in getting mothers to apply free protective covers to electrical wall outlets in their homes, even though the remainder of the educational experiment proved ineffective in changing often-repeated parental actions such as leaving matches within reach of young children.[24] In Sweden, wall plugs in all new housing units have "child-proof" covers.

At one hospital, realization that mouth burns in young children were not generally caused by biting through a "live" wire (as often stated on the hospital chart) but by sucking on the female end of an extension cord led to development of a nonconductive cuff that covers this critical junction.[21] In Denmark, a once-common source of electrical mouth burns was virtually eliminated after members of the burns units discovered that most electrical mouth burns in young children were caused by broken female plugs on the cords of a particular brand of vacuum cleaner. They approached the manufacturer and were told that new models were being made with unbreakable plugs and that few of the old, dangerous models were in use. Nurses visiting homes with young children, however, found that 29 per cent

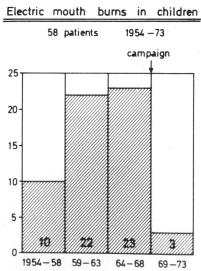

Figure 28–7. *Electric mouth burns. Results of a campaign against electric mouth burns caused by the electric cord of a vacuum cleaner. Ordinate: number of patients; abscissa: the period from 1954–1973 in 5-year periods. (From Sorensen, B.: J. Trauma 16:249, 1976.)*

had the old model vacuum cleaners, many of them with defective plugs. The physicians persuaded the firm to exchange the old plugs for new, safe ones. The press publicized the facts, 20,000 plugs were exchanged and a major source of mouth burns was practically eliminated[90] (Fig. 28-7).

Fatalities from electric current occur at highest rates in males age 15–34, with the preponderance occurring at work; contact between cranes or other machinery and high-tension wires is a common cause.[52]

SPORTS-RELATED INJURIES

The number of sports-related injuries each year is more than 2 million, with football, baseball and basketball each contributing about 400,000. These estimates are based on the Consumer Product Safety Commission's National Electronic Injury Surveillance System (NEISS), which collects information on product-related injuries from a sample of 119 emergency rooms.[101] To compare various sports in their risk of injury, the number of injuries must be related to the number of players and amount of exposure. The preeminence of football, for example, which accounts for almost two thirds of all sports injuries among high school males, is due partly to the large number of participants. According to the National Athletic Injury/Illness Reporting System (NAIRS), the college sports with the highest rates of significant injuries *per season and per 1000 males* are wrestling (380), volleyball (300), football (240), ice hockey (220), gymnastics (200), basketball (200) and lacrosse (170); among females, gymnastics (200) and basketball (150) are foremost.[72]

These rates do not necessarily reflect differences between sports in likelihood of *severe* injury. NAIRS, for example, defines "significant" injuries as those that involve fractures or dental injuries or preclude participation for a week or longer. Thus, they exclude such injuries as the repetitive minor blows to the boxer's head that result in cumulative and irreversible brain damage in many boxers.[100] Severe injuries, especially those that are fatal or permanently disabling, are relatively uncommon for most sports but merit special attention.

The incidence of permanent spinal cord injury from sports was studied in 7000 high schools and colleges for a 3-year period. The total number of such injuries was greatest for football (46 cases, compared to 13 for male gymnastics), but the rate per 1000 athletes was highest for gymnastics — four times the rate for football.[18] Physicians concerned about quadriplegia associated with trampoline use have taken the lead in advocating that trampolines be banned from school sports.

Sports equipment often determines the probability and type of injury. Ski injuries not only decreased but changed in their characteristics as boots and bindings changed. Between 1960 and 1973, lower extremity fractures decreased from 2.3 to 0.9 per 1,000 skier-days. Ankle fractures, which comprised 47 per cent of all fractures in the earlier period, dropped to 16 per cent as low, soft boots were replaced by high, stiff boots. Fractures of the shaft of the tibia, which now tend to occur at the level of the new boot tops, comprised 15 to 18 per cent of the fractures in the two periods; their severity warrants attention to the design of new ski equipment.[41] Ice hockey exemplifies the need for protective equipment: annually, about one player in 15 or 20 receives a facial injury, and by the eighth season of play 60 per cent have sustained one or more facial injuries. The value of mandatory full facial protection is illustrated by the lower rates of facial injuries among goalies, for whom facial protection is mandatory because of their greater risk of injury.[83]

Equipment, of course, can also *cause* injury, and the leading role of the stick in producing facial injury among hockey players has led to recommendations by physicians that the butt end be padded and the blade made broader.[83] Similarly, football helmets, which caused 12 per cent of all injuries sustained by 9000 high school players,[13] should be designed to reduce the risk of injury to other players (Table 28-2).

The sports *environment* often contributes unnecessarily to injuries. Not only the playing surface but its surroundings, such as the walls of polo and hockey rinks, can be modified to advantage. In football, it is estimated that 7 per cent of hospitalized offensive players had struck a fixed obstacle outside the playing field, and that some 95 per cent of such injuries could be prevented by establishing an 18-foot obstacle-free zone around the field.[34] A large proportion of injuries occurs in practices; in high school football, 34 per cent of all injuries occur in tackling drills alone, leading to recommendations for reduced-speed tackling drills as well as limited contact in other practice sessions.[13]

Specific plays or *maneuvers* are sometimes associated with a high incidence of injuries, as in the case of the cross-body block, which accounted for 54 per cent of 289 serious knee injuries among football players.[76] Knee injuries are the most common disabling football injury, and physicians may eventually be successful in eliminating this maneuver, just as they contributed to the outlawing of "spearing" and "butt-blocking," in which the initial impact is taken by the football player's head and often results in serious injury to the head or neck.

Compared with organized sports, informal recreation often poses even greater obstacles to injury prevention, as well as far greater risk of injury. In 1974, the 44 deaths among some 15,000 hang-gliding enthusiasts were about three times the annual number of deaths from football injuries, and represented a rate about 300 times the death rate for football players. Some of the protective equipment commonly used in organized sports needs to be extended to informal sports. Good helmets, for example, should replace the fashionable but less protective riding hat, since head injuries predominate among equestrian injuries. Of 154 patients admitted to the hospital for injuries related to horseback riding, one sustained a fatal skull fracture; 31, moderately severe brain injuries; 79, less serious concussions. Sequelae included post-traumatic epilepsy and hemiplegia. There were about 20 admissions per 1000 riding horses per year.[8] Mountain climbing, off-road motorcycling, and snowmobiling exemplify informal sports that combine high injury rates with remoteness from medical care, making timely medical treatment almost as difficult as prevention. For such activities, training the participants in life-saving skills deserves much greater emphasis than it presently receives.

Sports injuries have provided many surgeons with opportunities for prevention:

modification of rules, development and promotion of better equipment, improved training programs and emergency services all reflect the concerns and action of the medical community. Much of the progress in sports medicine results from addressing the problem of unnecessary *injuries* rather than concentrating on "accidents," human error and undesirable behavior. Extension of the same philosophy could do much to prevent injuries in the home, at work and on the highway.

INTENTIONAL INJURIES

Injuries that are self-inflicted or that result from interpersonal violence, arson, terrorist acts and war are major sources of morbidity and mortality in today's world. The increasing frequency of criminal violence has become a burdensome reality to urban emergency departments, and increased publicity has sensitized many physicians to the problems of child abuse, battered wives and sexual assault, yet there have been few studies addressed to the frequency, severity and prevention of nonfatal injuries inflicted in these situations. It is with the hope of stimulating such studies that intentional injuries are treated separately in this chapter.

The spectrum of injurious intent is illustrated by the law of homicide, in which involuntary manslaughter, voluntary manslaughter, and third-degree, second-degree and first-degree murder approximate points on a spectrum of increasing intent to kill. The mechanisms of injury and the injuries themselves, however, are the same regardless of intent. Moreover, the degree of intentionality has no bearing on many preventive strategies. Energy-attenuating steering columns can reduce injuries to the driver hit by a car traveling the wrong way on an expressway, the driver who crashes into a telephone pole while intoxicated and the driver who attempts suicide by crashing into a bridge abutment. Similarly, elimination of privately owned handguns would reduce the frequency of injury from firearms without regard to the intent of potential shooters.

Interpersonal Violence

The best national data on reported crimes come from the annual Uniform

Crime Reports (UCR), based on reports submitted to the Federal Bureau of Investigation by law enforcement agencies.[30] The UCR include aggravated assault, robbery, forcible rape, murder and several property crimes. Except for murder, a sizeable proportion of all offenses go unreported, so official statistics must be considered minimum estimates.

The frequency and correlates of bodily injury resulting from personal crime were studied in household surveys of victimization in eight United States cities. Of over 200,000 victims of personal crime (aggravated assault, robbery, rape and larceny from the person, and attempts to commit these offenses), 25 per cent had been injured. Of those injured, 8 per cent reported knife or gunshot wounds, 7 per cent broken bones or teeth, 7 per cent internal injuries or having been knocked unconscious, 3 per cent rape or attempted rape injuries, 78 per cent such minor injuries as bruises, black eyes, cuts or scratches and 13 per cent "other" injuries.* The proportions of personal crimes that resulted in injury were highest between midnight and 6 A.M., for crimes occurring in the victim's home, or when the offender had a weapon. Injury was more common when the offender was not a stranger; this partly explains the high frequency of injury in victimizations in the home, where nonstrangers are disproportionately involved. The age, sex and race of the offender were not important correlates of injury.[39]

Murders (excluding deaths caused by negligence or justifiable homicide) numbered 18,780† in 1976, or 8.8 per 100,000 United States population. Metropolitan areas have a higher murder rate than rural areas, which have a higher rate than cities outside metropolitan areas. For 10,847 murders in which there were a single offender and single victim and in which both were identified, 75 per cent of the victims were male and 25 per cent female; 52 per cent were black, 46 per cent white and 2 per cent of other races; 59 per cent involved males killing males, 22 per cent males killing females, 16 per cent females killing males and 2 per cent females killing females. In 91 per cent, the murderer

*Some of the victims suffered injuries in more than one category, so the percentages total more than 100.

†U.S. Vital statistics give the total number of homicides in 1976 as 19,554.[102]

and victim were of the same race. The victim and offender were relatives in 27 per cent of cases, friends, neighbors or acquaintances in 54 per cent and strangers in 18 per cent.[30]

Guns were used in 64 per cent of murders in the United States in 1976; 77 per cent of these were handguns, 9 per cent rifles, and 14 per cent shotguns. Thus, half of all murders were committed with handguns. Cutting and stabbing weapons were used in 18 per cent; personal weapons, e.g., fists, feet, in 6 per cent; blunt objects in 5 per cent and other weapons or means in 7 per cent. Marked increases in the homicide rate in United States cities from the early 1960's to the early 1970's were due almost entirely to increasing rates of homicide by firearm.[25] Handguns rather than long guns (rifles, shotguns) were predominantly involved in this homicide epidemic (Fig. 28–8).

Increasing numbers of privately owned handguns are associated with increasing homicide rates,[25] and there is evidence that elimination of privately owned handguns would substantially reduce the homicide rate.[110] Moreover, the rate of unintentional firearm injury would be reduced, especially among children. Approximately one fourth of the firearms in civilian hands in the United States are handguns,[74] but almost half of the gunshot wounds in children under 15 are due to handguns.[25]

Bullet design and velocity, the major determinants of gunshot wound severity, have important implications for the control of firearm injuries, whether intentional or unintentional. Despite the availability of relatively safe plastic ammunition for target shooting,[23] far more deadly ammuni-

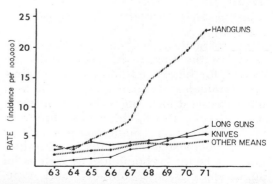

Figure 28–8. *Homicide rate by weapon used 1963– 1971. (From Fisher, J. C.: Homicide in Detroit: The role of firearms.* Criminology *14:387–400, Nov. 1976.)*

tion is commonly used. Advertisements and editorial content in hunting and gun magazines emphasize the "stopping power" or "kill power" of munitions, although these are irrelevant for target shooting. Distribution of safer ammunition is a public health measure that warrants evaluation.

Studies in various cities have repeatedly shown that 60–85 per cent of homicides occur on Friday, Saturday and Sunday and some two thirds between sunset and sunrise.[25] This is similar to the pattern of occurrence of aggravated assault, robbery and rape.[26, 75, 77] The pattern, which resembles that of other forms of violence such as fatal crashes, strongly suggests the contribution of alcohol use to these crimes. Supporting this belief is a study of people arrested during or immediately after felonies who were tested for alcohol: the great majority of those picked up by police for cuttings, other assaults and the carrying of concealed weapons had been drinking alcohol.[87]

It would be of interest to know whether the chances of surviving an injury of given severity were related to time of occurrence. In any case, it is clear that assaultive injuries, just as transportation injuries and falls, demand more resources from emergency medical systems during evening, night and weekend shifts than during conventional working hours. Wolfgang, in his classic study of Philadelphia homicides from 1948 to 1952, found that death of the victims occurred within 10 minutes for 48 per cent of shootings and 28 per cent of stabbings, and within the first hour for 71 per cent of shootings and 68 per cent of stabbings.[109] This suggests that improved emergency transportation might have a greater impact on the case fatality ratio of stab wounds than of gunshot wounds.

Approximately half of all homicides occur in the home; the proportions are higher for black victims, female victims and homicides between spouses. The next most frequent location is the public highway (streets, alleys, sidewalks), followed by bars and other commercial places.[25]

Low socioeconomic status is an important risk factor for homicide, as well as for aggravated assault, robbery and rape. Among the more remediable aspects of low socioeconomic status are housing conditions. Homicide rates are positively correlated with population density and with indicators of substandard housing.[12] Although no conclusions can yet be drawn about homicide, there is evidence that housing design has a marked effect on the rates of more common crimes: the robbery rate in housing projects, for example, is positively correlated with the height of the buildings.[73] Structures that maximize surveillance of streets, sidewalks, entryways, stairways and halls offer promise for reducing rates of personal crimes,[73] although domestic violence and those homicides that result from it cannot be expected to be greatly affected by improved surveillance alone.

This discussion of murder has made repeated reference to other offenses because murder is best understood as a subset of assaultive incidents. Thus, in 1976 there were 18,780 murders out of 986,570 reported violent crimes (aggravated assault, robbery, rape and murder), for a case fatality ratio of 20 deaths per 1000 reported violent crimes. This is approximately the same as the case fatality ratio for ruptured acute appendicitis, although assaultive incidents are far more common than appendicitis and result in 25 times as many deaths.[102]

Aggravated assault is defined as "the unlawful attack by one person upon another for the purpose of inflicting severe bodily injury usually accompanied by the use of a weapon or other means likely to produce death or serious bodily harm."[30] In 1976, 490,850 offenses were tabulated in UCR, for a rate of 2.3 per 1000 United States population. One third to one half of reported assault victims are hospitalized, and most of the others are also injured.[25] Aggravated assault is most common on the weekends, at night and during the summer; the rate is generally higher in metropolitan areas than in smaller cities and higher in smaller cities than in rural areas.[30, 77]

In one study, more than one half of the offenses occurred outdoors, an observation that probably indicates that reporting is most likely for public offenses; two thirds of offenses by females took place indoors, compared with two fifths of offenses by males. In 96 per cent of cases the offender and victim were of the same race, and in 60 per cent they were of the same sex. For offenses between males and females, the male attacked the female in 67 per cent.[77]

Zimring found that all but one of the 358 victims assaulted with knives were injured (69 per cent in the head, neck or torso; 31 per cent in the extremities), as compared with 87 per cent of victims assaulted with guns (49 per cent in the head, neck or torso; 38 per cent in the extremities).[110] In one victimization survey, 3 per cent of persons age 16 and older reported having been the victims of assault in 1970 (about 4.5 per cent of males, 2 per cent of females). Injury rates were even higher than suggested by UCR data: 3 to 4 per 1000 persons 16 and over had been injured with a weapon or severely injured (knocked unconscious, fractured bones or teeth, internal injury) without a weapon.[62] Another victimization survey showed that rates of aggravated assault in 1972 were highest for males, for nonwhites, for ages 16–19, and among those never married. Thirty-one per cent of the victims of simple and aggravated assault were injured, and 25 to 38 per cent of the injured received hospital care (60 to 86 per cent in emergency rooms, the remainder being admitted).[63]

Robbery is defined as "stealing or taking anything of value from the care, custody or control of a person, in his presence, by force or by threat of force."[30] In 1976, there were 420,210 offenses, including robbery attempts, for a rate of 2 per 1000 United States population. Robberies occur largely on the street (47 per cent) and in commercial and business establishments (26 per cent); 12 per cent occur in residences. Firearms were used in 43 per cent, knives and other cutting instruments in 13 per cent, other weapons in 8 per cent and personal weapons in 37 per cent. Robbery is most common in the winter and is much more common in metropolitan areas than in smaller cities or rural areas.[30] Studies based on police reports of robberies indicate that injuries were associated with 27–56 per cent. Of those injured, 25–46 per cent received slight or minor injuries and 54–75 per cent received injuries requiring medical attention.[19, 75]

Conklin noted that the more dangerous the weapon, the lower the proportion of robbery victims who were injured: injuries occurred among 9 per cent of those robbed

with firearms, 25 per cent with knives and 42 per cent by personal force.[19] Although Conklin interpreted this finding as indicating that offenders are less willing to fire a gun than to use personal force, it also seems likely that crimes involving no injury are more likely to be reported when a deadly weapon is involved.

The rate of robbery with injury to the victim was 5 to 8 per 1000 persons age 12 and over in the nation's five largest cities in 1972. Rates of robbery with injury were highest for males, for nonwhites, for ages 16–19 and for the lowest income group. Twenty-five per cent of the victims were injured and 23 to 32 per cent of the injured received hospital care (78 to 86 per cent in emergency departments, the remainder being admitted).[63]

Forcible rape is defined as "carnal knowledge of a female through the use of force or the threat of force."[30] The UCR reported 56,730 offenses in 1976, including assaults to commit forcible rape, for a rate of 0.6 per 1000 females in the United States. Rates estimated from surveys in the nation's five largest cities in 1972 are much higher: 2 to 5 per 1000 females age 12 and over.[63] The rate per 1000 females is more than twice as high in metropolitan areas as in other areas.[30] Reported rapes are most common in the summer, on weekends and between 8 P.M. and 2 A.M. Available evidence suggests that in approximately one half of reported rapes, the victim and the offender meet one another in the street and that in approximately one third, the victim is attacked in her home. It is noteworthy that in about half of reported cases, the rape does not take place where the participants met one another. It appears that generally the rapist either gains access to the victim's residence or else entices, coerces or forces her into going someplace with him. Strategies to prevent rape therefore include both those designed to prevent illegal entry and abduction, and those designed to intervene in sequences of interaction between men and women that require the cooperation of the potential victim.[26]

The frequency and severity of physical injury to rape victims is unknown. In the largest review of police records, 85 per cent of the 646 rape victims were treated forcefully. Of the entire group, 28 per cent were handled roughly, 25 per cent were beaten (but not brutally), 20 per cent were brutally beaten and 12 per cent choked. The more extreme degrees of force were more common when two or more offenders were involved and when the rape occurred outdoors.[2]

Studies of rape victims coming to medical attention show varying frequencies of injury. In a series of 2190 victims, 82 (4 per cent) had sustained severe physical injury (e.g., vaginal or vaginoperineal tears, multiple head injuries, stab wounds, fractures) and hundreds more required treatment of less severe injuries.[49] In another study, 11 per cent of 480 cases showed external evidence of trauma, ranging from small cuts to severe contusions and facial fractures. Gynecological injuries in 5 per cent ranged from laceration of the hymen to rupture of the cul-de-sac.[67] In a third study of 146 rape victims, 59 per cent had external signs of trauma and 39 per cent had signs of trauma on gynecological examination; 14 per cent required additional medical, surgical or orthopedic consultation.[16]

Violence in the family has been an area of growing concern.[94] Preliminary reports from a national survey indicate that the frequency of assaults within families is extremely high. Of the parental couples interviewed, 20 per cent admitted to having hit a child with some object, 4.2 per cent to having "beaten up" a child, and 2.9 per cent to actually using a knife or gun on a child at some time. About 1 per cent of husbands and wives admitted to having gone beyond slapping, kicking or throwing things at one another to the point of one partner being "beaten up" during the previous year, and about 5 per cent had been involved in such a beating at some time in the marriage. During the survey year, three fourths of children age 3–17 had assaulted a sibling, including kicking, biting or hitting with a fist (39 per cent), hitting with an object (36 per cent), "beating up" (14 per cent) and actually using a knife or gun (0.3 per cent).[96]

About 600 recognized murders each year involve parents killing their children. Kempe reported that the "battered child syndrome" accounted for roughly 25 per cent of all fractures seen in the first 2 years of life and 10 to 15 per cent of all trauma seen in the emergency department in children under 3 years of age.[57] Unpublished reports from specialized rape centers indicate that a substantial proportion of rapes involve victims (both male and female) under age 16, including infants and very young children. Injuries to multiple body surfaces, injuries in various stages of healing, cigarette burns, abrasions from ropes or gags and malnutrition are well-known signs of child abuse.[69] Available evidence indicates that 60 per cent of battered children who are returned home are battered again[88] and that the tendency for successive generations to perpetuate child abuse is not reduced by extensive medical and social help to battering parents. No study has shown convincingly that any treatment of battering parents is effective. Unless and until more effective intervention techniques are developed, temporary or permanent removal of an abused child or the abusing parent from the home is the safest strategy for preventing physical injury, but the relative risks of psychological harm must be carefully weighed. (This syndrome is also discussed in Chapter 24.)

A British study of 100 women who had received deliberate, severe and repeated demonstrable physical injuries from their husbands found that all had bruises caused by a fist; 59 per cent claimed they had also been kicked and 42 per cent said a weapon had also been used in the attack. Lacerations had been sustained at some time by 44 per cent, fractures of bones or teeth or dislocations by 36 per cent, strangulation attempts by 19 per cent and burns or scalds by 11 per cent.[35] In another British study, the pattern of soft tissue injuries in wife-beating cases was compared with other assaultive injuries sustained by women; those assaulted by husbands had a greater proportion of facial injuries, especially around the eyes.[33]

The literature on wife abuse emphasizes the need for intervention from professionals and social agencies but provides no evidence that such intervention is effective. A number of investigators advocate the provision of shelters for battered women and their children to give them temporary asylum. Of the 100 women studied by Gayford, 37 per cent admitted to "being violent" with their children and 54 per cent claimed that their husbands' violence had extended to the children.[36] Thus, separation of family members might protect more than one person. The problems of intentional injuries to husbands, siblings and elderly relatives are only beginning to receive attention[95] and are in need of systematic investigation.

Assaultive injuries in schools, although common enough to warrant research attention and preventive efforts, usually are excluded from data on crime, criminal victimization or child abuse, partly because fist fights and other assaultive acts between juveniles are so common that they are generally considered "normal" unless someone is hospitalized or killed. In the Seattle Public Schools there were 3.6 assaultive injuries per 1000 students during the 180-day 1969–1970 academic year. The rate was higher for junior high students (5.8) than for elementary school (3.4) or senior high (1.7) students. At each grade level, boys had an injury rate about five times as high as girls. Most injuries resulted from fighting (47 per cent), pushing (32 per cent), or throwing objects (15 per cent).[53] Nationwide estimates for student injuries are not available; the number of assaultive injuries to teachers is estimated at 75,000 annually,[10] or about 35 per 1000 teachers. Between 1970 and 1973 the frequency of homicide in schools increased by 18 per cent, assaults on students by 85 per cent, assaults on teachers by 77 per cent, robberies by 37 per cent and rapes and attempted rapes by 40 per cent.[10]

Self-inflicted Injury

Although it is frequently difficult or impossible to ascertain the degree of intentionality underlying a car crash, fall, poisoning or other injury-producing event, many deaths and injuries are attributed to suicidal intent. The legal need to differentiate suicides from homicides or accidents and the traditional emphasis on psychosocial determinants of suicide have led to the separation of statistics and research on self-inflicted injuries from those on other injuries. This separation tends to reinforce the false belief that injuries are either intentional or unintentional. Moreover, it inhibits meaningful injury control research and fosters the view that suicide prevention is a mental health problem.

Suicide is defined by the many coroners, medical examiners and other physicians whose opinions determine the manner of death recorded on death certificates; their various criteria are neither clear nor consistent.[28] In 1976, 26,832 suicides were recorded in the United States, making suicide the ninth leading cause of death in all age groups combined, with a rate of 12.5 per 100,000 population. The rate for males exceeds the rate for females in each age group and is about three times as high overall. The male rate increases with age; that for females peaks in the 45–54 age group. Suicide rates are generally higher among whites than among blacks, and variations in rates by age are more pronounced for whites.[37] The most tenable explanations for variations in suicide rates have to do with large social issues, such as employment, religion and family structure, that are not amenable to rapid or simple intervention.

Despite many published claims about the time of day that suicides occur, the time cannot be determine with sufficient accuracy to justify any useful conclusions.[9] Even the often cited maxim that hospital staff need to be especially watchful of depressed patients at the time of morning shift changes is probably derived from the discovery of hospital suicides at that time among patients who have not been properly checked throughout the night.

The most common means of committing suicide are firearms (14,700 deaths in 1976), poisoning with solids or liquids (3700), hanging (3700) and carbon monoxide poisoning using automotive exhaust (2000). For all means combined, there were 3300 more identified suicides in 1976 than in 1970; 90 per cent of the increase was accounted for by an increase in the number of suicides by firearms. In one study, the reasons for obtaining the firearms were determined for 26 of 35 suicides: 12 per cent were obtained for the purpose of committing suicide, 58 per cent for protection of self and family and the remainder for hunting or occupational reasons; 83 per cent of the 35 firearms used were handguns.[14] This and other evidence warrants measures to reduce the availability and lethality of firearms and ammunition and evaluation of their effect on the frequency and severity of all firearm injuries, including those self-inflicted.

Jumping from heights is a common means of suicide in some places, for example, San Francisco and East Harlem.[70, 85] Some countermeasures worthy of evaluation are building codes mandating controlled access to roofs and egress from windows, barriers to jumping or nets beneath bridges and overpasses and shrubbery or soft architectural components around the base of multistory buildings. As with strategies to prevent firearm injuries, poisoning, crashes and other potentially lethal events, measures to prevent suicide by jumping would also reduce unintentional injuries and deaths.

The effectiveness of "passive," automatic protection in preventing death regardless of intent was illustrated when the carbon monoxide content of piped gas supplied to homes in England was drastically reduced. Between 1964 and 1972, the death rate from unintentional carbon monoxide poisoning dropped from 1.8 to 0.2 per 100,000.[1] The number of suicides by coal gas poisoning, which had been the most common means of suicide, also dropped — from 87 to 12 per year in the city of Birmingham — without a compensating increase in suicide by other methods.[48] Thus, despite claims that persons intent on destruction of self or others will always find the means, it is clearly possible to control even self-inflicted injuries by controlling the means of producing injury.

Parasuicide is "a nonfatal act in which an individual deliberately causes self-injury or ingests a substance in excess of any prescribed or generally recognized therapeutic dosage."[60] The concept of parasuicide is preferable to the more traditional concepts of attempted suicide and suicidal gesture, for it avoids the problem of making inferences about the person's ultimate purpose. Unfortunately, studies of the epidemiology of nonfatal self-harm in the United States have generally attempted to assess the distribution of suicide attempts, and no consistent definition or method of ascertainment has been employed.

Weissman's review of the epidemiology of reported suicide attempts indicates that the incidence increased during the 1960's and that by the beginning of the 1970's the annual incidence was on the order of 2 to 3 per 1000 population, a figure that is nonetheless believed to be a low estimate. All ages except the youngest are represented among suicide attempters, but the highest incidence is in the 20–24 age group. About two thirds of attempters are females in most studies, but this may be because men more frequently attempt suicide in jail and are excluded from the usual data. Self-medication accounts for 70 to 90 per cent of reported attempts and wrist cutting about 10 to 12 per cent. Most methods of injury prevention that have been suggested amount to recommendations for broad social change.[106]

Firearm injuries are relatively rare among parasuicides because most attempts with firearms are successful. The best available data indicate that 79 per cent of suicidally inflicted gunshot wounds are fatal,[84] and that even for patients who reach neurosurgical attention, 70 per cent of self-inflicted gunshot wounds to the head are fatal.[38] A high case fatality ratio also applies to suicidal jumps from heights (99 per cent in jumps from the Golden Gate Bridge).[85]

Weissman reports that the New Haven study of suicide attempts indicated that pill ingestors, though having less suicidal intent and less psychiatric disturbance than attempters using more violent means, suffered the most serious medical effects and more frequently required medical (as opposed to psychiatric) hospitalization.[106] This finding, in conjunction with the popularity of pill ingestion as a method, underscores the importance of careful drug prescribing, especially to depressed or impulsive patients.

The risk of suicide following parasuicide appears to be approximately 1 to 2 per cent for each follow-up year.[60] Referral of parasuicide cases to psychiatric services is intended to help prevent further self-harm, but the success of psychiatric services in achieving this aim is unknown. Available evidence does not support the notion that suicide prevention centers have significant effect on the local suicide rate.[60, 64] Guidelines for hospital "suicide-proofing" have been offered but have not been implemented frequently enough. These include locating psychiatric units on lower floors, using shatter-proof glass and tamper-proof screens on all internal and external windows and use of break-away curtain and shower rods, minimal-length electrical cords and other measures.[11]

FORENSIC MEDICINE IN THE EMERGENCY DEPARTMENT

Beyond the immediate treatment of existing injuries, the physician attending victims of intentional injury has two opportunities for reducing the likelihood of further injuries. The first consists of enabling the identification, arrest and conviction of violent offenders through the preservation of physical evidence, documentation of injuries and cooperation with police and other authorities. The entrance wounds caused by bullets, knives, icepicks, scissors and so on provide important clues or corroboration as to the type and caliber or size of the weapon. Although it is rarely necessary to repair these superficial skin defects or to make surgical incisions through them, it is not uncommon for surgeons to do so, thereby destroying important evidence. Occasionally cases are seen in which attention seems to have been devoted to neatly suturing an entrance wound while the patient hemorrhaged internally.

The preservation of evidence in rape cases has received much attention in the past decade. Evidence should also be preserved in other cases of assaultive violence. For example, deposits of powder and other debris in and around gunshot wounds or the overlying clothing provide information as to the direction and distance of fire. From human bite wounds it is sometimes possible to identify the blood type of assailants and thereby eliminate some of the suspects. Fingernail scrapings, adherent hairs, fibers and trace materials that would ordinarily escape attention can all be essential evidence in a criminal case. Bullets should be handled with rubber-tipped forceps rather than with instruments that can deform the identifying lands and grooves. Rape evidence kits contain the kinds of specimen containers and labels that are needed (see Chapter 15). All of these types of evidence can usually be preserved without compromising the patient's treatment. In order that the chain of custody be maintained, specimens should never be left unattended and should be handed directly to the investigating officer in return for a receipt.

At the time of this writing, a technique is being perfected for the retrieval of fingerprints from human skin and from clothing. So far, this new laser technique requires that prints be obtained from living skin within a few hours. If the victim of a personal assault can pinpoint an area of clothing or skin that was touched by an assailant, protection of this surface and a call to the city or state police crime laboratory might be the critical element in identifying the assailant and obtaining a conviction.

The accurate description of the size and location of contusions, abrasions, lacerations and incised wounds, supplemented by photographs, can be extremely helpful in subsequent adjudication and may obviate the need for the physician's personal appearance in court.

The physician's second opportunity for reducing the likelihood of further injuries consists in attempts to intervene in patterns of recurrent violence. It has become standard practice in most university hospitals for suicide attempters to be seen by the psychiatric service prior to discharge. Now that physicians have become familiar with the battered child syndrome and with their legal duty to report child abuse, mechanisms need to be developed for the efficient referral of these patients to intervention programs. Other forms of intrafamilial violence, although not subject to mandatory reporting, appear to be least as recurrent as child abuse. The victims of extrafamilial violence vary in their risk of repeated injuries, but the multiple old scars characteristic of so many murder victims suggest that it might be useful to initiate intervention programs for persons surviving extrafamilial assaultive injuries.

Thus, despite the poor results of those intervention programs that have been adequately evaluated to date, increasing referral of affected families and individuals to various programs will be necessary to foster the continued development and evaluation of intervention strategies. Until such time as effective intervention programs are developed, surgical staff who treat victims of intentional violence should ensure that their patients have access to the best counseling services available.

CONCLUSION

Surgeons and other medical personnel dealing with trauma have a variety of opportunities to prevent injuries. They can make the observations and collect the data needed as a basis for better methods of injury prevention. More importantly, they can work with and influence decision makers such as legislators and regulators, manufacturers and designers — as well as the public — in initiation and support of policies and practices that will reduce injuries. Their experience in dealing with the tragedies of needless injuries makes them uniquely qualified to translate scientific knowledge into successful injury prevention strategies.

REFERENCES

1. Alphey, R. S., and Leach, S. J.: Accidental death in the home. R. Soc. Health J. 94:97, 1974.
2. Amir, M.: Patterns in Forcible Rape. Chicago, University of Chicago Press, 1971.
3. Baker, S. P.: Motor vehicle occupant deaths in young children. Pediatrics (In press, 1979).
4. Baker, S. P., O'Neill, B., Haddon, W., Jr., and Long, W. B.: The Injury Severity Score: A method for describing patients with multiple injuries and evaluating emergency care. J. Trauma 14:187, 1974.
5. Baker, S. P., and Schultz, R. C.: Recurrent problems in emergency room management of maxillofacial injuries. Clin. Plast. Surg. 2:65, 1975.
6. Baker, S. P., and Spitz, W. U.: Age effects and autopsy evidence of disease in fatally injured drivers. J.A.M.A. 214:1079, 1970.
7. Barancik, J. I., and Shapiro, M. A.: Pittsburgh Burn Study. Pittsburgh and Allegheny County, Pa., June 1, 1970–April 15, 1971. Washington, U.S. Consumer Product Safety Commission, May 1976. Available from NTIS, Arlington, Va., Pub. No. PB 250-737.
8. Barber, H. M.: Horse-play: Survey of accidents with horses. Br. Med. J. 3:532, 1973.
9. Barraclough, B. M.: Time of day chosen for suicide. Psychol. Med. 6:303, 1976.
10. Bayh, B.: Our Nation's Schools — A Report Card: "A" in School Violence and Vandalism. Preliminary Report to the Subcommittee to Investigate Juvenile Delinquency of the Committee on the Judiciary, U.S. Senate. Washington, U.S. Government Printing Office, 1975.
11. Benensohn, H. S., and Resnik, H. L. P.: Guidelines for "suicide-proofing" a psychiatric unit. Am. J. Psychother. 27:204, 1973.
12. Bensing, R. C., and Schroeder, O.: Homicide in an Urban Community. Springfield, Ill., Charles C Thomas, 1960.
13. Blyth, C. S., and Mueller, F. O.: Football Injuries. Minneapolis; McGraw-Hill, 1974.
14. Browning, C. H.: Epidemiology of suicide: Firearms. Compr. Psychiatry 15:549, 1974.
15. Buhr, A. J., and Cooke, A. M.: Fracture patterns. Lancet 1:531, 1959.
16. Burgess, A. W., and Holmstrom, L. L.: Rape: Victims of Crisis. Bowie, Md., Robert J. Brady Co., 1974.
17. Champion, H. R., Caplan, Y., Baker, S. P., Benner, C., Fisher, R. S., Cowley, R. A., and Gill, W.: Alcohol intoxication and serum osmolality. Lancet 2:1402, 1975.
18. Clarke, K. S.: A survey of sports-related spinal cord injuries in schools and colleges, 1973. J. Safety Res. 9:140, 1977.
19. Conklin, J. E.: Robbery and the Criminal Justice System. Philadelphia, J. B. Lippincott Co., 1972.
20. Cooke, C. H. Assessing Field Performance of VW Rabbit Passive Belt Knee Bolster Systems. 74–14 GR 156. Washington, National Highway Traffic Safety Administration, March 10, 1978.
21. Crikelair, G. F., and Dhaliwal, A. S.: The cause and prevention of electric burns of the mouth in children. Plast. Reconstr. Surg. 58:206, 1976.
22. DeHaven, H.: Mechanical analysis of survival in falls from heights of fifty to one hundred and fifty feet. War Med. 2:586, 1942.
23. DeMaio, V. J. M., and Spitz, W. U.: Variations in wounding due to unusual firearms and recently available ammunition. J. Forensic Sci. 17:377, 1972.
24. Dershewitz, R. S., and Williamson, J. W.: Prevention of childhood household injuries: A controlled clinical trial. Am. J. Public Health 67:1148, 1977.
25. Dietz, P. E.: Medical criminology and homicide control. Paper presented at the Ninth Annual Meeting of the American Academy of Psychiatry and the Law. Montreal, Canada, October 19–22, 1978.
26. Dietz, P. E.: Social factors in rapist behavior. In Rada, R. T. (ed.): Clinical Aspects of the Rapist. New York, Grune & Stratton, 1978, pp. 59–115.
27. Drysdale, W. F., Kraus, J. F., Franti, C. E., and Riggins, R. S.: Injury patterns in motorcycle collisions. J. Trauma 15:99, 1975.
28. Farberow, N. L., Mackinnon, D. R., and Nelson, F. L.: Suicide: Who's counting? Public Health Rep. 92:225, 1977.
29. Feck, G. A., Baptiste, M. S., and Tate, C. L., Jr.: An Epidemiologic Study of Burn Injuries and Strategies for Prevention. A study for the U.S. Public Health Service Center for Disease Control. Albany, New York State Department of Health, 1977.
30. Federal Bureau of Investigation: Uniform Crime Reports for the United States — 1976. Washington, U.S. Government Printing Office, 1977.
31. Fenner, H. A., Jr.: Testimony before the Senate Committee on Commerce, Science, and Transportation, Consumer Subcommittee, on Senate Concurrent Resolution 31 to Disapprove Safety Standard 208. September 9, 1977.
32. Flamm, E. S., Demopoulos, H. B., Seligman, M.

L., et al.: Ethanol potentiation of central nervous system trauma. J. Neurosurg. 46:328, 1977.

33. Fonseka, S.: A study of wife-beating in the Camberwell area. Br. J. Clin. Practice 28:400, 1974.

34. Garrick, J. G., Collins, G. S., and Requa, R. D.: Out of bounds in football: Player exposure to probability of football injury. J. Safety Res. 9:34, 1977.

35. Gayford, J. J.: Battered wives. Med. Sci. Law 15:237, 1975.

36. Gayford, J. J.: The plight of the battered wife. Intern. J. Environmental Studies 10:283, 1977.

37. Gibbs, J. P.: Sociological views of suicide. In Yochelson, L. (ed.): Symposium on Suicide. Washington, George Washington University Press, 1967, pp. 47–59.

38. Goodman, J. M., and Kalsbeck, J.: Outcome of self-inflicted gunshot wounds of the head. J. Trauma 5:636, 1965.

39. Gottfredson, M. R., and Hindelang, M. J.: Bodily injury in personal crimes. In Skogan, W. G. (ed.): Sample Surveys of the Victims of Crime. Cambridge, Mass., Ballinger, 1976, pp. 73–87.

40. Grubel, F.: Falls: A principal patient incident. Hospital Management 88:37, 1959.

41. Gutman, J., Weisbuch, J., and Wolf, M.: Ski injuries in 1972–1973: A repeat analysis of a major health problem. J.A.M.A. 230:1423, 1974.

42. Haddon, W., Jr.: Energy damage and the ten countermeasure strategies. J. Trauma 13:321, 1973.

43. Haddon, W., Jr.: A logical framework for categorizing highway safety phenomena and activity. J. Trauma 12:193, 1972.

44. Haddon, W., Jr.: Strategy in preventive medicine: Passive versus active approaches to reducing human wastage. J. Trauma 14:353, 1974.

45. Haddon, W., Jr., and Baker, S. P.: Injury control. In Clark, D., and MacMahon, B. (eds.): Preventive Medicine, 2nd ed., Boston, Little Brown & Co., (In press, 1979).

46. Haddon, W., Jr., Valien, P., McCarroll, J. R., and Umberger, C. J.: A controlled investigation of the characteristics of adult pedestrians fatally injured by motor vehicles in Manhattan. J. Chronic Dis. 14:655, 1961.

47. Hallel, T., and Naggan, L.: Parachuting injuries: A retrospective study of 83,718 injuries. J. Trauma 15:14, 1975.

48. Hassall, C., and Trethowan, W. H.: Suicide in Birmingham. Br. Med. J. 1:717, 1972.

49. Hayman, C. R., and Lanza, C.: Sexual assault on women and girls. Am. J. Obstet. Gynecol. 109:480, 1971.

50. Hongladarom, G. C.: Analysis of the Causes and Prevention of Injuries Attributed to Falls. A Study for the U.S. Public Health Service Center for Disease Control. Olympia, Wash., Washington State Department of Social and Health Services, 1977.

51. Insurance Institute for Highway Safety: Background Manual on the Passive Restraint Issue. Washington, Insurance Institute for Highway Safety, Watergate 600, 1977.

52. Iskrant, A. P., and Joliet, P. V.: Accidents and Homicide. Cambridge, Harvard University Press, 1968.

53. Johnson, C. J., Carter, A. P., Harlin, V. K., and Zoller, G.: Student injuries due to aggressive behavior in the Seattle Public Schools during the school year 1969–1970. Am. J. Public Health 64:904, 1974.

54. Jones, R. K., and Joscelyn, K. B.: 1977 Report on Alcohol and Highway Safety. (2 Volumes). U.S. Department of Transportation. Washington, Government Printing Office, 1978.

55. Joscelyn, K. B., and Maickel, R. P.: Report on an International Symposium on Drugs and Driving. Report No. DOT–HS–4–00994–75–1. Springfield, Va., National Technical Information Service, 1975.

56. Kelley, A. B., and Hebert, R.: Boobytrap! 16mm teaching film. New York, Harvest A-V, Inc., 1972.

57. Kempe, C. H.: Paediatric implications of the battered baby syndrome. Arch. Dis. Child. 46:28, 1971.

58. Klein, D., and Waller, J. A.: Causation, Culpability and Deterrence in Highway Crashes. U.S. Department of Transportation. Washington, Government Printing Office, 1970.

59. Kraus, J. F., Franti, C. E., Riggins, R. S., Richards, D., and Borhani, N. O.: Incidence of traumatic spinal cord lesions. J. Chronic Dis. 28:471, 1975.

60. Kreitman, N. (ed.): Parasuicide. New York, John Wiley & Sons, 1977.

61. Langwieder, K.: Collision characteristics and injuries to motorcylists and moped drivers. In Society of Automotive Engineers Proceedings of the 21st Stapp Car Crash Conference. Warrendale, Pa., Society of Automotive Engineers, 1977, pp. 261–301.

62. Law Enforcement Assistance Administration: Crimes and Victims: A Report on the Dayton-San Jose Pilot Survey of Victimization. Washington, U.S. Government Printing Office, 1974.

63. Law Enforcement Assistance Administration: Criminal Victimization Surveys in the Nation's Five Largest Cities: National Crime Panel Surveys of Chicago, Detroit, Los Angeles, New York, and Philadelphia. Washington, U.S. Government Printing Office, 1975.

64. Lester, D.: Suicide prevention centers: Data from 1970. J.A.M.A. 229:394, 1974.

65. Liedtke, A. J., and DeMuth, W. E.: Effects of alcohol on cardiovascular performance after experimental nonpenetrating chest trauma. Am. J. Cardiol. 35:243, 1975.

66. Lummis, M., and McSwain, N. E., Jr.: Impact of motorcycle helmet law repeal. Proceedings of the 21st Conference of the American Association for Automotive Medicine. Morton Grove, Ill., American Association for Automotive Medicine, 1977.

67. Massey, J. B., Garcia, C.-R., and Emich, J. P.: Management of sexually assaulted females. Obstet. Gynecol. 38:29, 1971.

68. McLoughlin, E., Clarke, N., Stahl, K., and Crawford, J. D.: One pediatric burn unit's experience with sleepwear-related injuries. J. Pediatr. 60:405, 1977.

69. McNeese, M. C., and Hebeler, J. R.: The abused child: A clinical approach to identification and management. *Ciba Symposium* 29:1, 1977.

70. Monk, M., and Warshauer, M. E.: Completed and attempted suicide in three ethnic groups. Am. J. Epidemiol. 100:333, 1974.

71. Moskowitz, H. (Guest editor): Special Issue on Drugs and Driving. Accid. Anal. Prev. 8:1, 1976.

72. National Safety Council: Accident Facts, 1977 edition. Chicago, National Safety Council, 1977. (Also, 1961 edition.)

73. Newman, O.: Defensible Space: Crime Prevention Through Urban Design. New York, Collier, 1973.

74. Newton, G. D., and Zimring, F. E.: Firearms and Violence in American Life: A Staff Report Submitted to the National Commission on the Causes and Prevention of Violence. Washington, U.S. Government Printing Office, 1968.

75. Normandeau, A.: Trends and patterns in crimes of robbery. Ph.D. dissertation, University of Pennsylvania, 1968.

76. Peterson, T. R.: The cross-body block, the major cause of knee injuries. J.A.M.A. 211:449, 1970.

77. Pittman, D. J., and Handy, W.: Patterns in criminal aggravated assault. J. Criminal Law, Criminology, and Police Science 55:462, 1974.

78. Pochin, E. E.: Occupational and other fatality rates. Community Health 6:2, 1974.

79. Reisinger, K. S., and Williams, A. F.: Evaluation of programs designed to increase the protection of infants in cars. Pediatrics 62:280, 1978.

80. Robertson, L. S.: An instance of effective legal regulation: Motorcyclist helmet and daytime headlamp use laws. Law and Society Review 10:467, 1976.

81. Robertson, L. S.: Estimates of motor vehicle seat belt effectiveness and use: Implications for occupant crash protection. Am. J. Public Health 66:859, 1976.

82. Robertson, L. S., and Baker, S. P.: Prior violation records of 1447 drivers involved in fatal crashes. Accid. Anal. Prev. 7:121, 1975.

83. Rontal, E., Rontal, M., Wilson, K., and Cram, B.: Facial injuries in hockey players. Laryngoscope 87:884, 1977.

84. Schneidman, E. S., and Farberow, N. L.: Statistical comparisons between attempted and committed suicides. *In* Farberow, N. L., and Schneidman, E. S. (eds.): The Cry for Help. New York, McGraw-Hill, 1961, pp. 19–47.

85. Seiden, R. H.: Suicide capital? A study of the San Francisco suicide rate. Bull. Suicidology 1–10, 1977.

86. Sheldon, J. H.: On the natural history of falls in old age. Br. Med. J. 2:1685, 1960.

87. Shupe, L. M.: Alcohol and crime: A study of the urine alcohol concentration found in 822 persons arrested during or immediately after the commission of a felony. J. Criminal Law, Criminology, and Police Science 44:661, 1954.

88. Skinner, A. E., and Castle, R. L.: 78 Battered Children: A Retrospective Study. London, National Society for the Prevention of Cruelty to Children, 1969.

89. Snyder, R. G., Foust, D. R., and Bowman, B. M.: Study of Impact Tolerance Through Free-Fall Investigation. UM–HSRI–77–8. Ann Arbor, Highway Safety Research Institute, 1977.

90. Sorensen, B.: Prevention of burns and scalds in a developed country. J. Trauma 16:249, 1976.

91. Spiegel, C. N.: Children can't fly: A program to prevent childhood morbidity and mortality from window falls. Am. J. Public Health 67:1143, 1977.

92. Stapp, J. P.: Effects of mechanical force on living tissues. I. Abrupt deceleration and windblast. J. Aviat. Med. 26:268, 1955.

93. States, J. D.: Case studies of racing accidents. *In* Society of Automotive Engineers Proceedings of 8th Stapp Car Crash Conference. Warrendale, Pa., Society of Automotive Engineers, 1968, pp. 251–258.

94. Steinmetz, S. K.: The Cycle of Violence: Assertive, Aggressive and Abusive Family Interaction. New York, Praeger, 1977.

95. Steinmetz, S. K.: Overlooked aspects of family violence: Battered husbands, battered siblings and battered elderly. Testimony prepared for the Committee on Science and Technology, U.S. House of Representatives, Feb. 15, 1978.

96. Straus, M. A., Gelles, R. J., and Steinmetz, S. K.: Violence in the American Family. (In press, 1979.)

97. Svanstrom, L.: Falls on stairs: An epidemiological accident study. Scand. J. Soc. Med. 2:113, 1974.

98. Thorson, J.: Pedal cycle accidents. Scand. J. Soc. Med. 2:12, 1974.

99. Tonge, J. I., O'Reilly, M. J., and Davison, A., et al.: Traffic-crash fatalities (1968–73); injury patterns and other factors. Med. Sci. Law 17:9, 1977.

100. Unterharnscheidt, F. J.: Head injury after boxing. Scand. J. Rehab. Med. 4:77, 1972.

101. U.S. Consumer Product Safety Commission. NEISS Data Highlights. 1:6, 2–3, Washington, Consumer Product Safety Commission, 1977.

102. U.S. National Center for Health Statistics: Monthly Vital Statistics Report: Advance Report, Final Mortality Statistics, 1976. Vol. 26, No. 11 Supplement. U.S. Department of Health, Education, and Welfare. Washington, U.S. Government Printing Office, 1978.

103. Waller, J. A.: Nonhighway injury fatalities. I. The roles of alcohol and problem drinking,

drugs, and medical impairment. II. Interaction of product and human factors. J. Chronic Dis. 25:33 and 47, 1972.

104. Waller, J. A., and Manheimer, D. I.: Nonfatal burns of children in a well-defined urban population. J. Pediatr. 63:863, 1964.

105. Wechsler, H., Kasey, E. H., Thum, D., and Demone, H. W.: Alcohol level and home accidents. Public Health Rep. 84:1043, 1969.

106. Weissman, M. M.: The epidemiology of suicide attempts, 1960 to 1971. Arch. Gen. Psychiatry 30:737, 1974.

107. Wigglesworth, E. C.: Occupational injuries: An exploratory analysis of successful Australian strategies. Med. J. Aust. 1:335, 1976.

108. Williams, A. F., and Zador, P. L.: Injuries to children in automobiles in relation to seating location and restraint use. Accid. Anal. Prev. 9:69, 1977.

109. Wolfgang, M. E.: Patterns in Criminal Homicide. Philadelphia, University of Pennsylvania Press, 1958.

110. Zimring, F.: Is gun control likely to reduce violent killings? University of Chicago Law Rev. 35:721, 1968.

CHAPTER 29

PSYCHIATRIC MANAGEMENT OF ACUTE TRAUMA

Chester W. Schmidt Jr., M.D.

INTRODUCTION

Nonfatal injuries are caused by accidents, assaults and suicide attempts. The scope of the public health problem involved is enormous. In this country accidents account for approximately 115,000 deaths, suicides for 22,000 deaths and homicides for 12,000 deaths — an amazing total of almost 150,000 deaths per year. There are 50,000,000 nonfatal injuries secondary to accidents of all types, approximately 200,000 injuries secondary to suicide attempts and probably at least a like number of injuries secondary to assaults. The estimated cost of accidents alone is in excess of $25 billion, of which $1.7 billion to $3 billion is spent for medical treatment.

All injuries are associated with some type of psychological reaction. Patients who are mentally healthy generally have the capacity to cope with the psychological stresses of injury. However, the manner in which an injury takes place, the nature of the injury and the parts of the body damaged and the current life circumstances of the patient are additional factors that affect a patient's psychological response to injury. The presence of a psychiatric disorder may occasionally play an etiological role in the events leading to an injury, but more often major psychiatric complications to trauma are the result of psychological reactions to injury.

Following an injury, the initial causes of psychological stress are pain, fear of loss of bodily function, fear of death and sometimes guilt associated with the events that led to the occurrence of the injury. All trauma patients are to some degree anxious and depressed, and they are often mildly agitated. Most patients are sufficiently hurt and frightened to be willing to place themselves in the hands of a physician to seek relief of their pain and repair of their body. Thus the initial surgical contact with trauma patients is determined by the surgical urgency of the injury and the patient's desire for relief and comfort. Psychiatric complications are more likely to occur following emergency surgical treatment, although there are exceptions to this statement. The purpose of this chapter is first, to alert trauma surgeons to the psychological and psychiatric issues that attend trauma, and second, to recommend procedures for the evaluation, diagnosis and management of those psychiatric disorders that occasionally accompany trauma.

THE ROLE OF THE PSYCHIATRIST IN MANAGEMENT OF TRAUMA

The role of the psychiatrist in emergency rooms or specialized trauma services is that of consultant to the surgeons who have primary responsibility for the patient. The psychiatrist is able to evaluate, diagnose and treat psychiatric disorders. Psychiatrists rarely take sole responsibility for the care of an injured patient during the emergency or immediate postoperative stages of treatment. Therefore, the management of the psychiatric aspects of any case are a collaborative effort between the surgeon who is primarily responsible for the patient and the psychiatrist who is the consultant. The effectiveness of the collaborative effort between these two physicians depends upon the confidence they have in each other. Psychiatrists who specialize in consultative psychiatry in general hospitals tend to be more effective consultants for two reasons: because they have more experience in the psychological problems of patients with surgical disorders and because by the nature of their consultative work they have developed a working relationship with the surgical staff. Highly specialized treatment centers such as shock-trauma, burn, intensive care and coronary care units include psychiatric consultants on their staff, thus incorporating the psychiatrists into the treatment team. Most general hospitals have no need for specialized psychiatric services, but a psychiatrist who specializes in hospital consultations or reserves some portion of his practice for hospital consultations is an important resource for surgeons in the management of trauma patients.

PSYCHIATRIC EVALUATION OF THE INJURED PATIENT

Methods of evaluating tissue damage of various body areas and organ systems of injured patients have been carefully outlined in the preceding chapters of this textbook. Assessment of the patient's mental state before, during and after surgical intervention should also be a routine examination. Each patient's psychological reaction to trauma can be evaluated for the severity of reaction or the apperaance of unusual reactions or diagnosable psychiatric conditions. The benefits of making a mental state assessment are (1) preventing severe stress reactions or psychiatric disorders, (2) minimizing the impact of those reactions or disorders if they do occur and (3) developing strategies to definitively treat those disorders when present.

The mental state examination is a method of systematically assessing a patient's mental condition. Detailed descriptions of complete mental state examinations are available in all textbooks of psychiatry. However, the elements of the mental state examination most useful for trauma surgeons would be composed of the following items:

Appearance: Grooming, motor activity (quiet versus agitated).

General level of consciousness: Alert, sleepy, stuporous, obtunded.

Orientation: The patient knows who he is, where he is and the date (day, month and year).

Speech: Ability to use customary syntax, slurring, inability to find the right word (meaning), pressured, mute.

Memory: Recent memory — knowledge of recent events, capacity to remember names of current treating physicians. Remote memory — ability to give history and present illness in proper historical sequence.

Attention and concentration: Ability to understand and follow directions.

Intelligence: Can be estimated from level of schooling achieved, vocational history, use of words.

Mood: Depressed, euphoric, neutral.

Affect: Displays of anger, anxiety, fear, humor. Display of affect is or is not consistent with the content of speech, thoughts and behaviors.

Perceptions: Presence of hallucinations (visual, auditory, somatic), delusions, paranoid ideas.

Suicidal thoughts: Statements or actions that indicate the patient wishes to harm or kill himself.

Homicidal or violent thoughts: Statements or actions that indicate patient wishes to harm or kill others.

Judgment: Capacity to understand the situation in which the patient finds himself and a demonstrated ability to comply with instructions and directions for care.

Much of the data for completing a brief mental state examination are available through observation during routine history taking. Only a few sections of the examination require specific questions. Some of these are: Do you hear voices? Have you ever had any visions or seen things that other people don't see? Are you experiencing suicidal thoughts now?

Case Illustrations

Case One. A 31-year-old male was admitted to the emergency department with a gunshot wound to the right shoulder. Vital signs were stable and bleeding controlled. His clothes were disheveled and he was moderately agitated; his speech was slightly slurred. He was alert, oriented in three spheres and his memory for both recent and remote events appeared intact. His intelligence was judged to be average. His mood was slightly depressed. The principal affects he displayed were anger and belligerence. He had no perceptual aberrations such as delusions or hallucinations, and he denied suicidal thoughts. He talked of killing "the bastard." During treatment he refused to follow instructions. His history was that he was drinking, was in a fight and was shot. The mental state examination indicated the probability of mild to moderate alcohol intoxication.

A blood alcohol level should be drawn. Information about the patient's drinking behavior should be obtained from the patient and from family members. During postsurgical care the nursing staff should be alerted to the possibility of withdrawal as well as a need for alcoholism evaluation and possibly alcoholism counseling.

Case Two. A 27-year-old separated female was admitted to the emergency department with third-degree burns of her right hand and forearm. She was slightly disheveled and almost mute. She occasionally mumbled something about God and punishment. She was alert and watched all that went on about her. Her orientation, memory and intelligence were difficult to assess. She denied hallucinations but talked of the devil, God and punishment in a disorganized fashion. She denied suicidal or homicidal ideation. She was compliant and followed instructions. Her mood appeared neutral and she showed no emotion. Her history was that the wound was self-inflicted when she had placed her hand on a stove burner. The mental state examination suggested a functional psychosis.

The patient and the family should be questioned about past psychiatric illness, the present treatment and whether the patient is currently taking any psychotro-

pic medications. Postemergency care arrangements should include a psychiatric evaluation. Even though the patient denied suicidal ideation, the likely presence of a psychosis and the bizarre manner in which she had burned herself requires that the patient be placed on suicidal precautions until the psychiatric evaluation is completed.

Case Three. A 17-year-old white single female was admitted to the emergency department with self-inflicted laceration of the right wrist. She was well groomed and attractive, but sobbing uncontrollably. She was alert and oriented in three spheres. Her memory was intact and her intelligence slightly above average. The patient denied hallucinations or delusions. The patient openly expressed the wish to die. She denied homicidal ideation. The patient complied reluctantly with the treatment procedures.

The fact that the patient has made a suicide attempt necessitates a psychiatric evaluation before she leaves the emergency department if she is to be discharged home. If admitted, she should be placed on suicidal precautions until a psychiatric evaluation is complete.

PAIN

Pain is a unique, subjective experience for every traumatized patient. Severe injury may produce a moderate amount of pain in one patient, while a minor injury may result in severe pain for another patient. Clinically there is a limited correlation between the amount of tissue damage and the intensity of pain experienced by patients. An explanation for this clinical observation is that the perception of pain is affected by the patient's psychological set, i.e., anxiety can aggravate pain. The events leading up to the injury, the parts of the body injured, fear of loss of function, fear of cosmetic disfigurement and fear of pain itself are some of the stressors that produce anxiety and that can enhance the intensity of pain. Thus, there are multiple stress factors that can create cycles of escalating pain followed by anxiety followed by pain, resulting in levels of pain that appear out of proportion to the amount of tissue damage.

If the subjective aspects of pain and

the role of anxiety as a potential enhancer of the experience of pain are fully appreciated by the surgeon, the control of pain is made much easier. So far as the patient is concerned, relief of pain is a very important issue. Successful relief of pain results in strong feelings of gratitude and trust toward the doctor who has provided that relief. Thus, based upon these observations and opinions, the following guidelines for management of pain are suggested.

1. The surgeon should have a sympathetic, nonjudgmental attitude toward the patient's experience of pain. Relief of pain should be a high priority aspect of patient care, and the surgeon should communicate to the patient his determination and ability to control pain.

2. Pain should be treated aggressively. Unless there are medical contraindications to the use of potent analgesics, there is no reason to practice brinksmanship by attempting to relieve pain with the less potent analgesics. Nothing will increase anxiety more than failure of pain medication to provide the promised relief. Failure to control or substantially reduce pain can on occasion initiate destructive angry, complaining interactions between the patient and the doctor about pain that can interfere with the doctor-patient relationship.

3. Avoid PRN orders for pain medication; the physician must remain in control of the treatment of pain. PRN orders place the patient in an inappropriate position of responsibility for determining his own medication needs. The patient should have the responsibility of reporting the effect of the medication on pain, but the physician must retain the responsibility of medical judgment for prescribing. PRN orders also place the nursing staff in an awkward position vis-a-vis the patient. Nursing staffs have a tendency to limit administration of pain medication and are especially wary of the use of narcotics. The nursing staff also tends to protect the surgeon from the demands and complaints of the patient. Once the patient becomes aware of these two facts of ward life, he immediately becomes fearful about the possibilities that he won't get the relief he needs even though orders have been written and that

the staff will not allow him access to the physician if his pain is not controlled. The effect of the patient's fretting over these two issues can markedly increase his anxiety and result in substantial increases in pain.

4. Orders for routine administration of pain medication are often indicated. However, the surgeon should personally monitor the effectiveness of the prescribed medication. Pain fluctuates; it is not a steady state. Therefore, the effectiveness of the prescribed pain medication should be monitored frequently by the surgeon. This process of monitoring will be very supportive for the patient and probably will reduce his need for pain medication.

5. Antianxiety medication such as diazepam (Valium) is helpful in controlling anxiety associated with pain in difficult cases. Diazepam can be administered in doses of 10 mg. by mouth three times a day for several days. Running orders of minor tranquilizers should be avoided.

In summary, the management of pain during the acute phases of treatment of traumatized patients is an important aspect of treatment that should receive high priority. Successful management during the acute phases of treatment may prevent a variety of complications associated with chronic pain during the rehabilitative phase of care.

CONFUSION, DELIRIUM AND POSTSURGICAL PSYCHOSIS

All three of these conditions are at times complications of trauma. Despite the potential seriousness of the conditions, clinicians do not agree on the meanings of the terms and there remain questions about the causes of each of the conditions. Confusion is manifested by defects in orientation to time, place and person. The clinical state is usually produced by insult to the central nervous system and reflects a degree of altered state of consciousness. A method of assessing the level of consciousness in relationship to craniocerebral injuries is discussed in Chapter 8. Confusion is also a symptom of delirium and is discussed within that context in the following paragraphs.

Delirium is defined by most clinicians as a disturbance in the sensorium or cognitive functions of the patient. This syndrome is usually reversible, although rare cases involving detectable cognitive defects persisting over extended periods of time have been reported. There are many causes of delirium, including craniocerebral injury, hypoxia, inadequate cerebral perfusion, increased intracranial pressure, fever, infectious brain disease, and neoplasms and degenerative diseases of the central nervous system. Delirium can result from toxic reactions to many drugs: corticosteroids, anticholinergics, anesthetic agents, sedative hypnotics, amphetamines and hallucinogens. Metabolic causes of delirium include hypernatremia, hyponatremia, hypercalcemia, hypocholemia, hyperthyroidism, hypothyroidism, hepatic decompensation, alkylosis and azotemia. A particular form of delirium, delirium tremens is caused by withdrawal from addicting sedative hypnotic drugs such as alcohol and barbiturates or barbiturate-like drugs.

The major symptoms of delirium are disorientation (principally time and place), impairment of memory and impairment of cognition. In addition, there are fluctuations of the patient's affect. Hallucinations when present are usually visual and are vivid, in that the patient is convinced he sees something or someone and can describe the visual hallucination in explicit detail. The predominant mood is one of fear and anxiety, accompanied by agitated behavior. The degree of agitation can be severe, accompanied by physical attacks on others, attempts to escape (even through windows) and suicide attempts.

Since delirium can be caused by a specific factor or combinations of factors, treatment begins with a search through the list just given for those specific causes. As the evaluation proceeds, the delirious patient must be protected from his own erratic or potentially destructive behavior. He should be placed in a room near the nurses' station where he can be conveniently and frequently observed by the staff. The window of the room should have a protective screen. If the staff is not able to observe the patient, then special nursing should be obtained. Sharp and other potentially dangerous objects should be removed from the room. Four-point restraints may be necessary but if used require close nursing supervision. A quiet, controlled environment should be maintained with attempts to keep the patient oriented to time, place and person. The number of staff who attend the patient should be limited and they should identify themselves with each contact. Night lights, visits by relatives, calendars, clocks, patient-controlled TV sets and simple and precise nursing routines are all helpful elements in the treatment program for re-establishing the patient's ability to orient himself and reduce confusion.

Correction or treatment of the specific cause will usually control delirium, but in those cases in which a specific cause cannot be found or the patient is severely agitated, phenothiazines or other neuroleptics may be used. Antipsychotics that can be given in parenteral form are especially useful because the delirious patient is often unable to take oral medication. Haloperidol (Haldol) has been increasingly recommended because it appears to have fewer hypotensive side effects than Thorazine and can be administered orally or parenterally in doses of 2.5 to 5 mg. every 4 hours, up to a total of 30 mg. during a 24-hour period. Geriatric patients may require a quarter or less of the usual adult dose. Sedative hypnotic drugs should be avoided because they may paradoxically exacerbate the delirious state. Chlordiazepoxide (Librium) is useful in the treatment of delirium tremens. The delirious state associated with withdrawal from barbiturates requires the implementation of a detoxification schedule. Antipsychotic drugs should not be used in the treatment of any addictive withdrawal states because the phenothiazines lower seizure threshold. Delirium resulting from toxic reactions to abuse of street drugs is responsive to treatment with medications depending upon the drug involved. Amphetamine intoxication responds well to haloperidol, 2.5 to 5 mg. q/4 hours up to 30 mg. per 24-hour period. Anticholinergics and antihistamine toxicity is usually short-lived, but in those patients with severe agitation or with severe hypopyrexia, physostigmine,

1 to 5 mg. IM or IV, will rapidly reverse peripheral and central effects of poisoning. Antipsychotics should be avoided because they potentiate toxicity. Hallucinogens such as lysergic acid diethylamide (LSD), phencyclidine hydrochloride (PCP) and dimethyltryptamine (DMT) are not thought to be responsive to specific chemotherapy. Reassurance, quiet and support, in combination with the measures already outlined for management of delirium, are recommended.

Postoperative psychoses or postoperative delirium is considered by some clinicians to be a specific syndrome. Other clinicians do not believe there are any significant differences in either the causes of or the clinical manifestations of either delirium or postoperative psychosis. However, allowing for the possibility of differences between the two conditions and because many trauma patients do require surgical procedures, a discussion of postsurgical psychosis is warranted.

Postoperative psychosis may begin as soon as a patient begins awakening from anesthesia, but more often develops 1 to 2 days after surgery. The signs and symptoms of postsurgical delirium are similar to general delirium. Some patients may be floridly delirious, others are not even identified as such because they display little unusual behavior. Specific etiological factors include infections of wound, urinary or respiratory tract; sedative-hypnotics, especially barbiturates; psychotropic medications; narcotics; withdrawal states from sedative-hypnotic agents and alcohol; operative stress; large amounts of blood transfusions and the many metabolic changes already listed as factors in causing delirium. Some other factors possibly unique to postsurgical delirium are pre-existing cardiovascular disease, certain types of ophthalmological surgery, advanced age, history of previous psychotic illness, history of previous neurotic illness, history of previous episode of delirium or postoperative psychosis and low socioeconomic status. Patients who are unconscious after sustaining trauma may be especially susceptible to both postsurgical confusion and delirium because they cannot be prepared for their surgical experience and

they awake not knowing where they are and what has happened to them. They have to fill in, with limited information, gaps in memory, plus adapting to their postoperative status. Treatment for postoperative delirium follows the same steps described in the treatment of delirium, beginning with a differential diagnosis to rule out specific causes followed by the general measures already discussed.

MANAGEMENT OF VIOLENT OR COMBATIVE PATIENTS

Patients who threaten or physically assault other patients and staff are extremely troublesome on any account, but especially so when they are being evaluated and treated for trauma. If a patient's violent behavior is not brought under control, a dangerous situation can develop that may result in further injury or death. Unfortunately, the violent patient is not a rare problem and therefore all emergency department personnel or trauma teams must be familiar with the principles of management of the violent patient. Common causes of violence or combativeness include confusion associated with head injury, alcohol intoxication, toxic reactions to medications or drugs of abuse, withdrawal reactions to alcohol or sedative hypnotics, delirium from any cause or combinations of any of these. Less common causes include states of anger associated with the events leading to trauma, temporal lobe epilepsy, paranoia associated with functional psychoses and certain personality disorders.

Management begins with physical control of the patient, but at the same time a differential diagnosis must be made to identify treatable causes of the violence. The staff's capacity to control combative patients depends on their experience, training and confidence in the medical leadership during the situation. If the staff members are caught off guard, are inexperienced or doubt their competency to manage violent patients, their anxiety will usually exacerbate an already bad situation. Continuing education of emergency department or trauma unit staffs should include a periodic review of management of the violent patient. In addition, a written protocol describing management steps is helpful. The following outline is suggested.

Policy on Management of Violent Patients

1. Attempts at verbal control are usually ineffective.
2. Armed patients should be left alone and the police called for assistance.
3. All efforts are to be made to protect the patient, the staff and innocent bystanders.

Procedure for Management of Violent Patients

1. The patient should be isolated so that family, friends and unnecessary staff leave the area.
2. The area around the patient should be cleared of all moveable equipment in order to reduce the possibility of injury.
3. Physical restraint is usually necessary and should be carried out by the largest male personnel available.
4. If sufficient male personnel are not available, other departments of the hospital should be called to obtain such personnel.
5. Each member of the staff who will be involved in the effort of physical restraint should be assigned a limb, and when the actual effort at restraint is attempted, efforts should be carried out rapidly and as humanely as possible. Continued or prolonged physical efforts increase the risk of injury to both patient and staff.
6. Medications for chemically restraining the patient should be mixed prior to the efforts to restrain the patient physically.
7. Medications recommended for rapid control are short-acting barbiturates such as sodium amytal 200 to 500 mg. in a 5 per cent solution given at 1 ml./min. Resuscitation and cardioversion equipment should be available. For prolonged control, intramuscular antipsychotics such as haloperidol 2.5 to 5 mg. given in divided doses to a total of 30 mg. over a 24-hour period are recommended.

Patients with head injury represent special problems during physical restraining because additional injury must be avoided. Restraint can be done with large pillows or with mattresses to protect the patient during the act of restraint. In those cases in which violence or combativeness is secondary to alcohol intoxication, protective isolation of the patient and watchful waiting is the best strategy, provided the surgical condition of the patient permits. As the blood al-

cohol level decreases, so does the level of violence. The factors that cause violence or combativeness are such that management should include a psychiatric consultation during the behavioral display, if feasible, but certainly as a follow-up.

MANAGEMENT OF THE SUICIDAL PATIENT

Unfortunately a remarkable number of patients are seen in emergency departments following suicide attempts but do not have psychiatric evaluation. Every patient who makes such an attempt, regardless of its degree of seriousness, should be psychiatrically evaluated. The evaluation should be done as soon as surgical intervention is completed and the patient is able to participate in the evaluation. Even minor suicide attempts or gestures may be the result of severe psychiatric disease. If psychiatric consultation is not readily available, the patient should be admitted to the hospital until a psychiatric evaluation can be carried out.

Patients who are admitted to the surgical service following a suicide attempt should be considered at risk until there is agreement between the surgeon and the psychiatric consultant that the patient is no longer suicidal. Suicidal patients who are admitted to a surgical service should be placed on suicide precautions.

An example of such a protocol and policy statement is as follows:

Policy on Suicide Precautions

1. The patient should be placed on suicide precautions when it is determined that he is a threat to his own life. This procedure can be initiated by the surgical staff, psychiatric liaison service or nursing staff responsible for the patient.
2. An order should be written on the patient's chart indicating the need for suicide precautions.
3. The unit is responsible for carrying out the outlined precautions. The nursing care plan should indicate in red letters: SUICIDE PRECAUTIONS.
4. Data on the patient on suicide precautions should be written in the shift report to facilitate communication of his mental state.
5. Consultation with the psychiatric liaison

service is a mandatory part of the evaluation in treatment of these patients.

6. The following procedure list should be located in the Procedure Manual on each unit. A copy of the procedure should be placed in the Kardex of each patient on suicide precautions.

Precautions for the Suicidal Patient

1. Place the patient on continued one-to-one care.
2. Locate the patient close to the nurses' station.
3. Assign the patient to a double room when feasible with protective screening on the window.
4. Confine the patient's activities to unit area.
5. Have the patient's unit activities supervised (bathing, toilet, smoking, etc.).
6. Keep potentially dangerous objects out of the patient's room (sharp objects, glass, matches, lighters, etc.).
7. Describe the condition of the patient and approaches to be utilized in the individual nursing care plan.
8. Check the patient's room for hazardous objects left by visitors (vases, razor blades, etc.).
9. Have the patient followed daily by the psychiatric liaison service.
10. The physician-in-charge should be notified of these precautions.

Most patients are suicidal for relatively short periods of time (24 to 48 hours). The psychiatric conditions most frequently associated with suicide attempts are affective disorders (depression), schizophrenia, alcoholism and delirium. Occasionally patients who develop postoperative delirium may become suicidal. In all instances the treatment of the psychiatric condition underlying the suicidal symptoms should be carried out collaboratively between the surgeon and the psychiatric consultant, with transfer of the patient to a psychiatric ward as soon as possible.

THE ROLE OF ALCOHOL IN THE CAUSATION OF INJURY

During the past several decades physicians who care for trauma patients have recognized the etiological role of alcohol in accidents, suicide attempts and criminal assaults. Depending on factors such as age, sex and means of injury, alcohol

may be an etiological factor in 30 to 50 per cent of trauma cases. Males in their second, third and fourth decades are very likely to have measurable blood alcohol levels at the time of their injury. Alcohol complicates the treatment of trauma patients in several ways. Moderate levels of intoxication may mask pain, obscure signs and symptoms of head injury and cause patients to be violent and combative. In addition, alcohol may act synergistically with anesthesia, analgesics and sedatives, causing unexpected depression of the central nervous system. Patients with hepatic damage secondary to alcohol abuse are at greater risk for surgical procedures.

The management problems associated with alcohol abuse can even extend beyond the phase of emergency care when withdrawal reactions develop during the postsurgical phase of care. Alcohol is so pervasive a complicating factor that the initial evaluation of all trauma patients should include an assessment of their use of alcohol. In instances of trauma involving children, the parents of the child should be assessed for alcohol use in order to determine if this was a contributing factor in the child's injury. The surgeon who is aware of the relationship between alcohol use and trauma, who obtains information about the patient's drinking habits, draws blood to test alcohol levels when indicated and is alert to withdrawal reactions, will certainly be in a position to reduce the complications caused by alcohol throughout all phases of trauma care.

THE ACCIDENT PRONE SYNDROME

Human factors, especially personality characteristics or traits of individuals involved in injuries, have been intensively studied for 6 decades in this country. Studies have been done of accidents involving the automobile and the airplane and of industrial accidents. The findings from many studies consistently show a relationship between the personality characteristics of aggressiveness and impulsivity and involvement in accident and injury. In addition, individuals involved in accidents are likely to be subject to a variety of psychiatric disorders, including abuse of alcohol. Although there are fewer studies to support this opinion, aggressiveness, impulsivity and alcohol abuse are very likely to be important human factors in the etiology of trauma related to assault.

From a psychiatric point of view, the personality traits associated with injury involvement are lifelong but vary in intensity and are modified by current life situation and stresses. Nevertheless, the presence of these traits predisposes certain individuals to an increased likelihood of injury at various points of time during their lives. There are other important human factors and epidemiological considerations that are discussed in Chapter 28, which defines additional high-risk groups.

The presence of these generally disagreeable personality characteristics has a clinical bearing on the management of trauma patients. Emergency treatment may be complicated by unruly, uncooperative and sometimes combative behavior stemming from these traits. In addition, such patients are more likely to have ingested alcohol, which exaggerates all of the personality-related complications already discussed at the time of their injury. Even during the rehabilitative phase of care, traits of aggressiveness and impulsivity may cause a variety of problems. These patients may have difficulty following the prescribed treatment regimens, they may not take medications as prescribed, they do not properly care for their dressings and they miss physical therapy sessions. In general their behavior often delays recovery.

Often, patients with maladaptive personality traits have made marginal social and vocational adjustments prior to their injury. If recovery is prolonged, these patients may have difficulty resuming their former levels of social and vocational function. Minor physical impairments can become incapacitating, resulting in disproportionate levels of vocational disability. Patients with these personality characteristics need early social work, psychological and psychiatric assessments, physical therapy, vocational rehabilitation, family counseling and/or

psychiatric treatment as indicated in order to foster speedy recovery and prevent disability.

INJURY PREVENTION

The surgeon occupies a unique and potentially vital role in the prevention of injury not only for his own patients but also for the public at large. The goal of primary prevention is to prevent future injuries. One means by which this goal can be accomplished is through the elimination of environmental hazards that produce injuries. A good example of primary prevention is "child-proof" containers, which protect children by making their environment more safe. Practicing surgeons have limited opportunity to participate in primary prevention, but one can never tell if treatment of the same type of injury in many patients by a surgeon might lead to an idea for preventing such an injury.

Secondary prevention reduces the consequences of injuries even though they continue to occur. The supplying of active (seatbelts) and passive (airbag) restraining equipment on automobiles is an example of a secondary preventive measure. Surgeons, because of the nature of their relationship with patients, are in a good position to encourage proper use of safety equipment. If so disposed, surgeons who see the tragedies associated with injury may even be inclined to support legislation that mandates community-wide safety measures (see Chapter 28).

Tertiary prevention reduces or minimizes the consequences of injuries that have already occurred. This is familiar ground for the trauma surgeon as he provides the best of surgical emergency care followed by the use of ancillary services such as physical therapy, social work and vocational rehabilitation. At the community level, tertiary prevention can be accomplished through programmatic development of regional emergency medical systems: specialized services including burn units, shock-trauma units, pediatric trauma units, electronic dispatching of ambulances, accident site telemetry and helicopter evacuation teams. Thus, surgeons involved in the care of trauma have multiple opportunities for participating in injury prevention.

RECOMMENDED READING

1. Howells, J. G. (ed.): Modern Perspectives in the Psychiatric Aspects of Surgery. New York, Brunner/Mazel, 1976.
   Chapter 4. The Accident Prone Syndrome
   Chapter 25. Psychiatry and the Management of an Accident Service
   Chapter 30. Psychiatry and Surgical Delirium
   Chapter 35. Accident Neurosis

2. Kissin, B., and Begleiter, H.: The Biology of Alcoholism: Vol. 4: Social Aspects of Alcoholism. New York, Plenum, 1977.
   Chapter 9. Alcohol and Unintentional Injury

3. Schnaper, N., and Cowley, R. W.: Overview: Psychiatric sequelae of multiple trauma. Am. J. Psychiatry 133:8, 1976

4. Shader, R. I. (ed.): Manual of Psychiatric Therapeutics. Boston, Little, Brown and Co. 1975.
   Chapter 7. Management of Violent Patients
   Chapter 12. Treatment of Dependence on Barbiturates and Sedative-Hypnotics
   Chapter 14. Treatment of the Alcohol Withdrawal Syndrome

INDEX

Abdominal injury, 429–477. See also
  *Duodenal injury; Gastric injury; Hepatic
  injury; Intestinal injury; Pancreatic
  injury; Splenic injury.*
  alcohol and, 438
  antibiotics, prophylactic, use in, 454
  background of, 429–430
  classification of, 430–431
  closed, 16–18
  corrosive gastritis in, 435–436
  diagnosis of, 439–448
    angiography in, 444–445
    auscultation in, 441
    hemorrhage in, 441
    intubation in, 441–442
    laboratory studies in, 442–445
    location of wound in, 439–440
    palpation in, 441
    paracentesis in, 445–448
    patient history in, 439
    pelvic examination in, 441
    peritoneal lavage in, 448
    physical examination in, 439–442
    rectal examination in, 441
    referred pain in, 441
    signs and symptoms in, 440–442
    sinography in, 445
    x-ray studies in, 442–444
  extra-abdominal complications in, 437–439
  foreign bodies in, ingested, 436
  iatrogenic causes of, 436–437
  management of, general, 453–454
  narcotics and, 438
  nonpenetrating, 434–436
    incidence of, 434
    treatment of, 452–453
  operation in, 454–456
  penetrating, 18–19, 431–434
    incidence of, 431
    treatment of, 449–452
  shock associated with, 438–439
  stab-induced, 432
    management of, 449–452
  treatment of, 448–456
    delayed, 438
Abdominal wall, injury to, 456
Abortion, induced, 491–493
  management of, 492–493
  spontaneous, 493
Acceleration injury, cervical, 230–231, 251
Accident-prone child, 753
Accident-prone syndrome, 829–830

Acetabular fracture, 620–621
Acromioclavicular dislocation, 628–629
Acute respiratory distress. See *Pulmonary
  insufficiency, post-traumatic.*
Adhesive strapping, in treatment of rib
  fracture, 383
Aggravated assault, 812–813
Air embolism, in tracheostomy, 367
Airway, maintenance of, in treatment of
  shock, 87
Airway obstruction. See also *Tracheostomy;
  Coniotomy.*
  in maxillofacial injury, 287–291
  in thoracic injury, 410–412
  partial, tracheostomy in, 289–290
  upper, in injury to larynx and trachea, 347
Akinesia, O'Brien, 261
  Van Lint, 261
Alcohol, in abdominal injury, 26–27, 438
  as risk factor in injury, 796–797
  role in causation of injury, 829
  management of trauma patient intoxicated
    with, 26–27
Allografting, in treatment of thermal injury,
  704
  split-thickness, as temporary wound
    closure, 758–759
Amniocentesis, for abortion, 493
Amniotic membrane dressing, in treatment of
  thermal injury, 704–705
Amphibionts, in thermal injury, 677
Amputation, in hand injury, 584–585
  of extremities, replantation of, 543–546
  of fingers, 585
  of thumb, 585
Analgesia and sedation, in injured patients,
  25–26
Anastomosis, end-to-end, arterial, 603
  nerve, 603
Anemia, and post-traumatic pulmonary
  insufficiency, 128
Anesthesia, in trauma, 102–113
  general, 108
    specific rules of, 108–111
  in hand injury, 563
  in vascular neck injury, 356
  local, 107
  regional, 107–108
  nerve block in, intercostal, 382–383
Anesthesia and operation, effects on
  post-traumatic pulmonary insufficiency,
  121–123